Drugs During Pregnancy and Lactation

Treatment Options and Risk Assessment

Third Edition

Drugs During Pregnancy and Lactation

Treatment Options and
Risk Assessment

Third Edition

Edited by
Christof Schaefer, Paul Peters, and Richard K. Miller

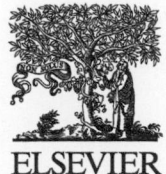

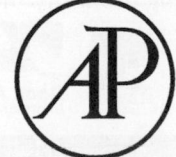

AMSTERDAM • BOSTON • HEIDELBERG • LONDON
NEW YORK • OXFORD • PARIS • SAN DIEGO
SAN FRANCISCO • SINGAPORE • SYDNEY • TOKYO
Academic Press is an imprint of Elsevier

Academic Press is an imprint of Elsevier
32 Jamestown Road, London NW1 7BY, UK
225 Wyman Street, Waltham, MA 02451, USA
525 B Street, Suite 1800, San Diego, CA 92101-4495, USA
The Boulevard, Langford Lane, Kidlington, Oxford OX5 1GB, UK

Third edition 2015

8th edition published in German under the title *Arzneimittel in Schwangerschaft & Stillzeit*

8th edition 2012 © Elsevier GmbH, Urban & Fischer Verlag, München

This 3rd English-language edition of the 8th edition of *Arzneimittel in Schwangerschaft & Stillzeit* by
Christof Schaefer, Horst Spielmann, Klaus Vetter and Corinna Weber-Schöndorfer is published by arrangement
with Elsevier GmbH, Urban and Fischer Verlag, Munich. The 3rd English-language edition is for the most part an
extension and update of this work.

ISBN 978-0-12-408078-2 (Drugs During Pregnancy and Lactation, 3rd English Edition)

ISBN 978-3-437-21203-1 (*Arzneimittel in Schwangerschaft & Stillzeit*, 8. Auflage 2012)

British Library Cataloguing-in-Publication Data
A catalogue record for this book is available from the British Library

Library of Congress Cataloging-in-Publication Data
A catalog record for this book is available from the Library of Congress

For information on all Academic Press publications
visit our website at www.store.elsevier.com

Typeset by TNQ Books and Journals

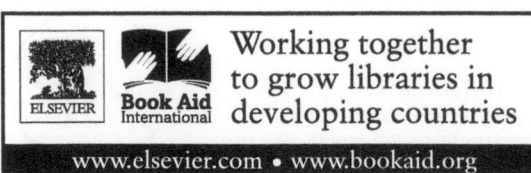

Contents

List of Contributors   xix
Preface   xxiii
Disclaimer   xxv

1   General commentary on drug therapy and drug risks in pregnancy
Paul Peters, Richard K. Miller and Christof Schaefer

1.1	Introduction	1
1.2	Development and health	2
1.3	Reproductive stages	3
1.4	Reproductive and developmental toxicology	4
1.5	Basic principles of drug-induced reproductive and developmental toxicology	8
1.6	Effects and manifestations	10
1.7	Pharmacokinetics of drugs in pregnancy	11
1.8	Mechanisms of developmental toxic agents	13
1.9	Causes of developmental disorders	14
1.10	Embryo/fetotoxic risk assessment and plausibility	15
1.11	Classification of drugs used in pregnancy	17
1.12	Paternal use of medicinal products	18
1.13	Communicating the risk of drug use in pregnancy	19
1.14	Risk communication prior to pharmacotherapeutic choice	20
1.15	Risk communication regarding the safety of drugs already used in pregnancy	21
1.16	Teratology information centers	21

2   Specific drug therapies during pregnancy

2.1   Analgesics, non-steroidal anti-inflammatory drugs (NSAIDs), muscle relaxants, and antigout medications
Heli Malm and Cornelia Borisch

2.1.1	Paracetamol (acetaminophen)	27
2.1.2	Acetylsalicylic acid	29
2.1.3	Pyrazolone compounds and phenylbutazone	32
2.1.4	Analgesic drug combination products and drugs used for osteoarthritis	33
2.1.5	Opioid agonists and antagonists and other centrally acting analgesics	34
2.1.6	Non-steroidal anti-inflammatory and antirheumatic drugs	41
2.1.7	Migraine therapy	46
2.1.8	Muscle relaxants and other analgesics	48
2.1.9	Antigout preparations	49

2.2   Allergy and hyposensitization therapy
Lee H. Goldstein, Corinna Weber-Schöndorfer and Matitiahu Berkovitch

2.2.1	Antihistamines (H_1-blocker)	59
2.2.2	Hyposensitization therapy	61
2.2.3	C1-Esterase inhibitor deficiency	61

2.3. Antiasthmatic and cough medication
*Lee H. Goldstein, Corinna Weber-Schöndorfer
and Matitiahu Berkovitch*

2.3.1	Selective β_2-adrenergic agonists	66
2.3.2	Inhaled corticosteroids (ICSs)	67
2.3.3	Theophylline	68
2.3.4	Leukotriene antagonists	69
2.3.5	Mast cell stabilizers (inhibitors)	69
2.3.6	Anticholinergics	70
2.3.7	Omalizumab and roflumilast	70
2.3.8	Expectorants and mucolytic agents	70
2.3.9	Antitussives	71
2.3.10	Non-selective β-adrenergic agonists	72

2.4. Nausea and vomiting in pregnancy
*Lee H. Goldstein, Corinna Weber-Schöndorfer
and Matitiahu Berkovitch*

2.4.1	Treatment options	76
2.4.2	Complementary treatment options	76
2.4.3	Pharmacological treatment options	78
2.4.4	Dopamine antagonists	81
2.4.5	Pyridoxine (vitamin B6)	83
2.4.6	Vitamin B1	84
2.4.7	Serotonin antagonists	85
2.4.8	Glucocorticoids	86
2.4.9	Other antiemetics	86

2.5. Gastro-intestinal medications, hypolipidemic agents and spasmolytics
Maurizio Clementi and Corinna Weber-Schöndorfer

2.5.1	Antacids	94
2.5.2	Sucralfate and pirenzepine	95
2.5.3	H_2 receptor antagonists	95
2.5.4	Proton pump inhibitors	96
2.5.5	Bismuth salts	97
2.5.6	*Helicobacter pylori* therapy	97
2.5.7	Digestives and carminatives	98
2.5.8	Atropine and other anticholinergic spasmolytics	98
2.5.9	Cholinergics	99
2.5.10	Constipation during pregnancy	99
2.5.11	Antidiarrheal agents	102
2.5.12	Medications for inflammatory bowel disease	103
2.5.13	Chenodesoxycholic acid and ursodeoxycholic acid	104
2.5.14	Lipid lowering agents	105
2.5.15	Appetite suppressants, weight loss medications, and obesity	108

2.6. Anti-infective Agents
Stephanie Padberg

2.6.1	Penicillins and β-lactamase inhibitors	116
2.6.2	Cephalosporins	117
2.6.3	Carbapenems and monobactams	117
2.6.4	Erythromycin and other macrolides	118
2.6.5	Clindamycin and lincomycin	119

2.6.6   Tetracyclines   120
2.6.7   Sulfonamides and trimethoprim   121
2.6.8   Quinolones   122
2.6.9   Nitrofurans and drugs for urinary tract infections   123
2.6.10   Nitroimidazole antibiotics   125
2.6.11   Aminoglycosides   125
2.6.12   Glycopeptide and polypeptide antibiotics   126
2.6.13   Other antibiotics   127
2.6.14   Tuberculosis and pregnancy   129
2.6.15   Local antibiotics   132
2.6.16   Malaria prophylaxis and treatment in pregnancy   132
2.6.17   Azole antifungals   139
2.6.18   Amphotericin B   141
2.6.19   Echinocandins   141
2.6.20   Flucytosine   142
2.6.21   Griseofulvin   142
2.6.22   Terbinafine   143
2.6.23   Topical antifungal agents   143
2.6.24   Anthelmintics   144
2.6.25   Herpes medications   147
2.6.26   Antiviral drugs for hepatitis   148
2.6.27   Antiviral drugs for influenza   150
2.6.28   Antiretroviral agents   151
2.6.29   Overview of the antiretroviral medications   152
2.6.30   Nucleoside and nucleotide reverse transcriptase
         inhibitors (NRTIs)   153
2.6.31   Non-nucleoside reverse transcriptase inhibitors (NNRTIs)   155
2.6.32   Protease inhibitors (PIs)   157
2.6.33   Entry inhibitors   160
2.6.34   Integrase inhibitors   161
2.6.35   Hyperthermia   162
2.6.36   Long-distance travel and flights   162

2.7.   Vaccines and immunoglobulins
        Benedikte-Noël Cuppers and Christof Schaefer

2.7.1   Thiomersal as a preservative for vaccines   178
2.7.2   Cholera vaccination   179
2.7.3   Diphtheria and tetanus vaccination   179
2.7.4   Haemophilus influenza B (HIB) vaccination   180
2.7.5   Hepatitis A and hepatitis B vaccination   180
2.7.6   HPV vaccination   180
2.7.7   Influenza vaccination   181
2.7.8   Measles and mumps vaccination   183
2.7.9   Meningococcal vaccination   183
2.7.10   Pertussis vaccination   184
2.7.11   Pneumococcal vaccination   184
2.7.12   Poliomyelitis vaccination   184
2.7.13   Rabies vaccination   185
2.7.14   Rubella vaccination   185
2.7.15   Tick-borne encephalitis vaccination   186
2.7.16   Typhoid vaccination   186
2.7.17   Varicella vaccination   187
2.7.18   Yellow fever vaccination   187
2.7.19   Immunoglobulins   188

2.8.   Heart and blood medications
       Fernanda Sales Luiz Vianna, Lavinia Schüler-Faccini and Corinna Weber-Schöndorfer

2.8.1	Arterial hypertension and pregnancy	194
2.8.2	α-Methyldopa	195
2.8.3	β-Receptor blockers	196
2.8.4	Calcium channel blockers	198
2.8.5	ACE inhibitors	199
2.8.6	Angiotensin II receptor blockers (ARBs; Sartans)	200
2.8.7	Dihydralazine	202
2.8.8	α-1 Blockers (peripherally acting adrenergic antagonists)	202
2.8.9	α-2 Blockers (centrally acting adrenergic antagonists)	203
2.8.10	Other antihypertensive medications	204
2.8.11	Pulmonary hypertension and pregnancy	205
2.8.12	Hypotension and antihypotensive drugs	207
2.8.13	Adrenergic agents	208
2.8.14	Cardiac glycosides	208
2.8.15	Antiarrhythmic medications	208
2.8.16	Coronary therapeutic drugs (cardiac vasodilators)	213
2.8.17	Vasocirculatory drugs and peripheral vasodilators	214
2.8.18	Diuretics	215

2.9.   Anticoagulants, thrombocyte aggregation inhibitors, fibrinolytics and volume replacement agents
       Janine E. Polifka and Juliane Habermann

2.9.1	Indications for anticoagulation	226
2.9.2	Heparins and danaparoid	227
2.9.3	Protamines	229
2.9.4	Thrombin-inhibitors	230
2.9.5	Factor Xa inhibitors	231
2.9.6	Inhibitors of thrombocyte aggregation	231
2.9.7	Vitamin K antagonists	233
2.9.8	Vitamin K	237
2.9.9	Fibrinolysis	238
2.9.10	Streptokinase	239
2.9.11	Antihemorrhagics	239
2.9.12	Other antihemorrhagics	240
2.9.13	Volume replacement substances and rheologics	241

2.10. Epilepsy and antiepileptic medications
       Christina Chambers and Christof Schaefer

2.10.1	Antiepileptic therapy	252
2.10.2	Antiepileptic and contraceptive drugs	253
2.10.3	Epilepsy and fertility	253
2.10.4	Frequency of seizures in pregnancy	254
2.10.5	Risk of malformations	254
2.10.6	Typical malformations and other anomalies	256
2.10.7	Pregnancy complications	256
2.10.8	Mental development dysfunction	257
2.10.9	"Damage mechanisms"	258
2.10.10	Folic acid and antiepileptic drugs	259
2.10.11	Vitamin K and antiepileptic drugs	259

2.10.12 Is epilepsy teratogenic? 260
2.10.13 Carbamazepine 260
2.10.14 Clobazam and clonazepam 263
2.10.15 Eslicarbazepine 264
2.10.16 Ethosuximide and other succinimides 264
2.10.17 Felbamate 265
2.10.18 Gabapentin 265
2.10.19 Lacosamide 266
2.10.20 Lamotrigine 267
2.10.21 Levetiracetam 268
2.10.22 Oxcarbazepine 269
2.10.23 Phenobarbital and primidone 270
2.10.24 Phenytoin 273
2.10.25 Pregabalin 274
2.10.26 Rufinamide 275
2.10.27 Sultiame 275
2.10.28 Tiagabine 275
2.10.29 Topiramate 276
2.10.30 Valnoctamide 277
2.10.31 Valproic acid 278
2.10.32 Vigabatrin 282
2.10.33 Zonisamide 283

2.11. Psychotropic drugs
Katherine L. Wisner and Christof Schaefer

2.11.1 Psychiatric disorder during pregnancy 294
2.11.2 Antidepressant treatment 294
2.11.3 Selective serotonin-reuptake-inhibitors (SSRI) 295
2.11.4 Tri- and tetracyclic antidepressants 302
2.11.5 Individual antidepressants 303
2.11.6 Antipsychotic treatment 313
2.11.7 Individual antipsychotic drugs 316
2.11.8 Lithium and other anti-manic agents 322
2.11.9 Anxiolytics, hypnotics, sedatives in general 324
2.11.10 Benzodiazepines 325
2.11.11 Zaleplon, zolpidem and zopiclone 327
2.11.12 Other anxiolytics and hypnotics 328
2.11.13 Psychoanaleptics 328
2.11.14 Anti-Parkinson drugs and restless legs syndrome 329

2.12. Immunosuppression, rheumatic diseases, multiple sclerosis, and Wilson's disease
Corinna Weber-Schöndorfer

2.12.1 Azathioprine/6-mercaptopurine 341
2.12.2 Selective immunosuppressants 342
2.12.3 Biologics 345
2.12.4 Multiple sclerosis 352
2.12.5 Interferons 354
2.12.6 Other immunostimulatory drugs 356
2.12.7 Transplantation 358
2.12.8 Drugs for rheumatic diseases 358
2.12.9 Drugs for Wilson's disease 363

2.13. Antineoplastic drugs
Jan M. Friedman and Corinna Weber-Schöndorfer

2.13.1 Malignancy and pregnancy 374
2.13.2 Breast cancer 376
2.13.3 Vinca alkaloids and analogs 377
2.13.4 Podophyllotoxin derivatives 377
2.13.5 Nitrosourea alkylators 378
2.13.6 Nitrogen mustard analog alkylators 378
2.13.7 Other alkylating agents 379
2.13.8 Cytotoxic anthracycline antibiotics 380
2.13.9 Other cytotoxic antibiotics 381
2.13.10 Folate antagonists 382
2.13.11 Purine antagonists 383
2.13.12 Pyrimidine antagonists 383
2.13.13 Taxanes and other cytostatic agents 385
2.13.14 Monoclonal antibodies 385
2.13.15 Platin compounds 386
2.13.16 Thalidomide and its analogs 387
2.13.17 Tyrosine kinase inhibitors 388
2.13.18 Antineoplastic drugs with endocrine effects 389
2.13.19 Other antineoplastic agents 390

2.14. Uterine contraction agents, tocolytics, vaginal therapeutics and local contraceptives
Gerard H.A. Visser and Angela Kayser

2.14.1 Prostaglandins 401
2.14.2 Oxytocin 403
2.14.3 Ergot alkaloids 404
2.14.4 Tocolytics in general 405
2.14.5 β₂-Sympathomimetics 406
2.14.6 Calcium antagonists 407
2.14.7 Magnesium sulfate 407
2.14.8 Oxytocin receptor antagonists 408
2.14.9 Prostaglandin antagonists 408
2.14.10 Other tocolytics 409
2.14.11 Vaginal therapeutics 409
2.14.12 Spermicide contraceptives 410
2.14.13 Intrauterine devices 410

2.15. Hormones
Asher Ornoy and Corinna Weber-Schöndorfer

2.15.1 Hypothalamic releasing hormones 414
2.15.2 Anterior pituitary hormones 415
2.15.3 Prolactin antagonists/dopamine agonists 416
2.15.4 Posterior pituitary hormones 417
2.15.5 Thyroid function and iodine supply during pregnancy 417
2.15.6 Hypothyroidism, triiodothyronine (T3) and thyroxin (T4) 418
2.15.7 Hyperthyroidism and thyrostatics 419
2.15.8 Glucocorticoids 423
2.15.9 Diabetes mellitus and pregnancy 426
2.15.10 Insulin 428
2.15.11 Oral antidiabetics (OAD) 430

2.15.12 Estrogens   434
2.15.13 Gestagens   435
2.15.14 Duogynon®   437
2.15.15 Diethylstilbestrol   437
2.15.16 Androgens and anabolics   438
2.15.17 Cyproterone and danazol   439
2.15.18 Mifepristone (RU486)   440
2.15.19 Clomiphene   440
2.15.20 Erythropoietin   441

2.16. General and local anesthetics and muscle relaxants
    Stefanie Hultzsch and Asher Ornoy
2.16.1 Halogenated inhalational anesthetic agents   452
2.16.2 Ether (diethyl ether)   454
2.16.3 Nitrous oxide   454
2.16.4 Xenon   454
2.16.5 Occupational exposure to anesthetic gases   454
2.16.6 Injection anesthetics   455
2.16.7 Local anesthetics   457
2.16.8 Muscle relaxants   460

2.17. Dermatological medications and local therapeutics
    Gudula Kirtschig and Christof Schaefer
2.17.1 Typical skin changes during pregnancy   468
2.17.2 Antiseptics and disinfectants   468
2.17.3 Glucocorticoids and non-steroid antiphlogistics   471
2.17.4 Astringents   471
2.17.5 Antipruritics and essential oils   472
2.17.6 Coal tar and slate oil preparations   472
2.17.7 Local immunomodulators as therapy for atopic eczema   473
2.17.8 Keratolytics   473
2.17.9 Retinoids for acne and psoriasis therapy   475
2.17.10 Ultraviolet light   479
2.17.11 Fumaric acid preparations   479
2.17.12 Biologicals   480
2.17.13 Wart therapeutics   480
2.17.14 Lithium   481
2.17.15 Lice medications   481
2.17.16 Anti-scabies   482
2.17.17 Vein therapeutics   483
2.17.18 Antihidrotica   483
2.17.19 Eflornithine, finasteride and minoxidil   484
2.17.20 Repellents   485
2.17.21 Cosmetics   485
2.17.22 Eye, nose and ear drops   486
2.17.23 Hemorrhoid medications   488
2.17.24 Vaginal therapeutics   488

2.18. Vitamins, minerals and trace elements
    Richard K. Miller and Paul Peters
2.18.1 Vitamin A (retinol)   494
2.18.2 Vitamin B_1 (thiamine)   496

2.18.3   Vitamin B_2 (riboflavin)   496
2.18.4   Vitamin B_3 (nicotinamide)   497
2.18.5   Vitamin B_6 (pyridoxine)   497
2.18.6   Vitamin B_{12} (cyanocobalamin)   497
2.18.7   Vitamin C (ascorbic acid)   498
2.18.8   Folic acid   498
2.18.9   Vitamin D group   501
2.18.10   Vitamin E (tocopherol)   502
2.18.11   Vitamin K   503
2.18.12   Multivitamin preparations   503
2.18.13   Iron   503
2.18.14   Calcium   504
2.18.15   Fluoride   505
2.18.16   Strontium   506
2.18.17   Biphosphonates and other osteoporosis drugs   506
2.18.18   Iodide   507
2.18.19   Trace elements   507

2.19. Herbs during pregnancy
Henry M. Hess and Richard K. Miller
2.19.1   The safety of herbs during pregnancy   511
2.19.2   Counseling a pregnant woman about herbs   512
2.19.3   General concepts regarding the use of herbs during pregnancy   513
2.19.4   Herbs used as foods   514
2.19.5   Essential oils that are safe during pregnancy   514
2.19.6   Herbs frequently used during pregnancy   514
2.19.7   Herbs controversially used during pregnancy   515
2.19.8   Herbs contraindicated during pregnancy   520

2.20. Diagnostic agents
Stefanie Hultzsch
2.20.1   Diagnostic imaging   527
2.20.2   Contrast media   531
2.20.3   Radioactive isotopes   534
2.20.4   Stable isotopes   536
2.20.5   Dyes   537
2.20.6   Other diagnostic agents   538

2.21. Recreational drugs
Sally Stephens and Laura M. Yates
Introduction   541
2.21.1   Alcohol   542
2.21.2   Caffeine and other xanthines   547
2.21.3   Tobacco and smoking   549
2.21.4   Drugs of abuse in general (excluding caffeine)   555
2.21.5   Sedating drugs   562

2.22. Poisonings and toxins
Laura M. Yates and Sally Stephens
2.22.1   The general risk of poisoning in pregnancy   575
2.22.2   Treatment of poisoning in pregnancy   576
2.22.3   Medicines   582

2.22.4	Animal toxins	590
2.22.5	Mushrooms	592
2.22.6	Other plant toxins	592
2.22.7	Bacterial endotoxins	592

2.23. Occupational, industrial and environmental agents
Susan M. Barlow, Frank M. Sullivan and Richard K. Miller

2.23.1	Solvent exposure in general	601
2.23.2	Formaldehyde and formalin	607
2.23.3	Photographic/printing chemicals	607
2.23.4	Pesticides	608
2.23.5	Phenoxyacetic acid derivatives and polychlorinated dibenzo-dioxins	612
2.23.6	Polychlorinated biphenyls	614
2.23.7	Chlorinated drinking water by-products	614
2.23.8	Metals	616
2.23.9	Hazardous waste landfill sites and waste incinerators	622
2.23.10	Radiation associated with the nuclear industry	623
2.23.11	Cell/mobile phones	625
2.23.12	Other sources of electromagnetic radiation	625
2.23.13	Electric shocks and lightning strikes	627

3   **General commentary on drug therapy and drug risk during lactation**
Ruth A. Lawrence and Christof Schaefer

3.1	The advantages of breastfeeding versus the risks of maternal medication	639
3.2	The passage of medications into the mother's milk	641
3.3	Infant characteristics	642
3.4	Milk plasma ratio	643
3.5	Amount of medication in the milk and relative dose	644
3.6	Toxicity of medications in the mother's milk	645
3.7	Medications that affect lactation	647
3.8	Breastfeeding support	648

4   **Specific drug therapies during lactation**

4.1. Analgesics, antiphlogistics and anesthetics
Maria Ellfolk and Stefanie Hultzsch

4.1.1	Paracetamol	653
4.1.2	Acetylsalisylic acid	654
4.1.3	Pyrazolone and phenylbutazone derivatives	655
4.1.4	Non-steroidal anti-inflammatory drugs (NSAID)	655
4.1.5	Selective COX-2 inhibitors	657
4.1.6	Other antirheumatics	658
4.1.7	Migraine medications	659
4.1.8	Opioids and opioid derivatives	660
4.1.9	Local anesthetics	664
4.1.10	Other medications used in connection with anesthesia	665
4.1.11	Myotonolytics and other analgesics	666
4.1.12	Gout therapy	666

4.2. Antiallergics, antiasthmatics and antitussives
Paul Merlob and Corinna Weber-Schöndorfer

4.2.1   Antihistamines (H_1-blocker)   671
4.2.2   Selective effective β_2-sympathomimetics   672
4.2.3   Inhalable corticosteroids (ICS)   673
4.2.4   Leukotrien-receptor antagonists   673
4.2.5   Theophylline   674
4.2.6   Mast cell inhibitors   674
4.2.7   Anticholinergics for asthma treatment   674
4.2.8   Omalizumab   675
4.2.9   Mucolytics, expectorants and cold remedies   675
4.2.10 Antitussives   675

4.3. Gastrointestinal drugs
Paul Merlob and Corinna Weber-Schöndorfer

4.3.1   Gastritis and ulcer medications   677
4.3.2   Peristaltic stimulators   679
4.3.3   Cholinergics   680
4.3.4   Anticholinergic spasmolytics   681
4.3.5   Laxatives   681
4.3.6   Agents used for chronic inflammatory bowel diseases   682
4.3.7   Antidiarrheals for acute diarrhea   683
4.3.8   Digestives and carminatives   683
4.3.9   Lipid reducers   683
4.3.10 Chenodeoxycholic acid and ursodeoxycholic acid   684
4.3.11 Appetite suppressants   684
4.3.12 Antiemetics   684

4.4. Anti-infectives
Stephanie Padberg

4.4.1   Penicillins, cephalosporins and other β-lactam antibiotics   688
4.4.2   Erythromycin and other macrolides   688
4.4.3   Tetracyclines   689
4.4.4   Sulfonamides and trimethoprim   689
4.4.5   Quinolones   690
4.4.6   Nitrofurans and drugs for urinary tract infections   690
4.4.7   Nitroimidazole antibiotics   691
4.4.8   Aminoglycosides   692
4.4.9   Glycopeptide and polypeptide antibiotics   692
4.4.10 Other antibiotics   692
4.4.11 Tuberculostatics   693
4.4.12 Local antibiotics   694
4.4.13 Antimalarial medication   695
4.4.14 Systemic antifungal agents   696
4.4.15 Topical antifungal agents   696
4.4.16 Anthelmintics   697
4.4.17 Antiviral agents   697

4.5. Vaccines and immunoglobulins
Ruth A. Lawrence and Mary Panse

4.5.1   Maternal immunization   705
4.5.2   Efficacy of immunization in breastfed infants   706

4.5.3   Hepatitis A vaccine   706
4.5.4   Hepatitis B vaccine   706
4.5.5   Human papillomavirus vaccine   707
4.5.6   Influenza vaccine   707
4.5.7   Polio vaccine   707
4.5.8   Rabies vaccine   708
4.5.9   Rubella vaccine   708
4.5.10   Smallpox vaccine   708
4.5.11   Typhoid vaccine   708
4.5.12   Immunoglobulins   709
4.5.13   CDC recommendations   709

4.6.   Cardiovascular drugs and diuretics
Paul Merlob and Corinna Weber-Schöndorfer
4.6.1   β-Receptor blockers   711
4.6.2   Hydralazine   713
4.6.3   α-Methyldopa   713
4.6.4   Calcium antagonists   714
4.6.5   ACE inhibitors   715
4.6.6   Angiotensin-II receptor-antagonists (sartan)   715
4.6.7   Other antihypertensives   716
4.6.8   Antihypotensives   717
4.6.9   Digitalis   717
4.6.10   Antiarrhythmics   717
4.6.11   Vasodilators and circulatory drugs   719
4.6.12   Diuretics   720

4.7.   Anticoagulants, thrombocyte aggregation inhibitors and fibrinolytics
Paul Merlob and Juliane Habermann
4.7.1   Heparin and danaparoid   725
4.7.2   Thrombin- and factor Xa-inhibitors   726
4.7.3   Thrombocyte aggregation inhibitors   726
4.7.4   Vitamin K-antagonists   727
4.7.5   Fibrinolytics   728
4.7.6   Antihemorrhagics   728
4.7.7   Volume expanders   728

4.8.   Antiepileptics
Paul Merlob and Christof Schaefer
4.8.1   Introduction   731
4.8.2   Individual antiepileptics   732

4.9.   Psychotropic drugs
Paul Merlob and Christof Schaefer
4.9.1   Introduction   743
4.9.2   Antidepressants   743
4.9.3   Individual antidepressants   745
4.9.4   Antipsychotic   755
4.9.5   Individual antipsychotic drugs   756
4.9.6   Lithium and other antimanic drugs   762
4.9.7   Anxiolytics, hypnotics and sedatives   764
4.9.8   Benzodiazepines   764

4.9.9	Zaleplon, zolpidem and zopiclone	767
4.9.10	Other anxiolytics, hypnotics and sedatives	767
4.9.11	Psychoanaleptics	768
4.9.12	Anti-Parkinson drugs	769

4.10. Immunomodulating and antineoplastic agents
Paul Merlob and Corinna Weber-Schöndorfer

4.10.1	Azathioprine and 6-mercaptopurine	775
4.10.2	Selective immune suppressants	776
4.10.3	Monoclonal antibodies (mAb) and other biologicals	777
4.10.4	Interferons	778
4.10.5	Other immune stimulants	779
4.10.6	Antineoplastics	779

4.11. Hormones and hormone antagonists
Gerard H.A. Visser and Corinna Weber-Schöndorfer

4.11.1	Pituitary and hypothalamic hormones	783
4.11.2	Methylergometrine (methylergonovine)	784
4.11.3	Bromocriptine and other prolactin inhibitors	785
4.11.4	Thyroid hormones and thyroid receptor antibodies (TRAb)	785
4.11.5	Thyrostatics	786
4.11.6	Iodine	787
4.11.7	Corticosteroids	788
4.11.8	Adrenaline	789
4.11.9	Insulin and oral antidiabetics	789
4.11.10	Estrogens, gestagens, and hormonal contraceptives	790
4.11.11	Androgens and anabolics	792
4.11.12	Cyproterone acetate and other sex-hormone inhibitors	792
4.11.13	Prostaglandins	793

4.12. Dermatological medication and local therapeutics
Christof Schaefer and Gudula Kirtschig

4.12.1	Topical applications and cosmetics	797
4.12.2	Essential oils	798
4.12.3	Retinoids and topicals for psoriasis, dermatitis and acne	798
4.12.4	Photochemotherapy and fumaric acid preparations	799
4.12.5	Wart removal medications	799
4.12.6	Medications for lice and scabies	799
4.12.7	Eye, nose and ear drops	800
4.12.8	Vein therapeutics and other local therapeutics	801
4.12.9	Vaginal therapeutics	801

4.13. Alternative remedies, vitamins, and minerals
Ruth A. Lawrence and Eleanor Hüttel

4.13.1	Alternative remedies and phytotherapeutics	803
4.13.2	Herbal galactogogues and antigalactogogues	805
4.13.3	Topical treatment for breast problems	807
4.13.4	Vitamins, minerals, and trace elements	808
4.13.5	Biphosphonates	808
4.13.6	Exercise	809
4.13.7	Glucose 6-phosphate-dehydrogenase deficiency	809

4.14. Contrast media, radionuclides and diagnostics
Stefanie Hultzsch

4.14.1	X-ray studies, ultrasound, and magnetic resonance imaging	813
4.14.2	Iodine-containing contrast media	813
4.14.3	Magnetic resonance contrast agents	815
4.14.4	Ultrasound contrast media	816
4.14.5	Radionuclides	816
4.14.6	Dyes	817
4.14.7	Other diagnostics	818

4.15. Infections during breastfeeding
Bernke te Winkel and Christof Schaefer

4.15.1	Common infections	822
4.15.2	Cytomegaly	822
4.15.3	Dengue virus	823
4.15.4	Hepatitis A	823
4.15.5	Hepatitis B	824
4.15.6	Hepatitis C	824
4.15.7	Hepatitis E	824
4.15.8	Herpes simplex	825
4.15.9	Herpes zoster (shingles), chicken pox (varicella)	825
4.15.10	HIV infection	826
4.15.11	Human T-lymphotropic virus (HTLV)	827
4.15.12	Influenza	827
4.15.13	Lyme disease	828
4.15.14	Methicillin-resistant *staphylococcus aureus* (MRSA)	828
4.15.15	Rotavirus	828
4.15.16	Tuberculosis	829
4.15.17	West Nile virus	830
4.15.18	Other infectious diseases	830

4.16. Recreational drugs
Mark Anderson and Marc Oppermann

4.16.1	Alcohol	835
4.16.2	Amphetamines	836
4.16.3	Caffeine	836
4.16.4	Cannabis	837
4.16.5	Cocaine	837
4.16.6	Nicotine	838
4.16.7	Opiates, including methadone	839
4.16.8	Other drugs	841

4.17. Plant toxins
Ruth A. Lawrence and Christof Schaefer

4.18. Industrial chemicals and environmental contaminants
Ruth A. Lawrence and Christof Schaefer

4.18.1	Persistent organochlorine compounds (pesticides, polychlorinated biphenyls and dioxins)	847
4.18.2	Mercury	851

4.18.3	Lead	853
4.18.4	Cadmium	855
4.18.5	Other contaminants	855
4.18.6	Breastfeeding despite environmental contaminants?	857
4.18.7	Breastfeeding and the workplace	858

Index   863

List of Contributors

MARK ANDERSON
Great North Children's Hospital, Newcastle upon Tyne, UK

SUSAN M. BARLOW
Harrington House, Brighton, East Sussex, UK

MATITIAHU BERKOVITCH
Clinical Pharmacology Unit and Teratogen Information Service, Assaf
Harofeh Medical Center, Tel Aviv University, Israel

CORNELIA BORISCH
Berlin Institute for Clinical Teratology and Drug Risk Assessment in
Pregnancy, Charité-University Clinic, Berlin, Germany

CHRISTINA D. CHAMBERS
Department of Pediatrics, University of California San Diego, La Jolla,
CA, USA

MAURIZIO CLEMENTI
Clinical Genetics Unit, Department of Women's and Children's Health,
University of Padova, Padova, Italy

BENEDIKTE-NOËL CUPPERS
Teratology Information Service, Lareb, Den Bosch, The Netherlands

MARIA ELLFOLK
Teratology Information Service, HUSLAB and Helsinki University
Central Hospital, Helsinki, Finland

JAN M. FRIEDMAN
Department of Medical Genetics, University of British Columbia,
Vancouver, Canada

LEE H. GOLDSTEIN
Clinical Pharmacology Unit, Haemek Medical Center, Tel Aviv
University, Tel Aviv, Israel

JULIANE HABERMANN
Berlin Institute for Clinical Teratology and Drug Risk Assessment in
Pregnancy, Charité-University Clinic, Berlin, Germany

HENRY M. HESS
Department of Obstetrics and Gynecology, University of Rochester
School of Medicine and Dentistry, Rochester NY, USA

STEFANIE HULTZSCH
Berlin Institute for Clinical Teratology and Drug Risk Assessment in
Pregnancy, Charité-University Clinic, Berlin, Germany

ELEANOR HÜTTEL
Berlin Institute for Clinical Teratology and Drug Risk Assessment in
Pregnancy, Charité-University Clinic, Berlin, Germany

ANGELA KAYSER
Berlin Institute for Clinical Teratology and Drug Risk Assessment in
Pregnancy, Charité-University Clinic, Berlin, Germany

GUDULA KIRTSCHIG
Department of Dermatology, VU Medical Centre, Amsterdam, The
Netherlands

RUTH A. LAWRENCE
Department of Pediatrics, University of Rochester School of Medicine
and Dentistry, Rochester, NY, USA

FERNANDA SALES LUIZ VIANNA
Teratogen Information Service, Medical Genetics Service, Hospital de
Clinicas de Porto Alegre, Porto Alegre, Brazil

HELI MALM
Teratology Information Service, HUSLAB and Helsinki University
Central Hospital, Helsinki, Finland

PAUL MERLOB
Beilinson Teratology Information Service (BELTIS) Department of
Neonatology, Rabin Medical Center, Schneider Children Hospital,
Petah Tikva, and Sackler School of Medicine, Tel-Aviv University,
Tel-Aviv, Israel

RICHARD K. MILLER
Department of Obstetrics and Gynecology, University of Rochester
School of Medicine and Dentistry, Rochester, NY, USA

MARC OPPERMANN
Berlin Institute for Clinical Teratology and Drug Risk Assessment in
Pregnancy, Charité-University Clinic, Berlin, Germany

ASHER ORNOY
Department of Medical Neurobiology, Hebrew University Hadassah
Medical School and Israeli Ministry of Health, Jerusalem, Israel

STEPHANIE PADBERG
Berlin Institute for Clinical Teratology and Drug Risk Assessment in
Pregnancy, Charité-University Clinic, Berlin, Germany

MARY PANSE
Berlin Institute for Clinical Teratology and Drug Risk Assessment in
Pregnancy, Charité-University Clinic, Berlin, Germany

PAUL PETERS
Department of Obstetrics, University Medical Center Utrecht, Utrecht,
The Netherlands

JANINE E. POLIFKA
Department of Pediatrics, University of Washington, Seattle, WA, USA

CHRISTOF SCHAEFER
Berlin Institute for Clinical Teratology and Drug Risk Assessment in
Pregnancy, Charité-University Clinic, Berlin, Germany

LAVINIA SCHÜLER-FACCINI
Teratogen Information Service, Medical Genetics Service, Hospital de Clinicas de Porto Alegre, Porto Alegre, Brazil

SALLY STEPHENS
UK Teratology Information Service (UKTIS), Newcastle upon Tyne Hospitals NHS Foundation Trust, Newcastle-upon-Tyne, UK

FRANK M. SULLIVAN
Harrington House, Harrington Road, Brighton, East Sussex, UK

GERARD H.A. VISSER
Department of Obstetrics, University Medical Center, Utrecht, The Netherlands

CORINNA WEBER-SCHÖENDORFER
Berlin Institute for Clinical Teratology and Drug Risk Assessment in Pregnancy, Charité-University Clinic, Berlin, Germany

BERNKE TE WINKEL
Teratology Information Service, Lareb, Den Bosch, The Netherlands

KATHERINE L. WISNER
Department of Psychiatry, Northwestern University, Feinberg School of Medicine, Chicago, IL, USA

LAURA M. YATES
UK Teratology Information Service (UKTIS), Newcastle upon Tyne Hospitals NHS Foundation Trust, Newcastle-upon-Tyne, UK

Preface

We wish to thank the readership for their suggestions and support of the second English edition. We were most appreciative that this textbook was not only available in the German language (eight editions with almost 80,000 copies), but also in Chinese and Russian. This third English edition with contributions from the experts in the field continues the tradition of integrating therapies for disease with drug selections during pregnancy and lactation. We hope that physicians, health care and cure providers will find that this expanded third English edition enhances their ability to answer the queries frequently asked by concerned women who are planning a pregnancy, are pregnant, or are breastfeeding regarding the risk of medicinal products for themselves, their unborn or breastfed infant.

We continue to focus the content of this volume for Family Medicine Physicians, Internists, Obstetricians, Pediatricians, Psychiatrists, Medical Geneticists, Dermatologists, Lactation Consultants, Midwives, Nurses, Pharmacists, Psychologists and Toxicologists among all health care providers. The third English edition features the most relevant information in regard to acceptable treatment options and allows readers to be confident in their capability to assess the risk of an inadvertent or required treatment/exposure.

As we have indicated in previous editions, aspects of drug counseling are inadequately supported by various sources of information such as the *Physician's Desk Reference*, package leaflets or pharmacotherapy handbooks. Formal drug risk classifications or statements such as "contraindicated during pregnancy" may even lead to a simplified perception of risk, e.g., an overestimation of the risk or simple fatalism, and withholding of essential therapy or the prescription of insufficiently studied and potentially risky drugs may result. This simplified perception of risk can also lead to unnecessary invasive prenatal diagnostic testing or even to a recommendation to terminate a wanted pregnancy. During lactation, misclassification of a drug risk may lead to the advice to stop breastfeeding, even though the drug in question is acceptable or alternatives appropriate for the breastfeeding period are available.

This book continues to be based on a survey of the literature on drug risks during pregnancy and lactation, as yet unpublished results of recent studies, and current discussions in professional societies dealing with clinical teratology and developmental toxicology. Similar to the German edition originally founded by Horst Spielmann, Berlin, this volume reflects accepted "good therapeutic practice" in different clinical settings. It is written for clinical decision-makers. Arranged according to treatment indications, the third English edition provides an overview of the relevant drugs in the referring medical specialty available today that might be taken by women of reproductive age. The volume's organization facilitates a comparative risk approach, i.e., identifying the drugs of choice for particular diseases or symptoms. In addition, recreational drugs, diagnostic procedures (X-ray), vaccinations, poisonings, workplace and environmental contaminants, herbs, supplements and breastfeeding during infectious diseases are discussed in detail.

The third English edition has been completely revised. The content has been adapted for an international readership. The contributing authors reflect expertise in a range of clinical specialties, e.g. dermatology, obstetrics, pediatrics, internal medicine, psychiatry and many others.

Moreover, most authors are active members of the teratology societies including the Organization of Teratogen Information Specialists (OTIS) and the European Network of Teratology Information Services (ENTIS).

We are grateful for the outstanding contributions from each of the authors. It should be noted that the editors and authors have agreed that the royalties from this volume will be donated to women's health services in areas of need. The royalties from the second English edition helped to support women's health clinics in Guatemala.

The Editors and Authors do express our appreciation to Kristine Jones, publishing editor, from Elsevier/Academic Press for providing support and advice. We thank Shannon Stanton for constant and diligent support during the developmental process and overseeing the transfer of chapters to production and Elizabeth Hormann and Ekkehard Kemmann for translation. Finally, the editors wish to express our appreciation to our families for providing us the time and support to complete this edition.

May the reader use this volume, both in print and electronically, to perform a risk assessment and to examine treatment options for specific diseases in women of reproductive age. By providing pre-pregnancy counseling, the editors and authors hope that inappropriate therapeutic, occupational and/or environmental exposures will be minimized.

Finally, we continue to welcome comments, recommendations and suggestions from our readers using this volume. Please do share your suggestions with us at the following email address: DrugPregLac@urmc.rochester.edu.*

Richard K Miller, Rochester, New York, USA
Christof Schaefer, Berlin, Germany
Paul Peters, Utrecht, Netherlands

---

* Do not use this email address for patient-related questions because it is not constantly monitored. If you have specific patient related questions, please contact the nearest MotherToBaby or ENTIS Teratogen Information Service. Thank you.

Disclaimer

Knowledge and best practice in this field are constantly changing. As new research and experience broaden our understanding, changes in research methods, professional practices, or medical treatment may become necessary.

Practitioners and researchers must always rely on their own experience and knowledge in evaluating and using any information, methods, compounds, or experiments described herein. In using such information or methods they should be mindful of their own safety and the safety of others, including parties for whom they have a professional responsibility.

With respect to any drug or pharmaceutical products identified, readers are advised to check the most current information provided (i) on procedures featured or (ii) by the manufacturer of each product to be administered, to verify the recommended dose or formula, the method and duration of administration, and interactions. It is the responsibility of practitioners, relying on their own experience and knowledge of their patients, to make diagnoses, to determine dosages and the best treatment for each individual patient, and to take all appropriate safety precautions.

To the fullest extent of the law, neither the Publisher nor the authors, contributors, or editors, assume any liability for any injury and/or damage to persons or property as a matter of products liability, negligence or otherwise, or from any use or operation of any methods, products, instructions, or ideas contained in the material herein.

General commentary on drug therapy and drug risks in pregnancy

1

Paul Peters, Richard K. Miller and Christof Schaefer

1.1	Introduction	1
1.2	Development and health	2
1.3	Reproductive stages	3
1.4	Reproductive and developmental toxicology	4
1.5	Basic principles of drug-induced reproductive and developmental toxicology	8
1.6	Effects and manifestations	10
1.7	Pharmacokinetics of drugs in pregnancy	11
1.8	Mechanisms of developmental toxic agents	13
1.9	Causes of developmental disorders	14
1.10	Embryo/fetotoxic risk assessment and plausibility	15
1.11	Classification of drugs used in pregnancy	17
1.12	Paternal use of medicinal products	18
1.13	Communicating the risk of drug use in pregnancy	19
1.14	Risk communication prior to pharmacotherapeutic choice	20
1.15	Risk communication regarding the safety of drugs already used in pregnancy	21
1.16	Teratology information centers	21

1.1   Introduction

Most prescribers and users of drugs are familiar with the precautions given concerning drug use during the first trimester of pregnancy. These warnings were introduced after the thalidomide disaster in the early 1960s. However, limiting the exercise of caution to the first 3 months of pregnancy is both shortsighted and effectively impossible – firstly, because chemicals can affect any stage of pre- or postnatal development; and secondly, because when a woman first learns that she is pregnant, the process of organogenesis has already long since begun (for example, the neural tube has closed). Hence, the unborn could already be inadvertently exposed to maternal drug treatment during the early embryonic period (Figure 1.1).

This book is intended for practicing clinicians, who prescribe medicinal products, evaluate environmental or occupational exposures in women who are or may become pregnant. Understanding the risks of

Drugs During Pregnancy and Lactation. http://dx.doi.org/10.1016/B978-0-12-408078-2.00001-9

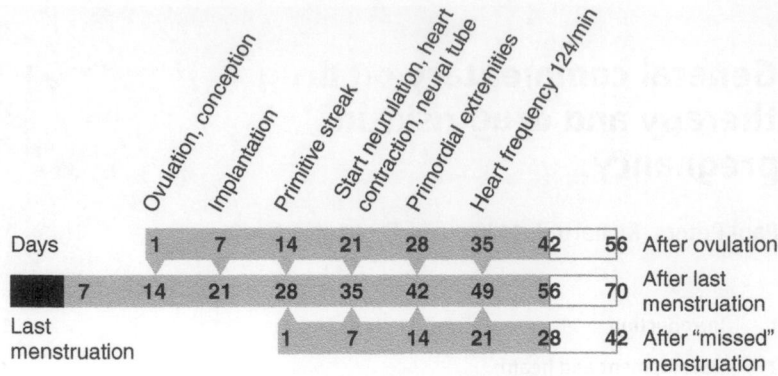

Figure 1 Timetable of early human development.

drug use in pregnancy has lagged behind the advances in other areas of pharmacotherapy. Epidemiologic difficulties in establishing causality and the ethical barriers to randomized clinical trials with pregnant women are the major reasons for our collective deficiencies. Nevertheless, since the recognition of prenatal vulnerability in the early 1960s, much has been accomplished to identify potential developmental toxicants such as medicinal products and to regulate human exposure to them. The adverse developmental effects of pharmaceutical products are now recognized to include not only malformations, but also growth restriction, fetal death and functional defects in the newborn.

The evaluation of human case reports and epidemiological investigations provide the primary sources of information. However, for many drugs and certainly new drugs (even more so in the case of chemicals) experience with human exposure is scarce, and animal experiments, *in vitro* tests, or information on related congeners provide the only basis for risk assessment. Registration authorities in different continents have mandated that medications potentially used in pregnant women must now be followed via pregnancy registries.

This book presents the current state of knowledge about the use of drugs during pregnancy. In each chapter, the information is presented separately for two different aspects of the problem: firstly, seeking a drug appropriate for prescription during pregnancy; and secondly, assessing the risk of a drug when exposure during pregnancy has already occurred.

1.2   Development and health

The care of pregnant women presents one of the paradoxes of modern medicine. Women usually require little medical intervention during a (uneventful) pregnancy. Conversely, those at high risk of damage to their own health, or that of their unborn, require the assistance of appropriate medical technology, including drugs. Accordingly, there are two classes of pregnant women; the larger group requires support but little intervention, while the other requires the full range of diagnostic and therapeutic measures applied in any other branch of medicine (Chamberlain 1991). Maternal illness demands treatment tolerated by the unborn. However, a normal pregnancy needs to avoid harmful drugs – both prescribed and over-the-counter, and drugs of abuse, including smoking and alcohol – as well as occupational and environmental exposure to potentially harmful chemicals. Obviously, sufficient and well-balanced nutrition is also essential. Currently, this set of positive preventive measures is by no means broadly guaranteed in either developing or industrial countries. When such primary preventive measures are neglected, complications of pregnancy and developmental disorders can result. Furthermore, nutritional deficiencies and toxic effects during prenatal life predispose the future adult to some diseases, such as schizophrenia (St Clair 2005), fertility disorders (Elias 2005), metabolic imbalances (Painter 2005), hypertension, non-insulin-dependent diabetes, and cardiovascular illnesses, as demonstrated by Barker (1998) and based upon epidemiological and experimental data. Studies of programming in fetal life are now on the agenda for medical research.

1.3   Reproductive stages

The different stages of reproduction are, in fact, highlights of a continuum. These stages concern a specific developmental time-span, each with its own sensitivity to a given toxic agent.

- *Primordial germ cells* are present in the embryo at about 1 month after the first day of the last menstruation. They originate from the yolksac-entoderm outside the embryo, and migrate into the undifferentiated primordia of gonads located at the medio-ventral surface of the urogenital ridges. They subsequently differentiate into oogonia and oocytes, or into spermatogonia. Toxic effects on primordial germ cells may cause infertility or mutagenic harm.
- *Oocytes* in postnatal life are at an arrested stage of the meiotic division. This division is reinitiated much later following birth, shortly before ovulation, and is finalized after fertilization with the expulsion of the polar bodies. Thus, all-female germ cells develop prenatally and no germ cells are formed after birth. Moreover, during a female lifespan approximately 400 oocytes undergo ovulation. All these facts make it possible to state that an 8-week pregnant mother of an unborn female is already prepared to be a grandmother! This implies that the oocytes are not only older than the female but also that they are being exposed to substances from prenatal time forward. As we have seen in Section 1.2, fetal programming during early stages of pregnancy might induce diseases in later adult life; such programming for toxicity might also be possibly focused upon oocytes.
- The embryonal *spermatogenic* epithelium, on the contrary, divides slowly by repeated mitoses, and these cells do not differentiate into spermatocytes and do not undergo meiosis in the prenatal period. Gonocytes exist in the neonatal testis and represent a transient population of male germ-line stem cells. It has been demonstrated that stem cell self-renewal and progeny production are probably controlled by the neighboring differentiated cells and extracellular matrix known as niches. The onset of meiosis in the male begins at puberty. Spermatogenesis continues throughout (reproductive) life. Even after chemotherapeutic treatment for example with anticancer drugs or radiation with destruction of spermatogonia, repopulation of the epithelium is possible with even a complete functional restitution. This is in contrast with oogonia after such chemotherapeutic treatment. When the complexity of sexual development and female and male gametogenesis is considered, it becomes apparent that pre- and postnatal drug exposures are special toxicological problems having different outcomes. The specificity of the male and

Pregnancy

1 General commentary on drug therapy and drug risks in pregnancy

female developmental processes also accounts for unique reactions to toxic agents, such as drugs, in both sexes.

■ After *fertilization* of the oocyte by one of the spermatozoa in the oviduct, there is the stage of cell division and transport of the blastocyst into the endocrine-prepared uterine cavity. After implantation, the bilaminar stage is formed and *embryogenesis* begins with beating heart and the functioning yolksac as a nutritional and excretion organ, followed by contact with the mother by the placenta. The next 7 weeks are a period of finely balanced cellular events, including proliferation, migration, association and differentiation, and programmed cell death, precisely arranged to produce tissues and organs from the genetic information present in each conceptus.

■ During this period of *organogenesis*, rapid cell multiplication is the rule. Complex processes of cell migration, pattern formation and the penetration of one cell group by another characterize these later stages.

■ Final morphological and functional development occurs at different times during *fetogenesis*, and is completed after birth.

■ *Postnatal adaptation* characterizes the passage from intra- into extra-uterine life with tremendous changes in, for example, circulatory and respiratory physiology (see also Table 1.1).

1.4   Reproductive and developmental toxicology

Reproductive toxicology is the subject area dealing with the causes, mechanisms, effects and prevention of disturbances throughout the entire reproductive cycle, including fertility induced by chemicals. Teratology (derived from the Greek word τερας which originally meant *star*; later meanings were *wonder, divine intervention* and, finally, *terrible vision, magic, inexplicability, monster*) is the science concerned with birth defects of a structural nature (dysmorphology). However, the terminology is not strict, since literature also recognizes "functional" teratogenic effects, such as fetal alcohol effects in the absence of alcohol-related birth defects and dysmorphology.

To understand the different definitions in this domain of toxicity the following explanations are helpful. Reproductive toxicology represents the harmful effects by agents on the progeny and/or impairment of male and female reproductive functions. *Developmental toxicity* involves any adverse effect induced prior to attainment of adult life. It includes the effects induced or manifested in the embryonic or fetal period, and those induced or manifested postnatally. *Embryo/fetotoxicity* involves any toxic effect on the conceptus resulting from prenatal exposure, including structural and functional abnormalities, and of postnatal manifestations of such effects. *Teratogenicity* is a manifestation of developmental toxicity, representing a particular case of embryo/fetotoxicity, by the induction or the increase of the frequency of structural disorders in the progeny.

The rediscovery of Mendel's laws about a century ago, and the knowledge that some congenital abnormalities were passed from parents to children, led to attempts to explain abnormalities in children based on genetic theory. However, Hale (1933) noticed that piglets born to sows fed a vitamin A-deficient diet were born without eyes. He rightly concluded that a nutritional deficiency leads to a marked disturbance of the internal factors, which control the mechanism of eye development. During a rubella epidemic in 1941, the Australian ophthalmologist, Gregg, observed that embryos exposed to the rubella virus often

Table 1.1 Reproductive stages: organs and functions potentially affected by toxicants

Reproductive stage	Female	Male	Possible endpoints
Germ cell formation	Oogenesis (occurs during fetal development of mother) Gene replication Cell division Egg maturation Hormonal influence on ovary Ovulation	Spermatogenesis Gene replication Cell division Sperm maturation Sertoli cell influence Hormonal influence on testes	Sterility, subfecundity, damaged sperm or eggs, chromosomal aberrations, menstrual effects, age at menopause, hormone imbalances, changes in sex ratio
Fertilization	Oviduct contractility secretions Hormonal influence on secretory and muscle cells Uterus contractility secretions Nervous system behavior libido	Accessory glands Sperm motility and nutrition Hormonal influence on glands Nervous system erection ejaculation behavior libido	Impotence, sterility, subfecundity, chromosomal aberrations, changes in sex ratio, reduced sperm function Impotence, sterility, subfecundity, chromosomal aberrations, changes in sex ratio, reduced sperm function
Implantation	Changes in uterine lining and secretions Hormonal influence on secretory cells		Spontaneous abortion, embryonic resorption, subfecundity, stillbirths, low birth weight
Embryogenesis	Uterus Yolksac placenta formation Embryo cell division, tissue differentiation, hormone production, growth		Spontaneous abortion, other fetal losses, birth defects, chromosomal abnormalities, change in sex ratio, stillbirths, low birth weight

(Continued)

1 General commentary on drug therapy and drug risks in pregnancy

Pregnancy

Table 1.1 (*Continued*)

Reproductive stage	Female	Male	Possible endpoints

Organogenesis	Placenta
	  nutrient transfer
	  hormone production
	  protection from toxic agents
	Embryo
	  organ development and differentiation growth
			Birth defects, spontaneous abortion, fetal defects, death, retarded growth and development, functional disorders (e.g. autism), transplacental carcinogenesis

Perinatal	Fetus
	  growth and development
	Uterus
	  Contractility
	  Hormonal effects
	  on uterine muscle cells
	  Maternal nutrition
			Premature births, births defects (particularly nervous system), stillbirths, neonatal death, toxic syndromes or withdrawal symptoms in neonates

Postnatal	Infant survival Lactation		Mental retardation, infant mortality, retarded development, metabolic and functional disorders, developmental disabilities (e.g. cerebral palsy and epilepsy)

displayed abnormalities, such as cataracts, cardiac defects, deafness and mental retardation (Gregg 1941). Soon after it was discovered that the protozoon *Toxoplasma*, a unicellular parasite, could induce abnormalities such as hydrocephaly and vision disturbances in the unborn. These observations proved undeniably that the placenta is not an absolute barrier against external influences.

Furthermore, from the early 1960s maternal exposure to the mild sedative *thalidomide*, marketed since 1957 in Germany appeared to be causing characteristic reduction deformities of the limbs, ranging from hypoplasia of one or more digits to the total absence of all limbs. An example of the thalidomide embryopathy is phocomelia: the structures of the hand and feet may be reduced to a single small digit, or may appear virtually normal but protrude directly from the trunk, like the flippers of a seal (phoca). Nowadays there exists some confusion and discussion about the discovery of thalidomide as human teratogen. The book "Dark Remedy: the Impact of Thalidomide and its Survival as a Vital Medicine" by Stephens (2009) explains in detail the events in 1961 and 1962. H.R. Wiedemann reported the first series of children with thalidomide-induced malformations in the 16 September 1961 Issue of the Med. Welt (in German). W.G. McBride placed a question in a 15-line Letter to the Editor published in the 16 December 1961 issue of the *Lancet* stating "... In recent month I have observed that the incidence of multiple severe abnormalities in babies delivered of women who were given the drug thalidomide ... bony development seems to be affected ... have any of your readers seen similar abnormalities who have taken this drug during pregnancy?" Following this letter, the Lancet editor inserted a statement indicating that the 2 December 1961 issue carried a statement from the Distillers Company Ltd. referring to "reports from two overseas sources possibly associating thalidomide with harmful effects on the foetus ... the company decided to withdraw from the market all its preparations containing thalidomide." On 6 January 1962 Widukind Lenz confirmed in a Letter to the *Lancet*: "I have seen 52 malformed infants whose mothers had taken "Contergan" (thalidomide) in early pregnancy ... since I discussed the aetiological role of "Contergan" ... at a conference with the producer on Nov. 18, 1961, I have received letters ... reporting 115 additional cases...".

This discovery of Wiedemann (1961), McBride (1961) and Lenz (1961) independently led to a worldwide interest in clinical teratology. In the Unites States Francis Kelsey, working at the FDA and being dissatisfied with the application for marketing of the product, prevented a catastrophe of unimaginable proportion (Kalter 2010, Kelsey 1988). Fifty years after the thalidomide disaster, the risk of drug-induced developmental disorders can be better delimited. To date there has been no sudden confrontation by a medicinal product provoking, as in the case of thalidomide, such devastating disorders. Drugs that nevertheless caused birth defects, such as retinoids, were known and expected, based upon animal experiments, to cause these conditions. Moreover, in general terms the prevalence of birth defects (3–4%) has not increased in the last half century, although substantially more substances have been marketed during these years. It should though be noted that it was not until the 1990s that autism was associated with thalidomide exposure very early in development before limb malformations would be induced (Strömland 1994).

Contrary to the assessment of drug-induced disorders and drugs of abuse, it is more difficult to indicate a risk from occupational chemical and physical exposure. In such situations, an individual risk assessment is nearly impossible since the information necessary for a pertinent evaluation is lacking, although Occupational Exposure Limits (OELs) or Threshold Limit Values (TLVs) and occupational precautions are important considerations (see Chapter 2.23).

Pregnancy

1 General commentary on drug therapy and drug risks in pregnancy

An essential aim of public health is prevention. Primary prevention of developmental disorders can be defined as an intervention to prevent the origin of a developmental disorder – for example, by rubella vaccination, or by correction of an aberrant lifestyle such as alcohol use. Moreover, primary prevention of developmental disorders can be achieved when a chemical substance is identified as a reproductive toxicant and either is not approved for marketing, or is approved with specific pregnancy labeling, restricted use or removed from the market. This is in contrast to secondary prevention of developmental disorders, which means the prevention of the birth of a child with a developmental defect – usually by termination of pregnancy. In this context, tertiary prevention of a developmental disorder indicates an early detection of a metabolic disorder so that, for example, in the case of phenylketonuria (PKU) as an intervention a special diet low in phenylanaline is indicated to prevent mental retardation (phenylpyruvic oligophrenia).

When thalidomide was recognized as being the causal factor of phocomelia, the removal of the drug from the market resulted in the disappearance of the embryopathy. However, it took at least 5 years before the association was made between the introduction of the teratogen and the extremely rare type of deformities. This event was also accompanied by a transient drastic avoidance of general drug intake by pregnant women.

Healthcare professionals and pregnant women must continue to develop a more critical approach to the use of drugs and exposure to chemicals, not only during pregnancy but also before pregnancy – or, even better, during the entire fertile period. Such a critical approach should result in avoiding many unnecessary and unknown risks.

These remarks imply that health professionals, couples planning to have children, and pregnant women must be informed about drugs proven to be safe, and the risks of wanted or unwanted exposures to chemicals as medications, environmental, including infections or occupational exposures.

1.5   Basic principles of drug-induced reproductive and developmental toxicology

Drugs that have the capacity to induce reproductive toxicity often can be identified before being marketed, based upon the outcome of laboratory animal experiments. The final conclusions can only become available through epidemiological studies after the product has been on the market for some time. The determination of whether a given medicinal product has the potentiality or capability to induce developmental disorders is essentially governed by four established fundamental principles (Wilson 1977). It can be stated that an embryo- and fetotoxic response depends upon exposure to: (1) a specific substance in a particular dose, (2) a genetically susceptible species, (3) a conceptus in a susceptible stage of development, and (4) by the mode of action of reproductive toxic drugs.

Principle 1

As in other toxicological evaluations, reproductive toxicity is governed by dose–effect relationships; the curve is generally quite steep. The dose–response is of the utmost importance in determining whether there is a true effect. Moreover, nearly every reproductive toxic drug that has been realistically tested has been shown to have a threshold, a "no-effect" level. Another aspect worth mentioning is the occasionally highly specific nature of the substance – for instance, thalidomide is a clear-cut teratogen in the human and specific species (rabbit), in contrast to its analogs, which were never proven to be developmental toxicants. Moreover, not only is the daily dose of importance to the result but also the route of exposure for a potential embryo/fetotoxic concentration of the drug.

Principle 2

Not all mammalian species are equally susceptible or sensitive to the reproductive/developmental toxic influence of a given chemical. The inter- and intraspecies variability may be manifested in several ways: a drug that acts in one species may have little or no effects in others; a reproductive/developmental toxicant may produce similar defects in various species, but these defects will vary in frequency; a substance may induce certain developmental disorders in one species that are entirely different from those induced in others. The explanation is that there are genetic differences such as in pharmacokinetics and/or in receptor sensitivity that influence the teratogenic response. This may be further modified by other environmental factors.

Principle 3

There exists a sensitive period for different effects, i.e. the developmental phase, during which originating, proliferating and differentiating cells and organs become susceptible to a given drug. This period may not be related to critical morphogenetic periods, but may, for example, be related to the appearance of specific receptors. This explains how, at an early stage of development, dysmorphology is induced by a substance, which, at the latter stage of the development, induces functional disorders such as those of the central nervous system. These stages are often called windows of susceptibility.

Principle 4

The pathogenesis and the final defects from developmental toxicity can be studied rather well. Knowledge about the early onset or the mechanisms associated with developmental toxicity of these agents is often absent. Mechanistic information is, however, essential to understanding how chemicals can perturb development, and is a critical component of the risk assessment. To improve the understanding of the mode of action of toxicants, including early repair mechanisms, critical molecular targets of the developmental processes should be identified. These targets are, among others: evolutionary conserved pathways of development; conserved molecular-stress and checkpoint pathways; and conserved toxicokinetic components, such as those involved in the transport and metabolism of toxicants. Different signaling pathways that operate in the development of the organs of model animals, such as the fruitfly, roundworm and zebrafish, also operate in the development of mammalian organs. Therefore, the effects of medicinal products on fundamental processes such as signaling can be detected. Because the same signaling pathways operating in the various kinds of organ development in mammals are more and more known, and will be even better known, a chemical's toxicological impact on these pathways can be predicted on the basis of the results in non-mammalian organisms and tested in mammals (Committee on Developmental Toxicology 2000).

Pregnancy

1 General commentary on drug therapy and drug risks in pregnancy

1.6   Effects and manifestations

A wide variety of responses characterizes developmental toxicity. Infertility, chromosomal and genetic disorders, spontaneous abortion, intrauterine death, prematurity, low birth weight, birth defects and functional disorders are the effects of such drug interference with the developmental and reproductive processes. The manifestation of a developmental or a reproductive toxicant can either be seen immediately after exposure, or will be expressed at a much later date. Interfering with male or female germ cell development might result in infertility, decreased sperm activity and/or libido, and impaired gametogenesis. The effects on the pre-implantation stage will cause early embryonic death, extra-uterine implantation, or delayed transport of the fertilized zygote. These last outcomes nuance the idea that at the early phase of development there exists a so-called "all or nothing effect".

A critical phase for the induction of structural malformations usually occurs during the period of organogenesis. In humans, this critical period extends from about 20–70 days after the first day of the last menstruation period, or from 1 week before the missed menstruation until the woman is 44 days late. It may be unwise to rely absolutely on this time period (Table 1.1). With physical agents such as X-rays used in laboratory animals, exposure can be limited exactly to a period of minutes to discover the exact sensitive period for inducing a specific disorder. However, with drugs and other chemicals, we are unsure about the time course of absorption, metabolism and excretion. In addition, the actual proximate teratogen may be a metabolite rather than the compound administered. If the moment of final differentiation of a particular organ is known with certainty, then a teratogen must have been present prior to that time, if it is presumed to be the causal agent of the malformation.

During the fetal period, the manifestations from toxicological interference are growth restriction, some forms of structural malformations, fetal death, functional impairment, and transplacental carcinogenesis. The period of organ and system maturation extends beyond the period of organogenesis, and even beyond the prenatal period. Therefore, the susceptible period for the induction of insults that may lead to functional deficits is much longer than that for the induction of gross structural defects. Functions affected by pre- and early postnatal exposure to chemicals include behavior, reproduction, endocrine function, immune competence, xenobiotic metabolism, learning capacity, and various other physiological functions.

Fetal tissues are intrinsically highly vulnerable to carcinogens because of their high rate of cellular proliferation. This phenomenon has been demonstrated in rats, mice, hamsters, rabbits, opossums, pigs, dogs, and monkeys. About 25 compounds and groups of chemicals and 10 industrial processes have been shown to induce carcinogenic effects in human beings. However, there is convincing epidemiological evidence of transplacental tumor-induction in humans for only one compound – diethylstilbestrol (DES). Exposure to DES *in utero* leads to the development of clear-cell adenocarcinoma of the vagina or cervix in about 1 in 1000 of those at risk. Moreover, DES is now a recognized female genital tract teratogen. The effects of exposure to DES *in utero* for males are known (e.g. short phallus); however, others (e.g. infertility) remain controversial (see also Chapter 2.15.15 for details).

1.7   Pharmacokinetics of drugs in pregnancy

Metabolism and kinetics of medicinal products are more complicated in pregnancy than otherwise. In general, the following pharmacokinetics influence the effective concentration of a drug or its metabolites:

- The uptake, distribution, metabolism and excretion by the mother (changes during pregnancy of some physiologic parameters influencing the metabolism of chemicals are summarized in Table 1.2);
- Passage and metabolism through the yolk sac and the placenta with its changing physiology;
- Distribution, metabolism and excretion by the embryo or fetus;
- Re-absorption and swallowing of substances by the unborn from the amniotic fluid.

Pregnancy induces many maternal physiological changes and adaptations, which can lead to clinically important reductions in the blood concentrations of certain medicinal products. The total body water increases by as much as 8 liters during pregnancy, which provides a substantially increased volume in which drugs can be distributed. During pregnancy, the intestinal, cutaneous and inhalatory absorption of chemicals changes due to a decreased peristalsis of the intestines and an increase in skin and lung blood flow. However, this has no consequences for the uptake of medicines from the intestinal tract. Serum proteins relevant to drug binding undergo considerable changes in concentration. Albumin, which binds acidic drugs and chemicals (such as phenytoin and aspirin), decreases in concentration by up to 10 g/L. The main implication of this change is in the interpretation of drug concentrations. The increased production of female hormones activates enzymes in the maternal liver, and this may result in a modified inactivation of medicinal and environmental agents. The renal plasma flow will have almost doubled by the last trimester of

Table 1.2 Changes during pregnancy of the pharmacokinetics of drugs

Resorption	
Gastrointestinal motility	↓
Lung function	↑
Skin blood circulation	↑
Distribution	
Plasma volume	↑
Body water	↑
Plasma protein	↓
Fat deposition	↑
Metabolism	
Liver activity	↑↓
Excretion	
Glomerular filtration	↑

Source: Loebstein (1997).

pregnancy, and drugs that are eliminated unchanged by the kidney are usually eliminated more rapidly; this change in renal clearance has been clinically important in only a few cases, and does not require adaptation of the dose of drugs in general (Loebstein 1997). Some drugs, such as anticonvulsants and theophylline derivatives, can undergo changes in distribution and elimination, which lead to ineffective treatment because of inadequate drug concentrations in the blood (Lander 1984).

Most studies of drug transfer across the maternal and embryonic/fetal barrier are concerned with the end of pregnancy. Little is known about the transport of substances in the early phases of pregnancy, in which, morphologically and functionally, both the yolk sac and the placenta develop and change in performance (Miller 2010, Carney 2004, Garbis-Berkvens 1987). Before birth when the placenta becomes more fibrotic it can be called both functionally and morphologically a geriatric organ, not representing the pharmacokinetics of, for example, the mid-term placenta. The placenta is essentially a lipid barrier between the maternal and embryonic/fetal circulations, like the lipid membrane of the gastrointestinal tract, allowing fat-soluble medicines to cross more easily than water-soluble. Hence, medicinal products that are taken orally and are well absorbed will pass the placental membranes. Drugs cross the placenta by passive diffusion, and a non-ionized drug of low molecular weight will cross the placenta more rapidly than a more polar drug. Given time, however, most drugs will achieve roughly equal concentrations on both sides of the placenta. Thus, the practical view to take when prescribing drugs during pregnancy is that the transfer of drugs to the fetus is inevitable. On the other hand, the placenta, like other organ barriers, contains efflux transporters that may prevent substantial transfer of particular substances to the fetus. The conclusion that equal and even higher concentrations of a (combination) of active substances can be present in the embryonic/fetal compartment is in fact dramatic. Since apart from exceptionally and specifically treating the unborn, these pharmacological effects upon the fetus are unwanted and need therefore to be defined as toxic. With such a high number of drugs used in pregnancy and so relatively few disorders observed postnatal, there has to be an already huge repair system in the fetus and newborn – even more realizing that there exists an absent or diminished metabolic, detoxifying and excretion system in the embryonic compartment.

Most drugs have a lower molecular weight than 600–800, and will therefore be able to cross the placenta. The notable exceptions to this rule are the conjugated steroid and peptide hormones such as insulin and growth hormone. However, larger molecules (e.g. vitamin B_{12} and immunoglobulins) do cross the placenta via specific receptor-mediated processes. It was shown that biologicals, such as TNF-α-Inhibitors cross the placenta during the second half of pregnancy and may reach therapeutic values in the newborn (see also Chapter 2.12).

In the third month of pregnancy, the fetal liver is already capable of activating or inactivating chemical substances through oxidation (Juchau 1989). In the fetal compartment the detoxification of drugs and their metabolites takes place at a low level, certainly in the first half of pregnancy. This aspect, among others – such as excretion in the amniotic fluid – makes it understandable that accumulation of biological active substances might take place in the fetal compartment. The (at that time not yet existing) blood–brain barrier in the fetus is another characteristic that might be important for the possible fetotoxic effects of chemicals.

Although fetal treatment is still an exception, it is of interest that in the case of prevention of vertical infections, such as HIV-1, at the time of a functioning circulation and kidney excretion, antibiotics (*penicillins*, *cephalosporins*) and *antiretrovirals* concentrate in the fetal compartment. Such depot effects are also enhanced by recirculation of the medicinal product through swallowing of the excreted antibiotics in the amniotic fluid, thus contributing to a great extent to the therapeutic effect. Obviously, this effect is lost when an early amniorrhexis (rupture of the membranes) occurs (Gonser 1995).

1.8 Mechanisms of developmental toxic agents

Although more information exists concerning the pathological history and final effects of developmental toxic agents, it is only recently that additional information has been known about the early onset and mechanisms of this interaction between the toxic agent and the different developmental stages and sensitivities. This leap forward is due to the insights provided by developmental molecular biology (Committee of Developmental Toxicology 2000):

■ *Receptor–ligand interactions.* Some chemicals interact directly with endogenous receptors for substances such as hormones, growth factors, cell-signaling molecules, and other endogenous compounds. They can activate the receptor inappropriately (agonists), inhibit the ability of the endogenous ligand to bind the receptor (antagonists), act in a manner that activates the receptor but produces a less than maximal response (partial agonist), or act in a way that causes a decrease from the normal baseline in an activity under the control of the receptor (negative agonist) or acts to permanent activate the receptor actions. Receptors can be broadly classified as cytosolic/nuclear or membrane bound. These receptors reside within the cell and have ligands that are small and generally hydrophobic so that they can pass easily through the cell membrane. After the ligand binds to these receptors, the complex translocates to the nucleus where it interacts directly with specific sequences of DNA to activate or inactivate the expression of special genes. Examples of these receptors are the estrogen, retinoic acid and benzodiazepine receptors. Membrane receptors are diverse and interact with a wide variety of molecules, from small molecules, such as glutamate and acetylcholine, and small proteins, such as insulin, to large proteins, such as Sonic Hedgehog (SHH) and Wnt. This binding of a ligand to a membrane receptor leads to a cascade of events within the cell membrane and cell known as signal transduction, which involves five or more steps. It is conceivable that developmental toxic agents could affect any of these steps.
■ *Covalent binding.* Covalent binding occurs when the exogenous molecule chemically reacts with an endogenous molecule (e.g. forming a DNA or protein adduct). Among the kinds of reactive chemicals are aldehydes, epoxides, free radicals, acylating agents, and alkylating agents. Exposure to these chemicals might then result in abnormal transcription or replication of DNA, or abnormal function of the adducted protein. An example of a developmental toxicant that forms both DNA and protein adducts in embryos is diphenylhydantoin.
■ *Peroxidation of lipids and proteins.* Some chemicals exist as free radicals or generate free radicals during their metabolism. Free radicals are highly reactive and will oxidize proteins or lipids, changing their structure. The developmental toxicity of niridazole appears to be entirely mediated by radical production (Barber 1993).

Pregnancy

1 General commentary on drug therapy and drug risks in pregnancy

- *Interference with sulfhydryl groups.* In some proteins, sulfhydryl groups are functional groups of the active (catalytic) site. Metals like mercury and cadmium are examples of developmental toxicants that cause oxidative stress and bind strongly to sulfhydryl groups and interfere with function.
- *Inhibition of protein function.* This is a broad category. Protein function occurs at catalytic sites (catalysis), regulatory sites (regulation of protein activity), macromolecule-binding sites (such as specific DNA binding), or protein-protein association sites (as in aggregation of ribosomal proteins).
- Some agents interfere with enzymes whose catalytic function is important in development, somewhat similar to an antagonist binding to a receptor. For example, methotrexate mimics a substrate of dihydrofolate reductase, and its inhibitory binding results in a functional folate deficiency causing developmental defects. Angiotensin-converting-enzyme (ACE) inhibitors are another example of agents that interfere with development by blocking enzyme action. These drugs block the conversion of angiotensin I to angiotensin II in the human fetus and neonate, needed to maintain renal perfusion and glomerular filtration. When angiotensin II levels are reduced in the fetus, glomerular filtration pressure and urine production are reduced, causing oligo-/anhydramnios, renal insufficiency, lung hypoplasia, joint contractures, skull hypoplasia and fetal/neonatal death.
- *Maternally mediated effects.* All of the mechanisms discussed above occur within the embryo/fetus. However, there are examples in which developmental toxicity is the consequence of toxicity in the mother. Effects on the embryo occur secondarily, as a result of actions on the pregnant mother.
- *Other mechanistic considerations.* There are other mechanisms that might be found to affect development. These might include such events as DNA intercalation, interaction with as yet unidentified targets, or complicated interactions that involve multiple changes, each of which is necessary – but not by itself sufficient – to initiate a pathogenic cascade (Committee of Developmental Toxicology 2000).

1.9   Causes of developmental disorders

Wilson (1977), during a presentation in Vienna in 1973, presented an estimate of the causes of developmental disorders (Table 1.3). His most important observation, that about two-thirds of the causes are of unknown etiology, is still of current importance. This lack of clear causal connections explains the problems faced in primary prevention of developmental disorders.

Table 1.3 presents the estimates from different sources (Nelson 1989, Kalter 1983, Wilson 1977). In addition, data are added from Saxony-Anhalt derived from a study of Rösch (2003) who meticulously analyzed the etiology of 4,146 children born with major malformations from her birth registry (1987–2000) with 143,335 births in the registration area. The registration was limited to live births up to the completion of the first week.

Medicinal products and other chemical substances are estimated to account for only a few percent of all developmental disorders, but they may play a more important role in the causation of defects through interaction with other (genetic) factors and maternal metabolic diseases. Table 1.4 presents an overview of the drugs and chemicals proven to be developmental toxicants in humans. Logan (2011) extensively reviewed the prevention of maternal infections leading to developmental disorders.

Table 1.3 Estimates of causes of developmental disorders (percentages)

	Wilson 1977	Kalter 1983	Nelson 1989	Rösch 2003
Monogenetic conditions	20	7.5	17.6	8.3
Chromosomal disorders	3–5	6.0	10.1	7.3
Environmental	8.5	5.0	6.1	2.0
Maternal infections		2.0		1.1
Maternal diabetes		1.4		0.1
Medicinal products		1.3		0.2
Other maternal conditions		0.3	2.9	0.6
Multifactorial and interactions	?	20	23	48.8
Unknown	65–70	61.5	43.2	33.6

1.10   Embryo/fetotoxic risk assessment and plausibility

There are different methods for assessing the embryo/fetotoxicity of medicinal products. The risk assessment process for new drugs is limited to experimental studies on laboratory animals. For drugs on the market, large epidemiological studies are of great value. In the case of thalidomide, more than 2 years passed before, in Germany, Lenz's early suspicions about the phocomelia were accepted (Lenz 1988). It is generally accepted that the predictive value of animal teratogenicity and reproductive toxicity tests is in extrapolating results of chemicals into terms of human safety; however, such predictions are still inadequate. Not all developmental toxic substances have been discovered by laboratory screening methods before they were used in humans and not all substances shown to be developmental toxicants in animals act as such in humans. There were discoveries made from case studies by "alert" clinicians, and not primarily from epidemiological studies. However, prospective cohort or retrospective case-control studies (see below) help to quantify risks.

In this respect, it is worth mentioning that in the 1970s collaboration was started among birth defects registries around the world. At present this International Clearinghouse for Birth Defects Monitoring Systems with its International Centre for Birth Defects Surveillance and Research in Rome (www.icbdsr.org) consists of programs monitoring several million newborns each year. Cooperative research is performed, but the main activity is the exchange of information collected within each program. The scope of this Clearinghouse includes fetal and childhood conditions of prenatal cause. A primary goal of the Clearinghouse is to detect changes in the incidence of specific malformations or patterns of malformations that may indicate the presence of chemicals (including medicinal hazards), to identify such hazards, and, if possible, eliminate them. Today, European and US registration authorities require new drugs or suspicious medications to have pregnancy registries developed to monitor prospectively the incidence of birth defects in such drug-exposed pregnant women.

Table 1.4 Medicinal products, chemicals and drugs of abuse with proven embryo/fetotoxic potential in humans

Agent	Indicating signs
Alcohol	Fetal alcohol syndrome/effects
Androgens	Masculinization
Antimetabolites	Multiple malformations
Benzodiazepines	Floppy infant syndrome
Carbamazepine	Spina bifida, multiple malformations
Cocaine	CNS, intestinal and kidney damage
Coumarin anticoagulants	Coumarin syndrome
Diethylstilbestrol	Vaginal dysplasia and neoplasms
Iodine overdose	Reversible hypothyroidism
Lead	Cognitive developmental retardation
Methyl mercury	Cerebral palsy, mental retardation
Misoprostol	Moebius-sequence, reduction defects of extremities
Penicillamine	Cutis laxa
Phenobarbital/primidone (anticonvulsive dose)	Multiple malformations
Phenytoin	Multiple malformations
Polychlorinated biphenyls	Mental retardation, immunological disorders, skin discoloration
Retinoids	Ear, CNS, cardiovascular, and skeletal disorders
Tetracycline (after week 15)	Discoloration of teeth
Thalidomide	Malformations of extremities, autism
Trimethadione	Multiple malformations
Valproic acid	Spina bifida, multiple malformations
Vitamin A (>25,000 IU/day)[1]	See retinoids

[1]Biologically, doses >5,000 IU/day are not required. The threshold for teratogenesis is much greater than 25,000 IU/day. Provitamin A = β-carotene harmless.
Note: Individual risk is dose- and time-dependent. The risk increases only two- to threefold at maximum with monotherapy or single administration of most substances in the list (see text). Never use this list for individual risk characterization or risk management! Drugs not mentioned in the list are not proven to be safe.

The process of assessing a reproductive or embryo/fetoxic effect of a drug includes the establishment of a biological plausibility and epidemiological evidence with the following criteria (according to Shepard 1994 and Wilson 1977):

- A sudden increase in the prevalence of a specific malformation is observed.
- An association is established between the introduction or an increased usage of a drug and an increased incidence of a specific malformation in a certain region and during a given time.

- Drug use must have taken place in the sensitive period (window) for the induction of that specific malformation.
- It must be established that the drug and not the condition for which the drug is prescribed causes the specific malformation.
- The drug or its metabolite suspected of causing the malformation has to be proven capable of reaching the embryo or fetus.
- The findings have to be confirmed by another independent study.
- The results of specific laboratory animal studies might support the epidemiological findings.

In reproductive epidemiology, the principle of causal analytical studies of birth defects is simple: compare the observed number of exposed pregnancies with an adverse outcome with the expected number. However, this implies that the rate of adverse outcomes of pregnancy in the population and the rate of exposure must be known.

The easiest possible technique is to study all pregnancies, prospectively. This demands large numbers, producing many problems (such as mistakes in data entry and dealing with confounders that co-vary both with the exposure and the outcome), and a known ascertainment rate (Källén 1988).

The second type of causal analytical studies is the cohort approach (either historical or prospective), when adverse reproductive outcome is studied in a group of women defined by a specific exposure situation. The outcome in the exposed group is compared either with the total population or with an unexposed control cohort. Such cohort studies make it possible to examine many different outcomes after a specific exposure; for example, spontaneous abortion, low birth weight, perinatal mortality, and different types of malformations.

The prolonged use of medicines during pregnancy occurs in cases of chronic diseases such as epilepsy, psychiatric illnesses, diabetes, and thyroid dysfunction. The registration of new drugs developed for conditions requiring treatment during pregnancy should be based on comparative clinical trials in which not only the therapeutic but also the teratogenic properties are examined.

As mentioned earlier, developmental disorders are not only manifested as structural malformations – other embryo/fetotoxic effects include:

- spontaneous abortions
- intrauterine growth retardation
- reversible functional postnatal effects, such as sedation, hypoglycemia, bradycardia, and withdrawal effects
- central nervous system disorders, from motility disturbances to learning disabilities; immunological and fertility and reproductive disorders

Most of these are not apparent at birth but will be manifested much later, which explains why the prevalence of developmental disorders is about 3% at birth and about 8% or more at the age of 5 years

1.11   Classification of drugs used in pregnancy

About 80% of pregnant women use prescribed or over-the-counter drugs. There is no doubt that even during pregnancy, drugs are often unjustifiably used. Healthcare professionals and pregnant women need to develop a more critical attitude to the use of drugs during pregnancy, or, more importantly, to the use of drugs during the fertile period, as well as exposures to occupational and environmental agents. These drugs and chemicals should only be taken or used when essential, thereby avoiding many unnecessary and unknown risks. The same obviously applies for social drugs like tobacco, alcohol, and addictive drugs.

Since 1984, drug risk classification systems have been introduced in the USA, Sweden and Australia. Classification is general, and of a "ready-made" fashion. The FDA classification as published in the Federal Register (2008) is resulting in revision of drug descriptions for pregnancy, now beginning to appear. In the EU, a specification of the medicinal products to be used in pregnancy has to be provided in the summary of product characteristics, including:

- facts regarding human experience and conclusions from preclinical toxicity studies which are of relevance for the assessment of risks associated with exposure during pregnancy
- recommendations on the use of the medicinal product at different times during pregnancy in respect of gestation
- recommendations on the management of the situation of an inadvertent exposure, where relevant.

However, there are intrinsic problems with these categorization systems. It is doubtful whether the texts in the drug inserts will be updated frequently enough, and the use of the wording "contraindication in pregnancy" might result in unnecessary terminations of pregnancy (Briggs 2003). Moreover, labeling for pregnancy generally does not include specific advice regarding when the drug is used inadvertently during pregnancy (see also later).

1.12   Paternal use of medicinal products

Husbands or partners are rarely, if ever, warned to avoid known embryo/fetotoxic medicinal products. Nevertheless, awareness is increasing that if males are exposed to reproductive toxic agents, these might damage their offspring. To date, no one is certain regarding the safety of substances that, after administration to males or via their occupational exposure, can cause birth defects.

Theoretically, there are three possible modes of action:

1. Substances such as cytostatics could damage the sperm itself genetically, or impair spermatogenesis or the maturation of sperm; it is also possible that the substance may become attached to sperm and transported during fertilization in the oocyte.
2. Agents in semen may undergo resorption through the vaginal mucosa, reaching the maternal circulation. However, drugs or their metabolites found in semen are mostly at a much lower concentration as in the patients' blood.
3. After conception agents may directly reach the embryo/fetus through the semen.

No one believes at this moment that drugs taken by males are major contributors to developmental disorders, but many (experimental) investigators have concluded that these medicinal products *could* cause such disorders (Colie 1993). Certainly, fertility disturbances are to be expected and have been reported with, for example, radiotherapy, cyclophosphamide, dibromochlorpropane, and lead (Friedman 2003, Sallmén 2003). Environmental agents with anti-androgenic or estrogenic activities, such as PCBs, dioxins and phthalates, are also incriminated in this respect (see review by Storgaard 2006). Causation cases have been mentioned with *mesalazine* in colitis ulcerosa (Chermesh 2004, Fisher 2004). Male occupational exposure to pesticides, heavy metals, organic solvents, radiation, and smoking (see Chapter 2.23) have also been associated with an increased risk of spontaneous abortions, developmental abnormalities and even childhood cancers (Aitken 2003). Acknowledging this possible cause of developmental toxicity should be considered when stimulating primary prevention of congenital disorders. The best (and indeed most hygienic) way to take precautions after conception during pregnancy is by the use of condoms when the man is taking medicinal products that are suspected to be harmful when ejaculated (chemotherapy) (Cordier 2008).

At present there are no data that justify elective termination of pregnancy (ETOP) because of paternal teratogenicity or to perform primary chromosome analysis after paternal exposure to cytoxic or mutagenic medicinal products. In theory, it is advisable to wait 2 spermatogenic cycles (about 6 months) after such treatment before conception is planned. However, clinical data are scarce to demonstrate a risk of disregard of this precautionary measure.

1.13   Communicating the risk of drug use in pregnancy

It is estimated that a pregnant woman takes about three to eight different drugs, partly as self-medication and partly prescribed. This average is not much different from the average drug use by nonpregnant women. There are, however, more questions about the safety of medicinal products used in pregnancy regarding the unborn – particularly in cases of unplanned pregnancies. In teratology counseling, a distinction must be made between the following three situations:

1. Risk communication before a pharmacotherapeutic choice has been made or before a pregnancy is initiated.
2. Risk communication regarding the safety of drugs used in pregnancy when drug exposure has already taken place.
3. Risk communication in the case where a child is born with a developmental disorder following drug use during pregnancy.

In the second situation, during pregnancy the question is whether or not fetal development is at risk, leading to discussion of whether additional (invasive) diagnostic procedures or even pregnancy termination may be considered. In the third situation feelings of guilt might be the motivation for asking about risk; however, this situation is also frequently of importance when medical geneticists ask for specific details of genetic or environmental causations. Moreover, these issues are the subject of much debate in cases of legal procedures.

In our experience, these three risk communication situations require different approaches, which are dealt with separately below.

The safety warnings provided on package inserts or other sources such as the *Physician's Desk Reference* are so general, sometimes outdated and, in some cases, even misleading that the prescribing physician cannot make a "tailor-made" choice for the patient on such a basis. In some cases, these texts are written primarily to protect the drug producers and registration authorities from potential liability. The phrase "contraindicated in pregnancy" is in some cases correctly applied to an embryo/fetotoxic product, but it may also mean that experience with this drug in pregnancy has not been sufficiently documented. Registration authorities and drug producers view drug risks differently from the clinician who is treating an individual patient. When, for example, a particular drug involves a relative risk (risk ratio) of only 1.2 (which is indeed a very low risk), it is not essential that the clinician communicates the risk to an individual patient. To the drug producer, however, the same risk value implies an additional 400 malformed children per 100,000 exposed pregnancies, considering a spontaneous malformation rate of 2%.

1.14   Risk communication prior to pharmacotherapeutic choice

Drug administration during pregnancy means that both the mother and unborn child are exposed. The drug or metabolite concentration may be even higher in the embryonic or fetal compartment than it is in the mother. The fetus as an "additional" patient therefore demands a strict pharmacotherapeutic approach, as it is imperative to try to restore maternal health without endangering the development of the child. In severe conditions, such as bronchial asthma, diabetes mellitus, epilepsy or particular communicable diseases, treatment is obligatory regardless of pregnancy. In contrast, inessential products such as antitussive preparations, "pregnancy-supporting" substances, and high doses of vitamins and minerals should not be prescribed or used, as their potential risks outweigh their unproven benefits.

The following rules of thumb are applicable when prescribing drugs:

■ Women of reproductive age must be asked, prior to drug prescription, whether an as-yet undetected pregnancy is possible, or whether they are planning a pregnancy. By the time a woman learns that she is pregnant, organogenesis has already progressed substantially.
■ In chronic treatment of women of reproductive age, the possibility of pregnancy must be considered. In the case of drugs with teratogenic potential, effective contraceptive measures must be discussed and implemented. Products proven to be safe in pregnancy are the drugs of first choice for long-term treatment during the reproductive years.
■ Some medicinal products (e.g. anticonvulsants) reduce the effectiveness of hormonal contraception.
■ In general, drugs that have already been in use for several years should be the preferred choice during reproductive age, provided that they have not been substantially suspected of carrying risk. These products usually involve greater safety in their therapeutic efficacy in the mother and tolerability by the fetus. On the contrary, recently introduced agents must be considered to be an unappraised risk; in many instances these products are also "pseudo-innovations" without any proven therapeutic advantage.
■ If possible, monotherapy is preferred.
■ The lowest effective dose should be prescribed.
■ Non-drug treatment should be considered.
■ The disease itself may be a greater fetotoxic risk than the appropriate drug therapy, as in diabetes mellitus. The same applies to severe psychic stress. An individual risk evaluation related to condition and treatment is necessary in these cases.

1.15   Risk communication regarding the safety of drugs already used in pregnancy

A pregnant woman who uses a medicinal product must be given an individual risk assessment, and advice should be sought from a specialized institution when the assessment is difficult. A potential at-risk exposure should be handled in the same manner as a genetic or chromosomal disorder in a family. In the latter case, a special consultation will take place. A well-grounded individual risk assessment can help to allay unnecessary fears and avoid unnecessary diagnostic intervention, or the termination of a wanted and healthy pregnancy. A detailed maternal medical (obstetric) history, including all (drug) exposures with precise description of treatment intervals during embryogenesis, is an obligatory prerequisite.

When drug exposure has already taken place during pregnancy, a different approach is required from that used in cases of planning future pharmacotherapy. The latter allows the calm and fully confident selection of a safe drug. However, when the treatment has already begun, the pregnant patient will mainly be concerned about any possible disorder of the unborn. These different cases therefore require different communication strategies. When drug exposure has already taken place, the consultant should avoid vague comments that increase anxiety. Experimentally derived results or unconfirmed hypotheses based on individual case reports should not be emphasized, as these could alarm the already anxious patient and perhaps lead to a drastic decision – for example, the termination of a wanted pregnancy based on a misinterpreted product warning such as "inadequately studied", "experimentally suspected" or "contraindicated in pregnancy". If no exposure-associated risk is known or strongly suspected, the woman should be given a straightforward answer: that there is no reason to worry about her pregnancy. In the case of a developmental toxicant the patient's physician should be provided with the relative risk, organ specificity, and recommended diagnostics.

For certain exposures, additional prenatal diagnostic procedures, in particular a detailed ultrasound examination, should be recommended. However, the intake of potentially embryo/fetotoxic substances does not require invasive diagnostic measures, such as intrauterine umbilical puncture, amniocentesis or chorion villous sampling. It is important to add that teratology information services frequently intervene to prevent the unjustified termination of wanted pregnancies.

1.16   Teratology information centers

In 1990, two networks of teratology information services were established – one in Europe (ENTIS, the European Network of Teratology Information Services, http://www.entis-org.eu/) and another in the Americas (OTIS, the Organization of Teratology Information Specialists, www.mothertobaby.org). A teratology information service provides health professionals and patients with "tailor-made" information relating to the pertinent situation, illness and chemical exposure of the individual involved (Schaefer 2011). These services also conduct prospective cohort follow-up studies. Pregnancy outcomes of counseled patients are essential to identify more precisely the risk of medicinal products.

Pregnancy

1 General commentary on drug therapy and drug risks in pregnancy

References

Aitken RJ, Sawyer D. The human spermatozoon – not waving but drowning. Adv Exp Med Biol 2003; 518: 85–98.

Barber CV, Fantel AG. The role of oxygenation in embryotoxic mechanisms of three bioreducible agents. Teratology 1993; 47: 209–223.

Barker DJP. Mothers, Babies and Health in Later Life, 2nd edn. Edinburgh: Churchill Livingstone, 1998.

Briggs GG, Freeman RK, Yaffe SJ. Classification of drugs for teratogenic risk: an anachronistic way of counseling: a reply to Merlob and Stahl. Birth Defects Res A 2003; 67: 207–8.

Carney EW, Scialli AR, Watson RE et al. Mechanisms regulating toxicant disposition to the embryo during early pregnancy: an interspecies comparison. Birth Defects Res C Embryo Today 2004; 72: 345–60.

Chamberlain G. ABC of antenatal care. Organisation of antenatal care. Br Med J 1991; 302: 647–50.

Chermesh I, Eliakim R. Mesalazine-induced reversible infertility in a young male. Dig Liver Dis 2004; 36: 551–2.

Colie CF. Male mediated teratogenesis. Reprod Toxicol 1993; 7: 3–9.

Committee on Developmental Toxicology NAS/NRC. Scientific Frontiers in Developmental Toxicology and Risk Assessment Washington, DC: National Research Council, 2000, pp. 10–25.

Cordier S. Evidence for a role of paternal exposures in developmental toxicity. Basic Clin Pharmacol Toxicol 2008; 102: 176–81.

Elias SG, van Noord PA, Peeters PH et al. Childhood exposure to the 1944–1945 Dutch famine and subsequent female reproductive function. Hum Reprod 2005; 20: 2483–8.

Federal Register. 2008, https://www.federalregister.gov/articles/2008/05/29/E8-11806/content-and-format-of-labeling-for-human-prescription-drug-and-biological-products-requirements.

Fisher JS. Environmental anti-androgens and male reproductive health: focus on phthalates and testicular dysgenesis syndrome. Reproduction 2004; 127: 305–15.

Friedman JM. Implications of research in male-mediated developmental toxicity to clinical counsellors, regulators, and occupational safety officers. Adv Exp Med Biol 2003; 518: 219–26.

Garbis-Berkvens JM, Peters PWJ. Comparative morphology and physiology of embryonic and fetal membranes. In: H Nau, WJ Scott (eds), Pharmacokinetics in teratogenesis, Vol. I. Boca Raton: CRC Press, 1987, pp. 13–44.

Gonser M, Stoll P, Kahle P. Clearance prediction and drug dosage in pregnancy. A clinical study on metildigoxin, and application to other drugs with predominant renal elimination. Clin Drug Invest 1995; 9: 197–205.

Gregg NM. Congenital cataract following German measles in mother. Trans Ophthalmol Soc Aust 1941; 3: 35–46.

Hale F. Pigs born without eyeballs. J Hered 1933; 24: 105–6.

Juchau MR. Bioactivation in chemical teratogenesis. Ann Rev Pharmacol Toxicol 1989; 29: 165–87.

Källén, B. Epidemiology of Human Reproduction Boca Raton: CRC Press, 1988.

Kalter H. Teratology in the Twentieth Century and Plus Ten, New York, Springer, 2010.

Kalter H, Warkany J. Congenital malformations. N Eng J Med 1983; 308: 424–31, 491–7.

Kelsey FO Thalidomide update: regulatory aspects. Teratology 1988, 38: 221–6.

Lander CM, Smith MT, Chalk JB et al. Bioavailability in pharmacokinetics of phenytoin during pregnancy. Eur J Clin Pharmacol 1984; 27: 105–10.

Lenz W. Kindliche Fehlbildungen nach Medikament während der Gravidität? Dtsch Med Wochenschr 1961; 86: 2555–6.

Lenz W. Thalidomide and Congenital Abnormalities. Lancet 6 January 1962; 45.

Lenz W. A Short History of Thalidomide Embryopathy. Teratology 1988; 38: 203–15.

Loebstein R, Lalkin A, Koren G. Pharmacokinetic changes during pregnancy and their clinical relevance. Clin Pharmacokinet 1997; 33: 328–43.

Logan S, Price L. Infectious disease in pregnancy. Obstet Gynaec Reprod Med 2011; 21:12 331-8.

McBride WG. Thalidomide and congenital abnormalities. Lancet 1961; ii: 1358.

Miller RK. Does the placenta protect against insult or is it the target? In Teratology Primer, Reston, VA: Teratology Society, 2010, pp. 9–14.

Nelson K, Holmes LB. Malformations due to presumed spontaneous mutations in newborn infants. N Engl J Med 1989; 320: 19–23.

Painter RC, Roseboom TJ, Bleker OP. Prenatal exposure to the Dutch famine and disease in later life: an overview. Reprod Toxicol 2005; 20: 345–52.

Rösch Chr. Aufgaben, Funktionen und Entwicklungperspektiven eines populationsbezogenen Fehlbildungsregisters in Deutschland (Habilitationsschrift – PhD thesis). Magdeburg, 2003.

Sallmén M, Liesivuori J, Taskinen H et al. Time to pregnancy among the wives of Finnish greenhouse workers. Scand J Work Environ Health 2003; 29: 85–93.

Schaefer C. Drug Safety in Pregnancy – Utopia or achievable prospect? Risk information, risk research, advocacy in Teratology Information Services. Congenit Anom (Kyoto) 2011; 51: 6–11.

Shepard TH. Letter: "proof" of teratogenicity. Teratology 1994; 50: 97.

Stephens T, Brynner R, Dark Remedy: the impact of thalidomide and its survival as a vital medicine. Basic Books, New York, 2009.

St Clair D, Xu M, Wang P et al. Rates of adult schizophrenia following prenatal exposure to the Chinese famine of 1959–1961. J Am Med Assoc 2005; 294: 557–62.

Storgaard L, Bonde JP, Olsen J. Male reproductive disorders in humans and prenatal indicators of estrogen exposure; a review of published epidemiological studies. Reprod Toxicol 2006; 21: 4–15.

Strömland K, Nordin V, Miller M, Akerström B, Gillberg C. Autism in thalidomide embryopathy: a population. Study. Dev. Med. Child Neurol. 1994; 36: 251–6.

Wiedemann HR. Hinweis auf eine derzeitige, Häufung hypo-und aplastischer Fehlbildunger der Gliedmassen. Med Welt. 1961; 37: 1863–6.

Wilson JD. Embryotoxicity of drugs to man. In: JD Wilson, FC Frazer (eds), Handbook of Teratology, Vol. 1. New York: Plenum Press, 1977, pp. 309–55.

Electronic databases offering an overview on published studies

Reprotox: Information database on environmental hazards to human reproduction and development. Reproductive Toxicology Center (RTC), 7831 Woodmont Ave, #375, Bethesda, MD 20814; telephone: +1 301/514–3081; Internet: http://reprotox.org

Teris: Teratogen Information System and the on-line version of Shepard's Catalog of Teratogenic Agents. University of Washington, TERIS Project, CHDD, Rm. 207 S. Bldg., Box 357920, Seattle WA 98195–7920. Fax +1-206/543-7921, Email: terisweb@u.washington.edu; Internet: http://depts.washington.edu/terisweb/teris/

Bumps: Bumps (best use of medicines in pregnancy) Evidence based information leaflets for women and their families on the fetal effects of specific medicines and chemicals, written by the UK Teratology Information Service: www.medicinesinpregnancy.org

Pregnancy

1 General commentary on drug therapy and drug risks in pregnancy

Specific drug therapies during pregnancy

2

by authors listed below

2.1 Analgesics, non-steroidal anti-inflammatory drugs (NSAIDs), muscle relaxants, and antigout medications (Heli Malm and Cornelia Borisch)   27

2.2 Allergy and hyposensitization therapy (Lee H. Goldstein, Corinna Weber-Schöndorfer and Matitiahu Berkovitch)   59

2.3 Antiasthmatic and cough medication (Lee H. Goldstein, Corinna Weber-Schöndorfer and Matitiahu Berkovitch)   65

2.4 Nausea and vomiting in pregnancy (Lee H. Goldstein, Corinna Weber-Schöndorfer and Matitiahu Berkovitch)   75

2.5 Gastro-intestinal medications, hypolipidemic agents and spasmolytics (Maurizio Clementi and Corinna Weber-Schöndorfer)   93

2.6 Anti-infective agents (Stephanie Padberg)   115

2.7 Vaccines and immunoglobulins (Benedikte-Noël Cuppers and Christof Schaefer)   177

2.8 Heart and blood medications (Fernanda Sales Luiz Vianna, Lavinia Schüler-Faccini and Corinna Weber-Schöndorfer)   193

2.9 Anticoagulants, thrombocyte aggregation inhibitors, fibrinolytics and volume replacement agents (Janine E. Polifka and Juliane Habermann)   225

2.10 Epilepsy and antiepileptic medications (Christina Chambers and Christof Schaefer)   251

2.11 Psychotropic drugs (Katherine L. Wisner and Christof Schaefer)   293

2.12 Immunosuppression, rheumatic diseases, multiple sclerosis, and Wilson's disease (Corinna Weber-Schöndorfer)   341

2.13 Antineoplastic drugs (Jan M. Friedman and Corinna Weber-Schöndorfer)   373

2.14 Uterine contraction agents, tocolytics, vaginal therapeutics and local contraceptives (Gerard H.A. Visser and Angela Kayser)   401

2.15 Hormones (Asher Ornoy and Corinna Weber-Schöndorfer)   413

2.16 General and local anesthetics and muscle relaxants (Stefanie Hultzsch and Asher Ornoy)   451

2.17 Dermatological medications and local therapeutics (Gudula Kirtschig and Christof Schaefer)   467

2.18 Vitamins, minerals and trace elements (Richard K. Miller and Paul Peters)   493

2.19 Herbs during pregnancy (Henry M. Hess and Richard K. Miller)   511

2.20 Diagnostic agents (Stefanie Hultzsch)   527

2.21 Recreational drugs (Sally Stephens and Laura M. Yates)   541

2.22 Poisonings and toxins (Laura M. Yates and Sally Stephens)   575

2.23 Occupational, industrial and environmental agents (Susan M. Barlow, Frank M. Sullivan and Richard K. Miller)   599

Please note that in the following chapters drugs are discussed under their generic names. For trade names, please refer to the *Physician's Desk Reference* or comparable pharmacopoeias of your country.

Analgesics, non-steroidal anti-inflammatory drugs (NSAIDs), muscle relaxants, and antigout medications

2.1

Heli Malm and Cornelia Borisch

2.1.1	Paracetamol (acetaminophen)	27
2.1.2	Acetylsalicylic acid	29
2.1.3	Pyrazolone compounds and phenylbutazone	32
2.1.4	Analgesic drug combination products and drugs used for osteoarthritis	33
2.1.5	Opioid agonists and antagonists and other centrally acting analgesics	34
2.1.6	Non-steroidal anti-inflammatory and antirheumatic drugs	41
2.1.7	Migraine therapy	46
2.1.8	Muscle relaxants and other analgesics	48
2.1.9	Antigout preparations	49

Most of the commonly used analgesics can also be used during pregnancy. *Paracetamol* (acetaminophen) is the first choice and is considered relatively safe in any trimester. *Acetylsalicylic acid* (ASA) in analgesic doses close to delivery may increase the risk of hemorrhage in both the mother and the infant, and should be avoided. Opiates should be prescribed only with compelling indications and their use should primarily be occasional. Of the non-steroidal anti-inflammatory drugs (NSAIDs), most experience is available for *ibuprofen* and *diclofenac*. Repeated use of NSAIDs should be avoided after the twenty-eighth week of pregnancy and use of cyclooxygenase (COX)-2 inhibitors should be avoided when planning pregnancy and throughout pregnancy. Acute migraine attacks can be treated with *sumatriptan* when conventional medication fails to be effective. The use of muscle relaxants is not recommended, while *probenecid* may be safely used in the rare cases of pregnant women needing lowering of uric acid.

2.1.1   Paracetamol (acetaminophen)

Pharmacology

Paracetamol is a centrally acting analgesic and antipyretic drug lacking anti-inflammatory properties. It acts by inhibiting central prostaglandin synthesis and by elevating pain threshold, but the exact mechanism of action is unknown. Paracetamol passes the placenta and fetal drug concentrations equal that of the mother (Roberts 1984).

Drugs During Pregnancy and Lactation. **http://dx.doi.org/10.1016/B978-0-12-408078-2.00002-0**

Toxicology

Paracetamol use during the first trimester was not associated with an increased risk of major overall or specific birth defects in a population-based, case-control study which included more than 11,000 case infants of whom more than 5,000 had been exposed prenatally to paracetamol mono-preparations (Feldkamp 2010). In that study, the risk for selected malformations, including neural tube defects and orofacial clefts, anotia or microtia, and gastroschisis decreased when paracetamol was used for a febrile illness, suggesting a beneficial effect in lowering temperature. According to all data published to date there is no indicative evidence that paracetamol is teratogenic in humans (Scialli 2010a).

Contrary to these reassuring findings, research in experimental studies has shown that prostaglandins are important in testosterone-dependent differentiation of the male genital tract (Gupta 1992), and a recent *ex vivo* study in cultured rat testes indicated that paracetamol, even in low concentrations, is a potent inhibitor of testosterone synthesis (Kristensen 2011). While testosterone is important in programming normal testis descent, low testosterone levels during a critical phase of development could consequently affect this event occurring in a later phase of pregnancy (Welsh 2008). Several studies based on this hypothesis have recently been published. Data on 47,400 male offspring, including 980 boys with a diagnosis of cryptorchidism confirmed from the patient register, were included in a study based on the Danish National Birth Cohort during the years 1996–2002 (Jensen 2010). Paracetamol exposure continuing for more than 4 weeks and occurring during the eighth- to fourteenth-gestation weeks was associated with cryptorchidism; however, no association remained when only cases needing operative treatment were included (Jensen 2010). In another study with possibly partly overlapping study material and including nearly 500 boys from Denmark and a cohort of nearly 1,500 boys from Finland, paracetamol use for 2 weeks or longer during the first and second trimester was associated with an increased risk of cryptorchidism in the Danish cohort, while no association was observed in the Finnish cohort (Kristensen 2011). Further, a population-based study from the Netherlands included more than 3,000 boys with follow-up visits until at least 6 months' of age, observed an association with paracetamol use during the fourteenth to twenty-second gestational weeks and cryptorchidism (Snijder 2012). Even if unconfirmed, together with the published experimental data, these findings are suggestive of a possible causal association.

Several epidemiological studies have observed an association between prenatal exposure to paracetamol and wheezing or asthma in offspring (Bakkeheim 2011, Perzanowski 2010, Garcia-Marcos 2009, Kang 2009, Rebordosa 2008, Shaheen 2002). The Avon Longitudinal Study, with prospectively collected exposure data, observed a statistically significant risk for childhood asthma after exposure to paracetamol during the latter half of pregnancy, while no risk was observed if exposure was before 20 gestational weeks (Shaheen 2002). The risk for persistent wheezing until age 7 was highest after exposure occurring in the first trimester in another population-based prospective cohort study (Rebordosa 2008), while a prospective study including 1,500 women observed a significantly lower risk for asthma at 6 years' of age after exposure to paracetamol during the first or third trimester (Kang 2009). Confounding by indication (e.g. maternal illness) and exposure to paracetamol during infancy remains a major concern when interpreting conflicting results (Henderson 2013). A recent meta-analysis of published studies and a recent review both concluded that prenatal exposure to paracetamol is associated with an increased risk of childhood asthma, but causation still remains to be established (Henderson 2013, Eyers 2011). The putative biological mechanisms that have been proposed to play a role in pathogenesis include epithelial cell damage caused by the toxic metabolite N-acetyl-p-benzoquinone imine (NAPQI), or by selective cyclooxygenase-2 (COX-2) inhibition, together with paracetamol-induced depletion of glutathione, an important antioxidant in the airways (Henderson 2013, Nuttall 2003). However, as the respiratory epithelium develops later in pregnancy, damage is not expected to occur during the first trimester (Scialli 2010b). Further, the capacity of the fetal liver to metabolize paracetamol to NAPQI is limited. To conclude, a causal association between prenatal paracetamol exposure and childhood wheezing has not been established, but neither can it be ruled out.

Use of paracetamol during pregnancy has also been associated in a single study with an increased risk of preeclampsia and thromboembolic diseases, both conditions in which reduction in prostacyclin production may play a role (Rebordosa 2010). Causality cannot be confirmed on the basis of this study. No association was observed between acetaminophen, ASA, or NSAID use during pregnancy and the risk for childhood leukemias (Ognjanovic 2011).

A Norwegian mother and child cohort study with siblings found an association between long-term use (>28 days) of paracetamol during pregnancy and several adverse neurodevelopmental outcomes at 3 years of age, including delayed motor development with externalizing and internalizing behaviors (Brandlistuen 2013). Another population-based study from Denmark linking prospectively collected data from maternal interviews together with hospital and prescription registers, and adjusting for several important confounders found an association between paracetamol use and hyperkinetic disorders (Liew 2014). Use of paracetamol for 20 weeks or more, and exposure during the second and third trimester showed the highest risk estimates, but use of 2–5 weeks was also associated with an increased risk (Liew 2014). The biological mechanism by which paracetamol might affect fetal neurodevelopment is not established, and causality cannot be confirmed on the basis of these observational studies. Further research should address the effect of dosing and the critical time window for neurodevelopmental outcomes, while focusing on a possible genetic susceptibility predisposing for the suspected adverse effects. The findings from these two studies should not change practice, but suggest that paracetamol should be used during pregnancy only when clearly indicated.

Regarding overdoses during suicide attempts see Chapter 2.22. Regarding the combination with Codeine see Section 2.1.5(C).

> **Recommendation.** Paracetamol is the analgesic and antipyretic of first choice during pregnancy, and can be used in any trimester when indicated.

2.1.2   Acetylsalicylic acid

Pharmacology

Acetylsalicylic acid (ASA), also known as aspirin, acts by irreversibly inhibiting the platelet cyclooxygenase (COX) enzyme, resulting in inhibition of platelet thromboxane A2 (TXA-2) synthesis. TXA-2 has vasoconstriction activity with increased platelet aggregation, and inhibition results in opposite effects, favorable in preventing arterial thrombosis. A dose of 160–325 mg is sufficient to nearly completely (90%) inhibit platelet COX enzyme, and this effect lasts for the platelet life span (7–10 days). Higher doses, however, also inhibit the synthesis of prostacyclin in blood vessel endothelial cells. Contrary to TXA-2, prostacyclin acts as a vasodilator and inhibits platelet aggregation. Prostacyclin also acts as a modulator in inflammatory processes. These dose-dependent effects of ASA are consequently reflected in different indications for use.

After oral intake, salicylates are quickly absorbed and reach the fetus via the placenta. Doses of 500 mg and higher close to delivery can significantly reduce fetal prostacyclin synthesis. In users, a 100 mg dose reduces thromboxane A2 synthesis but has no effect on prostacyclin synthesis. ASA is hydrolyzed to salicylic acid and further metabolized to glucuronide conjugates in the liver.

Use and effectiveness of low-dose ASA

Low doses (50–150mg/day) have been used during pregnancy to prevent several pregnancy complications. By reducing vasoconstriction and platelet aggregation, low-dose ASA could be beneficial in preventing pregnancy induced hypertension and preeclampsia. A randomized trial including more than 9,000 women assigned to take low-dose ASA (60 mg/day) or placebo, did not find a significantly reduced rate of preeclampsia or intrauterine growth retardation, but risk for preterm birth was significantly lower in the ASA group (the Collaborative Low-Dose Aspirin in Pregnancy Study, CLASP 1994). A decline in the rate of preeclampsia was also observed in women who had started ASA treatment prior to 20 weeks gestation. Low-dose aspirin was safe and there was no evidence of excess bleeding during delivery. A recently published meta-analysis reported that use of low-dose ASA was significantly associated with risk reduction for preeclampsia, intra-uterine growth retardation and preterm birth, but only if treatment was started at 16 weeks gestation or earlier (Bujold 2010). A more recent review and meta-analysis stated that low-dose ASA when initiated at or before 16 weeks reduces the risk of severe preeclampsia, while no effect to reduce the risk for mild preeclampsia has been confirmed (Roberge 2012).

The pathophysiology of preeclampsia includes impaired trophoblast invasion and abnormal placental development starting early in pregnancy. It is therefore biologically plausible that treatment, particularly during early gestation would be beneficial. The protective effect of low-dose ASA on hypertensive pregnancy complications, including pre-eclampsia and preterm delivery, however, could not be replicated in a meta-analysis based on individual patient data and investigating ASA use (100 mg/day). This study followed a group of women from the preconception stage, and focused on IVF pregnancies (Groeneveld 2013). The American College of Chest Physicians recommends low-dose ASA treatment starting from the second trimester for those who are at risk for pre-eclampsia (Bates 2012).

The possible benefits of low-dose ASA in treating women with recurrent unexplained miscarriages were investigated in a randomized prospective trial, which included nearly 300 women receiving either ASA alone (dose 80 mg/day), ASA and nadroparin (a low molecular weight heparin) or placebo. The treatment began as soon as a viable pregnancy could be demonstrated. There was no difference in live birth rates between the groups, indicating no beneficial effects of either treatment (Kaandorp 2010a). In patients with thrombophilia, the presence of antiphospholipid antibodies (APLA) is known to be associated with adverse pregnancy outcomes, including an increased risk of miscarriage (McNamee 2012). According to current guidelines by the British Committee for Standards in Haematology and the American College of Chest Physicians, women with APLAs who have experienced ≥3 miscarriages are recommended antenatal administration of heparin combined with low-dose aspirin throughout pregnancy (Bates 2012, Keeling 2012). Treatment should be started as soon as pregnancy has been confirmed (Keeling 2012).

Toxicology

In experimental studies, acetylsalicylic acid given in high doses to animals has been associated with developmental toxicity including structural malformations. Conflicting results regarding humans have been obtained in epidemiological settings. Population-based data from the Swedish Birth Registry did not observe an association between ASA use during early pregnancy and cardiovascular malformations (Källén 2003), and several other publications did not observe an increased risk of overall malformations (Kozer 2002). Three case-control studies observed an association between acetylsalicylic acid use in early pregnancy and a risk for gastroschisis (Draper 2008, Werler 2002, Martinez-Frias 1997); this was also reported in a meta-analysis by Kozer (2002). However, a further study by Werler (2009a) failed to repeat the previously observed association. Other malformations that have been associated with ASA use include limb reduction defects corresponding to the amniotic band syndrome (Werler 2009b), and holoprosencephaly (Miller 2010). Several limitations, including the potential for recall bias and confounding by indication, limit the relevance of these findings. An increased risk of cryptorchidism was observed in a Danish study after use of ASA in the first or second trimester; however, this association was statistically significant only when use had lasted for more than 2 weeks (Kristensen 2011). In another part of the same study assessing the risk in Finnish boys, no association was found between the use of mild analgesics and cryptorchidism. Neither was an association observed in a larger study from Denmark, with possibly partly overlapping study material (Jensen 2010). Further, mild analgesic use during the second trimester was associated with an increased risk for cryptorchidism but not for hypospadias in a Dutch population-based cohort study, but use of ASA was not specifically analyzed (Snijder 2012). No further conclusions can be drawn from these conflicting results. Another study did not find an association between the intake of acetaminophen, ASA, or NSAIDs during pregnancy and the risk for leukemia during childhood (Ognjanovic 2011).

In summary, according to currently available data it can be concluded that there is no serious evidence of teratogenic effects of ASA.

ASA use at the time of conception was associated with an increased risk for miscarriage in a prospective cohort study, including more than 1,000 women who were recruited as soon as a pregnancy test was positive (Li 2003). The rate of miscarriage was 23% in those exposed to ASA ($n = 22$) compared to 15% in non-exposed controls. As prostaglandins are important in the implantation process, drugs inhibiting prostaglandin synthesis, including ASA, could adversely affect this process. However, this association has not been confirmed, and miscarriage rates have been documented to be in this range normally without exposure to ASA.

A cohort study including more than 600 children exposed prenatally to low-dose ASA and born very preterm (prior to 33rd week of gestation), evaluated the neurodevelopment up to 5 years' of age. The study did not observe negative effects in the neurocognitive development of these children. Instead, the results suggested rather a protective effect for behavior abnormalities, including hyperactivity (Marret 2010). Regarding overdoses in suicide attempts, see Chapter 2.22.

Prior to parturition

A sensitivity of the ductus arteriosus to prostaglandin inhibitors increases from 28 gestation weeks onward. Repeated use of prostaglandin inhibitors, including ASA, can produce a narrowing or premature closure of the ductus, which in normal circumstances is not closed until soon after birth. This effect is both time- and dose-dependent, and was first documented with the use of another prostaglandin inhibitor, *indomethacin* (Section 2.1.6(A)). Individual susceptibility to prostaglandin inhibitors obviously varies, and repeated analgesic doses of ASA are best avoided after 28 weeks.

As prostaglandin inhibitors decrease uterine contractility, salicylates can prolong duration of pregnancy and labor by decreasing the activity of contractions. Consequently, salicylates have been used for tocolysis in the past. Because analgesic doses (500 mg and higher) increase the risk for bleeding, such dosing should be avoided beginning at least 2 weeks before the expected date of delivery. Risk for bleeding applies to the mother (increased bleeding during delivery) and the infant.

Low-dose ASA does not constrict the ductus arteriosus nor does it increase the risk for bleeding in the mother or the infant (CLASP 1994).

Recommendation. ASA is not an analgesic or anti-inflammatory medication of first choice during pregnancy. Paracetamol is preferable, or when anti-inflammatory therapy is indicated, ibuprofen or diclofenac are first-line options of the non-steroidal anti-inflammatory drugs (NSAIDs). ASA or NSAIDs should not be used routinely at analgesic or anti-inflammatory doses in the last third of pregnancy. Prolonged use after 28 weeks may lead to premature closure of the fetal ductus arteriosus. If repeated analgesic doses of ASA or NSAIDs are used after 28 weeks gestation, the ductal flow and amniotic fluid volume (adverse renal effects related to NSAID use, see Section 2.1.6) has to be regularly followed up with ultrasound. A single application of 500 mg of ASA close to the time of delivery can increase the bleeding tendency of the mother, the fetus and the newborn during delivery. Low-dose therapy with ASA can be used safely without limitations with appropriate indication.

2.1.3   Pyrazolone compounds and phenylbutazone

Pyrazolone compounds

Metamizol (dipyrone), *phenazone* and other *pyrazolone* compounds have largely lost their role as analgesics and antipyretics because of their potentially life threatening hematologic adverse effects, and have been replaced accordingly by pharmaceuticals with greater effectiveness and safety. Pyrazolone compounds are prostaglandin inhibitors, and as other drugs in this class, repeated use after 28 weeks gestation can cause premature closure of the fetal ductus arteriosus. Prostaglandin inhibitors can also affect fetal renal tubular function resulting in decreased amniotic fluid volume. There are two case reports describing the development of oligohydramnion in pregnant women taking high doses of metamizol shortly before the end of their pregnancy (Weintraub 2006, Catalan 1995). In the case presented by Weintraub, a reversible narrowing of the ductus arteriosus was also observed.

While experience of use during early pregnancy is limited, there has been no suggestion of an increased risk for malformations in humans after exposure to metamizol. A prospective follow-up study including more than 100 women treated in the first trimester with metamizol did not observe an increased risk for major malformations when compared to non-exposed controls (Bar-Oz 2005). Another prospective study from Brazil, which included more than 500 exposed pregnancies, observed no increased risk for malformations or perinatal complications, including preterm birth or low birth weight (da Silva Dal Pizzol 2009).

An increased risk of Wilm's tumor after prenatal exposure to metamizol was observed in a Brazilian study (Sharpe 1996). No other studies assessing the risk for this outcome have been published. In two retrospective case-control studies, metamizol use during pregnancy was more common among mothers with infants with acute leukemia than among mothers with healthy children (Alexander 2001). Contrary to these findings, a subsequent study did not observe a significant association between mothers' metamizol use and childhood leukemia (Pombo-de-Oliveira 2006).

Propyphenazone was not teratogenic in experimental testing in animals (rats). There are no data regarding propyphenazone or phenazone use during pregnancy in humans.

Phenylbutazone is a prostaglandin inhibitor with analgesic, antiinflammatory and antipyretic properties. Phenylbutazone has been used primarily in the treatment of ankylosing spondylitis and rheumatoid arthritis (RA). As with pyrazolone compounds, phenylbutazone is rarely used today because of potentially serious adverse effects related to its use (renal failure, hematologic effects, and potent accumulation with a biological half-life of 50 to 100 hours). Animal experiments have reported teratogenic effects. There are insufficient data regarding malformation risk in humans, but a major teratogenic potential appears unlikely. As an inhibitor of prostaglandin synthesis, phenylbutazone, like ASA and NSAIDs, can produce premature closure of ductus arteriosus when used in the last trimester, and potentially affect fetal renal function.

> **Recommendation.** Use of pyrazolone compounds and phenylbutazone should be avoided during pregnancy. Paracetamol is the analgesic of choice during pregnancy, in individual cases and also in combination with codeine when needed. Exposure during the first trimester to pyrazolone compounds or phenylbutazone is not an indication for specific diagnostic procedures. Close observation to assess ductal flow with Doppler echocardiography, and controlling amniotic fluid volume by ultrasound is advisable were these medications are used in repeated doses after the twenty-eighth week of pregnancy.

2.1.4   Analgesic drug combination products and drugs used for osteoarthritis

In principle, use of analgesic drug combination products should be avoided during pregnancy. Even if there is no established evidence for

Pregnancy

2.1 Analgesics, non-steroidal anti-inflammatory drugs (NSAIDs), muscle relaxants, and antigout medications

teratogenicity, the potential risks increase with the number of simultaneous use of different pharmaceuticals. The combination of paracetamol plus codeine represents an exception and can be used relatively safely in well-justified cases.

Ademethionine (S-adenosyl methionine), chondroitin sulfate, glucosamine, hyaluronic acid and *oxaceprol* are used primarily in the management of osteoarthritis (OA). Their mechanism of action is hypothesized to intervene in cartilage metabolism and consequently slow down or even arrest the disease process. Based on the slow onset of clinical effectiveness these substances have been labeled as "Slow Acting Drugs in Osteoarthritis" (SADOA) (Steinmeyer 2006). Evidence of effectiveness is inconclusive though (Madry 2011). One prospective study involved 54 women, of whom 34 were exposed to glucosamine in the first trimester, but did not observe malformations in offspring other than a scrotal hernia in one infant (Sivojelezova 2007). There are no data for ademetionine, hyaluronic acid, or oxaceprol use during pregnancy.

> **Recommendation.** Drugs used for osteoarthritis are best avoided during pregnancy but inadvertent exposure during a critical phase of development is no indication for specific measures.

2.1.5 Opioid agonists and antagonists and other centrally acting analgesics

The term opioid covers endogenous opioids, morphine and derivatives, and synthetic compounds capable of binding to opioid receptors (both agonists and antagonists). Opioids are centrally acting analgesics and can be compared in their effectiveness to morphine, the major opium alkaloid. Opioids can be grouped according to chemical structure into morphine analogs (*morphine, hydromorphone, codeine, oxycodone* and *naloxone*, the latter being an antagonist), *phenylpiperidines (pethidine (meperidine), fentanyl, alfentanil, remifentanil, sufentanil)*, methadone analogs (*methadone, propoxyphene*), and tebaine derivatives (*buprenorphine*). A grouping can also be made among the pure agonists (endorphins, morphine and opiates with similar effectiveness), pure antagonists (such as *naloxone* and *naltrexone*), and substances that exhibit both agonistic and antagonistic properties (such as buprenorphine, *nalorfin, pentazocine*).

Like morphine, opioid agonists can induce dependence and their use close to delivery can lead to respiratory depression and withdrawal symptoms in the newborn.

Short-term therapeutic use of opioids during pregnancy is viewed separately from abuse (Chapter 2.21).

► **A. Morphine and hydromorphone**

Morphine and hydromorphone have induced teratogenic effects at high doses in animals. While one case-control study has reported an increase in specific congenital anomalies, including heart defects and spina bifida associated with opioid use, morphine or hydromorphine were not included in the exposures (Broussard 2011). However, because opioids act by binding to the same receptors, these findings may bear relevance to all opioids. To date, there are no studies regarding teratogenicity of morphine or hydromorphine in clinical use, but there is no evidence that these agents, having been used for several decades, would be major teratogens.

Prenatal exposure to morphine can result in a decreased biophysical score in the fetus, including attenuation of breathing movements. This was described in a small study involving 10 pregnant women in the third trimester who were given one single intramuscular application of 10–15 mg morphine for pain control during fetal blood sampling. The authors hypothesized that the adverse effects could be related to placental vasculature contraction (Kopecky 2000). One case reported reduced flow in the umbilical and middle cerebral arteries, together with limited variability and decelerations in fetal heart rate at 27 gestational weeks after long-term use of morphine for severe pain. These changes normalized once the medication was changed to fentanyl (Collins 2005).

Additionally, one case report describing long-term use of intrathecal morphine to manage chronic pain reported a healthy newborn with normal Apgar values, no withdrawal symptoms, and normal development up to the age of 18 months (Oberlander 2000).

Exposure close to delivery may cause respiratory depression in the newborn, and long-term use of morphine and other opioids during pregnancy may produce withdrawal symptoms, including increased muscle tone, irritability and gastrointestinal symptoms (diarrhea). The presentation of withdrawal symptoms depends on the pharmacokinetics of the compound. For morphine, the onset of withdrawal symptoms is on average 1.5 days after birth (Bio 2011, Ebner 2007).

Recommendation. Morphine and hydromorphine use during pregnancy should be limited to special situations where no safer alternatives are available. Tapering off the medication should always be done gradually to avoid withdrawal symptoms in both the mother and the fetus. The newborn may exhibit respiratory depression if morphine is given shortly before delivery. With prolonged exposure, the newborn may present severe symptoms of withdrawal. In these cases the parturient should be referred to a center prepared for neonatal intensive care.

▶ **B.   Pethidine (meperidine) and meptazinol**

Pethidine is a potent analgesic drug, and has been used for decades during delivery for pain relief. Pethidine has been used with 50–100 mg intramuscular doses at an early-stage of delivery. The maximal effect for pain relief is reached at about 30–50 minutes after dose, and the effect lasts for 2–4 hours. Adverse effects in the mother are common and include sedation, nausea, decreased gastric emptying, and occasionally respiratory depression.

Toxicology

Little information on the use of pethidine in the first trimester is available and does not suggest a specific risk for malformations (Heinonen 1977). One case-control study observed an association between specific cardiovascular defects and opioid use, but no association with pethidine when individual opioids were analyzed separately (Broussard 2011).

Pregnancy

2.1 Analgesics, non-steroidal anti-inflammatory drugs (NSAIDs), muscle relaxants, and antigout medications

Pethidine passes the placenta and being slightly basic, may reach higher concentrations in the fetus than in the mother, and particularly so if the fetus is distressed and acidotic. In the fetus, breathing movements, oxygen saturation and heart rate variability are reduced after administration of pethidine to the mother (Reynolds 2011). Pethidine at low doses may induce metabolic acidosis in the newborn. A placebo-controlled study with nearly 400 women found that neonatal acidosis (pH <7.12) was more common if the mother had received 100 mg pethidine during the first stage of labor, and acidosis was most prevalent when the drug was given 5 hours prior to delivery (Sosa 2006). Neonatal pharmacological effects include respiratory depression, sedation, and poor sucking. The risk for neonatal pharmacologic effects increases with repeated doses and when given within 3–5 hours prior to birth (Reynolds 2011). Premature infants are more prone to severe symptoms. Pethidine-induced neonatal effects can be reversed by naloxone administration. The half-life of the parent compound and the active metabolite norpethidine in a newborn is prolonged to 13–23 hours and 2–3 days, respectively, due to immature drug metabolism. Neonatal symptoms may therefore continue for several days after birth.

Meptazinol has been used for labor analgesia as with pethidine, with similar effectiveness for pain relief during labor. However, no established advantages when compared to pethidine have been observed, while maternal side-effects may be more common after meptazinol use (Morrison 1987).

Recommendation. Pethidine (or *meptazinol*) may be used during labor after critical assessment, and when no signs of pre-existing fetal acidosis are present. Use is relatively contraindicated in premature births. Application during the first trimester is acceptable if no safer alternatives are available.

▶ **C.   Codeine and oxycodone**

Pharmacology

Codeine is a morphine derivative with less analgesic and sedative effects than morphine. Codeine is metabolized to morphine by the cytochrome P450 enzyme (CYP) 2D6. Inhibitors of this enzyme (such as *fluoxetine* and *citalopram*) can decrease or even abolish the effect of codeine. In addition, there are agonistic interactions between codeine and many other medications that must be considered when prescribing codeine. Codeine is available as single preparations, as an antitussive in cough medicines, and in analgesic combinations with paracetamol or ASA. As with other opioids, repeated use of codeine can lead to dependence.

Oxycodone is a semi-synthetic opium alkaloid with analgesic properties comparable to morphine. Oxycodone is indicated for management of postoperative pain or other severe pain treatment when opioid analgesics are needed. Both codeine and oxycodone pass through the placenta.

Toxicology

Individual studies using retrospective design have observed associations with codeine use and different organ-specific malformations, including congenital heart defects (Broussard 2011, Bracken 1981, Rothman 1979), orofacial clefts (Bracken 1981, Saxén 1975), and several other organ-specific malformations (Bracken 1981). In the most recent of these publications which included nearly 17,500 cases of children of whom 8,000 had a diagnosis of congenital heart disease, an increased risk of hypoplastic left heart syndrome was observed after opioid analgesic use (Broussard 2011). When analyzed on individual drug level, codeine use was associated with atrioventricular septal defects, left ventricular outflow tract defects, and hypoplastic left heart syndrome (Broussard 2011), however, the associations were based on unadjusted analyses due to a small number of affected cases. Contrary to these findings, a retrospective analysis of 141 children with congenital heart defects did not observe an association with maternal intake of codeine during the first trimester (Shaw 1992). Another retrospective study did not find an association between neural tube defects in 538 fetuses or children and codeine exposure during the first trimester (Shaw 1998). Further, the most recent study based on data from population registers in Norway did not find an increased risk of overall congenital anomalies in more than 600 exposed pregnancies with first-trimester exposure (Nezvalová-Henriksen 2012a, 2011). Considering the limitations in the study design in several of the published studies and the discrepant findings, no firm conclusions can be made about possible causality. To summarize, codeine use in early pregnancy is not expected to increase the rate of overall malformations, but a small risk for cardiovascular defects cannot be ruled out.

Much less data are available for *hydrocodone* and *oxycodone*. A small prospective study, published only in abstract, identified 40 pregnancies with exposure to hydrocodone and 78 exposed to oxycodone during the first trimester. There were six infants with a malformation in the hydrocodone group but no pattern of malformations (Schick 1996). As with codeine, a recently published case-control study observed an increased risk for specific cardiac defects after exposure to hydrocodone (atrioventricular septal defects, hypoplastic left heart syndrome, and further, Tetralogy of Fallot and pulmonary valve stenosis). Associations were also observed between hydrocodone exposure in early pregnancy and spina bifida, cleft palate, and gastroschisis, while oxycodone use was associated with an increased risk of pulmonary valve stenosis (Broussard 2011). Several limitations, including the retrospective study design predisposing to recall bias, the role of underlying maternal illness, and the small numbers of exposed case infants, all suggest that no conclusions about a causal association can be made on the basis of these results.

As with all opiate derivatives, treatment close to delivery can lead to neonatal respiratory depression and withdrawal symptoms.

Recommendation. Codeine may be used in pregnant women as an analgesic if clearly indicated, and primarily in combination with paracetamol. When possible, use should be restricted to short-term therapy. Codeine may be used on a short-term basis as an antitussive when agonizing, dry cough has failed to respond to other physical measures. In each case possible interaction with other medications and the potential of addiction need to be considered. Oxycodone is also acceptable under strict indication. Long-term use is limited to special situations only. Depending upon dose, timing and duration of exposure, the newborn may suffer from respiratory depression and withdrawal symptoms.

2.1 Analgesics, non-steroidal anti-inflammatory drugs (NSAIDs), muscle relaxants, and antigout medications   Pregnancy

▶ **D.   Fentanyl, alfentanil, remifentanil and sufentanil**

Fentanyl, *alfentanil*, *remifentanil* and *sufentanil* are synthetic phenylpip-eradine-opioids with pure agonistic activity and high analgesic potency. They are used in perioperative situations in anesthesia, and fentanyl is further used in severe chronic pain where less potent opioid treatments have failed. In these situations administration can occur by using resorib-lets, buccal films, nasal spray or transdermal patches.

Fentanyl has been reported to cross the placenta readily in early pregnancy (Cooper 1999, Shannon 1998). No teratogenicity has been observed in animal experiments. Systematic studies on fentanyl use in early pregnancy are lacking, but until now no suggestion of teratogenicity exists. Exposure close to delivery may produce respiratory depression in the newborn.

Two case reports describe the application of transdermal fentanyl patches throughout pregnancy. In the first case the dose was 125 µg/h. The full-term, healthy baby had normal Apgar scores, but after 24 hours developed symptoms of withdrawal including irritability and high-pitched crying (Regan 2000). The symptoms subsided within 4 days without any treatment. Neonatal fentanyl blood levels were one-third of the maternal values immediately after birth. Another case described a woman using 25 µg/h fentanyl patches to manage chronic pain due to systemic lupus erythematosus and fibromyalgia (Einarson 2009). A healthy boy was born full-term with no recorded symptoms of withdrawal, and meeting normal developmental milestones at 8 months of age.

Fentanyl is frequently applied during labor either by neuraxial techniques (epidural or intrathecal administration) or sometimes intravenously. In epidural and intrathecal analgesia the amount of fentanyl used is relatively small, and the risk for neonatal respiratory depression is consequently low (Reynolds 2011). Neuraxial analgesia, in general, offers favorable outcomes, e.g. reduced maternal stress, hyperventilation, and increased uterine vasodilatation (Reynolds 2011). For systemic administration, i.v. fentanyl can be administered by a patient-control analgesic (PCA) pump; however, when used systematically and in larger doses, respiratory depression in the neonate is more likely (Reynolds 2011, 2010). In a prospective, randomized, controlled study based on 12 pregnant women, five treated with PCA fentanyl and the seven controls treated with paracervical blockade, neonatal arterial oxyhemoglobin saturation was significantly lower in the fentanyl group, and prolonged, significantly decreased fetal oxyhemoglobin saturation was observed in one infant in the fentanyl exposure group, requiring *naloxone* treatment (Nikkola 2000). The prolonged desaturation was suggested to have been associated with fentanyl-induced hypoventilation, or possibly with respiratory muscle rigidity (Nikkola 2000). It has been suggested that when the interval from fentanyl dosing to delivery is sufficiently long (≥3 hours), the risk for neonatal respiratory depression appears to be small (Herschel, 2000). In another study, nearly 140 infants exposed prenatally to i.v. fentanyl 50–100 mcg hourly as needed for labor analgesia, did not suffer from respiratory depression or low Apgar score more often than unexposed controls (Rayburn 1989). The last fentanyl dose was given on average 112 minutes before delivery. However, large inter-individual differences exist in fentanyl pharmacokinetics, and neonatal monitoring after maternal opiate use during labor is essential. Further, fentanyl, as in other opioids, is a weak base and may accumulate in an acidotic fetus, thereby further jeopardizing fetal wellbeing. Accordingly, fentanyl should not be administered in situations where fetal acidosis is suspected or has been confirmed.

Fentanyl can occasionally cause neuromuscular side effects including primarily the respiratory muscles. Three case reports have described development of chest wall rigidity in the neonate after intrauterine exposure to fentanyl shortly before delivery; two of these cases were associated with systemic administration of fentanyl to the mother (Eventov-Friedman 2010, Lindemann 1998). One case was reported after intrathecal administration for labor analgesia (Bolisetty 1999). Spontaneous recovery occurred in two of the cases (Bolisetty1999, Lindemann 1998), while administration of naloxone resolved the symptoms in the third case (Eventov-Friedman 2010).

The compatibility of maternal i.v. alfentanil administration on the newborn appears to be similar to fentanyl. Alfentanil passes the placenta, umbilical vein alfentanil concentration being 30% of maternal plasma concentration (Cartwright 1989). In an investigation comparing PCA using fentanyl or alfentanil during the early phase of labor, no difference was observed in Apgar scores or other neonatal outcome parameters, while fentanyl provided somewhat better pain relief (Morley-Forster 2000).

Remifentanil is an ultra-short acting opioid, with a half-life of only 3 minutes. It is metabolized rapidly by blood and tissue esterases, and metabolism and excretion is not dependent on liver or kidney function. Remifentanil (i.v.) has been used for pain control during delivery and use may provide more reliable analgesia and higher Apgar scores than that obtained with pethidine (Reynolds 2011). As with other opioids used in labor analgesia, remifentanil use may also increase the risk for neonatal respiratory depression.

Sufantanil is used in epidural and spinal anesthesia during labor and has been reported to pass the placenta at term (Loftus 1995). While fetal bradycardy and late decelerations have been associated with sufentanil intrathecal administration in individual studies (Van de Velde 2004, 2001), neuraxial analgesia using opioids is nevertheless generally considered relatively safe for the newborn (Reynolds 2011, Capogna 2004).

No reports of teratogenic effects for alfentanil, remifentanil and sufentanil exposure during early pregnancy have been published, but data are insufficient for definitive conclusions.

Recommendation. Under strict indication, fentanyl and with compelling indications also other drugs in this group, may be used in any trimester of pregnancy. When administered close to delivery, risk for neonatal respiratory depression exists. Opioid use in obstetric analgesia should be avoided in cases with suspected or confirmed fetal acidosis, as exposure may further impair fetal well-being.

► E.   Other opioids and centrally acting non-opioid analgesics

Pentazocine is an opioid analgesic with a weak antagonistic effect, available in some European countries and in drug combination products together with *paracetamol* in the US. Pentazocine was sold in the US primarily during the 1980s in combination with the antihistamine *tripelennamine* under the name of "T's and Blues" which was used as, for example, a substitute for heroine. Animal teratology studies have been negative apart from a hamster study (Geber 1975). Limited experience in humans comes mainly from abuse and has not suggested an increased risk for malformations (DeBooy 1993, Little 1990). Intrauterine growth restriction and behavioral abnormalities have been associated with pentazocine abuse (Chasnoff 1983); however, the effects cannot always be differentiated from other illicit drug use or other lifestyle factors with a negative influence on

Pregnancy

2.1 Analgesics, non-steroidal anti-inflammatory drugs (NSAIDs), muscle relaxants, and antigout medications

pregnancy outcome. As with other opioids, exposure close to delivery may cause withdrawal symptoms and respiratory depression in the newborn.

Tilidine is another potent opioid analgesic, often used in combination with the opioid antagonist *naloxone*. Animal studies do not suggest teratogenicity but data in humans are lacking. Side effects are similar to other opioids and exposure close to delivery is expected to increase the risk for neonatal problems as discussed with other opioids.

Tramadol is a synthetic opioid analgesic mainly used in oral formulae for treatment of chronic pain and in parenteral forms for acute pain. The analgesic potency is similar to codeine. Tramadol is metabolized to *O-desmethyltramadol*, which is more potent in producing analgesia than the parent compound. In addition to binding to opioid receptors, tramadol also acts by inhibiting the uptake of serotonin. Tramadol crosses the placenta, with fetal drug concentrations similar to maternal concentrations (Claahsen-van der Grinten 2005). Animal experiments have not shown teratogenic effects. There are no reports of teratogenic effects in humans, but systematic studies on safety during pregnancy are few. One small prospective study of nearly 150 pregnant women was quoted not to have observed an increased risk for malformations in offspring exposed to tramadol in early pregnancy (Bloor 2012). Withdrawal symptoms after long-term therapy during pregnancy, and with relatively high doses (300–800 mg/day) have been described in case reports. Symptoms appeared between 24 hours and several days of age (Hartenstein 2010, O'Mara 2010, Willaschek 2009, Meyer 1997). Due to the dual mechanism of action of tramadol, the most suitable agent to treat neonatal tramadol withdrawal is uncertain but treatment with benzodiazepines, phenobarbital, opium tincture or clonidine has been successful in individual cases (Bloor 2012).

Parenterally administered opioids, including tramadol, offer limited benefit in controlling pain during labor. A recent Cochrane meta-analysis comparing intramuscularly administered tramadol to pethidine, found that pethidine was more effective in pain relief than tramadol while maternal side effects or neonatal problems did not differ between the groups (Ullman 2010).

The relatively abundant data on buprenorphine use during pregnancy in opioid dependence substitution treatment does not suggest teratogenic effects, while scarce or no data are available for meptazinol, nalbuphine or piritramide. Tapentadol is a recently introduced centrally acting synthetic opioid that acts by binding to opioid receptors, and also by inhibiting norepinephrine reuptake, and is indicated for use in chronic, moderate or severe pain in adults. According to the manufacturer, preclinical studies of tapentadol did not demonstrate teratogenic effects in rats or rabbits after intravenous and subcutaneous administration. There is no experience concerning use during pregnancy, neither for ziconotide and flupirtine, both which are centrally-acting non-opioid analgesics.

Recommendation. Individual drugs in this group with experience for use during pregnancy, such as tramadol or buprenorphine, may be used in pregnancy with compelling indication. Depending on duration and dose of treatment, all opioid agonists can cause respiratory depression in the newborn and withdrawal symptoms. Withdrawal symptoms are common after long-term exposure, as with substitution therapy, and can appear within days or weeks after delivery. For pain management, paracetamol (combined with codeine if needed), or ibuprofen until gestational week 28 are preferable. Inadvertent exposure to the more recently introduced agents such as ziconotide or tapentadol in the first trimester is not an indication for specific diagnostic procedures.

▶ **F.   Opioid antagonists: naloxone, naltrexone and nalorphine**

Naloxone and *naltrexone* are pure opioid antagonists with competitive action and high affinity to the opioid receptors. Naloxone is used also in newborns to reverse central nervous system and respiratory depression caused by maternal opioid use. By binding to the opioid receptors, naloxone displaces both opioid agonists and partial antagonists, such as pentazocine. Naloxone passes the placenta, and given close to delivery, unbound naloxone concentration is higher in the newborn than in the mother (Asali 1984). Administration of naloxone to a pregnant habitual opioid addict may induce withdrawal symptoms also in the fetus (Chapter 2.1.5C). Naltrexone is a more potent opioid antagonist than naloxone and with a longer duration of action, used in alcohol and opioid dependence. Nalorphine is a partial opioid antagonist rarely used today. Teratogenic effects have not been reported for any of these drugs in animal studies but systematic studies in humans are lacking.

Recommendation. Naloxone may be used under strict indications during pregnancy. However, acute withdrawal symptoms in the mother and the fetus are to be strictly avoided.

2.1.6   Non-steroidal anti-inflammatory and antirheumatic drugs

Pharmacology

The anti-inflammatory activity of NSAIDs is based on the inhibition of the cyclo-oxygenase (COX) enzyme, resulting in prostaglandin synthesis inhibition. At least two types of COX enzyme exist: the constitutional COX-1 is responsible for physiological prostanoid production, such as prostacyclin and TGE2, whereas COX-2 enzyme activity increases in pathological conditions such as inflammatory processes. COX-2 is expressed in the fetal kidney and appears to be essential for kidney development and function (Boubred 2006). COX-2 is also important in labor and NSAIDs with COX-2 activity have been used as tocolytic agents for treatment of preterm delivery. Commonly used NSAIDs include the propionic acid derivatives *ibuprofen, ketoprofen* and *naproxen*; the acetic acid derivatives *diclofenac, indomethacin, etodolac* and *ketorolac*; the oxicams *meloxicam* and *piroxicam*; the fenamates *mefenamic acid* and *tolfenamic acid*, and others including *nabumetone* and *nimesulide* (all non-selective COX-inhibitors); and the coxibes, including *celecoxib, parecoxib*, and *etoricoxib* (all selective COX-2 inhibitors). Most NSAIDs are highly bound to plasma proteins but nevertheless are transferred through the placenta. Data on placental passage are available for diclofenac, which passes the placenta readily during the first trimester with fetal diclofenac concentrations similar to maternal concentrations, while transfer of naproxen is somewhat limited in early pregnancy but increases with advancing pregnancy (Siu 2000). Indomethacin concentration in the fetus corresponds to maternal plasma concentrations in the third trimester (Moise 1990).

Pregnancy

2.1 Analgesics, non-steroidal anti-inflammatory drugs (NSAIDs), muscle relaxants, and antigout medications

Toxicology

Use of NSAID has been associated with an increased risk for luteinized unruptured follicle (LUF) syndrome. Follicular rupture is dependent on prostaglandins, and prostaglandin inhibition may consequently disturb this process. Repeated use of NSAIDs in the preovulatory phase of the menstrual cycle has been associated with an increased risk for LUF. In nearly 60 monitored cycles of patients with continuous NSAID use, LUF syndromes occurred in more than one-third of women compared to 3% in untreated women (Micu 2011). Of the LUF syndromes, 75% occurred in etoricoxib users and 15% in diclofenac users, while even high doses of ibuprofen (1,600 mg/day) did not prevent ovulation. The authors suggested that continuous periovulatory exposure to NSAIDs, and especially COX-2 selective NSAIDs should be avoided when planning pregnancy (Micu 2011).

NSAID use around conception has been associated with an increased risk of miscarriage. A prospectively conducted study recruiting more than 1,000 women with a positive pregnancy test, 53 (5%) of whom reported NSAID use, observed a nearly 2-fold risk for miscarriage in women having used naproxen or ibuprofen compared to non-users (Li 2003). The association was stronger when NSAID use started around conception, or if NSAID use lasted more than 1 week. ASA use at the time of conception was also associated with an increased risk, while paracetamol use was not. The authors suggested that suppression of prostaglandin biosynthesis could lead to abnormal implantation resulting in miscarriage. However, conclusive evidence on causal association is lacking.

There is no consistent evidence of increased malformation risk associated with NSAID use. Inhibition of prostaglandin synthesis after 28 gestation weeks may lead to premature closure of the ductus arteriosus (Botalli) and renal impairment in the fetus (see below).

▶ A.   Non-selective COX inhibitors

Congenital malformations

Ibuprofen has not been consistently teratogenic in experimental animal studies, but high doses have been associated with an increased risk of cardiac defects (Cappon 2003). In humans, individual studies have observed an association between ibuprofen use and specific birth defects, including gastroschisis and cardiac septal defects. Data from the National Birth Defects Prevention Study, with retrospectively assessed exposure data, observed an association between first trimester ibuprofen use and gastroschisis while no association was observed between ibuprofen exposure and *omphalocele* (Mac Bird 2009). Another retrospective, case-control study observed a marginally increased risk for gastroschisis after exposure to ibuprofen (Torfs 1996), while a similar association was not observed in a nested case-control study, which, nevertheless, observed an association between ibuprofen use and overall congenital anomalies (Ofori 2006). Further, a recent case-control study from the National Birth Defects Prevention Study reported an association between ibuprofen use and orofacial clefts, spina bifida, and anophthalmy or microphthalmy (Hernandez 2012). Methodological limitations in some of these studies include the retrospective study design, and further, the possible role of maternal illness, which could not be ruled out.

Contrary to these findings several large, population based studies including altogether nearly 10,000 exposed pregnancies, did not observe an increased risk for overall malformations (Nezvalová-Henriksen 2013a, Daniel 2012), or specific malformations, including cardiac malformations (Daniel 2012, Källén 2003) after exposure to ibuprofen in early pregnancy. A population-based study from Norway, based on maternal interview on exposures prospectively to delivery, observed a marginally increased risk of cardiac defects when infants were followed up until 18 months of age, but this finding was not statistically significant (Nezvalová-Henriksen 2013a). In summary, data gathered to date does not suggest an increased risk for malformations.

There are no documented reports about the use of *dexibuprofen*, the (S)-enantiomer of the racemate ibuprofen, but the effects may be expected to be comparable to ibuprofen.

Diclofenac has not been teratogenic in animal species including rodents and non-rodents. In humans, data are less abundant than for ibuprofen, but not suggestive of an increased risk for malformations. One study carried out prospectively by teratology information services included 145 first trimester exposures to diclofenac, and observed no pattern of defects among the seven offspring with a diagnosis of malformation (Cassina 2010). Further, a study from Israel based on dispensed medicines with over 1,300 exposed pregnancies (Daniel 2012), and a population-based study from Norway reporting 192 first trimester exposures (Nevlazova-Henriksen 2013a), did not observe an increased risk for congenital malformations.

Naproxen use was associated with orofacial clefts in a study based on Swedish registers with prospectively collected exposure data (Ericson 2001). Extending follow-up in the Swedish register data for three years observed an association of naproxene and cardiac malformations (Källén 2003). Oral clefts (cleft lip with or without cleft palate) were also associated with naproxen use in a National Birth Defects Prevention study based on retrospective exposure information (Hernandez 2012), as were other specific anomalies, including anophthalmy, isolated encephalocele and pulmonary valve stenosis. Contrary to these findings, no increased risk of overall major malformations was observed in a population-based study, including nearly 1,000 pregnancies with first trimester exposure to naproxen (Daniel 2012).

Another population-based study with 168 first trimester exposures, did not observe an increased risk of cardiovascular malformations when extending follow-up until 1.5 years of age (Nevlazová-Henriksen 2013a).

A register-based study from Israel analyzed 265 pregnancies exposed to etodolac and observed no increased risk for major malformations (Daniel 2012). The same study included 128 indomethacin exposures with no risk for major malformations. No other studies related to the first trimester are available; however, neither are there reports suggesting malformation risk associated with etodolac or indomethacin use.

For the other non-selective COX inhibitors (*ketoprofen, dexketoprofen, ketorolac, meloxicam, mefenamic acid, tolfenamic acid,* and *sulindak*), there are little or no data for use during the first trimester, nor reports suggested malformation risk.

Effects on the circulatory system and renal function in the fetus

Indomethacin and *sulindac* have been used for tocolysis, the primary mechanism is thought to be prostaglandin inhibition. However, fetal side effects have limited this use. NSAID use from 28 weeks of

Pregnancy

2.1 Analgesics, non-steroidal anti-inflammatory drugs (NSAIDs), muscle relaxants, and antigout medications

gestation onwards can lead to premature closure of the fetal ductus arteriosus (Botalli). Sensitivity to prostaglandin inhibitors increases with advancing pregnancy. Constriction of the ductus together with use of NSAIDs has already been observed in fetal echocardiography at the twenty-seventh gestational week, although not earlier; it occurs increasingly after 32 weeks and is reported to occur with indomethacin in 60–100% of cases if exposure occurs during week 34 (Moise 1993, 1988, Van den Veyver 1993). This effect can sometimes be reversed, and may spontaneously resolve itself within 1–2 days after cessation of therapy (Østensen 2004). Several cases have also been reported after nimesulide use in the third trimester; in some cases, after only one or two doses (Prefumo 2008, Paladini 2005). Even topical administration may affect ductal flow. A case report describes constriction of the ductus after local application of diclofenac gel during week 35 on the shoulder–neck region, together with a post-application adhesive patch containing *methylsalicylate, menthol* and *camphor* (Torloni 2006). Both narrowing of the ductus and a tricuspid insufficiency regressed within 5 days after cessation of therapy. Premature closure of the ductus arteriosus may lead to serious secondary pathology involving the right heart and pulmonary circulation, including pulmonary hypertension of the newborn (PPHN) (Gewillig 2009). A case report describes a full-term infant exposed to naproxen 220 mg twice daily during the last 4 days prior to birth, diagnosed with a closed ductus arteriosus and PPHN with hypertrophy of the right heart (Talati 2000). NSAID use in pregnancy has been associated with PPHN in several other case-reports (Siu 2004, Zenker 1998), and studies (Alano 2001, van Marter 1996). Contrary to these findings, a recent population-based case-control study including 377 PPHN cases and nearly 900 controls, observed a marginally protective effect of ibuprofen use any time during pregnancy (van Marter 2013). Inflammation may play an important role in the pathogenesis of PPHN, and the authors speculated that ibuprofen might have been protective because of its anti-inflammatory properties.

In addition to indomethacin, sulindac has been used to treat preterm delivery. Sulindac is a prodrug, metabolized in the liver to the active sulfide derivative. Despite earlier reports suggesting a more favorable profile than indomethacin, more recent studies have indicated that sulindac use is associated with similar fetal side-effects as use of other NSAIDS during the third trimester (Loudon 2003, Sawdy 2003). Further, a randomized, placebo-controlled trial failed to show efficacy of sulindac in inhibiting recurrent preterm birth in women primarily treated successfully with magnesium sulfate, but sulindac dose in this trial was low (100 mg/day) (Humphrey 2001).

Prostaglandins are necessary in maintaining renal blood flow and tubular function (Boubred 2006). Several reports have described renal failure in the fetus resulting from late second, or third trimester exposure to NSAIDs. The nephrotoxic effects are related to COX-2 inhibition, resulting in reduced renal perfusion of the kidney and an increase in circulatory vasopressin and angiotensin II activity (Antonucci, 2007, 2012, Benini 2004). Most of the reports concern indomethacin (Itabashi 2003, Butler-O'Hara 2002, Robin 2000, van der Heijden 1994, 1995) and nimesulide (a non-selective COX inhibitor with primary COX-2 inhibition activity) (Magnani 2004, Sawdy 2004, Balasubramanniam 2000, Holmes 2000, Peruzzi 1999). Naproxen use during the late second trimester has also been associated with oligohydramnion and renal tubular dysgenesis (Koklu 2006). In some cases, the renal effects as reflected in decreased amniotic fluid volume, have been reversible, in other cases the exposure has led to permanent renal damage or fetal death (review in Antonucci 2012, Boubred 2006).

Indomethacin, diclofenac and sulindac have all been successfully administered in cases of severe polyhydramnion without fetal side effects (Suzumori 2009, Jayagopal 2007, Rode 2007).

Necrotizing enterocolitis

Necrotizing enterocolitis (NEC) in a neonate is associated with significant morbidity and mortality. Antenatal use of NSAIDs, and especially indomethacin, has been associated with NEC in premature infants (Sood 2011, Amin 2007); however, a direct causal association has not been confirmed.

> **Recommendation.** Ibuprofen is the analgesic of choice second to paracetamol, and the anti-inflammatory agent of first choice until gestational week 28. Use of diclofenac is also possible. After 28 weeks of gestation, repeated use of NSAIDs should be avoided. If used repeatedly during the third trimester, ductal flow and amniotic fluid volume should be regularly evaluated by sonography.

▶ B.   Selective cyclooxygenase-2 (COX-2)-inhibitors

Pharmacology

Selective COX-2 inhibitors were developed to avoid the gastrointestinal side effects related to COX-1 inhibition. Those currently on the market include *celecoxib*, *etoricoxib* and *parecoxib*. The coxibes bind strongly to plasma proteins but no data on placental transfer are available. However, transplacental passage to some degree is expected due to the low molecular weight (Antonucci 2012).

Toxicology

Unruptured luteinized follicle (LUF) syndrome seems to be associated strongly with selective COX-2 inhibitors, and continuous use of coxibes should be avoided prior to ovulation (see "Toxicology", Section 2.1.6).

Animal studies have observed embryotoxic effects after exposure to etoricoxib and parecoxib, and teratogenic effects including cardiovascular malformations in rabbits after celecoxib exposure. There are no studies about the use of coxibes during early pregnancy in humans. COX-2 is constitutively expressed in the fetal kidney and appears to be essential for kidney development and function, and COX-2 knockout mice exhibit abnormal renal development (Boubred 2006, Norwood 2000, Dinchuk 1995). The circulatory and renal adverse effects discussed in association with the non-selective COX inhibitors are to be expected also with the selective COX-2 inhibitors. In particular, renal impairment and failure may be more strongly associated with COX-2 inhibition, as suggested by the several case reports described after nimesulide or indomethacin use, both drugs which, even if being non-selective COX -inhibitors, have a relative specificity to COX-2 inhibition.

A randomized trial including more than 100 women who were between 24 and 34 weeks gestation with preterm labor, were randomized in groups receiving either celecoxib 100 mg×2 or intravenous *magnesium sulfate*.

Celecoxib was as effective as magnesium sulfate in arresting labor for 48 hours (81 versus 87%) and no fetal adverse effects were observed (Borna 2007). Another randomized study including only 24 pregnant women failed to show differences in tocolytic efficacy between celecoxib or indomethacin (Stika 2002). In contrast to indomethacin, use of cele-coxib did not increase ductal flow velocity, but amniotic fluid volume was transiently decreased in both groups (Stika 2002). However, the numbers included were small and no conclusions about relative safety can be made on this basis. The fetotoxic effects described in association with the use of non-selective NSAIDs are to be expected also with the COX-2 selective NSAIDs.

> **Recommendation.** Selective COX-2 inhibitors are contraindicated during preg-nancy because of a lack of experience, and the potential fetal effects on kidney maturation and other adverse effects related to NSAIDs. Continuous use of selec-tive COX-2 inhibitors may prevent ovulation and should be avoided in the perio-vulatory phase. Inadvertent exposure during the first trimester is no indication for special diagnostic measures.

2.1.7   Migraine therapy

The prevalence of migraine among women of childbearing age can reach 30%, while symptoms improve in 50–80% of women during preg-nancy, and usually during the first trimester (Sances 2003). If significant improvement does not occur during the first trimester, further improve-ment during pregnancy is unlikely (Marcus 1999). Non-pharmaceutical interventions, such as nutritional and lifestyle habits might be important. Other measures that may be considered include acupuncture, relaxation techniques or cognitive behavior therapies.

The medications discussed below are in part presented in other sec-tions of this book in more detail.

▶ A.   Triptans (selective serotonin-agonists)

Triptans are selective 5-HT1 receptor agonists, indicated in severe migraine attacks. These drugs act by causing vasoconstriction primarily in the cranial blood vessels. However, vasoconstrictive effects outside the central nervous system are also possible. The relatively numerous data on triptans, mainly on *sumatriptan*, has so far not suggested an increased risk of malformations or other adverse fetal effects.

More than 3,000 pregnancies exposed to sumatriptan during the first trimester have been reported in the literature without any suggestion of teratogenicity. The Swedish pregnancy register, with partially prospec-tively collected exposure data, included 2,229 pregnancies exposed in early pregnancy, with no higher risk for malformations than in the gen-eral population (Källén 2011). Further, data collected prospectively by the manufacturer and including 480 pregnancies (Cunnington 2009), and data from the Norwegian population-based datasets and registers, including over 600 pregnancies but obviously partially overlapping study material, similarly failed to indicate an increase in the rate of congenital malformations (Nezvalová-Henriksen 2010, 2012b, 2013b).

Less experience is available for other triptans, but approximately 500 reported first trimester exposures to *zolmitriptan* and *rizatriptan* (Nezvalová-Henriksen 2013b, 2012b, 2010, Källén 2011), while data on other triptans are based on smaller numbers (Nezvalová-Henriksen 2013b, 2012b, 2010, Källén 2011, Cunnington 2009). No data are available for *frovatriptan*.

Triptan use during the second or third trimester in more than 1,200 women was associated with preterm birth and pre-eclampsia; however, a causal association cannot be confirmed on the basis of these results (Källén 2011). Maternal migraine *per se* is associated with pre-eclampsia and conditions predisposing to pre-eclampsia, such as gestational hypertension (Chen 2010, Facchinetti 2009) The Norwegian study (Nezvalová-Henriksen 2010, 2012b) observed an increased risk of atonic uterus in 229 women using triptans during the second or third trimester; however, triptan use only during the second trimester, but not during third trimester, was associated with excess postpartum bleeding in a larger study from the same authors with overlapping study material (Nezvalová-Henriksen 2013b). No other studies have reported such associations.

To summarize, for triptans, most data are available for sumatriptan. While it is not possible to give a final assessment for other triptans, a major risk with this group seems unlikely according to current data.

▶ **B.   Ergotamine derivatives**

The ergot alkaloids *ergotamine* and *dihydroergotamine* (DHE) act as partial agonists on the alpha-receptor inducing vasoconstriction. Prolonged vasoconstriction of the uterine vessels may impair uteroplacental blood flow, and ergot alkaloids also increase myometrial tone, which may further impair oxygenation.

Based on their pharmacokinetic properties, non-hydrogenated ergot alkaloids such as *ergotamine tartrate* are theoretically more likely than DHE to initiate uterine concentrations and expose the fetus to hypoxia. While impaired placental perfusion may lead to hypoxia or even death of the fetus, there are no conclusive data of an increased risk of malformations. The Swedish Birth Register data identified more than 500 pregnancies exposed to ergot alkaloids during the first trimester without an increased risk of malformations (Källén 2011). While ergotamine use was not associated with an increased overall malformation rate in a Hungarian case-controlled study which included nearly 10,000 children with congenital anomalies, an association was observed between maternal intake of ergotamines and neural tube defects (NTD) – however, exposure to ergotamine had occurred during the first trimester in only three of the cases (Czeizel 1989). In a subsequent conducted study of 1,202 infants with NTDs, five had been exposed during the first trimester to ergotamine (Medveczky 2004), with none exposed during the sensitive second gestational month.

Single cases with defects based on disruption of vascular development, and cases resulting in stillbirth have been described in association with ergotamine (Hughes 1988). There are also two case reports with Möbius syndrome (developmental anomaly of the cranial nerves) after exposure during the early pregnancy (Smets 2004, Graf 1997). Oxygen deprivation in the early stages of development has been associated with an increased risk of Möbius syndrome and autism, providing a biologically plausible explanation and suggesting true causality. Oxygen deprivation during later stages of

Pregnancy

2.1 Analgesics, non-steroidal anti-inflammatory drugs (NSAIDs), muscle relaxants, and antigout medications

pregnancy and preterm birth has also been associated with an increased risk of autism in offspring (Salmaso 2014, McGinnis 2013). A recent case-control study reported an increased risk of prematurity associated with dihydroergotamine use but no increased risk of major malformations (Bérard 2012).

Recommendation

Therapy of migraine attack during pregnancy
Metoclopramide is the recommended antiemetic of choice and considered safe in any trimester. Of analgesics, paracetamol (1 g × 3), paracetamol and codeine, or ibuprofen (800 mg × 3) or diclofenac (50 mg × 2–3) are all considered safe for use in migraine attack. Use of naproxen or ASA is also acceptable, as is caffeine combined to any of these drugs. Repeated use of NSAID drugs is best avoided after 28 gestational weeks, and ASA in analgesic doses should be further avoided close to delivery, and independently of length of gestation in cases of threatening premature labor (Section 2.1.2). Where treatment with these conventional agents fails, use of sumatriptan, or in compelling situations zolmitriptan or rizatriptan, is also acceptable. Ergot alkaloids are contraindicated in all trimesters.

Migraine prophylaxis
During pregnancy, treatment options for migraine prophylaxis include the beta-blockers *metoprolol*, *propranolol*, or when considered superior for symptom treatment, *bisoprolol*. Other drugs acceptable include tricyclic antidepressants (*amitriptylin*, *nortriptylin*). Anticonvulsant drugs should not be used during pregnancy for migraine prophylaxis. The same applies to drugs acting on the renin-angiotensin system (ACE inhibitors and ATII receptor antagonists), which are contraindicated, and to *flunarizine*, a calcium channel-blocking agent for which no experience during pregnancy is available.

2.1.8   Muscle relaxants and other analgesics

▶ A.   Baclofen, orphenadrine and tizanidine

Baclofen is a gamma-aminobutyric acid (GABA) derivative and acts as a specific agonist of central GABA-receptors. Intrathecal application throughout pregnancy has been reported in several cases for management of spastic paralysis without adverse outcome (Ali Sakr Esa 2009, Dalton 2008, Roberts 2003, Munoz 2000). Oral baclofen therapy throughout pregnancy has been described in two case reports with no structural malformations, but with withdrawal symptoms presenting as seizures on the 7th day in one infant (Ratnayaka 2001) and grunting, retracting and breathing difficulties shortly after delivery in the other (Moran 2004). If treatment with baclofen cannot be avoided, intrathecal application may be preferable, as the effective dose is several 10-fold lower than that used for oral preparations (Moran 2004).

Orphenadrine has indicated possible teratogenic potential in animal studies while *tizanidine* has not, but there are no data in humans.

▶ B.   Botulinum toxin and dantrolene

Limited experience on *botulinum toxin* use during pregnancy is based on approximately 20 cases and has not suggested specific risks to the fetus. In the majority of cases, the indication has been cervical dystonia (Aranda 2012). When injected locally, systemic exposure to the toxin is unlikely. Further, the few cases described in literature with botulinum toxin infection suggest that the toxin does not pass the placenta. Because of the very limited experience, however, botulinum toxin is not recommended during pregnancy unless used under very strict indications. Use in cosmetic purposes is contraindicated.

Very little is known about safety of *dantrolene* during pregnancy and no cases with first trimester exposure have been described. Because of serious side effects, including the circulatory and hematopoietic systems, use is restricted to rare cases of malignant hyperthermia. Dantrolene should not be used during pregnancy unless compelling indications are present.

> **Recommendation.** Aside from the emergency management of malignant hyperthermia with dantrolene, use of muscle relaxants during pregnancy should generally be avoided. Physical interventions and medication with anti-inflammatory agents are preferable. If necessary, the muscle relaxing effect of the well-studied diazepam may be used on a short-term basis. Intrathecal baclofen can be considered in severe chronic spasticity conditions refractory to standard therapy, such as in multiple sclerosis, post-traumatic spinal cord injuries, or in other spasticity conditions of central origin.

2.1.9   Antigout preparations

Gout is seldom encountered prior to menopause and treatment is, therefore, rarely needed in women during the reproductive years. Gout is caused by disturbed purine metabolism leading to increased levels of uric acid in blood and tissues. Between acute attacks, interval treatment is based on drugs increasing renal elimination of uric acid (*probenecid, benzpromarone*) or inhibiting uric acid synthesis (*allopurinol, febuxostat*), while acute attacks are treated with anti-inflammatory drugs (NSAIDs), intra-articular or systemic corticosteroids or colchicine. Hyperuricemia can also be caused by neoplasms or by aggressive chemotherapy.

▶ **A.   Interval treatment: probenecid, benzpromarone, allopurinol, febuxostat**

No safety studies of probenecid during pregnancy are available, but the drug has been used for decades without reports of specific adverse fetal effects, and is considered compatible for use during pregnancy when clearly indicated. As probenecid has no analgesic and anti-inflammatory activity, it is ineffective during an acute gout attack. There are no data for benzbromarone use during pregnancy. Benzbromarone use has been associated with severe, sometimes fatal hepatotoxicity in users.

Allopurinol is an uricostatic drug, which together with its major metabolite, *oxypurinol*, inhibits the enzyme xanthine oxidase needed in uric acid biosynthesis, thereby lowering uric acid levels in the blood. Uric acid is the end-product of purine metabolism. Allopurinol is structurally related to purine bases and a theoretical possibility exists that allopurinol or its metabolites are incorporated into the nucleic acid molecules of the embryo. However, neither *in vitro* nor *in vivo* experiments have

Pregnancy

2.1 Analgesics, non-steroidal anti-inflammatory drugs (NSAIDs), muscle relaxants, and antigout medications

shown evidence of carcinogenicity or mutagenicity. In experimental animal studies allopurinol was not teratogenic in rabbits or rats, while an increased rate of cleft palate was observed in mice exposed during organogenesis (Fujii 1972); human experience is limited. A recently published case report describes a newborn with multiple malformations after the mother had taken allopurinol throughout her pregnancy (Kozenko 2011). Further, a recent case series describes 31 pregnancies exposed to allopurinol in the first trimester. Even if the overall rate of spontaneous abortions and malformations in this small series was not higher than expected, one child was reported to have severe malformations including micropthalmia, cleft lip and palate, renal hypoplasia, low-set ears, hearing deficit, bilateral cryptorchidism and micropenis (Hoeltzenbein 2013). The pattern of anomalies was similar to those described by Kozenko (2011) and according to the authors, could be a signal for allopurinol teratogenicity, possibly mediated by the drug's capacity to interfere with purine metabolism. Use of allopurinol during the third trimester has not been associated with adverse outcomes, and antenatally administered allopurinol has even been proposed as a potential agent to prevent hypoxic-ischaemic brain injury because of the drug's capacity to prevent free radical formation, and thereby possibly reducing hypoxic-reperfusion damage (Kaandorp 2010b).

Febuxostat is a recently introduced uricostatic agent, blocking xanthine oxidase similarly as allopurinol. No teratogenicity was observed in animal studies but there are no data for use during pregnancy in humans.

Pegloticase and *rasburicase* catalyze the enzymatic oxidation of uric acid to allantoin, a water-soluble substance that is easily eliminated via the kidneys. Pegloticase is indicated for gout refractory to conventional treatment. Rasburicase is used for hyperuricemia caused by hematologic malignancies. There is no experience of either drug for use during pregnancy.

> **Recommendation.** Probenecid is the medication of choice during pregnancy for uric acid elimination. Allopurinol is relatively contraindicated. Pegloticase should not be used during pregnancy due to lack of experience. However, exposure of allopurinol or other referred medications during the first trimester is no indication to consider pregnancy termination. Treatment should be switched to probenecid, and ultrasound evaluations be offered to confirm normal fetal development.

▶ **B.   Treatment of acute attack, colchicine**

NSAIDs and intra-articular or systemic corticosteroids are the first treatment options for acute gout attack during pregnancy. Ibuprofen is the preferred drug of the NSAIDs but indomethacin may be more effective as it also increases the excretion of uric acid. For the general recommendations of NSAID use, see Section 2.1.6. Repeated use should be avoided after week 28 gestation.

Colchicine is an antimitotic agent extracted from the autumn crocus (*Colchicum autumnale*). Colchicine is effective in the prophylaxis and treatment of acute attacks and development of renal amyloidosis in patients suffering from the Familial Mediterranean Fever (FMF). Colchicine crosses the placenta. It possesses mutagenic and genotoxic properties and has been embryotoxic in a number of species. Mutagenic effects have been observed in lymphocytes in patients treated with colchicine.

In humans, teratogenic or other harmful effects on the pregnancy or on the embryo associated with colchicine have not been observed in several studies including more than 1,000 pregnancies. A recent study from Israel compared pregnancy outcome in nearly 200 women suffering from FMF and using colchicine with two reference groups: women with FMF but without colchicine treatment, and healthy controls. No significant differences in the rate of abortions or congenital malformations were observed among the three groups (Ben-Chetrit 2010). Likewise, a study including 238 colchicine-exposed women, the majority of them FMF patients, with exposure data collected prospectively to outcome did not observe an increased risk for malformations, or chromosomal anomalies, when compared to women with exposure to nonteratogens (Diav-Citrin 2010). Length of gestation was shorter, median birth weight lower, and prematurity more common in the colchicine group. The underlying disease *per se* may have influenced these outcomes.

The rate of chromosomal abnormalities or birth defects did not differ from the background rate among nearly 900 pregnancies exposed to maternal (2/3 of cases), or paternal (1/3) colchicine at the time of conception (Berkenstadt 2005). No increased risk for spontaneous abortion or congenital anomalies was observed in more than 200 offspring conceived during paternal colchicine treatment (Ben-Chetrit 2004). The authors concluded that paternal colchicine treatment need not be discontinued prior to conception. Also, maternal colchicine exposure at conception is presently not considered an indication for amniocentesis (Ben-Chetrit 2010).

Phenylbutazone has been used for the therapy of the acute gout attack. Serious adverse effects including hematological, endocrinological and cardiovascular effects have restricted its use, and phenylbutazone should not be used during pregnancy as safer alternatives are available (Section 2.1.3).

> **Recommendation.** Until the twenty-eighth gestational week, ibuprofen is the medication of first choice in the rare event of a gout attack during pregnancy. Intra-articular or systemic corticosteroids can be administered in any trimester. Colchicine use should be restricted to special situations. Long-term therapy with colchicine may be necessary even during pregnancy to treat Familial Mediterranean Fever. Colchicine therapy (either paternal or maternal) at conception or during the first trimester is not an indication to consider invasive diagnostic procedures or pregnancy termination. Ultrasound should be offered to confirm normal development of the fetus when the mother has been exposed. Biological agents targeting Interleukin-1beta blockade (*anakinra, canalizumab*) have shown efficacy in treatment of acute gout arthritis, but should as yet be avoided during pregnancy (Section 2.1.3).

References

Alano MA, Ngougmna E, Osrea EM et al. Analysis of antiinflammatory drugs in meconium and its relation to persistent pulmonary hypertension of the newborn. Pediatrics 2001; 107: 519–23.

Alexander FE, Patheal SL, Biondi A et al. Transplacental chemical exposure and risk of infant leukemia with MLL gene fusion. Cancer Res 2001; 61: 2542–6.

Ali Sakr Esa W, Toma I, Tetzlaff JE et al. Epidural analgesia in labor for a woman with an intrathecal baclofen pump. Int J Obst Anesth 2009; 18: 64–6.

Amin SB, Sinkin RA, Glantz JC Metaanalysis of the effect of antenatal indomethacin on neonatal outcomes. Am J Obstet Gynecol 2007; 197: 486, e1–10.

Antonucci R, Cuzzolin L, Arceri A et al. Urinary prostaglandin E2 in the newborn and infant. Prostag Oth Lipid M 2007; 84: 1–13.

Antonucci R, Zaffanello M, Puxeddu E et al. Use of non-steroidal anti-inflammatory drugs in pregnancy: impact on the fetus and newborn. Curr Drug Metab 2012; 13: 474–90.

Aranda MA, Herranz A, del Val J et al. Botulinum toxin A during pregnancy, still a debate. Eur J Neurol 2012; 19: e81–82.

Asali LA, Brown KF. Naloxone protein binding in adult and foetal plasma. Eur J Clin Pharmacol 1984; 27: 459–63.

Bakkeheim E, Mowinckel P, Carlsen KH et al. Paracetamol in early infancy: the risk of childhood allergy and asthma. Acta Paediatr 2011; 100: 90–6.

Balasubramaniam J. Nimesulide and neonatal renal failure. Lancet 2000; 355: 575.

Bar-Oz B, Clementi M, Di Giantonio E et al. Metamizol (dipyrone, optalgin) in pregnancy, is it safe? A prospective comparative study. Eur J Obstet Gynecol Reprod Biol 2005; 119: 176–9.

Bates SM, Greer IA, Middeldorp S et al. VTE, thrombophilia, antithrombotic therapy, and pregnancy: Antithrombotic Therapy and Prevention of Thrombosis, 9th ed. American College of Chest Physicians Evidence-Based Clinical Practice Guidelines. Chest 2012; 141: e691S–736S.

Ben-Chetrit E, Ben-Chetrit A, Berkun Y et al. Pregnancy outcomes in women with familial Mediterranean fever receiving colchicine: is amniocentesis justified? Arthritis Care Res 2010; 62: 143–8.

Ben-Chetrit E, Berkun Y, Ben-Chetrit E et al. The outcome of pregnancy in the wives of men with familial mediterranean fever treated with colchicine. Semin Arthritis Rheum 2004; 34: 549–52.

Benini D, Fanos V, Cuzzolin L et al. In utero exposure to nonsteroidal anti-inflammatory drugs: neonatal renal failure. Pediatr Nephrol (Berlin) 2004; 19: 232–4.

Bérard A, Kori S. Dihydroergotamine (DHE) use during gestation and the risk of adverse pregnancy outcomes. Headache 2012; 52: 1085–93.

Berkenstadt M, Weisz B, Cuckle H et al. Chromosomal abnormalities and birth defects among couples with colchicine treated familial Mediterranean fever. Am J Obstet Gynecol 2005; 193: 1513–6.

Bio LL, Siu A, Poon CY. Update on the pharmacologic management of neonatal abstinence syndrome. J Perinatol 2011; 31: 692–701.

Bloor M, Paech MJ, Kaye R. Tramadol in pregnancy and lactation. Int J Obstet Anesth 2012; 21: 163–7.

Bolisetty S, Kitchanan S, Whitehall J. Generalized muscle rigidity in a neonate following intrathecal fentanyl during caesarean delivery. Intensive Care Med 1999; 25: 1337.

Borna S, Saeidi FM. Celecoxib versus magnesium sulfate to arrest preterm labor: randomized trial. J Obstet Gynaecol Res 2007; 33: 631–4.

Boubred F, Vendemmia M, Garcia-Meric P et al. Effects of maternally administered drugs on the fetal and neonatal kidney. Drug Saf 2006; 29: 397–419.

Bracken MB, Holford TR. Exposure to prescribed drugs in pregnancy and association with congenital malformations. Obstet Gynecol 1981; 58: 336–44.

Brandlistuen RE, Ystrom E, Nulman I et al. Prenatal paracetamol exposure and child neurodevelopment: a sibling-controlled cohort study. Int J Epidemiol 2013; 42: 1702–13.

Broussard CS, Rasmussen SA, Reefhuis J. Maternal treatment with opioid analgesics and risk for birth defects. Am J Obstet Gynecol 2011; 204: 314.

Bujold E, Roberge S, Lacasse Y et al. Prevention of preeclampsia and intrauterine growth restriction with aspirin started in early pregnancy: a meta-analysis. Obstet Gynecol 2010; 116: 402–14.

Butler-O'Hara M, D'Angio CT. Risk of persistent renal insufficiency in premature infants following the prenatal use of indomethacin for suppression of preterm labor. J Perinatol 2002; 22: 541–6.

Capogna G, Camorcia M. Epidural analgesia for childbirth: effects of newer techniques on neonatal outcome. Paediatr Drugs 2004; 6: 375–86.

Cappon GD, Cook JC, Hurtt ME. Relationship between cyclooxygenase (COX) 1 and 2 selective inhibitors and fetal development when administered to rats and rabbits during the sensitive periods for heart development and midline closure. Birth Defects Res B 2003; 68: 47–56.

Cartwright DP, Dann WL, Hutchinson A. Placental transfer of alfentanil at caesarean section. Eur J Anaesthesiol 1989; 6: 103–9.

Cassina M, De Santis M, Cesari E et al. First trimester diclofenac exposure and pregnancy outcome. Reprod Toxicol 2010; 30: 401–4.

Catalan JL, Santonja J, Martinze L et al. Oligoamnios associated with the use of magnesium dipyrone. Med Clin (Barc) 1995; 104: 541–3.

Chasnoff IJ, Hatcher R, Burns WJ. Pentazocine and tripelennamine (T's and blue's): effects on the fetus and neonate. Devel Pharmacol Ther 1983; 6: 162–9.

Chen HM, Chen SF, Chen YH et al. Increased risk of adverse pregnancy outcomes for women with migraines: a nationwide population-based study. Cephalalgia 2010; 30: 433–8.

Claahsen-van der Grinten HL, Verbruggen I, van den Berg PP et al. Different pharmacokinetics of tramadol in mothers treated for labour pain and in their neonates. Eur J Clin Pharmacol 2005; 61: 523–9.

CLASP Collaborative Group. CLASP: a randomized trial of low-dose aspirin for the prevention and treatment of preeclampsia among 9364 pregnant women. Lancet 1994; 343: 619–29.

Collins LR, Hall RW, Dajani NK et al. Prolonged morphine exposure in utero causes fetal and placental vasoconstriction: a case report. J Matern Fetal Neonat Med 2005; 17: 417–21.

Cooper J, Jauniaux E, Gulbis B et al. Placental transfer of fentanyl in early human pregnancy and its detection in fetal brain. Br J Anaesth 1999; 82: 929–31.

Czeizel A. Teratogenicity of ergotamine. J Med Genet 1989; 26: 69–70.

Cunnington M, Ephross S, Churchill P. The safety of sumatriptan and naratriptan in pregnancy: what have we learned? Headache 2009; 49: 1414–22.

Dalton CM, Keenan E, Jarrett L et al. The safety of baclofen in pregnancy: intrathecal therapy in multiple sclerosis. Mult Scler 2008; 14: 571–2.

Daniel S, Matok I, Gorodischer R et al. Major malformations following exposure to nonsteroidal antiinflammatory drugs during the first trimester of pregnancy. J Rheumatol 2012; 39: 2163–9.

da Silva Dal Pizzol T, Schüler-Faccini L, Mengue SS. Dipyrone use during pregnancy and adverse perinatal events. Arch Gynecol Obstet 2009; 279: 293–7.

DeBooy VD, Seshia MM, Tenenbein M et al. Intravenous pentazocine and methylphenidate abuse during pregnancy. Maternal lifestyle and infant outcome. Am J Dis Child 1993; 147: 1062–5.

Diav-Citrin O, Shechtman S, Schwartz V. Pregnancy outcome after in utero exposure to colchicine. Am J Obstet Gynecol 2010; 203: 144, e1–6.

Dinchuk JE, Car BD, Focht RJ et al. Renal abnormalities and an altered inflammatory response in mice lacking cyclooxygenase II. Nature 1995; 378: 406–9.

Draper ES, Rankin J, Tonks AM et al. Recreational drug use: a major risk factor for gastroschisis? Am J Epidemiol 2008; 167: 485–91.

Ebner N, Rohrmeister K, Winklbaur B et al. Management of neonatal abstinence syndrome in neonates born to opioid maintained women. Drug Alcohol Depend 2007; 87: 131–8.

Einarson A, Bozzo P, Taguchi N. Use of a fentanyl patch throughout pregnancy. J Obstet Gynaecol Canada 2009; 31: 20.

Ericson A, Källén BAJ. Nonsteroidal anti-inflammatory drugs in early pregnancy. Reprod Toxicol 2001; 15: 371–5.

Eventov-Friedman S, Rozin I, Shinwell ES. Case of chest-wall rigidity in a preterm infant caused by prenatal fentanyl administration. J Perinatol 2010; 30: 149–50.

Eyers S, Weatherall M, Jefferies S et al. Paracetamol in pregnancy and the risk of wheezing in offspring: a systematic review and meta-analysis. Clin Exp Allergy 2011; 41: 482–9.

Facchinetti F, Allais G, Nappi RE et al. Migraine is a risk factor for hypertensive disorders in pregnancy: a prospective cohort study. Cephalalgia 2009; 29: 286–92.

Feldkamp ML, Meyer RE, Krikov S et al. Acetaminophen use in pregnancy and risk of birth defects: findings from the National Birth Defects Prevention Study. Obstet Gynecol 2010; 115: 109–15.

Fujii T, Nishimura H. Comparison of teratogenic action of substances related to purine metabolism in mouse embryos. Jpn J Pharmacol 1972; 22: 201–6.

Garcia-Marcos L, Sanchez-Solis M, Perez-Fernandez V et al. Is the effect of prenatal paracetamol exposure on wheezing in preschool children modified by asthma in the mother? Int Arch Allergy Immunol 2009; 149: 33–7.

Geber WF, Schramm LC. Congenital malformations of the central nervous system produced by narcotic analgesics in the hamster. Am J Obstet Gynecol 1975; 123: 705–13.

Gewillig M, Brown SC, De Catte L et al. Premature foetal closure of the arterial duct: clinical presentations and outcome. Eur Heart J 2009; 30: 1530–6.

Graf WD, Shepard TH. Uterine contraction in the development of Möbius syndrome. J Child Neurol 1997; 12: 225–7.

Groeneveld E, Lambers MJ, Lambalk CB et al. Preconceptional low-dose aspirin for the prevention of hypertensive pregnancy complications and preterm delivery after IVF: a meta-analysis with individual patient data. Hum Reprod 2013; 28: 1480–8.

Gupta C, Bentlejewski CA. Role of prostaglandins in the testosterone-dependent Wolffian duct differentiation of the fetal mouse. Biol Reprod 1992; 47: 1151–60.

Hartenstein S, Proquitté H, Bauer S et al. Neonatal abstinence syndrome (NAS) after intrauterine exposure to tramadol. J Perinat Med 2010; 38: 695–6.

Heinonen OP, Slone D, Shapiro S. Birth Defects and Drugs in Pregnancy. Publishing Sciences Group, Littleton, 1977.

Henderson AJ, Shaheen SO. Acetaminophen and asthma. Paediatr Resp Rev 2013; 14: 9–15.

Hernandez RK, Werler MM, Romitti P et al. Nonsteroidal antiinflammatory drug use among women and the risk of birth defects. Am J Obstet Gynecol 2012; 206: 228.

Herschel M, Khoshnood B, Lass NA. Role of naloxone in newborn resuscitation. Pediatrics. 2000; 106: 831–5.

Hoeltzenbein M, Stieler K, Panse M et al. Allopurinol Use during Pregnancy – Outcome of 31 Prospectively Ascertained Cases and a Phenotype Possibly Indicative for Teratogenicity. PLoS One 2013; 8: e66637.

Holmes RP, Stone PR. Severe oligohydramnios induced by cyclooxygenase-2 inhibitor nimesulide. Obstet Gynecol 2000; 96: 810–1.

Hughes HE, Goldstein DA. Birth defects following maternal exposure to ergotamine, beta blockers, and caffeine. J Med Genet 1988; 25: 396–9.

Humphrey RG, Bartfield MC, Carlan SJ et al. Sulindac to prevent recurrent preterm labor: a randomized controlled trial. Obstet Gynecol 2001; 98: 555–62.

Itabashi K, Ohno T, Nishida H. Indomethacin responsiveness of patent ductus arteriosus and renal abnormalities in preterm infants treated with indomethacin. J Pediatr 2003; 143: 203–7.

Jayagopal N, Sinha D, Bhatti NR. Use of sulindac in polyhydramnios. J Obstet Gynaecol 2007; 27: 850.

Jensen MS, Rebordosa C, Thulstrup AM et al. Maternal use of acetaminophen, ibuprofen, and acetylsalicylic acid during pregnancy and risk of cryptorchidism. Epidemiology 2010; 21: 779–85.

Kaandorp SP, Goddijn M, van der Post JA et al. Aspirin plus heparin or aspirin alone in women with recurrent miscarriage. N Engl J Med 2010a; 362: 1586–96.

Kaandorp JJ, Benders MJ, Rademaker CM et al. Antenatal allopurinol for reduction of birth asphyxia induced brain damage (ALLO-Trial); a randomized double blind placebo controlled multicenter study. BMC Pregnancy Childbirth 2010b; 10: 8.

Keeling D, Mackie I, Moore GW et al. Guidelines on the investigation and management of antiphospholipid syndrome. Br J Haematol 2012; 157: 47–58.

Källén BA, Nilsson E, Otterblad Olausson P. Delivery outcome after maternal use of drugs for migraine: a register study in Sweden. Drug Saf 2011; 34: 691–703.

Källén BA, Otterblad Olausson P. Maternal drug use in early pregnancy and infant cardiovascular defect. Reprod Toxicol 2003; 17: 255–61.

Kang EM, Lundsberg LS, Illuzzi JL et al. Prenatal exposure to acetaminophen and asthma in children. Obstet Gynecol 2009; 114: 1295–1306.

Koklu E, Gurgoze M, Akgun H et al. Renal tubular dysgenesis with atypical histology and in-utero exposure to naproxen sodium. Ann Trop Paediatr 2006; 26: 241–5.

Kopecky EA, Ryan ML, Barrett JFR, et al. Fetal response to maternally administered morphine. Am J Obstet Gynecol 2000; 183: 424–30.

Kozenko M, Grynspan D, Oluyomi-Obi T et al. Potential teratogenic effects of allopurinol: a case report. Am J Med Genet A 2011; 155: 2247–52.

Kozer E, Nikfar S, Costei A et al. Aspirin consumption during the first trimester of pregnancy and congenital anomalies: a meta-analysis. Am J Obstet Gynecol 2002; 187: 1623–30.

Kristensen DM, Hass U, Lesné L et al. Intrauterine exposure to mild analgesics is a risk factor for development of male reproductive disorders in human and rat. Hum Reprod 2011; 26: 235–44.

Li DK, Liu L, Odouli R. Exposure to non-steroidal anti-inflammatory drugs during pregnancy and risk of miscarriage: population based cohort study. BMJ 2003; 327: 1–5.

Liew Z, Ritz B, Rebordosa C et al. Acetaminophen Use During Pregnancy, Behavioral Problems, and Hyperkinetic Disorders. JAMA Pediatr 2014; doi:10.1001/jamapediatrics.2013.4914. Published online Feb 24.

Lindemann R. Respiratory muscle rigidity in a preterm infant after use of fentanyl during Caesarean section. Eur J Pediatr 1998; 157: 1012–3.

Little BB, Snell LM, Breckenridge JD et al. Effects of T's and blues abuse on pregnancy outcome and infant health status. Am J Perinatol 1990; 7: 359–62.

Loftus JR, Hill H, Cohen SE. Placental transfer and neonatal effects of epidural sufentanil and fentanyl administered with bupivacaine during labor. Anesthesiology 1995; 83: 300–8.

Loudon JA, Groom KM, Bennett PR. Prostaglandin inhibitors in preterm labour. Best Pract Res Clin Obstet Gynaecol 2003; 17: 731–44.

Mac Bird T, Robbins JM, Druschel C et al. Demographic and environmental risk factors for gastroschisis and omphalocele in the National Birth Defects Prevention Study. J Pediatr Surg 2009; 44: 1546–51.

Madry H, Grün UW, Knutsen G. Cartilage repair and joint preservation: medical and surgical treatment options. Dtsch Ärztebl Int 2011; 108: 669–77.

Magnani C, Moretti S, Ammenti A. Neonatal chronic renal failure associated with maternal ingestion of nimesulide as analgesic. Eur J Obstet Gynaecol Reprod Biol 2004; 116: 244–5.

Marcus DA, Scharff L, Turk D. Longitudinal prospective study of headache during pregnancy and postpartum. Headache 1999; 39: 625–32.

Marret S, Marchand L, Kaminski M et al. Prenatal low-dose aspirin and neurobehavioral outcomes of children born very preterm. Pediatrics 2010; 125: e29–34.

Martinez-Frias ML, Rodriguez-Pinilla E, Prieto L. Prenatal exposure to salicylates and gastroschisis: a case-control study. Teratology 1997; 56: 241–3.

McGinnis WR, Audhya T, Edelson SM. Proposed toxic and hypoxic impairment of a brainstem locus in autism. Int J Environ Res Public Health 2013; 10: 6955–7000.

McNamee K, Dawood F, Farquharson R. Recurrent miscarriage and thrombophilia: an update. Curr Opin Obstet Gynecol 2012; 24: 229–34.

Medveczky E, Puhó E, Czeizel EA. The use of drugs in mothers of offspring with neural-tube defects. Pharmacoepidemiol Drug Saf 2004; 13: 443–55.

Meyer FP, Rimasch H, Blaha B et al. Tramadol withdrawal in a neonate. Eur J Clin Pharmacol 1997; 53: 159–60.

Micu MC, Micu R, Ostensen M. Luteinized unruptured follicle syndrome increased by inactive disease and selective cyclooxygenase 2 inhibitors in women with inflammatory arthropathies. Arthritis Care Res (Hoboken) 2011; 63: 1334–8.

Miller EA, Rasmussen SA, Siega-Riz AM et al. Risk factors for non-syndromic holoprosencephaly in the National Birth Defects Prevention Study. Am J Med Genet C Semin Med Gen 2010; 154C: 62–72.

Moise KJ Jr, Huhta JC, Sharif DS et al. Indomethacin in the treatment of premature labor, effects on the fetal ductus arteriosus. N Engl J Med 1988; 319: 327–31.

Moise KJ Jr, Ou CN, Kirshon B et al. Placental transfer of indomethacin in the human pregnancy. Am J Obstet Gynecol 1990; 162: 549–54.

Moise KJ Jr. Effect of advancing gestational age on the frequency of fetal ductal constriction in association with maternal indomethacin use. Am J Obstet Gynecol 1993; 168: 1350–3.

Moran LR, Almeida PG, Worden S et al. Intrauterine baclofen exposure: a multidisciplinary approach. Pediatrics 2004; 114: e267–269.

Morley-Forster PK, Reid DW, Vandeberghe H. A comparison of patient-controlled analgesia fentanyl and alfentanil for labour analgesia. Can J Anaesth 2000; 47: 113–9.

Morrison CE, Dutton D, Howie H et al. Pethidine compared with meptazinol during labour. Anaesthesia 1987; 42: 7–14.

Munoz FC, Marco DG. Pregnancy outcome in a woman exposed to continuous intrathecal baclofen infusion. Ann Pharmacother 2000; 34: 956.

Nezvalová-Henriksen K, Spigset O, Nordeng H. Triptan exposure during pregnancy and the risk of major congenital malformations and adverse pregnancy outcomes: results from the Norwegian Mother and Child Cohort Study. Headache 2010; 50: 563–75.

Nezvalová-Henriksen K, Spigset O, Nordeng H. Effects of codeine on pregnancy outcome: results from a large population-based cohort study. Eur J Clin Pharmacol 2011; 67: 1253–61.

Nezvalová-Henriksen K, Spigset O, Nordeng HM. Erratum to: Effects of codeine on pregnancy outcome: results from a large population-based cohort study. Eur J Clin Pharmacol 2012a; 68: 1689–90.

Nezvalová-Henriksen K, Spigset O, Nordeng HM. Errata in: Triptan exposure during pregnancy and the risk of major congenital malformations and adverse pregnancy outcomes: results from the Norwegian mother and child cohort study. Headache 2012b; 52: 1319–20.

Nezvalová-Henriksen K, Spigset O, Nordeng H. Effects of ibuprofen, diclofenac, naproxen, and piroxicam on the course of pregnancy and pregnancy outcome: a prospective cohort study. Br J Obstet Gynaecol 2013a; 120: 948–59.

Nezvalová-Henriksen K, Spigset O, Nordeng H. Triptan safety during pregnancy: a Norwegian population registry study. Eur J Epidemiol 2013b; 28: 759–69.

Nikkola EM, Jahnukainen TJ, Ekblad UU et al. Neonatal monitoring after maternal fentanyl analgesia in labor. J Clin Monit Comput 2000; 16: 597–608.

Norwood VF, Morham SG, Smithies O. Postnatal development and progression of renal dysplasia in cyclooxygenase-2 null mice. Kidney Int 2000; 58: 2291–300.

Nuttall SL, Khan JN, Thorpe GH et al. The impact of therapeutic doses of paracetamol on serum total antioxidant capacity. J Clin Pharm Ther 2003; 28: 289–94.

Oberlander TF, Robeson P, Ward V et al. Prenatal and breast milk morphine exposure following maternal intrathecal morphine treatment. J Hum Lact 2000; 16: 137–42.

Ofori B, Oraichi D, Blais L et al. Risk of congenital anomalies in pregnant users of non-steroidal anti-inflammatory drugs: a nested case-control study. Birth Defects Res B Dev Reprod Toxicol 2006; 77: 268–79.

Ognjanovic S, Blair C, Spector LG et al. Analgesic use during pregnancy and risk of infant leukaemia: a Children's Oncology Group study. Br J Cancer 2011; 104: 532–6.

O'Mara K, Gal P, Davanzo C. Treatment of neonatal withdrawal with clonidine after long-term, high-dose maternal use of tramadol. Ann Pharmacother 2010; 44: 1342–4.

Østensen ME, Skomsvoll JF. Anti-inflammatory pharmacotherapy during pregnancy. Expert Opin Pharmacother 2004; 5: 571–80.

Paladini D, Marasini M, Volpe P. Severe ductal constriction in the third-trimester fetus following maternal self-medication with nimesulide. Ultrasound Obstet Gynecol 2005; 25: 357–61.

Peruzzi L, Gianoglio B, Porcellini MG et al. Neonatal end-stage renal failure associated with maternal ingestion of cyclo-oxygenase-type I selective inhibitor nimesulide as tocolytic. Lancet 1999; 354: 1615.

Perzanowski MS, Miller RL, Tang D et al. Prenatal acetaminophen exposure and risk of wheeze at age 5 years in an urban low-income cohort. Thorax 2010; 65: 118–23.

Pombo-de-Oliveira MS, Koifman S. Infant acute leukemia and maternal exposures during pregnancy. Cancer Epidemiol Biomarkers Prev 2006; 15: 2336–41.

Prefumo F, Marasini M, de Biasio P et al. Acute premature constriction of the ductus arteriosus after maternal self-medication with nimesulide. Fetal Diagn Ther 2008; 24: 35–8.

Ratnayaka BDM, Dhaliwal H, Watkin S. Neonatal convulsions after withdrawal of baclofen. Br Med J 2001; 323: 85.

Rayburn W, Rathke A, Leuschen MP et al. Fentanyl citrate analgesia during labor. Am J Obstet Gynecol 1989; 161: 202–6.

Rebordosa C, Kogevinas M, Sørensen HT et al. Pre-natal exposure to paracetamol and risk of wheezing and asthma in children: a birth cohort study. Int J Epidemiol 2008; 37: 583–90.

Rebordosa C, Zelop CM, Kogevinas M et al. Use of acetaminophen during pregnancy and risk of preeclampsia, hypertensive and vascular disorders: a birth cohort study. J Matern Fetal Neonat Med 2010; 23: 371–8.

Regan J, Chambers F, Gorman W et al. Neonatal abstinence syndrome due to prolonged administration of fentanyl in pregnancy. Br J Obstet Gynaecol 2000; 107: 570–2.

Reynolds F. The effects of maternal labour analgesia on the fetus. Best Pract Res Clin Obstet Gynaecol 2010; 24: 289–302.

Reynolds F. Labour analgesia and the baby: good news is no news. Int J Obstet Anesth 2011; 20: 38–50.

Roberge S, Giguère Y, Villa P et al. Early administration of low-dose aspirin for the prevention of severe and mild preeclampsia: a systematic review and meta-analysis. Am J Perinatol 2012; 29: 551–6.

Roberts AG, Graves CR, Konrad PE et al. Intrathecal baclofen pump implantation during pregnancy. Neurology 2003; 61: 1156.

Roberts I, Robinson MJ, Mughal MZ et al. Paracetamol metabolites in the neonate following maternal overdose. Br J Clin Pharmacol 1984; 18: 201–6.

Robin YM, Reynaud P, Orliaguet T et al. Renal tubular dysgenesis-like lesions and hypocalvaria. Report of two cases involving indomethacin. Pathol Res Pract 2000; 196: 791–4.

Rode L, Bundgaard A, Skibsted L et al. Acute recurrent polyhydramnios: a combination of amniocenteses and NSAID may be curative rather than palliative. Fetal Diagn Ther 2007; 22: 186–9.

Rothman KJ, Fyler DC, Goldblatt A et al. Exogenous hormones and other drug exposures of children with congenital heart disease. Am J Epidemiol 1979; 109: 433–9.

Salmaso N, Tomasi S, Vaccarino FM. Neurogenesis and Maturation in Neonatal Brain Injury. Clin Perinatol 2014; 41: 229–39.

Sances G, Granella F, Nappi R et al. Course of migraine during pregnancy and postpartum: a prospective study. Cephalalgia 2003; 23: 197–205.

Sawdy RJ, Lye S, Fisk NM et al. A double-blind randomized study of fetal side effects during and after short-term maternal administration of indomethacin, sulindac, and nimesulide for the treatment of preterm labour. Am J Obstet Gynecol 2003; 188: 1046–51.

Sawdy RJ, Groom KM, Bennett PR. Experience of the use of nimesulide, a cyclo-oxygenase-2 selective prostaglandin synthesis inhibitor, in the prevention of preterm labour in 44 high-risk cases. J Obstet Gynaecol 2004; 24: 226–9.

Saxén I. Associations between oral clefts and drugs taken during pregnancy. Int J Epidemiol 1975; 4: 37–44.

Schick B, Hom M, Tolosa J et al. Preliminary analysis of first trimester exposure to oxycodone and hydrocodone {Abstract}. Reprod Toxicol 1996; 10: 162.

Scialli AR, Ang R, Breitmeyer J et al. A review of the literature on the effects of acetaminophen on pregnancy outcome. Reprod Toxicol 2010a; 30: 495–507.

Scialli AR, Ang R, Breitmeyer J et al. Childhood asthma and use during pregnancy of acetaminophen. A critical review. Reprod Toxicol 2010b; 30: 508–19.

Shaheen SO, Newson RB, Sherriff A et al. Paracetamol use in pregnancy and wheezing in early childhood. Thorax 2002; 57: 958–63.

Shannon C, Jauniaux E, Gulbis B et al. Placental transfer of fentanyl in early human pregnancy. Hum Reprod 1998; 13: 2317–20.

Sharpe CR, Franco EL. Use of dipyrone during pregnancy and risk of Wilms' tumor. Brazilian Wilms' Tumor Study Group. Epidemiology 1996; 7: 533–5.

Shaw GM, Malcoe LH, Swan SH et al. Congenital cardiac anomalies relative to selected maternal exposures and conditions during early pregnancy. Eur J Epidemiol 1992; 8: 757–60.

Shaw GM, Todoroff K, Velie EM et al. Maternal illness, including fever and medication use as risk factors for neural tube defects. Teratology 1998; 57: 1–7.

Siu KL, Lee WH. Maternal diclofenac sodium ingestion and severe neonatal pulmonary hypertension. J Paediatr Child Health 2004; 40: 152–3.

Siu SSN, Yeung JHK, Lau TK. A study on placental transfer of diclofenac in first trimester of human pregnancy. Hum Reprod 2000; 15: 2423–5.

Sivojelezova A, Koren G, Einarson A. Glucosamine use in pregnancy: an evaluation of pregnancy outcome. J Womens Health (Larchmt) 2007; 16: 345–8.

Smets K, Zecic A, Willems J. Ergotamine as a possible cause of Möbius sequence: additional clinical observation. J Child Neurol 2004; 19: 398.

Snijder CA, Kortenkamp A, Steegers EA et al. Intrauterine exposure to mild analgesics during pregnancy and the occurrence of cryptorchidism and hypospadia in the offspring: the Generation R Study. Hum Reprod 2012; 27: 1191–1201.

Sood BG, Lulic-Botica M, Holzhausen KA et al. The risk of necrotizing enterocolitis after indomethacin tocolysis. Pediatrics 2011; 128: e54–62.

Sosa CG, Buekens P, Hughes JM et al. Effect of pethidine administered during the first stage of labor on the acid-base status at birth. Eur J Obstet Gynecol Reprod Biol 2006; 129: 135–9.

Steinmeyer J, Konttinen YT. Oral treatment options for degenerative joint disease – presence and future. Adv Drug Deliv Rev 2006; 58: 168–211.

Stika CS, Gross GA, Leguizamon G et al. A prospective randomized safety trial of celecoxib for treatment of preterm labour. Am J Obstet Gynecol 2002; 187: 653–60.

Suzumori N, Hattori Y, Kaneko S et al. Cytomegalovirus-associated acute hydramnios treated by amniocentesis and maternal indomethacin. Congenit Anom (Kyoto) 2009; 49: 274–5.

Talati AJ, Salim MA, Korones SB. Persistent pulmonary hypertension after maternal naproxen ingestion in a term newborn: a case report. Am J Perinatol 2000; 17: 69–71.

Torfs CP, Katz EA, Bateson TF et al. Maternal medications and environmental exposures as risk factors for gastroschisis. Teratology 1996; 54: 84–92.

Torloni MR, Cordioli E, Zamith MM. Reversible constriction of the fetal ductus arteriosus after maternal use of topical diclofenac and methyl salicylate. Ultrasound Obstet Gynecol 2006; 27: 227–9.

Ullman R, Smith LA, Burns E. Parenteral opioids for maternal pain relief in labour. Cochrane Database Syst Rev 2010; 8: CD007396.

Van de Velde M, Vercauteren M, Vandermeersch E. Fetal heart rate abnormalities after regional analgesia for labor pain: the effect of intrathecal opioids. Reg Anaesth Pain Med 2001; 26: 257–62.

Van de Velde M, Teunkens A, Hanssens M et al. Intrathecal sufentanil and fetal heart rate abnormalities: a double-blind, double placebo-controlled trial comparing two forms of combined spinal epidural analgesia with epidural analgesia in labor. Anesth Analg 2004; 98: 1153–9.

Van den Veyver IB, Moise KJ Jr, Ou CN et al. The effect of gestational age and fetal indomethacin levels on the incidence of constriction of the fetal ductus arteriosus. Obstet Gynecol 1993; 82: 500–3.

Van der Heijden BJ, Carlus C, Narcy F et al. Persistent anuria, neonatal death, and renal microcystic lesions after prenatal exposure to indomethacin. Am J Obstet Gynecol 1994; 171: 617–23.

Van der Heijden B, Gubler MC. Renal failure in the neonate associated with in utero exposure to non-steroidal anti-inflammatory agents. Pediatr Nephrol (Berlin) 1995; 9: 675.

Van Marter LJ, Leviton A, Allred EN. Persistent pulmonary hypertension of the newborn and smoking and aspirin and nonsteroidal antiinflammatory drug consumption during pregnancy. Pediatrics 1996; 97: 658–63.

Van Marter LJ, Hernandez-Diaz S, Werler MM et al. Nonsteroidal antiinflammatory drugs in late pregnancy and persistent pulmonary hypertension of the newborn. Pediatrics 2013; 131: 79–87.

Weintraub A, Mankuta D. Dipyrone-induced oligohydramnios and ductus arteriosus restriction. Isr Medic Assoc J 2006; 8: 722–3.

Welsh M, Saunders PT, Fisken M et al. Identification in rats of a programming window for reproductive tract masculinization, disruption of which leads to hypospadias and cryptorchidism. J Clin Invest 2008; 118: 1479–90.

Werler MM, Sheehan JE, Mitchell AA. Maternal medication use and risks of gastroschisis and small intestinal atresia. Am J Epidemiol 2002; 155: 26–31.

Werler MM, Mitchell AA, Moore CA et al. Is there epidemiologic evidence to support vascular disruption as a pathogenesis of gastroschisis? Am J Med Genet A 2009a; 149A: 1399–406.

Werler MM, Bosco JL, Shapira SK et al. Maternal vasoactive exposures, amniotic bands, and terminal transverse limb defects. Birth Defects Res A Clin Mol Teratol 2009b; 85: 52–7.

Willaschek C, Wolter E, Buchhorn R. Tramadol withdrawal in a neonate after long-term analgesic treatment of the mother. Eur J Clin Pharmacol 2009; 65: 429–30.

Zenker M, Klinge J, Krüger C et al. Severe pulmonary hypertension in a neonate caused by premature closure of the ductus arteriosus following maternal treatment with diclofenac: a case report. J Perinat Med 1998; 26: 231–4.

Allergy and hyposensitization therapy

2.2

Lee H. Goldstein, Corinna Weber-Schöndorfer and Matitiahu Berkovitch

2.2.1	Antihistamines (H₁-blocker)	59
2.2.2	Hyposensitization therapy	61
2.2.3	C1-Esterase inhibitor deficiency	61

Both antihistamines and glucocorticoids have demonstrated a lack of toxicity when used during pregnancy for the management of allergy symptoms. Some antihistamines are also administered with success in the treatment of hyperemesis gravidarum (Chapter 2.4) or as sleeping medication (Chapter 2.11). For glucocorticoids, see Chapters 2.3 and 2.15.

2.2.1   Antihistamines (H₁-blocker)

Pharmacology

Antihistamines competitively inhibit the interaction of histamine with histamine receptors. The release of histamine stimulates both the H_1-receptors present on the smooth muscles of many organs and the H_2-receptors of the gastric mucosa resulting in an increase in gastric secretion. Inhibition of H_1-receptors is key to antiallergenic therapy.

Orally administered H_1-antihistamines are well absorbed and metabolized in the liver by oxidation, and eliminated, only in traces unchanged, via the kidneys.

Older medications, still used in allergies have a minor but sometimes undesirable sedative effect. This group includes *azelastine, clemastine, cyproheptadine, dexchlorpheniramine, dimethindene, hydroxyzine, mizolastine* and *triprolidine*. For *meclozine, dimenhydrinate, diphenhydramine* and *doxylamine*, see Chapter 2.4.

The following medications belong to the newer, non-sedative antihistamines: *Cetirizine, desloratadine, ebastine, fexofenadine, levocetirizine, loratadine,* and *terfenadine. Rupatadine* was released in 2008, and *bilastine* in December 2010.

Astemizole and terfenadine not only have very long biological half-lives of 20–26 hours (astemizole metabolites for more than 9 days), but also significant cardiotoxic side effects, including cardiac arrhythmias. Thus, in most countries, astemizole and terfenadine have been recalled. Fexofenadine is the active metabolite of terfenadine.

The following antihistamines are available for local application: *Bamipine, chlorphenoxamine, levocabastine,* and the newer agents *epinastine* and *olopatadine*.

Chlorphenamine is only found in cold products.

Drugs During Pregnancy and Lactation. http://dx.doi.org/10.1016/B978-0-12-408078-2.00003-2

Toxicology

For both the sedative and evaluated non-sedative antihistamines, long practical experience, and in part, extensive studies, have failed to support an earlier suspicion that there might be teratogenic effects in humans (Källén 2002, Schardein 2000, Lione 1996).

In 1,230 pregnant women who ingested clemastine at least once during early pregnancy, no increase in malformations was noted (Källén 2002).

In the animal model, cyproheptadine displays a diabetogenic effect upon the fetal islet cells. Suggestions for a similar effect in humans are currently not available. Eight cases in the Swedish Birth Registry did not indicate signs of an embryotoxic effect when cyproheptadine was taken during the first trimester (Källén 2002).

There are experiences with more than 80 cases where hydroxyzine was used during pregnancy, all showing no abnormalities in the newborn (Diav-Citrin 2003, Einarson 1997). In a case report about anxiolytic therapy with 150 mg/d hydroxyzine at the end of pregnancy, the child born at 29 weeks developed tonic-clinic seizures 4 hours postpartum. Its plasma concentration 2 hours later was identical to the maternal values. The seizures were regarded as withdrawal symptoms. Six months later the neurologic development of the infant was normal (Serreau 2005).

Sixty-eight pregnancies exposed to chlorpheniramine identified one child with congenital hip dysplasia (Diav-Citrin 2003).

In an older study, the prevalence of retrolental fibroplasia was doubled in premature babies when antihistamines were administered during the last 2 weeks of pregnancy (Zierler 1986). Other investigators did not confirm this finding.

Cetirizine, a metabolite of hydroxyzine, is one of the relatively well-studied newer antihistamines with experiences in about 1,300 pregnancies (Anderka 2012, Djokanovic 2010, Weber-Schöndorfer 2008, Källén 2002) where no teratogenic risk has been observed.

Loratadine is the most popular non-sedative antihistamine used during pregnancy. An earlier suspicion that it might induce hypospadia could not be confirmed (Pedersen 2008). Today, it is the antihistamine of first choice for pregnant women backed by more than 5,000 pregnancies that were systematically followed-up in a number of investigations (Schwarz 2008). Desloratadine, a metabolite of loratadine has no published data in humans although it does not seem to be teratogenic in animal studies.

The children of more than 1,000 pregnant women treated with terfenadine did not display any increased malformation risk (Källén 2002, Diav-Citrin 2003).

A survey of first trimester did not identify an increased incidence of malformations in the offspring of 244 women who were exposed to triprolidine (Källén 2006).

Pregnancy-related experiences with the administration of ebastine, desloratadine, fexofenadine and levocetirizine (the active enantiomer of citirizine) are limited and based on a few (not exceeding 50) documented courses. No published human pregnancy experiences are available for azelastine, levocabastine dimethindene, mizolastine, ebastine, belastine rupatadine and the local antihistamines epinastine and olopatadine. The use of dermal, usually only affecting small areas, bamipine or chlorphenoxamine can be considered safe. Negative side effects of a local antiallergenic treatment (eye/nose) have not been reported for azelastine and levocabastine.

Treatment with systemic antihistamines, especially the sedative varieties, can lead to tremor and diarrhea until birth (Lione 1996).

> **Recommendation.** H$_1$-antihistamines may be used for the treatment of allergic diseases during pregnancy. Loratadine and cetirizine should be preferred as they are the best-investigated antihistamines. If a sedative effect is desired, clemastine, for example, may also be used.

2.2.2   Hyposensitization therapy

In the hyposensitization procedure, one starts with very small doses of the allergen and increases them gradually, either subcutaneously or orally. The immune system responds by producing blocking antibodies to bind the allergen before it reacts with sensitized mast cells. Thus, when after completion of the treatment there is exposure to the allergen, histamine release by the mast cells distinctly decreases and the allergic reaction attenuated. While hyposensitization has proved to be quite effective for hay fever and allergies to insect stings, it has been less successful for full-blown asthma.

Specific embryo- and fetotoxic effects are not to be expected (Metzger 1978). Allergen immunotherapy is not usually initiated during pregnancy because of concerns about potential adverse effects of systemic reactions and their resultant treatment on the fetus, mother, or both; such as fetal hypoxia, premature labor, and loss of the infant (Krishna 2011). If pregnancy occurs during the build-up phase, and the patient is receiving a dose that is unlikely to be therapeutic, discontinuation of immunotherapy should be considered. Allergen immunotherapy maintenance doses can be continued during pregnancy (Cox 2011).

> **Recommendation.** Allergen immunotherapy should not usually be initiated during pregnancy, but maintenance doses can be continued if necessary. If pregnancy occurs during the build-up phase, discontinuation of immunotherapy should be considered. Allergen immunotherapy maintenance doses can be continued during pregnancy.

2.2.3   C1-Esterase inhibitor deficiency

A C1-esterase inhibitor deficiency is characterized by the development of subcutaneous and submucosal edema of the skin, the respiratory tract, and the gastrointestinal tract. A distinction is made between a congenital form that is inherited in the autosomal dominant pattern, and an acquired angioedema, often caused by monoclonal B-cell diseases and C1-INH-autoantibodies, respectively. Triggers for angioedema include inflammatory foci (e.g. *Helicobacter pylori*-associated gastritis), trauma (including dental interventions), or medications (e.g. ACE-inhibitors, nonsteroidal anti-inflammatory drugs, estrogenic contraceptives) (Gompels 2005). C1-INH is important for the control of vascular permeability and plays a critical role in the initial activation phase of the complement system. A German study with 35 pregnancies included 22 women with hereditary angioedema. In 83% of these cases an increase in attacks of angioedema was observed during pregnancy, but it should be noted that in most cases patients with severe disease were involved (19).

Long-term prophylaxis is necessary only in a subset of the affected persons. In use were *danazol* that is, however, contraindicated during pregnancy (Chapter 2.15), and *tranexamic acid* Chapter 2.9). The latter may be administered in pregnancy after weighing up the pros and cons (see also the British consensus document, Gompels 2005). In pregnant women with a severe disease process, regular infusions with C1-INH concentrate may become necessary. For short-term prophylaxis, such as a visit to the dentist or during an acute angioedema attack, aside from tranexamic acid, C1-INH concentrate may also be given. Case series (Martinez-Saguer 2010) and single case reports support this approach as safe and effective during pregnancy and prior to birth.

Icatibant acetate is a synthetic selective bradykinin B_2-receptor competitive antagonist that has been approved by the European Medicines Agency (EMA) treatment of acute HAE-C1-INH attacks in patients 18 years or older. No specific secondary effects in female patients are known.

Ecallantide is a new potent, and specific plasma kallikrein inhibitor for the treatment of acute HAE-C1-INH attacks in patients 16 years or older. No specific secondary effects in female patients are known.

Recombinant human C1 esterase inhibitor (rhC1INH) is produced in transgenic rabbits and has been approved for the treatment of acute HAE-C1-INH attacks in patients 18 years or older. No specific secondary effects in female patients are known.

Conestat alfa represents an analog of the human C1-esterase inhibitor. It was released in 2010 and is derived from the milk of transgenic rabbits. No information exists on teratogenic potential or influence during pregnancy and lactation.

> **Recommendation.** C1-esterase inhibitor concentrate is the treatment of choice during pregnancy for C1-IN deficiency.

References

Anderka M, Mitchell AA, Louik C. Medications used to treat nausea and vomiting of pregnancy and the risk of selected birth defects. Birth Defects Res (Part A) 2012; 94: 22–30.

Cox L, Nelson H, Lockey et al. Allergen immunotherapy: a practice parameter third update. J Allergy Clin Immunol 2011; 127: S1–S55.

Diav-Citrin O, Shechtman S, Aharonovich A, et al. Pregnancy outcome after gestational exposure to loratadine or antihistamines: A prospective controlled cohort study. J Allergy Clin Immunol 2003; 111: 1239–43.

Djokanovic M, Moretti M, Boskovic, R. Fetal safety of cetirizine use in pregnancy – a prospective controlled cohort study {Abstract}. Birth Defects Research (Part A) 2010; 88: 438.

Einarson A, Bailey B, Jung G, et al. Prospective controlled study of hydroxyzine and cetirizine in pregnancy. Ann Allergy Asthma Immunol 1997; 78: 183–6.

Gompels MM, Lock RJ, Abinun M, et al. C1 inhibitor deficiency: consensus document. Clin Exp Immunol 2005; 139: 379–394. Review. Erratum in: Clin Exp Immunol 2005; 141: 189–90.

Källén B. Use of antihistamine drugs in early pregnancy and delivery outcome. J Matern Fetal Neonat Med 2002; 11: 146–152.

Källén B, Olausson PO. No increased risk of infant hypospadias after maternal use of loratadine in early pregnancy. Int J Med Sci 2006; 3: 106–7.

Krishna MT, Huissoon AP. Clinical immunology review series: an approach to desensitization. Clin Exp Immunol 2011 Feb; 163: 131–46.

Lione A, Scialli AR. The developmental toxicity of the H1-histamine antagonists. Reprod Toxicol 1996; 10: 247–55.

Martinez-Saguer I, Rusicke E, Aygören-Pürsün E, et al. Characterization of acute hereditary angioedema attacks during pregnancy and breast-feeding and their treatment with C1 inhibitor concentrate. Am J Obstet Gynecol 2010; 203: 131, e1–7.

Metzger WJ, Turner E, Patterson R. The safety of immunotherapy during pregnancy. J Allergy Clin Immunol 1978; 61: 268–74.

Pedersen L, Nørgaard M, Rothman KJ, et al. Loratadine during pregnancy and hypospadias. Epidemiology 2008; 19: 359–60.

Schardein JL. Chemically Induced Birth Defects. 4th edn. New York, Basel: Marcel Dekker, 2000.

Schwarz EB, Moretti ME, Nayak S, et al. Risk of hypospadias in offspring of women using loratadine during pregnancy: a systematic review and meta-analysis. Drug Saf 2008; 31: 775–88.

Serreau R, Komiha M, Blanc F, et al. Neonatal seizures with maternal hydroxyzine hydrochloride in late pregnancy. Reprod Toxicol 2005; 20: 573–4.

Weber-Schöndorfer C, Schaefer C. The safety of cetirizine during pregnancy. A prospective observational cohort study. Reprod Toxicol 2008; 26: 19–23.

Zierler S, Purohit D. Prenatal antihistamine exposure and retrolental fibroplasia. Am J Epidemiol 1986; 123: 192–6.

Antiasthmatic and cough medication

2.3

Lee H. Goldstein, Corinna Weber-Schöndorfer and Matitiahu Berkovitch

2.3.1	Selective β_2-adrenergic agonists	66
2.3.2	Inhaled corticosteroids (ICSs)	67
2.3.3	Theophylline	68
2.3.4	Leukotriene antagonists	69
2.3.5	Mast cell stabilizers (inhibitors)	69
2.3.6	Anticholinergics	70
2.3.7	Omalizumab and roflumilast	70
2.3.8	Expectorants and mucolytic agents	70
2.3.9	Antitussives	71
2.3.10	Non-selective β-adrenergic agonists	72

Bronchial asthma affects 4–12% of pregnant women worldwide. During pregnancy, asthma should be adequately treated not only for the benefit of the mother but also to safeguard proper fetal oxygenation. Severe, poorly treated asthma is associated with adverse perinatal outcomes (Murphy 2013, Murphy 2011), such as a higher risk of prematurity (Bakhireva 2008a), lower birth weight (Breton 2009) or small for gestational age (SGA) children (Firoozi 2010), preeclampsia (Rudra 2006), and other complications (Enriquez 2007). There is a debate about the possibility of a slight increase of some malformations (Lin 2012, Blais 2010), and also if the fetal gender can influence the course of asthma during pregnancy. Results are contradictory (Bakhireva 2008b, Baibergenova 2006). In a recently published meta-analysis, maternal asthma was associated with an increased risk of cleft lip but not with other major malformations (Murphy 2013). Maternal asthma can be associated with an increased offspring risk of infectious and parasitic diseases, diseases of the nervous system, ear, respiratory system, and skin (Tegethoff 2013).

The traditional classification of asthma based on symptoms with four categories (intermittent, persistent to a minor degree, medium degree, and severe degree) is only useful for untreated patients. It does not consider the impact of therapy, and is thus not able to help adjust treatment in the course of the disease. Three stages of asthma control have been defined:

- Controlled asthma
- Partially controlled asthma
- Uncontrolled asthma.

Drugs During Pregnancy and Lactation. http://dx.doi.org/10.1016/B978-0-12-408078-2.00004-4

The aim of asthma treatment is to obtain freedom from symptoms as much as possible ("controlled asthma"), with the least number of antiasthmatic drugs at the lowest possible dose. Outside pregnancy it is recommended to try to reduce asthma medication after 3 months of stabilization. This approach, however, should be very carefully applied in pregnant women (Schatz 2009). Pregnant women using long-term therapy should be seen monthly by their physician/specialist, or even more frequently if the asthma exacerbates or is inadequately controlled during pregnancy (Schatz 2009).

Pharmacotherapy and drug-free interventions (such as cessation of smoking and weight loss) are building blocks of asthma management. The step-wise approach for asthma therapy for adults applies, in principle, for pregnant women as well (see specific medication groups), starting with a rapidly effective β_2-adrenergic drug, and a short-acting beta agonist (SABA) used as inhaler when necessary. When this is inadequate, low-dose inhaled corticoids (ICS) or leukotriene modifiers are added as long-term medication. At the third level of therapy low dose ICSs are combined with LABA, leukotriene modifier or sustained release theophylline. The next level consists of ICSs at medium or high dose plus a long-acting beta agonist. Theophylline and/or leukotriene modifiers may become necessary. If all this fails, oral prednisolone or anti-IgE treatment should be used (Global Initiative for Asthma 2012). Other treatment options are of lesser importance in the outpatient care of adults, but will be presented here briefly.

2.3.1   Selective β_2-adrenergic agonists

β_2-adrenergic agonists induce a relaxation of the smooth muscle of blood vessels (vasodilatation), bronchi (bronchodilatation), and uterus as well as a rise in the blood levels of glucose, lipids, and ketones. An exclusively acting β_2-agonistic drug is not available; those listed here act primarily as β_2-agonists.

Because of rapid onset of action, good effectiveness, and low side-effect profile inhalative β_2-agonists should be chosen as medications on demand. They include: *fenoterol, albuterol, salbutamol,* and *terbutaline, levalbuterol, pirbuterol* and *reproterol*. About 10% of inhalative SABAs reach the bronchi directly, while the rest is swallowed and absorbed by the gastrointestinal tract (Martel 2007).

Albuterol is the best investigated drug for use during pregnancy (Bakhireva 2004, Schatz 2004) and it was well tolerated in most studies. A case-control study with 4,593 asthmatic pregnant women even detected a protective effect of SABA in pregnancy-induced hypertension (Martel 2007).

However, there are also results with converse outcomes. For instance, retrospective case-control studies found an association with gastroschisis (Lin 2008) and with heart defects (Lin 2009). An additional publication reported a slightly increased risk of cardiac defects (Källén 2007). In a large population based study, some association was found between bronchodilator and inhaled steroid use on omphalocele, esophageal atresia and anorectal atresia, although possibly due to the level of asthma severity (hypoxia) and not the asthma medications (Lin 2012). In another large database study, SABAs during the first trimester were not associated with an increased risk of congenital malformations (Eltonsy 2011). Terbutalin exposure has been associated with autism spectrum disorders of the offspring if used for more than 2 days in the third trimester, although larger studies are required to confirm this observation (Croen 2011).

Long-term acting β_2-adrenergic agonists or long-acting beta agonists (LABAs) should be applied exclusively in combination with corticoids; they include *formoterol* with its rapid onset, *salmeterol* and the new *indacaterol*. Experiences with these are limited; it can be assumed that they do not differ in their compatibility from SABAs, although some studies have found an association with first trimester exposure to LABA and cardiac malformations (Eltonsy 2011).

Oral and parenteral administration of beta agonists is limited to special situations. Currently available are salbutamol, terbutaline, *bambuterol*, *tulobuterol*, reproterol, and *clenbuterol*.

At sufficient dose all adrenergic agents can trigger tachycardia and arrhythmias, not only in the mother but also in the fetus. They can also increase glucose intolerance – an effect that needs to be taken into consideration in pregnant women with a diabetogenic metabolism. Terbutalin has been associated with autism spectrum disorders among the offspring (Croen 2011).

Experience in pregnancy with indacaterol have not been reported, and for bambuterol, clenbuterol, and tulobuterol they are inadequate. Yet, there are no indications that these drugs have teratogenic effects in humans.

> **Recommendation.** Adrenergic drugs are also part of asthma management in pregnancy. Inhalative drug of choice is the well-investigated short-acting albuterol as medication on demand. If the severity of asthma makes it necessary, the administration of the long-acting formoterol (together with an ICS) is the treatment of choice in pregnancy. The treatment steps outlined above should be observed. At the end of pregnancy, inhibition of uterine contractions and β_2-specific effects need to be taken into consideration.

2.3.2　Inhaled corticosteroids (ICSs)

Inhaled corticosteroids (ICSs) are part of any long-term treatment of asthma and should not be discontinued in pregnancy.

ICSs have anti-inflammatory, antiallergenic, and immunosuppressive activities and enhance the response of bronchial β-receptors. Available treatments are *budesonide*, an agent well-studied in pregnancy, as well as the following halogenated ICSs: *beclomethasone, fluticasone, mometasone*, and *ciclesonide* and *triamcinolone*.

Theoretical concerns about use of ICSs during pregnancy are based on the results of some studies of systemic use (Chapter 2.15). Studies of ICSs in thousands of pregnant women have been able to remove these doubts (Breton 2010, Rahimi 2006, Martel 2005, Bakhireva 2004). In a large population based study some association was found between bronchodilator and inhaled steroid use on omphalocele, esophageal atresia and anorectal atresia, although possibly due to the degree of asthma severity (hypoxia), and not the asthma medications (Lin 2012). Low to moderate doses of ICSs were not associated with an increased prevalence of perinatal outcomes such as low birth weight, preterm birth and small for gestational age (Cossette 2013), although there is still concern regarding high dose ICS therapy (Blais 2009). ICS therapy is known to have an inhibitory effect upon the maternal cortisol feedback regulation only when the fetus was female ($n = 38$) (Hodyl 2011); this needs to be explored in future studies. ICS therapy has been associated with offspring endocrine, metabolic, and nutritional disorders (Tegethoff 2012).

Pregnancy

2.3 Antiasthmatic and cough medication

Most experiences have been reported with budesonide (Norjavaara 2003), followed by beclometasone and fluticasone. At this point there is no evidence that the minimally investigated mometasone or ciclesonide would lead to different results.

In cases of severe asthma, or for the treatment of an asthma attack, glucocorticoids may also be used systemically (Chapter 2.15).

> **Recommendation.** According to the International Asthma Guidelines, ICS is the preferred treatment of choice for long-term therapy in pregnancy (Global Initiative for Asthma 2012). More thoroughly investigated substances such as budesonide are to be preferred.

2.3.3   Theophylline

Theophylline is a strong bronchial dilatator. Aside from theophylline, the related *aminophylline* is also available.

The plasma concentration of theophylline correlates closely with a bronchodilatative effect, but also has undesirable side effects. When the bronchial obstruction is less pronounced, theophylline is a less effective dilatator than β_2-agonists.

Theophylline has a mildly positive cardiac effect, and stimulates different parts of the central nervous system. It enhances the sensitivity of the breathing center for CO_2 and thus increases frequency and depth of breathing. This effect is used to prevent threatening apnea in premature infants; in these premature children the half-life is prolonged to more than 24 hours. There are no observations of negative sequelae on later childhood development.

Theophylline crosses the placenta. Because protein binding and clearance decrease during pregnancy and, despite an increase in the distribution volume, a reduction in the dose may become necessary in order to avoid side effects for both the mother and the child. Maternal serum concentrations of 8–12 µg/ml should not be exceeded during treatment.

Although theophylline has been shown to be teratogenic at high concentrations in the animal model, no embryotoxic effects have been observed in humans (Briggs 2011). Significant differences regarding birth parameters have not been noted when comparing inhalable β_2-adrenergic agonists, inhalable corticoids, and theophylline. The rate of side effects increased with the use of theophylline in pregnant women (Dombrowski 2004, Schatz 2004), consisting primarily of tremors, tachycardia, and vomiting. Such symptoms can also be exhibited by newborns exposed to theophylline *in utero*. For that reason, pregnant women should be treated with the lowest possible dose. Newborns need to be monitored for effects of theophylline therapy. Moreover, if treatment with theophylline continues until the end of pregnancy, uterine contractions may be inhibited.

> **Recommendation.** Theophylline may be used for the treatment of asthma throughout pregnancy. The therapeutic steps outlined by the Asthma Guidelines (Global Initiative for Asthma 2012) should be observed. To minimize maternal and neonatal side effects, treatment should aim for the lowest possible but still effective dose.

2.3.4　Leukotriene antagonists

Available leukotriene antagonists are *montelukast, pranlucast, zefirlucast* and *zilenton*.

Montelukast is the most studied leukotriene antagonist during pregnancy. Based on a pregnancy registry with first trimester exposure to montelukast, eight cases with malformations (two with limb defects) out of 200 cases were reported. Based on additional reports the FDA cautioned in 2009: "During worldwide marketing experience, congenital limb defects have been rarely reported in the offspring of women being treated with Singulair during pregnancy" (FDA on Montelukast 2009).

A study of the data from the Swedish Birth Registry failed to find an increase in the rate of malformations (Källén 2007). Similarly, a prospective study in the USA did not observe a specific teratogenic risk in children born after exposure to montelukast ($n = 72$) or zafirlukast ($n = 22$), when compared to SABA-exposed children or children of healthy mothers (Bakhireva 2007). This was confirmed in a Canadian study of 166 pregnancies with exposure during the first trimester. As only one infant in the study group displayed malformations and none in the two control groups, the quality of the data is dubious (Sarkar 2009). In a large retrospective insurance claims cohort study comprising approximately 12 million covered lives, and more than 277,000 pregnancies linked to a live-birth outcome, there were no events similar to the six post marketing surveillance events of limb reduction defects among the 1535 infants born to mothers in the montelukast cohort (Nelsen 2012).

Recommendation. Montelukast may be used during pregnancy where better-tried medications have not lead to a desired result. In doing so, the therapeutic steps outlined by the Asthma Guidelines (see above) need to be observed. When used during the first trimester, a follow-up sonographic examination should be offered to confirm normal fetal development.

2.3.5　Mast cell stabilizers (inhibitors)

When *cromoglicic acid* or *sodium cromoglicate* are supplied regularly, mast cells of the connective tissue lose their ability to release their stored histamine. As histamine leads to bronchial narrowing, cromoglicic acid is used for the prophylactic therapy of asthmatic (allergic) afflictions. Cromoglicic acid does not possess a direct bronchodilatatory effect and is not effective in the management of an acute attack. About 5–10% of a dose reaches the alveoli, the remainder is swallowed, and only 1% of it will be absorbed into the intestines. The effect becomes apparent after 3–5 days. Because of its limited effectiveness the drug has lost significance in asthma therapy.

Cromoglicic acid is also available for the management of allergic diseases of the nose, eye, and for food allergies. It has no embryotoxic effects, as confirmed by a large number of treated pregnant women (Briggs 2011). *Ketotifen* has not been sufficiently investigated regarding its prenatal compatibility. There is no suggestion of embryotoxicity in humans.

Pregnancy

2.3 Antiasthmatic and cough medication

> **Recommendation.** Cromoglicic acid may be used during pregnancy to prevent allergy or exercise-induced asthma. Ketotifen is not part of the standard therapy for asthma, but inadvertent use does not require intervention.

2.3.6   Anticholinergics

As anticholinergic agents, *ipratropium bromide* and *oxitropium bromide* are bronchodilators with modest activity, usually reserved for patients who are intolerant of beta agonists due to side effects such as tachycardia, etc. Teratogenicity has not been observed in animal models. There is insufficient experience in its use during pregnancy. Ipratropium has a longer market experience.

Tiotropium bromide is reserved for COPD and not for asthma patients, and there is no experience in pregnancy.

> **Recommendation.** Ipratropium bromide may be used for bronchodilatation during pregnancy when drugs of choice (SABA, ICS, LABA) are not sufficiently effective.

2.3.7   Omalizumab and roflumilast

Omalizumab is a monoclonal IgG1-κ-antibody that binds to the IgE receptor; it may be used in cases of severe allergic asthma where conventional medications have failed. The manufacturer indicates that omalizumab crosses the placenta, but experience during pregnancy has not been published.

The phosphodiesterase-4 inhibitor roflumilast is used for chronic-obstructive pulmonary disease; it has an anti-inflammatory effect and does not dilate the bronchi. There are no reported experiences in pregnancy although proved teratogenic in animals.

> **Recommendation.** The above-named substances are not drugs of choice during pregnancy. They should only be used if conventional therapies have been exhausted.

2.3.8   Expectorants and mucolytic agents

According to current experience, expectorants and mucolytic agents such as *acetyl cysteine*, *ambroxol*, and *bromhexine* may be used during pregnancy without a recognizable risk of a teratogenic effect. This also holds for high doses of *N-acetylcysteine (NAC)* when used as an antidote in acetaminophen intoxication (Chapter 2.22).

Investigations of human teratogenicity are also lacking for *carbocisteine*, *guaifenesin*; essential oils such as *eucalyptol*, and various phytopharmaceuticals such as extracts from *ivy leaves*, *thyme*, *buckhorn plantain* (*Plantago lanceolata*), and *marshmallow root*. Studies about their compatibility in pregnancy are also missing (Chapter 2.19).

The use of potassium iodide as an expectorant is therapeutically obsolete and contraindicated in pregnancy. In the past, the practice was to give patients a single therapeutic dose of 250–500 mg iodine. However, this is not to be confused with the modern recommended iodine substitution dose of 200 μg/day for pregnant women.

> **Recommendation.** If inhalation and fluid therapy fail, trial expectorants and mucolytic agents may be used during pregnancy. Potassium iodide is contraindicated.

2.3.9   Antitussives

Codeine (*methylmorphine*) is a morphine derivative with a strong inhibitory effect upon the coughing center. No other medication exceeds its antitussive effect. Because of its analgesic effect, codeine is also part of pain medication (see more in Chapter 2.1). It is not teratogenic, although it has been associated with acute caesarian delivery and postpartum hemorrhage (Nezvalová-Henriksen 2011). Longer and high-dose maternal intake at birth, can cause respiratory depression and opiate-typical withdrawal in the newborn (Chapter 2.21).

The opioid d*ihydrocodeine* is not well investigated, but can be regarded similarly as codeine.

Although *dextromethorphan* belongs to the opium alkaloids, it does not have analgesic and respiratory depressive effects at therapeutic doses, and its potential for dependency and abuse is low. The antitussive effect is similar to that of codeine. Based on animal experiments dextromethorphan was imputed to have a teratogenic potential in the late 1990s. However, based on experiences with more than 500 pregnancies, this suspicion has not been confirmed for humans (Martinez-Frias 2001).

The following medications have been insufficiently examined for prenatal risks in humans, but also have not shown any evidence of teratogenicity. *Noscapine* is a major alkaloid of opium. It has an antitussive but no analgesic effect and is weaker than codeine. Contrary to morphine, noscapine enhances respiration and dilates the bronchi. *Benproperine* is also a respiratory stimulant and it inhibits the coughing reflex in the afferent portion of the reflex arc. *Pentoxyverine* is a non-narcotic antitussive that acts centrally, while *levodropropizine* acts primarily peripherally.

> **Recommendation.** If physical measures have failed, and dry cough persists, codeine may be used as an antitussive during pregnancy for a short time. It may also be used during pregnancy as an analgesic (in combination with acetaminophen). In either situation, potential interactions with other medications and the possibility of abuse have to be taken into account. Depending on dose, time, and duration of its application, respiratory depression and withdrawal symptoms are possible side effects in the newborn.
>
> Dexomethorphan may be used as an antitussive, and dihydrocodeine is probably acceptable. The other medications mentioned should not be used as first choices during pregnancy.

Pregnancy

2.3 Antiasthmatic and cough medication

2.3.10   Non-selective β-adrenergic agonists

▶ **Orciprenaline and adrenaline (epinephrine)**

Orciprenaline (*metoproterenol*) is approved as injectable for the treatment of acute asthmatic attacks. As a non-selective β-adrenergic agonist it elicits an increased number of side effects. There is no known association with embryo- or fetotoxicity.

The use of catecholamines, such as *adrenaline* (*epinephrine*), is to be limited to emergencies, in general practice as well as in pregnancy. Adrenalin can be administered intravenously or as an aerosol, in the latter case as an inhalant or directly into the trachea. Oral application is ineffective as the intestinal tract will degrade it. Catecholamines cross the placenta but are to some degree enzymatically inactivated.

Because of the short half-time of 1–4 minutes and brief application, consequences are unlikely for the newborn. When catecholamines are used systemically, it cannot be ruled out that they may not decrease placental perfusion.

Local anesthetics used by the dentist to which epinephrine has been added are quite safe however.

> **Recommendation.** Orciprenaline and adrenalin are used in emergency situations only. An exposure does not justify a risk-based pregnancy termination or invasive diagnostic interventions (Chapter 1.13). A follow-up sonographic examination may be considered. The amounts of epinephrine present in some local anesthetics can be considered as harmless.

▶ **Other adrenergic agonists**

The bronchodilatator *ephedrine* is no longer of therapeutic relevance; it is only available in a combination medication for colds. Ephedrine has both α- and β-adrenergic effects. *Pseudoephedrine* and *phenylephedrine* have α-agonistic activity.

All three agonists are vasoconstrictors. They did not show teratogenic activity in prospective studies. Some retrospective case-control studies suggested an association between disruptive malformations such as gastroschisis, intestinal atresia, and hemifacial microsomia and systemic application of pseudoephedrine (Werler 2006). In some case studies a link to certain malformations was noted with other adrenergic agonists as well. Even if this would be proven to be causally related, the individual risk appears to be rather small due to the rare occurrence of such defects.

Decongestants during the second or third trimester have been associated with less preterm delivery (Hernandez 2010).

> **Recommendation.** Combination drugs with ephedrine, pseudoephedrine, and phenylephedrine should not be used during pregnancy. If (inadvertently) used systemically during the first trimester, a follow-up sonography may be considered, more so with long-term exposure.

References

Baibergenova A, Thsabane L, Akhtar-Danesh N et al. Is fetal gender associated with emergency department visits for asthma during pregnancy? J Asthma 2006; 43: 293-9.

Bakhireva LN, Jones KL, Johnson DL et al. Pregnancy outcome among women who have asthma and use asthma medications. Birth Defects Res A 2004; 70: 418-29.

Bakhireva LN, Jones KL, Schatz M et al. Organization of Teratology Information Specialists Collaborative Research Group: Safety of leukotriene receptor antagonists in pregnancy. J Allergy Clin Immunol 2007; 119: 618-25.

Bakhireva LN, Schatz M, Jones KL et al. Organization of Teratology Information Specialists Collaborative Research Group: Asthma control during pregnancy and the risk of preterm delivery or impaired fetal growth. Ann Allergy Asthma Immunol 2008a; 101: 137-43.

Bakhireva LN, Schatz M, Jones KL et al. OTIS Collaborative Research Group: Fetal sex and maternal asthma control in pregnancy. J Asthma 2008b; 45: 403-7.

Blais L, Beauchesne MF, Lemière C et al. High doses of inhaled corticosteroids during the first trimester of pregnancy and congenital malformations. J Allergy Clin Immunol 2009; 124: 1229-34.

Blais L, Kettani FZ, Elftouh N et al. Effect of maternal asthma on the risk of specific congenital malformations: A population-based cohort study. Birth Defects Res A Clin Mol Teratol 2010; 88: 216-22.

Breton MC, Beauchesne MF, Lemière C et al. Risk of perinatal mortality associated with asthma during pregnancy. Thorax 2009; 64: 101-6.

Breton MC, Beauchesne MF, Lemière C et al. Risk of perinatal mortality associated with inhaled corticosteroid use for the treatment of asthma during pregnancy. J Allergy Clin Immunol 2010; 126: 772-7.

Briggs GG, Freeman RK, Yaffe SJ. Drugs in Pregnancy and Lactation. 9th edn. Baltimore: Williams & Wilkins 2011.

Cossette B, Forget A, Beauchesne MF et al. Thorax 2013; 68: 724-30.

Croen LA, Connors SL, Matevia M et al. Prenatal exposure to β_2-adrenergic receptor agonists and risk of autism spectrum disorders. Neurodev Disord 2011; 3: 307-15.

Dombrowski MP, Schatz M, Wise R. Randomized trial of inhaled beclomethason dipropionate versus theophylline for moderate asthma during pregnancy. Am J Obstet Gynecol 2004; 190: 737-44.

Eltonsy S, Forget A, Blais L. Beta2-agonists use during pregnancy and the risk of congenital malformations. Birth Defects Res A Clin Mol Teratol 2011; 91: 937-47.

Enriquez R, Griffin MR, Carroll KN et al. Effect of maternal asthma and asthma control on pregnancy and perinatal outcomes. J Allergy Clin Immunol 2007; 120: 625-30.

FDA on Montelukast 2009, www.accessdata.fda.gov/drugsatfda_docs/label/2009/020829s0 51_020830s052_021409s028lbl.pdf.

Firoozi F, Lemière C, Ducharme FM et al. Effect of maternal moderate to severe asthma on perinatal outcomes. Respir Med 2010; 104: 1278-87.

Global Initiative for Asthma. Global strategy for asthma management and prevention: updated December 2012, http://www.ginasthma.org/uploads/users/files/GINA_Report_ 2012.pdf.

Hernandez RK, Mitchell AA, Werler MM. Decongestant use during pregnancy and its association with preterm delivery. Birth Defects Res A Clin Mol Teratol 2010; 88: 715-21.

Hodyl NA, Stark MJ, Osei-Kumah A, et al. Fetal glucocorticoid-regulated pathways are not affected by inhaled corticosteroid use for asthma during pregnancy. Am J Respir Crit Care Med 2011; 183: 716-22.

Källén B, Otterblad Olausson P. Use of anti-asthmatic drugs during pregnancy. 3. Congenital malformations in the infant. Eur J Clin Pharm 2007; 63: 383-8.

Lin S, Herdt-Losavio M, Gensburg L et al. Maternal asthma, asthma medication use, and the risk of congenital heart defects. Birth Defects Res A Clin Mol Teratol 2009; 85: 161-8.

Lin S, Munsie JP, Herdt-Losavio ML et al. National Birth Defects Prevention Study: Maternal asthma medication use and the risk of gastroschisis. Am J Epidemiol 2008; 168: 73-9.

Lin S, Munsie JP, Herdt-Losavio ML et al. National Birth Defects Prevention Study. Maternal asthma medication use and the risk of selected birth defects. Pediatrics 2012; 129: e317-24.

Martel MJ, Rey E, Beauchesne MF et al. Use of inhaled corticosteroids during pregnancy and risk of pregnancy-induced hypertension: nested case-control study. BMJ 2005; 330: 230-3.

Pregnancy

2.3 Antiasthmatic and cough medication

Martel MJ, Rey E, Beauchesne MF et al. Use of short-acting beta2-agonists during pregnancy and the risk of pregnancy-induced hypertension. J Allergy Clin Immunol 2007; 119: 576–82.

Martinez-Frias ML, Rodriguez-Pinilla E. Epidemiologic analysis of prenatal exposure to cough medicines containing dextromethorphan: no evidence of human teratogenicity. Teratology 2001; 63: 38–41.

Murphy VE, Namazy JA, Powell H et al. A meta-analysis of adverse perinatal outcomes in women with asthma. BJOG 2011; 118: 1314–23.

Murphy VE, Wang G, Namazy JA et al. The risk of congenital malformations, perinatal mortality and neonatal hospitalisation among pregnant women with asthma: a systematic review and meta-analysis. BJOG 2013; 120: 812–22.

Nelsen LM, Shields KE, Cunningham ML et al. Congenital malformations among infants born to women receiving montelukast, inhaled corticosteroids, and other asthma medications. J Allergy Clin Immunol 2012; 129: 251–4, e1–6.

Nezvalová-Henriksen K, Spigset O, Nordeng H. Effects of codeine on pregnancy outcome: results from a large population-based cohort study. Eur J Clin Pharmacol 2011; 67: 1253–61.

Norjavaara E, de Verdier MG. Normal pregnancy outcomes in a population-based study including 2,968 pregnant women exposed to budesonide. J Allergy Clin Immunol 2003; 111: 736–42.

Rahimi R, Nikfar S, Abdollahi M. Meta-analysis finds use of inhaled corticosteroids during pregnancy safe: a systematic meta-analysis review. Hum Exp Toxicol 2006; 25: 447–52.

Rudra CB, Williams MA, Frederick IO et al. Maternal asthma and risk of preeclampsia: a case-control study. J Reprod Med 2006; 51: 94–100.

Sarkar M, Koren G, Kalra S et al. Montelukast use during pregnancy: a multicentre, prospective, comparative study of infant outcomes. Eur J Clin Pharmacol 2009; 65: 1259–64.

Schatz M, Dombrowski MP. Clinical practice. Asthma in pregnancy. Review. N Engl J Med 2009; 360: 1862–9.

Schatz M, Dombrowski MP, Wise R et al. The relationship of asthma medication use to perinatal outcomes. J Allergy Clin Immunol 2004; 113: 1040–5.

Tegethoff M, Greene N, Olsen J et al. Inhaled glucocorticoids during pregnancy and offspring pediatric diseases: a national cohort study. Am J Respir Crit Care Med 2012; 185: 557–63.

Tegethoff M, Olsen J, Schaffner E et al. Asthma during pregnancy and clinical outcomes in offspring: a national cohort study. Pediatrics 2013; 132: 483–91.

Werler MM. Teratogen update: pseudoephedrine. Birth Defects Res A Clin Mol Teratol 2006; 76: 445–52.

Nausea and vomiting in pregnancy

2.4

Lee H. Goldstein, Corinna Weber-Schöndorfer and
Matitiahu Berkovitch

2.4.1	Treatment options	76
2.4.2	Complementary treatment options	76
2.4.3	Pharmacological treatment options	78
2.4.4	Dopamine antagonists	81
2.4.5	Pyridoxine (vitamin B6)	83
2.4.6	Vitamin B1	84
2.4.7	Serotonin antagonists	85
2.4.8	Glucocorticoids	86
2.4.9	Other antiemetics	86

More than half (50–80%) of pregnant women suffer from nausea and vomiting (NVP), also known as morning sickness – although symptoms may persist the whole day. Usually limited to the first trimester, NVP may continue throughout the entire pregnancy.

NVP may range from mild discomfort to hyperemesis gravidarum, causing severe vomiting and nausea, weight loss, severe dehydration, metabolic compromise and in severe cases can be fatal. The death of the famous Charlotte Brontë, author of *Jane Eyre*, in 1855 of suspected morning sickness and hyperdemesis gravidarum, reflects the potential severity of NVP, and the fact that the opinion at that time was that no therapy was considered necessary, as it was attributed solely to psychological factors, and as such was not treated medically. However, more recent discussions have suggested that tuberculosis with secondary Addison's disease could better explain her signs and symptoms (Weiss 1991, Rhodes 1972). Nevertheless, NVP may pose a serious socioeconomic burden as 25% of the women suffering from it miss work as a result of their symptoms (Vellacott 1988). Hyperemesis gravidarum occurs in 1 in 200 pregnancies, although women who have suffered hyperemesis gravidarum in earlier pregnancies increases the risk to 15% (Trogstad 2005).

The pathogenesis of NVP has been attributed to multiple factors such as elevated levels of β-hCG, prostaglandin levels (by relaxing the gastro-esophageal sphincter), gastric dysrhythmia, vitamin B6 deficiency, hyperolfaction, and *Helicobacter pylori*. Psychological factors (depression, anxiety, eating disorders), were once thought to be the only etiology of NVP, but might in fact be a result of the NVP. A genetic predisposition has been suggested based on the concordance in monozygotic twins, variation within ethnic groups, and the fact that siblings and mothers of patients with NVP are more likely to have had NVP themselves (Goodwin 2002).

NVP has been postulated to protect the embryo by encouraging the mother to avoid potentially harmful or teratogenic foods and beverages (Furneaux 2001, Profet 1992, Hook 1976). For women suffering NVP, it may be reassuring to know that it is associated with less chance of spontaneous abortions, and a reduced risk of congenital heart defects (Boneva 1999).

Women whose past pregnancies were complicated by severe forms of NVP or hyperemesis gravidarum may benefit by pre-emptive therapy, initiated as soon as the patient becomes aware of her pregnancy and before the symptoms of NVP appear. Twenty-five women with severe NVP in previous pregnancies were administered anti-emetic therapy before symptoms became evident, and the dosage of the anti-emetic therapy was gradually increased as the NVP emerged. The severity of the NVP was significantly reduced in comparison to a group of women with the same maternity history of severe NVP in previous pregnancies, who initiated anti-emetic treatment only when the nausea and vomiting appeared (Koren 2004).

2.4.1   Treatment options

The treatment options for NVP range from conservative measures such as reassurance and diet manipulation in the mildly symptomatic women, to drug therapy, and if necessary in severe and intractable cases, total parenteral nutrition or even therapeutic pregnancy termination. One Cochrane review on the treatment options found a lack of high-quality evidence to back up any of the interventions (Matthews 2014).

▶ **Drug free treatments**

Diet manipulations

Dietary measures are often suggested for the mildly symptomatic woman, although little evidence supports these measures. Women may benefit from frequent and small meals, with high carbohydrate and low fat content. Salty foods may be tolerated better in the morning, and sour or tart beverages may be better tolerated than water (Quinlan 2003).

Severe intractable hyperemesis gravidarum is occasionally treated by total parenteral nutrition and intravenous fluids.

2.4.2   Complementary treatment options

Complementary therapy has become very popular in Western countries, and many people prefer complementary or natural therapy more than medical therapy believing that "natural" treatment is less harmful. Pregnant women and their doctors are especially reluctant to use medicinal therapy during pregnancy, especially during the first trimester when symptoms of the NVP and hyperemesis gravidarum are worse, and so may prefer alternative therapy.

The following sections present a review on the various alternative therapies available for NVP, and the evidence, if any, of efficacy and safety.

▶ Acupuncture and acupressure

Acupuncture is a popular form of Chinese medicine, based on the notion that vital life energy (*qi*) flows through dozens of paths (meridians) throughout the human body. Illness is thought to be the result of obstructed or misdirected energy flow, and stimulation of acupoints within the meridian system is believed to restore health by correcting this energy flow. By inserting very thin needles 5 mm deep under the skin, different organs can be influenced via the meridians. Many acupoints influence the upper gastrointestinal tract, but the acupoint studied most by western scientists is the P6 (*Nei Guan*), located on the anteromedial aspect of the forearm, at a three finger distance from the wrist crease, between the palmaris longus and flexor carpi radialis tendons. This point can be activated using needles (acupuncture) or pressure (acupressure) by applying an acupressure band. The summary evidence for benefits of acupressure or acupuncture in alleviating symptoms of NVP remains mixed and inconclusive. Acupuncture seems ineffective in treating NVP (Matthews 2014, Smith 2009).

▶ Hypnosis

Hypnotherapy may be used as an adjunct to medical therapy in patients with NVP or hyperemesis gravidarum. In a study of 138 patients hospitalized with refractory hyperemesis gravidarum, 88% stopped vomiting after one to three sessions of medical hypnosis (Simon 1999, Fuchs 1994). The hypnotic state induces a deep state of psychological relaxation, with a corresponding decrease in sympathetic tone. Symptoms associated with hyper-sympathetic arousal tend to remit. The patient might be given suggestions during the hypnotic state to relax their stomach and throat muscles, causing their nausea, gagging and vomiting to subside. A recent review of the evidence for hypnotherapy in NVP concluded that although promising, the quality of current evidence is insufficient to establish if hypnosis is an effective treatment for hyperemesis gravidarum (McCormack 2010).

▶ Ginger

Ginger is used in Asian and Indian medicine to treat nausea, indigestion, diarrhea, stomach-ache and flatulence, and is used with caution for treating NVP. It has been found effective in the treatment of motion sickness and postoperative nausea (Bone 1990, Mowry 1982). Ginger antiemetic effect is attributed to an increase in gastric tone and peristalsis via anticholinergic and antiserotonergic pathways (Wilkinson 2000).

Concern has been expressed regarding the safety of ginger's use by pregnant women due to the mutagenic activity of 6-gingerol, one of the constituents of ginger. The whole rhizome however, is not mutagenic due to the substance *zingerone* that suppresses the mutagenic activity of 6-gingerol (Nakamura 1982). Ginger has been claimed to inhibit platelet aggregation and, theoretically, could affect testosterone receptor binding and

Pregnancy

2.4 Nausea and vomiting in pregnancy

sex steroid differentiation of the fetus; however, no clinical evidence has suggested that this is the case (Borrelli 2005, Guh 1995, Backon 1991, Murphy 1988). Numerous trials have tested the efficacy of ginger in comparison to *placebo, pyridoxine* and *dimenhydranate* (Ensiyeh 2009, Chittumma 2007, Smith 2004, Portnoi 2003, Willetts 2003, Vutyavanich 2001). In a recent review of the randomized controlled trials of ginger for NVP, ginger was reported to be more effective than placebo and as effective as pyridoxine, without serious side effects, in both ambulatory and hospitalized pregnant women with NVP, although all the trials were short-term (3 weeks) and most of the participants were in their second or third trimester. Ginger improved symptoms of nausea, but did not significantly reduce the number of vomiting episodes (Viljoen 2014, Ding 2013). Ginger is not without risk; the recommended dose is 1,000 mg per day for NVP, but the recommended daily dose should not exceed 4 g, due to uterine stimulating effects (Borrelli 2005), which could adversely affect the pregnancy. High doses of ginger may also aggravate pre-existing conditions, such as cholelithiasis (Hardy 2004), or contribute to cardiac arrhythmia, CNS depression and heartburn (Westfall 2004). Caution should be exercised when combining ginger with hypoglycemic and antiplatelet drugs or herbs, due to a theoretical interaction, worsening the side effects of these agents (insulin, aspirin, ginseng, garlic, etc.), and with proton pump inhibitors or H_2-blockers due to increased production of gastric acid (Ding 2013).

Exacerbation of the symptoms of NVP after taking ginger may also be associated with the Yin–Yang principle of the traditional Chinese medicine; ginger is considered a Yang or hot remedy, and would help women with deficient Yang energy or Qi. The NVP of Qi deficient women is characteristically worse in the morning and improves after eating and resting. NVP of women with excess Yang energy characteristically report nausea at other times of the day that worsens after meals. These women would benefit, according to the Chinese traditional medicine, by a Yin or "cool" remedy such as peppermint (Tiran 2002).

In summary, ginger is efficient for NVP, and has not as yet been associated with developmental disorders; however, larger trials are needed (see also Chapter 2.19 for additional information about Ginger).

Recommendation. Complementary therapies for treating NVP, such as acustimulation, hypnosis and ginger have proved in some cases to be efficient, although more large-scale studies are needed. Complementary therapy is often expensive and difficult to obtain reliably, but may be a good solution for women who are reluctant to use pharmacological therapy for NVP.

2.4.3   Pharmacological treatment options

▶ Antihistamines (H₁ blockers)

First- and second-generation antihistamines are an effective and safe treatment for nausea and vomiting in pregnancy, and are usually first-line drugs for treatment of both NVP and hyperemesis gravidarum. The antihistamines that are indicated for nausea and vomiting are: *buclizine, cyclizine, dimenhydranate, diphenhydramine, doxylamine, hydroxyzine* and *meclizine*. The drawback of the first-generation antihistamines are their sedative effects. However, the fact that they have been on the market for so long, with no evidence of adverse effects on the newborn, is very reassuring. The newer antihistamines such as meclizine are also safe and less sedating. A large meta-analysis of 24 studies with more than 200,000 participating women showed no increased risk for major malformations; on the contrary, it seemed that the use of antihistamines for NVP might even be protective (Seto 1997). Another large prospective study on antihistamine use in the first trimester of more than 18,000 infants, failed to demonstrate any adverse effect on the birth outcome. The outcome of the pregnancies was more favorable than the controls with respect to preterm births, low birth weight and perinatal death (Källén 2002).

▶ Buclizine

A piperazine derivative antihistamine which acts centrally, and via the labyrinthine apparatus, to suppress nausea and vomiting. There is very little evidence supporting use during pregnancy, although probably safe according to a single study of 44 women treated with buclizine (Heinonen 1977), as are the other related antihistamines such as cyclizine and meclizine.

▶ Cyclizine

A piperazine derivative antihistamine with anticholinergic properties that exerts its anti-emetic effect via direct effects on the labyrinthine apparatus, the chemoreceptor trigger zone, and possibly by increasing the muscular tone of the lower esophagus. Milkovich (1976) reported no increased malformation rate among 111 offspring of mothers taking the drug during the first 84 days of pregnancy.

▶ Dimenhydrinate

Dimenhydrinate is the chlorotheophylline salt of diphenhydramine, that inhibits labyrinthine stimulation and the vestibular system. Dimenydranate is safe during early pregnancy (Mazzota 2000, Seto 1997, Lione 1996), and was further confirmed in a very large retrospective case-control study which included 22,843 infants with major birth anomalies (Czeizel 2005). As with diphenhydramine, dimenhydrinate should be avoided during the third trimester due its potential to stimulate uterine contractions (Brost 1996).

▶ Diphenhydramine

An ethanolamine antihistamine that acts by competitively antagonizing histamine at the H1 histamine receptor. Diphenhydramine is a first-generation antihistamine mainly used as a sedative, although safe and effective as an anti-emetic during pregnancy (Mazzota 2000). Combined with metoclopramide diphenhydramine is also effective in hyperemesis gravidarum (Reichmann 2012).

In a recent case control study (Gilboa 2009), diphenhydramine was associated with birth defects but the association was weak, and the authors concluded that their results should be used for hypotheses generation only. The National Birth Defects Prevention Study (NBDPS), a multi-site population-based case-control study, found no association between diphenhydramine and cleft lip, cleft palate, neural tube defects or hypospadias (Anderka 2012). Diphenhydramine has oxytocin-like effects, especially when given intravenously or in an overdose, and may cause uterine contractions (Brost 1996) and therefore should not be given during the third trimester.

▶ Doxylamine

An antihistamine, doxylamine was marketed with *pyridoxine* alone or together with *dicyclomine* (an antispasmodic), was marketed worldwide to millions of pregnant women as an effective treatment for NVP. In the mid-1970s, limb and various gastrointestinal malformations were suspected to be associated with the combination (Donnai 1978, Smithells 1978), and doxylamine was withdrawn from the market in the USA and in Europe. Subsequently, extensive prospective and retrospective studies failed to confirm this suspicion (Brent 1995, McKeigue 1994). A few years later, the risk of malformation was reassessed and showed unambiguously that there is no evidence of a teratogenic effect (Brent 2003, Kutcher 2003). Also, in a comparative trial, a therapy using a higher dose failed to show any negative effects on the pregnancies (Atanackovic 2001).

A comparative study of the neurophysiologic development of children between the ages of 3–7 failed to find any significant differences between those who had been exposed to doxylamine/pyridoxine *in utero* ($n = 45$), those whose mothers had untreated morning sickness ($n = 45$), and those whose mothers had no nausea or vomiting in pregnancy ($n = 29$) (Nulman 2009).

Today, doxylamine is available as a single agent drug for sleeping medications in most countries. In Canada, it has again become the most important medication for morning sickness. To obtain new approval in the USA, a controlled double-blind study was conducted comparing a combination medication with 10 mg doxylamine plus 10 mg pyridoxine (2 to a maximum of 4 tablets daily) ($n = 131$) versus a placebo ($n = 125$) (Koren 2010). Doxylamine plus pyridoxine were superior to the placebo, as could be expected.

▶ Meclizine

A piperazine antihistamine with anticholinergic and antiemetic activity. The antiemetic effects appear to be related to inhibition of the emetic center in the brain stem, vestibular nucleus and labyrinth. The onset of effect is 1 hour, but the effect is prolonged, usually 24 hours once daily dosing is appropriate. The first study proving efficacy of meclizine in the treatment of nausea and vomiting of pregnancy was published by Diggory (1962). Since then there have been four placebo-controlled studies confirming meclizine's high effectiveness for emesis/hyperemesis (Arznei-Telegramm 2009).

While in rats meclizine has a teratogenic effect, several studies with large numbers have not shown any evidence of a malformation risk in humans (Källén 2003, Seto 1997, Lione 1996, Heinonen 1977). A Swedish study involving more than 18,000 women treated with meclizine during the first trimester, and more than 1,200 with the antihistamine cyclizine, did not detect any increase in malformation rates (Asker 2005). The national birth defect prevention study showed that maternal treatment with meclizine during the first trimester of pregnancy reported more frequently than expected in 575 mothers of infants with isolated cleft palate (odds ratio = 12.7, 95% CI 2.9–55.7; Gilboa 2009). The authors suggested that their findings might only "warrant further investigation," since the observed elevated associations were part of multiple weak associations investigated, and based on an analysis of retrospective, self-reported data.

Recommendation. First- and second-generation antihistamines are a safe and effective treatment for NVP. Doxylamine should be first choice, preferably combined with vitamin B6 (Diclectin, if available), otherwise second generation antihistamines such as Meclizine should be used due to the sedative effects of the first generation antihistamines.

2.4.4   Dopamine antagonists

The dopamine antagonists used to treat NVP are *domperidone, droperidol, metoclopramide, phenothiazines* and *trimethobenzamide*.

▶ **Domperidone**

Not teratogenic in animals (Shepard 1992), but studies are scarce with regard to examining its safety in pregnancy or efficacy in emesis or hyperemesis gravidarum. Safety has been demonstrated in a small trial of 120 women in their first trimester using domperidone for gastrointestinal complaints. Fetal outcomes which included major malformations, gestational age at birth, birth weight and length, head circumference at birth, and 1- and 5-min Apgar score were similar to that of a control group (Choi 2013). Domperidone should not be administered intravenously as it has been associated with severe cardiac arrhythmias.

▶ **Droperidol**

The most recent dopamine antagonist to join the pharmacologic regimens used to treat severe NVP and/or hyperemesis gravidarum, droperidol belongs to the family of butyrophenones, is more potent than phenothiazines, and is used by anesthesiologists to treat postoperative nausea. The only published trial in the first trimester, combined droperidol with *diphenhydramine* in 80 women with hyperemesis gravidarum. In comparison to another group exposed to various anti-emetics, the combination of droperidol and diphenhydramine shortened the length of hospitalization, and reduced the chance of readmission (Nageotte 1996). There has been no association between droperidol and congenital malformations (Magee 2002), but there is a small risk of the mother developing prolonged QT syndrome, which can lead to a potentially fatal arrhythmia. There is a black box warning associated with its use in all patients, and The American College of Obstetricians and Gynecologists (ACOG Practice Bulletin 2004) recommends that this medication be used with caution.

Pregnancy

2.4 Nausea and vomiting in pregnancy

▶ Metoclopramide (MCP)

An effective anti-emetic that acts both centrally (dopamine blockade in the chemoreceptor trigger zone, decreasing sensitivity of the visceral nerves that transmit GI impulses to the central emetic center), and peripherally by stimulating motility of the upper gastrointestinal tract, and increasing the lower esophageal sphincter basal tone.

It counteracts some of the physiological changes during pregnancy that may lead to nausea or vomiting, such as decreased lower esophageal sphincter tone (Van Thiel 1977) and decreased propulsive motility time, as well as increased transit time of the small intestine.

Extrapyramidal symptoms are undesirable side effects. After ingestion MCP is well resorbed and rapidly reaches the fetus. Relatively little work has been done to investigate MCP's effectiveness for vomiting in pregnancy. Nevertheless, it is being used for this indication in many countries (Bsat 2003). In a newer randomized double-blind study promethazine i.v. (25 mg every 8 hours) was compared to MCP i.v. (10 mg every 8 hours) in pregnant women with hyperemesis. The therapeutic effectiveness in 73 and 76 patients, respectively, was similar, while the side effect profile of MCP was more favorable (Tan 2010). A retrospective cohort study compared 130 pregnant women with hyperemesis, who received MCP and diphenhydramine i.v. with a historical group of 99 patients who had been treated with droperidol and diphenhydramine i.v. The new protocol with MCP and diphenhydramine decreased vomiting more effectively and showed less maternal side effects. Nausea and duration of hospitalization were comparable in both groups (Lacasse 2009). Continuous subcutaneous administration of metoclopramide has been tried in several trials, and although it seems efficacious and comparable to continuous subcutaneous odansetron, there is not enough evidence to recommend this modality of treatment (Reichmann 2012).

As to the safety of MCP, three studies with 3,458, 884, and 175 pregnant women, respectively, all treated with MCP during the first trimester, failed to detect an increased rate of abnormalities in the children who had been exposed in utero (Matok 2009, Asker 2005, Berkovitch 2002). This was also seen in a study that examined prescription protocols and birth registry data (Sorensen 2000). In the National Birth Defects Prevention Study (Anderka 2012), maternal use of metoclopramide during the first trimester of pregnancy was not significantly associated with cleft lip, cleft palate or hypospadias. Children who had been exposed prenatally were found to display normal development up to the age of 4 years (Martynshin 1981).

The USA Food and Drug Administration in 2009 mandated a black box warning for metoclopramide due to reports of tardive dyskinesia, particularly with high dose and long-term use (US Food and Drug Administration 2009). Metoclopramide should not be given at a dose exceeding 10 mg three times a day or for longer than 3 months.

▶ Phenothiazines

Chlorpromazine, perphenazine, prochlorperazine, promethazine and *trifluoperazine.* Phenothiazines such as prochlorperazine and chlorpromazine are dopamine antagonists, and inhibit vomiting by inhibiting the chemoreceptor trigger zone along with a direct action on the gastrointestinal tract D_2-receptors. Their attenuating and dissociating effect may be desirable in hyperemesis.

Long-term experiences have not shown teratogenic effects for promethazine (e.g. Anderka 2012, Asker 2005, Källén 2002, Magee 2002) or of any other phenothiazines, although there have been case reports of cleft palate, skeletal, limb, and cardiac abnormalities with its use (Gill 2007).

Phenothiazines significantly decrease NVP (Mazzota 2000, Fitzgerald 1955, Lask 1953), although the Cochrane collaboration has not confirmed this as yet in the absence of placebo controlled trials (Matthews 2014). In a study comparing promethazine (25 mg × 3/day) with metoclopramide (10 mg × 3/day), 150 women at their first hospitalization for hyperemesis gravidarum were randomized. Promethazine and metoclopramide had similar therapeutic effects but the adverse effects profile was better with metoclopramide (Tan 2010).

▶ Thiethylperazine

Used as an antiemetic primarily in Switzerland and Eastern Europe with no evidence of risk for the fetus. In a retrospective case-control study no evidence of an increased overall malformation risk was found, but a weak association between *thiethylperazine* and an increased risk of cleft lip and palate in children who had been exposed *in utero* was evident (Puhó 2007, Czeizel 2003). In contrast, in a Swedish study the malformation rate in 137 children who had been exposed during the first trimester was 1.1% – a rate within normal limits (Asker 2005).

▶ Trimenthobenzamide

Pooling the results of three dated studies (two cohorts and one case control) there was no increased risk for malformations, and in comparison to placebo alone or in combination with pyridoxine, *trimenthobenzamide* significantly improved symptoms of NVP (Magee 2002). Two recently published articles demonstrated teratogenic potential in rats, developing growth failure, neurological and hepatic damage, so caution should be exercised in respect to this antiemetic (Fazliogullari 2012, Goksu Erol 2011).

> **Recommendation.** Dopamine antagonists are widely used for treatment of NVP, especially in countries where *diclectin* or *bendectin* are unavailable. Metoclopramide seems safe and efficacious, has less of the sedating properties of the phenothiazines, and should probably be first choice of the dopamine antagonists.

2.4.5   Pyridoxine (vitamin B6)

Pyridoxine has been empirically recommended for NVP for more than 40 years, although no association has ever been found between pyridoxine levels and NVP (Schuster 1985). Pyridoxine requirements increase during pregnancy, although low serum concentrations are usually normal until the second or third trimester.

Proof of efficacy was obtained in two large trials showing a significant reduction of nausea and number of vomiting episodes (Vutyavanich 1995, Sahakian 1991). The first trial showed efficacy in severe NVP only, but the second trial, larger and more adequately

Pregnancy

2.4 Nausea and vomiting in pregnancy

resourced, showed efficacy in both moderate and mild NVP. Pyridoxine was administered for 3–5 days, with the maximum benefit achieved during the first 3 days of treatment. The beneficial effect appeared to diminish over time (Vutyavanich 1995). A randomized placebo-controlled trial examined the effect of pyridoxine in women with hyperemesis. The study group ($n = 47$) received *metoclopramide*, i.v. rehydration, plus 3×20 mg pyridoxine, and the control group ($n = 45$) only metoclopramide and i.v. rehydration. The pyridoxine group did not fare better than the controls (Tan 2009). Twenty-nine women with NVP, treated with a combination of B6 (100 mg daily) and *doxylamine* (25–50 mg daily), were compared in a case control study to 29 women treated with metoclopramide due to moderate to severe NVP. There was no difference in response to antiemetic therapy between groups (Ashkenazi-Hoffnung 2013).

It is important to note that large doses of pyridoxine are neurologically detrimental in nonpregnant patients, and therefore, maximum doses of 80 mg a day are warranted (Schaumburg 1983). Many years of experience in North America with combination drugs containing doxylamine and pyridoxine, indicate that there is no evidence of teratogenicity. A case control study from the National Birth Defects Prevention Study did not find an association between use of pyridoxine for the nausea and vomiting of pregnancy and facial clefts, neural tube defects, or hypospadias (Anderka 2012) (see Chapter 2.18.5).

Recommendation. An amount of 40 mg/day initially and a maximum of 80 mg/day vitamin B6 is recommended. If vitamin B6 alone is not successful, then combined with the antihistamine doxylamine (10 mg), a combination similar to Diclectin (available in Canada), may improve the efficacy. This formulation was also previously marketed as Bendectin, which has been proved safe for use during pregnancy, even though in the past the safety of use during pregnancy was questioned in the United States. Lately a delayed release combination of Diclegis (10 mg doxylamine succinate and 10 mg pyridoxine hydrochloride) has been approved by the FDA for marketing in the USA (Madjunkova 2014).

2.4.6   Vitamin B1

Vitamin B1 (*thiamin*) has no antiemetic properties, although it should be kept in mind especially for those cases of hyperemesis gravidarum with vomiting for more than 3 weeks. Thiamin deficiency has been described in 20 cases causing memory loss, ataxia, nystagmus, visual disturbances, permanent neurological case and even maternal death (Gardian 1999) (see Chapter 2.18.2).

Recommendation. Consider treatment with Vitamin B1 as an adjunctive to other antiemetic therapy for prolonged hyperemesis gravidarum. Give 100–500 mg intravenous thiamine for 3 days, and then maintenance of 2–3 mg daily. Intravenous dextrose should not be given without prior administration of thiamine, as the metabolism of the dextrose consumes the remaining B1 and may worsen symptoms.

2.4.7 Serotonin antagonists

▶ **Ondansetron**

Ondansetron is a selective serotonin antagonist, used for treating chemotherapy-induced nausea and vomiting. Ondansetron binds to the serotonin receptors located on the vagal neurons lining the gastrointestinal tract, and block signaling to the vomiting center in the brain, thus preventing nausea and vomiting.

Although widely used for severe cases of NVP, there is inconsistent data regarding efficacy and fetal safety as it crosses the placenta (Siu 2006).

Regarding efficacy, it was not superior in two comparison studies: in one study ondansetron ($n = 15$) was compared to *promethazine* ($n = 15$; Arznei-Telegramm 2009); in the other subcutaneous ondansetron ($n = 521$) was compared to *metoclopramide* ($n = 355$; Klauser 2011). Case descriptions noted successful intravenous application where other medications had failed in severe hyperemesis gravidarum between weeks 6–30 (Siu 2002, World 1993, Guikontes 1992).

Fetal safety was first addressed in a prospective trial, where 176 pregnant women treated with ondansetron were compared with two different control groups (Einarson 2004). Control Group 1 consisted of pregnant women treated with other antiemetics, primarily doxylamine plus pyridoxine, or metoclopramide, phenothiazines, or ginger. Control Group 2 did not suffer from nausea, and did not use any or only harmless medications. There were no statistically significant differences between these groups in terms of pregnancy outcome and health of the newborns, although this study was resourced to detect a 5-fold difference in major malformations.

A recent large multicenter case control study of major birth malformations, including 4,524 cases and 5,859 controls, detected a 2-fold increased risk of cleft palate associated with ondansetron taken for NVP in the first trimester of pregnancy (odds ratio 2.37 [95% CI 1.28–4.76]) (Anderka 2012). In a large historical cohort study, from a Danish registry, which included 608,385 pregnancies with 1,970 exposures to ondansetron – there was no association of adverse fetal outcomes such as major malformations, abortion, premature delivery, stillbirth, etc. No cases of cleft palate were reported. Pasternak (2013) and Colvin (2012) reported 251 pregnancies of women prescribed ondansetron during pregnancy, and found no evidence for an increased risk of major birth defects among the offspring in a population-linked study.

The FDA has issued a warning of QT prolongation and cardiac arrhythmias associated with Ondansetron. Given that patients with hyperemesis gravidarum may have other risk factors of QT prolongation, such as hypokalemia and hypomagnesaemia, this medication should be administered as a last resort after other medications have failed (Koren 2012).

Other serotonin antagonists such as *dolasetron*, *granisetron* and *palonosetron* exist, although there is no safety data in human pregnancies and sparse data of animal pregnancy.

> **Recommendation.** Ondansetron should be used only if other anti-emetics fail due to the inconsistency of safety studies and possible side effects. The use of a serotonin antagonist in itself is not an indication for either invasive diagnostic procedures or termination of pregnancy. A detailed fetal ultrasound should be obtained if used in the first trimester.

Pregnancy

2.4 Nausea and vomiting in pregnancy

2.4.8   Glucocorticoids

Corticosteroids have been proposed to modify the chemoreceptor trigger zone in the brain, and are used to control nausea and emesis associated with chemotherapy (Italian Group for Antiemetic Research 2000).

Corticosteroids are currently used to treat intractable hyperemesis gravidarum, the most extreme form of NVP. These patients have severe nausea and vomiting causing weight loss, dehydration and occasionally requiring hospitalization. In the first randomized trial examining intramuscular ACTH versus placebo in 32 women with hyperemesis gravidarum, no difference in response between both groups was observed (Ylikorkala 1979). A number of randomized controlled studies have since been published. Twenty-five patients were randomized to receive 40 mg prednisolone daily versus placebo. The only difference between the groups was the sense of well-being that improved in the prednisolone group (Nelson-Piercy 2001). In a randomized double blind trial that compared parenteral, followed by oral corticosteroids versus placebo for treatment of intractable hyperemesis gravidarum, the corticosteroids had no effect on the hyperemesis gravidarum and did not reduce recurrent hospitalizations (all patients were treated with promethazine and metoclopramide in addition) (Yost 2003). When compared with promethazine, however, a short course of methylprednisolone was more effective than promethazine (Safari 1998). Treatment with oral prednisolone promptly resolved symptoms if given specifically to the subset of patients with the more severe hyperemesis, defined as weight loss of >5% (Moran 2002). In another prospective double-blind study each group of 20 pregnant women with the most severe hyperemesis, received either 300 mg of hydrocortisone i.v. daily (after 3 days the dose was reduced), or alternatively 10 mg metoclopramide i.v. three times daily. The women in the hydrocortisone group fared significantly better (Bondok 2006).

The safety of glucocorticoid exposure during pregnancy is controversial, see Chapter 2.15.

> **Recommendation.** Corticosteroids may be an effective therapy for severe intractable hyperemesis gravidarum, associated with dehydration. Their use in itself is an indication neither for invasive diagnostic procedures, nor for termination of pregnancy.

2.4.9   Other antiemetics

Alizapride stimulates gastrointestinal peristalsis and is used primarily prior to radiation or chemotherapy; its antiemetic effect is based on a blockage of dopaminergic receptors of the vomiting center. There are no reports about its application during pregnancy.

The same holds for *aprepitant* and *fosaprepitant*, the latter a prodrug of the former. Both are new forms of antiemetics used in oncology that belong to the neurokinin-1 receptor antagonists.

> **Recommendation.** Antiemetics discussed in this section should only be used if drugs recommended in the previous sections have failed.

Summary

Nausea and vomiting, a common predicament in early pregnancy has various treatment options ranging from diet and lifestyle modifications, to pharmacological and complementary therapy. Patients can be reassured of the benign nature of their condition, and should be encouraged to use the various treatment options that have been proved to be efficacious with little risk to the fetus.

References

ACOG Practice Bulletin. Nausea and vomiting of pregnancy. Obstet Gynecol 2004; 103: 803–14.

Anderka M, Mitchell AA, Louik C et al. Medications used to treat nausea and vomiting of pregnancy and the risk of selected birth defects. Birth Defects Res A Clin Mol Teratol 2012; 94: 22–30.

Arznei-Telegramm. Anti-emetic therapy for vomiting during pregnancy (in German). 2009; 40: 87–9.

Ashkenazi-Hoffnung L, Merlob P, Stahl B et al. Evaluation of the efficacy and safety of bi-daily combination therapy with pyridoxine and doxylamine for nausea and vomiting of pregnancy. Isr Med Assoc J 2013; 15: 23–6.

Asker C, Norstedt Wikner B, Källén B. Use of antiemetic drugs during pregnancy in Sweden. Eur J Clin Pharmacol 2005; 61: 899–906.

Atanackovic G, Navioz Y, Moretti ME et al. The safety of higher than standard dose of doxylamine-pyridoxine (Diclectin) for nausea and vomiting of pregnancy. J Clin Pharmacol 2001; 41: 842–5.

Backon J. Ginger in preventing nausea and vomiting of pregnancy: a caveat due to its thromboxane synthetase activity and effect on testosterone binding. Eur J Obstet Gynecol Reprod Biol 1991; 42: 163–4.

Berkovitch M, Mazzota P, Greenberg R et al. Metoclopramide for nausea and vomiting of pregnancy: a prospective multicenter international study. Am J Perinatology 2002; 19: 311–6.

Bondok RS, El Sharnouby NM, Eid HE et al. Pulsed steroid therapy is an effective treatment for intractable hyperemesis gravidarum. Crit Care Med 2006; 34: 2781–3.

Bone ME, Wilkinson DJ, Young JR et al. Ginger root- a new antiemetic. The effect of ginger root on postoperative nausea and vomiting after major gynecological surgery. Anaesthesia 1990; 45:669–71.

Boneva RS, Moore C, Botto L et al. Nausea during pregnancy and congenital heart defects: a population-based case-control study. Am J Epidemiol 1999; 149: 717–25.

Borrelli F, Capasso R, Aviello G et al. Effectiveness and safety of ginger in the treatment of pregnancy-induced nausea and vomiting. Obstetrics and Gynecology 2005; 105: 849–856.

Brent R. Bendectin and birth defects: hopefully, the final chapter. Birth Defects Res A 2003; 67: 79–87.

Brent RL. Bendectin. Review of the medical literature of a comprehensively studied human non-teratogen and the most prevalent teratogen-litigen. Reprod Toxicol 1995; 59: 337–49.

Brost BC, Scardo JA, Newman RB. Diphenhydramine overdose during pregnancy: lessons from the past. Am J Obstet Gynecol 1996; 175: 1376–7.

Bsat FA, Hoffman DE, Seubert DE. Comparison of three outpatient regimens in the management of nausea and vomiting in pregnancy. J Perinatol 2003; 23: 531–5.

Chittumma P, Kaewkiattikun K, Wiriyasiriwach B. Comparison of the effectiveness of ginger and vitamin B6 for treatment of nausea and vomiting in early pregnancy: A randomized double-blind controlled trial. J Med Assoc Thai 2007; 90: 15–20.

Choi JS, Han JY, Ahn HK et al. Fetal and neonatal outcomes in women taking domperidone during pregnancy. J Obstet Gynaecol 2013; 33: 160–2.

Colvin L, Slack-Smith L, Stanly F et al. Pregnancy outcomes in women dispensed Ondansetron in pregnancy. Birth Defects research (Part A): Clinical molecular Teratology 2012; 94: 404–6.

Czeizel AE, Vargha P. A case-control study of congenital abnormality and dimenhydrinate usage during pregnancy. Arch Gynecol Obstet 2005; 271: 113–8.

Czeizel AE, Vargha P. Case-control study of teratogenic potential of thiethylperazine, an anti-emetic drug. BJOG 2003; 110: 497–9.

Diggory PLC, Tomkinson JS. Nausea and vomiting in pregnancy. A trial of meclozine dihydrochloride with and without pyridoxine. Lancet 1962; 2: 370–92.

Ding M, Leach M, Bradley H. The effectiveness and safety of ginger for pregnancy-induced nausea and vomiting: a systematic review. Women and Birth 2013; 26: e26–30.

Donnai D, Harris K. Unusual fetal malformations after antiemetics in early pregnancy. BMJ 1978; 1: 691–2.

Einarson A, Meltepe C, Navioz Y et al. The safety of ondansetron for nausea and vomiting of pregnancy: a prospective comparative study. Br J Obstet Gynecol 2004; 111: 940–3.

Ensiyeh J, Sakineh MA. Comparing ginger and vitamin B6 for the treatment of nausea and vomiting in pregnancy: a randomised controlled trial. Midwifery 2009; 25: 649–53.

Fazliogullari Z, Karabulut AK, Uysal II et al. Investigation of developmental toxicity and teratogenicity of antiemetics on rat embryos cultured in vitro. Anat Histol Embryol 2012; 42: 239–46.

Fitzgerald JPB. The effect of promethazine in nausea and vomiting of pregnancy. NZ Med J 1955; 54: 215–8.

Fuchs K, Paldi E, Abramovici H et al. Treatment of hyperemesis gravidarum. Am J Clin Hypn 1994; 37: 1–11.

Furneaux EC, Langley-Evans AJ, Langley-Evans SC. Nausea and vomiting of pregnancy: an endocrine basis and contribution to pregnancy outcome. Obstet Gynecol Surv 2001; 56: 775–82.

Gardian G, Voros E, Jardanhazy T et al. Wernicke's encephalopathy induced by hyperemesis gravidarum. Acta Neurol Scand 1999; 99: 196–8.

Gilboa SM, Strickland MJ, Olshan AF et al. National Birth Defects Prevention Study: use of antihistamine medications during early pregnancy and isolated major malformations. Birth Defects Res A Clin Mol Teratol 2009; 85: 137–50.

Gill S, Einarson A. The safety of drugs for the treatment of nausea and vomiting of pregnancy. Expert Opin Drug Saf 2007; 6: 685–94.

Goksu Erol AY, Gokcimen A, Ozdemir O. Growth failure, tardive dyskinesia, megacolon development, and hepatic damage in neonatal rats following exposure to trimethobenzamide in utero. J Matern Fetal Neonatal Med 2011; 24: 1176–80.

Goodwin TM. Nausea and vomiting of pregnancy: an obstetric syndrome. Am J Obstet Gynecol 2002; 186: S184–9.

Guh JH, Ko FN, Jong TT et al. Antiplatelet effect of gingerol isolated from Zingiber officinale. J Pharm Pharmacol 1995; 47: 329–32.

Guikontes E, Spantideas A, Diakakis J. Ondansetron and hyperemesis gravidarum. Lancet 1992; 340: 1223.

Hardy M, Udani J. Does ginger help with symptoms of nausea in early pregnancy? Alternative Therapies in Women's Health 2004; 6: 25–9.

Heinonen OP, Slone D, Shapiro S. Birth Defects and Drugs in Pregnancy. Littleton/USA: Publishing Sciences Group, 1977.

Hook EB. Changes in tobacco smoking and ingestion of alcohol and caffeinated beverages during early pregnancy: are these consequences, in part, of feto-protective mechanisms diminishing maternal exposure to embryotoxins? In: Kelly S, Hook EB, Janrich DT, Porter IH, editors. Birth defects: risks and consequences. New York: Academic Press; 1976, pp. 173–83.

Italian Group for Antiemetic Research. Dexamethasone alone or in combination with ondansetron for the prevention of delayed nausea and vomiting induced by chemotherapy. N Engl J Med 2000; 342: 1554–9.

Källén B. Use of antihistamine drugs in early pregnancy and delivery outcome. J Matern Fetal Neonatal Med 2002; 11: 146–52.

Källén B, Mottet I. Delivery outcome after the use of meclozine in early pregnancy. Eur J Epidemiol 2003; 18: 665–9.

Klauser CK, Fox NS, Istwan N et al. Treatment of severe nausea and vomiting in pregnancy with subcutaneous medications. Am J Perinatol 2011; 28: 715–21.

Koren G, Clark S, Hankins GD et al. Effectiveness of delayed-release doxylamine and pyridoxine for nausea and vomiting of pregnancy: a randomized placebo controlled trial. Am J Obstet Gynecol 2010; 203: 571.e1–7.

Koren G, Maltepe C. Pre-emptive therapy for severe nausea and vomiting of pregnancy and hyperemesis gravidarum. J Obstet Gynecol 2004; 24: 530–3.

Koren G. Motherisk update. Is ondansetron safe for use during pregnancy? Can Fam Physician 2012; 58: 1092–3.

Kutcher JS, Engle A, Firth J et al. Bendectin and birth defects. II: Ecological analyses. Birth Defects Res A 2003; 67: 88–97.

Lacasse A, Lagoutte A, Ferreira E et al. Metoclopramide and diphenhydramine in the treatment of hyperemesis gravidarum: effectiveness and predictors of rehospitalisation. Eur J Obstet Gynecol Reprod Biol 2009; 143: 43–9.

Lask S. Treatment of nausea and vomiting of pregnancy with anti-histamines. Br Med J 1953; 1: 652–3.

Lione A, Scialli A. The developmental toxicity of the H1 histamine antagonists. Reprod Toxicol 1996; 10: 247–55.

Madjunkova S, Maltepe C, Koren G. The delayed-release combination of doxylamine and pyridoxine for the treatment of nausea and vomiting of pregnancy. Paediatr Drugs 2014 [Epub ahead of print].

Magee LA, Mazzotta P, Koren G. Evidence-based view of safety and effectiveness of pharmacology therapy for nausea and vomiting of pregnancy (NVP). Am J Obstet Gynecol 2002; 186: S256–61.

Martynshin MIa, Arkhangel'skiĭ AE. Experience with metoclopramide therapy in early pregnancy toxicosis. Akush Ginekol 1981; 57: 44–5.

Matok I, Gorodischer R, Koren G et al. The safety of metoclopramide use in the first trimester of pregnancy. N Engl J Med 2009; 360: 2528–35.

Matthews A, Haas DM, O'Mathúna DP et al. Interventions for nausea and vomiting in early pregnancy. Cochrane Database Syst Rev 2014; 3: Art. No. CD007575.

Mazzota P, Magee LA. A risk-benefit assessment of pharmacological and non-pharmacological treatment for nausea and vomiting of pregnancy. Drugs 2000; 59: 781–800.

McCormack D. Hypnosis for hyperemesis gravidarum. J Obstet Gynaecol 2010; 30: 647–53.

McKeigue PM, Lamm SH, Linn S et al. Bendectin and birth defects: a meta-analysis of the epidemiologic studies. Teratology 1994; 50: 27–37.

Milkovich L, Van den Berg BJ. An evaluation of the teratogenicity of certain antinauseant drugs. Am J Obstet Gynecol 1976; 125: 244–8.

Moran P, Taylor R. Management of hyperemesis gravidarum: the importance of weight loss as a criterion for steroid therapy. Q J Med 2002; 95: 153–8.

Mowry DB, Clayson DE. Motion sickness ginger and psychophysics. Lancet 1982; 1: 655–7.

Murphy PA. Alternative therapies for nausea and vomiting of pregnancy. Obstet Gynecol 1988; 91: 149–55.

Nageotte MP, Briggs GC, Towers CV et al. Droperidol and diphenhydramine in the management of hyperemesis gravidarum. Am J Obstet Gynecol 1996; 174: 1801–6.

Nakamura H, Yamatoto T. Mutagen and antimutagen in ginger, Zingiber officinale. Mut Res 1982; 103: 119–26.

Nelson-Piercy Fayers P, De Sweit M. Randomized, double blind, placebo-controlled trial of corticosteroids for the treatment of hyperemesis gravidarum. Br J Obstet Gynecol 2001; 108: 9–15.

Nulman I, Rovet J, Barrera M et al. Long-term neurodevelopment of children exposed to maternal nausea and vomiting of pregnancy and diclectin. J Pediatr 2009; 155: 45–50.

Pasternak B, Svanström H, Hviid A. Ondansetron in pregnancy and risk of adverse fetal outcomes. N Engl J Med 2013; 368: 814–23.

Portnoi G, Chng LA, Karimi-Tabesh L et al. Prospective comparative study of the safety and effectiveness of ginger for the treatment of nausea and vomiting in pregnancy. Am J Obstet Gynecol 2003; 189: 1374–7.

Profet M. Pregnancy sickness as adaptation: a deterrent to maternal ingestion of teratogens. In: Barlow JH, Cosmides L, Tooby J, editors. The Adapted Mind: Evolutionary Psychology and The Generation of Culture. New York: Oxford University Press; 1992, pp. 327–65.

Puhó EH, Szunyogh M, Métneki J et al. Drug treatment during pregnancy and isolated orofacial clefts in Hungary. Cleft Palate Craniofac J 2007; 44: 194–202.

Quinlan JD, Hill DA. Nausea and vomiting of pregnancy. Am Fam Physician 2003; 68: 121–8.

Reichmann JP, Kirkbride MS. Reviewing the evidence for using continuous subcutaneous metoclopramide and ondansetron to treat nausea & vomiting during pregnancy. Manag Care 2012; 21: 44–7.

Pregnancy

2.4 Nausea and vomiting in pregnancy

Rhodes P. A Medical Appraisal of the Brontës. Brontë Society Transactions 1972; 16: 101–9.

Safari HR, Fassett MJ, Souter IC et al. The efficacy of methylprednisolone in the treatment of hyperemesis gravidarum: A randomized, double blind, controlled study. Am J Obstet Gynecol 1998; 179: 921–4.

Sahakian V, Rouse D, Sipes S et al. Vitamin B6 is effective therapy for nausea and vomiting of pregnancy: a randomized, double blind, placebo-controlled trial. Obstet Gynecol 1991; 78: 33–6.

Schaumburg H, Kaplan J, Windebank A et al. Sensory neuropathy from pyridoxine abuse: A new megavitamin syndrome. N Engl J Med 1983; 309: 445–8.

Schuster K, Baily LB, Dimperio D et al. Morning sickness and vitamin B6 status of pregnant women. Hum Nutr Clin Nutr 1985; 39: 75–9.

Seto A, Einarson T, Koren G. Pregnancy outcome following first trimester exposure to antihistamines: meta-analysis. Am J Perinatol 1997; 14: 119–24.

Shepard TH. Catalogue of Teratogenic Agents. 7th edn, Baltimore: John Hopkins University Press, 1992.

Simon E. Hypnosis in the treatment of hyperemesis gravidarum. Am Fam Physician 1999; 60: 56.

Siu SS, Chan MT, Lau TK. Placental transfer of ondansetron during early human pregnancy. Clin Pharmacokinet 2006; 45: 419–23.

Siu SS, Yip SK, Cheung CW et al. Treatment of intractable hyperemesis gravidarum by ondansetron. Eur J Obstet Gynecol Reprod Biol 2002; 105: 73–4.

Smith CA, Cochrane S. Does acupuncture have a place as an adjunct treatment during pregnancy? A review of randomized controlled trials and systematic reviews. Birth 2009; 36: 246–53.

Smith C, Crowther C, Willson K et al. A randomized controlled trial of ginger to treat nausea and vomiting in pregnancy. Obstet Gynecol 2004; 103: 639–45.

Smithells RW, Shepard S. Fetal malformation after debendox in early pregnancy. BMJ 1978; 1: 1055–6.

Sorensen HT, Nielsen GL, Christensen K et al. Birth outcome following maternal use of metoclopramide. The Euromap study group. Br J Clin Pharmacol 2000; 49:264–8.

Tan PC, Khine PP, Vallikkannu N et al. Promethazine compared with metoclopramide for hyperemesis gravidarum: a randomized controlled trial. Obstet Gynecol 2010; 115: 975–81.

Tan PC, Yow CM, Omar SZ. A placebo-controlled trial of oral pyridoxine in hyperemesis gravidarum. Gynecol Obstet Invest 2009; 67: 151–7.

Tiran D. Nausea and vomiting in pregnancy: safety and efficacy of self-administered complimentary therapies. Complement Ther Nurs Midwifery 2002; 8: 191–6.

Trogstad LI, Stoltenberg C, Magnus P et al. Recurrence risk in hyperemesis gravidarum. BJOG 2005; 112: 1641–5.

US Food and Drug Administration. Boxed warning and risk mitigation strategy for metoclopramide; 2009. http://www.fda.gov/NewsEvents/Newsroom/PressAnnouncements/2009/ucm149533.htm.

Van Thiel DH, Gavaler JS, Joshi SN et al. Heartburn of pregnancy. Gastroenterology 1977; 72: 666–8.

Vellacott ID, Cooke EJ, James CE. Nausea and vomiting in early pregnancy. Int J Obstet Gynecol 1988; 27: 57–62.

Viljoen E, Visser J, Koen N et al. A systematic review and meta-analysis of the effect and safety of ginger in the treatment of pregnancy associated nausea and vomiting. Nutr J 2014; 13: 20.

Vutyavanich T, Kraisarin T, Ruangsri RA. Ginger for nausea and vomiting in pregnancy: Randomized, double masked, placebo-controlled trial. Obstet Gynecol 2001; 97: 577–82.

Vutyavanich T, Wontra-ngan S, Ruangsri R. Pyridoxine for nausea and vomiting of pregnancy: A randomized, double blind, placebo-controlled trial. Am J Obstet Gynecol 1995; 173: 881–4.

Weiss G. The Death of Charlotte Brontë, Obstet Gynecol 1991; 78: 4: 705–7.

Westfall R. Use of antiemetic herbs in pregnancy: women's choices, and the question of safety and efficacy. Complement Ther Nurs Midwifery 2004; 10: 30–6.

Wilkinson J. What do we know about herbal morning sickness treatments? A literature survey. Midwifery 2000; 16: 224–8.

Willetts KE, Ekangaki A, Eden JA. Effect of ginger extract on pregnancy induced nausea: a randomized controlled trial. Aus and New Zealand J of Obstet Gynecol 2003; 43: 139–44.

World MJ. Ondansetron and hyperemesis gravidarum. Lancet 1993; 341: 185.

Ylikorkala O, Kauppila A, Ollanket ML. Intramuscular ACTH or placebo in the treatment of hyperemesis gravidarum. Acta Obstet Gynecol Scand 1979; 58: 453–5.

Yost NP, McIntire DD, Wians FH et al. A randomized, placebo-controlled trial of corticosteroids for hyperemesis due to pregnancy. Obstet Gynecol 2003; 102: 1250–4.

Gastro-intestinal medications, hypolipidemic agents and spasmolytics

2.5

Maurizio Clementi and Corinna Weber-Schöndorfer

2.5.1	Antacids	94
2.5.2	Sucralfate and pirenzepine	95
2.5.3	H₂ receptor antagonists	95
2.5.4	Proton pump inhibitors	96
2.5.5	Bismuth salts	97
2.5.6	*Helicobacter pylori* therapy	97
2.5.7	Digestives and carminatives	98
2.5.8	Atropine and other anticholinergic spasmolytics	98
2.5.9	Cholinergics	99
2.5.10	Constipation during pregnancy	99
2.5.11	Antidiarrheal agents	102
2.5.12	Medications for inflammatory bowel disease	103
2.5.13	Chenodeoxycholic acid and ursodeoxycholic acid	104
2.5.14	Lipid lowering agents	105
2.5.15	Appetite suppressants, weight loss medications, and obesity	108

Gastrointestinal symptoms are common in pregnancy. Approximately 50% of women manifest episodes of heartburn. This is a consequence of the gastro-esophageal reflux due to the physiological reduction in the tone of both the stomach wall and the gastro-esophageal junction. In most cases, symptoms are controlled by a modification in the patient's diet and lifestyle. However, if a pharmacologic therapy is needed, antacids are the first choice. If antacids are ineffective, then H2 receptor antagonists and Proton Pump Inhibitors (PPIs) may also be used (*ranitidine* and *omeprazole*, respectively, are the best investigated medications of these two groups). In the case of a *Helicobacter pylori* infection, the triple therapy including omeprazole, amoxicillin and clarithromycin can be prescribed during pregnancy when indicated.

Constipation is another common condition in pregnancy, especially in the third trimester; it is usually a consequence of pressure being exerted by the uterus on the intestine, and high levels of progesterone, which reduce the contractility of the intestinal smooth muscle. If adequate hydration and a diet rich in fiber are not sufficiently effective, bulking agents may be used. After the bulking agents, lactulose and macrogol are the drugs of choice during pregnancy.

Drugs During Pregnancy and Lactation. http://dx.doi.org/10.1016/B978-0-12-408078-2.00006-8

In cases of acute diarrhea during pregnancy, priority is to be given to symptomatic therapy with fluid replacement and balancing of electrolytes. With the exception of infections that require a specific antibiotic treatment, it is rare that acute diarrhea requires a treatment that would exceed dietetic measures. In such cases, charcoal and apple pectin can be safely used; loperamide may be used, for short periods, but only in selected cases.

The management of inflammatory bowel diseases (IBD) is more complex. Generally, in order to reduce complications, pregnancy should ideally be initiated when the disease is not active, and it is very important to promptly recognize and adequately treat any exacerbations of disease during gestation. Aminosalicylic acid preparations, in particular *mesalazine*, are the drugs of first choice in the treatment of IBD. When necessary, local or systemic corticosteroids, azathioprine or 6-mercaptopurine may also be used. Other drugs should be considered only if the aforementioned agents have failed.

In the case of gestational cholestasis, a disorder characterized by generalized pruritus that usually occurs in the second and third trimester, the drug of first choice is ursodeoxycholic acid (UDCA).

Another very complex scenario is the management of hyperlipidemia in pregnancy. When prescribing a possible lipid-lowering therapy, the physiological increase of cholesterol and triglyceride levels in pregnancy should be taken into consideration, which is essential for fetal development, and risks and benefits should be balanced. Initial treatment should consist of a proper diet and a reduction and/or control of body weight. Only in severe and selected cases, should drug therapy be considered after the first trimester of pregnancy. Moreover, obese women require expert pregnancy management and appetite suppressants are contraindicated during pregnancy.

2.5.1   Antacids

Antacids are basic compounds, which neutralize hydrochloric acid in the gastric secretions.

The following are currently available as single drugs: *sodium bicarbonate*, *aluminum phosphate*, *calcium carbonate* and *carbaldrate* that have an effect similar to *aluminum hydroxide*. The latter is mainly offered as combination drugs.

Hydrotalcite, *magaldrate*, and *almasilate* contain fixed combinations of aluminum- and magnesium-containing antacids.

In addition, there are combination drugs of various compositions; e.g. of *calcium carbonate* and *magnesium salts*, of a substance that contains aluminum such as *algeldrate* combined with magnesium salts, and of combinations containing *alginic acid* or *licorice root extracts* (see Chapter 2.19).

Aluminum hydroxide and *aluminum phosphate* neutralize the stomach acid forming aluminum chloride. Up to 20% of an oral dose can be absorbed. Elimination takes place primarily via the kidneys. Animal tests indicate that absorbed aluminum salts also reach the fetus. While occasionally it has been argued that aluminum absorbed from antacids could possibly lead to functional derangements of the central nervous system or the kidneys of the fetus, no clinical evidence of this has been found.

In the presence of gastric hydrochloric acid, *alginic acid* or *alginate* form a viscous gel that "floats" on the gastric contents, acts as a mechanical barrier, and thus reduces the gastro-esophageal reflux. A study with 150 pregnant women indicates effectiveness and safety during the second and third trimester (Lindow 2003). Another multicenter, prospective study did not suggest an increased risk of negative outcomes for exposure during the second and third trimester (Strugala 2012).

Calcium carbonate neutralizes hydrochloric acid by forming calcium chloride, carbon dioxide, and water. About 15–30% of the orally ingested dose is absorbed. Patients with normal kidney function are not in danger of hypercalcemia when taking medications with calcium carbonate in therapeutic doses. Excessive calcium intake from antacids, combined with mineral preparations and considerable daily milk consumption, can result in the rare milk-alkali syndrome during pregnancy (e.g. Bailey 2008, Ennen 2006, Gordon 2005). Therefore, the maximum daily intake of elementary calcium should not exceed 1.5 g (corresponding to 3.75 g calcium carbonate).

Hydrotalcite releases magnesium and aluminum ions depending on the gastric pH.

The use of *sodium bicarbonate* can lead to a metabolic alkalosis.

There is no evidence that any of the discussed antacids is linked to teratogenicity.

> **Recommendation.** Antacids may be used throughout pregnancy. Fixed combinations of aluminum- and magnesium salts as well as combination drugs should be preferred. The recommended therapeutic doses are not to be exceeded.

2.5.2   Sucralfate and pirenzepine

Sucralfate is composed of a water-insoluble aluminum-saccharose compound. It adheres to the surface of ulcers, protects the mucosa, and is virtually not absorbed.

Pirenzepine is an anticholinergic drug, presumably only acting on the stomach, where inhibits the muscarinic M1 acetylcholine receptor. About up to 25% of an oral dose is absorbed. Experiences in pregnancy are too limited to allow a precise risk assessment, but there are also no indications of a specific teratogenic effect.

> **Recommendation.** Sucralfate may be used at any time during pregnancy. Pirenzepine, however, should not be prescribed.

2.5.3   H$_2$ receptor antagonists

Cimetidine, famotidine, ranitidine, nizatidine and *roxatidine* enhance the healing of gastric and duodenal ulcers by blocking histamine H$_2$ receptors in the gastric mucosa that induce the secretion of hydrochloric acid.

In some animal species *cimetidine* induced weak androgenic effects (Pereira 1987); however, there have been no reports of disruption in gender development in children who had been exposed *in utero*. A case report from Turkey describes a pregnant woman who developed a marked increase in her transaminase levels by taking ranitidine during the first trimester; after the medication was discontinued levels decreased (Kantarçeken 2006).

The current experience during the first trimester to exposure of ranitidine in about 1,700 women, of *famotidine* in almost 1,000, and of *cimetidine* in about 800 argues against a teratogenic potential in humans (Matok 2010, Gill 2009b, Garbis 2005, Ruigomez 1999, Källén 1998, Magee 1996). The number and types of malformations were similar in both study and control populations. Also, premature birth and intrauterine growth retardation were not seen more frequently in the exposed groups.

Extensive experience is available for the management of symptoms during late pregnancy. While *nizatidine* and *roxatidine* are not under suspicion at the moment, they have been inadequately examined, with each drug so far having been reported in only 15 published pregnancies (Garbis 2005).

To reduce the risk of aspiration at the time of a caesarean section *ranitidine* and *cimetidine* have been applied; they are generally well tolerated by the mother and her fetus.

Recommendation. H$_2$ receptor antagonists may be used during pregnancy. Ranitidine is the best investigated medication and should be preferred.

2.5.4   Proton pump inhibitors

PPIs such as *omeprazole, esomeprazole,* an isomer of omeprazole, *lansoprazole, pantoprazole* and *rabeprazole* block the enzyme H$^+$/K$^+$-ATPase, which is critical for the secretion of gastric acid.

About 6,000 pregnant women who used PPIs during their first trimester have so far been documented (reported in, for example, Erichsen 2012, Pasternak 2010, Gill 2009a, Diav-Citrin 2005, Källén 1998, Källén, 2001).

Omeprazole is by far the most extensively tested PPI, followed by *pantoprazole, lansoprazole* and *esomeprazole,* each with experiences of about 500–1,000 pregnancies. None of the studies indicated an increased risk of malformations; other problems were also not described. One study (Colvin 2011) has suggested that premature births might be more common after PPI use, although this does not appear to be biologically plausible. *Rabeprazole* has not been adequately examined. So far there are no indications of any fetotoxic effects.

An association between intrauterine exposure to acid-blocking medications and childhood asthma was found in a study that linked and analyzed a number of Swedish registers. While the normal prevalence is 3.7%, the study noted a prevalence of childhood asthma of 5.6% after exposure. Medications used were PPIs, H$_2$ receptor antagonists, drugs for the treatment of *Helicobacter pylori,* and sucralfate; antacids were not included as they are available over-the-counter (Dehlink 2009). Another study evaluating 197,060 singletons born between 1996 and 2008 in northern Denmark observed that prenatal exposure to PPIs and H$_2$ receptor antagonists was associated with an increased risk of asthma (Andersen 2012).

Recommendation. Proton pump inhibitors may be prescribed during pregnancy. Omeprazole is the medication of choice of this group.

2.5.5   Bismuth salts

Bismuth salts used previously as an antidiarrheal agent have regained some popularity since the discovery of a link between the occurrence of gastric and duodenal ulcers and an infection with the bacterium *Helicobacter pylori*. Bismuth salts have an antibacterial effect on *Helicobacter pylori*. Experiences in pregnancy are too limited to allow a risk assessment. So far there is no indication of a teratogenic effect in humans.

> **Recommendation.** Bismuth salts are relatively contraindicated in pregnancy.

2.5.6   *Helicobacter pylori* therapy

In the last decades the treatment of *Helicobacter pylori* has fundamentally changed the management of gastric and duodenal ulcers and of atrophic gastritis. The so-called triple therapy with PPIs, *clarithromycin*, and *amoxicillin* or *metronidazole*, has become standard since it was recommended by consensus conferences held around the world. Although some studies conducted in Asia have confirmed a high eradication rate (>80%), other studies have shown a reduction in efficacy due to the increase in *Helicobacter pylori* resistance to clarithromycin (O'Connor 2013, Malfertheiner 2012). According the European Consensus Guidelines on *Helicobacter pylori* therapy (Maastricht IV/Florence Consensus Report, Malfertheiner 2012) clarithromycin-containing treatments are recommended for first-line empirical treatment only in areas of low clarithromycin resistance. Moreover, treatment regimens using amoxicillin and clarithromycin are equivalent. In areas of high clarithromycin resistance, bismuth-containing quadruple therapies are recommended for first-line empirical treatment (*omeprazole-bismuth-metronidazole-tetracycline*, Malfertheiner 2012). In areas where bismuth is not available, the so-called sequential treatment (5-day period with PPI and amoxicillin, followed by a 5-day period with PPI-clarithromycin-metronidazole) or a non-bismuth quadruple treatment (amoxicillin-clarithromycin-metronidazole-PPI) is recommended (Malfertheiner 2012).

> **Recommendation.** Triple therapy can be undertaken during pregnancy when indicated; *omeprazole* is the medication of choice among PPIs. *Amoxicillin* can be safely used during pregnancy and there is no evidence of increased risks of birth defects after prenatal therapy with macrolides, such as *clarithromycin* (see Chapter 2.6). Although human data do not indicate an increased risk, the application of *metronidazole* should be carefully considered during the first trimester of pregnancy.
>
> Bismuth-containing quadruple therapies are not recommended during pregnancy since bismuth salts are relatively contraindicated (see section 2.5.5) and *tetracyclines* are contraindicated after the fifteenth week of gestation (see Chapter 2.6).

Pregnancy

2.5 Gastro-intestinal medications, hypolipidemic agents and spasmolytics

2.5.7   Digestives and carminatives

Indigestion has many possible causes. A combination of *citric acid* and *pepsin-proteinase* is available when the stomach is not producing enough hydrochloric acid.

Agents such as *pancreatin* with lipases, amylases, and proteases (trypsin and chymotrypsin), mostly derived from the pancreas of pigs, are used to treat disorders of the exocrine function of the pancreas and for cystic fibrosis. *Tilactase*, a lactase obtained from *Aspergillus oryzae*, is used to treat lactose intolerance. The gastrointestinal tract absorbs neither pancreatin nor tilactase.

Simeticone, the active form of *dimeticone*, defoams the gas-liquid mixture responsible for meteorism and thus facilitates the progressing movement within the intestinal tract. It is not absorbed and is well tolerated during pregnancy.

There are no detailed studies in animals or humans concerning the use of these agents during pregnancy. No embryotoxic damage has been observed as yet, and it is unlikely, based upon the mode of action, that these agents would be teratogenic.

> **Recommendation.** The aforementioned digestives and carminatives may be used during pregnancy.

2.5.8   Atropine and other anticholinergic spasmolytics

Atropine is a classic parasympatholytic agent that inhibits the action of acetylcholine by competitively blocking muscarine receptors. *Atropine* reaches concentrations in the fetus equivalent to those in the mother within a few minutes (Kivado 1977). Fetal cardiac frequency may increase after systemic application. It is used, among others, as a spasmolytic, a premedication in surgical and endoscopic procedures (for secretory inhibition), as an antidote for the treatment of poisoning from acetylcholinesterase inhibitors, and as a mydriatic agent.

Atropine-like belladonna alkaloids and their quaternary ammonium derivatives or their synthetic analogs are used for a number of indications. The mechanism of action of these parasympatholytics corresponds to that of atropine. When applied systemically, atropine-like effects on the fetus cannot be excluded.

Butylscopolamine is the most widely used spasmolytic agent. Orally it is poorly absorbed. Two case reports describe that, after the intravenous administration of *butylscopolamine*, eclamptic seizures occurred in two pregnant women who suffered from preeclampsia (Kobayashi 2002).

Methantheline is available for treating hyperhidrosis, irritable bladder, and gastrointestinal cramps.

There are no systematic investigations of the toxicity during pregnancy of these agents and of related spasmolytics such as *darifenacin, fesoterodine, glycopyrronium bromide, hymecromone, mebeverine, oxybutynin, propiverine, tolterodine, trospium chloride, flavoxate* and *solifenacin*. However, specific embryotoxic effects in humans have not been observed so far (Raghavan 2008, Samuels 2007, Ure 1999).

> **Recommendation.** Anticholinergic agents including atropine may be used throughout pregnancy under a stringent indication. If applied systemically it has to be considered that there can be fetal side effects (e.g. upon the cardiac frequency). Butylscopolamine is the spasmolytic of choice in this medication group. Also, for certain forms of bladder incontinence the widely used oxybutryn appears to be acceptable. The diagnostic application of a mydriatic agent is harmless. A diarrhea attack should not be treated routinely with anticholinergics.

2.5.9   Cholinergics

Many case reports on the use of cholinesterase inhibitors such as *pyridostigmine* and *neostigmine* in pregnancy have been published. Both cross the placenta. Primarily *pyridostigmine* has been used for the treatment of the autoimmune disease myasthenia gravis. Based on these experiences, cholinergics have no teratogenic potential in humans. The myasthenic symptoms observed in 10–15% of babies born to mothers with myasthenia gravis are caused by the placental transfer of receptor-blocking antibodies and not by medication.

There is insufficient data on the use of cholinergic *anethole trithione* for the treatment of dry mouth, *ambenonium, bethanechol, carbachol, distigmine, edrophonium*, and the antidote *physostigmine* during pregnancy. Nevertheless, teratogenic problems are unlikely, specifically for the widely used drugs carbachol, distigmine, and physostigmine.

For treatment of the Lambert-Eaton myasthenic syndrome 3,4-*diaminopyridine* (approved as *amifampridine*) is used; it is not a cholinergic but a potassium channel blocker. Few case reports on its application in pregnancy have been published, indicating that it is well tolerated (Pelufo-Pellicer 2006).

> **Recommendation.** Under appropriate indications neostigmine, pyridostigmine, distigmine, carbachol, and physostigmine may be used during pregnancy. If another medication of this group has been used during the first trimester, fetal ultrasound may be offered.

2.5.10   Constipation during pregnancy

Constipation refers to infrequent defecation with hardened feces, whereby a bowel movement every three days may still be normal. Up to 40% of all pregnant women may complain of symptoms of constipation. Hormonal changes during pregnancy lead to relaxation of the smooth muscle of the intestines and thus increase the gastrointestinal transit time. The enhanced absorption of water and electrolytes during pregnancy also favors constipation. Dietary habit changes and diminished activity during pregnancy may be additional causative factors.

The first therapeutic step should be to improve the situation by using foods rich in fiber and adequate liquids (about 2 liters per day), and by increasing physical activity. When these measures are not successful, it may become necessary to use laxatives to accelerate transit time within the intestinal tract.

Efforts need to be made to counteract habituation to these agents and an evolving abuse that could follow with higher doses, such as the loss of water, electrolyte imbalance, and, in the late stage of pregnancy, uterine contractions which could endanger the fetus.

▶ Bulking agents

Non-absorbable substances that increase their volume when absorbing water enhance intestinal peristalsis. This group of laxatives includes food items with a high content of cellulose such as *linseed*, *wheat bran* and *wheat germ*, as well as *agar-agar, guar gum, carboxymethyl cellulose, methyl cellulose, sterculia*, and *psyllium seed husks* (*Plantago ovata*). They are all deemed safe during pregnancy.

▶ Osmotic laxatives

Lactulose, a hard to cleave disaccharide with an osmotic effect, and its analog, *lactitol*, are widely used and well tolerated when taken in moderation. The poorly absorbed sugar alcohols *sorbitol* and *mannitol* have a similar effect when used orally or rectally, but are less tested and rarely available as laxatives.

Macrogol has a high molecular weight and acts as a laxative by increasing the liquid contents of the intestine. It is not absorbed enterally and is well tolerated.

Saline laxatives such as *sodium sulfate* (Glauber's salt) and *magnesium sulfate* (Epsom salt) have decreased in importance. Potassium–sodium tartrate, magnesium citrate, potassium bitartrate, and potassium citrate are also used. All of them act osmotically. Isotonic solutions are recommended because hypertonic solutions have the disadvantage that they remove significant quantities of fluid from the body.

Generally, magnesium sulfate can inhibit contractions, but when given orally as a laxative this effect is barely detectable. Magnesium sulfate is primarily contraindicated in pregnant women with diseases of the heart, circulation, and kidneys, as in these situations the absorption of magnesium ions brings on an additional burden. When using sodium sulfate at normal dosing, the absorption of sodium ions is negligible.

▶ Triarylmethanes

The triarylmethane derivatives *bisacodyl* and *sodium picosulfate* work as laxatives by stimulating the peristalsis of the colon.

About up to 5% of bisacodyl can be absorbed. Neither of the two agents has been shown to have teratogenic or specific fetotoxic effects.

▶ Anthraquinone derivatives

Anthraquinone derivatives with a laxative effect can be found in a number of plants: *Senna leaves* or *fruits, rhubarb root, alder tree bark, cascara bark* and *aloe* (see Chapter 2.19). The laxative effect is elicited by direct stimulation of the musculature of the colon. Anthraquinone derivatives are present as glycosides. After the sugar part has been cleaved off in the intestine it is absorbed to some degree and eliminated through urine (discoloration!). Anthraquinones are apparently not teratogenic. It is debatable whether they have a stimulating effect upon the uterine musculature, also if there is a risk of meconium release in the fetus triggered directly by aloe's active ingredient *aloin*.

Therefore, anthraquinone derivates are to be avoided during pregnancy.

▶ Castor oil

Lipases in the small intestine release ricinoleic acid from *castor oil*, which irritates the mucosa and thus leads to a laxative effect. Castor oil is a purging agent with a drastic effect not suited for long-term therapy. In humans no specific embryotoxic effects are known. Some authors caution that it may trigger uterine contractions. In the context of a "natural" initiation of labor it has been used mixed with, for instance, orange juice.

A single application of castor oil is acceptable if really needed. However, castor oil should not be used in the last trimester as it could possibly enhance uterine contractions.

▶ Lubricants

Viscous paraffin oil, *paraffinum subliquidum*, inhibits the absorption of fat-soluble vitamins (e.g. vitamin K) and can therefore interfere with fetal development. The fact that small amounts are absorbed and can trigger granulomatous reactions, as well as the risk of pulmonary damage after aspiration (lipoid pneumonia), limit the therapeutic value of viscous paraffin in general. It is contraindicated in pregnancy.

Docusate is an anionic detergent that increases lubrication for the contents in the colon. While interfering with the functioning of the intestinal mucosa docusate increases the absorption of some medications. Further, there is a report of a newborn that displayed a clinically evident hypomagnesemia after the mother had taken a high dose of docusate (Schindler 1984).

Bonapace and Fisher (1998) did not find an increased risk of malformations when docusate was used during pregnancy. Docusate is mainly available in combination with glycerol.

Glycerol is available even for infants in a rectal application. It is a trivalent alcohol that increases the stimulation to defecate. An osmotic effect leads to the secretion of water into the intestinal lumen resulting in a softening of the stool.

As a mono-preparation glycerol is harmless and to be preferred to its combination with docusate.

▶ Other medications for constipation

There are no reported experiences in pregnancy with *methylnaltrexone* that is available for subcutaneous injection for patients with constipation due to opioids, and with *prucalopride*, a selective serotonin receptor (5-HT4) agonist.

Pregnancy

2.5 Gastro-intestinal medications, hypolipidemic agents and spasmolytics

> **Recommendation.** If the conversion to a diet rich in fiber is not sufficiently effective, bulking agents may be used. After the bulking agents, lactulose and macrogol are the drugs of choice during pregnancy. If those fail, a short-term application of bisacodyl is acceptable. Also, glycerol may be used rectally, when indicated. Sodium picosulfate, sodium sulfate, and mannitol and sorbitol rectally are acceptable. Restraint is advised in the use of docusate and magnesium sulfate.
>   Anthraquinone derivatives, paraffin, and, if possible, castor oil are not to be used.

2.5.11   Antidiarrheal agents

In cases of acute diarrhea during pregnancy, priority is to be given to symptomatic therapy with fluid replacement and balancing of electrolytes. If infectious enteritis has an invasive course (bloody stools, high fever), diagnostic clarification is mandatory and antibiotic treatment may be necessary.

Diphenoxylate is available for inhibiting intestinal motility. It is a pethidine derivative, which reacts with opiate receptors, but it does not have analgesic properties.

Loperamide is related to diphenoxylate with respect to structure and action. Only a small portion of it is absorbed. In a prospective study of 105 pregnant women who took loperamide (89 of them exposed in the first trimester), no evidence of teratogenic effects was seen. Notable, however, was that the birth weight of newborns was on average 200 g lower than controls when mother were continuously treated (Einarson 2000). An analysis of data of the Swedish Birth Registry with 638 loperamide-treated pregnant women noted a slightly increased risk of malformation, but, as the author admits, exposure time, duration and application dosage were not, or were only partially, known. The statistically elevated risk for hypospadia, placenta previa, high birth weight and caesarean section was considered to be a random event due to multitesting (Källén 2008).

Racecadotril, a prodrug of tiorphan, works by inhibiting a cell membrane peptidase (enkephalinase) as an antisecretory agent in the intestine. There are no reports about its use in pregnancy.

Regarding *tannin* and *albumin tannate*, agents that are not appreciably absorbed, there are no indications of specific embryotoxic effects, but also hardly any documented pregnancy experiences.

Medical charcoal, apple pectin and similar agents do not present a danger for the pregnancy.

Oral *ethacridine lactate* is effective primarily locally in the intestine at a local level, and almost none of it is absorbed. It has astringent and antibacterial effects and some spasmolytic activity. As little of it becomes biologically available, an increased risk for malformation appears to be unlikely.

> **Recommendation.** It is rare that acute diarrhea requires a treatment that would exceed dietetic measures. Charcoal and apple pectin are safe. If it really becomes necessary to impede intestinal motility any further, loperamide may be used, preferably after the first trimester. Oral intake of albumin tannate and ethacridine lactate is likely to be harmless.

2.5.12   Medications for inflammatory bowel disease

Crohn's disease and *ulcerative colitis* are the major exponents of IBD, a group of potentially disabling disorders characterized by chronic or relapsing inflammation within the gastrointestinal tract which is often associated with the involvement of other organs. The flare-up risk of IBD during pregnancy usually depends on the disease status at conception: if before or at conception the patient was in remission, the course of the pregnancy generally takes a favorable direction and flare-ups are usually mild and responsive to medical treatment. An active disease increases the risk of miscarriage, premature birth, low birth weight, and perinatal complications. Naturally, exacerbations need to be treated during pregnancy in order to improve the pregnancy outcome. In view of the risk-benefit ratio the therapy has to be determined for each patient based on the individual course (Pedersen 2013, Bortoli 2011, Mowat 2011, Dignass 2010, van der Woude 2010, Cassina 2009, Travis 2008). This applies also for a therapy during the remission phase of an unplanned pregnancy.

The following medications are available:

- corticoids, such as rectal or oral budesonide or systemic prednisone, prednisolone and methylprednisolone (see Chapter 2.15)
- 5-aminosalicylic acid (5-ASA) preparations: mesalazine, olsalazine, balsalazide and sulfasalazine (see below)
- the immuno-suppressive azathioprine/6-mercaptopurine/thioguanine (see Chapter 2.12)
- biologic agents such as infliximab, adalimumab, etanercept, certolizumab and natalizumab (see Chapter 2.12)
- low-dose methotrexate (see Chapter 2.12)
- selective immunosuppressants (see Chapter 2.12) may be considered as back-up drugs.

Other drugs usually used in the treatment of IBD are antibiotics, PPIs and probiotics. The antibiotics metronidazole, ciprofloxacin and clarithromycin may be used during pregnancy if necessary (see Chapter 2.6). *Omeprazole* is the PPI of first choice (see Section 2.5.4). *Probiotics* derived from, for example, *Escherichia coli*, *Lactobacillus* and *Bifidobacterium* spp. have not been investigated but can be considered safe because they are not adsorbed.

Salazosulfapyridine or *sulfasalazine*, a combination drug with a sulfonamide and 5-ASA, has been the drug of choice for ulcerative colitis for a long time. Concerns that the sulfonamide, when given prenatally, might favor kernicterus in the newborn are theoretically plausible, but practically insignificant. Sulfasalazine is also an inhibitor of dihydrofolate reductase.

In most cases the anti-inflammatory portion of sulfasalazine, 5-ASA, is equally effective in the management of IBD as a single drug *mesalazine* and is currently a first-line drug in the treatment of IBD. *Olsalazine* is a double molecule consisting of two mesalazine parts and is used to prevent recurrences of IBDs. The compatibility with embryonic development is similar as that of mesalazine. *Balsalazide* is a pro-drug and is metabolized to 5-ASA in the colon.

Sulfasalazine and mesalazine have been well investigated; fewer data are available for olsalazine and balsalazide. Up to now, no animal and human studies have demonstrated a consistent teratogenic effect of these drugs. Many varied experiences support that sulfasalazine and mesalazine are well tolerated by mother and fetus throughout

Pregnancy

2.5 Gastro-intestinal medications, hypolipidemic agents and spasmolytics

pregnancy. Studies on 157, 165, and 123 pregnant women (Nørgård 2007, Diav-Citrin 1998, Marteau 1998) failed to detect an increased developmental risk. A meta-analysis including seven studies on the tolerance of the 5-ASA substances sulfasalazine, mesalazine, balsalazide, and olsalazine with 642 exposed pregnancies did not find an increased risk when compared to 1,158 pregnant women with IBD who were not treated with medication. There was no increase in miscarriages, premature births, and low birth weights (Rahimi 2008). One small study on the effects of topic 5-ASA during pregnancy did not show an increase of congenital anomalies or poor pregnancy outcomes (Bell 1997).

A case report of a newborn with renal functional disturbances whose mother had taken 2–4 g/d mesalazine from the third to the fifth month has been published (Colombel 1994). The authors' suggestion that this was caused by 5-ASA's prostaglandin antagonism has not been accepted by others. While up to 50% of orally given mesalazine is adsorbed, only small amounts cross the placenta and reach the fetus. This may also explain why so far no cases of premature closure of the ductus arteriosus have been observed when treatment took place after the 30th gestational week. On the other side, a publication described similar concentrations of mesalazine in maternal and umbilical blood (Christensen 1994).

Paternal exposure: Sulfasalazine may lead to a reversible reduction in the number and motility of sperm (e.g. Toovey 1981, Toth 1979).

Recommendation. An Inflammatory bowel disease requires treatment accordingly with its degree of intensity in the pregnancy. Flare-ups of the disease activity should be treated appropriately since they have been associated with fetal and maternal adverse effects. Mesalazine is the drug of choice for treatment of IBD and has to be dosed as high as medically necessary.

Olsalazine may be prescribed, too. Sulfasalazine is more useful in cases of extra-intestinal manifestations.

Corticosteroids may be used during pregnancy, locally or systemically, when indicated (see Chapter 2.15). Azathioprine may also be taken during pregnancy when it becomes necessary. The same holds for 6-mercaptopurine and, in a more limited way, for 6-thioguanine. Biological agents such as infliximab and adalimumab are only to be used when the aforementioned agents have failed (see Chapter 2.12); their use specifically during the second trimester should be critically assessed as they easily cross the placenta. Methotrexate and mycophenolate mofetil are contraindicated.

2.5.13   Chenodeoxycholic acid and ursodeoxycholic acid

Chenodeoxycholic acid and *ursodeoxycholic acid* (UDCA) or a combination of both are usually used in the treatment of cholesterol-containing gallstones, chronic cholestatic liver diseases and intrahepatic cholestasis of pregnancy.

The formation of gallstones with cholesterol is favored during pregnancy presumably due to a lessened contractility of the gall bladder. This effect is apparently not due to the also observed increase on the cholesterol concentration in the biliary fluid (Braverman 1980). Ursodeoxycholic acid (UDCA) is effective in cases of hepatocellular damage induced by bile acid, thus foremost in cholestatic diseases such as primary biliary cirrhosis. Continuous therapy will be necessary as it is a symptomatic treatment.

At the time of writing, there have been no definite studies on the use of UDCA during the first trimester of pregnancy, and no reports of embryotoxicity have been reported. In the Berlin TIS databank there are 55 pregnancies with UDCA exposure during the first trimester and no malformations were observed. So far, only four cases have been published with exposure during the first trimester (Zamah 2008, Korkut 2005). Malformations and liver damage have been observed in animal experiments when these medications were administered; a corresponding finding has not been observed in humans.

Meaningful investigations assessing the safety of UDCA during the second part of pregnancy are present, most of all for the management of gestational cholestasis (e.g. Joutsiniemi 2013, Bacq 2012, Binder 2006, Liu 2006, Glantz 2005, Roncaglia 2004).

A comparative study of 84 women with gestational cholestasis taking either UDCA or *cholestyramine* indicated marked advantages for the use of UDCA. It decreased itching more effectively, resulted in less prematurity, and brought liver values to lower levels (Kondrackiene 2005). UDCA treatment is able to prevent intrauterine death from gestational cholestasis.

There is no documented experience with the use of chenodeoxycholic acid in pregnancy.

Recommendation. Chenodeoxycholic acid and UDCA should be avoided during the first three months of pregnancy. If a patient conceives during therapy, the medication should be discontinued, if possible. Exceptions are chronic cholestatic liver diseases, such as primary biliary cirrhosis, that may have to be treated throughout pregnancy with UDCA. Gestational cholestasis may be treated with UDCA. After exposure during the first trimester, a follow-up sonogram may be offered to verify normal fetal development.

2.5.14   Lipid lowering agents

▶ **Clofibric acid derivatives and analogs**

Fibrates are lipid reducer drugs that act on the triglycerides and, to a limited extent, on cholesterol. In the treatment of hypercholesterolemia fibrates represent an outdated treatment approach; the superiority of statins has been documented. Treatment with fibrates is further compromised by suspected carcinogenicity, hepatotoxicity, and immune reactions. Moreover, as the fetus has a diminished ability to conjugate glucuronides, it is possible that toward the end of pregnancy fibrates accumulate in the fetus.

Pharmacologically and toxicologically *bezafibrate, etofibrate, fenofibrate, ciprofibrate* and *gemfibrozil* appear similar to *clofibrate* that has been withdrawn from the market in several countries because of severe side effects.

Gemfibrozil is useful (as a back-up medication) for the management of severe hypertriglyceridemia and combined hypertriglyceridemia and hypercholesterolemia, more so when there is a high risk for pancreatitis.

A pregnant woman who developed a pancreatitis with severe hyperlipidemia has been treated successfully with fenofibrate (weeks 32–35) delivering a healthy boy (Whitten 2011).

Experiences with the above-mentioned medications are inadequate for a risk assessment. However, there is no evidence of a significant teratogenic potential in humans.

> **Recommendation.** Fibrates should not be prescribed during pregnancy.

▶ Statins

Statins are cholesterol reducers, which inhibit the 3-hydroxy-3-methylglutaryl coenzyme A (HMG-CoA) reductase, an enzyme critical for the cholesterol biosynthesis. *Atorvastatin, fluvastatin, lovastatin, simvastatin,* and *pitavastatin* are lipophilic drugs, while *pravastatin* and *rosuvastatin* are hydrophilic. *Cerivastatin* was removed from the market in 2001 as it leads to severe rhabdomyolysis, sometimes with lethal outcome.

Indisputably, statins have a beneficial effect in secondary prevention in patients who have manifested a cardiovascular disease. Less clear is the situation regarding their use for primary prevention. Thus, a recent meta-analysis failed to find a reduction in the mortality when statins were used in patients without preexisting cardiovascular disease (Ray 2010).

There are theoretical concerns about the use of these medications in pregnancy, when an undisturbed cholesterol synthesis is important. A number of malformations, such as holoprosencephaly, other central nervous system (CNS) malformations, and limb defects (Edison 2004), have been observed in newborns prenatally exposed to simvastatin and other lipophilic statins. Since the binding of cholesterol to the sonic hedgehog homolog (SHH) protein is necessary for normal embryogenesis, it has been debated if the above-mentioned malformations are connected to a defective pathway of SHH protein. Moreover, there is some suspicion that statins can influence the development of the embryo and fetus by blocking the synthesis of cholesterol.

Apart from an analysis of 70 retrospective case reports of the American Food and Drug Administration (FDA) (Edison 2004) where CNS and limb abnormalities were discussed as a possible risk – although doubted by other authors (e.g. Gibb 2005) – there are no other studies suggesting a risk of embryonic/fetal development.

Positive experiences with the use of statins during pregnancy covers more than 600 women exposed to them. One manufacturer reports about 225 prospectively ascertained pregnancies where simvastatin or lovastatin was used. Retrospective case reports were also analyzed (Pollack 2005). They did not reveal an increased risk of malformations, nor did two prospective studies with 64 (Taguchi 2008) and 249 (Winterfeld 2013) pregnant women exposed in the first trimester. An investigation with registry data of 64 pregnancies with exposure to statins did not find an increased risk when compared to a fibrate group and a control group with affected women not taking any medication (Ofori 2007). Evaluation of the data of the National Birth Defect Prevention Study and the Slone Epidemiology Center

Birth Defects Study failed to reveal a malformation pattern (Petersen 2008). In these studies children displayed malformations, and 13 and 9, respectively, had been exposed to statins, but none displayed holoprosencephaly or other CNS abnormalities or limb malformations. The methods applied to collect the data in different studies and their low case numbers do not allow a reliable assessment of risk. However, the data do not suggest that statins are teratogenic in humans.

When interpreting these data it should be recognized that the mothers have significant comorbidity, such as obesity, diabetes mellitus, hypertension, and preeclampsia.

> **Recommendation.** Statins used for primary prevention should be discontinued when planning a pregnancy, or at the very latest when a (unplanned) pregnancy is diagnosed, as the therapeutic benefit still has not been proven, and harm for the mother is not to be expected when therapy is withheld during the duration of her pregnancy. However, for women with severe metabolic disease an individual decision should be made weighting risks and benefits. If statins were prescribed for secondary prophylaxis after a cardiovascular event, they may be continued in pregnancy as well, if this is deemed necessary. In this case, proven medications such as simvastatin are to be preferred. After statin exposure during the first trimester, a detailed fetal ultrasound should be offered to ascertain normal fetal development.

▶ Colestyramine

Colestyramine, also cholestyramine, is an anion exchange resin that is not adsorbed by the gastrointestinal tract. It binds with bile acids forming an insoluble complex that is eliminated with the feces. As a result serum cholesterol and low-density lipoproteins are reduced. Colestyramine is used in the treatment of dyslipidemia, chronic cholestatic liver diseases and intrahepatic cholestasis of pregnancy. *Ursodeoxycholic acid*, however, is more effective in the treatment of hitching due to gestational cholestasis (Kondrackiene 2005).

Case reports with colestyramine do not show any signs of teratogenicity (Landon 1987). This is further supported by a recommendation of the manufacturer to use colestyramine as a washout therapy (3× daily 8 g over 11 days) when there had been an accidental *leflunomide* treatment during pregnancy. In the largest prospective study assessing the compatibility of leflunomide in the first trimester, 61 pregnant women had received colestyramine (Cassina 2012, Chambers 2010). Evidently, it was well tolerated when taken for a short time.

Moreover, there is a theoretical risk for fetuses because colestyramine binds not only to bile acids but also to other lipophilic agents such as fat-soluble vitamins and medications. Two case reports describe severe brain hemorrhage in fetuses after exposure to colestyramine and discuss a vitamin K deficiency due to the pharmacologic therapy of the mother (Sadler 1995, and from unpublished own data).

Other bile acid sequestrants that are not adsorbed by the gastrointestinal tract are *colestipol* and *colesevelam*. These medications have not been sufficiently studied for pregnancy effects, but there have not, as yet, been indications of specific teratogenic effects. As with the related agent cholestyramine, they can bind and impede the absorption of a variety of nutrients.

Pregnancy

2.5 Gastro-intestinal medications, hypolipidemic agents and spasmolytics

> **Recommendation.** When UDCA cannot be used for the treatment of gestational cholestasis, colestyramine may be used. When absolutely necessary, colestyramine may also be used to lower a high lipid level. If given for a longer time, the need for the supply of fat-soluble vitamins has to be considered, although these have to be taken at a different time from colestyramine. A washout therapy may be conducted when leflunomide has been used.

▶ Other lipid-lowering drugs

Fish oil contains the omega-3 fatty acids (eicosapentaenoic, docosahexaenoic and linoleic acids) that are thought to reduce triglyceride levels. The mechanism of action remains unclear and the effectiveness in terms of any reduction of vascular problems is unproven.

Nicotinic acid, a water-soluble B-vitamin, and its derivative *acipimox* are used in the treatment of hypertriglyceridemia but their mechanism of action has not been fully explained. Nicotinic acid often triggers a flush, and to control this side effect, a combination drug with *Laropiprant* and nicotinic acid has been released. Laropiprant is a prostaglandin D2 receptor 1 antagonist that has its own side effect profile. It has not yet been tested whether this therapy has a positive effect upon cardiovascular endpoints.

Ezetimibe selectively inhibits the intestinal resorption of cholesterol from food and bile. It may be used in combination with statins, when these are not effective alone. There is some concern that the combination of these two cholesterol-lowering drugs could lead to a higher incidence of myopathy and hepatitis with elevations of transaminases.

Lomitapide is a new medication used in the treatment of homozygous familial hypercholesterolemia as a single drug or in association with other lipid reducers; it reduces the serum cholesterol levels inhibiting the microsomal triglyceride transfer protein (MTTP), which is necessary for very low-density lipoprotein (VLDL) assembly. Experiences in pregnancy are not available for the above-mentioned drugs.

> **Recommendation.** Fish oil preparations lack proof of effectiveness and are not recommended. The other lipid-lowering agents mentioned here should not be prescribed as they lack safety data.

2.5.15   Appetite suppressants, weight loss medications, and obesity

Amfepramone (*diethylpropion*), *clobenzorex*, *fenproporex*, *mefenorex*, *norpseudoephedrine* (*cathine*), *phentermine* and *phenylpropanolamine* are sympathomimetic drugs and belong to the class of appetite suppressants.

Most anorectics have been taken off the market in Europe, even *dexfenfluramine* worldwide, because of cardiac side effects. On the basis of experimental results, and single case observations, concerns have been repeatedly expressed about the use of appetite suppressants in pregnancy. It has been pointed out that these drugs have a similar potential as amphetamines in reducing vascular perfusion that theoretically could lead to vascular disruption-related birth defects. Some authors discuss embryotoxic damage such as neural tube defects which could be caused by disturbances in temperature regulation or ketoacidosis induced by weight loss (Robert 1992). A study by the European Network of Teratology Information Services (ENTIS) with 168 pregnancies primarily exposed to dexfenfluramine did not reveal any teratogenic properties of appetite suppressants (Vial 1992).

Approval of the serotonin- and noradrenaline-reuptake inhibitor *sibutramine* was withdrawn in 2010 as this agent is structurally related to amphetamines that present a negative risk-benefit profile, namely increased cardiovascular incidences and little reduction in weight. A case series with 52 pregnant women (de Santis 2006), and publications of over 10 and 2 pregnancies, respectively (Einarson 2004, Kardioglu 2004), did not display a specific risk when it was used in the first trimester.

Orlistat, a lipase inhibitor, is a weight-loss drug little of which is absorbed by the gastrointestinal tract, making it unlikely that it will induce teratogenic effects. There is a case reported by Kalyoncu (2005) that discusses the birth of a healthy mature girl after exposure until the eighth gestational week.

Obesity increases worldwide and occurs more commonly in younger people. According to the latest estimates in European Union countries, overweight (BMI $\geq$25 kg/m^2) affects 30–60% of adult women, and obesity (BMI $\geq$30 kg/m^2) affects 9–30% of adult women (European Commission 2010, WHO, IASO).

According to a study in the USA from 2007/2008, 34% of women in the age group of 20–39 years are obese (BMI $\geq$30 kg/m^2) and 18.9% have a BMI $\geq$35 kg/m^2 with increasing tendency (Carmichael 2010).

Depending on the amount of the obesity there is a 2- to 3-fold increased risk of neural tube defects while the link to other malformations remains unclear (Agopian 2013, Gao 2013, McMahon 2013, Yang 2012, Carmichael 2010). Cardiac malformation, cleft lip and palate, anorectal atresia, hydrocephalus, and limb defect are 1.2–1.7 times more common according to a meta-analysis (Carmichael 2010).

In obese women complications of pregnancy increase with the BMI, such as hypertension, preeclampsia, gestational diabetes, fetal and neonatal macrosomia, caesarean sections, shoulder dystocia, fetal hypoxia, and neonatal infections; such problems were also noted in obese pregnant women without diabetic metabolic problems (Blomberg 2013, Bonnesen 2013, Cnattingius 2013, Minsart 2013, Catalano 2012, Marshall 2012, HAPO Study Cooperative Research Group 2010, American Dietetic Association 2009).

Recommendation. Obese women require expert pregnancy management. Appetite suppressants are contraindicated during pregnancy. Accidental use does not justify a risk-based pregnancy termination (see Chapter 1.13). In the case of abuse or long-term use during pregnancy, as well as after a considerable loss of weight in early pregnancy, a detailed fetal ultrasound is recommended to evaluate morphologic development; screening for neural tube defects using maternal serum or amniotic fluid α-fetoprotein can be considered.

References

Agopian AJ, Tinker SC, Lupo PJ et al. Proportion of neural tube defects attributable to known risk factors. Birth Defects Res A Clin Mol Teratol 2013; 97: 42–6.
American Dietetic Association; American Society of Nutrition, Siega-Riz AM, King JC. Position of the American Dietetic Association and American Society for Nutrition: obesity, reproduction, and pregnancy outcomes. J Am Diet Assoc 2009; 109: 918–27.

Andersen AB, Erichsen R, Farkas DK et al. Prenatal exposure to acid-suppressive drugs and the risk of childhood asthma: a population-based Danish cohort study. Aliment Pharmacol Ther 2012; 35: 1190–8.

Bacq Y, Sentilhes L, Reyes HB et al. Efficacy of ursodeoxycholic acid in treating intrahepatic cholestasis of pregnancy: a meta-analysis. Gastroenterology 2012; 143: 1492–501.

Bailey CS, Weiner JJ, Gibby OM et al. Excessive calcium ingestion leading to milk-alkali syndrome. Ann Clin Biochem 2008; 45: 527–9.

Bell CM, Habal FM. Safety of topical 5-aminosalicylic acid in pregnancy. Am J Gastroenterol 1997; 92: 2201–2.

Binder T, Salaj P, Zima T et al. Randomized prospective comparative study of ursodeoxycholic acid and S-adenosyl-L-methionine in the treatment of intrahepatic cholestasis of pregnancy. J Perinat Med 2006; 34: 383–91.

Blomberg M. Maternal obesity, mode of delivery, and neonatal outcome. Obstet Gynecol 2013; 122: 50–5.

Bonapace ES Jr, Fisher RS. Constipation and diarrhea in pregnancy. Gastroenterol Clin North Am 1998; 27: 197–211.

Bonnesen B, Secher NJ, Møller LK et al. Pregnancy outcomes in a cohort of women with a preconception body mass index >50 kg/m². Acta Obstet Gynecol Scand 2013; 92: 1111–4.

Bortoli A, Pedersen N, Duricova D et al. Pregnancy outcome in inflammatory bowel disease: prospective European case-control ECCO-EpiCom study, 2003–2006. Aliment Pharmacol Ther 2011; 34: 724–34.

Braverman DZ, Johnson ML, Jern E. Efects of pregnancy and contraceptive steroids on gallbladder function. N Engl J Med 1980; 302: 362–4.

Carmichael SL, Rasmussen SA, Shaw GM. Prepregnancy obesity: a complex risk factor for selected birth defects. Birth Defects Res A Clin Mol Teratol 2010; 88: 804–10.

Cassina M, Fabris L, Okolicsanyi L et al. Therapy of inflammatory bowel diseases in pregnancy and lactation. Expert Opin Drug Saf 2009; 8: 695–707.

Cassina M, Johnson DL, Robinson LK et al. Pregnancy outcome in women exposed to leflunomide before or during pregnancy. Arthritis Rheum 2012; 64: 2085–94.

Catalano PM, McIntyre HD, Cruickshank JK et al. The hyperglycemia and adverse pregnancy outcome study: associations of GDM and obesity with pregnancy outcomes. Diabetes Care 2012; 35: 780–6.

Chambers CD, Johnson DL, Robinson LK et al., and the Organization of Teratology Information Specialists Collaborative Research Group. Birth outcomes in women who have taken leflunomide during pregnancy. Arthritis Rheum 2010; 62: 1494–503.

Christensen LA, Rasmussen SN, Hansen SH. Disposition of 5-aminosalicylic acid and N-acetyl-5-aminosalicyclic acid in fetal and maternal body fluids during treatment with different 5-aminosalicylic acid preparations. Acta Obstet Gynecol Scand 1994; 7: 399–402.

Cnattingius S, Villamor E, Johansson S et al. Maternal obesity and risk of preterm delivery. JAMA 2013; 309: 2362–70.

Colombel JF, Brabant G, Gubler MC et al. Renal insufficiency in infant: side-effect of prenatal exposure to *mesalazine*? Lancet 1994; 344: 620–1.

Colvin L, Slack-Smith L, Stanley FJ et al. Dispensing patterns and pregnancy outcomes in women dispensed proton pump inhibitors during pregnancy (Abstract). Birth Defects Res A 2011; 91: 334.

Dehlink E, Yen E, Leichtner AM et al. First evidence of a possible association between gastric acid suppression during pregnancy and childhood asthma: a population-based register study. Clin Exp Allergy 2009; 39: 246–53.

De Santis M, Straface G, Cavaliere AF et al. Early first-trimester sibutramine exposure: pregnancy outcome and neonatal follow-up. Drug Saf 2006; 29: 255–9.

Diav-Citrin O, Park YH, Veerasuntharam G et al. The safety of mesalamine in human pregnancy: a prospective controlled cohort study. Gastroenterology 1998; 114: 23–8.

Diav-Citrin O, Arnon J, Shechtman S et al. The safety of proton pump inhibitors in pregnancy: a multicentre prospective controlled study. Aliment Pharmacol Ther 2005; 21: 269–75.

Dignass A, Van Assche G, Lindsay JO et al. The second European evidence-based Consensus on the diagnosis and management of Crohn's disease: Current management. J Crohns Colitis 2010; 4: 28–62.

Edison RJ, Muenke M. Mechanistic and epidemiologic considerations in the evaluation of adverse birth outcomes following gestational exposure to statins. Am J Med Gen 2004; 131A: 287–98.

Einarson A, Bonari L, Sarkar M et al. Exposure to sibutramine during pregnancy: a case series. Eur J Obstet Gynecol Reprod Biol 2004; 116: 112.

Einarson A, Mastroiacovo P, Arnon J et al. Prospective, controlled, multicentre study of loperamide in pregnancy. Can J Gastroenterol 2000; 14: 185–7.

Ennen CS, Magann EF. Milk-alkali syndrome presenting as acute renal insufficiency during pregnancy. Obstet Gynecol 2006; 108 (3 Pt 2): 785–6.

Erichsen R, Mikkelsen E, Pedersen L et al. Maternal use of proton pump inhibitors during early pregnancy and the prevalence of hypospadias in male offspring. Am J Ther 2012 Feb 3 [Epub ahead of print].

European Commission. Strategy for Europe on nutrition, overweight and obesity related health issues. Implementation Progress Report 2010. http://ec.europa.eu/

Gao LJ, Wang ZP, Lu QB et al. Maternal overweight and obesity and the risk of neural tube defects: a case-control study in China. Birth Defects Res A Clin Mol Teratol 2013; 97: 161–5.

Garbis H, Elefant E, Diav-Citrin O et al. Pregnancy outcome after exposure to ranitidine and other H2-blockers. A collaborative study of the European Network of Teratology Information Services. Reprod Toxicol 2005; 19: 453–8.

Gibb H, Scialli AR. Statin drugs and congenital anomalies. Am J Med Gen 2005; 135 A: 230–1.

Gill SK (A), O'Brien L, Einarson TR et al. The safety of proton pump inhibitors (PPIs) in pregnancy: a meta-analysis. Am J Gastroenterol 2009; 104: 1541–5.

Gill SK (B), O'Brien L, Koren G. Th safety of histamine 2 (H2) blockers in pregnancy: a meta-analysis. Dig Dis Sci 2009; 54: 1835–8.

Glantz A, Marschall HU, Lammert F et al. Intrahepatic cholestasis of pregnancy: a random-ized controlled trial comparing dexamethasone and ursodeoxycholic acid. Hepatology 2005; 42: 1399–405.

Gordon MV, McMahon LP, Hamblin PS. Life-threatening milk-alkali syndrome resulting from antacid ingestion during pregnancy. Med J Aust 2005; 182: 350–1.

HAPO Study Cooperative Research Group. Hyperglycaemia and Adverse Pregnancy Out-come (HAPO) Study: associations with maternal body mass index. BJOG 2010; 117: 575–84.

IASO, International Association for the Study of Obesity. http://www.iaso.org/

Joutsiniemi T, Timonen S, Leino R et al. Ursodeoxycholic acid in the treatment of intrahe-patic cholestasis of pregnancy: a randomized controlled trial. Arch Gynecol Obstet 2013 {Epub ahead of print}.

Källén BAJ. Delivery outcome after the use of acid-suppressing drugs in early pregnancy with special reference to omeprazole. Br J Obstet Gynaecol 1998; 105: 877–81.

Källén BAJ. Use of omeprazole during pregnancy – no hazard demonstrated in 955 infants exposed during pregnancy. Eur J Obstet Gynecol Reprod Biol 2001; 96: 63–8.

Källén B, Nilsson E, Otterblad Olausson P. Maternal use of loperamide in early pregnancy and delivery outcome. Acta Paediatri 2008; 97: 541–5.

Kalyoncu NI, Yaris F, Kadioglu M et al. Pregnancy outcome following exposure to orlistat, ramipril, glimepiride in a woman with metabolic syndrome. Saudi Med J 2005; 26: 497–9.

Kantarçeken B, Cetinkaya A, Bülbüloğlu E et al. Severe liver enzyme elevation due to single-dose ranitidine in a pregnant woman. Turk J Gastroenterol 2006; 17: 242–3.

Kardioglu M, Ulku C, Yaris F et al. Sibutramine use in pregnancy: report of two cases. Birth Defects Res A 2004; 70: 545–6.

Kivado I, Saari-Roski S. Placental transmission of atropine at full term pregnancy. Br J Anaesth 1977; 49: 1017–21.

Kobayashi T, Sugimura M, Tokunaga N et al. Anticholinergics induce eclamptic seizures. Semin Thromb Hemost 2002; 28: 511–4.

Kondrackiene J, Beuers U, Kupcinskas L. Efficacy and safety of ursodeoxycholic acid versus cho-lestyramine in intrahepatic cholestasis of pregnancy. Gastroenterology 2005; 129: 894–901.

Korkut E, Kisacik B, Akcan Y et al. Two successive pregnancies after ursodeoxycholic acid therapy in a previously infertile woman with antimitochondrial antibody-negative primary biliary cirrhosis. Fertil Steril 2005; 83: 761–3.

Landon MB, Soloway RD, Freedman LJ et al. Primary sclerosing cholangitis and pregnancy. Obstet Gynecol 1987; 69: 457.

Lindow SW, Regnell P, Sykes J et al. An open-label, multicentre study to assess the safety and efficacy of a novel reflux suppressant (Gaviscon Advance) in the treatment of heartburn during pregnancy. Int J Clin Pract 2003; 57: 175–9.

Liu Y, Qiao F, Liu H et al. Ursodeoxycholic acid in the treatment of intraheptic cholestasis of pregnancy. J Huazhong Univ Sci Technolog Med Sci 2006; 26: 350–2.

Magee LA, Inocencion G, Kamboj L et al. Safety of first trimester exposure to histamine H2-blockers. A prospective cohort study. Dig Dis Sci 1996; 41: 1145–9.

Malfertheiner P, Megraud F, O'Morain CA et al. Management of *Helicobacter pylori* infection – the Maastricht IV/Florence Consensus Report. Gut 2012; 61: 646–64.

Marshall NE, Spong CY. Obesity, pregnancy complications, and birth outcomes. Semin Reprod Med 2012; 30: 465–71.

Marteau P, Tennenbaum R, Elefant E et al. Foetal outcome in women with inflammatory bowel disease treated during pregnancy with oral *mesalazine* microgranules. Aliment Pharmacol Ther 1998; 12: 1101–8.

Matok I, Gorodischer R, Koren G et al. The safety of H(2)-blockers use during pregnancy. J Clin Pharmacol 2010; 50: 81–7.

McMahon DM, Liu J, Zhang H et al. Maternal obesity, folate intake, and neural tube defects in offspring. Birth Defects Res A Clin Mol Teratol 2013; 97: 115–22.

Minsart AF, Buekens P, De Spiegelaere M et al. Neonatal outcomes in obese mothers: a population-based analysis. BMC Pregnancy Childbirth 2013; 13: 36.

Mowat C, Cole A, Windsor A et al. Guidelines for the management of inflammatory bowel disease in adults. Gut 2011; 60: 571–607.

Nørgård B, Pedersen L, Czeizel AE et al. Therapeutic drug use in women with Crohn's disease and birth outcomes: a Danish nationwide cohort study. Am J Gastroenterol 2007; 102: 1406–13.

O'Connor A, Molina-Infante J, Gisbert JP et al. Treatment of *Helicobacter pylori* Infection 2013. Helicobacter 2013; 18 (Suppl 1): 58–65.

Ofori B, Rey E, Bérard A. Risk of congenital anomalies in pregnant users of statin drugs. Br J Clin Pharmacol 2007; 64: 496–509.

Pasternak B, Hviid A. Use of proton-pump inhibitors in early pregnancy and the risk of birth defects. N Engl J Med 2010; 363: 2114–23.

Pedersen N, Bortoli A, Duricova D et al. The course of inflammatory bowel disease during pregnancy and postpartum: a prospective European ECCO-EpiCom Study of 209 pregnant women. Aliment Pharmacol Ther 2013; 38: 501–12.

Pelufo-Pellicer A, Monte-Boquet E, Romá-Sánchez E et al. Fetal exposure to 3,4-diaminopyridine in a pregnant woman with congenital myasthenia syndrome. Ann Pharmacother 2006; 40: 762–6.

Pereira OC. Some effects of cimetidine on the reproductive organs of rats. Gen Pharmacol 1987; 18: 197–9.

Petersen EE, Mitchell AA, Carey JC, Werler MM, Louik C, Rasmussen SA, National Birth Defects Prevention Study. Maternal exposure to statins and risk for birth defects: a case-series approach. Am J Med Genet A. 2008 Oct 15; 146A: 2701–5.

Pollack PS, Shields KE, Burnett DM et al. Pregnancy outcomes after maternal exposure to simvastatin and lovastatin. Birth Defects Res A 2005; 73: 888–96.

Raghavan R. The effect of hyoscine butyl bromide on the first stage of labour in term pregnancies. BJOG 2008; 115: 1064; author reply 1064–5.

Rahimi R, Nikfar S, Rezaie A et al. Pregnancy outcome in women with inflammatory bowel disease following exposure to 5-aminosalicylic acid drugs: a meta-analysis. Reprod Toxicol 2008; 25: 271–5.

Ray KK, Seshasai SR, Erqou S et al. Statins and all-cause mortality in high-risk primary prevention: a meta-analysis of 11 randomized controlled trials involving 65,229 participants. Arch Intern Med 2010; 170: 1024–31.

Robert E. Handling surveillance types of data on birth defects and exposures during pregnancy. Reprod Toxicol 1992; 6: 205–9.

Roncaglia N, Locatelli A, Arreghini A et al. A randomised controlled trial of ursodeoxycholic acid and S-adenosyl-L-methionine in the treatment of gestational cholestasis. BJOG 2004; 111: 17–21.

Ruigomez A, Garcia Rodriguez LA, Cattaruzzi C et al. Use of cimetidine, omeprazole, and ranitidine in pregnant women and pregnancy outcomes. Am J Epidemiol 1999; 150: 476–81.

Sadler LC, Lane M, North R. Severe fetal haemorrhage during treatment with cholestyramine for intrahepatic cholestasis of pregnancy. Br J Obstet Gynaecol 1995; 102: 169–70.

Samuels LA, Christie L, Roberts-Gittens B et al. The effect of hyoscine butyl bromide on the first stage of labour in term pregnancies. BJOG 2007; 114: 1542–6.

Schindler AM. Isolated neonatal hypomagnesemia associated with maternal overuse of stool softener. Lancet 1984; 2: 822.

Strugala V, Bassin J, Swales VS et al. Assessment of the safety and efficacy of a raft-forming alginate reflux suppressant (liquid Gaviscon) for the treatment of heartburn during pregnancy. ISRN Obstet Gynecol 2012; 2012: 481870.

Taguchi N, Rubin ET, Hosokawa A et al. Prenatal exposure to HMG-CoA reductase inhibitors: effects on fetal and neonatal outcomes. Reprod Toxicol 2008; 26: 175–7.

Toovey S, Hudson E, Hendry WF et al. Sulphasalazine and male infertility: Reversibility and possible mechanism. Gut 1981; 22: 445–51.

Toth A. Reversible toxic effect of salicylazosulfapyridine on semen quality. Fertil Steril 1979; 1: 538–40.

Travis SP, Stange EF, Lémann M et al. European evidence-based Consensus on the management of ulcerative colitis: Current management. J Crohns Colitis 2008; 2: 24–62.

Ure D, James KS, McNeill M et al. Glycopyrrolate reduces nausea during spinal anaesthesia for caesarean section without affecting neonatal outcome. Br J Anaesth 1999; 82: 277–9.

van der Woude CJ, Kolacek S, Dotan I et al. European evidenced-based consensus on reproduction in inflammatory bowel disease. J Crohns Colitis 2010; 4: 493–510.

Vial T, Robert E, Carlier P et al. First-trimester in utero exposure to anorectics: a French collaborative study with special reference to dexfenfluramine. Intern J Risk Saf Med 1992; 3: 207–14.

Whitten AE, Lorenz RP, Smith JM. Hyperlipidemia-associated pancreatitis in pregnancy managed with fenofribrate. Obstet Gynecol 2011; 117 (2 Pt 2): 517–9.

WHO, World Health Organization. Regional Office for Europe. http://www.euro.who.int

Winterfeld U, Allignol A, Panchaud A et al. Pregnancy outcome following maternal exposure to statins: a multicentre prospective study. BJOG 2013; 120: 463–71.

Yang W, Carmichael SL, Tinker SC et al. Association between weight gain during pregnancy and neural tube defects and gastroschisis in offspring. Birth Defects Res A Clin Mol Teratol 2012; 94: 1019–25.

Zamah AM, El-Sayed YY, Milki AA. Two cases of cholestasis in the first trimester of pregnancy after ovarian hyperstimulation. Fertil Steril 2008; 90: 1202, e7–10.

Anti-infective Agents

Stephanie Padberg

2.6

2.6.1	Penicillins and β-lactamase inhibitors	116
2.6.2	Cephalosporins	117
2.6.3	Carbapenems and monobactams	117
2.6.4	Erythromycin and other macrolides	118
2.6.5	Clindamycin and lincomycin	119
2.6.6	Tetracyclines	120
2.6.7	Sulfonamides and trimethoprim	121
2.6.8	Quinolones	122
2.6.9	Nitrofurans and drugs for urinary tract infections	123
2.6.10	Nitroimidazole antibiotics	125
2.6.11	Aminoglycosides	125
2.6.12	Glycopeptide and polypeptide antibiotics	126
2.6.13	Other antibiotics	127
2.6.14	Tuberculosis and pregnancy	129
2.6.15	Local antibiotics	132
2.6.16	Malaria prophylaxis and treatment in pregnancy	132
2.6.17	Azole antifungals	139
2.6.18	Amphotericin B	141
2.6.19	Echinocandins	141
2.6.20	Flucytosine	142
2.6.21	Griseofulvin	142
2.6.22	Terbinafine	143
2.6.23	Topical antifungal agents	143
2.6.24	Anthelmintics	144
2.6.25	Herpes medications	147
2.6.26	Antiviral drugs for hepatitis	148
2.6.27	Antiviral drugs for influenza	150
2.6.28	Antiretroviral agents	151
2.6.29	Overview of the antiretroviral medications	152
2.6.30	Nucleoside and nucleotide reverse transcriptase inhibitors (NRTIs)	153
2.6.31	Non-nucleoside reverse transcriptase inhibitors (NNRTIs)	155
2.6.32	Protease inhibitors (PIs)	157
2.6.33	Entry inhibitors	160
2.6.34	Integrase inhibitors	161
2.6.35	Hyperthermia	162
2.6.36	Long-distance travel and flights	162

Infections may be hazardous to the health of the mother, the course of pregnancy, and the unborn child. They can lead to premature labor or premature rupture of membranes and thereby increase the risk for spontaneous abortion and prematurity. Furthermore, certain germs can pass to the unborn child and harm it directly. Therefore, an anti-infective treatment which should be both effective and safe for the mother and the unborn child is often required. The use of penicillins and older cephalosporins is well documented and considered to be safe. Consequently, they are the drug of choice during pregnancy. In selected cases of bacterial resistance or intolerance to first-line antibiotics, other anti-infective agents might be recommended. Especially for life-threatening infections, a therapy with not so well-tried agents might be needed. The potential benefit of treatment in such cases most often outbalances the potential risk for the unborn child.

Drugs During Pregnancy and Lactation. http://dx.doi.org/10.1016/B978-0-12-408078-2.00007-X

2.6.1   Penicillins and β-lactamase inhibitors

Penicillins belong to the β-lactam antibiotics. They inhibit cell-wall synthesis in bacteria and have bactericidal properties. The group of penicillins includes *amoxicillin, ampicillin, azidocillin, bacampicillin, benzylpenicillin (penicillin G), carbenicillin, cloxacillin, dicloxacillin, flucloxacillin, mezlocillin, oxacillin, phenoxymethylpenicillin (penicillin V), piperacillin, pivmecillinam, propicillin,* and *ticarcillin.*

Penicillins cross the placenta and can be detected in the amniotic fluid. In thousands of studied pregnancies over the past decades, no indications were seen to show that treatment with penicillins is embryo- or fetotoxic (e.g. Cooper 2009, Jepsen 2003, Dencker 2002, Czeizel 2000a, 2001a). Nevertheless, a few studies have discussed an association with cleft palate and maternal use of amoxicillin or ampicillin (Lin 2012, Puhó 2007). Lin (2012) discussed an absolute cleft risk of 2–4 per 1,000, a quite modest increase compared to the background risk. Mølgaard-Nielsen (2012) could not find an increased risk for oral clefts after intrauterine amoxicillin exposure; but they saw an increased risk for cleft palate after pivmecillinam exposure in the third month. In one investigation of more than 2,000 pregnant women exposed to pivmecillinam – more than 500 of them in the first trimester – found neither an increased malformation rate nor other abnormalities in the newborns (Vinther Skriver 2004). Pregnant women who are treated with penicillin for syphilis may develop the Jarisch-Herxheimer reaction – a febrile reaction, often with headache and myalgia. Fetal monitoring is recommended in such cases, as uterine contractions may occur (Myles 1998). The carboxypenicillins carbenicillin and ticarcillin also did not show any adverse effects in animal experiments, but experience in humans is very limited.

Clavulanic acid, sulbactam, and *tazobactam* are β-lactamase inhibitors that are prescribed in combination with a penicillin. Fixed combinations are for example, clavulanic acid plus ampicillin, sulbactam plus ampicillin and tazobactam plus piperacillin. Sultamicillin is an orally available prodrug of ampicillin and sulbactam that is rapidly cleaved in the body into both components. So far as studied, β-lactamase inhibitors cross the placenta and reach the fetus in relevant quantities. Malformations have not been observed in animal experiments or in humans (Berkovitch 2004, Czeizel 2001a).

In a large, randomized multicenter trial, the prenatal use of ampicillin and clavulanic acid was associated with a significant increase in the occurrence of neonatal necrotizing enterocolitis (Kenyon 2001); other studies could not confirm this concern (Ehsanipoor 2008).

The clearance of penicillin and β-lactamase inhibitors is increased during pregnancy, leading to a discussion that it might be necessary to adjust dose and administration intervals during pregnancy (Heikkilä 1994). Muller (2008) failed to observe any relevant differences in the pharmacokinetics when studying 17 women who received amoxicillin for premature rupture of membranes.

Recommendation. Penicillins belong to the antibiotics of choice during pregnancy. Where bacterial resistance studies are indicated, penicillins may be combined with clavulinic acid, sulbactam, or tazobactam.

2.6.2   Cephalosporins

Like penicillins, cephalosporins belong to the β-lactam antibiotics. They inhibit the cell wall synthesis of bacteria and have a bactericidal effect. Cephalosporins are classified according to their antimicrobial activity.

Cephalosporins of the first generation include *cefadroxil, cefazolin, cephalexin, cephalotin,* and *cephradine.* To the second generation belong *cefaclor, cefamandole, cefdinir, cefditoren, cefmetazole, cefotetan, cefotiam, cefoxitin, cefprozil, cefuroxime,* and the carbacephem *loracarbef* that is related to the cephalosporins. The third generation contains *cefdinir, cefditoren, cefixim, cefoperazone, cefotaxime, cefpodoxim, ceftazidime, ceftibuten, ceftizoxime,* and *ceftriaxone.* Cefepime and cefpirome are fourth generation cephalosporins. The new cephalosporins *ceftaroline* and *ceftobiprole* have been assigned to the fifth generation, and are indicated for severe infections with methicillin-resistant staphylococci (MRSA) and other multi-resistant germs.

Cephalosporins cross the placenta and are detectable in the amniotic fluid at bactericidal concentrations. Elimination in pregnant women is faster, and it may be necessary to adjust dosage (Heikkilä 1994). According to observations so far, e.g. about cefuroxim during the first trimester (Berkovitch 2000), cephalosporins do not cause teratogenic problems at therapeutic doses (Czeizel 2001b). Normal physical and mental development has been confirmed in children up to the age of 18 months, where mothers had been treated with cefuroxim during pregnancy (Manka 2000).

> **Recommendation.** Like penicillins, cephalosporins belong to the antibiotics of choice during pregnancy. Whenever possible, well established cephalosporins should be used preferentially, e.g., cefaclor, cefalexin, and cefuroxim.

2.6.3 Carbapenems and monobactams

Like all β-lactam antibiotics, carbapenems and monobactams inhibit bacterial cell wall synthesis and thus are bactericidal. Generally, they are well tolerated and act as broad-spectrum antibiotics. The carbapenems include *doripenem, ertapenem, meropenem,* and *imipenem.* Imipenem can only be obtained in combination with *cilastin* which itself has no antimicrobic activity. Cilastin specifically inhibits the enzyme dehydropeptidase-1 and blocks the rapid degradation of imipenem. Aztreonam is the first monobactam available for clinical applications.

As far as is known, both carbapenems and monobactams cross the placenta and reach the fetus in relevant quantities (Heikkilä 1992). Animal studies and human experience do not show malformations or other undesirable effects; however, systematic investigations have not been conducted. Specifically, there are hardly any experiences in pregnancy with the newer carbapenems – doripenem and ertapenem.

> **Recommendation.** Aztreonam, imipenem, and meropenem may be used when resistance testing indicates that they are needed. Doripenem and ertapenem should only be used in pregnancy when no alternatives are available.

Pregnancy

2.6 Anti-infective Agents

2.6.4   Erythromycin and other macrolides

Pharmacology

Erythromycin and other macrolides inhibit bacterial protein synthesis and are bacteriostatic. Macrolides are primarily applied in the treatment of infections with Gram-positive germs, but are also effective against *Haemophilus influenzae* and intracellular pathogens such as chlamydia. Macrolides offer an alternative for patients with penicillin allergy.

Erythromycin is the oldest medication of this group. Its resorption can be delayed in the third trimester. Gastrointestinal side effects can lead to lower than therapeutic plasma concentrations, resulting in treatment failure (Larsen 1998). Only 5–20% of the maternal erythromycin concentration is obtained in the fetus. Therefore, erythromycin is not a sufficiently reliable drug for fetal or amniotic infections.

The newer macrolide antibiotics *azithromycin, clarithromycin, dirithromycin, josamycin, midecamycin, roxithromycin* and *troleandomycin* have a similar antibacterial spectrum as erythromycin, but to some degree less gastrointestinal side effects. *Spiramycin* is used for toxoplasmosis in the first trimester.

Telithromycin is the first ketolide antibiotic for clinical use. It is structurally related to erythromycin.

Toxicology

Erythromycin has always been considered a safe and effective antibiotic during pregnancy. Data on several thousand first trimester exposures do not support an association between erythromycin and congenital malformations (e.g. Czeizel 1999a). However, an analysis of the data from the Swedish Birth Registry showed a weakly significant increase in malformations in 1,844 children whose mothers took erythromycin in early pregnancy compared to offspring whose mothers used phenoxymethylpenicillin (Källén 2005a). This was based on an increased rate of cardiovascular malformations, especially ventricular and atrial septal defects. An update of the Swedish data verified an association between the use of erythromycin during early pregnancy and cardiovascular defects (Källén 2014). An increased incidence of pyloric stenosis was discussed by the same author (Källén 2005a). This observation after intrauterine exposure in the first trimester is biologically not plausible; but it should be mentioned that a link has been suggested between a neonatal treatment with erythromycin during the first two weeks and the development of pylorus stenosis (e.g. Mahon 2001). Other studies have failed to find a higher rate of septum defects, pyloric stenosis or other malformations (Bahat Dinur 2013, Lin 2013, Romøren 2012, Malm 2008, Cooper 2002, Louik 2002). In summary, the experiences argue against an increased embryo- and fetotoxic risk for erythromycin.

There are several reports of maternal hepatotoxic changes when *erythromycin estolate* was administered in the second half of pregnancy. These women developed a cholestatic icterus during the second week of treatment that abated within weeks when the treatment was discontinued, without evidence of permanent damage or signs of fetal compromise (e.g. McCormack 1977).

Azithromycin, clarithromycin and *roxithromycin* have also been studied in several publications without any indication of embryo- or fetotoxic effects (Bar-Oz 2012, Bar-Oz 2008, Chun 2006, Sarkar 2006, Drinkard 2000, Einarson 1998). In the case of clarithromycin, there was some initial concern as animal experiments demonstrated teratogenic effects, and for instance, in some studies cardiovascular defects were induced in rats. Recently a Danish cohort study based on a prescription register observed an increased risk of miscarriage after clarithromycin in early pregnancy, but no increased risk for major malformations (Andersen 2013a).

Experience with *dirithromycin, josamycin, midecamycin, spiramycin*, and *troleandomycin* is very limited (Czeizel 2000b). Spiramycin has been used in many first trimesters for the treatment of toxoplamosis. Although these reports did not focus on a possible teratogenic effect, numerous normal births after spiramycin exposure are reassuring.

There is no published experience with the use of the ketolide *telithromycin* in the first trimester. The animal experiments did not show that this agent is teratogenic.

A local treatment with macrolides is quite safe for the fetus. Yet, because resistance develops quickly and allergies are frequent, macrolides should be used with some reservation.

> **Recommendation.** Erythromycin, clarithromycin, azithromycin, and roxithromycin may be used in pregnancy when the resistance spectrum requires them, or in cases of an allergy to penicillin. Because of hepatotoxicity, erythromycin estolate should not be given during the second and third trimester. Spiramycin is the treatment of choice for toxoplasmosis in the first trimester. Telithromycin and other makrolides should only be given during pregnancy when no alternatives are available.

2.6.5   Clindamycin and lincomycin

Clindamycin and *lincomycin* belong to the lincosamide group. They inhibit bacterial protein synthesis and can be bactericidal or bacteriostatic depending on concentration and sensitivity. After an oral dose the resorption is almost complete. About half of the maternal concentration can be attained in the umbilical veins. There were no signs of embryo- or fetotoxic effects in several hundred pregnant women treated with lincomycin at different points in pregnancy (Czeizel 2000c, Mickal 1975). There were also no problems found for clindamycin. Pseudomembranous enterocolitis is a dangerous maternal complication of clindamycin treatment that may also happen after vaginal application.

Pregnancy complications due to bacterial vaginosis are not sufficiently preventable by vaginal clindamycin therapy (Joesoef 1999). It should be noted though, that other investigators found a reduction in late abortions and prematurity when treating several hundred patients with oral clindamycin for an abnormal vaginal flora (Ugwumadu 2003).

> **Recommendation.** Clindamycin and lincomycin should only be used when penicillins, cephalosporins and macrolides have failed. Clindamycin should not be routinely used after dental procedures.

Pregnancy

2.6 Anti-infective Agents

2.6.6   Tetracyclines

Pharmacology

The bacteriostatic effect of *tetracyclines* is based on an inhibition of the bacterial protein synthesis. These broad-spectrum antibiotics, especially tetracycline itself, form stable chelates with calcium ions. The standard agent today is *doxycycline*. *Minocycline* is especially lipophilic and displays a somewhat wider antibacterial spectrum than doxycycline. The older derivatives such as *oxytetracycline* and tetracycline are now rarely used as they are poorly resorbed.

Chlortetracycline, demeclocycline, and *meclocycline* are only used as local agents.

Tigecycline is a minocycline derivative that belongs to the glycylcyclines; it has a very broad-spectrum and is especially effective against multi-resistant pathogens such as MRSA.

Toxicology

Tetracyclines cross the placenta. According to current knowledge an increased risk of malformation is not expected when tetracyclines are used (Cooper 2009, Czeizel 1997). The results of a population-based case-control study suggested that oxytetracycline was associated with an increased incidence of congenital malformations (Czeizel 2000d). However, the number of cases in this study was small, and there are no other studies confirming this suspicion. A Danish cohort study found an association between oral clefts and maternal tetracycline exposure in the second month, but this result was based on only two exposed cases (Mølgaard-Nielsen 2012).

From the sixteenth week of pregnancy when fetal mineralization takes place, tetracyclines can bind to calcium ions in developing teeth and bones. In the 1950s numerous publications described the brown/yellow discoloration of teeth in children who were prenatally exposed to tetracyclines. Such dental discoloration is the only proven prenatal side effect of tetracyclines in humans. Under discussion were also enamel defects leading to an increased risk of caries, inhibition of the growth of the long bones, specifically the fibula and further, cataracts due to depositions into the lens. As doxycycline has a weaker affinity to calcium ions than the older tetracyclines, the risk appears to be lower for doxycycline exposures.

A discoloration of milk teeth is not to be expected prior to the sixteenth week of gestation. Even thereafter, at worst, only the first molars of the permanent teeth would be affected when the usual therapeutic regimens if current dosings are adhered to. A bigger risk for the described development abnormalities can possibly expected with higher tetracycline doses during the second and third trimester that are necessary, for example, in malaria treatment.

In the past, the use of tetracyclines, especially in high doses or via intravenous administration in the second half of pregnancy, has been associated with severe maternal hepatic toxicity (e.g. Lewis 1991). In most cases these were patients with kidney problems whose serum concentrations were markedly above the therapeutic range.

No untoward effects have been described in pregnant women who applied tetracyclines locally during pregnancy.

There is a lack of experience with *tigecycline*; no statement can be made about its tolerance in pregnancy.

> **Recommendation.** All tetracyclines are contraindicated after the fifteenth gestational week. Prior to this, they are antibiotics of second choice. Doxycycline should be preferred in such cases. Inadvertent use of tetracyclines, even after the fifteenth week, is not an indication for termination of pregnancy (Chapter 1.15). If really necessary, a local application to a small area may be conducted throughout pregnancy. Tigecyclin is reserved for special situations when sufficiently tested antibiotic are not effective.

2.6.7   Sulfonamides and trimethoprim

Pharmacology

Sulfonamides have a bacteriostatic effect by inhibiting bacterial folic acid synthesis. Important representatives of this group are *sulfadiazine, sulfadoxine, sulfalene, sulfamerazine, sulfamethizole* and *sulfamethoxazole*. For local application *silver sulfadiazine* is used for burn injuries and *sulfacetamide* for eye infections.

Sulfonamides attain 50–90% of the maternal concentration in the fetus and compete with bilirubin for binding sites on albumin. Today, sulfonamides are seldom used as monotherapy because their spectrum is limited and resistance develops rapidly. Combined with a folate antagonist such as *trimethoprim* or *pyrimethamine* (Section 2.6.16), sulfonamides are indicated among others in the treatment of toxoplasmosis and malaria. The fixed combination of the sulfonamide sulfamethoxazole and trimethoprim is available as *co-trimoxazole*. Both agents in this combination are not subject to pregnancy-induced variation in clearance that would require dose modifications. Trimethoprim is effective as a monotherapy in uncomplicated urinary tract infections with sensitive pathogens.

Toxicology

To date, there are no indications that sulfonamides, trimethoprim, and their combinations have a teratogenic potential in humans (Nørgård 2001, Czeizel 1990). An embryotoxic potential has been discussed from time to time, because antagonists to folic acid can lead to malformations in animal experiments, and in humans the spontaneous incidence of neural tube defects (spina bifida) can be decreased by the administration of folic acid during early pregnancy (Chapter 2.18). The fact that human folic acid reductase is much less sensitive to trimethoprim than the bacterial enzyme, could explain that teratogenic problems have so far not been documented in humans when antibiotics with folic acid antagonists were used.

Trimethoprim has been used for many decades in pregnant women. At present, there is an ongoing discussion concerning the association between the use of folic acid antagonists and an increased risk of congenital malformations. A retrospective case-control study discusses the causal relationship between treatment with trimethoprim and other folic acid antagonists, and the development of neural tube defects, cardiovascular abnormalities, cleft lip and palate, and urinary tract anomalies (Hernandez-Diaz 2000). Authors' views on a preventative dose of multivitamin and folic acid preparations vary. Additional case-control studies, some of them with notable methodological problems, found weakly significant evidence for the development of cardiovascular defects, urinary tract anomalies, anencephaly, limb defects, and orofacial clefts (e.g. Mølgaard-Nielsen 2012, Crider 2009, Czeizel 2001c). An increased risk for preterm birth and low birth weight has also been observed after exposure to trimethoprim/sulfamethoxazole (Santos 2011, Yang 2011). A Danish cohort study based on a prescription register found a doubling of the hazard of miscarriage after trimethoprim exposure in the first trimester (Andersen 2013b). Based on the same prescription register, an increased risk of heart and limb defects was observed after preconceptional exposure (during the 12 weeks before conception) to trimethoprim (Andersen 2013c). Beside methodological problems, such an association seems unlikely because a short-term therapy with trimethoprim does not usually lead to a relevant folic acid deficiency as a possible cause for birth defects. Trimethoprim and sulfonamides are not drugs of first choice, but they exhibit no established teratogens. According to current knowledge the teratogenic risk of a trimethoprim and sulfonamide therapy is negligible. Actually, there are no sufficiently convincing arguments to support the recommendation of an additional folic acid administration during an antibiotic therapy with the discussed medications, see Chapter 2.18.8 for additional discussion concerning folic acid usage.

Extensive, generally reassuring experiences in the use of co-trimoxazole for common urinary tract infections during pregnancy, do not include the conclusion that this medication is safe when used at a much higher dose for opportunistic infections such as a Pneumocystis pneumonia in the context of an HIV infection. So far, there have been no reports of malformations when such therapy was used in pregnant women.

There are no systematic studies about the local application of sulfonamides during pregnancy.

Neonatal toxicity
As sulfonamides compete with bilirubin for binding sites with plasma proteins, it has been argued that the risk of neonatal kernicterus is increased when sulfonamides are given at the end of gestation. With current surveillance, the danger of kernicterus is not tangible. However, a rise in bilirubin, especially in premature infants, cannot be excluded when sulfonamides have been used until birth. A Danish population-based study could not find an association between sulfamethoxzole exposure near term and an increased risk of neonatal jaundice (Klarskov 2013).

> **Recommendation.** Sulfonamides, trimethoprim, and co-trimoxazole are antibiotics of second choice throughout pregnancy. If high dose co-trimoxazole is used for a Pneumocystis pneumonia during the first trimester, based on theoretical grounds, folic acid should be supplemented and a detailed ultrasound examination should be offered to ascertain the normal development of the fetus. If a premature birth is threatening, sulfonamides should be avoided in view of the bilirubin levels of the newborn. A short-term local treatment is acceptable, especially if the site is small.

2.6.8   Quinolones

Quinolones inhibit the bacterial enzymes topoisomerase II and IV that are important for the nucleic acid metabolism of bacteria. Quinolones have a high affinity for cartilage and bone tissue which is highest in immature cartilage.

Pipemidic acid and *nalidixid acid* belong to the group of older quinolones. They have been displaced by the newer fluoroquinolones. The most important *fluoroquinolones* include *ciprofloxacin, enoxacin, levofloxacin, moxifloxacin, norfloxacin,* and *ofloxacin*. Several substances have been removed from the market because of severe side effects. *Garenoxacin, lomefloxacin, pefloxacin, rosoxacin,* and *sparfloxacin* are still available in some countries. *Gatifloxacin* and *nadifloxacin* are only used as local agent.

Quinolones cross the placenta and are found in the amniotic fluid at low concentrations.When moxifloxacin is used about 8% of the maternal serum concentration can be measured in the amniotic fluid, and with lovofloxacin about 16% (Ozyüncü 2010).

Quinolones have not been found to be teratogenic in animals but severe, irreversible damage to joint cartilages was noted in young dogs treated after birth with quinolones (e.g. Gough 1992). Such alterations have not been described in prenatally exposed children. Many publications failed to show indications of joint cartilage damage or an increased risk of malformations (Bar-Oz 2009, Cooper 2009, Larsen 2001, Loebstein 1998, Schaefer 1996, Berkovitch 1994). One study expressed concern that the prenatal use of fluoroquinolones may be associated with an increased risk of bone malformations (Wogelius 2005). Although not resembling each other, in three out of four birth defects the skeleton was affected. However, in this study of 130 women who redeemed a prescription for fluoroquinolones during the first trimester, or 30 days before conception, the total malformation rate was not increased (Wogelius 2005). In a prospective cohort study with 949 women who were exposed to a fluorquinolone during the first trimester, neither the rate of major birth defects, nor the risk of spontaneous abortion were increased compared to a control group (Padberg 2014). Altogether, most data are available for norfloxacin and ciprofloxacin and, to a lesser extent, for levofloxacin, moxifloxacin, ofloxacin and pefloxacin. There are few or no data for the other fluoroquinolones.

There have been no reports of undesirable side effects after topical use of quinolones during pregnancy.

> **Recommendation.** Quinolones are antibiotics of second choice during pregnancy. In well-founded situations, when better studied antibiotics are ineffective, those quinolones that are well documented may be preferred such as norfloxacin or ciprofloxacin. A detailed ultrasound examination may be offered after exposure with the other fluoroquinolones during the first trimester. Local treatment with quinolones is acceptable throughout pregnancy.

2.6.9 Nitrofurans and drugs for urinary tract infections

Nitrofurantoin is a chemotherapeutic agent for drug-resistant urinary tract infections (UTIs) and for the prevention of recurrent UTIs. It acts as a bacteriostatic, but is also bactericidal at higher concentrations. Details of its mechanism of action remain to be clarified. After an oral dose, therapeutic effective levels are attained only in the urinary tract.

Several publications do not support an association between nitrofurantoin and congenital malformations (Nordeng 2013, Goldberg 2013,

Czeizel 2001d, Ben David 1995), although in a number of studies, some of them with methodological faults, weakly significant findings were noted for craniosysnostosis, ophthalmic malformations, oral clefts, and cardiovascular defects (Crider 2009, Källén 2005b, Källén 2003). A case-control study observed an increased risk of craniosynostosis after intrauterine exposure to nitrosatable drugs (Gardner 1998).

As nitrofurantoin lowers the activity of glutathione reductase, discussions arise periodically as to whether an intrauterine exposure could trigger a fetal hemolysis. Bruel (2000) reported a mature newborn with hemolytic anemia whose mother took nitrofurantoin during the last gestational month. Nitrofurantoin is often used during pregnancy, and fetal hemolysis has not been commonly observed; therefore, a relevant risk is not likely. However, Nordeng (2013) observed an increased risk of neonatal jaundice after maternal nitofurantoin treatment in the last 30 days before delivery.

There is a case report of a pregnant woman who developed a toxic hepatitis after having been exposed to nitrofurantoin in her thirty-sixth week (Aksamija 2009). In another case a woman took nitrofurantoin in her thirty-third week and was interpreted to present a gestational nitrofurantoin-induced pneumonia (Mohamed 2007).

The nitrofurantoin derivative *nifuroxazide* is used for the treatment of diarrhea. There are no documented reports of its tolerance in pregnancy nor evidence of effectiveness.

Nifurtimox is a nitrofuran used for treatment of Chagas disease. Experience for pregnancy is very limited and the World Health Organization recommends that nifurtimox should not be taken by pregnant women (WHO 2013a). One study about safety included 14 pregnant women, but did not give information about the pregnancy outcome (Schmid 2012).

For local treatment the nitrofurans *furazolidone, nitrofural*, and *nifuratel* are available. There has been no evidence of embryo- or fetotoxic risk in local applications. The use of local nitrofurans, especially as vaginal therapy, remains controversial and needs to be critically assessed not only during pregnancy.

Methenamine is a UTI medication that releases the antiseptic *formaldehyde* into the urine. *Methenamine mandelate* had been used for chronic UTIs due to *E. coli* and unproblematic germs. Effectiveness and tolerance of the agent remain controversial. Embryo- or fetotoxic problems have not been reported.

There are no reports about the use of the hydroxy-quinolone derivative *nitroxoline* in pregnancy.

▶ Fosfomycin

Fosfomycin is a broad-spectrum antibiotic that is bactericidal by inhibiting the synthesis of the bacterial cell wall. It is used as an intravenous injectable and as a reserve antibiotic in severe infections such as osteomyelitis. *Fosfomycin tromethamine* is an orally taken salt of fosfomycin used for the treatment of uncomplicated UTIs. Some authors also recommend the oral use during pregnancy (e.g. Falagas 2010, Bayrak 2007). These studies, however, are primarily focused on the effectiveness of fosfomycin tromethamine, not on the risk for the newborn. Overall, the experience argues against a teratogenic and fetotoxic potential in humans.

> **Recommendation.** Nitrofurantoin can be given during pregnancy to treat urinary tract infections when the antibiotics of choice have been ineffective. If possible, it should be avoided towards the end of pregnancy. The use of nifuroxazide, nifurtimox, local nitrofurans, methenamine, and nitroxoline should be avoided during pregnancy.
>
> When the antibiotics of choice in pregnancy cannot be used, fosfomycin tromethamine may be used to treat urinary tract infections in pregnancy. The intravenous application of fosfomycin should be restricted to severe bacterial infections with problematic germs.

2.6.10   Nitroimidazole antibiotics

Nitroimidazoles are effective bactericidal agents against anaerobes and protozoa. They are converted into metabolites that impede intracellular bacterial DNA synthesis. The main representative of the nitroimidazoles is *metronidazole*. Metronidazole is now being recommended by some investigators for the treatment of bacterial vaginosis in pregnancies at high risk for preterm delivery, as a strategy to decrease this risk (review by Joesoef 1999). Others, however, failed to notice an improvement in the incidence of prematurity (Shennan 2006, Andrews 2003, Klebanoff 2001).

After oral and intravenous administration, concentrations as high as those in the mother are reached in the embryo/fetus. Significant systemic absorption occurs after vaginal application, exposing the fetus as well. The pharmacokinetic profile of metronidazole did not change at the different time points assessed during pregnancy, and did not differ from nonpregnant patients (Wang 2011).

Like all nitroimidazoles, metronidazole displays an experimentally mutagenic and cancerogenic potential (review by Dobias 1994) that has not been confirmed in humans. An investigation that ranged over 20 years did not show any indication of an increased risk of cancer when metronidazole was used (Beard 1988).

On the basis of over 3,000 analyzed pregnancies, it can be stated that metronidazole has no teratogenic potential in humans (e.g. Koss 2012, Diav-Citrin 2001, Czeizel 1998). Suggestions from the Hungarian Malformation Registry of a link between vaginal therapy with metronidazole and miconazole during the second and third month, and an increased appearance of syndactylies and hexadactylies have not been confirmed by other investigators (Kazy 2005a).

Nimorazole and *tinidazole*, both registered for the treatment of trichomonas infections, amebiasis, and bacterial vaginosis, cannot be evaluated sufficiently because of the lack of human data – the same applies to *ornidazole*. So far, there are no reports of human teratogenicity.

> **Recommendation.** Metronidazol may be used in pregnancy when indicated. A single oral dose of 2 g is preferable to vaginal administration spread over several days, particularly as there are doubts about the effectiveness of the vaginal application. A parenteral administration is only indicated for a serious anaerobic infection. Metronidazole is to be preferred to the less examined nitroimidazoles.

2.6.11   Aminoglycosides

The aminoglycoside antibiotics *amikacin, framycetin, gentamicin, kanamycin, neomycin, netilmicin, paromomycin, ribostamycin, streptomycin,* and *tobramycin* inhibit protein synthesis and are bactericidal primarily for Gram-negative germs. After oral administration only a minimal portion of aminoglycosides is resorbed. After parenteral administration of about 20–40% of the maternal plasma concentration is detectable in the fetus. *Spectinomycin* is an aminocyclitol antibiotic closely related to the aminoglycosides.

Oto- and nephrotoxic side effects are also known to occur in nonpregnant patients when aminolgycosides are used parenterally. There are case reports about the parenteral use of kanamycin and streptomycin during pregnancy describing auditory problems, even deafness, in children exposed *in utero* (e.g. Jones 1973, Conway 1965, Robinson 1964). A similar case was reported in connection with gentamicin (Sánchez Sainz-Trápaga 1998). An investigation of the hearing ability of 39 children whose mothers had received gentamicin intravenously during pregnancy found no deficiencies. This argues against a major ototoxic risk of gentamicin when used in pregnancy (Kirkwood 2007).

Theoretically, a fetal nephrotoxic risk exists because aminoglycosides concentrate in the fetal kidneys. A case report about a connatal kidney dysplasia after maternal gentamicin therapy (Hulton 1995) does not prove a clinically relevant human risk, nor does a case of a hydronephrosis and suspected stenosis at the uteropelvic junction with lethal outcome, where the mother had been treated for UTI first with *ciprofloxacin* and then with gentamicin at weeks 4–5 (Yaris 2004).

Except for these case reports, studies argue against a high oto- or nephrotoxic risk of gentamicin in the fetus and newborn. There has been no increase in the observation of malformations (Czeizel 2000e). No untoward effects have been described with aminoglycosides as local treatment during pregnancy.

Experience with *spectinomycin* is insufficient to analyze a risk in pregnancy.

> **Recommendation.** Aminoglycosides should only be used parenterally in life-threatening infections with difficult Gram-negative pathogens and when first-choice antibiotics fail. The serum levels need to be monitored regularly during the treatment. A risk-based termination of pregnancy or invasive diagnostic are not required (Chapter 1.15). If the parenteral therapy had been extensive, renal function should be monitored in the neonate and an auditory test should be performed. If local or oral application of aminoglycosides is indicated, they can be given because systemic absorption is minimal by these routes.

2.6.12   Glycopeptide and polypeptide antibiotics

▶ Glycopeptide antibiotics

The glycopeptides *vancomycin* and *teicoplanin* are bactericidal only for Gram-positive pathogens by inhibiting their cell wall synthesis. They are considered reserve antibiotics to be used against MSRA and multiresistant enterococci. To avoid the development of resistance, their application should be critically appraised, and possibly limited only to fighting problematic pathogens. Oral glycopeptides are hardly resorbed. This is useful when treating pseudomembranous enterocolitis with vancomycin. However, in this situation metronidazole (Section 2.6.10) should be considered as an alternative, as vancomycin therapy is more expensive, and to prevent the selection for vancomycin-resistant enterococci.

Vancomycin crosses the placenta reaching the fetus in relevant quantities (Laiprasert 2007). It has not shown teratogenic effects in animal studies. Experience with treatment in human pregnancy is limited to a few case reports. There were no observations of malformations, kidney damage, or hearing deficits (Reyes 1989).

Experience with teicoplanin and the new lipoglycopeptides *dalbavancin*, *oritavancin* and *telavancin* is insufficient to analyze a risk in pregnancy. *In vitro* telavancin crosses the human placenta, with fetal concentrations reaching less than 3% of maternal concentrations (Nanovskaya 2012).

> **Recommendation.** Glycopeptides should only be used in cases of life-threatening bacterial infections; vancomycin should then be preferred.

▶ **Lipopeptide antibiotics**

Daptomycin belongs to a new class of cyclic lipopeptides and is effective exclusively against Gram-positive bacteria. It works by interfering with the bacterial cell membrane and protein synthesis, and is indicated to treat complicated infections with difficult pathogens. In animal experiments, daptomycin crossed the placenta and was not teratogenic. Two children whose mothers took daptomycin in the fourteenth and twenty-seventh weeks were unremarkable (Stroup 2010, Shea 2008).

> **Recommendation.** The use of daptomycin is limited to cases of life-threatening bacterial infections.

▶ **Polypeptide antibiotics**

Polymyxins belong to the polypeptide antibiotics that are bactericidal by interfering with the transport mechanism of the cell wall. While the polymyxin *colistin* is today mostly used locally, it can also be applied parenterally where there is an infection with multi-resistant Gram-negative germs. In patients with mucoviscidosis it is used as an inhalative. Enterally colistin is not resorbed; therefore its oral administration is used to selectively decontaminate the intestinal tract.

The polypeptide antibiotics *bacitracin*, *polymyxin B*, and *tyrothricin* are used locally. Only limited experience is available in the application of polypeptide antibiotics during pregnancy and do not indicate a substantial risk (Kazy 2005b).

> **Recommendation.** The parental use of colistin is limited to cases of life-threatening bacterial infections. The local and oral application of polypeptide antibiotics need to be critically assessed.

2.6.13   Other antibiotics

▶ **Chloramphenicol**

Chloramphenicol and *Tiamphenicol* inhibit bacterial protein synthesis and have bacteriostatic activity. Chloramphenicol is relatively toxic, and can cause severe agranulocytosis. It crosses the placenta well and can reach therapeutic concentrations in the fetus. In premature and term births it may lead to the grey baby syndrome. Chloramphenicol can reach toxic levels in the neonate even when only the mother has been treated. There have been no suggestions of malformations (Czeizel 2000f).

Experience with thiamphenicol is insufficient to analyze a risk in pregnancy.

> **Recommendation.** The systemic use of chloramphenicol and thiamphenicol is contraindicated throughout pregnancy. Exceptions are life-threatening maternal infections that do not respond to less toxic antibiotics. When systemic treatment is absolutely necessary before birth, it is important to observe the newborn for toxic symptoms. A local application is also to be avoided during pregnancy.

▶ Dapsone

Dapsone, used among other indications against leprosis, apparently has no teratogenic potential (e.g. Lush 2000, Bhargava 1996). However, cases of hemolytic anemia have been reported in mothers and newborns. As dapsone bears a structural similarity to the sulfonamides, it has been argued that it might compete with bilirubin for protein binding, and thus could lead to hyperbilirubinemia in the newborn.

> **Recommendation.** During pregnancy, dapsone should be reserved for specific indications. If treatment took place in the first trimester, a detailed ultrasound examination should be offered to ascertain the normal development of the fetus.

▶ Fidaxomicin

Fidaxomicin is a macrocyclic antibiotic which is approved for the treatment of infections with Clostridium difficile. Enterally fidaxomicin is very poorly resorbed. No experiences have been reported about its use during pregnancy.

> **Recommendation.** Fidaxomicin should be avoided in pregnancy. If treatment took place in the first trimester, a detailed ultrasound examination should be offered to ascertain the normal development of the fetus.

▶ Linezolid

Linezolid is a member of the oxazolidinone class, a new group of antibiotics. It acts bactericidally by inhibiting bacterial protein synthesis and is indicated in the treatment of multi-resistant pathogens. There is just one case report about the use of linezolid during pregnancy. After intrauterine exposure from gestational weeks 14 to 18 a healthy infant was delivered at term (Mercieri 2010).

> **Recommendation.** With the lack of experience, linezolid should only be used for severe infections with problematic germs. If treatment took place in the first trimester, a detailed ultrasound examination should be offered to ascertain the normal development of the fetus.

▶ Pentamidine

The antiprotozoal agent *pentamidine*, among others effective in Pneumocystis pneumonia, has not been evaluated sufficiently in pregnancy to estimate its embryotoxic potential for humans. Usually it can be replaced by other antibiotics, e.g. *co-trimoxazole* (Section 2.6.7).

> **Recommendation.** Pentamidine is to be reserved in pregnancy for special situations when better tested antibiotics are not effective. If treatment took place in the first trimester, a detailed ultrasound examination should be offered to ascertain the normal development of the fetus.

▶ Rifaximin

Rifaximin is an antibiotic to treat travelers' diarrhea. There is not enough experience regarding its use in pregnancy. Minimal enteral resorption and negative animal testing suggest that a high embryotoxic risk is unlikely.

> **Recommendation.** If possible, rifaximin should be avoided during pregnancy.

▶ Streptogramins

Streptogramins are a group of cyclic peptide antibiotics that inhibit, like *macrolides* and *lincosamides*, the synthesis of bacterial proteins. They are derivatives of the naturally occurring *pristinamycin*. The later developed derivatives *quinupristin* and *dalfopristin* are used in a fixed combination. Streptogramins should only be applied as reserve antibiotics for infections with highly resistant Gram-positive germs. Reports about use in pregnancy have not been available.

> **Recommendation.** Streptogramins are to be avoided during pregnancy. If treatment took place in the first trimester, a detailed ultrasound examination should be offered to ascertain the normal development of the fetus.

2.6.14   Tuberculosis and pregnancy

Active tuberculosis (TB) requires treatment in pregnancy, as the disease endangers not only the mother, but also the fetus. Pregnancy does not seem to affect the course of TB. The prevalence of congenital TB is less than 1% where no treatment is initiated. Lin (2010) investigated 761 newborns of mothers who had received treatment for TB during the gestation. Their children were smaller and had lower birth weights than the control group of children of healthy mothers.

There are slight differences in the recommendations of the different organizations in the world, such as the WHO (2010a), the International Union against Tuberculosis and Lung Disease (IUATLD), and several national organizations (e.g. Blumberg 2003). Treatment considerations depend on disease status and drug resistance. First-line drugs for the treatment of TB during pregnancy are *isoniazid* (+*pyridoxine*), *rifampicin, ethambutol* and *pyrazinamide*. These standard medications have not shown teratogenic or fetotoxic effects in humans (e.g. Bothamley 2001). As far as we know today, TB drugs reach the fetus in relevant quantities. An increasing development of resistance makes it harder to choose the right medication in pregnancy. Pregnant women with multidrug-resistant TB (MDR-TB) may also require second-line antituberculous

Pregnancy

2.6 Anti-infective Agents

drugs; the necessity for treatment should be weighed against the risk for the fetus on an individual base. Current experiences in the management of MDR-TB argue against a high risk of the reserve drugs for the newborn (Drobac 2005, Shin 2003). Streptomycin, however, should be avoided because of its ototoxic potential.

▶ Ethambutol

Ethambutol is a bacteriostatic drug used against tuberculosis. It can cross the placenta, but the risk of congenital malformations when used during pregnancy appears to be low. There are no reports indicating that ethambutol can cause ocular toxicity in the fetus, as it does in adults, when given in higher doses.

> **Recommendation.** Ethambutol is a first-line drug for treatment of tuberculosis during pregnancy.

▶ Isoniazid

Isoniazid (INH) has proven to be a highly effective drug against many strains of mycobacterium, and can be used for tuberculous prophylaxis and for treatment of an active disease during pregnancy. Although INH can cross the placenta, it does not appear to be teratogenic, even when given during the first trimester. The older literature contains case reports of different malformations and neurological damages in prenatally exposed children. INH intake, lack of pyridoxine, co-medication, and even the TB disease itself was blamed. Newer publications did not confirm a teratogenic risk (e.g. Taylor 2013, Czeizel 2001e). In summary, experiences speak against a major risk. INH increases pyridoxine metabolism, which may be responsible for CNS toxicity. To prevent a possible vitamin B6 deficiency, INH should be given during pregnancy in combination with *pyridoxine*.

> **Recommendation.** Isoniazid is a first-line drug for treatment of tuberculosis during pregnancy. It needs to be given together with pyridoxine.

▶ Pyrazinamide

Pyrazinamide (PZA) is an antibiotic with specific effectiveness against Mycobacterium tuberculosis. As its structure resembles nicotinamide, it is assumed that it intervenes with the nucleic acid metabolism of the bacterial cell. PZA has effective bactericidal properties. Systematic studies of its tolerance in pregnancy are lacking. So far, there has been no evidence of embryo- or fetotoxic effects in humans. The use of PZA during pregnancy is recommended in several guidelines (e.g. WHO 2010a). The American Thoracic Society recommends in its guidelines to hold PZA as a reserve drug during pregnancy, as there are currently insufficient data about its teratogenicity (Blumberg 2003). If PZA is not used, treatment may be prolonged.

> **Recommendation.** Pyrazinamide may be used during pregnancy to treat active TB.

▶ Rifampicin

Rifampicin also called *rifampin*, inhibits bacterial RNA polymerase and is effective as a bactericidal agent against different pathogens, particularly mycobacteria. Rifampicin can cross the placenta. In animal experiments, teratogenic effects were seen with doses 5–10 times higher than in human treatment. Because rifampicin inhibits DNA-dependent RNA polymerase, there has been concern that it might interfere with fetal development. Until now, no reports in the literature have confirmed this fear. There is apparently no increased risk of malformations. A long-term therapy of the mother could result in inhibition of vitamin K synthesis, and result in a higher bleeding tendency in neonates.

> **Recommendation.** Rifampicin is a first-line drug for treatment of tuberculosis during pregnancy. When used near term the newborn should receive an extended vitamin K prophylaxis (Chapter 2.9). Regarding other infections such as MRSA, rifampicin should only be administered when the drugs of first choice for pregnancy cannot be used.

▶ Streptomycin

Streptomycin is an aminoglycoside that is used parenterally in the treatment of TB. It is bactericidal, particularly affecting germs that proliferate extracellularly. Its ototoxicity can also hurt the fetus (Section 2.6.11).

> **Recommendation.** Streptomycin is contraindicated during pregnancy because of its ototoxic properties. Inadvertent exposure does not require risk-based termination of pregnancy or invasive diagnostic procedures, but hearing tests should be performed after birth (Chapter 1.15).

▶ Other tuberculostatics

Aside from the above discussed first-line drugs for TB, reserve medications are available and used in cases of resistance or intolerance.

No systematic studies exist on the tolerance of *4-aminosalicylic acid (p-aminosalicylic acid*; PAS). So far, no evidence for embryo- or fetotoxic effects has been found in humans (e.g. Lowe 1964). *Capreomycin, ethionamide, protionamide, rifabutin, rifapentine, thioacetazone,* and *terizidone,* a prodrug of *cycloserine,* are all second-line agents used internationally for MDR-TB. The extent of documented experiences in pregnancy is limited, and insufficient for a differentiated risk assessment. Single case reports argue against a high teratogenic risk of these drugs (e.g. Lessnau 2003, Drobac 2005).

For additional reserve drugs for multi-resistant TB such as *amikacin,* see Section 2.6.11, and diverse quinolones, see Section 2.6.8; for other anti-infective agents, view the relevant sections of this chapter.

Pregnancy

2.6 Anti-infective Agents

> **Recommendation.** The reserve drugs discussed here should only be used for multi-resistant tuberculosis when standard therapy is not indicated. An inadvertent exposure during pregnancy does not require a risk-based termination or invasive diagnostic, but a detailed ultrasound examination should be carried out (Chapter 1.15).

2.6.15   Local antibiotics

Generally, each external antibiotic treatment needs to be examined carefully to see whether or not the bacterial infection is more effectively treated with systemic medication. The potential of local treatment is often overestimated. Further, with topical therapy, sensitization and resistance development need to be considered.

Fusafungine has bacteriostatic and anti-inflammatory effects and is used as a spray for the treatment of infections of the nose and throat area. There is insufficient experience about its application in pregnancy.

Fusidic acid is an antibiotic that is almost exclusively used externally; its prenatal tolerance has not been examined systematically, although the medication has been available for a long time. It has a narrow spectrum of effectiveness against Gram-positive bacteria (staphylococci) and is not recommended for an untargeted treatment.

Mupirocin is primarily bacteriostatic, affecting staphylococci and streptococci by inhibiting bacterial protein synthesis. It is especially used as a nasal ointment to eliminate MRSA. Mupirocin has not been examined systematically, but there is no evidence of undesirable effects in pregnancy.

Retapamulin is the first representative of the pleuromutilins that is approved for human treatment. It is applied as an ointment for short-term treatment of superficial skin infections. Retapamulin inhibits bacterial protein synthesis and is bacteriostatic, primarily for Gram-positive germs. Systemic resorption is minimal with topical use, but nevertheless, as experience in pregnancy has been limited, its application needs to be critically examined.

Taurolidine is an antimicrobial solution that can be used for lavage in peritonitis and for the prevention of infections with catheters. As a bactericidal agent, its mechanism of action is only partially clarified. There are no reported experiences in pregnancy.

See the corresponding sections for the local application of *aminoglycosides* (Section 2.6.11), *chloramphenicol* (Section 2.6.13), *quinolones* (Section 2.6.8), *macrolides* (Section 2.6.4), *nitrofurans* (Section 2.6.9), *nitroimidazoles* (Section 2.6.10), *polypeptide* antibiotics (Section 2.6.12), *sulfonamides* (Section 2.6.7), and *tetracyclines* (Section 2.6.6).

> **Recommendation.** Externally used antibiotics are not suspected to be teratogenic. Nevertheless, the application of local antibiotics needs to be critically assessed. Antibiotics that are safe when used systemically may also be used locally. If another local antibiotic is absolutely necessary, it may be used in pregnancy.

2.6.16   Malaria prophylaxis and treatment in pregnancy

Apart from pregnant women living in malaria areas, pregnant women are increasingly traveling to tropical countries and need a suitable malaria prophylaxis. Increased resistance of malaria pathogens make it more difficult to suggest a general recommendation. The guidelines of tropical medicine should be followed, also in pregnancy, according to the travel destination. Especially difficult is the management of malaria tropica caused by *Plasmodium falciparum*. Pregnancy enhances the clinical severity of falciparum malaria, especially in the primiparous and non-immune woman. Pregnancy alters a woman's immunity to malaria, making her more susceptible to malaria infection and increasing the risk of illness, severe anaemia, and death. Maternal malaria increases the risk of spontaneous abortion, stillbirth, prematurity, and low birth weight, and thus results in excess infant mortality (e.g. Bardaji 2011, Shulman 2003). Therefore, mosquito-bite prevention, prophylaxis, and treatment of malaria should not be shortened or omitted in an ongoing pregnancy. Traveling to areas with multidrug-resistant malaria should be avoided if possible.

The choice of drug for malaria prophylaxis and treatment during pregnancy depends on the local pattern of antimalarial drug resistance, the severity of the malaria, and the degree of pre-existing immunity. It is important to be well informed about the current recommendations for prophylaxis and treatment of malaria in the area to be visited. For travelers to malaria-endemic areas, a general recommendation is difficult because of increasing resistances. Depending on the drug, the chemoprophylaxis must be continued for up to 4 weeks after leaving the malarial region.

For women living in falciparum-endemic areas with stable transmission, the World Health Organization recommends the use of insecticide-treated nets (ITNs) and *intermittent preventive treatment* (IPT) with sulfadoxine-pyrimethamine during pregnancy (WHO 2013b, Nyunt 2010). IPT reduces maternal malaria episodes, maternal anaemia, placental parasitaemia, low birth weight, and neonatal mortality (review by McClure 2013). A prompt diagnosis and effective treatment of malaria infections is vital.

Although data from prospective studies are limited *quinine, chloroquine, proguanil,* and *clindamycin* (Section 2.6.5) are considered safe during early pregnancy. Pregnant women in the first trimester with uncomplicated malaria tropica should be treated with quinine plus clindamycin (if available) (WHO 2010b). For the second and third trimester the World Health Organization recommends *artemisinin* derivatives. The choice of combination partner is difficult because of limited information.

Reserve medications include the following: *amodiaquine, atovaquone, dapsone* (Section 2.6.13), *lumefantrine, mefloquine, piperaquine,* and *pyrimethamine* plus *sulfadoxine. Doxycycline* is contraindicated after the sixteenth gestational week (Section 2.6.6). *Halofantrine* and *primaquine* should be avoided. See the relevant sections of this chapter about the specific active substrates.

During gestation plasma concentrations of many antimalaria agents are lower and their elimination is enhanced. This can result in treatment failure. Thus, in each patient dose and dose interval need to be assessed individually.

Recommendation. Generally, the physician should discuss with a patient if the trip to a tropical region could be postponed (Section 2.6.36). The risk of exposure can be reduced by long clothes, mosquito netting, and repellents. In no case should medications be denied for prophylaxis or treatment on behalf of a pregnancy, as the potential risk for the unborn child predominates. If medications with inadequate pregnancy experience are used in the first trimester, a detailed ultrasound examination should be offered. A risk-based termination is not justified when the above-described medications have been used in pregnancy (Chapter 1.15).

Pregnancy

2.6 Anti-infective Agents

▶ **Amodiaquine**

Amodiaquine, like *chloroquine*, belongs to the group of 4-aminoquino-lines. It can cause severe side effects such as liver damage and agranulo-cytosis, and for this reason, is unsuitable for prophylaxis. Its use is limited as a reserve medication for malaria. There has been no evidence of teta-togenicity (review by Thomas 2004), but experiences are limited. With regard to early pregnancy, only single case reports have been published. One study found only mild maternal side effects in 450 pregnant women who had been treated in the second or third trimester. An increase in miscarriages, prematurity, stillbirth, or malformations was not observed (Tagbor 2006).

> **Recommendation.** Amodiaquine may be used as a reserve medication for the treatment of malaria.

▶ **Artemisinin derivatives**

Artemisinin and its derivatives *artemether, artemotil, artesunate*, and *dihydroartemisinin*, are increasingly used against malaria as *Plasmodium falciparum* has developed resistance to other drugs. These compounds combine rapid blood schizonticide activity with a wide therapeutic index. Artemisinins should be given as combination therapy to protect them from resistance. Typical combinations of such *artemisinin-based combination therapy* (ACT) are artemether plus *lumefantrine*, artesunate plus *amodiaquine*, artesunate plus *mefloquine*, artesunate plus *sulfadoxine-pyrimethamine*, and dihydroartemisinin plus *piperaquine*

First trimester experiences with the use of artemisinin derivatives are limited. A number of studies contain data of more than 250 pregnant women treated with an artemisinin derivative during the first trimester, without showing evidence of a teratogenic risk (Mosha 2014, Adam 2009, Clark 2009, WHO 2006). Manyando (2010) more commonly found umbilical hernias in an additional 140 children whose mothers had been treated with artemether and lumefantrine. After 12 months most of these hernias were not detectable anymore.

There are experiences with more than 1,500 pregnant women who used artemisinin derivatives in the second and third trimester (e.g. Piola 2010, Bounyasong 2001, Deen 2001, McGready 2001, Phillips-Howard 1996). In summary, these studies did not find an increased risk in miscarriages, stillbirths, and malformations. To some degree the artemisisin derivatives were better tolerated by pregnant women, and were more effective than treatments of the control group. As plasma levels of artemether are decreased during pregnancy, it has been suggested that the dose and the dose interval may have to be adjusted (e.g. Tarning 2013, Morris 2011).

These reassuring data led the WHO (2010b) to recommend using artemisinin derivatives as medications of choice for malaria tropica in the second and third trimester. It does not specify what combination is recommended in the context of ACT. During the first trimester, based on a lack of experiences, the WHO views artemisinin derivatives as reserve medications that should not be withheld in an individual case where needed.

> **Recommendation.** Artemisinin derivatives may be used in the second and third trimester. In the first trimester they are reserve medications for the treatment of malaria.

▶ Atovaquone

Atovaquone is a broad-spectrum anti-protozoal drug that is also used in Pneumocystis pneumonia. Monotherapy quickly leads to resistance, thus it is combined with *proguanil* when used for malaria prophylaxis and treatment.

Experience with atovaquone is limited in pregnancy. A Danish cohort study based on a prescription register with 149 women exposed during their first trimester to atovaquone, 93 of them exposed at any time in weeks 3 through 8 after conception, found no increased risk for birth defects (Pasternak 2011). When used in the second and third trimester, small studies observed no adverse effects (McGready 2005, Na-Bangchang 2005). Available data are insufficient for a differentiated risk assessment, but do not suggest a teratogenic risk. McGready (2003) discusses the need of a dose adjustment as clearance increases and levels decrease during pregnancy.

> **Recommendation.** Atovaquone may be used as a reserve medication for the treatment of malaria.

▶ Chloroquine

Chloroquine, an antimalaria drug of the group of 4-aminoquinolines, works well and effectively as a schizonticidal drug against the erythrocytic forms of all types of plasmodia. Today though, almost all pathogens of the potentially lethal malaria tropica have become resistant to this rather well tolerated, and for many decades, useful medication. Resistance has also been noted for *Plasmodium vivax*, the pathogen of the less severe malaria tertiana. *Plasmodium ovale* and *plasmodium malariae* still remain mainly sensitive to chloroquine.

Chloroquine is not embryo- and fetotoxic when used at the usual dose for malaria prophylaxis or for a three-day treatment of a typical malaria attack (McGready 2002, Phillips-Howard 1996). Current evidence does not suggest fetal ocular toxicity when chloroquine was used as antimalarian medication during pregnancy (review by Osadchy 2011). Lee (2008) examined 12 pregnant women and nonpregnant controls, and did not find any changes in the pharmacokinetics or the serum level of chloroquine.

The anti-inflammatory properties of chloroquine are used also for antirheumatic therapy (Section 2.12.8). Antirheumatic doses of chloroquine are higher than those used for malaria prevention.

> **Recommendation.** Chloroquine may be used throughout pregnancy for the prophylaxis and treatment of malaria. If chloroquine resistance of the parasite is likely or has been demonstrated, other drugs must be used.

Pregnancy

2.6 Anti-infective Agents

▶ Halofantrine

Halofantrine has a rapid schizonticidal effect upon the erythrocytic forms of those plasmodia that are resistant to chloroquine and other antimalarials. Halofantrine prolongs the QT interval in the EKG. Becauses it can provoke life-threatening cardiac arrhythmias in patients with heart disease, or in conjunction with other arrhythmogenic medications, halofantrine is no longer recommended. The limited experiences in pregnancy allow no differentiated risk analysis.

> **Recommendation.** Halofantrine is only to be used in cases of acutely threatening malaria that cannot be managed with better tested and less toxic drugs. When cardiac problems are an issue, other antimalaria medications must be used.

▶ Lumefantrine

Lumefantrine belongs to the group of arylamine alcohols like quinine, mefloquine, and halofantrine. *Artemether* plus lumefantrine is currently a popular artemisinin-based combination therapy. Few experiences are available regarding its application in the first trimester without showing evidence of a teratogenic risk (e.g. Mosha 2014). For the second and third trimester, studies with several hundred patients have been reported and do not indicate a major risk (Piola 2010, McGready 2008). Manyando (2010) found only a mild increase in umbilical hernias in 140 children whose mothers took artemether and lumefantrine during the first trimester. Most of these had disappeared when follow-up examination was conducted 12 months later. In summary, current experiences do not suggest a major embryo- or fetotoxic risk of lumefantrine. During pregnancy, the plasma concentration is lower and the elimination enhanced, thus increasing the risk of treatment failure (e.g. Tarning 2009, McGready 2008).

> **Recommendation.** Lumefantrine may be used as a reserve medication for the treatment of malaria.

▶ Mefloquine

Mefloquine displays an effective and rapid activity against the erythrocytic forms of all plasmodia. Current experiences with more than 2,000 treated pregnant women, several hundred of them in the first trimester, do not suggest a teratogenic or fetotoxic potential in humans (e.g. Schlagenhauf 2012, Bounyasong 2001, McGready 2000).

One single study of the use of mefloquine has been debated as finding an increased rate of stillbirths. This study compared 200 pregnant women who received mefloquine for malaria, and found them to have a significantly higher rate of stillbirth than those who had been treated with quinine and other antimalarials (Nosten 1999). Other studies, however, have not confirmed this risk, and mefloquine has been an established medication in pregnancy for some time.

> **Recommendation.** Mefloquine may be used throughout pregnancy for the prophylaxis and treatment of malaria if there is no resistance.

▶ **Piperaquine**

A fixed oral combination of the bisquinolone *piperaquine* and *dihydroartemisinin* (DHP) is a new and promising artemisinin-based combination therapy. The mechanism of action of piperaquine is unknown. An Indonesian observational study detected a higher rate of abortion after first trimester exposure to dihydroartemisinin-piperaquine (Poespoprodjo 2014). This observation was based on five abortions among eight pregnancies (63%). The same study found a lower risk of perinatal mortality after dihydroartemisinin-piperaquine in the second and third trimester compared to quinine-based regimens. The limited experiences in pregnancy allow no differentiated risk analysis. No significant pharmacokinetic differences between pregnant and nonpregnant women were reported in two small studies (Adam 2012, Hoglund 2012).

> **Recommendation.** Piperaquine may be used as a reserve medication for the treatment of malaria.

▶ **Primaquine**

Primaquine, an 8-aminoquinoline derivative, is effective against the intrahepatic permanent forms of *Plasmodium vivax* and *Plasmodium ovale*. It is used for the complete elimination of pathogens in combination with a blood schizontocide for the erythrocytic parasites. Primaquine should not be used in pregnancy because of the potential risk of hemolytic effects in the fetus. As yet, there are no studies that permit a well-grounded risk assessment. However, there is no substantial evidence for a teratogenic potential in humans (Phillips-Howard 1996).

> **Recommendation.** Primaquine is not a therapeutic option during pregnancy. A prophylactic elimination of hepatic spores should usually be postponed for a time after birth.

▶ **Proguanil**

Proguanil, an older medication for malaria prophylaxis belonging to the folic acid antagonists, is experiencing a renaissance as it has become useful in the face of increasing chloroquine resistance. Most often it is applied in combination with the synergistic *atovaquone*. There is no evidence of an embryotoxic potential in humans (e.g. Pasternak 2011, McGready 2005). McGready (2003) discuss the need to adjust the dose as clearance is increased and blood levels decreased during pregnancy.

> **Recommendation.** Proguanil may be used throughout pregnancy for prophylaxis and treatment of malaria provided there is no resistance.

▶ **Pyrimethamine/sulfadoxine**

Pyrimethamine is an inhibitor of folic acid synthesis that is also used in the treatment of toxoplasmosis and Pneumocystis pneumonia. In malaria

Pregnancy

2.6 Anti-infective Agents

treatment it is only applied in combination with another folic acid antagonist such as *sulfadoxine* (Section 2.6.7). This particular combination is used for *intermittent preventive treatment* (IPT) during pregnancy. However, increasing resistance has started to limit the effectiveness of this popular combination (Newman 2003).

As animal experiments indicated embryotoxic effects, concerns had been raised about the use of these folic acid antagonists in early pregnancy. Numerous investigations, however, have not demonstrated an increased malformation risk in humans (e.g. Manyando 2010, Phillips-Howard 1996).

Some studies suggest that pregnancy adversely alters the pharmacokinetics of pyrimethamine and sulfadoxine (e.g. Karunajeewa 2009, Green 2007). As data are inconsistent, a general recommendation about dose adjustments in pregnancy is difficult. When sulfadoxine-pyrimethamine is given in early pregnancy, it should be supplemented by folic acid until the tenth week. The WHO recommends 0.4–0.5 mg per day, as a co-administration of high dose (5 mg daily) compromises the efficacy of sulfadoxine-pyrimethamine in pregnancy (WHO 2010b).

> **Recommendation.** Pyrimethamine in combination with sulfadoxine may be administered for the treatment of malaria. For toxoplasmosis it is the drug of choice when combined with a long-term sulfonamide, especially after the first trimester. When pyrimethamine is given in early pregnancy, it should be supplemented with folic acid, see also Chapter 2.18.8.

▶ Quinine

Quinine is the oldest antimalarial agent. It works well and effectively as a schizonticidal drug against the erythrocytic forms of all Plasmodium species. Despite a relatively high toxicity and a narrow therapeutic range, it is used again increasingly in the treatment of chloroquine-resistant malaria. In combination with clindamycin (Section 2.6.5) its effectiveness is increased. Concentrations in the fetus are just as high as in the mother, and are potentially toxic.

In some case reports it was observed that children had auditory or visual defects after the use of quinine in pregnancy. However, in those cases considerably higher doses had been administered than currently in use. There is no evidence of an increased risk of abortion or preterm delivery with the use of a standard dosage of quinine for treatment of acute malaria (Phillips-Howard 1996). These findings were confirmed by other studies with several hundred pregnant women exposed during the first trimester, where no increased rates of spontaneous abortion, congenital malformations, stillbirth or low birth weight were found (e.g. Adam 2004b, McGready 2002).

Quinine increases the secretion of insulin (Elbadawi 2011). Especially in the last part of pregnancy, severe maternal hypoglycaemia has been induced by quinine therapy. Due to the risk of hypoglycemia, the WHO (2010b) guidelines prefer to use an artemisinin combination for the management of malaria tropica from the second trimester on. A study of the metabolism of quinine in pregnant and nonpregnant women failed to show significant pharmacokinetic differences. The authors concluded that dose adjustment is not necessary during pregnancy (Abdelrahim 2007). Induction of contractions with high doses of quinine cannot be excluded.

Quinine is a component of some analgesic compounds and of certain beverages, although in lower and apparently nonembryotoxic doses.

Recommendation. Despite its toxicity, quinine belongs to the drugs of choice when dealing with chloroquine-resistant malaria tropica in pregnancy. In this situation the potential risk of treatment is much smaller for the fetus than the danger of a severe maternal disease. Attention needs to be paid to possible maternal hypoglycemia. Even though embryotoxic effects due to quinine in analgesic compounds are not to be expected, these agents should be avoided because they do not conform to good therapeutical practice. The same holds for the regular or excessive consumption of quinine drinks.

2.6.17   Azole antifungals

▶ **Azole antifungals for systemic use**

Azole derivatives inhibit the ergosterol biosynthesis, thereby causing disturbances in the permeability and functions of the fungal cell membrane. Azole antifungals include two broad classes, imidazoles and triazoles. In animal experiments azole antifungals cross the placenta and are teratogenic at high doses.

With regard to the use of the triazole derivative *fluconazole* in pregnancy, there was a report of three children (two of them siblings) with craniofacial, skeletal, and cardiac malformations, similar to those seen in animal studies (Pursley 1996). Because of meningitis, their mother had used high doses of fluconazole (400–800 mg daily) through or beyond the first trimester on a long-term basis. Additional case reports have described two births involving craniofacial, limb, and cardiac defects in two mothers who used fluconazole (Lopez-Rangel 2005, Aleck 1997). Those cases shared some characteristics with the Antley–Bixler syndrome.

However, there was no evidence of an increased risk of malformation in a prospective cohort study with 226 women exposed during the first trimester (Mastroiacovo 1996). In several other studies, first trimester exposure to low-dosage regimens of fluconazole for vaginal candidiasis did not appear to cause an increased risk of malformations (e.g. Jick 1999, Campomori 1997, Inman 1994).

Danish cohort studies based on a prescription register also could not find an increased risk of birth defects after first trimester exposure in several thousand pregnant women (Nørgaard 2008, Sørensen 1999). An extended analysis of the Danish data observed an increased risk for tetralogy of Fallot based on seven cases (prevalence 0.1%) compared to unexposed pregnancies (OR 3.16; 95% CI 1.49–6.71). The rate of major birth defects was not increased (Mølgaard-Nielsen 2013). In most cases the low and single dose consisted of 150 mg fluconazole usually used for a vaginal yeast infection.

Itraconazole is a triazole derivative with wide-spectrum activity. There has been no evidence of teratogenicity in prospective studies examining several hundred women with first trimester exposure (e.g. de Santis 2009, Bar-Oz 2000); most of the exposures were short-term. A Danish register analysis did not find an increased risk of birth defects among 687 women with a first trimester prescription of itraconazole (Mølgaard-Nielsen 2013).

Pregnancy

2.6 Anti-infective Agents

The imidazole derivative *ketoconazole* is usually avoided in systemic use because it is poorly tolerated and has many suitable alternatives. Ketoconazole is administered on occasion for the treatment of Cushing syndrome as it inhibits steroid synthesis. Theoretically, by decreasing testosterone synthesis, it might impede the sexual development of male foetuses; however, this has not been described. Ketoconazole has been used in several cases in pregnancy with good maternal and fetal outcome (e.g. Boronat 2011, Berwaerts 1999, Amado 1990). A retrospective study from data of the Hungarian Malformation Registry based on 18 exposed subjects shows no evidence of an increased risk of malformations after systemic use of ketoconazole (Kazy 2005c). An analysis of a Danish register did not observe a significantly increased risk of birth defects among 72 pregnant women with a prescription for this agent during first trimester (Mølgaard-Nielsen 2013).

For *posaconazole* and *voriconazole* which are used for aspergillosis and other invasive mycoses, information is lacking about use during pregnancy. There is only one published case report of a normal child, born after voriconazole treatment of the mother in the second and third trimester (Shoai Tehrani 2013).

> **Recommendation.** If a systemic treatment with an azole derivative becomes absolutely necessary, fluconazole and itraconazole are to be preferred as the better-tested medications. If possible, treatment should start after the first trimester. An inadvertent exposure during pregnancy does not require a risk-based termination or invasive diagnostic, but a detailed ultrasound examination should be carried out (Chapter 1.15).

► Azole antifungals for topical use

A multitude of poorly resorbed topical azole derivatives are available for the treatment of superficial fungal infections. The drugs of this group that had been introduced first, namely *clotrimazole* and *miconazole*, are most thoroughly investigated for use in pregnancy. Regarding clotrimazole, there are extensive studies about the treatment of vaginal yeast infections that do not indicate an embryotoxic potential (e.g. Czeizel 1999b, King 1998). Also, there is no suggestion that there is an increase in miscarriages. Czeizel (2004a) noted a decrease in prematurity when vaginosis was treated locally with clotrimazole. Experiences with several thousand pregnant women are available for miconazole (e.g. Czeizel 2004b, McNellis 1977). A suggestion by the Hungarian Malformation Registry about a link between vaginal therapy with miconazole plus metronidazole during the second and third gestational month, and an increase in syndactyly and hexadactyly, has not been substantiated by other studies (Kazy 2005a).

An Israeli report describes two cases of severe skeletonal anomalies after the use of *bifonazole* that are reminiscent of anomalies seen after systemic use of fluconazole. In the first case, bifonazole was taken orally from week 6 to 16, in the second case 500 mg/d vaginally throughout pregnancy and clearly at a higher dose than recommended (Linder 2010). At dose levels which are reached with nomally recommended topical application no teratogenic risks have been noted, yet systematic studies are lacking.

For *ketoconazole* see above (azole antifungals for systemic use).

Clearly less experience has been collected about the local applications of *butoconazole, croconazole, econazole, fenticonazole, isoconazole, omoconazole, oxiconazole, sertaconazole, sulconazole, terconazole,* and *tioconazole.* Teratogenic effects have not been observed (King 1998). This was confirmed for vaginal econazole treatment in a study of 68 pregnant patients (Czeizel 2003a).

> **Recommendation.** Clotrimazole and miconazole belong to the local antifungal medications of choice in pregnancy. The other azole derivates are antimycotic drugs of second choice.

2.6.18   Amphotericin B

Amphotericin B is a broad-spectrum antifungal agent of the polyene group. It binds to ergosterol at the cell membrane of fungi and disturbs cell wall permeability. It can be used intravenously, orally, and locally. With oral application, it is poorly resorbed and thus has only a local effect in the intestinal tract. Conventional amphotericin B given parenterally has a number of side effects, primarily nephrotoxicity. Newer lipid formulations of amphotericin B such as liposomal amphotericin B are characterized by a markedly better tolerance and less nephrotoxicity.

Amphotericin passes the placenta. Relevant plasma concentrations could be measured in a newborn, although the mother had taken her last dose four months prior (Dean 1994). This could be due to placental accumulation or delayed elimination by the fetal kidneys.

Several case reports do not indicate an increased risk of malformations with amphotericin B (e.g. Costa 2009, Ely 1998, King 1998). More than 10 pregnancy courses with liposomal amphotericin B also argue against an embryo- or fetotoxic risk (e.g. Mueller 2006, Pagliano 2005, Pipitone 2005). These experiences are insufficient for a differentiated risk assessment.

As resorption is minimal with oral or local use, a risk appears unlikely.

> **Recommendation.** Amphotericin B should only be used parenterally in cases of serious disseminated fungal infections. The liposomal formulation may be preferred. If treatment took place in the first trimester, a detailed ultrasound examination should be offered to ascertain the normal development of the fetus. Oral and local use of amphotericin B is acceptable in pregnancy.

2.6.19   Echinocandins

Echinocandins are a new antifungal medication group. These parenteral synthetic lipopeptides inhibit the synthesis of $1,3-\beta$-D-glucan, a key ingredient of the fungal cell wall. *Anidulafungin, caspofungin,* and *micafungin* are currently approved.

In animal experiments echinocandins cross the placenta. There have been no reports of their use in pregnancy. Yalaz (2006) described the successful postnatal application of caspofungin in a dystrophic premature newborn of the twentieth-seventh gestational week.

Recommendation. As there is insufficient data regarding the use of echinocandins in pregnancy, they should only be used where no alternatives are available and the mycosis is life-threatening. If treatment took place in the first trimester, a detailed ultrasound examination should be offered to ascertain the normal development of the fetus.

2.6.20   Flucytosine

Flucytosine is effective against *Cryptococcus neoformans* and many Candida species. It inhibits the DNA synthesis. Within the mycotic cell flucytosine is partially converted into the cytostatic 5-fluorouracil. To a smaller degree this reaction has to be expected in humans as well. Due to a high incidence of resistance, flucytosine should only be administered in combination with another antifungal drug such as amphotericin B.

In animal experiment, fluycytosine has a teratogenic effect at doses below those used in humans. As yet, no malformations have been reported in humans; however, there is, as yet, no published experience with the use of flucytosine in the first trimester. Case reports about application in the second and third trimester for dangerous disseminated cryptococcosis have not shown evidence of fetal damage (e.g. Ely 1998).

Recommendation. Flucytosine should only be used for life-threatening disseminated fungal infections during pregnancy. As it is not indicated as a monotherapy, it needs to be assessed critically if its use as a second mycotic drug is really necessary. If treatment took place in the first trimester, a detailed ultrasound examination should be offered to ascertain the normal development of the fetus.

2.6.21   Griseofulvin

Griseofulvin is an organically derived antifungal agent that is used orally for several weeks against fungal infections of the skin, hair and nails. As it is deposited within the keratin, it is especially suited for the management of fungal infections of nail mykoses.

In animal experiments griseofulvin is teratogenic and, at high doses, cancerogenic. It crosses the placenta at term (Rubin 1965). One publication, based on birth defects data, reported two pairs of conjoined twins after the use of griseofulvin in early pregnancy (Rosa 1987). This observation could not be confirmed in other publications (Knudsen 1987, Metneki 1987). A population based case-control study with some 31 exposed pregnant women did not demonstrate an increased risk of malformations (Czeizel 2004c). These experiences are insufficient for a differentiated risk assessment.

Recommendation. As griseofulvin is not used to treat life-threatening fungal infections, its application in pregnancy should be avoided. If treatment took place in the first trimester, a detailed ultrasound examination should be offered to ascertain the normal development of the fetus.

2.6.22   Terbinafine

Terbinafine is used for both oral and topical treatment of fungal infections of the nails and other dermatophytoses. A prospective study reported on 54 pregnant women exposed to terbinafine which showed no evidence of a teratogenic potential (Sarkar 2003). Of these women 24 were exposed during the first trimester and 26 had an oral exposure. These data are insufficient for a differentiated risk analysis. When used topically, less than 5% is resorbed making a risk unlikely.

> **Recommendation.** Terbinafine should be avoided during pregnancy as safety data are lacking and fungal nail infections do not require urgent treatment. If treatment took place in the first trimester, a detailed ultrasound examination should be offered to ascertain the normal development of the fetus. A topical application is likely to be harmless.

2.6.23   Topical antifungal agents

Regarding the topical use of azole derivatives such as *clotrimazole* and *miconazole*, see Section 2.6.17; for amphotericin B, Section 2.6.18; and for terbinafine, Section 2.6.22.

Nystatin is an antifungal drug from the polyene group. Like the closely related amphotericin B it binds with ergosterol of the mycotic cell wall and interferes with its function. Nystatin is an effective local antifungal drug for candidiasis of the skin or mucosa. When taken orally, it is poorly resorbed and only works locally in the intestinal tract. The indication for intestinal cleansing needs to be critically assessed in immunocompromized patients.

Nystatin is used frequently, and there is no evidence of embryo- or fetotoxic effects (e.g. King 1998). A population-based case control study did not show an increased risk of malformation after first trimester exposure. When treatment was performed in the second and third trimester, slightly more cases of hypospadia were noted (Czeizel 2003b). However, a low resorption rate, methodological weaknesses of the study, and the low number of only 106 pregnant women place the result in question.

A retrospective study of the Hungarian malformation register, with 160 exposed subjects, did not reveal signs of an increased risk of malformation when *natamycin* was applied vaginally (Czeizel 2003c). Based on the same register, a case-control study discussed a possible association between cardiovascular malformations and maternal use of *tolnaftate* in pregnancy (Czeizel 2004d). This observation was based on 26 exposed cases, of which four cases had varying types of cardiac defects (OR 3.1, 95%; CI 1.0–9.7). These data are insufficient for a differentiated risk analysis.

Amorolfine, butenafine, ciclopirox, haloprogin, naftifin, and *tolciclate* are insufficiently investigated with regard to prenatal human toxicity. As yet, there is no substantial indication for an increased risk of malformations after local use.

> **Recommendation.** Nystatin, like clotrimazole and miconazole is an antifungal drug of choice during pregnancy. Where possible, these drugs should be preferred. External treatment with amorolfine, butenafine, ciclopirox, haloprogin, natamycin, naftifin, tolciclate, and tolnaftate should be avoided during pregnancy.

Pregnancy

2.6 Anti-infective Agents

2.6.24   Anthelmintics

More than 2 billion people are infected with helminths worldwide. Soil-transmitted helminths have been recognized as an important public health problem in many developing countries. Severe hookworm and other helminth infections during pregnancy may cause anemia, reduced birth weight and increased perinatal mortality. A routine application of anthelmintics during the second and third trimester for women in areas endemic for hookworm infection has been suggested, with the argument that this may improve maternal anemia, birth weight, and neonatal mortility (e.g. WHO 2013c, Christian 2004). However, a randomized placebo-controlled study showed no advantage for newborns whose pregnant mothers had received albendazole or praziquantel (Webb 2011). Recently, it has been discussed if routine anthelmintic treatment during pregnancy might lead to an increased risk for allergies in infancy (Mpairwe 2011).

▶ **Benzimidazole anthelmintics**

The benzimidazole derivatives *albendazole, flubendazole, mebendazole, thiabendazole,* and *triclabendazole* inhibit the uptake of glucose and thereby kill the parasites. In animal experiments benzimidazole derivative with anthelmintic activity showed teratogenic effects.

Albendazole and *mebendazole* are poorly resorbed from the gastrointestinal tract, except when there is an inflammation. However, enteral absorption may be increased due to high-fat diet. Mebendazole is a highly effective and well tolerated anthelmintic drug used against nematodes (such as pinworms, roundworms, whipworms, and hookworms). There have been reports describing children with various malformations after *in utero* exposure to mebendazole, but a distinct pattern of malformations could not be discerned (review by Schardein 2000). An increased risk of congenital malformations was not observed in a study of over 400 pregnant women exposed to mebendazole in the first trimester (de Silva 1999). This was confirmed in a controlled prospective study covering 192 first trimester exposed pregnant women (Diav-Citrin 2003). Another study with 48 first trimester exposures also found no increased risk for malformations or miscarriages (McElhatton 2007). Although numbers are too small for any definite conclusion, mebendazole does not appear to represent a major teratogenic risk. Significantly more experience has been collected with exposure during the second and third trimester showing no evidence of a fetal risk (e.g. Gyorkos 2006).

Albendazole is a newer, highly effective broad-spectrum anthelmintic which combined with operative interventions has become the treatment of choice for alveolar and cystic echinococcosis. Limited experience in the first trimester has not shown evidence of a major risk (Gyapong 2003, Cowden 2000). There are several thousand pregnancies with the use of albendazole in the second or third trimester without any obvious adverse reactions reported (e.g. Webb 2011, Ndyomugyenyi 2008).

Two abstracts from Korea which reported the outcome of 16 pregnant women after the first trimester exposure to *flubendazole* showed no evidence of a teratogenic potential (Choi 2008, 2005). However, the data is insufficient for a differentiated risk assessment.

There are no reports of *thiabendazole* and *triclabendazole* use during human pregnancies.

Recommendation. Mebendazole may be used during pregnancy to treat relevant worm diseases. Albendazole may be used in cases of echinococcosis. The other benzimidazole anthelmintics should only be used with a compelling indication, and when more established anthelmintics are ineffective. After first trimester exposure a detailed ultrasound examination should be offered to ascertain the normal development of the fetus.

▶ Ivermectin

Ivermectin is a broad-spectrum anthelmintic agent which is mainly used in humans in the treatment of onchocerciasis (river blindness), lymphatic filiriasis and strongyloidiasis. It is also effective against other worm infections and some epidermal parasitic skin diseases, such as scabies. Ivermectin is well resorbed after oral administration. Animal experiments do not suggest a teratogenic potential, although at maternally toxic exposures malformations were noted in rodents. A number of case reports describing accidental treatments during the first trimester have not shown malformations in the children (Gyapong 2003, Chippaux 1993, Pacque 1990). However, data are insufficient for a differentiated risk assessment. A study encompassing more than 100 women who took ivermectin during the second trimester found no significant anomalies in the newborns (Ndyomugyenyi 2008).

Recommendation. With a compelling indication ivermectin may be used in pregnancy. After first trimester exposure a detailed ultrasound examination should be offered to ascertain the normal development of the fetus.

▶ Niclosamide

Niclosamide is an anthelmintic that is effective against tapeworms (cestodes). It affects the energy metabolism of the parasites and is practically not resorbed by the intestinal tract. This agent had been used extensively in the past and is not suspected to cause malformations, but has not been systematically studied in humans.

Recommendation. Niclosamide may be given during pregnancy to treat relevant tapeworm infections. Application in the first trimester needs to be critically assessed as tapeworm infections are generally not a great hazard to the mother or unborn child. After first trimester exposure, a detailed ultrasound examination should be offered to ascertain the normal development of the fetus.

▶ Praziquantel

Praziquantel is a highly effective broad-spectrum anthelmintic agent against many trematodes and cestodes. It is mainly used for the treatment of schistosomiasis (bilharziosis). No teratogenicity has been reported in animal studies. Over the last decades millions of pregnant women have been inadvertently treated with praziquatel during routine anthelmintic programs without an obvious adverse reactions reported. A few publications

Pregnancy

2.6 Anti-infective Agents

also found no evidence of a teratogenic potential after mothers had been treated in the first trimester (Adam 2004a, Paparone 1996). In a study from Uganda encompassing more than 1,000 pregnant women, treatment with praziquantel in the second and third trimester was not associated with an increase in adverse outcomes (Ndibazza 2010). The WHO (2002) recommends the use of praziquantel for schistosomiasis during pregnancy.

> **Recommendation.** Praziquantel should be reserved for specific severe indications like schistosomiasis. Usually for other indications better-established anthelmintics are available. After first trimester exposure a detailed ultrasound examination should be offered to ascertain the normal development of the fetus.

▶ Pyrantel

Pyrantel is a broad-spectrum anthelmintic that acts by inhibition of cholinesterase, causing spastic paralysis and subsequent death of the parasite. No teratogenicity has been reported in animal studies. Pyrantel is poorly absorbed from the gastrointestinal tract. Published experience on its use during pregnancy is not sufficient to determine risk.

> **Recommendation.** Pyrantel should be avoided in pregnancy because better tested alternatives are available for all indications. After first trimester exposure a detailed ultrasound examination should be offered to ascertain the normal development of the fetus.

▶ Pyrvinium

Pyrvinium is effective against pinworms (enterobius). After oral administration it is hardly absorbed. Therefore, it is unlikely to reach the fetus in relevant amounts. There are no reports of embryo- or fetotoxic effects. However, there has been no published experience with the use of pyrvinium during pregnancy. A Danish cohort study based on prescription registers identified 1606 women redeeming a prescription for pyrvinium (449 during first trimester). The pregnancy outcome was not considered in this article (Torp-Pedersen 2012).

> **Recommendation.** Pyrvinium may be used during pregnancy.

▶ Other anthelmintics

Diethylcarbamazine is used for the treatment of filiriasis and onchocercosis. No teratogenicity was reported in animal studies. No publications regarding its use during human pregnancies have been located.

Levamisole is used as anthelmintic and as an immunomodulator. A retrospective study with data from the Hungarian Malformation Registry based on 14 subjects (four first trimester exposures), shows no evidence of an increased risk of malformations after use of levamisole (Kazy 2004).

Oxamniquine is used for the treatment of schistosomiasis. No experiences have been reported about its use during pregnancy.

> **Recommendation.** Diethylcarbamazine, levamizole and oxamniquine should be avoided during pregnancy as better tested alternatives are available for most indications. After first trimester exposure a detailed ultrasound examination should be offered to ascertain the normal development of the fetus.

2.6.25   Herpes medications

▶ **Herpes medication for systemic use**

A number of closely related nucleoside analogs are used against viruses of the herpes group. They are effective by blocking the viral DNA polymerase. The affinity of the nucleoside analogs are much lower to human than to viral DNA polymerase.

The standard agent of this group is *acyclovir* which is used against the varicella-zoster virus (VZV) and herpes simplex virus (HSV) type 1 and 2. The manufacturer's case collection contains over 1,000 women treated systemically with acyclovir during pregnancy, 756 of them during the first trimester; with no evidence of embryo- or fetotoxic risk (Stone 2004). A study of a Danish Registry with 1,561 women with prescriptions in the first trimester, showed no increased risk after acyclovir (Pasternak 2010). Although these studies had some methodological weaknesses, the experiences argue against the risk of acyclovir in pregnancy.

Valacyclovir, the prodrug of acyclovir, is converted quickly and completely to acyclovir in the body. Orally it is distinctly better resorbed than acyclovir of which only about 20% is resorbed. The manufacturer did not find an increased risk of malformation in 56 women who had received valacyclovir during pregnancy, 14 of these during the first trimester (Glaxo Wellcome 1997). Also, the above cited study of the Danish Registry did not show evidence of embryo- or fetotoxic risk in 299 pregnancies, in which the mother filled a prescription for valacyclovir during the first trimester (Pasternak 2010).

Ganciclovir and its prodrug *valganciclovir* are effective in cytomegalus virus infections (CMV). In animal experiment, teratogenic effects were only seen with plasma levels that were twice as high as those recommended in human therapy. There are a few case reports describing normal pregnancy outcome after the first trimester treatment during early pregnancy (Pescovitz 1999). Puliyanda (2005) describes a successful oral treatment with ganciclovir for an intrauterine CMV infection after the 22nd week. These experiences are insufficient to evaluate the safety of ganciclovir in pregnancy.

Famciclovir is quickly converted after enteral resorption into the virostatic *penciclovir*. Neou (2004) reported a newborn whose mother took 250 mg famciclovir daily in her fifth week. The boy who succumbed to a severe neonatal infection had a hypoplastic thymus, a mild stenosis of the pulmonary valve, an ostium secundum defect, and an enlarged liver with stenotic extrahepatic biliary ducts. A retrospective study of data from the Danish Birth Registry contained 26 women who took oral famciclovir during the first trimester, and showed no increase in the malformation rate (Pasternak 2010).

There is insufficient data about the use in pregnancy for *brivudine*, *cidofovir*, *foscarnet*, and *fomivirsen*. In animal experiments, small doses of foscarnet sodium trigger skeletal anomalies in rats and rabbits.

No experience is reported for the combination therapy of *dimepranol* and *inosine* that is used to stimulate the immune system against viruses of the herpes group.

> **Recommendation.** If an antiviral therapy is indicated for a severe maternal disease, or to protect the fetus from an intrauterine infection, acyclovir or valacyclovir should be used as the best evaluated medication whenever possible. The other antiviral agents are only indicated in infections where they have a therapeutic advantage over acyclovir. After the application of one of the less well examined drugs during first trimester, a detailed ultrasound examination should be offered to ascertain the normal development of the fetus.

▶ Herpes medication for local use

Acyclovir, foscarnet, ganciclovir, idoxuridine, penciclovir, trifluridine, and *tromantadine* are locally applied in HSV infections. None of these agents has been suspected to give rise to teratogenic effects.

Acyclovir may be used in pregnancy systemically and is harmless in local application. In the above cited Danish Registry study 2,850 women had used acyclovir and 118 women penciclovir locally during the first trimester, and no increased malformation risk was noted (Pasternak 2010). The other agents lack studies about local application.

Docosanol is a newly approved agent for topical application in herpetic cold sores. The mechanism of action is unknown. There has been no experience about its use in pregnancy; however, a risk is unlikely with its minimal resoption.

The local application of *zinc sulfate* and of patches containing hydrocolloid particles is harmless in pregnancy.

> **Recommendation.** Where indicated, local remedies for herpes may be used during pregnancy. Drying agents and patches for herpes are harmless. Where possible, acyclovir should be preferred as the best evaluated antiviral drug.

2.6.26 Antiviral drugs for hepatitis

▶ Antiviral drugs for hepatitis B

Nucleoside/nucleotide analogs and α-interferon (Chapter 2.12) are used for the management of chronic hepatitis B. A general therapeutic recommendation cannot be made for pregnancy as data are inadequate. Experience so far did not reveal serious signs of teratogenic or fetotoxic damage in humans. If there is a very active Hepatitis B or cirrhosis, antiviral treatment might be considered. Passive–active immunoprophylaxis of infants have reduced mother-to-child-transmissions. However, in high viremic mothers immunoprophylaxis might fail. No consensus has been reached if pregnant women who are HBsAg positive, and highly viremic should be treated in the third trimester to prevent a perinatal transmission to the infant (e.g. Pan 2012).

For lamivudine and tenofovir see Section 2.6.30.

Adefovir dipivoxil, the prodrug of adefovir, is an orally-administered nucleotide analog. No teratogenicity has been reported in animal studies. The Antiretroviral Pregnancy Registry (2013) received reports of 48 births after a maternal adefovir dipivoxil regimen in the first trimester. No birth defects were observed in the infants.

Entecavir has shown teratogenic effects in animal studies where, in high doses, more vertebral and tail malformations occurred. Of 55 infants whose mothers were exposed to entecavir during first trimester, two babies were born with birth defects (no details available) (Antiretroviral Pregnancy Registry 2013). One case report describes a healthy baby born after entecavir exposure for 32 days in the second trimester (Kakogawa 2011).

Telbivudine raised no suspicions for teratogenicity in animal experiments. Among 86 pregnancies of women who received *telbivudine* before or in early pregnancy the abortion rate was 7.9%. Fifty mothers delivered 52 infants. One pregnancy was terminated because of cleft lip and palate and one infant showed right ear accessories, no other birth defects were reported (Liu 2013). In the Antiretroviral Pregnancy Registry (2013) no birth defects were observed in 10 infants after first trimester exposure to telbivudine.

In a prospective study, 136 infants were born after maternal treatment with telbivudine in late pregnancy to prevent perinatal transmission. Exposure took place from the twentieth to thirty-second gestational week until at least 1 month after delivery. There were no significant differences in infant outcomes compared to a control group. No serious adverse events were noted in the infants (Han 2011). There is an ongoing discussion as to whether telbivudine should be given to women with a high virus load during late pregnancy to prevent intrauterine transmission (review by Deng 2012).

▶ **Ribavirin**

The nucleoside analog *ribavirin* inhibits both DNA- and RNA-viruses, displaying a relatively broad antiviral spectrum experimentally. Among other applications, it is used to treat respiratory syncytial virus (RSV) infections in infants, and, combined with *α-interferon* (Chapter 2.12), against hepatitis C.

Ribavirin has teratogenic and mutagenic effects in animal experiments. Nine women who were treated during the second half of pregnancy for severe measles delivered healthy infants (Atmar 1992). A woman treated for SARS (severe acute respiratory syndrome) in the first trimester with ribavirin by injection for 3 days gave birth to a normal child (Rezvani 2006). In its Pregnancy Registry, the manufacturer noted eight women with ribavirin exposure in the first trimester, and 77 women with exposure within 6 months of the last menstrual period (Roberts 2010). The authors found no evidence of a teratogenic risk for humans.

In summary, current data is insufficient for a risk assessment for ribavirin. An embryo- or fetotoxic risk is not apparent with the available case reports.

Paternal exposure

The level of ribavirin is twice as high in seminal fluid as in sperm. There has been no increased risk of malformations after paternal ribavirin treatment and interferon in 20 pregnancies reported as case reports (review by Hofer 2010), and 110 pregnancies of the Ribavirin Pregnancy Registry (Roberts 2010). These numbers are inadequate to assess a possible risk after paternal exposure.

▶ **Other antiviral drugs for hepatitis C**

The protease inhibitors *boceprevir*, *simeprevir* and *telaprevir* have been approved for the treatment of chronic hepatitis C. There are no

Pregnancy

2.6 Anti-infective Agents

experiences with their use in pregnancy. The same applies to *sofosbuvir* – a recently approved polymerase inhibitor for the treatment of chronic hepatitis C.

> **Recommendation.** Ribavirin and the other antiviral agents discussed here should only be used during pregnancy when compellingly indicated. Treatment during the first trimester is not a justification for a risk-based termination of pregnancy (Chapter 1.15). In such a situation a detailed ultrasound examination should be offered to ascertain normal fetal development.

2.6.27   Antiviral drugs for influenza

▶ **Amantadine**

Amantadine enhances dopamine activity at the receptor and thus is also used as an antiparkinson drug. As an antiviral medication, it inhibits the membrane protein hampering the ability of the virus to enter the cell nucleus. Because of rapid resistance and frequent neurologic side effects, it is not recommended any more as an antiviral agent. For amantadin in Parkinson disease, see Chapter 2.11.

▶ **Neuraminidase inhibitors**

The neuraminidase inhibitors *oseltamivir, peramivir* and *zanamivir* are used to treat patients whose influenza requires therapy.

Oseltamivir has not shown teratogenic effects in animal studies. A prospective investigation at two Japanese centers did not see an increase in malformations where 90 women had been treated in the first trimester (review by Tanaka 2009). Another study involving 137 exposed offspring, 18 of them in the first trimester, also did not find a higher risk (Greer 2010). The manufacturer, too, noticed no increased risk in 115 women who had used oseltamivir during pregnancy, 44 of these during the first 3 months (Donner 2010). One study with 81 pregnant women exposed to oseltamivir, 24 in the first trimester, found an increased risk of late transient hypoglycaemia compared to an unexposed control group. No other increased risks of adverse birth outcomes among the infants have been observed. One child had a ventricular septal defect. This was the only major malformation after exposure in the first trimester (Svensson 2011). Another publication included 619 pregnant women exposed to oseltamivir, 159 of them in first trimester. The overall rate of major malformation after first trimester exposure was 1.3% (Saito 2013). In a French publication, a total of 337 mothers received at least one prescription of oseltamivir during pregnancy. One congenital heart defect was observed among 49 infants who were exposed during first trimester. No significant association between adverse fetal outcomes and exposure to oseltamivir during pregnancy could be found (Beau 2014). Dunstan (2014) could also find no signs of embryo- or fetotoxic effects in 27 exposed pregnant women. No birth defects were observed in eight first trimester exposures. A population-based retrospective cohort study analyzed data from 1,237 women who received oseltamivir during pregnancy. Compared to a control group, there were no associations between maternal use of oseltamivir with preterm birth and low Apgar score. Women who took oseltamivir during pregnancy were less likely to have a small for gestational age infant. However, birth defects and time of exposure were not mentioned (Xie 2013).

Two studies looked into the pharmacokinetics of oseltamivir and its active metabolite oseltamivir carboxylate during gestation. Greer (2011) compared the pharmacokinetics of 10 pregnant women in each group during the last trimester and found no significant differences. Beigi (2011) examined the pharmacokinetcs in 16 pregnant women (average gestational age 24.6 weeks) in comparison to 23 nonpregnant women, and found the pregnant group to have lower oseltamivir carboxylate level. However, it remains unclear if the dose needs to be adjusted during pregnancy.

Zanamivir is applied by inhalation and very little is resorbed. No teratogenicity was found in animal experiments. A case series study from Japan reported 50 infants born after intrauterine zanamivir exposure, 15 of them were exposed in the first trimester. No malformations have been observed (Saito 2013). A prospective surveillance study did not provide a case that use of zanamivir in pregnancy is associated with an increased risk of adverse pregnancy outcomes among 180 women exposed to zanamivir during pregnancy. No major malformations were reported in 37 zanamivir first trimester exposures (Dunstan 2014). Experience and the presence of low systemic concentrations, make it unlikely that there is an increased embryo- or fetotoxic risk.

Experience during pregnancy with *peramivir* is insufficient for a risk assessment.

> **Recommendation.** If indicated, neuraminidase inhibitors oseltamivir and tanamivir may be used in pregnancy. Peramivir should be avoided. Amantadine is no longer recommended for the treatment of influenza. When used during the first trimester, a detailed ultrasound examination should be offered to ascertain normal fetal development.

2.6.28   Antiretroviral agents

The aim of *antiretroviral therapy* (ART) during pregnancy is the prevention of a vertical transmission of the *human immunodeficiency virus* (HIV) from mother to child, and also the optimal management of the HIV-infected mother, whereby unwanted side effects are to be kept at a minimum for her and the child. ART in pregnancy has become an integral part in the prophylaxis of HIV transmission after data revealed the protective effect of perinatal prophylaxis, with the nucleoside analog reverse transcriptase inhibitor (NRTI) *zidovudine* that could prevent a possible vertical transmission during the last trimester and labor (Connor 1994). National and international guidelines recommend a standard therapy for both nonpregnant and pregnant HIV-infected women take a combination of at least three antiretroviral medications (EACS 2013, OARAC 2012, WHO 2010c). This *highly active antiretroviral therapy* (HAART) typically consists of two NRTIs and either a protease inhibitor (PI), or a non-nucleoside analog reverse transcriptase inhibitor (NNRTI). The intention is that the suppression of the plasma HIV load (HIV-RNA) should be as close to <50 copies/mL at least by the end of the pregnancy. When an effective HAART is applied during pregnancy and lactation, the HIV rate of transmission can be decreased from its former levels of

Pregnancy

2.6 Anti-infective Agents

20–30% to <1% (Townsend 2008, Warszawski 2008). The decision of what regimen to use is already complicated in nonpregnant patients, but more so in pregnancy. How to balance individual needs and risks should be considered, especially in view of the timing of the start of treatment, a possible interruption of therapy during the first trimester in women already under treatment, and the selection of appropriate antiretroviral medications.

The risks from intrauterine exposure to combinations of antiretroviral agents are difficult to assess, as data are limited concerning the pharmakinetics and the developmental toxicity for most of the drugs. There is no data about the long-term toxicity of the exposure to intrauterine retroviral substances. Information about the safety of retroviral drugs in pregnancy are limited to experiments in animals, single case reports, a few clinical studies, and analyses of registries such as the Antiretroviral Pregnancy Registry (2013) in the USA that contains most of the information about the safety of antiviral substances in pregnancy.

2.6.29   Overview of the antiretroviral medications

Five groups of antiviral substances are distinguished:

1. Nucleoside and nucleotide reverse transcriptase inhibitors (NRTIs): *abacavir, didanosine, emtricitabine, lamivudine, stavudine, tenofovir,* and *zidovudine.*
2. Non-nucleoside reverse transcriptase inhibitors (NNRTIs): *delavirdine, efavirenz, etravirine, nevirapine,* and *rilpivirine.*
3. Protease inhibitors (PIs): *atazanavir, darunavir, fosamprenavir, indinavir, lopinavir, nelfinavir, ritonavir, saquinavir,* and *tipranavir.*
4. Entry inhibitors: *enfuvirtide* and *maraviroc.*
5. Integrase inhibitors: *raltegravir, dolutegravir* and *elvitegravir.*

Data currently available do not allow for a summarizing differentiated risk analysis for antiretroviral medications in pregnancy. With the exception of efavirenz, there have been no serious signs of teratogenic or fetotoxic damages in humans (e.g. Watts 2011, ECS 2003). Prospectively documented pregnancies do not demonstrate a higher risk of malformations and, like retrospective case reports, fail to reveal any distinct pattern of anomalies. When antiretroviral agents are used in the first trimester, the embryotoxic risk appears to be generally small (Phiri 2014, Floridia 2013, Antiretroviral Pregnancy Registry 2010, Joao 2010). Nevertheless, substances that might be embryotoxic should be eschewed in early pregnancy. Common side effects in children treated *in utero* or after birth with zidovudine or antiretroviral combinations consist of hematologic problems, especially anemias and neutropenias (Dryden-Peterson 2011, Feiterna-Sperling 2007, Le Chenadec 2003). It is being debated if antiretroviral treatment with or without protease inhibitors favors prematurity (Chen 2012, Patel 2010, Kourtis 2007, Cotter 2006, Tuomala 2005). The maternal risks of therapy are discussed with the specific medications.

The medical treatment of HIV infection during pregnancy is a prime example for the need to sometimes utilize insufficiently tested medications – because of the acute danger for mother and child. In individual cases it needs to be critically assessed if an ongoing or maternally indicated treatment is absolutely necessary during the time of embryogenesis, or if it can be temporarily suspended.

Recommendation. Antiretroviral medications may be used in pregnancy. Specific risks for the prophylaxis of transmission and the therapy of maternal HIV infection need to be observed. The choice of medication and the timing of treatment have to be decided on an individual basis. When choosing medications it should be noted that some of the retroviral substances should be avoided during pregnancy, if possible. This concerns efavirenz (teratogenic effects) and the combination stavudine/didanosine (lactic acidosis). For newer medications such as maraviroc, raltegravir and etravirine, few or no data are available concerning their use in pregnancy. Caution is called for when nevirapine is used in women with CD4 cell counts of <250/mm mm^3 (hepatotoxicity). If nevirapine is used during pregnancy, transaminases need to be checked regularly, especially during the first 18 weeks of treatment; also, clinical symptoms are to be watched. The short-term use of nevirapine for transmission prophylaxis does not seem to carry a similar risk.

When exposure occurs during the first trimester, a detailed ultrasound examination should be offered to ascertain the normal development of the fetus. It is recommended that the pregnant patient is cared for in a specialized center. Physicians should report pregnancies involving the use of HIV medications shortly after diagnosis to the Antiviral Pregnancy Registry (www.APRegistry.com).

2.6.30   Nucleoside and nucleotide reverse transcriptase inhibitors (NRTIs)

Data from clinical studies during pregnancy in women are available for *abacavir, didanosine, emtricitabine, lamivudine, stavudine, tenofovir,* and *zidovudine*. With the exception of didanosine, the NRTIs showed comparable levels in the maternal serum, and the umbilical cord blood suggested an easy placental passage (Pacifici 2005). Having an affinity to mitochondrial γ-DNA polymerases, NRTIs can induce mitochondrial dysfunction. The greatest risk for mitochondrial toxicity is exhibited *in vitro* for didanosine, stavudine, and zidovudine. The question if a perinatal NRTI exposure could lead to mitochondrial problems in children is currently under discussion; a final consensus has not been reached (Benhammou 2007, Blanche 1999).

Lamivudine and zidovudine are the NRTIs that should be preferred during pregnancy because of extensive experience. Abacavir, emtricitabine and tenofovir are alternative NRTIs which also might be used. Didanosine and stavudine should only be used in special circumstances (OARAC 2012).

▶ **Abacavir**

Abacavir can lead to skeletal anomalies when given to rats at a high dosage. There is no evidence of teratogenicity in humans. Abacavir readily crosses the placenta (Chappuy 2004). Data from the Antiretroviral Pregnancy Registry (2013) with 27 birth defects in 905 cases, indicate a malformation rate of 3.0% after exposure during the first trimester, similarly as seen in the general population of the USA.

▶ **Didanosine**

In animal experiments *didanosine* given at high doses did not show teratogenic effects. Didanosine crosses the placenta only in limited

Pregnancy

2.6 Anti-infective Agents

amounts (Wang 1999). The data of the Antiretroviral Pregnancy Registry (2013) show a slightly increased malformation rate after first trimester exposure at 4.8% (20 of 416 births), in comparison to 2.7% in the general US population. However, no distinct pattern of birth defects has been discovered. In a study where 14 HIV infected women were treated at 26–36 weeks with didanosine, neither maternal nor neonatal side effects were noted (Wang 1999). Cases of lethal lactic acidosis have been described in pregnant women treated with a combination of stavudine and didanosine (Mandelbrot 2003, Sarner 2002). Due to the risk of fatal lactic acidosis, combination treatment with didanosine and stavudine should only be used in cases where no alternatives are available (Bristol-Myers Squibb 2001).

▶ Emtricitabine

Emtricitabine has not shown evidence of teratogenicity in animal experiments or in humans. It crosses the placenta readily (Stek 2012, Hirt 2009b). Among cases of first trimester exposures reported to the Antiretroviral Pregnancy Registry (2013), the prevalence of birth defects was 2.4% (34 of 1,400 births), similar to the rate in the general US population.

▶ Lamivudine

Lamivudine, one of the best evaluated NRTIs, is also approved for the treatment of chronic hepatitis B. Levels measured in the umbilical cord blood correspond to those of the mother. Data from the Antiretroviral Pregnancy Registry (2013) indicate an unsuspicious malformation rate of 3.1% (136 of 4,360 births). A larger study to prevent perinatal transmission was conducted in France where 445 pregnant women received zidovudine and lamivudine after gestational week 31, and their newborns were also given the combination for 6 weeks (Mandelbrot 2001). In this study newborns displayed significant side effects that included lethal mitochondriopathies. However, lamivudine and zidovudine are medications that are preferred in pregnancy because of extensive experience.

▶ Stavudine

There is no evidence that *stavudine* leads to teratogenic effects in animal experiments or humans. Stavudine crosses the placenta easily (Chappuy 2004). The malformation rate after exposure in the first trimester is 2.6% (21 of 805 births) according to data from the Antiretroviral Pregnancy Registry (2013), thus similar as in the general US population (2.7%). Good tolerance of a staduvine–lamivudine combination has been described in a small phase I/II study with 14 mother–child pairs (Wade 2004). Cases of lethal lactic acidosis have been described in pregnant women treated with a combination of stavudine and didanosine (Mandelbrot 2003, Sarner 2002). Due to the risk of a fatal lactic acidosis, combination treatment with didanosine and stavudine should only be used in cases where no alternatives are available (Bristol-Myers Squibb 2001).

▶ **Tenofovir**

In animal experiments, offspring of monkeys that received high doses of *tenofovir* have a decreased fetal growth rate and diminished fetal bone density (Tarantal 2002). During pregnancy tenofovir crosses the placenta easily (Flynn 2011, Hirt 2009a). There is no evidence that tenofovir is teratogenic in humans. According to the data of the Antiretroviral Pregnancy Registry (2013) the malformation rate after exposure during the first trimester is 2.3% (46 of 1,982 births), similar to the 2.7 % rate in the general US population. In clinical studies HIV patients, primarily children, displayed decreased bone density when treated with tenofovir. The clinical significance of these findings is still unclear. One study did not reveal any risk for adverse effects of *in utero* tenofovir exposure in 141 pregnant women (Gibb 2012). However, tenofovir should be used with caution during pregnancy, because of the risk of fetal bone changes and the paucity of other data about its pregnancy-related risks.

▶ **Zidovudine**

Zidovudine, also known as *azidothymidine* (AZT), is the oldest antiviral drug used for antiretroviral therapy. It readily crosses the placenta. In rats, maternal toxic doses lead to an increased malformation rate during organogenesis, an effect not seen with lower doses. There are no signs of teratogenicity in humans. According to data from the Antiretroviral Pregnancy Registry (2013) the malformation rate of 3.2% (129 of 4,000 births) was not significant higher than that of the general US population. The application of zidovudine has been well studied in pregnancy and is considered to be safe in regard to short-term and medium-term toxicities. A common side effect, when zidovudine is used in the perinatal period, is a transient anemia in newborns (Sperling 1998, Connor 1994). A follow-up study of 234 children who had been exposed to zidovudine *in utero* did not display any physical, immunological, or cognitive anomalies. The median age of children at the time of last follow-up was 4.2 years (range, 3.2–5.6 years) (Culnane 1999). Also, there was no evidence of an increased risk for neoplasia in more than 700 children after pre- and perinatal exposure (Culnane 1999, Hanson 1999). There are no data regarding long-term toxicity, especially for cancerogenicity.

2.6.31 Non-nucleoside reverse transcriptase inhibitors (NNRTIs)

Data from clinical studies about the safety in human pregnancy for NNRT is are limited. *Nevirapine* is the agent that should be preferred if a NNRTI is required during pregnancy. *Efavirenz* might be used in special circumstances. For *etravirine* and *rilpivirine* the data are insufficient to recommend use during pregnancy (OARAC 2012). *Delavirdine* is not recommended as part of an initial therapy.

▶ **Delavirdine**

Delavirdine caused an increased incidence of ventricular septal defects in rats. Experience in humans is limited to 11 births after first

Pregnancy

2.6 Anti-infective Agents

trimester exposure reported to the Antiretroviral Pregnancy Registry (2013). Although no birth defects have been observed, these data allow no differentiated risk analysis. Most guidelines do not recommend delavirdine as a part of antiretroviral regimens for initial treatment of HIV infection because of inferior efficacy.

► Efavirenz

In animal experiments *efavirenz* showed evidence of teratogenicity. Three of 20 prenatally exposed cynomolgus monkeys showed malformations when plasma levels were similar to the therapeutic levels in humans. Anencephaly with unilateral anophthalmia was observed in one fetus, microphthalmia in another, and cleft palate in a third. There are case reports in humans about neural tube defects in children whose mothers had received efavirenz during the first trimester (de Santis 2002, Fundaro 2002). According to the data of the Antiretroviral Pregnancy Registry (2013) the malformation rate of 2.3% (18 of 766 births) after first trimester exposure is comparable to the background rate of 2.7% in the general US population. The 18 birth defects included one infant with myelomeningocele. Another child was born with anophthalmia, severe facial cleft and amniotic banding. In total, the Antiretrorviral Pregnancy Register received six retrospective reports of neural tube defects; four of them were exposed to efavirenz.

A meta-analysis, including nine prospective studies together with 1,132 live births, did not detect an increased risk of overall birth defects after exposure to an efavirenz-containing regimen during the first trimester. Including retrospective studies, one neural tube defect was reported in 1,256 live births (Ford 2010). An update of this meta-analysis which included 181 additional subjects had similar results (Ford 2011).

In contrast to these reassuring findings, another study analyzes data of 1,112 infants born between 2002 and 2007. A significantly increased risk of congenital anomalies after exposure to efavirenz during first trimester was observed. Six of 47 infants with first trimester exposure to efavirenz had congenital anomalies (adj.OR 2.84, 95%; CI: 1.13–7.16) (Knapp 2012). However, the six observed major and minor defects (patent foramen ovale, gastroschisis, postaxial polydactyly, Arnold-Chiari malformation, talipes equinovarus, plagiocephaly), do not present a distinct pattern.

With the available published experience, the British HIV Association guidelines panels concluded that there are insufficient data to support the former position and furthermore recommend that efavirenz can be both continued and commenced in pregnancy (Taylor 2012). However, the United State guidelines are more restrictive. They recommend that an efavirenz-based regimen may be continued in women who present for antenatal care in the first trimester, provided the regimen produces virologic suppression (OARAC 2012).

► Etravirine

Animal experiments have not shown that *etravirine* is teratogenic. Experience in pregnancy is limited to case reports (Jaworsky 2010, Furco 2009). According to the data of the Antiretroviral Pregnancy Registry (2013) no birth defects were reported in 39 infants born after first trimester exposure to etravirine. Experiences are insufficient to analyze a possible risk in pregnancy.

▶ **Nevirapine**

There is no evidence in animal experiments or human experience that *nevirapine* is teratogenic. Nevirapine crosses the placenta easily and attains levels in the neonate that correspond to those of the mother (Benaboud 2011, Mirochnick 1998). According to the data of the Antiretroviral Pregnancy Registry (2013) the malformation rate after first trimester exposure is 2.9% (31 of 1,061 births), which is no higher than that of the general US population.

Studies indicate that viral transmission is blocked when 200 mg p.o. nevirapine is given to the mother at the beginning of labor, and the newborn receives a single dose of 2 mg/kg 48 to 72 hours after delivery (Guay 1999). There is a high risk of developing viral resistance even after a single dose (low resistance barrier and long half-life of nevirapine), thus nevirapine should only be administered in a combination regimen.

Reports have been published describing single cases of liver toxicity in pregnant women who took nevirapine (e.g. Knudtson 2003). This event is often rash-associated and potentially fatal. Liver toxicity is primarily observed in patients with higher CD4 cell counts (>250/mm³); in these patients the risk of symptomatic hepatic events is twelve times greater than in women with lower CD4 cell counts (<250/mm³). Studies indicate that pregnancy *per se* is a risk factor for liver toxicity. Pregnant patients using HAART that includes nevirapin have no higher risk of hepatotoxicity than those who use HAART without nevirapine (Ouyang 2010, Ouyang 2009). These data suggest that the risk of liver toxicity of nevirapine is similar in pregnant and nonpregnant patients. However, if nevirapine is used in pregnancy, physicians should be aware of hepatotoxicity.

▶ **Rilpivirine**

Animal experiments failed to show that *rilpivirine* is teratogenic. In the Antiretroviral Pregnancy Registry (2013) no birth defects were reported in 31 infants born after first trimester exposure to rilpivirine. One publication describes two healthy infants after rilpivirine exposure during pregnancy (Colbers 2014). Experiences are insufficient to analyze a possible risk in pregnancy.

2.6.32   Protease inhibitors (PIs)

PIs are being used increasingly in pregnancy. They are recommended in regimens combined with two NRTI drugs. PI therapy can lead to the disturbance of glucose tolerance and even to the manifestation or exacerbation of diabetes mellitus. It remains unclear if pregnancy itself increases the risk even further. Generally, PIs pass the placenta poorly (Gingelmaier 2006, Marzolini 2002, Mirochnick 2002). Therefore, fetal toxicity would seem to be unlikely.

Lopinavir/ritonavir and *atazanavir* with low-dose ritonavir boosting are the preferred PIs during pregnancy. Alternative PIs include ritonavir-boosted *saquinavir* and *darunavir*. *Indinavir* and *nelfinavir* should only be used in special circumstances. Data is too limited to recommend the routine use of *fosamprenavir* and *tipranavir* in pregnant women (OARAC 2012).

▶ **Atazanavir**

Atazanavir has not shown evidence of teratogenicity in animal experiments or human experience. According to the data of the Antiretroviral Pregnancy Registry (2013), the malformation rate of 2.2% (19 of 878 births) after first trimester exposure is comparable to the rate of 2.7% in the general US population. A number of studies are available, including pharmacokinetic evaluations in pregnant women using HAART with atazanavir (Mirochnick 2011, Ripamonti 2007). Some experts recommend an increased dose in late pregnancy. The umbilical cord blood of neonates shows atazanavir levels of 13–16% of those seen in the maternal serum. Atazanavir inhibits the uridin glucuronosyl transferase that metabolizes indirect bilirubin. Thus, as a common side effect, atazanavir treatment may lead to higher indirect bilirubin levels. While case numbers are relatively small, investigations showed that neonates of atazanavir-treated mothers did not show pathological elevations of indirect bilirubin. (Mirochnick 2011, Ripamonti 2007).

▶ **Darunavir**

Darunavir did not demonstrate evidence of teratogenicity in animal experiments. Some case reports demonstrated a limited placental transfer. Like with other PIs a reduction in plasma levels has been observed in late pregnancy (Pinnetti 2010). In the Antiretroviral Pregnancy Registry (2013) five birth defects were reported in 212 infants born after first trimester exposure to rilpivirine (prevalence 2.4%). Few experiences about its use in pregnancy are available (e.g. Jaworsky 2010, Ivanovic 2010). These data are insufficient for a differentiated risk assessment.

▶ **Fosamprenavir**

In animal experiments no evidence was found that *fosamprenavir* leads to teratogenicity. Human data about its use in pregnancy are very limited. Transplacental passage analyzed in seven cases was relatively high compared to other PIs. The authors detected a median ratio of 0.27 of cord blood to maternal amprenavir level (the active metabolite of fosamprenavir) (Cespedes 2013). One publication did not report adverse effects in nine infants after intrauterine exposure to fosamprenavir (Martorell 2010). Two birth defects among 102 births were reported to the Antiretroviral Pregnancy Registry (2013) after first trimester exposure to fosamprenavir. These data are insufficient for a differentiated risk assessment.

▶ **Indinavir**

Evidence for teratogenicity is not evident for *indinavir* in animal experiments or human reports. Little of indinavir crosses the placenta (Mirochnick 2002). According to the data of the Antiretroviral Pregnancy

Registry (2013) the malformation rate of 2.4% (7 of 289 births) after first trimester exposure is comparable to that in the general US population. These data are insufficient for a differentiated risk assessment. There is a theoretical concern that physiologic hyperbilirubinemia might be exacerbated due to indinavir.

▶ Lopinavir/ritonavir

Lopinavir is used in conjunction with its pharmacological booster ritonavir. In animal experiments with high doses of lopinavir, rats displayed evidence of embryotoxicity with an increased rate of miscarriages, less fetal viability, lower fetal weight, and skeletal changes. These problems were not apparent in rabbits. There is no evidence of teratogenicity in humans. Like most PIs, lopinavir/ritonavir crosses the placenta poorly (Gingelmaier 2006). According to the data of the Antiretroviral Pregnancy Registry (2013) the malformation rate is 2.3% (26 of 1,125 births) after first trimester exposure, and thus not increased in comparison to the general US population. Studies with HIV-infected pregnant women indicate that the treatment with lopinavir/ritonavir is well tolerated. Pharmacokinetic investigations show lower plasma levels, primarilty in the last trimester (Best 2010). It is unclear if pregnant women require a higher dose or just a continuation of the PI standard therapy. A report of 50 infants who received lopinavir/ritonavir after birth observed an association with transient adrenal dysfunction in the infants (Simon 2011). A systematic review about the safety and efficacy of lopinavir/ritonavir during pregnancy included nine studies involving 2,675 pregnant women. No concerns with the use of these agents were suggested (Pasley 2013).

▶ Nelfinavir

Nelfinavir did not display evidence of teratogenicity in animal experiments. According to the data of the Antiretroviral Pregnancy Registry (2013), the malformation rate is 3.9% (47 of 1,211 births) after first trimester exposure which is a modest evaluation compared to the general population (2.7%). No distinct pattern of birth defects defects has been discovered. In studies with HIV-infected pregnant women it was noted that a small amount crosses the placenta (Bryson 2008, Mirochnick 2002). When nelfinavir is used as an unboosted PI in pregnant women who need treatment for HIV, it is inferior to newer, low-dose ritonavir boosted PIs, but is useful as an alternative PI in combination with 2 NRTIs for the prophylaxis of HIV transmission. However, nevirapine should only be used under special circumstances during pregnancy.

▶ Ritonavir

Ritonavir should be used in combination with other PIs as a low-dose booster to increase levels of a second PI. Only a small amount crosses the placenta (Mirochnick 2002). There is no evidence that ritonavir is teratogenic in animal experiments or humans. According to the data of the Antiretroviral Pregnancy Registry (2013) the malformation rate is 2.3% (52 of 2,260 births) after first trimester exposure, thus similar to the general US population.

Pregnancy

2.6 Anti-infective Agents

▶ **Saquinavir**

Saquinavir has not demonstrated evidence of teratogenicity in animal experiments or human experience. Like with other PIs only small amounts of the drug cross the placenta (Mirochnick 2002). Pharmacokinetic studies indicate that the newer tablet formulation that has replaced the former capsule formulation, leads to plasma concentrations similar to nonpregnant patients (van der Lugt 2009). Thus, it is not necessary to adjust the doses in pregnancy. Seven birth defects among 182 first trimester exposures were reported to the Antiretroviral Pregnancy Registry (2013). These data are insufficient for a differentiated risk assessment.

▶ **Tipranavir**

Tipranavir shows no teratogenicity in animal experiments. There are no data about its ability to cross the placenta. Aside from single case reports of pregnant patients with multiple resistances (Weizsaecker 2011, Wensing 2006), there are no other data about the use of tipranavir in pregnancy. No birth defects were reported to the Antiretroviral Pregnancy Registry (2013) among four first trimester exposures to tipranavir. Experiences are insufficient to analyze a possible risk in pregnancy.

2.6.33   Entry inhibitors

Entry inhibitors are antiretroviral agents that inhibit viral binding or fusion of HIV to the cell, either by inhibition of the fusion of the viral capsule with the cell membrane or by blocking CD4- or co-receptors. Data about the use of *enfuvirtide* or *maravorioc* during pregnancy are insufficient to recommend their use during pregnancy (OARAC 2012).

▶ **Enfuvirtide**

In animal experiments no evidence was observed that *enfuvirtide* is teratogenic. A number of single case reports suggest that enfuvirtide apparently does not cross the placenta (Weizsaecker 2011, Brennan-Benson 2006). According to the data of the Antiretroviral Pregnancy Registry (2013) no birth defects have been reported among 20 first trimester exposure to enfuvirtide. Thus, it can be assumed that the risk of fetal toxicity is likely to be small. Enfuvirtide may be used in pregnant women with multi-resistant HIV in combination with other potent agents as a therapeutic option, but current experience in pregnancy is very limited.

▶ **Maraviroc**

Maraviroc is a CCR5 inhibitor that is used to treat pretreated HIV-infected adults in combination with other antiretroviral medications, when exclusively CCR5-tropic HIV type-1 have been proven to be present. Animal experiments using rats and rabbits did not show evidence of teratogenicity for maraviroc. There are no data indicating to what degree maraviroc crosses the placenta. While there has been no indication that the use of maraviroc leads to a higher rate of malignancy, a theoretical concern remains based on the method of its action. Maraviroc should only be used when the benefit justifies the potential fetal risk. There is a lack of data about its application in pregnancy. Among 13 cases with first trimester exposure reported to the Antiretroviral Pregnancy Registry (2013) no birth defects have been observed.

2.6.34   Integrase inhibitors

Integrase inhibitors block integrase, a HIV-coded enzyme, and thereby HIV replication. The use of *raltegravir* during pregnancy can be considered in special circumstances when preferred and alternative agents cannot be used (OARAC 2012). There is insufficient data for the new integrase inhibitors *dolutegravir* and *elvitegravir*.

▶ Dolutegravir

In animal experiments no evidence was seen that *dolutegravir* is teratogenic. Placental transfer has been described in animals. No experiences have been reported about its use during human pregnancy. There are also no reports about the use of dolutegravir to the Antiretroviral Pregnancy Registry (2013).

▶ Elvitegravir

Elvitegravir is combined with *colbicistat* which has no known antiretroviral activity. Colbicistat is a pharmacokinetic enhancer which inhibits enzymes that metabolize elvitegravir. Animal studies of elvitegravir have shown no evidence of teratogenicity. Only one report about the use of elvitagravir during the first trimester has been reported to the Antiretroviral Pregnancy Registry (2013). No birth defects were observed in this case.

▶ Raltegravir

Development studies in rats and rabbits did not show *raltegravir* to be teratogenic. However, there was a slightly increased incidence of supernumerary ribs in the offspring of rats that had received raltegravir at doses about 4.4 times higher than those recommended in human treatment. Potential human risks are not known at this time. According to the few data about its use during pregnancy, raltegravir crosses the placenta well (McKeown 2010). In a case series of five women raltegravir was well tolerated (Taylor 2011). Three birth defects were observed among 141 pregnant women with first trimester exposures reported to the Antiretroviral Pregnancy Registry (2013). Because experience is increasing, the United States guidelines recommend allowing a regimen including raltegravir in special circumstances, when preferred and alternative agents cannot be used (OARAC 2012). However, the data on the use of raltegravir during pregnancy allow no differentiated risk analysis.

Pregnancy

2.6 Anti-infective Agents

2.6.35   Hyperthermia

More than 30 years ago animal experiments demonstrated that an increase in the body temperature can cause malformations (review by Graham 2005, Edwards 1995, Miller 2013). This problem has also been discussed for humans. Neural tube defects, in particular (Suarez 2004, Shaw 1998), but also kidney, heart and abdominal wall defects (Abe 2003, Chambers 1998), have been reported in association with febrile infections in early pregnancy, even though the overall malformation risk is absent or only mildly increased. Moretti (2005) performed a meta-analysis about the risk of neural tube defects and hyperthermia. They included 15 studies with 1,719 cases and found a significant correlation (OR 1.9; 95%; CI 1.61–2.29), both in the nine case-control studies and the six cohort studies. Lowering fever in pregnant women seems to reduce the risk (Suarez 2004).

It has been debated if the use of sauna, electric blankets, or other factors that bring about a short-term increase in body temperature could lead to similar effects as high fever (Suarez 2004). In Finland, where this issue had been investigated repeatedly, visits to saunas occur frequently during pregnancy and is considered safe. The use of electric blankets and heated water beds has not shown, in other investigations, that they are linked to an increased malformation risk.

One study observed that children between the ages of 5 and 12 had more frequent emotional and cognitive deficits where there were reports about high fever during the second and third trimester (Dombrowski 2003).

In summary, it appears that there is a slightly higher risk of malformations when high fever (>39°C and >24 hours) occurs, especially during the first 4 weeks after conception.

> **Recommendation.** If there is an infection with high fever, especially during early pregnancy, the fever should be controlled with acetaminophen (paracetamol) or ibuprofen (Chapter 2.1). Ibuprofen should not be taken after 28 gestational weeks. Non pharmacological measures of fever control such as cool wrappings, and sufficient fluid intake should also be considered. In cases of high fever episodes in early pregnancy, a detailed ultrasound examination should be offered to ascertain the normal development of the fetus. A fever episode does not justify a risk-based termination of pregnancy (Chapter 1.15). Visits to a sauna should be limited to less than 10 minutes, and hot or long baths need to be avoided as well as other sources that can overheat the body.

2.6.36   Long-distance travel and flights

During long-distance travel and flights during pregnancy, a number of potential risks need to be considered:

- Prevention of infections (malaria prophylaxis, see Section 2.6.16.; vaccinations, see Chapter 2.7).
- The risk of other infections (fever, fluid loss), and required therapy.
- During long-distance flights:
  - risks of thrombosis
  - ionizing cosmic radiation

- decrease of the partial oxygen pressure equivalent to an altitude of 2,500 m
- dry air.
■ Physical and psychological stress.

Specific developmental anomalies have not been found in pregnant women undergoing vaccinations or recommended malaria prophylaxis, nor were such problems seen as a result of long-distance flights.

However, it needs to be noted that the stress of a long-distance trip, especially in predisposed women, might increase the risk of miscarriage. Also, aside from typical infectious diseases, "common" infections may be more prevalent due to altered hygienic standards in the destination country. The accompanying dehydration, fever, or other complications may also endanger the fetus.

The dose of cosmic radiation on a long-distance flight varies markedly – depending on solar activity. Yet, according to current knowledge, no doses are reached that are high enough to lead to an increased risk of malformations.

> **Recommendation.** The need for long distance travel, especially to tropical destinations, by pregnant women should be critically evaluated. Women with a history of miscarriage should preferably postpone their journey. A well-tolerated long-distance journey is no indication to expand prenatal diagnostic interventions.

References

Abdelrahim II, Adam I, Elghazali G et al. Pharmacokinetics of quinine and its metabolites in pregnant Sudanese women with uncomplicated Plasmodium falciparum malaria. J Clin Pharm Ther 2007; 32: 15–19.

Abe K, Honein MA, Moore CA. Maternal febrile illnesses, medication use, and the risk of congenital renal anomalies. Birth Defects Res A Clin Mol Teratol 2003; 67: 911–8.

Adam I, Elwasila el T, Homeida M. Is praziquantel therapy safe during pregnancy? Trans R Soc Trop Med Hyg 2004a; 98: 540–3.

Adam I, Elhassan EM, Omer EM et al. Safety of artemisinins during early pregnancy, assessed in 62 Sudanese women. Ann Trop Med Parasitol 2009; 103: 205–10.

Adam I, Idris HM, Elbashir MI. Quinine for chloroquine-resistant falciparum malaria in pregnant Sudanese women in the first trimester. East Mediterr Health J 2004b, 10: 560–5.

Adam I, Tarning J, Lindegardh N et al. Pharmacokinetics of piperaquine in pregnant women in Sudan with uncomplicated Plasmodium falciparum malaria. Am J Trop Med Hyg 2012; 87: 35–40.

Aksamija A, Horvat G, Habek D et al. Nitrofurantoin-induced acute liver damage in pregnancy. Arh Hig Rada Toksikol 2009; 60: 357–61.

Aleck KA, Bartley DL. Multiple malformation syndrome following fluconazole use in pregnancy: report of an additional patient. Am J Med Genet 1997; 72: 253–6.

Amado JA, Pesquera C, Gonzalez EM et al. Successful treatment with ketoconazole of Cushing's syndrome in pregnancy. Postgrad Med J 1990; 66: 221–3.

Andersen JT, Petersen M, Jimenez-Solem E et al. Clarithromycin in early pregnancy and the risk of miscarriage and malformation: a register based nationwide cohort study. PloS One 2013a; 8: e53327.

Andersen JT, Petersen M, Jimenez-Solem E et al. Trimethoprim use in early pregnancy and the risk of miscarriage: a register-based nationwide cohort study. Epidemiol Infect 2013b; 141: 1749–55.

Andersen JT, Petersen M, Jimenez-Solem E et al. Trimethoprim Use prior to Pregnancy and the Risk of Congenital Malformation: A Register-Based Nationwide Cohort Study. Obstet Gynecol Int 2013c: 364526.

Andrews WW, Sibai BM, Thom EA et al. Randomized clinical trial of metronidazole plus erythromycin to prevent spontaneous preterm delivery in fetal fibronectin-positive women. Obstet Gynecol 2003; 101: 847–55.

Pregnancy

2.6 Anti-infective Agents

Antiretroviral Pregnancy Registry Steering Committee. Antiretroviral Pregnancy Registry International Interim Report for 1 January 1989 through 31 July 2013. Wilmington, NC: Registry Coordinating Center 2013. Available from URL: www.APRegistry.com (accessed on 20–3–2014).

Atmar RL, Englund JA, Hammill H. Complications of measles during pregnancy. Clin Infect Dis 1992; 14: 217–26.

Bahat Dinur A, Koren G, Matok I et al. Fetal safety of macrolides. Antimicrob Agents Chemother 2013; 57: 3307–11.

Bar-Oz B, Diav-Citrin O, Shechtman S et al. Pregnancy outcome after gestational exposure to the new macrolides: a prospective multi-center observational study. Eur J Obstet Gynecol Reprod Biol 2008; 141: 31–4.

Bar-Oz B, Moretti ME, Bishai R et al. Pregnancy outcome after in utero exposure to itraconazole: a prospective cohort study. Am J Obstet Gynecol 2000; 183: 617–20.

Bar-Oz B, Moretti ME, Boskovic R et al. The safety of quinolones – a meta-analysis of pregnancy outcomes. Eur J Obstet Gynecol Reprod Biol 2009; 143: 75–8.

Bar-Oz B, Weber-Schoendorfer C, Berlin M et al. The outcomes of pregnancy in women exposed to the new macrolides in the first trimester: a prospective, multicentre, observational study. Drug Saf 2012; 35: 589–98.

Bardaji A, Sigauque B, Sanz S et al. Impact of malaria at the end of pregnancy on infant mortality and morbidity. J Infect Dis 2011; 203: 691–9.

Bayrak O, Cimentepe E, Inegol I et al. Is single-dose fosfomycin trometamol a good alternative for asymptomatic bacteriuria in the second trimester of pregnancy? Int Urogynecol J Pelvic Floor Dysfunct 2007; 18: 525–9.

Beard CM, Noller KL, O'Fallon WM et al. Cancer after exposure to metronidazole. Mayo Clin Proc 1988; 63: 147–53.

Beau AB, Hurault-Delarue C, Vial T et al. Safety of oseltamivir during pregnancy: a comparative study using the EFEMERIS database. BJOG 2014; doi: 10.1111/1471-0528.12617 [Epub ahead of print].

Beigi RH, Han K, Venkataramanan R et al. Pharmacokinetics of oseltamivir among pregnant and nonpregnant women. Am J Obstet Gynecol 2011; 204: S84–S88.

Ben David S, Einarson T, Ben DY et al. The safety of nitrofurantoin during the first trimester of pregnancy: meta-analysis. Fundam Clin Pharmacol 1995; 9: 503–7.

Benaboud S, Ekouevi DK, Urien S et al. Population pharmacokinetics of nevirapine in HIV-1-infected pregnant women and their neonates. Antimicrob Agents Chemother 2011; 55: 331–7.

Benhammou V, Tardieu M, Warszawski J et al. Clinical mitochondrial dysfunction in uninfected children born to HIV-infected mothers following perinatal exposure to nucleoside analogues. Environ Mol Mutagen 2007; 48: 173–8.

Berkovitch M, Diav-Citrin O, Greenberg R et al. First-trimester exposure to amoxycillin/clavulanic acid: a prospective, controlled study. Br J Clin Pharmacol 2004; 58: 298–302.

Berkovitch M, Pastuszak A, Gazarian M et al. Safety of the new quinolones in pregnancy. Obstet Gynecol 1994; 84: 535–8.

Berkovitch M, Segal-Socher I, Greenberg R et al. First trimester exposure to cefuroxime: a prospective cohort study. Br J Clin Pharmacol 2000; 50: 161–5.

Berwaerts J, Verhelst J, Mahler C et al. Cushing's syndrome in pregnancy treated by ketoconazole: case report and review of the literature. Gynecol Endocrinol 1999; 13: 175–82.

Best BM, Stek AM, Mirochnick M et al. Lopinavir tablet pharmacokinetics with an increased dose during pregnancy. J Acquir Immune Defic Syndr 2010; 54: 381–8.

Bhargava P, Kuldeep CM, Mathur NK. Antileprosy drugs, pregnancy and fetal outcome. Int J Lepr Other Mycobact Dis 1996; 64: 457–8.

Blanche S, Tardieu M, Rustin P et al. Persistent mitochondrial dysfunction and perinatal exposure to antiretroviral nucleoside analogues. Lancet 1999; 354: 1084–9.

Blumberg HM, Burman WJ, Chaisson RE et al. American Thoracic Society/Centers for Disease Control and Prevention/Infectious Diseases Society of America: treatment of tuberculosis. Am J Respir Crit Care Med 2003; 167: 603–62.

Boronat M, Marrero D, Lopez-Plasencia Y et al. Successful outcome of pregnancy in a patient with Cushing's disease under treatment with ketoconazole during the first trimester of gestation. Gynecol Endocrinol 2011; 27: 675–7.

Bothamley G. Drug treatment for tuberculosis during pregnancy: safety considerations. Drug Saf 2001; 24: 553–65.

Bounyasong S. Randomized trial of artesunate and mefloquine in comparison with quinine sulfate to treat P. falciparum malaria pregnant women. J Med AssocThai 2001; 84: 1289–99.

Brennan-Benson P, Pakianathan M, Rice P et al. Enfurvitide prevents vertical transmission of multidrug-resistant HIV-1 in pregnancy but does not cross the placenta. AIDS 2006; 20: 297–9.

Bristol-Myers Squibb Company. Healthcare Provider Important Drug Warning Letter. 2001. http://www.fda.gov/Safety/MedWatch/SafetyInformation/SafetyAlertsforHumanMedicalProducts/ucm173947.htm (accessed on 20-3-2014).

Bruel H, Guillemant V, Saladin-Thiron C et al. Hemolytic anemia in a newborn after maternal treatment with nitrofurantoin at the end of pregnancy. Arch Pediatr 2000; 7: 745–7.

Bryson YJ, Mirochnick M, Stek A et al. Pharmacokinetics and safety of nelfinavir when used in combination with zidovudine and lamivudine in HIV-infected pregnant women: Pediatric AIDS Clinical Trials Group (PACTG) Protocol 353. HIV Clin Trials 2008; 9: 115–25.

Campomori A, Bonati M. Fluconazole treatment for vulvovaginal candidiasis during pregnancy. Ann Pharmacother 1997; 31: 118–9.

Cespedes MS, Castor D, Ford SL et al. Steady-state pharmacokinetics, cord blood concentrations, and safety of ritonavir-boosted fosamprenavir in pregnancy. J Acquir Immune Defic Syndr 2013; 62: 550–4.

Chambers CD, Johnson KA, Dick LM et al. Maternal fever and birth outcome: a prospective study. Teratology 1998; 58: 251–7.

Chappuy H, Treluyer JM, Jullien V et al. Maternal-fetal transfer and amniotic fluid accumulation of nucleoside analogue reverse transcriptase inhibitors in human immunodeficiency virus-infected pregnant women. Antimicrob Agents Chemother 2004; 48: 4332–6.

Chen JY, Ribaudo HJ, Souda S et al. Highly active antiretroviral therapy and adverse birth outcomes among HIV-infected women in Botswana. J Infect Dis 2012; 206: 1695–705.

Chippaux JP, Gardon-Wendel N, Gardon J et al. Absence of any adverse effect of inadvertent ivermectin treatment during pregnancy. Trans R Soc Trop Med Hyg 1993; 87: 318.

Choi JS, Han JY, Ahn HK et al. Fetal outcome after exposure to antihelminthics albendazole and flubendazole during early pregnancy {Abstract}. Birth Defects Res A Clin Mol Teratol 2005; 73: 349.

Choi JS, Han JY, Ahn HK et al. Fetal outcome after exposure to flubendazole during pregnancy {Abstract}. Birth Defects Res A Clin Mol Teratol 2008; 82: 381.

Christian P, Khatry SK, West KP Jr. Antenatal anthelmintic treatment, birthweight, and infant survival in rural Nepal. Lancet 2004; 364: 981–3.

Chun JY, Han JY, Ahn HK et al. Fetal outcome following roxithromycin exposure in early pregnancy. J Matern Fetal Neonatal Med 2006; 19: 189–192.

Clark RL. Embryotoxicity of the artemisinin antimalarials and potential consequences for use in women in the first trimester. Reprod Toxicol 2009; 28: 285–96.

Colbers A, Gingelmaier A, van der Ende M et al. Pharmacokinetics, safety and transplacental passage of rilpivirine in pregnancy: two cases. AIDS 2014; 28: 288–90.

Connor EM, Sperling RS, Gelber R et al. Reduction of maternal-infant transmission of human immunodeficiency virus type 1 with zidovudine treatment. Pediatric AIDS Clinical Trials Group Protocol 076 Study Group. N Engl J Med 1994; 331: 1173–80.

Conway N, Birt BD. Streptomycin in pregnancy: effect on the foetal ear. Br Med J 1965; 2: 260–3.

Cooper WO, Ray WA, Griffin MR. Prenatal prescription of macrolide antibiotics and infantile hypertrophic pyloric stenosis. Obstet Gynecol 2002; 100: 101–6.

Cooper WO, Hernandez-Diaz S, Arbogast PG et al. Antibiotics potentially used in response to bioterrorism and the risk of major congenital malformations. Paediatr Perinat Epidemiol 2009; 23: 18–28.

Costa ML, Souza JP, Oliveira Neto AF et al. Cryptococcal meningitis in HIV negative pregnant women: case report and review of literature. Rev Inst Med Trop Sao Paulo 2009; 51: 289–94.

Cotter AM, Garcia AG, Duthely ML et al. Is antiretroviral therapy during pregnancy associated with an increased risk of preterm delivery, low birth weight, or stillbirth? J Infect Dis 2006; 193: 1195–201.

Cowden J, Hotez P. Mebendazole and albendazole treatment of geohelminth infections in children and pregnant women. Pediatr Infect Dis J 2000; 19: 659–60.

Crider KS, Cleves MA, Reefhuis J et al. Antibacterial medication use during pregnancy and risk of birth defects: National Birth Defects Prevention Study. Arch Pediatr Adolesc Med 2009; 163: 978–5.

Culnane M, Fowler M, Lee SS et al. Lack of long-term effects of in utero exposure to zidovudine among uninfected children born to HIV-infected women. Pediatric AIDS Clinical Trials Group Protocol 219/076 Teams. JAMA 1999; 281: 151–7.

Pregnancy

2.6 Anti-infective Agents

Czeizel A. A case-control analysis of the teratogenic effects of co-trimoxazole. Reprod Toxicol 1990; 4: 305–13.

Czeizel AE, Rockenbauer M. Teratogenic study of doxycycline. Obstet Gynecol 1997; 89: 524–8.

Czeizel AE, Rockenbauer M. A population based case-control teratologic study of oral metronidazole treatment during pregnancy. Br J Obstet Gynaecol 1998; 105: 322–7.

Czeizel AE, Rockenbauer M, Sorensen HT et al. A population-based case-control teratologic study of oral erythromycin treatment during pregnancy. Reprod Toxicol 1999a; 13: 531–6.

Czeizel AE, Toth M, Rockenbauer M. No teratogenic effect after clotrimazole therapy during pregnancy. Epidemiology 1999b; 10: 437–40.

Czeizel AE, Rockenbauer M, Olsen J et al. Oral phenoxymethylpenicillin treatment during pregnancy. Results of a population-based Hungarian case-control study. Arch Gynecol Obstet 2000a; 263: 178–181.

Czeizel AE, Rockenbauer M, Olsen J et al. A case-control teratological study of spiramycin, roxithromycin, oleandomycin and josamycin. Acta Obstet Gynecol Scand 2000b; 79: 234–7.

Czeizel AE, Rockenbauer M, Sorensen HT et al. A teratological study of lincosamides. Scand J Infect Dis 2000c; 32: 579–580.

Czeizel AE, Rockenbauer M. A population-based case-control teratologic study of oral oxytetracycline treatment during pregnancy. Eur J Obstet Gynecol Reprod Biol 2000d; 88: 27–33.

Czeizel AE, Rockenbauer M, Olsen J et al. A teratological study of aminoglycoside antibiotic treatment during pregnancy. Scand J Infect Dis 2000e; 32: 309–13.

Czeizel AE, Rockenbauer M, Sorensen HT et al. A population-based case-control teratologic study of oral chloramphenicol treatment during pregnancy. Eur J Epidemiol 2000f; 16: 323–7.

Czeizel AE, Rockenbauer M, Sorensen HT et al. Augmentin treatment during pregnancy and the prevalence of congenital abnormalities: a population-based case-control teratologic study. Eur J Obstet Gynecol Reprod Biol 2001a; 97: 188–92.

Czeizel AE, Rockenbauer M, Sorensen HT et al. Use of cephalosporins during pregnancy and in the presence of congenital abnormalities: a population-based, case-control study. Am J Obstet Gynecol 2001b; 184: 1289–96.

Czeizel AE, Rockenbauer M, Sorensen HT et al. The teratogenic risk of trimethoprim-sulfonamides: a population based case-control study. Reprod Toxicol 2001c; 15: 637–46.

Czeizel AE, Rockenbauer M, Sorensen HT et al. Nitrofurantoin and congenital abnormalities. Eur J Obstet Gynecol Reprod Biol 2001d; 95: 119–26.

Czeizel AE, Rockenbauer M, Olsen J et al. A population-based case-control study of the safety of oral anti-tuberculosis drug treatment during pregnancy. Int J Tuberc Lung Dis 2001e; 5: 564–8.

Czeizel AE, Kazy Z, Vargha P. A population-based case-control teratological study of vaginal econazole treatment during pregnancy. Eur J Obstet Gynecol Reprod Biol 2003a; 111: 135–40.

Czeizel AE, Kazy Z, Puho E. A population-based case-control teratological study of oral nystatin treatment during pregnancy. Scand J Infect Dis 2003b; 35: 830–5.

Czeizel AE, Kazy Z, Vargha P. A case-control teratological study of vaginal natamycin treatment during pregnancy. Reprod Toxicol 2003c; 17: 387–91.

Czeizel AE, Fladung B, Vargha P. Preterm birth reduction after clotrimazole treatment during pregnancy. Eur J Obstet Gynecol Reprod Biol 2004a; 116: 157–63.

Czeizel AE, Kazy Z, Puho E. Population-based case-control teratologic study of topical miconazole. Congenit Anom (Kyoto) 2004b; 44: 41–5.

Czeizel AE, Metneki J, Kazy Z et al. A population-based case-control study of oral griseofulvin treatment during pregnancy. Acta Obstet Gynecol Scand 2004c; 83: 827–31.

Czeizel AE, Kazy Z, Puho E. Tolnaftate spray treatment during pregnancy. Reprod Toxicol 2004d; 18: 443–4.

de Silva NR, Sirisena JL, Gunasekera DP et al. Effect of mebendazole therapy during pregnancy on birth outcome. Lancet 1999; 353: 1145–9.

de Santis M, Carducci B, De Santis L et al. Periconceptional exposure to efavirenz and neural tube defects. Arch Intern Med 2002; 162: 355.

De Santis M, Di Gianantonio E, Cesari E et al. First-trimester itraconazole exposure and pregnancy outcome: a prospective cohort study of women contacting teratology information services in Italy. Drug Saf 2009; 32: 239–44.

Dean JL, Wolf JE, Ranzini AC et al. Use of amphotericin B during pregnancy: case report and review. Clin Infect Dis 1994; 18: 364–8.

Deen JL, von Seidlein L, Pinder M et al. The safety of the combination artesunate and pyrimethamine-sulfadoxine given during pregnancy. Trans R Soc Trop Med Hyg 2001; 95: 424–8.

Dencker BB, Larsen H, Jensen ES et al. Birth outcome of 1886 pregnancies after exposure to phenoxymethylpenicillin in utero. Clin Microbiol Infect 2002; 8: 196–201.

Deng M, Zhou X, Gao S et al. The effects of telbivudine in late pregnancy to prevent intrauterine transmission of the hepatitis B virus: a systematic review and meta-analysis. Virol J 2012; 9: 185.

Diav-Citrin O, Shechtman S, Arnon J et al. Pregnancy outcome after gestational exposure to mebendazole: a prospective controlled cohort study. Am J Obstet Gynecol 2003; 188: 282–5.

Diav-Citrin O, Shechtman S, Gotteiner T et al. Pregnancy outcome after gestational exposure to metronidazole: a prospective controlled cohort study. Teratology 2001; 63: 186–92.

Dobias L, Cerna M, Rossner P et al. Genotoxicity and carcinogenicity of metronidazole. Mutat Res 1994; 317: 177–94.

Dombrowski SC, Martin RP, Huttunen MO. Association between maternal fever and psychological/behavior outcomes: a hypothesis. Birth Defects Res A Clin Mol Teratol 2003; 67: 905–10.

Donner B, Niranjan V, Hoffmann G. Safety of oseltamivir in pregnancy: a review of preclinical and clinical data. Drug Saf 2010; 33: 631–42.

Drinkard CR, Shatin D, Clouse J. Postmarketing surveillance of medications and pregnancy outcomes: clarithromycin and birth malformations. Pharmacoepidemiol Drug Saf 2000; 9: 549–56.

Drobac PC, del Castillo H, Sweetland A et al. Treatment of multidrug-resistant tuberculosis during pregnancy: long-term follow-up of 6 children with intrauterine exposure to second-line agents. Clin Infect Dis 2005; 40: 1689–92.

Dryden-Peterson S, Shapiro RL, Hughes MD et al. Increased risk of severe infant anemia after exposure to maternal HAART, Botswana. J Acquir Immune Defic Syndr 2011; 56: 428–36.

Dunstan H, Mill A, Stephens S et al. Pregnancy outcome following maternal use of zanamivir or oseltamivir during the 2009 influenza A/H1N1 pandemic: a national prospective surveillance study. BJOG 2014; doi: 10.1111/1471-0528.12640 [Epub ahead of print].

EACS: European AIDS Clinical Society. Europeans Guidelines for treatment of HIV-infected adults in Europe, version 7.0. 2013. Available from URL: www.eacsociety.org (accessed on 20-3-2014).

Edwards MJ, Shiota K, Smith MS et al. Hyperthermia and birth defects. Reprod Toxicol 1995; 9: 411–25.

Ehsanipoor RM, Chung JH, Clock CA et al. A retrospective review of ampicillin-sulbactam and amoxicillin + clavulanate vs cefazolin/cephalexin and erythromycin in the setting of preterm premature rupture of membranes: maternal and neonatal outcomes. Am J Obstet Gynecol 2008; 198: e54–e56.

Einarson A, Phillips E, Mawji F et al. A prospective controlled multicentre study of clarithromycin in pregnancy. Am J Perinatol 1998; 15: 523–5.

Elbadawi NE, Mohamed MI, Dawod OY et al. Effect of quinine therapy on plasma glucose and plasma insulin levels in pregnant women infected with Plasmodium falciparum malaria in Gezira state. East Mediterr Health J 2011; 17: 697–700.

Ely EW, Peacock JE Jr, Haponik EF et al. Cryptococcal pneumonia complicating pregnancy. Medicine (Baltimore) 1998; 77: 153–67.

ECS: European Collaborative Study. Exposure to antiretroviral therapy in utero or early life: the health of uninfected children born to HIV-infected women. J Acquir Immune Defic Syndr 2003; 32: 380–7.

Falagas ME, Vouloumanou EK, Togias AG et al. Fosfomycin versus other antibiotics for the treatment of cystitis: a meta-analysis of randomized controlled trials. J Antimicrob Chemother 2010; 65: 1862–77.

Feiterna-Sperling C, Weizsaecker K, Buhrer C et al. Hematologic effects of maternal antiretroviral therapy and transmission prophylaxis in HIV-1-exposed uninfected newborn infants. J Acquir Immune Defic Syndr 2007; 45: 43–51.

Floridia M, Mastroiacovo P, Tamburrini E et al. Birth defects in a national cohort of pregnant women with HIV infection in Italy, 2001–2011. BJOG 2013; 120: 1466–75.

Flynn PM, Mirochnick M, Shapiro DE et al. Pharmacokinetics and safety of single-dose tenofovir disoproxil fumarate and emtricitabine in HIV-1-infected pregnant women and their infants. Antimicrob Agents Chemother 2011; 55: 5914–22.

Pregnancy

2.6 Anti-infective Agents

Ford N, Calmy A, Mofenson L. Safety of efavirenz in the first trimester of pregnancy: an updated systematic review and meta-analysis. AIDS 2011; 25: 2301–04.

Ford N, Mofenson L, Kranzer K et al. Safety of efavirenz in first-trimester of pregnancy: a systematic review and meta-analysis of outcomes from observational cohorts. AIDS 2010; 24: 1461–70.

Fundaro C, Genovese O, Rendeli C et al. Myelomeningocele in a child with intrauterine exposure to efavirenz. AIDS 2002; 16: 299–300.

Furco A, Gosrani B, Nicholas S et al. Successful use of darunavir, etravirine, enfuvirtide and tenofovir/emtricitabine in pregnant woman with multiclass HIV resistance. AIDS 2009; 23: 434–5.

Gardner JS, Guyard-Boileau B, Alderman BW et al. Maternal exposure to prescription and non-prescription pharmaceuticals or drugs of abuse and risk of craniosynostosis. Int J Epidemiol 1998; 27: 64–7.

Gibb DM, Kizito H, Russell EC et al. Pregnancy and infant outcomes among HIV-infected women taking long-term ART with and without tenofovir in the DART trial. PloS Med 2012; 9: e1001217.

Gingelmaier A, Kurowski M, Kastner R et al. Placental transfer and pharmacokinetics of lopinavir and other protease inhibitors in combination with nevirapine at delivery. AIDS 2006; 20: 1737–43.

Glaxo Wellcome. Acyclovir pregnancy registry and valacyclovir pregnancy registry: Interim report for 1 June 1984 through 31 December 1997, Glaxo Wellcome Research Triangle Park, NC USA 1997.

Goldberg O, Koren G, Landau D et al. Exposure to nitrofurantoin during the first trimester of pregnancy and the risk for major malformations. J Clin Pharmacol 2013; 53: 991–5.

Gough AW, Kasali OB, Sigler RE et al. Quinolone arthropathy – acute toxicity to immature articular cartilage. Toxicol Pathol 1992; 20: 436–49.

Graham JM Jr. Marshall J. Edwards: discoverer of maternal hyperthermia as a human teratogen. Birth Defects Res A Clin Mol Teratol 2005; 73: 857–64.

Green MD, van Eijk AM, van Ter Kuile FO et al. Pharmacokinetics of sulfadoxine-pyrimethamine in HIV-infected and uninfected pregnant women in Western Kenya. J Infect Dis 2007; 196: 1403–08.

Greer LG, Leff RD, Rogers VL et al. Pharmacokinetics of oseltamivir according to trimester of pregnancy. Am J Obstet Gynecol 2011; 204: S89–S93.

Greer LG, Sheffield JS, Rogers VL et al. Maternal and neonatal outcomes after antepartum treatment of influenza with antiviral medications. Obstet Gynecol 2010; 115: 711–6.

Guay LA, Musoke P, Fleming T et al. Intrapartum and neonatal single-dose nevirapine compared with zidovudine for prevention of mother-to-child transmission of HIV-1 in Kampala, Uganda: HIVNET 012 randomised trial. Lancet 1999; 354: 795–802.

Gyapong JO, Chinbuah MA, Gyapong M. Inadvertent exposure of pregnant women to ivermectin and albendazole during mass drug administration for lymphatic filariasis. Trop Med Int Health 2003; 8: 1093–1101.

Gyorkos TW, Larocque R, Casapia M et al. Lack of risk of adverse birth outcomes after deworming in pregnant women. Pediatr Infect Dis J 2006; 25: 791–4.

Han GR, Cao MK, Zhao W et al. A prospective and open-label study for the efficacy and safety of telbivudine in pregnancy for the prevention of perinatal transmission of hepatitis B virus infection. J Hepatol 2011; 55: 1215–21.

Hanson IC, Antonelli TA, Sperling RS et al. Lack of tumors in infants with perinatal HIV-1 exposure and fetal/neonatal exposure to zidovudine. J Acquir Immune Defic Syndr Hum Retrovirol 1999; 20: 463–7.

Heikkilä A, Erkkola R. Review of beta-lactam antibiotics in pregnancy. The need for adjustment of dosage schedules. Clin Pharmacokinet 1994; 27: 49–62.

Heikkilä A, Renkonen OV, Erkkola R. Pharmacokinetics and transplacental passage of imipenem during pregnancy. Antimicrob Agents Chemother 1992; 36: 2652–5.

Hernandez-Diaz S, Werler MM, Walker AM et al. Folic acid antagonists during pregnancy and the risk of birth defects. N Engl J Med 2000; 343: 1608–14.

Hirt D, Urien S, Ekouevi DK et al. Population pharmacokinetics of tenofovir in HIV-1-infected pregnant women and their neonates (ANRS 12109). Clin Pharmacol Ther 2009a; 85: 182–9.

Hirt D, Urien S, Rey E et al. Population pharmacokinetics of emtricitabine in human immunodeficiency virus type 1-infected pregnant women and their neonates. Antimicrob Agents Chemother 2009b; 53: 1067–73.

Hofer H, Donnerer J, Sator K et al. Seminal fluid ribavirin level and functional semen parameters in patients with chronic hepatitis C on antiviral combination therapy. J Hepatol 2010; 52: 812–6.

Hoglund RM, Adam I, Hanpithakpong W et al. A population pharmacokinetic model of piperaquine in pregnant and non-pregnant women with uncomplicated Plasmodium falciparum malaria in Sudan. Malar J 2012; 11: 398.

Hulton SA, Kaplan BS. Renal dysplasia associated with in utero exposure to gentamicin and corticosteroids. Am J Med Genet 1995; 58: 91–3.

Inman W, Pearce G, Wilton L. Safety of fluconazole in the treatment of vaginal candidiasis. A prescription-event monitoring study, with special reference to the outcome of pregnancy. Eur J Clin Pharmacol 1994; 46: 115–8.

Ivanovic J, Bellagamba R, Nicastri E et al. Use of darunavir/ritonavir once daily in treatment-naive pregnant woman: pharmacokinetics, compartmental exposure, efficacy and safety. AIDS 2010; 24: 1083–4.

Jaworsky D, Thompson C, Yudin MH et al. Use of newer antiretroviral agents, darunavir and etravirine with or without raltegravir, in pregnancy: a report of two cases. Antivir Ther 2010; 15: 677–80.

Jepsen P, Skriver MV, Floyd A et al. A population-based study of maternal use of amoxicillin and pregnancy outcome in Denmark. Br J Clin Pharmacol 2003; 55: 216–21.

Jick SS. Pregnancy outcomes after maternal exposure to fluconazole. Pharmacotherapy 1999; 19: 221–2.

Joao EC, Calvet GA, Krauss MR et al. Maternal antiretroviral use during pregnancy and infant congenital anomalies: the NISDI perinatal study. J Acquir Immune Defic Syndr 2010; 53: 176–85.

Joesoef MR, Schmid GP, Hillier SL. Bacterial vaginosis: review of treatment options and potential clinical indications for therapy. Clin Infect Dis 1999; 28: S57–S65.

Jones HC. Intrauterine ototoxicity. A case report and review of literature. J Natl Med Assoc 1973; 65: 201–3, 215.

Kakogawa J, Sakurabashi A, Sadatsuki M et al. Chronic hepatitis B infection in pregnancy illustrated by a case of successful treatment with entecavir. Arch Gynecol Obstet 2011; 284: 1595–6.

Källén BA, Otterblad OP. Maternal drug use in early pregnancy and infant cardiovascular defect. Reprod Toxicol 2003; 17: 255–61.

Källén BA, Otterblad OP, Danielsson BR. Is erythromycin therapy teratogenic in humans? Reprod Toxicol 2005a; 20: 209–14.

Källén BA, Robert-Gnansia E. Maternal drug use, fertility problems, and infant craniostenosis. Cleft Palate Craniofac J 2005b; 42: 589–93.

Källén BA, Danielsson BR. Fetal safety of erythromycin. An update of Swedish data. Eur J Clin Pharmacol 2014; 70: 355–60.

Karunajeewa HA, Salman S, Mueller I et al. Pharmacokinetic properties of sulfadoxine-pyrimethamine in pregnant women. Antimicrob Agents Chemother 2009; 53: 4368–76.

Kazy Z, Puho E, Czeizel AE. Levamisole (Decaris) treatment during pregnancy. Reprod Toxicol 2004; 19: 3.

Kazy Z, Puho E, Czeizel AE. The possible association between the combination of vaginal metronidazole and miconazole treatment and poly-syndactyly population-based case-control teratologic study. Reprod Toxicol 2005a; 20: 89–94.

Kazy Z, Puho E, Czeizel AE. Parenteral polymyxin B treatment during pregnancy. Reprod Toxicol 2005b; 20: 181–2.

Kazy Z, Puho E, Czeizel AE. Population-based case-control study of oral ketoconazole treatment for birth outcomes. Congenit Anom (Kyoto) 2005c; 45: 5–8.

Kenyon SL, Taylor DJ, Tarnow-Mordi W. Broad-spectrum antibiotics for preterm, prelabour rupture of fetal membranes: the ORACLE I randomised trial. ORACLE Collaborative Group. Lancet 2001; 357: 979–88.

King CT, Rogers PD, Cleary JD et al. Antifungal therapy during pregnancy. Clin Infect Dis 1998; 27: 1151–60.

Kirkwood A, Harris C, Timar N et al. Is gentamicin ototoxic to the fetus? J Obstet Gynaecol Can 2007; 29: 140–5.

Klarskov P, Andersen JT, Jimenez-Solem E et al. Short-acting sulfonamides near term and neonatal jaundice. Obstet Gynecol 2013; 122: 105–10.

Klebanoff MA, Carey JC, Hauth JC et al. Failure of metronidazole to prevent preterm delivery among pregnant women with asymptomatic Trichomonas vaginalis infection. N Engl J Med 2001; 345: 487–93.

Knapp KM, Brogly SB, Muenz DG et al. Prevalence of congenital anomalies in infants with in utero exposure to antiretrovirals. Pediatr Infect Dis J 2012; 31: 164–70.

Knudsen LB. No association between griseofulvin and conjoined twinning. Lancet 1987; 2: 1097.

Knudtson E, Para M, Boswell H et al. Drug rash with eosinophilia and systemic symptoms syndrome and renal toxicity with a nevirapine-containing regimen in a pregnant patient with human immunodeficiency virus. Obstet Gynecol 2003; 101: 1094–7.

Koss CA, Baras DC, Lane SD et al. Investigation of metronidazole use during pregnancy and adverse birth outcomes. Antimicrob Agents Chemother 2012; 56: 4800–05.

Kourtis AP, Schmid CH, Jamieson DJ et al. Use of antiretroviral therapy in pregnant HIV-infected women and the risk of premature delivery: a meta-analysis. AIDS 2007; 21: 6 07–15.

Laiprasert J, Klein K, Mueller BA et al. Transplacental passage of vancomycin in noninfected term pregnant women. Obstet Gynecol 2007; 109: 1105–10.

Larsen B, Glover DD. Serum erythromycin levels in pregnancy. Clin Ther 1998; 20: 971–7.

Larsen H, Nielsen GL, Schonheyder HC et al. Birth outcome following maternal use of fluoroquinolones. Int J Antimicrob Agents 2001; 18: 259–62.

Le Chenadec J, Mayaux MJ, Guihenneuc-Jouyaux C et al. Perinatal antiretroviral treatment and hematopoiesis in HIV-uninfected infants. AIDS 2003; 17: 2053–61.

Lee SJ, McGready R, Fernandez C et al. Chloroquine pharmacokinetics in pregnant and nonpregnant women with vivax malaria. Eur J Clin Pharmacol 2008; 64: 987–92.

Lessnau KD, Qarah S. Multidrug-resistant tuberculosis in pregnancy: case report and review of the literature. Chest 2003; 123: 953–6.

Lewis JH. Drug hepatotoxicity in pregnancy. Eur J Gastroenterol Hepatol 1991; 3: 883–91.

Lin HC, Lin HC, Chen SF. Increased risk of low birthweight and small for gestational age infants among women with tuberculosis. BJOG 2010; 117: 585–90.

Lin KJ, Mitchell AA, Yau WP et al. Maternal exposure to amoxicillin and the risk of oral clefts. Epidemiology 2012; 23: 699–705.

Lin KJ, Mitchell AA, Yau WP et al. Safety of macrolides during pregnancy. Am J Obstet Gynecol 2013; 208: 221–8.

Linder N, Amarilla M, Hernandez A et al. Association of high-dose bifonazole adminis-tration during early pregnancy and severe limb reduction defects in the newborn. Birth Defects Res A Clin Mol Teratol 2010; 88: 201–4.

Liu M, Cai H, Yi W. Safety of telbivudine treatment for chronic hepatitis B for the entire pregnancy. J Viral Hepat 2013; 20: 65–70.

Loebstein R, Addis A, Ho E et al. Pregnancy outcome following gestational exposure to fluo-roquinolones: a multicenter prospective controlled study. Antimicrob Agents Chemother 1998; 42: 1336–9.

Lopez-Rangel E, Van Allen MI. Prenatal exposure to fluconazole: an identifiable dysmor-phic phenotype. Birth Defects Res A Clin Mol Teratol 2005; 73: 919–23.

Louik C, Werler MM, Mitchell AA. Erythromycin use during pregnancy in relation to pyloric stenosis. Am J Obstet Gynecol 2002; 186: 288–90.

Lowe CR. Congenital defects among children born to women under supervision or treat-ment for pulmonary tuberculosis. Br J Prev Soc Med 1964; 18: 14–16.

Lush R, Iland H, Peat B et al. Successful use of dapsone in refractory pregnancy-associated idiopathic thrombocytopenic purpura. Aust NZ J Med 2000; 30: 105–7.

Mahon BE, Rosenman MB, Kleiman MB. Maternal and infant use of erythromycin and other macrolide antibiotics as risk factors for infantile hypertrophic pyloric stenosis. J Pediatr 2001; 139: 380–4.

Malm H, Artama M, Gissler M et al. First trimester use of macrolides and risk of major malformations {OTIS Abstract}. Birth Defects Res Part A Clin Mol Teratol 2008; 82: 412.

Mandelbrot L, Kermarrec N, Marcollet A et al. Case report: nucleoside analogue-induced lactic acidosis in the third trimester of pregnancy. AIDS 2003; 17: 272–3.

Mandelbrot L, Landreau-Mascaro A, Rekacewicz C et al. Lamivudine-zidovudine combina-tion for prevention of maternal-infant transmission of HIV-1. JAMA 2001; 285: 2083–93.

Manka W, Solowiow R, Okrzeja D. Assessment of infant development during an 18-month follow-up after treatment of infections in pregnant women with cefuroxime axetil. Drug Saf 2000; 22: 83–8.

Manyando C, Mkandawire R, Puma L et al. Safety of artemether-lumefantrine in pregnant women with malaria: results of a prospective cohort study in Zambia. Malar J 2010; 9: 249.

Martorell C, Theroux E, Bermudez A et al. Safety and efficacy of fosamprenavir in human immunodeficiency virus-infected pregnant women. Pediatr Infect Dis J 2010; 29: 985.

Marzolini C, Rudin C, Decosterd LA et al. Transplacental passage of protease inhibitors at delivery. AIDS 2002; 16: 889–93.

Mastroiacovo P, Mazzone T, Botto LD et al. Prospective assessment of pregnancy outcomes after first-trimester exposure to fluconazole. Am J Obstet Gynecol 1996; 175: 1645–50.

McClure EM, Goldenberg RL, Dent AE et al. A systematic review of the impact of malaria prevention in pregnancy on low birth weight and maternal anemia. Int J Gynaecol Obstet 2013; 121: 103–9.

McCormack WM, George H, Donner A et al. Hepatotoxicity of erythromycin estolate during pregnancy. Antimicrob Agents Chemother 1977; 12: 630–5.

McElhatton P, Stephens S. Preliminary data on exposure to mebendazole during pregnancy (Abstract). Reprod Toxicol 2007; 24: 62.

McGready R, Ashley EA, Moo E et al. A randomized comparison of artesunate-atovaquone-proguanil versus quinine in treatment for uncomplicated falciparum malaria during pregnancy. J Infect Dis 2005; 192: 846–53.

McGready R, Brockman A, Cho T et al. Randomized comparison of mefloquine-artesunate versus quinine in the treatment of multidrug-resistant falciparum malaria in pregnancy. Trans R Soc Trop Med Hyg 2000; 94: 689–93.

McGready R, Cho T, Keo NK et al. Artemisinin antimalarials in pregnancy: a prospective treatment study of 539 episodes of multidrug-resistant Plasmodium falciparum. Clin Infect Dis 2001; 33: 2009–16.

McGready R, Stepniewska K, Edstein MD et al. The pharmacokinetics of atovaquone and proguanil in pregnant women with acute falciparum malaria. Eur J Clin Pharmacol 2003; 59: 545–52.

McGready R, Tan SO, Ashley EA et al. A randomised controlled trial of artemether-lumefantrine versus artesunate for uncomplicated plasmodium falciparum treatment in pregnancy. PLoS Med 2008; 5: e253.

McGready R, Thwai KL, Cho T et al. The effects of quinine and chloroquine antimalarial treatments in the first trimester of pregnancy. Trans R Soc Trop Med Hyg 2002; 96: 180–4.

McKeown DA, Rosenvinge M, Donaghy S et al. High neonatal concentrations of raltegravir following transplacental transfer in HIV-1 positive pregnant women. AIDS 2010; 24: 2416–8.

McNellis D, McLeod M, Lawson J et al. Treatment of vulvovaginal candidiasis in pregnancy. A comparative study. Obstet Gynecol 1977; 50: 674–8.

Mercieri M, Di RR, Pantosti A et al. Critical pneumonia complicating early-stage pregnancy. Anesth Analg 2010; 110: 852–4.

Metneki J, Czeizel A. Griseofulvin teratology. Lancet 1987; 1: 1042.

Mickal A, Panzer JD. The safety of lincomycin in pregnancy. Am J Obstet Gynecol 1975; 121: 1071–4.

Miller MW, Church CC. Arrhenius thermodynamics and birth defects: chemical teratogen synergy. Untested, testable, and projected relevance. Birth Defects Res C 2013; 99: 50–60.

Mirochnick M, Fenton T, Gagnier P et al. Pharmacokinetics of nevirapine in human immunodeficiency virus type 1-infected pregnant women and their neonates. Pediatric AIDS Clinical Trials Group Protocol 250 Team. J Infect Dis 1998; 178: 368–74.

Mirochnick M, Best BM, Stek AM et al. Atazanavir pharmacokinetics with and without tenofovir during pregnancy. J Acquir Immune Defic Syndr 2011; 56: 412–9.

Mirochnick M, Dorenbaum A, Holland D et al. Concentrations of protease inhibitors in cord blood after in utero exposure. Pediatr Infect Dis J 2002; 21: 835–8.

Mohamed A, Dresser GK, Mehta S. Acute respiratory failure during pregnancy: a case of nitrofurantoin-induced pneumonitis. CMAJ 2007; 176: 319–20.

Mølgaard-Nielsen D, Hviid A. Maternal use of antibiotics and the risk of orofacial clefts: a nationwide cohort study. Pharmacoepidemiol Drug Saf 2012; 21: 246–53.

Mølgaard-Nielsen D, Pasternak B, Hviid A. Use of oral fluconazole during pregnancy and the risk of birth defects. N Engl J Med 2013; 369: 830–9.

Moretti ME, Bar-Oz B, Fried S et al. Maternal hyperthermia and the risk for neural tube defects in offspring: systematic review and meta-analysis. Epidemiology 2005; 16: 216–9.

Morris CA, Onyamboko MA, Capparelli E et al. Population pharmacokinetics of artesunate and dihydroartemisinin in pregnant and non-pregnant women with malaria. Malar J 2011; 10: 114.

Mosha D, Mazuguni F, Mrema S et al. Safety of artemether-lumefantrine exposue in first trimester of pregnancy: an observational cohort. Malar J 2014; 13: 197.

Mpairwe H, Webb EL, Muhangi L et al. Anthelminthic treatment during pregnancy is associated with increased risk of infantile eczema: randomized-controlled trial results. Pediatr Allergy Immunol 2011; 22: 305–12.

Pregnancy

2.6 Anti-infective Agents

Mueller M, Balasegaram M, Koummuki Y et al. A comparison of liposomal amphotericin B with sodium stibogluconate for the treatment of visceral leishmaniasis in pregnancy in Sudan. J Antimicrob Chemother 2006; 58: 811–5.

Muller AE, Dorr PJ, Mouton JW et al. The influence of labour on the pharmacokinetics of intravenously administered amoxicillin in pregnant women. Br J Clin Pharmacol 2008; 66: 866–74.

Myles TD, Elam G, Park-Hwang E et al. The Jarisch-Herxheimer reaction and fetal monitoring changes in pregnant women treated for syphilis. Obstet Gynecol 1998; 92: 859–64.

Na-Bangchang K, Manyando C, Ruengweerayut R et al. The pharmacokinetics and pharmacodynamics of atovaquone and proguanil for the treatment of uncomplicated falciparum malaria in third-trimester pregnant women. Eur J Clin Pharmacol 2005; 61: 573–82.

Nanovskaya T, Patrikeeva S, Zhan Y et al. Transplacental transfer of vancomycin and telavancin. Am J Obstet Gynecol 2012; 207: 331–6.

Ndibazza J, Muhangi L, Akishule D et al. Effects of deworming during pregnancy on maternal and perinatal outcomes in Entebbe, Uganda: a randomized controlled trial. Clin Infect Dis 2010; 50: 531–40.

Ndyomugyenyi R, Kabatereine N, Olsen A et al. Efficacy of ivermectin and albendazole alone and in combination for treatment of soil-transmitted helminths in pregnancy and adverse events: a randomized open label controlled intervention trial in Masindi district, western Uganda. Am J Trop Med Hyg 2008; 79: 856–63.

Neou P, Gyftodemou Y, Valti E et al. Famciclovir exposure during organogenesis {Abstract}. Reprod Toxicol 2004; 18: 742.

Newman RD, Parise ME, Slutsker L et al. Safety, efficacy and determinants of effectiveness of antimalarial drugs during pregnancy: implications for prevention programmes in Plasmodium falciparum-endemic sub-Saharan Africa. Trop Med Int Health 2003; 8: 488–506.

Nordeng H, Lupattelli A, Romoren M et al. Neonatal outcomes after gestational exposure to nitrofurantoin. Obstet Gynecol 2013; 121: 306–13.

Nørgaard M, Pedersen L, Gislum M et al. Maternal use of fluconazole and risk of congenital malformations: a Danish population-based cohort study. J Antimicrob Chemother 2008; 62: 172–6.

Nørgård B, Czeizel AE, Rockenbauer M et al. Population-based case control study of the safety of sulfasalazine use during pregnancy. Aliment Pharmacol Ther 2001; 15: 483–6.

Nosten F, Vincenti M, Simpson J et al. The effects of mefloquine treatment in pregnancy. Clin Infect Dis 1999; 28: 808–15.

Nyunt MM, Adam I, Kayentao K et al. Pharmacokinetics of sulfadoxine and pyrimethamine in intermittent preventive treatment of malaria in pregnancy. Clin Pharmacol Ther 2010; 87: 226–34.

OARAC (Working group of the office of AIDS research advisory council), Panel on Treatment of HIV-Infected Pregnant Women and Prevention of Perinatal Transmission. Recommendations for Use of Antiretroviral Drugs in Pregnant HIV-1-Infected Women for Maternal Health and Interventions to Reduce Perinatal HIV Transmission in the United States. 2012. Available from URL: http://aidsinfo.nih.gov/guidelines (accessed on 20–3–2014).

Osadchy A, Ratnapalan T, Koren G. Ocular toxicity in children exposed in utero to antimalarial drugs: review of the literature. J Rheumatol 2011; 38: 2504–08.

Ouyang DW, Brogly SB, Lu M et al. Lack of increased hepatotoxicity in HIV-infected pregnant women receiving nevirapine compared with other antiretrovirals. AIDS 2010; 24: 109–14.

Ouyang DW, Shapiro DE, Lu M et al. Increased risk of hepatotoxicity in HIV-infected pregnant women receiving antiretroviral therapy independent of nevirapine exposure. AIDS 2009; 23: 2425–30.

Ozyüncü O, Beksac MS, Nemutlu E et al. Maternal blood and amniotic fluid levels of moxifloxacin, levofloxacin and cefixime. J Obstet Gynaecol Res 2010; 36: 484–7.

Pacifici GM. Transfer of antivirals across the human placenta. Early Hum Dev 2005; 81: 647–54.

Pacque M, Munoz B, Poetschke G et al. Pregnancy outcome after inadvertent ivermectin treatment during community-based distribution. Lancet 1990; 336: 1486–9.

Padberg S, Wacker E, Meister R et al. Observational Cohort Study of Pregnancy Outcome after First-Trimester Exposure to Fluoroquinolones. Antimicrob. Agents Chemother 2014; 58: 4392–98.

Pagliano P, Carannante N, Rossi M et al. Visceral leishmaniasis in pregnancy: a case series and a systematic review of the literature. J Antimicrob Chemother 2005; 55: 229–33.

Pan CQ, Duan ZP, Bhamidimarri KR et al. An algorithm for risk assessment and intervention of mother to child transmission of hepatitis B virus. Clin Gastroenterol Hepatol 2012; 10: 452–9.

Paparone PW, Menghetti RA. Case report: neurocysticercosis in pregnancy. NJ Med 1996; 93: 91–4.

Pasley MV, Martinez M, Hermes A et al. Safety and efficacy of lopinavir/ritonavir during pregnancy: a systematic review. AIDS Rev 2013; 15: 38–48.

Pasternak B, Hviid A. Use of acyclovir, valacyclovir, and famciclovir in the first trimester of pregnancy and the risk of birth defects. JAMA 2010; 304: 859–66.

Pasternak B, Hviid A. Atovaquone-proguanil use in early pregnancy and the risk of birth defects. Arch Intern Med 2011; 171: 259–60.

Patel K, Shapiro DE, Brogly SB et al. Prenatal protease inhibitor use and risk of preterm birth among HIV-infected women initiating antiretroviral drugs during pregnancy. J Infect Dis 2010; 201: 1035–44.

Pescovitz MD. Absence of teratogenicity of oral ganciclovir used during early pregnancy in a liver transplant recipient. Transplantation 1999; 67: 758–9.

Phillips-Howard PA, Wood D. The safety of antimalarial drugs in pregnancy. Drug Saf 1996; 14: 131–45.

Phiri K, Hernandez-Diaz S, Dugan KB et al. First Trimester Exposure to Antiretroviral Therapy and Risk of Birth Defects. Pediatr Infect Dis J 2014 [Epub ahead of print].

Pinnetti C, Tamburrini E, Ragazzoni E et al. Decreased plasma levels of darunavir/ritonavir in a vertically infected pregnant woman carrying multiclass-resistant HIV type-1. Antivir Ther 2010; 15: 127–9.

Piola P, Nabasumba C, Turyakira E et al. Efficacy and safety of artemether-lumefantrine compared with quinine in pregnant women with uncomplicated Plasmodium falciparum malaria: an open-label, randomised, non-inferiority trial. Lancet Infect Dis 2010; 10: 762–9.

Pipitone MA, Gloster HM. A case of blastomycosis in pregnancy. J Am Acad Dermatol 2005; 53: 740–1.

Poespoprodjo JR, Fobia W, Kenangalem E, Lampah DA, Sugiarto P, Tjitra E, Anstey NM, and Price RN. Dihydroartemisinin-piperaquine treatment of multidrug resistant falciparum and vivax malaria in pregnancy. PLoS One 2014; 9: e84976

Puhó EH, Szunyogh M, Metneki J et al. Drug treatment during pregnancy and isolated orofacial clefts in Hungary. Cleft Palate Craniofac J 2007; 44: 194–202.

Puliyanda DP, Silverman NS, Lehman D et al. Successful use of oral ganciclovir for the treatment of intrauterine cytomegalovirus infection in a renal allograft recipient. Transpl Infect Dis 2005; 7: 71–4.

Pursley TJ, Blomquist IK, Abraham J et al. Fluconazole-induced congenital anomalies in three infants. Clin Infect Dis 1996; 22: 336–40.

Reyes MP, Ostrea EM Jr, Cabinian AE et al. Vancomycin during pregnancy: does it cause hearing loss or nephrotoxicity in the infant? Am J Obstet Gynecol 1989; 161: 977–81.

Rezvani M, Koren G. Pregnancy outcome after exposure to injectable ribavirin during embryogenesis. Reprod Toxicol 2006; 21: 113–5.

Ripamonti D, Cattaneo D, Maggiolo F et al. Atazanavir plus low-dose ritonavir in pregnancy: pharmacokinetics and placental transfer. AIDS 2007; 21: 2409–15.

Roberts SS, Miller RK, Jones JK et al. The Ribavirin Pregnancy Registry: Findings after 5 years of enrollment, 2003–2009. Birth Defects Res A Clin Mol Teratol 2010; 88: 551–9.

Robinson GC, Cambon KG. Hearing loss in infants of tuberculous mothers treated with streptomycin during pregnancy. N Engl J Med 1964; 271: 949–51.

Romøren M, Lindbaek M, Nordeng H. Pregnancy outcome after gestational exposure to erythromycin – a population-based register study from Norway. Br J Clin Pharmacol 2012; 74: 1053–62.

Rosa FW, Hernandez C, Carlo WA. Griseofulvin teratology, including two thoracopagus conjoined twins. Lancet 1987; 1: 171.

Rubin A, Dvornik D. Placental transfer of griseofulvin. Am J Obstet Gynecol 1965; 92: 882–3.

Saito S, Minakami H, Nakai A et al. Outcomes of infants exposed to oseltamivir or zanamivir in utero during pandemic (H1N1) 2009. Am J Obstet Gynecol 2013; 209: 130–9.

Pregnancy

2.6 Anti-infective Agents

Sánchez Sainz-Trápaga C, Gutierrez FR, Ibanez RC et al. Relationship between a case of severe hearing loss and use of gentamycin in the pregnant mother. An Esp Pediatr 1998; 49: 397–8.

Santos F, Sheehy O, Perreault S et al. Exposure to anti-infective drugs during pregnancy and the risk of small-for-gestational-age newborns: a case-control study. BJOG 2011; 118: 1374–82.

Sarkar MS, Rowland K, Koren G. Pregnancy outcome following gestational exposure to terbinafine: A prospective comparative study [OTIS Abstract]. Birth Defects Res A Clin Mol Teratol 2003; 67: 390.

Sarkar M, Woodland C, Koren G et al. Pregnancy outcome following gestational exposure to azithromycin. BMC Pregnancy Childbirth 2006; 6: 18.

Sarner L, Fakoya A. Acute onset lactic acidosis and pancreatitis in the third trimester of pregnancy in HIV-1 positive women taking antiretroviral medication. Sex Transm Infect 2002; 78: 58–9.

Schaefer C, Amoura-Elefant E, Vial T et al. Pregnancy outcome after prenatal quinolone exposure. Evaluation of a case registry of the European Network of Teratology Information Services (ENTIS). Eur J Obstet Gynecol Reprod Biol 1996; 69: 83–9.

Schardein JL. Chemically Induced Birth Defects. 4th ed. Marcel Dekker, New York, Basel 2000.

Schlagenhauf P, Blumentals WA, Suter P et al. Pregnancy and fetal outcomes after exposure to mefloquine in the pre- and periconception period and during pregnancy. Clin Infect Dis 2012; 54: e124–31.

Schmid C, Kuemmerle A, Blum J et al. In-hospital safety in field conditions of nifurtimox eflornithine combination therapy (NECT) for T.B. gambiense sleeping sickness. PLoS Negl Trop Dis 2012; 6: e1920.

Shaw GM, Todoroff K, Velie EM et al. Maternal illness, including fever and medication use as risk factors for neural tube defects. Teratology 1998; 57: 1–7.

Shea K, Hilburger E, Baroco A et al. Successful treatment of vancomycin-resistant Enterococcus faecium pyelonephritis with daptomycin during pregnancy. Ann Pharmacother 2008; 42: 722–5.

Shennan A, Crawshaw S, Briley A et al. A randomised controlled trial of metronidazole for the prevention of preterm birth in women positive for cervicovaginal fetal fibronectin: the PREMET Study. BJOG 2006; 113: 65–74.

Shin S, Guerra D, Rich M et al. Treatment of multidrug-resistant tuberculosis during pregnancy: a report of 7 cases. Clin Infect Dis 2003; 36: 996–1003.

Shoai Tehrani M, Sicre de Fontbrune F, Roth P et al. Case report of exposure to voriconazole in the second and third trimesters of pregnancy. Antimicrob Agents Chemother 2013; 57: 1094–5.

Shulman CE, Dorman EK. Importance and prevention of malaria in pregnancy. Trans R Soc Trop Med Hyg 2003; 97: 30–5.

Simon A, Warszawski J, Kariyawasam D et al. Association of prenatal and postnatal exposure to lopinavir-ritonavir and adrenal dysfunction among uninfected infants of HIV-infected mothers. JAMA 2011; 306: 70–8.

Sørensen HT, Nielsen GL, Olesen C et al. Risk of malformations and other outcomes in children exposed to fluconazole in utero. Br J Clin Pharmacol 1999; 48: 234–8.

Sperling RS, Shapiro DE, McSherry GD et al. Safety of the maternal-infant zidovudine regimen utilized in the Pediatric AIDS Clinical Trial Group 076 Study. AIDS 1998; 12: 1805–13.

Stek AM, Best BM, Luo W et al. Effect of pregnancy on emtricitabine pharmacokinetics. HIV Med 2012; 13: 226–35.

Stone KM, Reiff-Eldridge R, White AD et al. Pregnancy outcomes following systemic prenatal acyclovir exposure: Conclusions from the international acyclovir pregnancy registry, 1984–1999. Birth Defects Res A Clin Mol Teratol 2004; 70: 201–7.

Stroup JS, Wagner J, Badzinski T. Use of daptomycin in a pregnant patient with Staphylococcus aureus endocarditis. Ann Pharmacother 2010; 44: 746–9.

Suarez L, Felkner M, Hendricks K. The effect of fever, febrile illnesses, and heat exposures on the risk of neural tube defects in a Texas-Mexico border population. Birth Defects Res A Clin Mol Teratol 2004; 70: 815–9.

Svensson T, Granath F, Stephansson O et al. Birth outcomes among women exposed to neuraminidase inhibitors during pregnancy. Pharmacoepidemiol Drug Saf 2011; 20: 1030–4.

Tagbor H, Bruce J, Browne E et al. Efficacy, safety, and tolerability of amodiaquine plus sulphadoxine-pyrimethamine used alone or in combination for malaria treatment in pregnancy: a randomised trial. Lancet 2006; 368: 1349–56.

Tanaka T, Nakajima K, Murashima A et al. Safety of neuraminidase inhibitors against novel influenza A (H1N1) in pregnant and breastfeeding women. CMAJ 2009; 181: 55–8.

Tarantal AF, Castillo A, Ekert JE et al. Fetal and maternal outcome after administration of tenofovir to gravid rhesus monkeys (Macaca mulatta). J Acquir Immune Defic Syndr 2002; 29: 207–20.

Tarning J, Kloprogge F, Dhorda M et al. Pharmacokinetic properties of artemether, dihydroartemisinin, lumefantrine, and quinine in pregnant women with uncomplicated plasmodium falciparum malaria in Uganda. Antimicrob Agents Chemother 2013; 57: 5096–103.

Tarning J, McGready R, Lindegardh N et al. Population pharmacokinetics of lumefantrine in pregnant women treated with artemether-lumefantrine for uncomplicated Plasmodium falciparum malaria. Antimicrob Agents Chemothem 2009; 53: 3837–46.

Taylor AW, Mosimaneotsile B, Mathebula U et al. Pregnancy outcomes in HIV-infected women receiving long-term isoniazid prophylaxis for tuberculosis and antiretroviral therapy. Infect Dis Obstet Gynecol 2013: 195637.

Taylor GP, Clayden P, Dhar J et al. British HIV Association guidelines for the management of HIV infection in pregnant women 2012. HIV Med 2012; 13: 87–157.

Taylor N, Touzeau V, Geit M et al. Raltegravir in pregnancy: a case series presentation. Int J STD AIDS 2011; 22: 358–60.

Thomas F, Erhart A, D'Alessandro U. Can amodiaquine be used safely during pregnancy? Lancet Infect Dis 2004; 4: 235–9.

Torp-Pedersen A, Jimenez-Solem E, Andersen JT et al. Exposure to mebendazole and pyrvinium during pregnancy: a Danish nationwide cohort study. Infect Dis Obstet Gynecol 2012: 769851.

Townsend CL, Cortina-Borja M, Peckham CS et al. Low rates of mother-to-child transmission of HIV following effective pregnancy interventions in the United Kingdom and Ireland, 2000–2006. AIDS 2008; 22: 973–81.

Tuomala RE, Watts DH, Li D et al. Improved obstetric outcomes and few maternal toxicities are associated with antiretroviral therapy, including highly active antiretroviral therapy during pregnancy. J Acquir Immune Defic Syndr 2005; 38: 449–73.

Ugwumadu A, Manyonda I, Reid F et al. Effect of early oral clindamycin on late miscarriage and preterm delivery in asymptomatic women with abnormal vaginal flora and bacterial vaginosis: a randomised controlled trial. Lancet 2003; 361: 983–8.

van der Lugt J, Colbers A, Molto J et al. The pharmacokinetics, safety and efficacy of boosted saquinavir tablets in HIV type-1-infected pregnant women. Antivir Ther 2009; 14: 443–50.

Vinther Skriver M, Nørgaard M, Pedersen L et al. Pivmecillinam and adverse birth and neonatal outcomes: a population-based cohort study. Scand J Infect Dis 2004; 36: 733–7.

Wade NA, Unadkat JD, Huang S et al. Pharmacokinetics and safety of stavudine in HIV-infected pregnant women and their infants: Pediatric AIDS Clinical Trials Group protocol 332. J Infect Dis 2004; 190: 2167–74.

Wang Y, Livingston E, Patil S et al. Pharmacokinetics of didanosine in antepartum and postpartum human immunodeficiency virus-infected pregnant women and their neonates: an AIDS clinical trials group study. J Infect Dis 1999; 180: 1536–41.

Wang X, Nanovskaya TN, Zhan Y et al. Pharmacokinetics of metronidazole in pregnant patients with bacterial vaginosis. J Matern Fetal Neonatal Med 2011; 24: 444–8.

Warszawski J, Tubiana R, Le CJ et al. Mother-to-child HIV transmission despite antiretroviral therapy in the ANRS French Perinatal Cohort. AIDS 2008; 22: 289–99.

Watts DH, Huang S, Culnane M et al. Birth defects among a cohort of infants born to HIV-infected women on antiretroviral medication. J Perinat Med 2011; 39: 163–70.

Webb EL, Mawa PA, Ndibazza J et al. Effect of single-dose anthelmintic treatment during pregnancy on an infant's response to immunisation and on susceptibility to infectious diseases in infancy: a randomised, double-blind, placebo-controlled trial. Lancet 2011; 377: 52–62.

Weizsaecker K, Kurowski M, Hoffmeister B et al. Pharmacokinetic profile in late pregnancy and cord blood concentration of tipranavir and enfuvirtide. Int J STD AIDS 2011; 22: 294–5.

Pregnancy

2.6 Anti-infective Agents

Wensing AM, Boucher CA, van Kasteren M et al. Prevention of mother-to-child transmission of multi-drug resistant HIV-1 using maternal therapy with both enfuvirtide and tipranavir. AIDS 2006; 20: 1465–7.

WHO. Report of the WHO informal consultation on the use of praziquantel during pregnancy/lactation and albendazole/mebendazole in children under 24 months. Available from: http://whqlibdoc.who.int/hq/2003/WHO_CDS_CPE_PVC_2002.4.pdf, 2002 (accessed on 14-3-2014).

WHO. Assessment of the safety of artemisinin compounds in pregnancy. Report of two joint informal consultations convened in 2006. Available from: http://whqlibdoc.who.int/publications/2007/9789241596114_eng.pdf, 2006 (accessed on 14-3-2014).

WHO. Guidelines for treatment of tuberculosis, 2010a. Available from: http://whqlibdoc.who.int/publications/2010/9789241547833_eng.pdf?ua=1 (accessed on 12-3-2014).

WHO. Guidelines for the treatment of malaria, 2010b. Available from: http://whqlibdoc.who.int/publications/2010/9789241547925_eng.pdf (accessed on 14-3-2014).

WHO. Antiretroviral drugs for treating pregnant women and preventing HIV infection in infants: recommendations for a public health approach, 2010c version. Available from: http://whqlibdoc.who.int/publications/2010/9789241599818_eng.pdf (accessed on 14-3-2014).

WHO. Chagas disease (American trypanosomiasis), 2013a. Available from: http://www.who.int/mediacentre/factsheets/fs340/en/index.html (accessed on 12-3-2014).

WHO. Malaria in pregnant women, 2013b. Available from: http://who.int/malaria/areas/high_risk_groups/pregnancy/en (accessed on 12-3-2014).

WHO. Soil-transmitted helminth infections; Fact sheet No. 366, 2013c; Updated June 2013. Available from: http://www.who.int/mediacentre/factsheets/fs366/en"http://www.who.int/mediacentre/factsheets/fs366/en (accessed on 17-3-2014).

Wogelius P, Norgaard M, Gislum M et al. Further analysis of the risk of adverse birth outcome after maternal use of fluoroquinolones. Int J Antimicrob Agents 2005; 26: 323–6.

Xie HY, Yasseen AS III, Xie RH et al. Infant outcomes among pregnant women who used oseltamivir for treatment of influenza during the H1N1 epidemic. Am J Obstet Gynecol 2013; 208: 293–7.

Yalaz M, Akisu M, Hilmioglu S et al. Successful caspofungin treatment of multidrug resistant Candida parapsilosis septicaemia in an extremely low birth weight neonate. Mycoses 2006; 49: 242–5.

Yang J, Xie RH, Krewski D et al. Exposure to trimethoprim/sulfamethoxazole but not other FDA category C and D anti-infectives is associated with increased risks of preterm birth and low birth weight. Int J Infect Dis 2011; 15: e336–e341.

Yaris F, Kesim M, Kadioglu M et al. Gentamicin use in pregnancy. A renal anomaly. Saudi Med J 2004; 25: 958–9.

Vaccines and immunoglobulins

2.7

Benedikte-Noël Cuppers and Christof Schaefer

2.7.1	Thiomersal as a preservative for vaccines	178
2.7.2	Cholera vaccination	179
2.7.3	Diphtheria and tetanus vaccination	179
2.7.4	Haemophilus influenza B (HIB) vaccination	180
2.7.5	Hepatitis A and hepatitis B vaccination	180
2.7.6	HPV vaccination	180
2.7.7	Influenza vaccination	181
2.7.8	Measles and mumps vaccination	183
2.7.9	Meningococcal vaccination	183
2.7.10	Pertussis vaccination	184
2.7.11	Pneumococcal vaccination	184
2.7.12	Poliomyelitis vaccination	184
2.7.13	Rabies vaccination	185
2.7.14	Rubella vaccination	185
2.7.15	Tick-borne encephalitis vaccination	186
2.7.16	Typhoid vaccination	186
2.7.17	Varicella vaccination	187
2.7.18	Yellow fever vaccination	187
2.7.19	Immunoglobulins	188

Vaccines protect pregnant women against serious infectious diseases through activation of the immune system. The induced antigen-specific antibodies are actively transferred through the placenta and protect her child as well. There are three types of vaccines: live viral or bacterial vaccines, inactivated vaccines or toxoids. There is no evidence that vaccines have embryo- or fetotoxic effects. Also, live vaccines have not been shown to induce fetal infections, the risks for the fetus seems theoretical. The range of reported experiences differs for various vaccines. Generally, routine vaccinations should be conducted before or after a pregnancy. Even though the risk of a fetal infection is more of a theoretical concern, vaccinations with live vaccines should be avoided during pregnancy. If, however, there is an obvious risk of exposure, a vaccination during

Drugs During Pregnancy and Lactation. http://dx.doi.org/10.1016/B978-0-12-408078-2.00008-1

pregnancy (view the specific vaccines) should be performed for the benefit of mother or child. An accidental vaccination during pregnancy is never a reason to consider the pregnancy at risk, or even to discuss a termination. Also immunoglobulins may be used in pregnancy for appropriate indications.

While official vaccination recommendations vary in detail concerning management during pregnancy; the US-American Center for Disease Control and Prevention (CDC) provides clear guidelines (www.cdc.gov/vaccines/pubs/preg-guide.htm). It recommends (April 2013) that all pregnant women in the USA undergo an influenza vaccination, even during the first trimester. The CDC recommends vaccinations specifically against hepatitis A and B, rabies and meningococcus under the appropriate indications. It does not place any limitations. The CDC also recommends that during each pregnancy, women should be administered a dose of tetanus-diphtheria-pertussis (Tdap), irrespective of the woman's prior history of receiving Tdap. Tdap given to pregnant women will stimulate the development of maternal antipertussis antibodies, which will pass through the placenta, likely providing the newborn with protection against pertussis in early life. It will also protect the mother from pertussis around the time of delivery, making her less likely to become infected and transmit pertussis to her infant. In September 2012, the Department of Health of the UK also recommended that all pregnant women should be offered pertussis vaccination in the third trimester of pregnancy. There is substantial interest in maternal immunization as a means to protect young infants against infections. Not only for pertussis, but also for influenza and tetanus, vaccinations during pregnancy could play an important role in preventing these serious infections in infants.

When discussing the risks of tropical vaccinations and malaria prophylaxis during pregnancy in the context of long-distance travel, the general risks of long-distance travel should also be discussed (Chapter 2.6). Whenever a vaccination is actually indicated, it needs to be given during pregnancy as well.

2.7.1   Thiomersal as a preservative for vaccines

Thiomersal and ethylmercury (ca. 5 μg) are present in a number of vaccines to aid preservation and have been discussed as a potential safety risk (Bigham and Copes 2005, Clements 2003, DeStefano 2002). For example, recently in the connection with the formulation of 2009 H1N1 influenza vaccines. However, quantities of ethylmercury are small, especially when only a single dose is given as is typical for vaccines. Thiomersal contains a different form of mercury (e.g. ethylmercury), which is different from environmental methylmercury accumulated in fish. Ethyl mercury does not accumulate in the body, and is metabolized and removed from the body much faster than methylmercury. Currently, there is no clear evidence that prenatal exposure of a vaccine with thiomersal has adverse effects, including neurodevelopmental disorders like autism. In addition, the continuous increase in the number of cases of autism diagnosed in the USA despite removal of thiomersal from most vaccines, strongly argues against a causal association between thiomersal in vaccines and autism (Global Advisory Committee on Vaccine Safety 2012). The WHO recommends thiomersal-containing vaccines for the so-called Third World, because they are more easily made available (especially if refrigeration is problematic), less expensive, safer, and more effective (Bigham 2005).

2.7.2   Cholera vaccination

Cholera vaccine is an inactivated vaccine and contains *vibrios* of the serotypes Inaba and Ogawa. In a mass vaccination campaign in Zanzibar in 2009 where 196 pregnant women were inadvertently vaccinated (Hashim 2012), there were no differences in birth outcomes between the exposed and unexposed pregnancies. There are no other studies concerning the use of this vaccine during pregnancy. Protection by this vaccination is incomplete and of short duration. For this reason vaccination is no longer recommended for most travelers. The antibiotic therapy of cholera can be performed during pregnancy. Noteworthy is that the pathogens have a high resistance to antibiotics. All people (including pregnant women) in areas where cholera is occurring, or has occurred, should observe five basic cholera prevention recommendations: (1) drink and use disinfected water; (2) wash your hands often; (3) use latrines; (4) clean up safely; and (5) cook or boil food, keep it covered, eat it hot and peel fruits and vegetables. Pregnant women who have to travel to an endemic region need to adhere rigorously to these precautions ("Boil it, cook it, peel it or forget it").

> **Recommendation.** If compelling reasons are indicated, vaccination can be performed during pregnancy.

2.7.3   Diphtheria and tetanus vaccination

Tetanus-diphtheria vaccines are inactivated bacterial vaccines that contain the relevant toxoids. There are no indications of embryotoxic properties in these vaccines, which have been extensively used for many decades (also in pregnant women). Large case control studies conducted in Hungary (Czeizel 1999) and Latin America (Silveira 1995), failed to detect any teratogenic effects of tetanus toxoid. Catindig (1996) noted that between 1980 and 1994 annual vaccinations increased in the Philippines by more than a factor of 10, and there was no increase in miscarriages. The suspicion by Heinonen (1977) linking an increased risk for *pectus excavatum* and club foot with tetanus toxoid has not been confirmed and appears to be anecdotal. Tetanus/diphtheria toxoid have been administered worldwide to pregnant women to prevent neonatal tetanus, which is associated with a high infant mortality; large studies examining the use of tetanus toxoid during pregnancy have not reported clinically significant severe adverse events (CDC 2013). If necessary, tetanus vaccinations should be refreshed during pregnancy to prevent maternal disease and neonatal tetanus. Reports about *tetanus neonatorum* in countries with inadequate vaccine protection support the urgency of the vaccination; for example, China (incidence of *tetanus neonatorum* is 0.16/1,000 live born, only 12% of mothers have been vaccinated (Chai 2004)) and Turkey (Kalaca 2004). Generally, the basic immunization is completed during childhood; thereafter, every 10 years a booster should be given, even during pregnancy.

Pregnancy

2.7 Vaccines and immunoglobulins

> **Recommendation.** If protection is inadequate, a pregnant woman should be vaccinated against tetanus (and diphtheria).

2.7.4   Haemophilus influenza B (HIB) vaccination

There are no systematic studies of the prenatal toxicity of this inactivated vaccine. It is possible that after vaccination in the third trimester, maternal antibodies may cross the placenta and protect the infant from potentially life-threatening infections (Glezen 1999); corresponding antibodies have been also detected 3 and 6 months postnatally in breast milk, when the vaccination had been given between gestational weeks 34 and 36.

> **Recommendation.** Vaccination can be given to pregnant women. To date, no recommendations have been made to protect the newborn by vaccination during late pregnancy.

2.7.5   Hepatitis A and hepatitis B vaccination

Hepatitis B vaccine is an inactivated virus vaccine derived from HB surface antigen. There is limited information about the use of hepatitis B vaccine during pregnancy. About 300 pregnancies with vaccinations at various times have been studied, and there is no increased risk of adverse outcomes demonstrated (Sheffield 2011, Reddy 1994, Grosheide 1993, Levy 1991, Ayoola 1987). Almost 90% of the mothers who demonstrated seroconversion after vaccination during pregnancy, developed protective antibodies that could be demonstrated in the umbilical blood (Sheffield 2011, Ingardia 1999). Passive transfer of the antibodies occurred in most of the newborns, but they disappeared rapidly in the infants (Ingardia 1999, Reddy 1994, Ayoola 1987). There are no reports that demonstrate adverse effects of hepatitis B vaccine during the course of pregnancy; however, the data are limited.

Hepatitis A vaccines use an inactivated form of hepatitis A virus. Systematic studies of the use of hepatitis A vaccine in pregnancy are not available. A small case series reports 29 pregnant women who were vaccinated with hepatitis A vaccine. While no adverse effects were apparent, methodical flaws limit the validity of the study (D'Acremont 2008). In an abstract, 23 pregnancies exposed to hepatitis A vaccine did not indicate an increased risk in adverse outcomes (Wilson 2010). So far, there have been no adverse effects with the use of hepatitis A vaccine in pregnancy; however, data are limited.

> **Recommendation.** Pregnant women at risk of acquiring hepatitis are recommended to undergo a vaccination.

2.7.6   HPV vaccination

The human papilloma virus (HPV) vaccine contains inactivated virus. There are two vaccines available, a bivalent (HPV2), and a quadrivalent

(HPV4) vaccine. HPV2 protects against HPV 16 and 18, HPV4 protects against HPV 6/11/16 and 18. In two clinical trials with HPV2 ($n = 1786$), there was no higher risk for spontaneous abortion after HPV vaccination before pregnancy (Wacholder 2010). Only 488 pregnancies occurred within 90 days of receiving the vaccine. In five clinical studies with HPV4 vaccine, 2008 pregnancies were followed for outcome, including those that occurred before, during or after vaccine exposure (Garland 2009). A registry maintained by the manufacturers reports more than 500 pregnancies that started 30 days or less after the administration of the quadrivalent HPV vaccine (Dana 2009), and no adverse effects were seen in the pregnancies or the offspring. However, results of such data collections have methodological flaws and are to be viewed with caution. To some degree, data have been published repeatedly.

> **Recommendation.** HPV vaccines should not be routinely administered during pregnancy. An accidental vaccination carries no consequences, but booster injections should be given after completion of the pregnancy.

2.7.7   Influenza vaccination

The influenza vaccine usually administered today is inactivated and trivalent. It contains three influenza virus strains that are expected to affect individuals during the upcoming winter. In many countries, including the USA and UK, vaccination against influenza is recommended for pregnant women. It can be administered at any time during pregnancy. Pregnant women are at an increased risk of serious illness, and complications from influenza can result in more frequent as well as longer hospitalizations for respiratory infections. The risk increases with trimester, the highest risk being in the third trimester. This holds for both seasonal and pandemic influenza (Liu 2013, Beigi 2012, Mosby 2011). Vaccination against influenza provides satisfactory immunity in pregnant women and reduces the risk of respiratory complications. Transplacental passage of maternal antibodies also protects the newborn.

Because inactivated influenza vaccine has been routinely administered to pregnant women in the USA since the 1950s, there is vast experience with its use during pregnancy. Studies during the last decades with thousands of women, which evaluated the safety of influenza vaccine just before, or during pregnancy, demonstrate no evidence of embryo- or fetotoxic effects of the vaccine (Bednarczyk 2012, Munoz 2012). In a retrospective cohort study of 8,690 vaccinated pregnant women (439 in the first trimester), there was no increase in major malformation rates. They did observe a decrease in the overall stillbirth rate (Sheffield 2012). In addition, adverse event data from the USA and Canada are available concerning the use of seasonal trivalent influenza vaccine in pregnant women. Moro (2011) reported that the US American Vaccine-Adverse Event Reporting System (VAERS) registered only 148 adverse events in pregnant women after influenza vaccination from 1990 through 2009. The reporting rate of spontaneous abortion was 1.9 per million pregnant women vaccinated. However, the well-known marked underreporting seen with such a method of collecting data diminishes the relevance and importance of this report. A case control study utilizing data from six health care organizations in the Vaccine Safety Datalink found no statistically significant increase in spontaneous abortion in the 4 weeks after vaccination (Irving 2013). In a retrospective, observational cohort also using data from the Vaccine Safety Datalink sites, no increased risks for adverse obstetric events was observed (Kharbanda 2013).

An investigation in Bangladesh noted 36% less respiratory illness with fever among 172 pregnant women vaccinated with inactivated influenza vaccine when compared to a control group of women. Also, the children of the vaccinated mothers had 29% less infection up to 24 weeks postpartum. The reduction was even greater for children for lab-confirmed influenza infections, namely 63% (Zaman 2008). Maternal influenza immunization had a substantial protective effect in both mothers and in their young infants.

During the 2009 H1N1 influenza pandemic, the Strategic Group of Experts on Immunization (SAGE) of the World Health Organization recommended that pregnant women should be vaccinated, especially during the second and third trimester, as they were at a higher risk of severe and lethal forms of infection. The 2009 H1N1 vaccines available were with (AS03 or MF59) or without adjuvants. The vaccine recommended for pregnant women differed among countries depending upon the perception of vaccine safety, efficacy, and operational issues related to vaccine production. Tens of thousands of pregnant women were vaccinated during the pandemic. There was an extensive monitoring of pregnancies which resulted in the development of substantial experience with these vaccines. Over 110,000 vaccinated pregnancies have been documented in numerous publications from Europe, United States, Asia and South America. In these publications almost 41,000 women were vaccinated with non-adjuvanted vaccine (Chavant 2013, Fell 2012, Oppermann 2012, Huang 2011), over 60,000 women with AS03-adjuvanted 2009 H1N1 vaccine (Håberg 2013, Källén 2012, Oppermann 2012, Pasternak 2012, Sammon 2012), and more than 10,000 pregnancies with MF-59-adjuvanted 2009 H1N1 vaccine (Rubinstein 2013, Heikkinen 2012, Huang 2011). Only a small number of the women were vaccinated during the first trimester. The adverse events described were similar to those in the general population and were mainly mild. Vaccination during pregnancy did not result in an increased risk of adverse perinatal events or congenital malformations. Some studies even suggested a lower risk for preterm birth, low birth weight and fetal death. As relatively few women were vaccinated in the first trimester, the ability to assess the impact of vaccination on rates of congenital malformations is limited. Because the use of adjuvants in pregnancy had not been well studied in clinical trials, there were concerns about the safety during pregnancy. Specific concerns were about the squalen-containing adjuvant AS03, as it could not be excluded that it would systematically enhance a Th1 (T1 helper cell) immunity, which is reduced during pregnancy. This could potentially result in placental dysfunction and a higher risk of preeclampsia, as a disturbed Th1/Th2 regulation has been discussed for some time as a cause of placental dysfunction (Mor 2010, Trowsdale 2006, Saito 2003). However, studies did not find any adverse effect of the AS03- or MF59-adjuvanted A/H1N1 vaccines on the ongoing pregnancy, or on the health of the mother, the fetus, or the newborn (Håberg 2013, Rubinstein 2013, Heikkinen 2012, Källén 2012, Oppermann 2012, Pasternak 2012, Sammon 2012, Huang 2011).

Since 2003 there has been a live-attenuated influenza vaccine (LAIV) on the market. LAIV is contraindicated in pregnancy. However, inadvertent use during pregnancy is no reason for termination of the pregnancy (Toback 2012).

In summary, no study to date has demonstrated adverse consequences following seasonal or pandemic influenza vaccination in pregnancy. These results provide reassurance when offering influenza vaccination to all pregnant women.

> **Recommendation.** Vaccination of women who are or will be pregnant during the flu season is recommended. Vaccination can occur in any trimester.

2.7.8   Measles and mumps vaccination

Measles and mumps vaccines should be avoided during pregnancy because they are live attenuated virus vaccines and theoretically, fetal infection with the attenuated vaccines might occur. Infection with wild-type measles during pregnancy has been associated with miscarriage, prematurity and perinatal death in infected pregnancies. Cases of first trimester mumps followed by adverse fetal outcome have also been reported but are inconclusive. There have been no indications that measles or mumps infections during pregnancy cause birth defects in the child (Enders 2007).

There is insufficient documented experience following the use of these vaccines during pregnancy. However, there have been no suggestions of developmental toxicity in humans. Some publications are focused on rubella vaccinations, but utilize data from rubella-measles combination vaccines, e.g. three studies with about 300 pregnant women who underwent mass vaccinations in Iran (see Section 2.7.13). Thus, theoretical concerns for a risk using this live vaccine during pregnancy have not been confirmed. Although this finding is reassuring, it should be stated that the data are limited.

> **Recommendation.** Neither vaccine should be administered during pregnancy because, theoretically, fetal infection with the live attenuated vaccines might occur. While, generally, there is no indication to perform a measles and mumps vaccination during pregnancy, an accidental vaccination does not require any further intervention.

2.7.9   Meningococcal vaccination

Meningococcal vaccine contains non-conjugated or conjugated polysaccharides of the groups A, C, Y, and W-135. It has been in use for decades and has not demonstrated fetotoxicity when given to pregnant women, primarily during the last trimester (Letson 1998). Protective antibodies have been demonstrated to cross the placenta. A study investigated 157 women who were vaccinated in the third trimester comparing them to a control group. It found that significantly higher levels of IgA and IgG, respectively, were present in the breast milk for up to three months, and in the serum of the newborns up to 6 months after birth (Shahid 2002). Currently, C-conjugated vaccines are preferred. They are also given to infants and result in a better immune response than the polysaccharide vaccines. In the conjugated variety, parts of the bacterial wall are additionally bound to a protein.

Pregnancy

2.7 Vaccines and immunoglobulins

> **Recommendation.** If clearly necessary, meningococcal vaccination may be conducted during pregnancy.

2.7.10   Pertussis vaccination

Pertussis vaccine is offered as a triple vaccine with tetanus and diphtheria (Tdap). It is being debated if the application of the acellular pertussis vaccine (aP) to the mother during pregnancy results in increased protection of the newborn through transmission of maternal antibodies. Because of the increase in incidences of pertussis in infants, immunization of pregnant women with pertussis vaccine is proposed (Leuridan 2013, Lindsey 2013, Bechini 2012). Maternal vaccination against pertussis is recommended in the United Kingdom and United States (CDC 2013), with new studies indicating their efficacy. Systematic studies are lacking about the safety of Tdap during pregnancy; however, case series and reports do not indicate a risk. At present in Canada and the USA, two clinical trials of acellular pertussis vaccines administered during the third trimester of pregnancy are underway.

> **Recommendation.** Pregnant women may be vaccinated with pertussis vaccine. Vaccination in the second and third trimester is the most effective.

2.7.11   Pneumococcal vaccination

There are two types of pneumococcal vaccine: unconjugated and conjugated polysaccharide vaccines. Both are inactivated vaccines. Pneumoccocal vaccination during pregnancy was proposed to be the way of preventing pneumococcal disease during the first month of life. However, experience with 280 pregnancies showed no evidence that pneumococcal vaccination during pregnancy reduces the risk of neonatal infection (Chaithongwongwatthana 2012). Mothers were vaccinated in the third trimester. There were no adverse effects on the pregnancy or on the health of the newborn.

> **Recommendation.** Pregnant women may be vaccinated for pneumococcal pneumonia if necessary.

2.7.12   Poliomyelitis vaccination

There are two types of polio vaccine, an inactivated and a live attenuated polio vaccine. Today, only the inactivated polio vaccine is used in Europe and the USA; it needs to be given parenterally. The formerly used oral polio vaccine (Sabin) contained live attenuated poliomyelitis viruses. Even with this live vaccine, no increased risk of malformations or miscarriages were observed when studies were conducted with mass vaccinations in Finland and Israel involving approximately 15,000 pregnant women (Harjulehto-Mervaala 1995, Ornoy 1993). While systematic studies are missing, today's inactivated polio vaccine is not expected to lead to adverse effects in the unborn.

> **Recommendation.** Pregnancy is not a contraindication for a necessary polio vaccination with the inactivated vaccine. If there has been a break in vaccination protection, a booster should be given in the interest of mother and child using today's inactivated vaccine.

2.7.13   Rabies vaccination

The rabies vaccine is an inactivated vaccine derived from cell cultures of human or chick embryo origin. Today's vaccine is much better tolerated than earlier preparations. Case reports and series regarding the active and/or passive immunization with more than 330 pregnant women demonstrate no adverse effects (Huang 2013, Toovey 2007, Chutivongse 1995). Maternal antibodies appear to cross the placenta.

> **Recommendation.** Because rabies is a disease with a lethal outcome, a pregnant woman bitten by an animal suspected to be carrying rabies has to be immunized with vaccine and immunoglobulin.

2.7.14   Rubella vaccination

The rubella vaccination is conducted with an attenuated live vaccine that is also present in the combination vaccines with measles and mumps (MMR). The wild-type rubella viruses are highly teratogenic. A rubella infection during pregnancy, especially during the first trimester, can result in miscarriage, stillbirths, and congenital rubella syndrome (CRS). The main clinical manifestations of CRS are eye defects (cataract, glaucoma, retinopathy), deafness, congenital heart defects and central nervous system (CNS) defects (mental retardation, microcephaly). Other possible effects are growth restriction, hepatosplenomegaly and thrombocytopenia (Dontigny 2008). Because rubella vaccine contains live rubella virus, immunization is contraindicated shortly before and during pregnancy.

A case report of a child with congenital cataract after maternal vaccination was not confirmed by another investigator (Fleet 1974). In another situation, the suspicion of rubella embryopathy after a maternal vaccination could be refuted by the demonstration of the presence of a wild-type virus (da Silva e Sá 2011). In a number of studies, data were analyzed covering more than 4,000 women who had been vaccinated from 3 months prior to conception and up to pregnancy. Data were collected from women in Germany, Sweden, England, Latin America, Iran and North America, some of them were already seropositive (Soares 2011, Nasiri 2009, Namaei 2008, Badilla 2007, Hamkar 2006, Enders 2005, Bar-Oz 2004). There were no cases of CRS after inadvertent exposure to rubella vaccine shortly before or during pregnancy, nor was there an association with other adverse effects.

No differences were seen in important developmental markers of 94 children (up to 1 year) of women who had received a vaccination in early pregnancy, or within 3 months prior to pregnancy, and their controls (Bar-Oz 2004). Also, a study from Iran did not detect clinical sequelae in the children from approximately 120 mothers who had no prior immunity (Hamkar 2006); in two other Iranian studies, 166 women were vaccinated shortly before or after conception. No signs of CRS were found in the neonates, or IgM in the cord blood (Nasiri 2009, Namaei 2008). An investigation from Costa Rica (Badilla 2007) examined about 1,000 women who had been vaccinated during pregnancy or 1 month before. They did not find anomalies in regard to malformations, miscarriages, birth weight, and prematurity when comparing seronegative and seropositive mothers. In the majority of women who completed the follow-up, the immune status was unknown. During a mass vaccination campaign in Brazil, 2,332 susceptible women were vaccinated shortly before or during pregnancy. No children were born with CRS (Soares 2011).

Rubella-specific IgM antibodies can be documented in the cord blood of offspring of about 0–6% of women who had received the rubella vaccination during early pregnancy (Soares 2011, Hamkar 2006, Enders 2005, CDC 1989). A persistent subclinical infection was diagnosed in one case (Hofmann 2000). In none of the children with rubella IgM antibodies was CRS detected.

In summary, there has not been a single case of a rubella embryopathy as a result of a maternal vaccination, regardless if mothers were seronegative or had a preexisting (residual) immunity.

> **Recommendation.** A rubella vaccination should not be planned immediately before or during pregnancy. Current experiences argue against a risk of a rubella embryopathy as a result of vaccination. Thus, an accidental vaccination is no rationale for termination or invasive diagnostic steps. An individual decision should be made, if, as an exception, a seronegative woman with a high risk of exposure should be vaccinated during pregnancy.

2.7.15   Tick-borne encephalitis vaccination

No evidence has been noted in smaller case studies that vaccination with tick-borne encephalitis vaccine containing inactivated viruses leads to embryotoxic effects in humans (e.g. Paulus 2006, personal communication). Systematic studies about its safety in pregnancy have not been published.

> **Recommendation.** The indication for vaccination during pregnancy requires critical assessment.

2.7.16   Typhoid vaccination

Two typhoid vaccines are available, one a parenteral inactivated version, the other an oral formulation with live bacteria. A typhoid septicemia during pregnancy increases the risk of miscarriage. Therefore, protection for pregnant women is advisable, especially when staying for a longer time in affected countries. A study of 18 pregnant women who received the live vaccine during the first trimester (Mazzone 1994), and another report with 174 accidentally vaccinated women during pregnancy (Brooking 2003), did not reveal any specific abnormalities.

> **Recommendation.** If indicated, a pregnant woman may receive a vaccination.

2.7.17   Varicella vaccination

A first infection with varicella during the first half of the pregnancy can harm the embryo and fetus in about 1% of cases. Congenital varicella syndrome is characterized by cutaneous scarring in a dermatome distribution and/or hypoplasia of an extremity. Additional manifestations may include low birth weight, microcephaly, localized muscular atrophy, ocular anomalies, and neurological abnormalities (Mandelbrot 2012). Infants born to women who develop varicella within the period of 5 days before, to 2 days after, delivery are at risk of neonatal varicella, which may be severe. This has not been observed when varicella vaccine is used during pregnancy. Varicella vaccine is a live attenuated viral vaccine. The manufacturer Merck collected 737 prospectively documented pregnancies, including 163 cases of live births of women who had been definitely seronegative prior to vaccination. The data revealed no evidence of a varicella embryopathy, higher malformation rates, or higher miscarriage rates. Also 65 retrospective case reports (Merck Pregnancy Registry for Varivax 2008) showed no varicella embryopathies. Although the results are reassuring, data are limited.

> **Recommendation.** Vaccination should not be administered during pregnancy. An accidental vaccination requires no further intervention.

2.7.18   Yellow fever vaccination

The yellow fever vaccine contains a live attenuated virus. Vaccination during pregnancy with this vaccine is contraindicated because of the (theoretical) risk of fetal infection. One case report describes a yellow fever infection in a newborn in connection with a vaccination during the first trimester (Tsai 1993). This has not been confirmed by other publications. A study of 101 pregnant women who were vaccinated, four in the first, and 89 in the third trimester, did not reveal developmental anomalies in the offspring up to ages 3–4 (Nasidi 1993). Another rather small retrospective study with 39 pregnant women indicates a non-significant increased miscarriage rate (Nishioka 1998). A study of 58 women who were vaccinated during the first trimester did not report congenital infections or evidence of teratogenicity (Robert 1999). Cavalcanti (2007) examined 304 prenatally exposed Brazilian children and compared them with a reference population: there was no increase in major malformations; minor dysmorphism were significantly more frequent, especially pigmented nevi. The authors suspect that this is due to a bias of clinical evaluation. The follow-up period of the exposed children was much longer (up to 1 year) than for the reference population (only during the neonatal period). Another study from the same institute describes that neither PCR-positive findings, nor IgM, was found at birth and that >98% of the vaccinated mothers were IgG-positive. About 20% of mothers report mild side effects with vaccination, e.g. fever and joint pain (Suzano 2006). A careful examination reveals that the mother–child pairs of this study are also contained in the publication by Cavalcanti (2007). In summary, the overall experiences with more than 500 vaccinated pregnant women speak against an appreciable developmental risk of this live vaccine. Although this finding is reassuring, it should be underlined that most reported series have been small in number.

> **Recommendation.** Yellow fever vaccine is not recommended during pregnancy. However, a pregnant woman who undertakes unavoidable travel to an endemic region has to be vaccinated even in the first trimester, because disease caused by yellow fever is life-threatening.

2.7.19   Immunoglobulins

Immunoglobulin preparations contain primarily immunoglobulin G (IgG) antibodies derived from pooled human plasma. The extent of placental passage of IgG antibodies depends on the gestational age, dose, duration of treatment, and type of the administered agent. Immunoglobulins are used for different maternal and fetal indications; for example, for antibody deficiency, infectious diseases (especially for prevention), autoimmune diseases (to treat maternal disease), and management of fetal medical symptoms such as fetal heart block as a result of maternal lupus erythematosus.

Both immunoglobulins and hyperimmune sera against specific infections are not, as far as we know today, embryotoxic (review in Briggs 2011).

A study of 93 children of mothers who had received gamma globulin to prevent hepatitis during pregnancy, describes significantly more changes in the epidermal ridges of the fingertips of prenatally exposed children (Ross 1996). These changes that can hardly be classified as malformations were only seen when exposure occurred during the first 162 days of pregnancy. The same author reports two children with duodenal stenosis and a para-esophageal hiatal hernia, respectively, whose mothers had received gamma globulin during the first trimester (Ross 1995). This anecdotal report has not been confirmed by other authors.

In summary, immunoglobulins for specific infections are not considered to be embryotoxic. Nonspecific risks caused by human blood products, such as transmission of viral infections and anaphylactic reactions, cannot be completely excluded and could indirectly endanger the fetus as well.

> **Recommendation.** If indicated, standard immunoglobulins may be given during pregnancy.

References

Ayoola EA, Johnson AO. Hepatitis B vaccine in pregnancy: immunogenicity, safety and transfer of antibodies to infants. Int J Gynaecol Obstet 1987; 25: 297–301.

Badilla X, Morice A, Avila-Aguero ML et al. Fetal risk associated with rubella vaccination during pregnancy. Pediatr Infect Dis J 2007; 26: 830–5.

Bar-Oz B, Levichek Z, Moretti ME et al. Pregnancy outcome following rubella vaccination: a prospective controlled study. Am J Med Genet A 2004; 130A: 52–4.

Bechini A, Tiscione E, Boccalini S et al. Acellular pertussis vaccine use in risk groups (adolescents, pregnant women, newborns and health care workers): a review of evidences and recommendations. Vaccine 2012; 30: 5179–90.

Bednarczyk RA, Adjaye-Gbewonyo D, Omer SB. Safety of influenza immunization during pregnancy for the fetus and the neonate. Am J Obstet Gynecol 2012; 207: S38–46.

Beigi RH. Influenza during pregnancy: a cause of serious infection in obstetrics. Clin Obstet Gynecol 2012; 55: 914–26.

Bigham M, Copes R. Thiomersal in vaccines: balancing the risk of adverse effects with the risk of vaccine-preventable disease. Drug Saf 2005; 28: 89–101.

Brooking JL, Kitchin NR. Inadvertent vaccination during pregnancy: Summary of Aventis Pasteur product data reported directly to Aventis Pasteur MSD UK, during the period 1995–2002. Pharmacoepidemiol Drug Saf 2003; 12: S212–3.

Briggs GG, Freeman RK, Yaffe SJ. *Drugs in Pregnancy and Lactation*, 9th edn. Lippincott Williams and Wilkins, 2011.

Catindig N, Abad-Viola G, Magboo F. Tetanus toxoid and spontaneous abortions: is there epidemiological evidence of an association? Lancet 1996; 348: 1098–9.

Cavalcanti DP, Salomão MA, Lopez-Camelo J et al. Campinas group of yellow fever immunization during pregnancy: early exposure to yellow fever vaccine during pregnancy. Trop Med Int Health 2007; 12: 833–7.

Centers for Disease Control and Prevention (CDC). Updated recommendations for use of tetanus toxoid, reduced diphtheria toxoid, and acellular pertussis vaccine (Tdap) in pregnant women – Advisory Committee on Immunization Practices (ACIP), 2012. MMWR Morb Mortal Wkly Rep 2013 Feb 22; 62: 131–5.

Centers for Disease Control and Prevention (CDC). Rubella vaccination in pregnancy. United States, 1971–1988. Morb Mort Weekly Rep 1989; 38: 289–93.

Chai F, Prevots DR, Wang X et al. Neonatal tetanus incidence in China, 1996–2001, and risk factors for neonatal tetanus, Guangxi province, China. Int J Epidemiol 2004; 33: 551–7.

Chaithongwongwatthana S, Yamasmit W, Limpongsanurak S et al. Pneumococcal vaccination during pregnancy for preventing infant infection. Cochrane Database Syst Rev 2012; 7: CD004903.

Chavant F, Ingrand I, Jonville-Bera AP et al. The PREGVAXGRIP Study: a cohort study to assess foetal and neonatal consequences of in utero exposure to vaccination against A(H1N1)v2009 influenza. Drug Saf 2013; 36. 455–65.

Chutivongse S, Wilde H, Benjavongkulchai M et al. Postexposure rabies vaccination during pregnancy: effect on 202 women and their infants. Clin Infect Dis 1995; 20: 818–20.

Clements CJ. The evidence for the safety of thiomersal in newborn and infant vaccines. Vaccine 2003; 22: 1854–61.

Czeizel AE, Rockenbauer M. Tetanus toxoid and congenital anomalies. Int J Gynaecol Obstet 1999; 64: 253–8.

D'Acremont V, Tremblay S, Genton B. Impact of vaccines given during pregnancy on the offspring of women consulting a travel clinic: a longitudinal study. J Travel Med 2008; 15: 77–81.

Dana A, Buchanan KM, Goss MA et al. Pregnancy outcomes from the pregnancy registry of a human papillomavirus type 6/11/16/18 vaccine. Obstet Gynecol 2009; 114: 1170–8.

da Silva e Sá GR, Camacho LA, Stavola MS et al. Pregnancy outcomes following rubella vaccination: a prospective study in the state of Rio de Janeiro, Brazil, 2001–2002. J Infect Dis 2011; 204: S722–8.

DeStefano F. MMR vaccine and autism: a review of the evidence for a causal association. Mol Psychiatry 2002; 7: 51–2.

Dontigny L, Arsenault MY, Martel MJ et al. Society of Obstetricians and Gynecologist of Canada. Rubella in pregnancy. J Obstet Gynaecol Can 2008; 30: 152–68.

Pregnancy

2.7 Vaccines and immunoglobulins

Enders G. Akzidentelle Rötelnschutzimpfungen um den Zeitpunkt der Konzeption und in der Frühschwangerschaft. BundesgesundheitsblGesundheitsforschGesundheitsschutz 2005; 48: 685–6.

Enders M, Biber M, Exler S. Measles, mumps and rubella virus infection in pregnancy. Possible adverse effects on pregnant women, pregnancy outcome and the fetus. Bundesgesundheitsblatt Gesundheitsforschung Gesundheitsschutz 2007 Nov; 50: 1393–8.

Fell DB, Sprague AE, Liu N et al. Better Outcomes Registry & Network (BORN) Ontario. H1N1 influenza vaccination during pregnancy and fetal and neonatal outcomes. Am J Public Health 2012; 102: e33–40.

Fleet WF Jr, Benz EW Jr, Karzon DT et al. Fetal consequences of maternal rubella immunization. JAMA 1974; 227: 621–7.

Garland SM, Ault KA, Gall SA et al. Quadrivalent Human Papillomavirus Vaccine Phase III Investigators: Pregnancy and infant outcomes in the clinical trials of a human papillomavirus type 6/11/16/18 vaccine: a combined analysis of five randomized controlled trials. Obstet Gynecol 2009; 114: 1179–88.

Glezen WP, Alpers M. Maternal immunization. Clin Inf Dis 1999; 28: 219–24.

Global Advisory Committee on Vaccine Safety, June 2012. Wkly Epidemiol Rec 2012; 87: 281–7.

Grosheide PM, Schalm SW, van Os HC et al. Immune response to hepatitis B vaccine in pregnant women receiving post-exposure prophylaxis. Eur J Obstet Gynecol Reprod Biol 1993; 50: 53–8.

Håberg SE, Trogstad L, Gunnes N et al. Risk of fetal death after pandemic influenza virus infection or vaccination. N Engl J Med 2013; 368: 333–40.

Hamkar R, Jalilvand S, Abdolbaghi MH et al. Inadvertent rubella vaccination of pregnant women: evaluation of possible transplacental infection with rubella vaccine. Vaccine 2006; 24: 3558–63.

Harjulehto-Mervaala T, Hovi T, Aro T et al. Oral poliovirus vaccination and pregnancy complications. Acta Obstet Gynecol Scand 1995; 74: 262–5.

Hashim R, Khatib AM, Enwere G et al. Recombinant Cholera Toxin B Subunit, Killed Whole-Cell (rBS-WC) Oral Cholera Vaccine in Pregnancy. PLoS Negl Trop Dis 2012 July; 6: e1743

Heikkinen T, Young J, van Beek E et al. Safety of MF59-adjuvanted A/H1N1 influenza vaccine in pregnancy: a comparative cohort study. Am J Obstet Gynecol 2012; 207: 177, e1–8.

Heinonen OP, Slone S, Shapiro S. Immunizing agents. In: Birth Defects and Drugs in Pregnancy. Littleton/USA: Publishing Sciences Group 1977: 314–321.

Hofmann J, Kortung M, Pustowoit B et al. Persistent fetal rubella vaccine virus infection following inadvertent vaccination during early pregnancy. J Med Virol 2000; 61: 155–8.

Huang G, Liu H, Cao Q et al. Safety of post-exposure rabies prophylaxis during pregnancy: a follow-up study from Guangzhou, China. Hum Vaccin Immunother 2013; 9: 177–83.

Huang WT, Chen WC, Teng HJ et al. Adverse events following pandemic A (H1N1) 2009 monovalent vaccines in pregnant women – Taiwan, November 2009–August 2010. PLoS One 2011; 6: e23049.

Ingardia CJ, Kelley L, Lerer T et al. Correlation of maternal and fetal Hepatitis B antibody titers following maternal vaccination in pregnancy. Am J Perinatol 1999; 16: 129–32.

Irving SA, Kieke BA, Donahue JG et al. Vaccine Safety Datalink. Trivalent inactivated influenza vaccine and spontaneous abortion. Obstet Gynecol 2013 Jan; 121: 159–65.

Kalaca S, Yalcin M, Simsek YS. Missed opportunities for tetanus vaccination in pregnant women, and factors associated with seropositivity. Public Health 2004; 118: 377–82.

Källén B, Olausson PO. Vaccination against H1N1 influenza with Pandemrix® during pregnancy and delivery outcome: a Swedish register study. BJOG 2012; 119: 1583–90.

Kharbanda EO, Vazquez-Benitez G, Lipkind H et al. Vaccine Safety Datalink Team. Inactivated influenza vaccine during pregnancy and risks for adverse obstetric events. Obstet Gynecol 2013 Sep; 122: 659–67.

Leuridan E, Hoang Thi Thu H, Duc Anh D et al. Pertussis vaccination and pregnancy. Clin Infect Dis 2013; 57: 147–2.

Letson GW, Little JR, Ottman J et al. Meningococcal vaccine in pregnancy: an assessment of infant risk. Pediatr Infect Dis J 1998; 17: 261–3.

Levy M, Koren G. Hepatitis B vaccine in pregnancy: maternal and fetal safety. Am J Perinatol 1991; 8: 227–32.

Lindsey B, Kampmann B, Jones C. Maternal immunization as a strategy to decrease susceptibility to infection in newborn infants. Curr Opin Infect Dis 2013; 26: 248–53.

Liu SL, Wang J, Yang XH et al. Pandemic influenza A(H1N1) 2009 virus in pregnancy. Rev Med Virol 2013; 23: 3–14.

Mandelbrot L. Fetal varicella – diagnosis, management, and outcome. Prenat Diagn 2012; 32: 511–8.

Mazzone T, Celestini E, Fabi R et al. Oral typhoid vaccine and pregnancy. Reprod Toxicol 1994; 8: 278–9.

Merck Pregnancy Registry for Varivax: The 14th Annual Report, 2008 Covering the period from approval (March 17, 1995) through March 16, 2011. Information available at: http://www.merckpregnancyregistries.com/varivax.html

Mor G, Cardenas I. The immune system in pregnancy: a unique complexity. Am J Reprod Immunol 2010; 63: 425–33.

Moro PL, Broder K, Zhcteyeva Y et al. Adverse events in pregnant women following administration of trivalent inactivated influenza vaccine and live attenuated influenza vaccine in the Vaccine Adverse Event Reporting System, 1990–2009. Am J Obstet Gynecol 2011; 204: 146.e1–7.

Mosby LG, Rasmussen SA, Jamieson DJ. 2009 pandemic influenza A (H1N1) in pregnancy: a systematic review of the literature. Am J Obstet Gynecol 2011; 205: 10–8.

Munoz FM. Safety of influenza vaccines in pregnant women. Am J Obstet Gynecol 2012; 207: S33–7.

Namaei MH, Ziaee M, Naseh N. Congenital rubella syndrome in infants of women vaccinated during or just before pregnancy with measles-rubella vaccine. Indian J Med Res 2008; 127: 551–4.

Nasidi A, Monath TP, Vanderberg J et al. Yellow fever vaccination and pregnancy: a four-year prospective study. Trans R Soc Trop Med Hyg 1993; 87: 337–9.

Nasiri R, Yoseffi J, Khajedaloe M et al. Congenital rubella syndrome after rubella vaccination in 1–4 weeks periconceptional period. Indian J Pediatr 2009; 76: 279–82.

Nishioka SDA, Nunes-Araujo FRF, Pires WP et al. Yellow fever vaccination during pregnancy and spontaneous abortion: A case-control study. Trop Med Internat Health 1998; 3: 29–33.

Oppermann M, Fritzsche J, Weber-Schoendorfer C ct al. A-(H1N1)v 2009: A controlled observational prospective cohort study on vaccine safety in pregnancy. Vaccine 2012; 30: 4445–52.

Ornoy A, Ben Ishai PB. Congenital anomalies after oral poliovirus vaccination during pregnancy. Lancet 1993; 341: 1162.

Pasternak B, Svanström H, Mølgaard-Nielsen D et al. Risk of adverse fetal outcomes following administration of a pandemic influenza A(H1N1) vaccine during pregnancy. JAMA 2012; 308: 165–74.

Reddy PA, Gupta I, Ganguly NK. Hepatitis-B vaccination in pregnancy: safety and immunogenic response in mothers and antibody transfer to neonates. Asia Oceania J Obstet Gynaecol 1994; 20: 361–5.

Robert E, Vial T, Schaefer C ct al. Exposure to yellow fever vaccine in early pregnancy. Vaccine 1999; 17: 283–5.

Ross L. Congenital anomalies in two infants born after gestational gamma-globulin prophylaxis. Acta Paediatr 1995; 84: 1436–7.

Ross LJ. Dermatoglyphics in offspring of women given gamma globulin prophylaxis during pregnancy. Teratology 1996; 53: 285–91.

Rubinstein F, Micone P, Bonotti A et al. Influenza A/H1N1 MF59 adjuvanted vaccine in pregnant women and adverse perinatal outcomes: multicentre study. BMJ 2013; 346: f393.

Saito S, Sakai M. Th1/Th2 balance in preeclampsia. J Reprod Immunol 2003; 59: 161–73.

Shahid NS, Steinhoff MC, Roy E et al. Placental and breast transfer of antibodies after maternal immunization with polysaccharide meningococcal vaccine: a randomized, controlled evaluation. Vaccine 2002; 20: 2404–9.

Sammon CJ, Snowball J, McGrogan A et al. Evaluating the hazard of foetal death following H1N1 influenza vaccination; a population based cohort study in the UK GPRD. PLoS One 2012; 7: e51734.

Sheffield JS, Greer LG, Rogers VL et al. Effect of influenza vaccination in the first trimester of pregnancy. Obstet Gynecol 2012; 120: 532–7.

Sheffield JS, Hickman A, Tang J et al. Efficacy of an accelerated hepatitis B vaccination program during pregnancy. Obstet Gynecol 2011; 117: 1130–5.

Silveira CM, Caceres VM, Dutra MG et al. Safety of tetanus toxoid in pregnant women: A hospital-based case-control study of congenital anomalies. Bull WHO 1995; 73:605–608.

Soares RC, Siqueira MM, Toscano CM et al. Follow-up study of unknowingly pregnant women vaccinated against rubella in Brazil, 2001–2002. J Infect Dis 2011; 204: S729–36.

Suzano CE, Amaral E, Sato HK et al. The effects of yellow fever immunization (17DD) inadvertently used in early pregnancy during a mass campaign in Brazil. Vaccine 2006; 24: 1421–6.

Toovey S. Preventing rabies with the Verorab vaccine: 1985–2005 Twenty years of clinical experience. Travel Med Infect Dis 2007; 5: 327–48.

Trowsdale J, Betz AG. Mother's little helpers: mechanisms of maternal-fetal tolerance. Nat Immunol 2006; 7: 241–6.

Tsai TF, Paul R, Lynberg MC et al. Congenital yellow fever virus infection after immunization in pregnancy. J Infect Dis 1993; 168: 1520–3.

Wacholder S, Chen BE, Wilcox A et al. Risk of miscarriage with bivalent vaccine against human papillomavirus (HPV) types 16 and 18: pooled analysis of two randomised controlled trials. BMJ 2010; 340: c712.

Wilson G, Stephens S, Jones D et al. Preliminary data on the use of hepatitis A and B vaccines during pregnancy {Abstract}. ENTIS Congress 2010 Barcelona.

Zaman K, Roy E, Arifeen SE et al. Effectiveness of maternal influenza immunization in mothers and infants. N Engl J Med 2008; 359: 1555–64. Erratum in: N Engl J Med 2009; 360: 648.

Heart and blood medications

2.8

Fernanda Sales Luiz Vianna, Lavinia Schüler-Faccini
and Corinna Weber-Schöndorfer

2.8.1	Arterial hypertension and pregnancy	194
2.8.2	α-Methyldopa	195
2.8.3	β-Receptor blockers	196
2.8.4	Calcium channel blockers	198
2.8.5	ACE inhibitors	199
2.8.6	Angiotensin II receptor blockers (ARBs; Sartans)	200
2.8.7	Dihydralazine	202
2.8.8	α-1 Blockers (peripherally acting adrenergic antagonists)	202
2.8.9	α-2 Blockers (centrally acting adrenergic antagonists)	203
2.8.10	Other antihypertensive medications	204
2.8.11	Pulmonary hypertension and pregnancy	205
2.8.12	Hypotension and antihypotensive drugs	207
2.8.13	Adrenergic agents	208
2.8.14	Cardiac glycosides	208
2.8.15	Antiarrhythmic medications	208
2.8.16	Coronary therapeutic drugs (cardiac vasodilators)	213
2.8.17	Vasocirculatory drugs and peripheral vasodilators	214
2.8.18	Diuretics	215

Profound hemodynamic changes take place during pregnancy. The blood volume starts to expand at the fifth gestational week, and by the end of pregnancy it has increased by 50%. Vascular resistance and blood pressure decrease, while the resting pulse increases by 10–20 beats/min. This results in a 30–50% rise of the cardiac output. Normally, during the second trimester, blood pressure decreases, and then rises again in the last trimester – up to the level before pregnancy or higher. During birth, cardiac output and blood pressure rise even further. Generally, 1–3 days after birth hemodynamic levels are back to pre-pregnancy levels, sometimes normalization may take 1 week (Oakley 2003).

While heart diseases are infrequent during pregnancy (<1%), hypertonic and hypotonic blood pressure problems requiring intervention are much more common.

2.8.1   Arterial hypertension and pregnancy

The management of arterial hypertension differs greatly between pregnant and nonpregnant women. One reason is that certain antihypertensive agents are clearly harmful for the fetus – e.g. ACE inhibitors or angiotensin II receptor antagonists (sartans) during the fetal period (second and third) trimester – while others have not been sufficiently examined regarding their safety. Also, the aims of therapy differ.

Outside pregnancy the main objective of treatment is to lower the risk of cardiovascular sequelae such as heart attack or stroke. This risk reduction has been proven for thiazide diuretics (also for chlortalidone and indapamide), β-blockers, calcium antagonists, ACE inhibitors and sartans. In nonpregnant patients these medications belong to the drugs of first choice whereby each type of agent has its own advantages and disadvantages. Thus, people with diabetes or a high risk of diabetes should not usually receive β-blockers, diuretics, or combinations.

During pregnancy the main objective of antihypertensive management is to lower the risk of maternal complications during gestation and to ascertain the normal development of the fetus. The goal is to lower the risk for preeclampsia, placental abruption, prematurity and intrauterine growth retardation.

The following types of hypertension are distinguished in pregnancy:

- *Chronic arterial hypertension*: diagnosed before, during, and after pregnancy.
- *Gestational hypertension*: develops after the twentieth gestational week, no proteinuria, and disappears within 6 weeks after birth. About half of these patients develop preeclampsia.
- *Preeclampsia and eclampsiay*: Proteinuria (>300 mg/24 hours) and first appearance of hypertension with possible edema.
- *Superimposed gestational hypertension*: preeclampsia in pregnant patients with chronic hypertension, seen in 20–25% of pregnant women with chronic hypertension.

A blood pressure reading of 140/90 mmHg marks the border to hypertension during pregnancy. There is controversy surrounding the issue of when pregnant women should be treated, and if women who already have lower blood pressure elevations would benefit from a therapeutic intervention. This discussion is partially based upon the results of a meta-analysis that showed that a lowering of the mean blood pressure by 10 mmHg during pregnancy decreased the birth weight by 145 g. This reduction did not correlate with the type of antihypertensive medication or with the duration of treatment (Von Dadelszen 2000). A pathophysiologic explanation for this finding might be that lowering of the pressure compromises utero-placental perfusion and thereby leads to a loss of weight (see also de Swiet 2000).

A pilot study investigating the issue at what level of diastolic pressure arterial hypertension should be treated during pregnancy finds only minor differences between tight and less tight blood pressure control when looking at maternal complications and fetal outcomes (Magee 2007).

A population-based retrospective cohort study investigated 100,029 deliveries; of those 1,964 were babies born to mothers who experienced hypertension during pregnancy, with 620 neonates exposed to at least one antihypertensive medication. The authors found a higher rate of intrauterine growth restriction, small for gestational age, and preterm deliveries between both the treated and untreated groups, concluding that not only medication, but also hypertension itself is an independent risk factor for perinatal adverse outcomes (Orbach 2013).

However, a large trial is still needed to identify optimal blood pressure goals and therapy of non-severe maternal hypertension in pregnancy (Magee 2011). Despite many studies and experiences there are still no uniform recommendations for pregnant women. *Methyldopa* remains the first line medication for long-term therapy of chronic hypertension during pregnancy. *Metoprolol, nifedipine*, and, with some reservation, *dihyralazine/hydralazine* are also considered to be well studied.

Blood pressure situations caused by preeclampsia that are more dangerous for mother and fetus are usually best managed with oral nifedipine or urapidil or, with reservations, dihyralazine/hydralazine IV. Also β-receptor blockers may be given, among them the well-studied labetalol.

2.8.2   α-Methyldopa

Pharmacology

α-*Methyldopa* is a centrally acting antihypertensive agent that is well resorbed and has a half-life of two hours. Cardiac functioning, especially output, is not altered, while peripheral resistance is lowered. Independent of IV or oral application, methyldopa becomes clinically effective after 60–90 minutes. The effect lasts for about 10–12 hours. Methyldopa crosses the placenta.

Toxicology

A group of 242 children who were exposed during the first trimester showed a normal pattern for frequency and types of malformations (quoted by Briggs 2011). Another investigation indicated that the head circumference was decreased by 1.3 cm in those newborns whose mothers had received methyldopa between weeks 16 and 20. The controls consisted of children of untreated hypertensive mothers (Moar 1978). This statistically significant result was no longer present at the ages of 6 and 12 months. No anomalies of mental development were apparent in these children at the ages of 4, 5, and 7.5 years. The authors could not explain why only the newborns of mothers treated between weeks 16 to 20 demonstrated a decreased cranial circumference. Fidler (1983) and co-workers did not observe a decrease of skull growth. Normal neurocognitive development was also observed in the study of Chan (2010), comparing exposed children to labetolol with those exposed to methyldopa, and a healthy population control group. A small non-significant decrease in IQ of children exposed to methyldopa was observed, but the authors explained this as a result of lower maternal IQs. A systematic review of neurodevelopmental effects of maternal hypertension and its treatments reinforces the need of the treatment, since no risk is identified with methyldopa therapy and/or labetolol, while hypertension itself can in fact affect development (Koren 2013).

In a few cases hepatotoxic effects were observed in pregnant patients taking methyldopa during pregnancy (e.g. Slim 2010, Smith 1995).

A lowering of the blood pressure by 4–5 mmHg was seen in newborns whose mothers had used methyldopa prior to birth; this effect had no clinical relevance (Whitelaw 1981). We received reports of three newborns that after having been exposed until birth displayed tremor, shaking, and irritability during their first three days. These symptoms were likely to be side effects and disappeared within a few days.

In an *in vitro* examination, methyldopa did not exhibit an influence on the vascular resistance of the umbilical artery (Houlihan 2004). Günenç (2002) analyzed the effect of methyldopa in 24 women with preeclampsia using Doppler sonography. The medication reduced the vascular resistance of the uterine artery, but not of the umbilical arteries or the fetal medial cerebral artery.

> **Recommendation.** α-Methyldopa is one of the oldest antihypertensive drugs that is well tolerated by mother and child during pregnancy. It is the medication of choice for hypertension in pregnancy.

2.8.3   β-Receptor blockers

β-Receptor blockers inhibit the interaction of the neurotransmitters noradrenaline and adrenaline on the β-receptors of the relevant target organ. The heart contains primarily β1-receptors.

β1-selective agents are *atenolol, acebutolol, betaxolol, bisoprolol, celiprolol, esmolol, nebivolol, metoprolol,* and *talinolol*. Most of these are used for the treatment of hypertension, and some for other indications.

The non-selective β-blockers include *carteolol, oxprenolol, penbutolol, pindolol, propranolol, timolol,* and the antiarrhythmic agent *sotalol* (discussed in Section 2.8.17).

Labetalol has an additional α-receptor blocking component. Hardly any experience is found with the use of carvedilol, an α1- and non-selective β-receptor blocker (more on β-receptor blockers in Chapter 2.17.22 Ophthalmic Medications).

β-Receptor blockers cross the placenta and have no teratogenic effect as far as is known (e.g. Diav-Citrin 2011, Nakhai-Pour 2010). These experiences refer primarily to the well-studied systemic β-blockers such as atenolol, bisoprolol, labetalol, metoprolol, and propranolol.

Using data from the Swedish Birth Registry a study compared 1,418 women without diabetes under various hypertensive drugs with 1,046, 842 women without hypertension and diabetes in early pregnancy. The risk of prematurity and small for gestational age (SGA) births was increased in the heterogeneous total group of users of hypertensive drugs, and major malformations were slightly increased (OR 1.63; 95% CI 1.26–2.12). No medication-specific risks or malformations were seen for subjects exposed to β-blockers (monotherapy $n = 798$) or to other hypertensive drugs (Lennestål 2009).

More undesirable effects have been reported with atenolol than with any other β-blocker. It is unresolved if this represents a specific effect of this agent, or if atenolol has been studied more closely, and those results might show up with all β-blockers (Magee 2003). Reports indicate a lower weight of the placenta, intrauterine growth retardation (IUGR), and a lower birth weight (Tabacova 2003a). Bayliss (2002) examined 491 pregnant women with hypertension in regard to the birth weight. As controls served 189 untreated women and patients treated with, among others, calcium antagonists ($n = 14$). The result is interesting, yet its validity limited by the low case number: Newborns whose mothers had taken *atenolol* since conception or during the first trimester until birth (*n* − 10) displayed a significantly lower birth weight. However, the use of atenolol during the second trimester did not show this effect. Independent of the type of hypertensive drug, a superimposed hypertension (second or third trimester) resulted in a lower birth weight. The use of IV labetalol is increasing, especially in a hypertensive crisis during pregnancy. Although there are reports of low birth weight associated with the use of this medication, most studies agree that it does not seem to offer greater risks in pregnancy (Xie 2013).

One report described a child with a retroperitoneal fibromatosis with compression of the medulla leading to a later scoliosis; this was linked to maternal treatment with atenolol. The authors consider that this association should be mentioned, as similar results had been described in adults after the use of atenolol (Satgé 1997).

Pathophysiologically β-receptor blockers, especially perhaps atenolol, could decrease placental perfusion and lead to IUGR and lower placental and birth weight. A causative factor could be that β-blockers increase the tonus of the uterus, but also their hypoglycemic activity has been discussed. As these problems can be induced by severe hypertension alone, the disease itself has to be considered as a co-factor as a minimum.

When considering the effects of the medication upon intrauterine growth, a distinction should be made between severe and lighter forms of maternal hypertension (Section 2.8.1). A meta-analysis of the side effects of antihypertensive drugs in lighter forms of hypertension found that the subgroup using β-receptor blockers only displayed a trend towards a lower birth weight (see Magee 2011).

A neonatal β-receptor blockage due to maternal treatment can lead to hypoglycemia and a decrease in heart frequency. Respiratory depression has been observed in newborns when propranolol is given IV just prior to a caesarean delivery (review by Briggs 2011); this, however, is an unusual event.

Some authors discuss the discontinuation of medication 24–48 hours prior to birth. This approach, though, cannot be recommended, because the maternal blood pressure increases during labor, and the generally mild side effects of a β-blocker in the newborn subside without sequelae within 48 hours. Nevertheless, obstetricians and pediatricians should be aware of the maternal medication.

The postnatal growth during the first year of life and other developments of the children do not appear to be affected (Reynolds 1984). This is confirmed in a later investigation of 32 children who had been exposed to labetalol *in utero*. At the age of 3–7 years they were compared with two control groups (Chan 2010). While in this study the "Labetalol Children" had slightly better results than the "Methyldopa Children," a Dutch study group found different results: Children with intrauterine exposure to labetalol (*n* = 58) had a higher tendency to develop attention deficit hyperactivity disorder (ADHD) than methyldopa-exposed offspring (Pasker-de Jong 2010).

Recommendation. β-receptor blockers belong to the antihypertensive drugs of choice during pregnancy. Well-tested agents such as metoprolol and labetalol should be preferred. If possible, atenolol should be avoided, mainly due to risk of prematurity, SGA and IUGR. When the treatment continues during labor with any β-blocker, perinatal effects may be encountered, such as a decrease in pulse frequency and hypoglycemia.

2.8.4   Calcium channel blockers

Most calcium channel blockers (CCBs) are approved for the management of hypertension, the majority for the treatment of coronary heart disease, and some as antiarrhythmic agents. *Nifepidine* is also used off-label as a tocolytic (Chapter 2.14.6).

In regard to use in pregnancy, *nifedipine* and *verapamil* are the best evaluated CCBs, followed by *amlodipine* and *diltiazem*.

Experience with the following agents is inadequate and at best limited to a few single case reports: *felodipine, gallopamil, isradipine, lercanidipine* (a vaso-selective blocker), *manidipine, nicardipine, nilvadipine, nisoldipine*, and *nitrendipine*. The CCB *nimodipine* is used to manage severe hypertension in pregnancy. In a Cochrane meta-analysis the drug was found to be useless (Duley 2006).

Contrary to the animal experience, there is no evidence that CCBs reduce utero-placental perfusion in humans. Magee (1996) observed no increased risks of malformations in 78 pregnancies (nifedipine $n = 34$, verapamil $n = 32$, diltiazem $n = 10$), but saw a higher rate of miscarriages and an earlier delivery. The birth weight of the newborns tended to be lower. These effects were, according to the authors, not caused by the medication. Also, Sørensen (1998) found no evidence of teratogenicity in 25 children exposed during the first trimester. An analysis of data of the Hungarian Malformation Registry found no evidence of limb defects or a higher malformation risk in general (Sørensen 2001) after exposure to nifedipine, verapamil, or felodipine. Another publication presented 56 retrospective reports concerning undesirable side effects after exposure to nifedipine – most during the second or third trimester (Tabacova 2002). Malformations were noted in 15 cases, four of these on the extremities, and among them one case with a defect of the end phalanges and a syndactyly. However, as the timing of the exposure had not been indicated, nifedipine cannot be causally linked to the problem. Also, a retrospective analysis does not allow an assessment of the frequency of malformations.

A prospective multi-center study with 299 women treated in the first trimester did not demonstrate an increase in malformations or an accumulation of more limb defects. Agents used included nifedipine ($n = 76$) and verapamil ($n = 62$), less common were diltiazem ($n = 41$) and amlodipine ($n = 38$). Significant differences were noted in the increased rate of premature births when compared to the controls. Further, there was a tendency toward a lower birth weight for premature as well as term births. These effects could be explained by the type and severity of the usually underlying placental disorder and not the medication (Weber-Schoendorfer 2008).

Nifedipine showed a faster response in a clinical trial that compared the effectiveness of nifedipine administered orally and intravenously administered labetalol for acute blood pressure control in hypertensive emergency of pregnancy in 60 pregnant women; this study identified no serious adverse maternal or perinatal side effects (Shekhar 2013).

Bortolus (2000) followed 94 children exposed to nifedipine during pregnancy at the age of 18 months. They did not differ from the 96 controls (children born from mothers not treated) in gross or fine motor measures, hearing, vision or language, based on maternal response to questionnaires. The use of sublingual nifedipine can lead to a rapid blood pressure fall (Hata 1995).

Verapamil used to manage fetal supraventricular tachycardia (Section 2.8.15) can induce hyperprolactinemia and galactorrhea.

In summary, current publications about CCBs do not suggest that there is an appreciable teratogenic risk in humans.

> **Recommendation.** After methyldopa and metoprolol calcium channel block-
> ers belong to the antihypertensive drugs of choice in pregnancy. Tested medica-
> tions such as nifedipine are to be preferred. The oral administration of the rapidly
> resorbed nifedipine belongs to the medications of choice in the emergency treat-
> ment of hypertension. Nifedipine should not be given in combination with mag-
> nesium IV.

2.8.5   ACE inhibitors

ACE inhibitors (ACEI) reduce activity of the angiotensin-converting
enzyme and lower blood pressure; they can also be used in cases of cardiac
failure, coronary disease, and diabetic nephropathy. Their effectiveness
is based essentially on a suppression of the plasma renin-angiotensin-
aldosterone system. ACE inhibitors have not shown teratogenic properties, but are fetotoxic. Experience covering more than 1,000 pregnant
women with exposure during the first trimester has been published as
case reports, case series, and analytic studies. In a somewhat older case
series with more than 200 pregnant women treated during the first trimester no clear evidence was seen concerning human teratogenicity (e.g.
Burrows 1998, Bar 1997, Feldkamp 1997). This result was confirmed by a
new two-center study with 224 ACEI-treated pregnancies that were compared with two control groups, one managed with other antihypertensive
drugs and the other a cohort of healthy pregnant women (Diav-Citrin
2011). The women treated with ACEI or angiotensin antagonists ($n = 28$)
had a less favorable profile: they tended to be older and suffered more
from diabetes. The investigation found, in both antihypertensive cohorts,
more premature births and a significantly lower, yet still normal birth
weight. Karthikeyan (2011) analyzed 71 ACEI-exposed pregnancies as
well as data of the United Kingdom Adverse Drug Reaction Reporting
System. They did not find an association with major malformations in
either case.

A methodologically somewhat flawed prescription study was published in 2006, the results of which had not been seen by other investigators, namely an increased risk for heart septum defects ($n = 7$) and
for CNS anomalies (Cooper 2006). Quite unusually, a coloboma was
counted as a CNS anomaly. A Finnish registry study of 137 pregnant women indicated a slightly increased rate of malformation after
ACEI exposure (corrected OR 2,20; 95% CI 1.19–4.08) and suggested
that this was related to maternal diabetes (Malm 2008). Data of the
Swedish Birth Registry showed 1,418 women without diabetes but intake
of various antihypertensive drugs during early pregnancy. Their data were
compared to those of 1,046,843 pregnant women without diabetes and
hypertension. The corrected odds ratio for cardiovascular defects, especially septum defects, was higher overall in the hypertensive group with
2.59 (95% CI 1.92–3.51). This result applied to both the ACEI ($n = 157$)
and the β-blocker subgroups ($n = 1,013$). The authors judged the effect
not to be related to the medications (Lennestål 2009).

It has been known for some time that during the second part of pregnancy ACEIs can lead to reduced placental circulation (de Moura 1995),
fetal hypotension, oligohydramnios, and neonatal anuria requiring dialysis
(Murki 2005, Filler 2003, Lavoratti 1997). Such developmental problems
have also been seen in animal experiments when high doses were used.
The following pathophysiologic mechanism is considered to be at work:
fetal kidney and urine production starts at the end of the first trimester.

Pregnancy

2.8 Heart and blood medications

ACEIs reduce the vascular tonus of renal vessels resulting in fetal renal compromise with longer exposure. The result of a decreased perfusion is lower urine production with oligohydramnios and eventually renal failure and anuria. In addition, hypoplasia of skull bones, contractures, and pulmonary hypoplasia have been noted. The case reports were supported by data from an analysis of conspicuous pregnancy courses after use of enalapril that had been reported to the FDA (Tabacova 2003b).

There are case reports that oligohydramnios subsides once ACIS had been discontinued (e.g. Muller 2002). Concerning later sequelae, there are reports of four children who had been anuric postnatally after ACEI exposure during the third trimester, but recovered fully during the first three months of life. Later, during childhood or adolescence three of the four children developed renal insufficiency with proteinuria, and some also developed arterial hypertension (Laube 2007, Guron 2006).

Since 1992 a so-called black box inscription warns against the administration of ACEIs during the second part of pregnancy in the USA. Nevertheless, the exposure rate tripled in a comparison of the late 1980s to 2003 (Bowen 2008).

> **Recommendation.** ACEIs are contraindicated in the second and third trimester, except for the management of severe conditions that do not respond to other treatments. An accidental application during pregnancy requires an immediate change to one of the recommended antihypertensive drugs. A follow-up sonography can be offered. If treatment occurs for a longer time during the second or third trimester, oligohydramnios should be excluded, and the newborn should be watched for his or her renal function and possible hypotension.

2.8.6   Angiotensin II receptor blockers (ARBs; Sartans)

Candesartan, eprosartan, irbesartan, losartan, olmesartan, telmisartan, and *valsartan* block the AT1 receptor selectively and competitively so that the formation of angiotensin II is inhibited. *Azilsartan* was approved as a new drug in the USA in 2011. Sartans are utilized to treat hypertension and cardiomyopathy. In patients with diabetic nephropathy the agents reduce proteinuria and increase the glomerular filtration rate.

Angiotensin II receptor blockers (ARBs) have not shown teratogenicity, but are fetotoxic.

Experiences covering more than 200 women with exposure in the first trimester are primarily found in case series or subgroups within antihypertensive drug studies. A follow-up study of 37 pregnancies with first trimester exposure reports about 30 live births and two pregnancies with major malformations, one of them was terminated because of exencephaly (Schaefer 2003). Serreau (2005) present 10 pregnancies with the exposure to sartans, seven of them until the thirteenth gestational week. The six live births did not display any malformations. In a case series with five children who had been exposed to ARBs *in utero*, one child with a negative family history showed a sixth right finger and a sixth left toe (Gersak 2009). A two-center study failed to find malformations in 28 pregnant women who had used ARBs in the first trimester (Diav-Citrin 2011). A further study investigated the effect of antihypertensive medications on the risk of cardiac malformation using the data of the Swedish Birth Registry. It detected 45 ARB-exposed pregnancies, 45 of these exclusively treated with sartans, and none of the offspring showed a cardiac anomaly (Lennestål 2009). When the results of the Diabetic Retinopathy Candesartan Trials (DIRECT) Program were analyzed, at least 40 women were identified who had taken candesartan during the first trimester. In none of their offspring was a malformation found (Porta 2011).

During use in the second and third trimester similar risks are present as with the ACE inhibitors. About 40 case reports describe oligo- and anhydramnios, renal dysfunction including anuria, pulmonary hypoplasia, and contractions of the extremities, hypoplasia of the skull, stillbirths and neonatal deaths (e.g. Oppermann 2011, Hünseler 2011, Alwan 2005, Schaefer 2003).

There have been reports of five children who had been exposed until, or during, the third trimester and developed a thrombosis *in utero* or an obliteration of the inferior vena cava, respectively. In one case, thrombosis of both renal veins was described (Oppermann 2011, Bakkum 2006). The pathogenesis has not been clarified; decreased renal blood flow may be of importance.

Oligohydramnios and compromised renal function may partially or completely reverse after medication has been discontinued (e.g. Munk 2010, Bos-Thompson 2005, Berkane 2004). In these publications, medication change occurred twice in the twenty-second and once in the twenty-fourth gestational week. However, a series of 20 cases of pregnant women exposed to ARB identified a poor neonatal outcome associated with oligohydramnios due to these agents, even when the medication was discontinued (Spaggiari 2012).

No studies have been undertaken so far as to whether children who have been exposed to sartans *in utero* may develop late sequelae such as kidney disease and hypertension, as seen in some children after ACEI exposure.

An analysis of 28 prospectively studied pregnancies with ARB exposure past the thirteen gestational week found that related fetal disease developed only when treatment continued past the twentieth week. The risk of oligohydramnios as the first visible sign of a sartan fetopathy was 31% in this scenario (Oppermann 2011).

A systematic review comparing neonatal outcomes between ARBs exposed babies with ACEIs showed poorer outcomes in the ARBs exposed group, and included renal failure, oligohydramnios, death, arterial hypotension, intrauterine growth retardation, respiratory distress syndrome, pulmonary hypoplasia, hypocalvaria, limb defects, persistent patent ductus arteriosus, or cerebral complications. The long-term outcome is described as positive in only 50% of the exposed children. The authors propose the term "fetal renin-angiotensin system blockade syndrome" to describe the related clinical findings (Bullo 2012).

Recommendation. Angiotensin II receptor blockers are contraindicated in the second and third trimester, except when for management of severe and otherwise untreatable diseases. When accidental treatment has occurred during pregnancy, therapy should be immediately changed to one of the recommended antihypertensive agents. A follow-up sonography can be offered. If treatment lasts longer, particularly past 20 weeks, oligohydramnios has to be excluded and fetal development needs to be followed by sonography. In this situation the neonate should be watched for his or her kidney function and possible hypotension.

Pregnancy

2.8 Heart and blood medications

2.8.7   Dihydralazine

Dihydralazine, an antihypertensive agent with central and peripheral action, belongs to the medications that have been used in pregnancy the longest. Eighty percent is resorbed and after oral administration the liver inactivates about 2/3. The half-life is 2–8 hours.

There are hardly any documented experiences about its use in the first trimester. A higher risk of malformation has not been observed (Briggs 2011).

Most investigations describe its application in the third trimester. In a few cases it was noted that patients with preeclampsia developed some liver toxicity (Hod 1986).

A pseudo-lupus syndrome has been known for some time to be a possible side effect of dihydralazine. Thus, a case description should be mentioned with a lupus-like syndrome in mother and offspring; the newborn died (Yemini 1989).

In a meta-analysis Magee (2003) examined maternal, fetal, and perinatal sequelae of the use of *hydralazine* in cases of severe hypertension – typically in the second or third trimester. As a comparison, the examined studies usually utilized nifedipine or labetalol. Three newer randomized studies compared hydralazine or dihydralazine with *labetalol* (Vigil-de Gracia 2006), *urapidil* (Wacker 2006) and *diazoxid* (Hennessy 2007). While results vary, it can be concluded that dihydralazine should not be the medication of first choice for the management of severe gestational hypertension.

> **Recommendation.** Dihydralazine may be used for gestational hypertension, intravenously even in hypertensive emergencies. However, it is no longer considered as a medication of first choice.

2.8.8   α-1 Blockers (peripherally acting adrenergic antagonists)

Urapidil, prazosin, bunazosin, doxazosin, and terazosin belong to the peripherally effective α-1 adrenergic receptor blockers.

Urapidil can be given orally or by IV injection. It is used foremost in the management of emergency hypertensive situations during pregnancy. In a comparative clinical study, Schulz (2001) concluded that urapidil represents an equally effective alternative to dihydrazaline in preeclamptic women. This is confirmed by another study with 42 patients. Side-effects and control, however, were better with urapidil (Wacker 2006). Urapidil is recommended as an alternative to dihydralazine in the management of preeclampsia. Compared to dihydralazine it may have the advantage that it does not increase the intracranial pressure. One case report notes a temporary respiratory depression in a premature infant of the thirtyfifth week in conjunction with high levels of urapidil in his urine (Vanhaesebrouck 2009).

Prazosin crosses the placenta. Few publications from the 1980s describe that it is well tolerated in late pregnancy. There is no evidence of a teratogenic potential, but reports are not well documented. Even less documented experiences are available for *bunazosin, doxazosin,* and *terazosin*. In the management of hypertension of nonpregnant patients, these agents are typically used as medications of second choice and combined with other antihypertensive drugs; they are primarily useful in men with an accompanying prostatic hyperplasia.

> **Recommendation.** Urapidil IV is useful in the emergency management of hypertension in pregnancy. Prazosin should only be used during the second or third trimester, when antihypertensive medications of first choice have failed. When α-1 blockers have been used during the first trimester, a follow-up sonography may be offered to confirm normal fetal development.

2.8.9   α-2 Blockers (centrally acting adrenergic antagonists)

Clonidine is an antihypertensive drug that works primarily at a central point of action. Seventy-five percent of it is bioavailable, while its half-life lasts 8.5 hours. Due to metabolic changes pregnant women have a higher clearance (Buchanan 2009). Clonidine is no longer of importance in today's management of hypertension. Occasionally it is given to alcoholics in intensive care as an IV injection in order to ease acute withdrawals. It has also lost its role as an antiglaucoma agent in ophthalmology. Sometimes clonidine is used during delivery by the anesthesiologist (Chapter 2.16.7).

A study with 66 women who received clonidine after their sixteenth gestational week demonstrated an effective lowering of blood pressure, but also a reduction of cardiac output; and in 31 of the 66 there was no reduction of the peripheral resistance resulting in a lower birth weight (Rothberger 2010).

There is no evidence that clonidine has a dangerous teratogenic potential; there are reports of more than 200 pregnancies indicating its effectiveness and tolerance (Horvath 1985). Boutroy (1988) describe a temporary hypertension in some newborns interpreted to present a form of withdrawal symptom. Huisjes (1986) examined children at the age of about six years whose mothers had been treated during pregnancy with a mono-therapy of clonidine. They exhibited hyperactivity and sleeping disorders somewhat more frequently than controls. The finding of this small study resembles those of animal experiments, but has so far not been verified by other clinical studies.

Moxonidine belongs to the group of centrally acting α-receptor agonists. A well-founded risk analysis cannot be made due to the lack of documented experience.

Reserpine is an orally well resorbed, centrally and peripherally effective sympatholytic that has lost much of its former importance. Prior to its use as an antihypertensive agent, it had been used extensively in psychiatry. When reserpine was administered during the last trimester, occasionally it was observed that the newborn had respiratory problems and difficulties in drinking (Czeizel 1988).

> **Recommendation.** Clonidine, moxonidine, and reserpine are no longer part of the armamentarium of antihypertensive management. They should not be used during pregnancy. However, if used during the first trimester, a follow-up sonography may be offered.

Pregnancy

2.8 Heart and blood medications

2.8.10   Other antihypertensive medications

Phenoxybenzamine, an α-adrenergic blocker, is used in the management of pheochromocytoma and neurogenic bladder. Published experiences about first trimester use are lacking. Case reports of use later in pregnancy do not describe developmental problems (e.g. Luk 2009).

Minoxidil is a vasodilator that has an antihypertensive effect. It is also used for alopecia. Case reports with various malformations and a case of hypertrichosis in a newborn that regressed spontaneously within 3 months do not allow for a differentiated risk assessment (Chapter 2.17.19).

Sodium nitroprusside belongs to the fast-acting vasodilators. It is used exclusively in intensive care medicine as an IV agent. Nitroprusside crosses the placenta easily. It reaches the same level in the fetus as in the maternal organism. Both metabolize it quickly to cyanide and thiocyanate resulting in a toxic potential. Experiences refer to 22 patients with 25 exposed fetuses, of which five were born as stillbirths. Eighteen pregnant women had been treated for severe hypertension and four for an intracranial aneurysm. In part, the course of these diseases and their management was described inadequately (Sass 2007).

Magnesium sulfate IV continues to be a basic component in the management of preeclampsia with hyperreflexia; it dampens neuromuscular hyperreflexia by blocking calcium. As in most such situations the delivery is planned, and treatment is generally short-term for pre-, peri-, and postnatal stabilization. Regarding the discussion, if use of magnesium lowers the blood pressure, it is now recognized that it does not and should not be used anymore for that purpose (Duley 2006).

Aliskiren is a newly developed renin inhibitor that blocks the conversion of angiotensinogen to angiotensin-I and lowers the levels of angiotensin-I and -II. Concluding studies, which would enable an assessment about the applicability of this drug, are not yet available. It appears that the degree of blood pressure decrease is moderate. There have been no reports about its use in pregnancy, but it stands to reason that renin blockers have similar problems as ACE inhibitors and sartans and could lead to renal dysfunction and oligohydramnios.

Diazoxide no longer has a role in the management of hypertension. It has been approved for the treatment of hypoglycemia due to different causes. After an oral dose it is resorbed fully and crosses the placenta. Hyperuricemia, water retention, and inhibition of uterine contractions have been observed in pregnant women, while newborns have shown alopecia, increased lanugo, and delayed bone development (Milner 1972).

> **Recommendation.** Phenoxybenzamine may be used for the treatment of pheochromocytoma in pregnancy. Sodium nitroprusside should be reserved for selected cases that cannot be managed otherwise. Diazoxide and minoxidil should be avoided. Aliskiren is contraindicated in pregnancy. An accidental intake is not an indication for a risk-based termination of pregnancy or for invasive diagnostic tests (Chapter 1.15). When any of the drugs mentioned here have been used in the first trimester, including Aliskiren, a follow-up sonography should be performed to verify the normal development of the fetus.

2.8.11 Pulmonary hypertension and pregnancy

Pulmonary hypertension (PH) and pulmonary arterial hypertension (PAH) are general terms for diseases marked by a permanent elevation of the resistance of the pulmonary arteries. Pulmonary hypertension is characterized by an elevation of the mean pressure of the pulmonary artery of >25 mmHg at rest and >30 mmHg under exertion. Aside from idiopathic forms, there are a number of underlying diseases that can lead to PH.

Management consists of treatment of the underlying disorders, symptomatic interventions such as nasal oxygen, anticoagulation, diuretics, possibly digitalis, calcium antagonists, and specific medications to prevent permanent damage to the pulmonary vessels.

The physiologic circulatory changes during pregnancy result in a worsening of the PAH which, without therapy, would result in a high maternal mortality of 30–50% (Weiss 1998; Systematic assessment of 125 pregnancy courses from 1978 to1996). For this reason, pregnancy is generally discouraged. Also, a PAH may be first diagnosed during pregnancy, while late pregnancy and postpartum are the most dangerous periods related to this condition. Pregnant women with PAH should be managed in specialized centers. Mortality is then clearly reduced (e.g. Kiely 2010; Analysis of 10 pregnancies from author's own center from 2002 to 2009: one patient died four weeks after delivery). A series of 30 cases of pregnant women with PH identified a maternal mortality rate of 16.7% and fetal/neonatal mortality was 13%. Only two of these underwent specific therapy for PAH, but the authors did not mention the medication used or the exact outcome for exposed fetuses (Ma 2012). However, in an erratum to this publication this omission was corrected, indicating as medication (nitric oxide, prostacyclin analogs, bosentan or sildenafil) (Ma 2013). The overall maternal mortality was 16.7% in puerperium, and there were four fetal/neonatal deaths (13%). No other factors were identified including mode of anaesthesia, mode of delivery, and categories and severity of PH, as significant predictors of mortality. They concluded that the maternal mortality in parturients with PH is high and women with PH who become pregnant warrant a multidisciplinary approach.

In the following section medications are presented to manage PAH but have relatively little documented experience in pregnancy.

► **Endothelin receptor antagonists (ERAs)**

The three ERAs that are approved to be marketed can all cause liver damage. *Sitaxsentan* was removed from the market at the end of 2010 because of severe liver toxicity.

Bosentan is bound to 98% to plasma albumen, has a half-life of about 5 hours, and binds specifically to endothelin receptors that cause vasoconstriction, fibrosis, cell proliferation, and remodeling. Bosentan is able to block these events to some degree.

Bosentan has shown teratogenicity in rats when plasma concentrations exceeded 1.5 times the therapeutic human level. Malformations of the head, face, and eyes were observed. As the connection appeared plausible, the USA and some member-states of the EU started a similar pregnancy prevention program, such as for isotretinoin (Segal 2005), although at this time, there is no direct evidence of human teratogenicity. However, the current experience is too limited to exclude a risk.

There are three case reports: (1) After a complicated pregnancy with an inadvertent intake of bosentan and *sildenafil* until delivery at 30 weeks, the newborn female was growth-retarded but did not display malformations. She thrived initially but then succumbed to an RS viral infection at the age of 6 months (Molelekwa 2005). (2) Elliot (2005) describe a dramatic pregnancy with exposure to bosentan and *warfarin* until week 6/7, followed by a change in therapy using *iloprost* as an inhalant and *heparin*. Cardiac arrest occurred after week 25. After a successful reanimation, the patient's iloprost use was changed to IV application. One week later she was surgically delivered of a boy who developed well after overcoming his prematurity problems. (3) The third case describes a woman with systemic lupus erythematosus and associated PH for which she used bosentan and *phenprocoumon* until week 5, also continuously sildenafil and various immunosuppressants. Phenprocoumon was replaced by heparin, and bosentan by iloprost after week 35. The patient was delivered of a healthy infant at 37 weeks (Streit 2009).

Ambrisentan has teratogenic effects in preclinical animal testing, but there is no reported experience with human pregnancy.

▶ Phosphodiesterase inhibitors

Phosphodiesterase type 5 is found in the corpus callosum of the penis as well as in the pulmonary vessels. In PAH, inhibition of the phosphoesterase will lead to a vasodilatation of the pulmonary vessels and, to some degree, in the major circulation.

There are currently six case reports about *sildenafil*. Lacassie (2004) reports about a 24-year-old woman with Eisenmenger syndrome who took sildenafil from gestational weeks 7 to 9 then stopped and, as symptoms got worse, resumed the therapy between week 31 to 36. Further medication consisted of *diltiazem*, and after week 32 of *l-arginine*. A healthy boy was born after 36 weeks. Two pregnancy courses with continuous sildenafil treatment have been reported under bosentan (Streit 2009, Molelekwa 2005). Goland (2010) describes two pregnant women who received sildenafil and IV *epoprostenol* in the last trimester and were delivered of healthy children by caesarean section. Finally, a pregnancy with a favorable outcome for mother and baby was described in a woman with PH, human immunodeficiency virus (HIV) and an atrial septal defect who was exposed to sildenafil, among other agents, before delivery (Ng 2012).

In an off-label application, sildenafil has been used with little success in patients with recurrent abortions (Jerzak 2008), *in vitro* fertilization (Jerzak 2010), and preeclampsia (Downing 2010, Samangaya 2009). However, no negative effects were reported concerning the fetus. With success it had been used in 10 pregnancies with severe growth retardation (von Dadelszen 2011).

There are no reported experiences about the use of *tadalafil* in pregnancy.

▶ Prostacyclin analogs

Currently three prostacyclin analogs are in use for the management of PAH: *Epoprostenol*, *treprostinil* and *iloprost*. They inhibit the aggregation of thrombocytes, dilate vessels, and reduce the remodeling of vessels.

Epoprostenol is an unstable, synthetic prostacyclin analog that needs to be infused continuously as its half-life is only 3 minutes. Moodley (1992) describes almost 50 patients with epoprostenol treatment for preeclampsia in late pregnancy. They noted only complications from prematurity, but none typical for medication. At least 14 pregnant women with PAH taking epoprostenol, some of them already during the first trimester, displayed no drug-specific embryo- or fetotoxic side effects (e.g. Garabedian 2010, Goland 2010, Bendayan 2005, Avdalovic 2004, Bildirici 2004, Geohas 2003, Stewart 2001, Badalian 2000). Another case of exposure to epoprostenol from the twenty-third week of gestation showed a course without postpartum complications. However, the baby died at 11 days of life. The autopsy revealed normal cardiac chambers with probe patent foramen ovale and patent ductus arteriosus. The death was attributed to sudden infant death syndrome (SIDS) (Timofeev 2013). Although as a comment the diagnosis of SIDS should not be given to the sudden death of an infant that is not predicted by medical history and remains unexplained after a thorough forensic autopsy.

Treprostinil is marketed as a subcutaneous infusion and it is also available for IV and inhalative applications. There are no reported experiences about its use in pregnancy. In animal experiments it did not show teratogenicity in rats and rabbits.

The stable synthetic prostacycline analog *iloprost* is offered as an IV injectable and as an inhalant for thromboangiitis obliterans and advanced stages of PAH. Six case descriptions of its use in PAH, among them one during the first trimester, do not show negative effects on the prenatal development (e.g. Streit 2009, Elliot 2005). Shorter toes have only been observed in rats but not in other animals; they are not considered a teratogenic effect, but caused by hypoperfusion (Battenfeld 1995). Iloprost as an inhalant was successfully applied in four very small premature infants with persisting PH and well tolerated (Eifinger 2008).

Recommendation. Pulmonary arterial hypertension during pregnancy is afflicted with a high maternal mortality; a multidisciplinary team in a specialized center should manage it. The treatment that appears most effective should be chosen. When different options are under discussion, the application of an endothelin receptor antagonist should be avoided during the first trimester. The use of PH medications does not justify a risk-based termination (Chapter 1.15); however, serial follow-up sonograms should monitor fetal development.

2.8.12 Hypotension and antihypotensive drugs

In principle, hypotension is without clinical significance during the course of pregnancy. This applies especially to the not infrequent circulatory deregulation in gestation. Treatment consists primarily of compression stockings, gymnastics of the legs prior to getting up, cold water applications, and brush massages. Coffee, too, is allowed within reason. Usually, medication is not indicated in cases of arterial hypotension or circulatory deregulation.

2.8.13   Adrenergic agents

The adrenergic agents *etilefrine, amezinium metilsulfate*, and *midodrine* have been used to treat low blood pressure.

Regarding *dihydroergotamine mesylate*, see Chapter 2.1.14.

In animal experiments adrenergic agents are able to reduce uterine blood flow. A teratogenic effect has not been observed in humans, when therapeutic doses were used. However, experiences have been too limited to exclude an increased risk for malformations.

> **Recommendation.** Named agents should be avoided during the first trimester. If there was an exposure during organogenesis, such exposure does not justify a termination. A follow-up sonogram can be offered to ascertain normal fetal development. If significant symptoms during the fetal period (second and third trimester) require medical therapy for low blood pressure, adrenergic drugs may be used. Medications with longer experience, such as etilefrine, are to be preferred. Combination drugs should be avoided.

2.8.14   Cardiac glycosides

Pharmacology

The intestinal resorption of *digitoxin* is about 90–100% while that of *metildigoxin* and *acetyldigoxin* is about 80%. Metildigoxin is demethylated in the liver, while acetyldigoxin is deacetylated in the intestinal mucosa. Digoxin is eliminated primarily via the kidneys and *digitoxin* via the liver. The half-life of digoxin is about 40 hours, while that of digitoxin on average 7 days. Digoxin is a metabolite of digitoxin.

All digitalis glycosides are able to cross the placenta; the fetal placenta concentration corresponds to the maternal one. Myocardial sensitivity appears to be lower in the fetus than in the adult. During the first trimester, digitalis is not a teratogen according to published experiences (Aselton 1985). Toxic effects in the fetus have not been observed when digitalis glycosides were used at therapeutic doses. Many case reports describe how well they are tolerated, when tachycardia of the pregnant women or the fetus is treated.

> **Recommendation.** During pregnancy digitalis glycosides may be used to manage cardiac failure and maternal or fetal arrhythmias. In cases of fetal tachycardia, they are the antiarrhythmics of first choice (Chapter 1.6 and Section 2.8.15).

2.8.15   Antiarrhythmic medications

A distinction needs to be made between the treatment of arrhythmias of both the mother and the fetus. In the former a possibly minimal low transplacental passage is desirable, while in the latter a sufficiently adequate passage is necessary to manage the fetus via the mother. Generally, supraventricular and ventricular extrasystoles do not require therapy in mother and fetus.

► **Antiarrhythmic therapy of the pregnant woman**

It is rare that women with a healthy heart will develop "classical" tachycardia for the first time in pregnancy. When supraventricular tachycardia, atrial flutter or fibrillation, and ventricular tachycardia lead to unstable hemodynamics, a cardioversion is indicated as in the cases of ventricular flutter or fibrillations. This treatment will not affect the fetus that is outside of the voltage field and has a high cardiac response threshold. If the woman is in a stable hemodynamic state, a cardiac conversion can be attempted with medication. Another indication for antiarrhythmic agents is the prevention of recurrences. Bombelli (2003) reports three pregnant women with supraventricular tachycardia not responding to treatment who underwent a successful catheter ablation during the third trimester. However, the radiation exposure during such an intervention needs to be considered as a risk.

Pregnant women with continuous bradycardia requiring treatment are managed with pacemakers.

► **Antiarrhythmic therapy of the fetus**

Fetal tachycardia

In about 0.4–0.6% of pregnancies the fetus develops (mostly supraventricular) tachycardia (>180 beats/min), typically in the second or third trimester. Most of these fetuses have no visible cardiac malformation. With longer duration the fetus may develop cardiac failure or a myopathy with pleural and pericardial effusion, ascites, and edema. Fetal hydrops refers to a condition where fluids are overfilling two or more compartments; it may precede intrauterine death.

In most cases the mother is medicated to treat the fetus. Thus, potential side effects concerning the mother need to be considered. Moreover, it is possible that an antiarrhythmic drug leads to an arrhythmogenic effect resulting in ventricular fibrillation in the fetus and his or her demise.

Because of effectiveness and safety, *digoxin* is the drug of first choice. If, however, a hydrops has already developed, it is unlikely that an adequate concentration of digoxin will reach the fetus (e.g. Maeno 2009). For such a scenario it has been proposed to inject digoxin IM directly into the fetal thigh (e.g. Cuneo 2008). An application into the umbilical cord could facilitate a fetal demise and should be avoided. In a series of 27 fetuses treated with a combination of digoxin and *flecainide*, the authors concluded that this treatment is effective for fetal supraventricular tachycardia (96% response rate and 81.4% restoration of sinus rhythm). In all, 26 treated infants were delivered alive, but one pregnancy was terminated for non-cardiac causes; there were no intrauterine deaths due to tachycardia and none of the pregnant women developed proarrhythmia (Uzun 2012).

If this approach fails *sotalol* – especially for atrial flutter – and/or *flecainide* may be used, combined with or without digitalis (Maeno 2009, Doherty 2003, Oudijk 2003).

In certain situations of fetal tachycardia, some authors prefer *amiodarone* (see also below) instead of flecainide after digoxin and sotalol. They indicate a high success rate and point out that it is rare to encounter fetal hypothyroidism (due to the high iodine content of the

Pregnancy

2.8 Heart and blood medications

medication) (Cuneo 2008). This, however, applies only to a short therapy of up to 1-week duration. In other case reports a high degree of effectiveness was also noted, but temporary hypothyroidism and struma were present in 43% of the children (Pézard 2008).

Experiences with other antiarrhythmic agents are very limited. The application of *verapamil* is generally not supported (e.g. Oudijk 2002). *Adenosine* has rarely been used as a direct injection into the umbilical vein. It can lead to fetal bradycardy. When medication is not successful, in certain situations an early delivery has been proposed to allow a postnatal cardioversion. In general, "fetal" antiarrhythmic therapy is well tolerated by women with a healthy heart.

Fetal bradycardia

A fetal bradycardia (<100 beats/min) is usually due to an atrioventricular (AV) block. It may be linked to fetal cardiac malformations or can occur in otherwise healthy fetuses due to the transplacental passage of maternal autoantibodies, often SSA-AK (Ro-AK). A maternal connective tissue disease has often not yet been diagnosed at that point (Maeno 2009). The bradycardia is initially compensated by an increase in the stroke volume; a heart frequency of <55/min appears to be hemodynamically insufficient (Eronen 2001). The resulting heart failure can lead to a fetal hydrops. Fetal bradycardia with a heart defect and hydrops obviously has a poor prognosis.

Treatment option demands sympathicomimetic drugs (e.g. *ritodrine, salbutamol, terbutaline*) to increase heart frequency, and, in cases of autoimmune-related heart blocks, the application of halogenated steroids provided the AV block is not yet complete. The administration of *betamethasone* or *dexamethasone* to the mother is guided by the concept that her autoantibodies cause an inflammation of the AV node and the myocardium leading to fibrosis. The result of this is an AV block, an endocardial fibrosis, and a dilatative cardiomyopathy that may not become apparent until after birth. The use of fluorided glucocorticoids is under discussion, as a sizable number of fetuses with a congenital heart block survive without anti-inflammatory therapy and the risks of treatment have to be balanced against the risk of a heart block (e.g. Lopes 2008 and comments). This notion is relevant for the issue of when to start treatment. Only one group proposes that a first-degree heart block is an indication for therapy (Rein 2009). Treatment consists of, e.g. 8 mg *dexamethasone* daily, corresponding to a fetal dose of 0.05 mg per kg body weight. It starts usually when the diagnosis is entertained, typically between weeks 19 and 24, and continues until birth (Hutter 2010). As in about 10% of cases oligohydramnios developed (Hutter 2010, Saleeb 1999, Vesel 2004), a pediatric cardiology team from Toronto modified the regimen for relatively uncomplicated courses by giving 8 mg per day only for 2 weeks, then 4 mg/d, and after 38 weeks 2 mg/d. An AV block that starts after the thirty-second week may not require treatment provided there is no cardiac malformation, no fibrosis, and the fetal heart frequency is at least 50–55 beats/min (Hutter 2010). The application of IV immunoglobulins to the mother to reduce her antibody burden has been attempted for prophylaxis (Friedman 2010) and also therapeutically but without convincing results. In some cases a preterm delivery can be contemplated to implant a pacemaker early enough.

Pharmacology and toxicology

Antiarrhythmic drugs are classified into different classes and used for diverse forms of arrhythmia:

- Class IA antiarrhythmics belong to the chinidin type. They include *chinidin* proper, as well as *ajmaline, disopyramide,* and *prajmalium bitartrate.*
- Class IB antiarrhythmics include substances related to *lidocaine* such as *mexiletine,* and also the *teratogenic phenytoin* only approved for epilepsy.
- Class IC antiarrhythmics contain *flecainide* and *propafenone.*
- Class II antiarrhythmics comprise the β-receptor blockers.
- Class III antiarrhythmics encompass *amiodarone,* and the β-receptor blocker *sotalol* as well as *dronedarone.*
- Class IV antiarrhythmics involve the calcium channel blockers *verapamil, gallopamil,* and *diltiazem.*

The nucleoside adenosine is not captured in any of the classic antiarrhythmic classes, likewise *ipratropium bromide* and *vernakalant.*

Class IA antiarrhythmics

Chinidin is almost fully resorbed after oral intake and reaches its maximum serum level in 1–4 hours. The liver, the rest via the kidneys, excretes about 80%. As a vagal antagonist chinidin increases heart frequency despite a depressing action on the pacemaker cells. Chinidin is one of the oldest antiarrhythmic drugs and does not appear to have a teratogenic potential. It crosses the placenta and reaches levels in the fetus as high as in the mother. It has been successfully used both for maternal and fetal treatments. With antiarrhythmic dosing the known stimulation of uterine contractions is not to be expected.

Disopyramide, too, is said to stimulate uterine contractions (Briggs 2011) and crosses the placenta. There are no reports of malformations. Data are insufficient about the tolerance of ajmaline and prajmalium.

Class IB antiarrhythmics

Most of the extensive experiences with *lidocaine* in pregnancy come from anesthesia. When used to manage arrhythmias, it needs to be administered parenterally as the oral dose is not sufficiently effective (Cuneo 2003) describes a fetus with Q-T prolongation on the EKG who displayed ventricular tachycardias and an intermittent AV block. He was successfully treated with lidocaine. A teratogenic effect has not been described in humans. Lidocaine crosses the placenta readily and, if its levels are high, can lead to CNS depression in the neonate (its use during labor is discussed in Chapter 2.16.7). A study from France reports a completely different application, namely, the use of lidocaine to induce feticide. Fetuses (between week 20 and 36) with various malformations received via the umbilical vein first sufentanil (5 μg), then 7 to 30 mL lidocaine (1%) resulting in a cardiac asystole (Senat 2003).

Phenytoin is a teratogenic anticonvulsive drug (Chapter 2.10.24).

Class IC antiarrhythmics

Many case reports document the effectiveness of *flecainide* in the treatment of fetal tachycardias (Walsh 2008, Krapp 2002). Especially when the fetus has already developed a hydrops, it is superior to *digitalis glycosides*. A tight monitoring of maternal serum levels is recommended to keep fetal levels low enough to minimize side effects (Rasheed 2003). In contrast to animal experiments, no evidence of teratogenicity has been found in humans, yet the data are very limited for first trimester use (e.g. Villanova 1998). *Propafenone* has not been sufficiently studied in pregnancy. The manufacturer reports about more than 30 pregnancies under propafenone that do not suggest a noteworthy prenatal risk.

Class II antiarrhythmics

See Section 2.8.3 for β-receptor blockers.

Class III antiarrhythmics

Amiodarone has a very long elimination half-life of approximately 40 days. To avoid fetal exposure, the medication would have to be discontinued several months prior to conception. The following fetal side effects have been seen more frequently: fetal bradycardia and connatal hypothyroidism due to the high (39%) iodine content (Lomenick 2004, Grosso 1998). In some situations it was reported that thyroxine was injected into the amnion as a substitute. Five of 26 children who had been treated *in utero* were found to have hypothyroidism at birth. A sixth child whose treatment with amiodarone was continued after birth developed hypothyroidism at the age of 3 months (Strasburger 2004). Bartalena (2001) analyzed 64 previously published cases. In 56 situations a maternal indication led to the treatment. Transient hypothyroidism was diagnosed in a dozen children, in two cases linked with a struma. In another publication transient hypothyroidism and struma were described in 43% of the children (Pézard 2008). Discrete neurological anomalies were seen in some of the intrauterine exposed children, also in euthyroid ones leading to the hypothesis that amiodarone may have a direct neurotoxic effect (Bartelena 2001). One case report describes a marked developmental delay in a child who had been exposed to amiodarone and *digoxin* for a fetal indication from gestational weeks 26 to 35 and again, postnatally, to amiodarone and propranolol for 24 months. There was no hypothyroidism at any time, and other causes had been excluded (Mikovic 2010). On occasion, a Q-T prolongation has been observed in the neonatal EKG. Intrauterine growth retardation has been noted, but it remains unclear to what degree amiodarone, accompanying drugs (usually β-receptor blockers), or the underlying disease contributed. Most children do not show problems. Children who have been followed past the neonatal period did not display recognizable functional deficits related to hypothyroidism (Magee 1999). Experience with amiodarone in the first trimester is limited to about 20 exposed pregnancies that were not suspicious (Briggs 2011).

Sotalol crosses the placenta with ease and is a potent antiarrhythmic drug for the management of fetal tachycardias. In a case study of 18 fetuses with tachycardia it was noted that the drug accumulated in the amniotic fluid, but not the fetus itself. Thirteen of fourteen fetuses treated with sotalol alone responded with a restoration of normal sinus rhythm, two had recurrences, and in one case the fetus died. Two of the four fetuses who were treated additionally with digoxin had a successful treatment (Oudijk 2003). Other case reports about the treatment of maternal or fetal arrhythmias do not show a significant prenatal toxic risk. However, when treatment continues until birth, symptoms of a β-receptor blockage may be encountered in the newborn such as bradycardia and hypoglycemia (Section 2.8.3).

Dronedarone is a new benzofuran; it does not contain iodine and is otherwise closely related to amiodarone. It represents a multi-channel inhibitor to prevent non-permanent atrial fibrillation. There have been no reports of its use in pregnancy.

Class IV antiarrhythmics

Regarding the CCBs verapamil and diltiazem see Section 2.8.4. Current experiences in humans do not indicate evidence of teratogenic effects. No reports about the tolerance of *gallopamil* are available.

Adenosine has a very brief half-fife of less than 2 seconds and has to be given IV. Current experiences in pregnancy and in the treatment of fetal arrhythmias do not suggest fetotoxic effects (Hasdemir 2009, Hubinont 1998).

Electrocardioversion and implanted defibrillators appear not to cause fetal side effects (e.g. Lin 2008). The cardiac threshold of the fetal heart is relatively high, and, in addition, the fetus lies outside of the voltage field and the electric current (Joglar 1999).

> **Recommendation.** As antiarrhythmic agents can also trigger arrhythmias, the indication for their use needs to be assessed critically. Medications of choice for the treatment of the pregnant patients are in Class IA chinidin, in Class IB lidocaine, in Class IC propafenone and, also in the second and third trimester, flecainide. In Class II well-tested β-receptor blockers should be preferred. If a Class III antiarrhythmic drug is required, sotalol should be chosen. In Class IV verapamil and diltiazem are acceptable; the same with adenosine.

Phenytoin is contraindicated, as it is a teratogen. If one of the medications was used that is not a primary recommendation, or if such a medication is necessary, a termination is not justified on a risk-based rationale. With the exception of the well-studied β-receptor blockers and CCBs, a follow-up sonography should be offered to patients with exposure during the first trimester to verify a normal fetal development. If amiodarone was applied, the development of a prenatal struma needs to be excluded by a sonogram, and the fetus and neonate should be checked for possible hypothyroidism. Supraventricular tachycardias of the fetus are foremost treated with digitalis glycosides. A secondary option is a trial with sotalol or flecainide. Amiodarne is at best a reserve medication, when other antiarrhythmic drugs have failed.

2.8.16   Coronary therapeutic drugs (cardiac vasodilators)

The nitrates *isosorbide mononitrate, isosorbide dinitrate, nitroglycerine* or *glyceryl trinitrate,* and *pentaerithritol tetranitrate* have been approved for the treatment of angina pectoris and, in some cases, of myocardial infarction. They are also used for other indications: for biliary colics, as a tocolytic agent in obstetrics (e.g. Smith 2007, 2010), for the initiation of labor (e.g. Nunes 2006), for preeclampsia (e.g. Manzur-Verástegui 2008), and other conditions.

A toxic effect upon the fetus has not been observed, but the rate of maternal side effects is high. A study to assess cervix length and the presence of cervical gland area in ultrasounds performed before and after the administration of vaginal isosorbide mononitrate for cervical ripening in pregnancy indicated for labor induction had to be discontinued due to adverse effects, such as nausea, dizziness, dyspnea, and vomiting (Hatanaka 2012). A randomized study comparing glyceryl trinitrite ($n = 81$) and β-sympathomimetics ($n = 75$) as tocolytic agents failed to see any developmental differences in children at the age of 18 months (Gill 2006). Experiences with use in the first trimester are limited.

Few relevant studies cover other coronary drugs such as *ivabradine, molsidomine, ranolazine*, and *trapidil*.

There is one case report on the use of *ivabradine* in the first trimester because of an acute heart attack; a healthy child was born later (Babic 2011). *Trapidil* was compared to a placebo in a study of 180 women with a higher risk of preeclampsia between weeks 22 and 38 (according to Dodd 2010). Specific side effects were not noted.

> **Recommendation.** Nitrates may be used in pregnancy provided they are used for the right indication. Use of other coronary drugs does not require a risk-based termination or any additional diagnostic interventions; see also Chapter 1.15.

2.8.17   Vasocirculatory drugs and peripheral vasodilators

The medications discussed here are primarily used to treat acute hearing loss, dizziness, and intermittent claudication. Before prescribing these agents to pregnant patients, it should be ascertained that their use is necessary and based on evidence. This applies particularly to hearing loss.

No studies on first trimester tolerance exist for *pentoxifylline* and *naftidrofuryl*. Past clinical experiences and pharmacology make it unlikely that these agents have an appreciable teratogenic potential.

There is no evidence that *Ginkgo biloba* is teratogenic, but it has not been studied extensively and as a nutraceutical the composition and effectiveness, let alone the indication, is doubtful. An increased malformation risk is not expected for *hydroxyethyl starch* (Chapter 2.9.13).

Flunarizine and *cinnarizine* are CCBs and have antihistamine properties. Experience in pregnancy is limited (e.g. Weber-Schoendorfer 2008); signs of harmful effects have not been reported. No documented experiences are available for the histamine analog *betahistine* which is supposed to improve the microcirculation in the inner ear.

Relevant experiences are lacking for the following medications that have been approved for treatment of peripheral arterial obstructions: the prostaglandin *alprostadil* inhibiting the aggregation of thrombocytes and has a vasodilatatory effect, and the heparinoid *pentosan polysulfate* that displays anticoagulatory and fibrinolytic properties. The same holds for the vasodilatator buflomedil (not approved in the USA). The European Medicines Agency's (EMA) Committee for Medicinal Products for Human Use (CHMP) concluded that the benefits of buflomedil do not outweigh its risks, and has recommended that all marketing authorizations for medicines containing *buflomedil* should be suspended throughout the European Union (EU). The reason being that this product has serious neurologic and cardiac side effects.

> **Recommendation.** If really needed and better-examined alternatives are not available, flunarizine may be used in pregnancy. If treatment with a vasocirculatory drug must be done, pentoxifylline should be preferred. Alprostdil should be avoided, as it is a prostaglandin. Use of any of the not-recommended drugs does not justify a risk-based termination (Chapter 1.15). In case of doubt, a follow-up sonography may be offered to ascertain normal fetal development.

2.8.18   Diuretics

Only in rare cases are diuretics indicated during pregnancy, e.g. pulmonary edema or cardiac insufficiency.

In recent years indications have changed and differ from nonpregnant patients. With a better understanding of the pathophysiology of preeclampsia, diuretics are no longer used to treat hypertension, edema and, especially, preeclampsia. Diuretics can reduce the plasma volume resulting in decreased placental perfusion that further compromises fetal support.

▶ **Thiazide diuretics**

This group belongs to *hydrochlorothiazide*, available as a monopreparation, and its analogs *chlortalidone* and *xipamide*.

Mefruside, bendroflumethiazide and *clopamide* are only present in combination preparations. *Indapamide* and *bemetizide* are sulfonamide derivatives that are pharmacologically related to thiazides.

The effectiveness of these drugs is based on the inhibition of the resorption of sodium and chloride in the distal tubules. At the beginning of therapy this leads to a decrease in plasma volume, loss of potassium, and inhibition of the excretion of uric acid.

Benzothiazides are well resorbed in the intestinal tract and excreted unchanged in urine. They cross the placenta. If administered during labor, the neonate may encounter electrolyte changes (hyponatremia, hypokalemia), thrombocytopenia, and a reactive hypoglycemia (due to a diabetogenic effect on the mother). Further, delay in labor has been described because of an inhibitory effect upon the smooth musculature.

Experiences with more than 5,000 pregnant women treated during the second and/or third trimester does not reveal fetotoxic effects (Collins 1985). Yet with a lack of efficacy and a better understanding of the pathophysiology, use of thiazide diuretics has become obsolete.

Hydrochlorothiazide is the best-examined drug of the group. A study of 567 women treated during the first trimester did not show an increase in specific anomalies or a higher rate of malformations in general (review by Briggs 2011).

Similarly, a study of 46 newborns that had been exposed to indapamide during the first trimester demonstrated no suspicious pattern for frequency and type of malformations (review by Briggs 2011).

Danish and Scottish birth registries contain 315 and 73 pregnancies, respectively, with exposure to diuretics (Olesen 2001), 263 of these involving thiazides. Thirty-five women who had been treated during the first trimester had offspring with malformations. The birth weight was described to be significantly lower when diuretics were used, and earlier deliveries were more common. The study, however, has some methodological flaws.

▶ **Loop diuretics**

Furosemide, bumetanide, piretanide, and *torasemide* belong to the loop diuretics and are natriuretic.

Furosemide given orally is well resorbed and excreted almost unchanged with urine and feces. Its effect decreases after 2–4 hours. In the mother, furosemide can decrease the intrauterine volume and diminish uteroplacental perfusion, compromising fetal support. This, however, was not evident in 10 intrauterine exposed children (Sibai 1984). In the fetus, it may lead briefly to a stimulation of urine production. In 21 pregnant women who received 20 mg furosemide daily after the first trimester the volume of cardiac output decreased while peripheral resistance increased to compensate. Blood pressure and pulse frequency remained stable (Carr 2007). As it is mediated by prostaglandin E2, it is debatable whether it could inhibit the physiologic occlusion of the *ductus arteriosus* in the premature offspring and thus lead to respiratory distress. The frequency of congenital malformations was slightly increased (5.1%) in 350 newborns who had been exposed during the first trimester; a specific pattern was not discernible (Briggs 2011). An ototoxic effect has been described, especially in combination with aminoglycosides (e.g. Brown 1991).

When *bumetanide* was used in the first trimester in a group of 44 pregnant patients, two children were born with cardiac malformations (cited by Briggs 2011). No relevant experiences are available at a sufficient extent for the loop diuretics *piretanide* and *torasemide*. A specific teratogenic effect has not been recognized in any of the named medications.

Danish and Scottish birth registries contain 315 and 73 pregnancies, respectively, with exposure to diuretics (Olesen 2001), 83 and 31, respectively, involving loop diuretics. Malformations were noted in five of 43 pregnant women treated during the first trimester. The birth weight was higher by 105 g in the Danish subgroup. This finding could also be explained by a greater prevalence of diabetes (10.3%). Early delivery was more common. The study, however, has some methodological flaws.

▶ **Aldosterone antagonists**

Spironolactone and its metabolite *potassium canrenoate*, available for IV injection, are the prime representatives of the aldosterone antagonists. Their effectiveness is based on the inhibition of receptors for aldosterone and other mineralocorticoids at the tubular cells. Gynecomastia may develop in treated men.

In contrast to the diuretics discussed above, spironolactone retains potassium. Thus hyperkalemia is a typical side effect. In animal experiments carcinogenic properties have been observed, but no evidence has indicated that these observations are clinically relevant. No specific malformations were noted in 31 newborns exposed during the first trimester (Briggs 2011). A case report describes a woman who used spironolactone in two pregnancies and delivered three healthy children (1 boy, 2 girls). The children developed normally also in view of antiandrogenic side effects, the oldest child having been followed up to age 13 (Groves 1995).

Eplerenone, another aldosterone antagonist, is applied as a co-medication to reduce the risk of cardiovascular morbidity and mortality in patients with left ventricular dysfunction and clinical signs of heart failure after a recent heart attack. One case report describes the birth of a healthy girl after continuous maternal treatment of a Gitelman syndrome with eplerenone (Morton 2011). In a case of primary aldosteronism during pregnancy, treatment with eplerenone in the latter half of pregnancy did not identify signs of feminization in the male fetus exposed (Cabassi 2012).

► **Amiloride and triamterene**

Amiloride and the weak folic acid antagonist *triamterene* belong to the potassium-sparing diuretics whose effectiveness is due to their influence on the tubular transport. In contrast to spironolactone, they are not aldosterone antagonists.

In a report on newborns exposed during the first trimester to *triamterene* in 318 cases and to amiloride in 28 cases, an accumulation of specific malformations was not noted (cited by Briggs 2011). Additional single reports about amiloride show normal newborns when mothers had been treated for Bartter syndrome, Gitelman syndrome, and Conn syndrome (Mascetti 2011, Al-Ali 2007, Deruelle 2004, Almeida 1989).

A specific teratogenic effect of amiloride or triamterene has not been noted.

> **Recommendation.** Diuretics are not part of the standard treatment for gestational hypertension and edema. Their application is limited to special indications. Hydrochlorothiazide is the drug of choice. Furosemide, too, may be used to manage heart or kidney failure. For longer treatments it is necessary to monitor electrolytes and hematocrit levels and to exclude the development of oligohydramnios. When treatment continues until birth, the newborn needs to be observed for possible hypoglycemia. Other diuretics should be avoided, if possible, or are applicable in unusual indications. None of the medications justify a risk-based termination or invasive diagnostic interventions (Chapter 1.15).

References

Al-Ali NA, El-Sandabesee D, Steel SA et al. Conn's syndrome in pregnancy successfully treated with amiloride. J Obstet Gynaecol 2007; 27: 730–1.

Almeida OJ, Spinnato JA. Maternal Bartter's syndrome and pregnancy. Am J Obstet Gynecol 1989; 160: 1225–6.

Alwan S, Polifka JE, Friedman JM. Angiotensin II receptor antagonist treatment during pregnancy. Birth Defects Res Part A 2005; 73: 123–30.

Aselton PA, Jick H, Milunsky A et al. First-trimester drug use and congenital disorders. Obstet Gynecol 1985; 65: 451–5.

Avdalovic M, Sandrock C, Hoso A et al. Epoprostenol in pregnant patients with secondary pulmonary hypertension Treat Respir Med 2004; 3: 29–34.

Babic Z, Gabric ID, Pintaric H. Successful primary percutaneous coronary intervention in the first trimester of pregnancy. Catheter Cardiovasc Interv 2011; 77: 522–5.

Badalian SS, Silverman RK, Aubry RH et al. Twin pregnancy in a woman on long-term epoprostenol therapy for primary pulmonary hypertension. J Reprod Med 2000; 45: 149–52.

Bakkum JN, Brost BC, Johansen KL et al. In utero losartan withdrawal and subsequent development of fetal inferior vena cava thrombosis. Obstet Gynecol 2006; 108: 739–40.

Bar J, Hod M, Merlob P. Angiotensin-converting enzyme inhibitors use in the first trimester of pregnancy. Int J Risk Safety Med 1997; 10: 23–6.

Bartalena L, Bogazzi F, Braverman LE et al. Effects of amiodarone administration during pregnancy on neonatal thyroid function and subsequent neurodevelopment. J Endocrinol Invest 2001; 24: 116–30.

Pregnancy

2.8 Heart and blood medications

Battenfeld R, Schuh W, Schöbel C. Studies on reproductive toxicity of iloprostin rats, rabbits and monkeys. Toxicol Lett 1995; 78: 223–34.

Bayliss H, Churchill D, Beevers M et al. Anti-hypertensive drugs in pregnancy and fetal growth: evidence for "pharmacological programming" in the first trimester? Hypertens Pregnancy 2002; 21: 161–74.

Bendayan D, Hod M, Oron G et al. Pregnancy outcome in patients with pulmonary arterial hypertension receiving prostacyclin therapy. Obstet Gynecol 2005; 106: 1206–10.

Berkane N, Carlier P, Verstraete L et al. Fetal toxicity of valsartan and possible reversible adverse side effects. Birth Defects Res A 2004; 70: 547–9.

Bildirici I, Shumway JB. Intravenous and inhaled epoprostenol for primary pulmonary hypertension during pregnancy and delivery. Obstet Gynecol 2004; 103: 1102–5.

Bombelli F, Lagona F, Salvati A et al. Radiofrequency catheter ablation in drug refractory maternal supraventricular tachycardias in advanced pregnancy. Obstet Gynecol 2003; 102: 1171–3.

Bortolus R, Ricci E, Chatenoud L et al. Nifedipine administered in pregnancy: effect on the development of children at 18 months. BJOG 2000; 107: 792–4.

Bos-Thompson MA, Hillaire-Buys D, Muller F et al. Fetal toxic effects of angiotensin II receptor antagonists: case report and follow-up after birth. Ann Pharmacother 2005; 39: 157–61.

Boutroy MJ, Gisonna CR, Legagneur M. Clonidine: placental transfer and neonatal adaption. Early Hum Dev 1988; 17: 275–86.

Bowen ME, Ray WA, Arbogast PG et al. Increasing exposure to angiotensin-converting enzyme inhibitors in pregnancy. Am J Obstet Gynecol 2008; 198: 291.e1–5.

Briggs GG, Freeman RK, Yaffe SJ. Drugs in Pregnancy and Lactation, 9th edn, Baltimore: Williams & Wilkins 2011.

Brown DR, Watchko JF, Sabo D. Neonatal sensorineural hearing loss associated with furosemide: a case-control study. Dev Med Child Neurol 1991; 33: 816–23.

Bullo M, Tschumi S, Bucher B et al. Pregnancy outcome following exposure to angiotensin-converting enzyme inhibitors or angiotensin receptor antagonists: a systematic review. Hypertension 2012; 60: 444–50.

Buchanan ML, Easterling TR, Carr DB et al. Clonidine pharmacokinetics in pregnancy. Drug Metab Dispos 2009; 37: 702–5.

Burrows RF, Burrows EA. Assessing the teratogenic potential of angiotensin-converting enzyme inhibitors in pregnancy. Aust NZ J Obstet Gynaecol 1998; 38: 306–11.

Cabassi A, Rocco R, Berretta R et al. Eplerenone use in primary aldosteronism during pregnancy. Hypertension 2012; 59: e18–9.

Carr DB, Gavrila D, Brateng D et al. Maternal hemodynamic changes associated with furosemide treatment. Hypertens Pregnancy 2007; 26: 173–8.

Chan WS, Korenm G, Barrera M et al. Neurocognitive development of children following in-utero exposure to labetalol for maternal hypertension: a cohort study using a prospectively collected database. Hypertens Pregnancy 2010; 29: 271–83.

Collins R, Yusuf S, Peto R. Overview of randomised trials of diuretics in pregnancy. BMJ (Clin Res Ed) 1985; 290: 17–23.

Cooper WO, Hernandez-Diaz S, Arbogast PG et al. Major congenital malformations after first-trimester exposure to ACE inhibitors. N Engl J Med 2006; 354: 2443–51.

Cuneo BF Treatment of fetal tachycardia. Heart Rhythm 2008; 5: 1216–8.

Cuneo BF, Ovadia M, Strasburger JF et al. Prenatal diagnosis and in utero treatment of torsades de pointes associated with congenital long QT syndrome. Am J Cardiol 2003; 91: 1395–8.

Czeizel A. Reserpine is not a human teratogen. J Med Genet 1988; 25: 787.

De Moura R, Lopes MA. Effects of captopril on the human foetal placental circulation: an interaction with bradykinin and angiotensin I. Br J Clin Pharmacol 1995; 39: 497–501.

Deruelle P, Dufour P, Magnenant E et al. Maternal Bartter's syndrome in pregnancy treated by amiloride. Eur J Obstet Gynecol Reprod Biol 2004; 115: 106–7.

De Swiet M. Maternal blood pressure and birthweight. Lancet 2000; 355: 81–2.

Diav-Citrin O, Shechtman S, Halberstadt Y et al. Pregnancy outcome after in-utero exposure to angiotensin converting enzyme inhibitors or angiotensin receptor blockers. Reprod Toxicol 2011; 31: 540–5.

Dodd JM, McLeod A, Windrim RC et al. Antithrombotic therapy for improving maternal or infant health outcomes in women considered at risk of placental dysfunction. Cochrane Database Syst Rev 2010; 6: CD006780.

Doherty G, Bali S, Casey F. Fetal hydrops due to supraventricular tachycardia-successful outcome in a difficult case. Ir Med J 2003; 96: 52–3.

Downing J. Sildenafil for the treatment of preeclampsia. Hypertens Pregnancy 2010; 29: 248–50; author reply, 251–2.

Duley L, Henderson-Smart DJ, Meher S. Drugs for treatment of very high blood pressure during pregnancy. Cochrane Database Syst Rev 2006; 3: CD001449.

Eifinger F, Sreeram N, Mehler K et al. Aerosolized iloprost in the treatment of pulmonary hypertension in extremely preterm infants: a pilot study. Klin Pädiatr 2008; 220: 66–9.

Elliot CA, Stewart P, Webster VJ et al. The use of iloprost in early pregnancy in patients with pulmonary arterial hypertension. Eur Respir J 2005; 26: 168–73.

Eronen M, Heikkila P, Teramo K. Congenital complete heart block in the fetus: hemodynamic features, antenatal treatment, and outcome in six cases. Pediatr Cardiol 2001; 22: 385–92.

Feldkamp M, Jones KL, Ornoy A. From the Centers for Disease Control and Prevention: Postmarketing surveillance for angiotensin-converting enzyme inhibitor use during the first trimester of pregnancy – United States, Canada, and Israel, 1987–1995. JAMA 1997; 277: 1193–4.

Fidler J, Smith V, Fayers P et al. Randomized controlled comparative study of methyldopa and oxprenolol in treatment of hypertension in pregnancy. BMJ (Clin Res) 1983; 18: 1927–30.

Filler G, Wong H, Condello AS et al. Early dialysis in a neonate with intrauterine lisinopril exposure. Arch Dis Child Fetal Neonatal Ed 2003; 88: F154–6.

Friedman DM, Llanos C, Izmirly PM et al. Evaluation of fetuses in a study of intravenous immunoglobulin as preventive therapy for congenital heart block: Results of a multi-center, prospective, open-label clinical trial. Arthritis Rheum 2010; 62: 1138–46.

Garabedian MJ, Hansen WF, Gianferrari EA et al. Epoprostenol treatment for idiopathic pulmonary arterial hypertension in pregnancy. J Perinatol 2010; 30: 628–31.

Geohas C, McLaughlin VV. Successful management of pregnancy in a patient with Eisenmenger syndrome with epoprostenol. Chest 2003; 124: 1170–3.

Gersak K, Cvijic M, Cerar LK. Angiotensin II receptor blockers in pregnancy: a report of five cases. Reprod Toxicol 2009; 28: 109–12.

Gill A, Madsen G, Knox M et al. Neonatal neurodevelopmental outcomes following tocolysis with glycerol trinitrate patches. Am J Obstet Gynecol 2006; 195: 484–7.

Goland S, Tsai F, Habib M et al. Favorable outcome of pregnancy with an elective use of epoprostenol and sildenafil in women with severe pulmonary hypertension. Cardiology 2010; 15: 205–8.

Grosso S, Berardi R, Cioni M et al. Transient neonatal hypothyreoidism after gestational exposure to amiodarone: a follow-up of two cases. J Endocrinol Invest 1998; 21: 699–702.

Groves TD, Corenblum B. Spironolactone therapy during human pregnancy. Am J Obstet Gynecol 1995; 172: 1655–6.

Günenç O, Çiçek N, Gorkemli H et al. The effect of methyldopa treatment on uterine, umbilical and fetal middle cerebral artery blood flows in preeclamptic patients. Arch Gynecol Obstet 2002; 266: 141–4.

Guron G, Mölne J, Swerkersson S et al. A 14-year-old girl with renal abnormalities after brief intrauterine exposure to enalapril during late gestation. Nephrol Dial Transplant 2006; 21: 522–5.

Hasdemir C, Musayev O, Alkan MB et al. Termination of idiopathic sustained monomorphic ventricular tachycardia by intravenous adenosine in a pregnant woman. Europace 2009; 11: 1560–1.

Hata T, Manabe A, Hata K et al. Changes in blood velocities of fetal circulation in association with fetal heart rate abnormalities: effect of sublingual administration of nifedipine. Am J Perinat 1995; 12: 80–1.

Hatanaka AR, Moron AF, Auxiliadora de Aquino MM et al. Interruption of a study of cervical ripening with isosorbide mononitrate due to adverse effects. Clin Exp Obstet Gynecol 2012; 39: 175–80.

Hennessy A, Thornton CE, Makris A et al. A randomised comparison of hydralazine and mini-bolus diazoxide for hypertensive emergencies in pregnancy: the PIVOT trial. Aust N Z J Obstet Gynaecol 2007; 47: 279–85.

Hod M, Friedman S, Schoenfeld A et al. Hydralazine-induced hepatitis in pregnancy. Int J Fertil 1986; 31: 352–5.

Pregnancy

2.8 Heart and blood medications

Horvath JS, Phippard A, Korda A. Clonidine hydrochloride, a safe and effective antihypertensive agent in pregnancy. Obstet Gynecol 1985; 66: 634–8.

Houlihan DD, Dennedy MC, Ravikumar N et al. Anti-hypertensive therapy and the fetoplacental circulation: effects on umbilical artery resistance. J Perinat Med 2004; 32: 315–9.

Hubinont C, Debauche C, Bernard P et al. Resolution of fetal tachycardia and hydrops by a single adenosine administration. Obstet Gynecol 1998; 92: 718.

Huisjes HJ, Hadders-Algra M, Touwen BCL. Is clonidine a behavioural teratogen in the human? Early Hum Dev 1986; 41: 43–8.

Hünseler C, Paneitz A, Friedrich D et al. Angiotensin II receptor blocker induced fetopathy: 7 cases. Klin Pädiatr 2011; 223: 10–4.

Hutter D, Silverman ED, Jaeggi ET. The benefits of transplacental treatment of isolated congenital complete heart block associated with maternal anti-Ro/SSA antibodies: a review. Scand J Immunol 2010; 72: 235–41.

Jerzak M, Kniotek M, Mrozek J et al. Sildenafil citrate decreased natural killer cell activity and enhanced chance of successful pregnancy in women with a history of recurrent miscarriage. Fertil Steril 2008; 90: 1848–53.

Jerzak M, Niemiec T, Nowakowska A et al. First successful pregnancy after addition of enoxaparin to sildenafil and etanercept immunotherapy in woman with fifteen failed IVF cycles – case report. Am J Reprod Immunol 2010; 64: 93–6.

Joglar JA, Page RL. Treatment of cardiac arrhythmias during pregnancy. Drug Safe 1999; 20: 85–94.

Karthikeyan VJ, Ferner RE, Baghdadi S et al. Are angiotensin-converting enzyme inhibitors and angiotensin receptor blockers safe in pregnancy: a report of ninety-one pregnancies. J Hypertens 2011; 29: 396–9.

Koren G. Systematic review of the effects of maternal hypertension in pregnancy and antihypertensive therapies on child neurocognitive development. Reprod Toxicol 2013; 39: 1–5.

Kiely DG, Condliffe R, Webster V et al. Improved survival in pregnancy and pulmonary hypertension using a multiprofessional approach. BJOG 2010; 117: 565–74.

Krapp M, Baschat AA, Gembruch U et al. Flecainide in the intrauterine treatment of fetal supraventricular tachycardia. Ultrasound Obstet Gynecol 2002; 19: 158–64.

Lacassie HJ, Germain AM, Valdés G et al. Management of Eisenmenger syndrome in pregnancy with sildenafil and L-arginine. Obstet Gynecol 2004; 103: 1118–20.

Laube GF, Kemper MJ, Schubiger G et al. Angiotensin-converting enzyme inhibitor fetopathy: long-term outcome. Arch Dis Child Fetal Neonatal Ed 2007; 92: F402–3.

Lavoratti G, Seracini D, Fiorini P et al. Neonatal anuria by ACE inhibitors during pregnancy. Nephron 1997; 76: 235–6.

Lennestål R, Otterblad Olausson P, Källén B. Maternal use of antihypertensive drugs in early pregnancy and delivery outcome, notably the presence of congenital heart defects in the infants. Eur J Clin Pharmacol 2009; 65: 615–25.

Lin CH, Lee CN. Atrial fibrillation with rapid ventricular response in pregnancy. Taiwan J Obstet Gynecol 2008; 47: 327–9.

Lomenick JP, Jackson WA, Backeljauw PF. Amiodarone-induced neonatal hypothyreoidism: a unique form of transient early-onset hypothyreoidism. J Perinatol 2004; 24: 397–9.

Lopes LM, Tavares GM, Damiano AP et al. Perinatal outcome of fetal atrioventricular block: one-hundred-sixteen cases from a single institution. Circulation 2008; 118: 1268–75.

Luk A, Ma RC, Lam CW et al. A 21-year-old pregnant woman with hypertension and proteinuria. PLoS Med 2009; 6: e1000037.

Ma L, Liu W, Huang Y. Perioperative management for parturients with pulmonary hypertension: experience with 30 consecutive cases. Front Med 2012; 6: 307–10.

Ma L, Liu W, Huang Y. Perioperative management for parturients with pulmonary hypertension: experience with 30 consecutive cases. Erratum in Front Med 2013; 7: 395.

Maeno Y, Hirose A, Kanbe T et al. Fetal arrhythmia: prenatal diagnosis and perinatal management. J Obstet Gynaecol Res 2009; 35: 623–9.

Magee LA, Abalos E, von Dadelszen P et al. CHIPS Study Group. How to manage hypertension in pregnancy effectively. Br J Clin Pharmacol 2011; 72: 394–401.

Magee LA, Cham C, Waterman EJ et al. Hydralazine for treatment of severe hypertension in pregnancy: meta-analysis. BMJ 2003; 327: 955–60.

Magee LA, Nulman I, Rovet JF et al. Neurodevelopment after in utero amiodarone exposure. Neurotoxicol Teratol 1999; 21: 261–5.

Magee LA, Schick B, Donnenfeld AE et al. The safety of calcium channel blockers in human pregnancy: a prospective, multicenter cohort study. Am J Obstet Gynecol 1996; 174: 823–8.

Magee LA, von Dadelszen P, Chan S et al. CHIPS Pilot Trial Collaborative Group. CHIPS Pilot Trial Collaborative Group: The Control of Hypertension in Pregnancy Study pilot trial. BJOG 2007; 114: 770, e13–20.

Malm H, Artama M, Gissler M et al. First trimester use of ACE-inhibitors and risk of major malformations. Reprod Toxicol 2008; 26: 67.

Manzur-Verástegui S, Mandeville PB, Gordillo-Moscoso A et al. Efficacy of nitroglycerine infusion versus sublingual nifedipine in severe pre-eclampsia: a randomized, triple-blind, controlled trial. Clin Exp Pharmacol Physiol 2008; 35: 580–5.

Mascetti L, Bettinelli A, Simonetti GD et al. Pregnancy in inherited hypokalemic salt-losing renal tubular disorder. Obstet Gynecol 2011; 117: 512–6.

Mikovic Z, Karadzov N, Jovanovic I et al. Developmental delay associated with normal thyroidal function and long-term amiodarone therapy during fetal and neonatal life. Biomed Pharmacother 2010; 64: 396–8.

Milner RDG, Chouksey SK. Effects of fetal exposure to diazoxide in man. Arch Dis Child 1972; 47: 537–43.

Moar CA, Jeffries MA. Neonatal head circumference and the treatment of maternal hypertension. Br J Obstet Gynaecol 1978; 85: 933–7.

Molelekwa V, Akhter P, McKenna P et al. Eisenmenger's syndrome in a 27 week pregnancy-management with bosentan and sildenafil. Ir Med J 2005; 98: 87–8.

Moodley J, Gouws E. A comparative study of the use of epoprostenol and dihydralazine in severe hypertension in pregnancy. Br J Obstet Gynaecol 1992; 99: 727–30.

Morton A, Panitz B, Bush A. Eplerenone for Gitelman syndrome in pregnancy. Nephrology (Carlton) 2011; 16: 349.

Muller PR, James A. Pregnancy with prolonged fetal exposure to an angiotensin-converting enzyme inhibitor. J Perinatol 2002; 22: 582–4.

Munk PS, von Brandis P, Larsen AI. Reversible fetal renal failure after maternal treatment with Candesartan: a case report. Reprod Toxicol 2010; 29: 381–2.

Murki S, Kumar P, Dutta S et al. Fatal neonatal renal failure due to maternal enalapril ingestion. J Matern Fetal Neonatal Med 2005; 17: 235–7.

Nakhai-Pour HR, Rey E, Bérard A. Antihypertensive medication use during pregnancy and the risk of major congenital malformations or small-for-gestational-age newborns. Birth Defects Res B Dev Reprod Toxicol 2010; 89: 147–54.

Ng WP, Yip WL. Successful maternal fetal outcome using nitric oxide and sildenafil in pulmonary hypertension with atrial septaldefect and HIV infection. Singapore Med J 2012; 53: e3–5.

Nunes FP, Campos AP, Pedroso SR et al. Intravaginal glyceryl trinitrate and dinoprostone for cervical ripening and induction of labor. Am J Obstet Gynecol 2006; 194: 1022–6.

Oakley C, Child A, Jung B. Expert consensus document on management of cardiovascular diseases during pregnancy. Eur Heart J 2003; 24: 761–81.

Orbach H, Matok I, Gorodischer R et al. Hypertension and antihypertensive drugs in pregnancy. AJOG 2013; 208: 301, e1–6.

Olesen C, de Vries CS, Thrane N et al. EuroMAP Group. Effect of diuretics on fetal growth: a drug effect or confounding by indication? Pooled Danish and Scottish cohort data. Br J Clin Pharmacol 2001; 51: 153–7.

Oppermann M, Padberg S, Schaefer C. Angiotensin II-receptor 1-antagonists during 2nd or 3rd trimester: Evaluation of a case series from the Berlin Institute for Clinical Teratology and Drug Risk Assessment in Pregnancy {Abstract}. Reprod Toxicol 2011; 31: 264.

Oudijk MA, Ruskamp JM, Ambachtsheer BE, et al. Drug treatment of fetal tachycardias. Pediatr Drugs 2002; 4: 49–63.

Oudijk MA, Ruskamp JM, Ververs TF et al. Treatment of fetal tachycardia with sotalol: transplacental pharmacokinetics and pharmacodynamics. J Am Coll Cardiol 2003; 42: 765–70.

Pasker-de Jong PC, Zielhuis GA, van Gelder MM et al. Antihypertensive treatment during pregnancy and functional development at primary school age in a historical cohort study. BJOG 2010; 117: 1080–6.

Pézard PG, Boussion F, Sentilhes L et al. Fetal tachycardia: a role for amiodarone as first- or second-line therapy? Arch Cardiovasc Dis 2008; 101: 619–27.

Porta M, Hainer JW, Jansson SO et al. On behalf DIRECT Study Group. Exposure to candesartan during the first trimester of pregnancy in type 1 diabetes: experience from the placebo-controlled diabetic retinopathy candesartan trials. Diabetologia 2011; 54: 1298–303.

Rasheed A, Simpson J, Rosenthal E. Neonatal ECG changes caused by supratherapeutic flecainide following treatment for fetal supraventricular tachycardia. Heart 2003; 89: 70.

Pregnancy

2.8 Heart and blood medications

Rein AJ, Mevorach D, Perles Z et al. Early diagnosis and treatment of atrioventricular block in the fetus exposed to maternal anti-SSA/Ro-SSB/La antibodies: a prospective, observational, fetal kinetocardiogram-based study. Circulation 2009; 119: 1867–72.

Reynolds B, Butters L, Evans J et al. First year of life after the use of atenolol in pregnancy associated hypertension. Arch Dis Child 1984; 59: 1061–3.

Rothberger S, Carr D, Brateng D et al. Pharmacodynamics of clonidine therapy in pregnancy: a heterogeneous maternal response impacts fetal growth. Am J Hypertens 2010; 23: 1234–40.

Saleeb S, Copel J, Friedman D. Comparison of treatment with fluorinated glucocorticoids to the natural history of autoantibody-associated congenital heart block: retrospective review of the research registry for neonatal lupus. Arthritis Rheum 1999; 42: 2335–45.

Samangaya RA, Mires G, Shennan A. A randomised, double-blinded, placebo-controlled study of the phosphodiesterase type 5 inhibitor sildenafil for the treatment of preeclampsia. Hypertens Pregnancy 2009; 28: 369–82.

Sass N, Itamoto CH, Silva MP et al. Does sodium nitroprusside kill babies? A systematic review. Sao Paulo Med J 2007; 125: 108–11.

Satgé D, Sasco AJ, Col JY et al. Antenatal exposure to atenolol and retroperitoneal fibromatosis. Reprod Toxicol 1997; 11: 539–41.

Schaefer C. Angiotensin II-receptor-antagonists: further evidence of fetotoxicity but not teratogenicity. Birth Defects Res A 2003; 67: 591–4.

Schulz M, Wacker J, Bastert G. Auswirkungen von Urapidil in der antihypertensiven Therapie bei Präeklampsie auf die Neugeborenen. Zentralbl Gynäkol 2001; 123: 529–33.

Segal ES, Valette C, Oster L et al. Risk management strategies in the postmarketing period: safety experience with the US and European bosentan surveillance programmes. Drug Saf 2005; 28: 971–80.

Senat MV, Fischer C, Bernard JP et al. The use of lidocaine for fetocide in late termination of pregnancy. BJOG 2003; 110: 296–300.

Serreau R, Luton D, Macher MA et al. Developmental toxicity of the angiotensin II type 1 receptor antagonists during human pregnancy: a report of 10 cases. BJOG 2005; 112: 710–2.

Shekhar S, Sharma C, Thakur S et al. Oral nifedipine or intravenous labetalol for hypertensive emergency in pregnancy: a randomized controlled trial. Obstet Gynecol 2013; 122: 1057–63.

Sibai BM, Grossman RA, Grossman HG. Effects of diuretics on plasma volume in pregnancies with long-term hypertension. Am J Obstet Gynecol 1984; 150: 831–5.

Slim R, Ben Salem C, Hmouda H et al. Hepatotoxicity of alpha-methyldopa in pregnancy. J Clin Pharm Ther 2010; 35: 361–3.

Smith GN, Guo Y, Wen SW et al. Canadian Preterm Labor Nitroglycerin Trial Group. Canadian Preterm Labor Nitroglycerin Trial Group: Secondary analysis of the use of transdermal nitroglycerin for preterm labor. Am J Obstet Gynecol 2010; 203: 565.e1–6.

Smith GN, Piercy WN. Methyldopa hepatotoxicity in pregnancy: a case report. Am J Obstet Gynecol 1995; 172: 222–4.

Smith GN, Walker MC, Ohlsson A et al. Canadian Preterm Labour Nitroglycerin Trial Group: Randomized double-blind placebo-controlled trial of transdermal nitroglycerin for preterm labor. Am J Obstet Gynecol 2007; 196: 37.

Sørensen HT, Czeizel AE, Rockenbauer M et al. The risk of limb deficiencies and other congenital abnormalities in children exposed in utero to calcium channel blockers. Acta Obstet Gynecol Scand 2001; 80: 397–401.

Sørensen HT, Steffensen FH, Olesen C et al. Pregnancy outcome in women exposed to calcium channel blockers:. Reprod Toxicol 1998; 12: 383–4.

Spaggiari E, Heidet L, Grange G et al. Renin-Angiotensin System Blockers Study Group, Muller F: Prognosis and outcome of pregnancies exposed to renin-angiotensin system blockers. Prenat Diagn 2012; 32: 1071–6.

Stewart R, Tuazon D, Olson G et al. Pregnancy and primary pulmonary hypertension. Chest 2001; 119: 973–5.

Strasburger JF, Cuneo BF, Michon MM et al. Amiodarone therapy for drug-refractory fetal tachycardia. Circulation 2004; 109: 375–9.

Streit M, Speich R, Fischler M. Successful pregnancy in pulmonary arterial hypertension associated with systemic lupus erythematosus: a case report. J Med Case Reports 2009; 3: 7255.

Tabacova SA, Kimmel CA, McCloskey CA. Developmental abnormalities reported to FDA in association with nifedipine treatment in pregnancy {Abstract}. Teratology 2002; 65: 368.

Tabacova SA, Kimmel CA, Wall K et al. Atenolol developmental toxicity: animal-to-human comparisons. Birth Defects Res A 2003a; 67: 181–92.

Tabacova SA, Little R, Tsong Y. Adverse pregnancy outcomes associated with maternal enalapril antihypertensive treatment. Pharmacoepidemiol Drug Saf 2003b; 12: 633–46.

Timofeev J, Ruiz G, Fries M et al. Intravenous epoprostenol for management of pulmonary arterial hypertension during pregnancy. AJP Rep 2013; 3: 71–4.

Uzun O, Babaoglu K, Sinha A et al. Rapid control of foetal supraventricular tachycardia with digoxin and flecainide combination treatment. Cardiol Young 2012; 22: 372–80.

Vanhaesebrouck S, Hanssens M, Allegaert K. Neonatal transient respiratory depression after maternal urapidil infusion for hypertension. Eur J Pediatr 2009; 168: 221–3.

Vesel S, Mazić U, Blejec T et al. First-degree heart block in the fetus of an anti-SSA/Ro-positive mother: reversal after a short course of dexamethasone treatment. Arthritis Rheum 2004; 50: 2223–6.

Vigil-de Gracia P, Lasso M, Ruiz E. Severe hypertension in pregnancy: hydralazine or labetalol. A randomized clinical trial. Eur J Obstet Gynecol Reprod Biol 2006; 128: 157–62.

Villanova C, Muriago M, Nava F. Arrhythmogenic right ventricular dysplasia: pregnancy under flecainide treatment. G Ital Cardiol 1998; 28: 691–3.

Von Dadelszen P, Dwinnell S, Magee LA et al. Research into Advanced Fetal Diagnosis and Therapy (RAFT) Group. Research into Advanced Fetal Diagnosis and Therapy (RAFT) Group: Sildenafil citrate therapy for severe early-onset intrauterine growth restriction. BJOG 2011; 118: 624–8.

Von Dadelszen P, Ornstein MP, Bull SB et al. Fall in mean arterial pressure and fetal growth restriction in pregnancy hypertension: a meta-analysis. Lancet 2000; 355: 87–92.

Wacker JR, Wagner BK, Briese V et al. Antihypertensive therapy in patients with pre-eclampsia: A prospective randomized multicentre study comparing dihydralazine with urapidil. Eur J Obstet Gynecol Reprod Biol 2006; 127: 160–5.

Walsh CA, Manias T, Patient C. Atrial fibrillation in pregnancy. Eur J Obstet Gynecol Reprod Biol 2008; 138: 119–20.

Weber-Schoendorfer C, Hannemann D, Meister R et al. The safety of calcium channel blockers during pregnancy: a prospective, multicenter, observational study. Reprod Toxicol 2008; 261: 24–30.

Weiss BM, Zemp L, Seifert B et al. Outcome of pulmonary vascular disease in pregnancy: a systematic overview from 1978 through 1996. J Am Coll Cardiol 1998; 31: 1650–7.

Whitelaw A. Maternal methyldopa treatment and neonatal blood pressure. BMJ 1981; 283: 471.

Xie RH, Guo Y, Krewski D et al. Trends in using β-blockers and methyldopa for hypertensive disorders during pregnancy in a Canadian population. Eur J Obstet Gynecol Reprod Biol 2013; 171: 281–5.

Yemini M, Shoham (Schwartz) Z, Dgani R et al. Lupus-like syndrome in a mother and newborn following administration of hydralazine: a case report. Eur J Obstet Gynaecol Reprod Biol 1989; 30: 193–7.

Pregnancy

2.8 Heart and blood medications

Anticoagulants, thrombocyte aggregation inhibitors, fibrinolytics and volume replacement agents

2.9

Janine E. Polifka and Juliane Habermann

2.9.1	Indications for anticoagulation	226
2.9.2	Heparins and danaparoid	227
2.9.3	Protamines	229
2.9.4	Thrombin-inhibitors	230
2.9.5	Factor Xa inhibitors	231
2.9.6	Inhibitors of thrombocyte aggregation	231
2.9.7	Vitamin K antagonists	233
2.9.8	Vitamin K	237
2.9.9	Fibrinolysis	238
2.9.10	Streptokinase	239
2.9.11	Antihemorrhagics	239
2.9.12	Other antihemorrhagics	240
2.9.13	Volume replacement substances and rheologics	241

During pregnancy, the risk for venous thromboembolism (VTE) is substantially increased. Antithrombotic therapy is indicated for the prevention and treatment of VTE, but such treatment is challenging because these medications have the potential to cause adverse effects in the developing fetus. The possibility of increased maternal bleeding is also an important consideration when these medications are used prior to surgical intervention or delivery. Low molecular weight heparins are the drugs of choice in the prevention and treatment of VTE during pregnancy because they have fewer side effects and cross the placenta poorly, if at all. The embryotoxicity of vitamin K antagonists, particularly that of *warfarin*, is well-known. Warfarin and other related coumarins have been found to produce a characteristic pattern of malformations, such as nasal hypoplasia, stippled epiphyses, and growth retardation in the children of women who took these drugs during pregnancy. The greatest period of susceptibility is between the 8th and 12th weeks postconception although, because of their long half-lives, discontinuation of treatment or substitution with heparin at 6 weeks post conception is recommended to avoid embryonic exposure. Also, usage during the second and third trimesters has been associated with growth restriction and behavioral dysfunction. Congenital anomalies have been reported among infants born to mothers who were treated with *dipyridamole* during pregnancy, but the rate of anomalies reported in these studies is small and the pattern of anomalies is inconsistent. No teratogenic effects have been reported in case studies of infants whose mothers had been treated during pregnancy with streptokinase, a plasminogen activator. At present, there is limited experience with the use of novel oral anticoagulants, such as *dabigatran*, *rivaroxaban*, and *apixaban* during pregnancy. Use of these and other related drugs that have insufficient teratology data should be considered on a case-by-case basis. The aim of this chapter is to provide the clinician with a review of the known teratogenic effects of currently used antithrombotic agents as well as recommendations for their appropriate use during pregnancy.

2.9.1   Indications for anticoagulation

During normal pregnancy, the concentrations of nearly all coagulation factors progressively rise in response to higher estrogen levels along with a decrease in the activity of coagulation inhibitors (e.g. antithrombin). These changes result in reduced fibrinolytic potential due to increased levels of plasminogen activator inhibitors (PAI) produced by the placenta and a hypercoagulable state of pregnancy that does not return to normal until approximately 8 weeks after delivery (Goland 2012). This increase in coagulation tendency appears to reflect a physiological need for effective coagulation during delivery after separation of the placenta. However, a consequence of these changes in hemostasis and fibrinolysis is an increased risk of VTE that is five times more frequent during pregnancy and occurs in 0.2% of cases (Nelson 2007, Dizon-Townson 2002).

Thrombophilia is a group of inherited or acquired coagulation disorders that is associated with an increased risk of thrombotic events such as VTE and pulmonary embolism. Commonly inherited thrombophilia include the Factor V Leiden mutation, the prothrombin G20210A gene mutation, methylenetetrahydrofolate reductase polymorphism, and deficiencies of antithrombin, protein C and protein S. Antiphospholipid syndrome belongs to the acquired thrombophilia (McNamee 2012). Growing evidence suggests that thrombophilia is associated with an increased risk of adverse pregnancy outcomes, such as early and late pregnancy loss, preeclampsia, placental abruption, and intrauterine growth restriction (IUGR) (Pierangeli 2011). However, the absolute risk of VTE and serious adverse pregnancy outcomes remains low. Universal agreement regarding the necessity and effectiveness of antithrombotic therapy during pregnancy has not been established to date because of the lack of reliable data (McNamee 2012). A prior thrombotic event or thrombophilia is not currently viewed by all clinicians as an indication for thromboprophylaxis during pregnancy (see Section 2.9.2). Most recommendations include the following indications:

- Thromboprophylaxis in patients with an established increased risk, including patients with malignancies, postoperative patients, long-term immobilization.
- Prevention and treatment of VTE.
- Prevention and treatment of systemic embolism in patients with valvular heart disease and/or mechanical heart valves.
- Prevention of pregnancy loss in women with antiphospholipid antibodies and previous pregnancy losses.

2.9.2   Heparins and danaparoid

▶ **Heparin**

Pharmacology

Heparin is a chain-linked, sulfated glycosaminoglycan, that is found naturally in the body and is produced by basophils and mast cells. Heparins prevent thrombus formation and limit thrombus extension by binding to lysine sites on antithrombin III and producing a conformational change that accelerates the rate at which antithrombin III neutralizes the hemostatic enzymes, thrombin (factor IIa) and factor Xa. Decreased levels of antithrombin III lead to resistance to heparin. When heparin is administered in low doses for prophylaxis, it is mainly factor Xa that is neutralized; in higher therapeutic doses, thrombin will also be neutralized. Heparins can initiate plasminogen activator release by endothelial cells, and this accounts for their fibrinolytic activity. *Unfractionated heparin* (UFH) has a molecular weight ranging from 5,000–30,000 daltons (Da). It inhibits factors IIa and Xa equally well. *Low molecular weight heparins* (LMWH) are fragments of the native heparin molecule with molecular weights that range between 1,000–10,000 Da. They have a different anticoagulant profile and are less able to catalyze the inhibition of thrombin relative to factor Xa due to their shorter chain lengths, which range between 5–17 monosaccharides.

Heparin is the strongest organic acid which exists in the body. The strong negative charge of heparin is important for the inhibition of coagulation. The formation of chemical salts with organic cations, such as *protamine* (Section 2.9.3), quickly overrides the actions of heparin.

UFH has a short half-life of 1–2 hours. Due to its strong negative charge and high molecular weight UFH is not absorbed in the gut. Consequently, heparin must be administered intravenously or subcutaneously. This is also true for LMWHs, such as *certoparin, dalteparin, enoxaparin, nadroparin, reviparin* and *tinzaparin*. LMWH are increasingly preferred to UFH for thromboprophylaxis as well as for the treatment of VTE and in the pregnant patient. Their advantage lies in a longer half-life requiring only one or two injections per day, better bioavailability (85%) and their association with a lower incidence of osteoporosis, allergy, and heparin-induced thrombocytopenia (HIT). Greer (2005) analyzed all studies published to the end of 2003 for the use of LMWH during pregnancy. They extracted data on VTE recurrence and adverse side effects from almost 2,800 pregnancies and found that LMWH were both safe and effective when used to treat VTE during pregnancy. Bleeding events and allergic skin reactions occurred in almost 2% and osteoporotic bone fractures in 0.04% of the cases. The authors did not find a single case of HIT. In addition, 95% of the pregnancies resulted in a live-born infant.

The long-term therapy with UFH has been associated with an increased risk of heparin-induced bone loss and osteoporotic fracture. Depending on the dose and duration of use, LMWH may have less influence on bone metabolism than UFH and therefore cause less bone loss, although not all studies have confirmed this effect (Lefkou 2010, Casele 2006). The decrease in bone loss observed in some of the studies may be related to maternal supplementation with calcium during treatment. More studies are needed before the true incidence of heparin-induced osteoporosis in pregnant women can be determined. Long-term anticoagulant therapy is associated with an increased risk of bleeding; however, the risk associated with the use of heparin is relatively low, around 2% (Greer 2005, Lepercq 2001, Lindqvist 2000, Sanson 1999).

Pregnancy

2.9 Anticoagulants, thrombocyte aggregation inhibitors, fibrinolytics and volume replacement agents

Prolonged anticoagulation therapy increases the risk for spinal hematoma formation, especially following neuraxial blockade (Butwick 2010). Guidelines for neuraxial blockade and thromboembolic prophylaxis have been established in a number of countries (Butwick 2010, Gogarten 2007). These guidelines specify the interval of time that the medications should be discontinued prior to puncture or removal of a catheter in order to avoid bleeding complications. Timing intervals vary among the different guidelines, but generally the interval of time that is recommended is two times the elimination half-life of the drug that is administered. Accordingly, prophylactic doses of UFH should be discontinued at least 4 hours prior to neuraxial blockade or catheter withdrawal and therapeutic doses of UFH should be discontinued at least 6 hours before blockade or catheter removal. Since LMWH have longer half-lives, prophylactic or therapeutic treatment with these drugs should be stopped 12 or 24 hours, respectively, before neuraxial blockade or catheter removal (Gogarten 2007). A study of 284 pregnant women who were treated with enoxaparin for an average of 251days found that the rate of hemorrhagic complications during delivery was not significantly increased when enoxaparin was discontinued at least 12 hours beforehand (Maslovitz 2005).

Toxicology

Placental transfer of UFH or LMWH is expected to be minimal due to their high molecular weight and negative charge (Dimitrakakis 2000, Schneider 1995, Mätzsch 1991). This has been confirmed by studies that have failed to find detectable levels of UFH or LMWH in samples from the umbilical cord vein after administration to pregnant women or in the fetal circulation following dual perfusion of an isolated placental lobule (Harenberg 1993, Bajoria 1992). The frequency of malformations or other adverse effects did not appear to be increased in more than 20 clinical studies of infants whose mothers were treated with either LMWH or UFH for various periods of time during pregnancy (Andersen 2010, Serrano 2009, Winger 2009, Badawy 2008, Fawzy 2008, Bauersachs 2007, Deruelle 2007, Kominiarek 2007, Voke 2007, James 2006, Rowan 2003, Bar 2000, Chan 2000, Sørensen 2000, Hanania 1994, Sbarouni 1994, Ginsberg 1989a, 1989b) On the other hand, major birth defects were reported in seven (11%) of 65 infants whose mothers had been given a prescription for heparin during the first trimester of pregnancy in a surveillance study of Michigan Medicaid recipients (Rosa, cited in Briggs 2011); the expected rate of birth defects was 5%. Four of the malformed infants had cardiovascular defects. The possible contribution of confounding factors in this study, such as maternal use of other drugs and underlying maternal disease, is not known. Congenital *aplasia cutis* has been reported in two infants whose mothers were given tinzaparin during pregnancy (Sharif 2005). Whether the association observed in these two case reports is causal or coincidental is unknown.

To date, heparin-induced alteration of the fetal coagulation system has been demonstrated in a sheep model (Andrew 1992), but not in humans; although subdural hemorrhages of prenatal onset were reported in one infant whose mother took dalteparin for deep vein thrombosis during pregnancy (Bauder 2009). It is feasible, then, that transplacental passage of LMWH may occur on rare occasions, as in pregnancies complicated by preterm delivery and placental abnormalities. In one study of 693 newborns whose mothers had received enoxaparin during pregnancy, there were 10 (1.4%) children with hemorrhages; none were thought to be treatment related (Lepercq 2001).

▶ **Danaparoid**

Danaparoid is a mixture of low-molecular-weight sulfated glycosami-noglycans. It is sometimes considered a LMWH, but is chemically distinct from heparin. Danaparoid is categorized in the class of heparinoids because it contains the structurally related *heparan sulfate* (84%), *dermatan sulfate* (12%) and a small amount of *chondroitin sulfate* (4%). Danaparoid catalyzes the inactivation of factor Xa via antithrombin and heparin-cofactor II. Its anti-factor Xa activity is considerably greater than its anti-thrombin activity. It is used for the prophylaxis and treatment of deep vein thrombosis in situations when heparin should not be used; for example, in patients with immune-mediated (type II) heparin-induced thrombocytopenia. Danaparoid shows a slight serological cross reactivity (5%) with heparin-induced antibodies with a frequency of clinical cross reactions of approximately 3%.

Examinations of human cord blood and experimental data in animals do not demonstrate a significant placental transfer of danaparoid (Greinacher 1993, Peeters 1986). No teratogenicity was observed among 87 pregnancies exposed to danaparoid (Ebina 2011, Magnani 2010, Gerhardt 2009, Myers 2003). Maternal treatment with danaparoid occurred in the first trimester of pregnancy in 61% of these pregnancies. To date, direct fetal toxicity has not been reported. The risk to the embryo or fetus associated with maternal use of danaparoid during pregnancy is unclear at this time.

> **Recommendation.** Heparins are by appropriate indication the method of choice for anticoagulation during pregnancy. In practice, the use of LMWH has by far replaced that of UFH which is reserved for special indications. In cases of heparin intolerance (allergic reactions, HIT II) or resistance it is appropriate to use danaparoid as an alternative anticoagulant. The potential for increased bleeding is an important consideration prior to surgical interventions and prior to delivery.

2.9.3   Protamines

Pharmacology and toxicology

Protamines are simple (alkaline) proteins found in the sperm of several species. Protamine-HCl and protamine sulfate are agents that are used intravenously to reverse the effects of heparin prior to surgical procedures or for the treatment of heparin overdose. They are basic polypeptides that neutralize the strongly negatively charged heparin by complexing with it to form a stable salt. Protamine-heparin complexes have no inhibitory effect on coagulation. The ability of protamines to neutralize heparin varies with heparin chain length. Short chain fragments cannot be neutralized with protamine, resulting in incomplete neutralization of anti-factor Xa activity. This explains why protamine has weaker effectiveness against LMWH than UFH. Protamines are also mixed with insulin formulations and administered subcutaneously to prolong the glucose-lowering activity of insulin. No data has been published regarding the embryo- or fetotoxic effects of protamine. However, in animal studies, protamines have been found to inhibit angiogenesis (Taylor 1982) and, therefore, may pose a risk to the developing embryo. There are two case reports of neonatal bradycardia, hypotension and hypotonicity after maternal administration of protamine prior to delivery (Boyle 2007, Wittmaack 1994). These effects are similar to side effects that have been reported in adults following administration of protamine.

> **Recommendation.** Protamines can be used acutely during pregnancy in cases of heparin overdose. However, continual/chronic use of protamines during pregnancy is not recommended because there are no data to support such usage.

2.9.4   Thrombin-inhibitors

Compounds such as *lepirudin and desirudin* are recombinant hirudin derivatives that directly inhibit free and fibrin-bound thrombin and block its activity. *Bivalirudin, argatroban,* and *dabigatran etexilate* are synthetic thrombin inhibitors. Hirudin and its derivatives are bivalent direct thrombin inhibitors that bind to both the active site and exosite 1. Bivalirudin binds reversibly to thrombin, so its inhibitory effect is transient resulting in a diminished risk of major bleeding. Argatroban and dabigatran etexilate are univalent direct thrombin inhibitors that bind only to the active site of thrombin (Di Nisio 2005). Dabigatran etexilate was the first new oral direct thrombin inhibitor to be approved for long-term anticoagulant treatment (Coppens 2012). Direct thrombin inhibitors are used in cases of heparin intolerability, such as heparin-induced thrombocytopenia. Bivalirudin is used in acute coronary syndrome together with *acetylsalicylic acid* (ASA) and *clopidogrel* in patients who undergo a percutaneous coronary intervention. Dabigatran etexilate is used for thromboprophylaxis in patients after hip replacement or knee replacement and prevention of strokes in atrial fibrillation. No information regarding the use of bivalirudin, desirudin, or dabigatran etexilate in pregnancy has been published.

Ten case reports describe healthy infants born to women who were treated with lepirudin or argatroban at different times during pregnancy (Tanimura 2012, Darki 2011, Ekbatani 2010, Chapman 2008, Taniguchi 2008, Young 2008, Furlan 2006, Harenberg 2005, Mehta 2004, Huhle 2000). Exposure during the first trimester occurred in four of the reported cases. Although one of the children was born with a patent foramen ovale and small ventricular septal defect, maternal treatment with argatroban is unlikely to have caused these defects since exposure did not occur until the third trimester (Young 2008).

> **Recommendation.** The above-mentioned medications should only be prescribed during pregnancy if they are urgently needed, i.e. with heparin intolerance (allergic skin reactions, HIT II) and in the absence of safer alternatives. Caution is required when using thrombin inhibitors prior to surgery or during the intrapartum period because of an increased risk of maternal hemorrhage.

2.9.5   Factor Xa inhibitors

A new class of anticoagulants inhibits thrombin generation by selectively inhibiting factor Xa, a trypsin-like serine protease that converts pro-thrombin to its active form, thrombin. The first product of this class of substances was the synthetically manufactured *fondaparinux*. In contrast to heparin, it is not a mixture of substances and is a chemically defined substance with a molecular mass of 1,728 Da. It consists of the minimal pentasaccharide sequence of heparin that selectively binds to antithrom-bin III, but does not bind and inactivate thrombin itself. Consequently, the risk for HIT II is much lower. It is administered parenterally in the treatment of venous thromboembolism, unstable angina and acute myocardial infarction. In an *in vitro* human dually perfused cotyledon model, there was no crossing of the placenta (Lagrange 2002). However, one study of four mother–child pairs found levels of fondaparinux in the umbilical cord blood following maternal treatment with fondaparinux that were 10% of those found in maternal plasma (Dempfle 2004). The clinical relevance of this slight transfer across the placenta is not known, and no adverse effects were observed in the infants. As many as 48 normal infants have been reported to be born to women who were treated with fondaparinux during pregnancy. Exposures to fondaparinux occurred in the first trimester of pregnancy in 26 (54%) of the infants (Nagler 2012, Hajj-Chahine 2010, Schapkaitz 2007). Several other direct factor Xa inhibitors have been developed for use in the prophylaxis of venous thromboembolism after elective hip or knee replacement or for the prevention of stroke in nonvalvular atrial fibrillation and secondary venous thromboembolism. These include *rivaroxaban, apixaban*, and *edoxaban*. In contrast to fondaparinux, these agents are administered orally. Currently there is no specific antidote to reverse the effects of the new oral anticoagulants. No data are available regarding the use of these substances during pregnancy.

> **Recommendation.** If urgently needed during pregnancy, e.g., with heparin incompatibility (allergic skin reactions, HIT II) or cross-reaction with danaparoid, it is acceptable to use fondaparinux for anticoagulation. Because no information is available on the use of rivaroxaban and apixaban during pregnancy, these medications should be administered in pregnancy only if conservative therapy is ineffective. If an exposure occurs inadvertently during the first trimester of pregnancy, ultrasound evaluation can be offered to confirm the normal development of the fetus. The potential for excessive bleeding when these medications are used has to be taken into account prior to surgical procedures and delivery.

2.9.6   Inhibitors of thrombocyte aggregation

Antiplatelet drugs inhibit thrombocyte aggregation and decrease thrombus formation. The thienopyridine adenosine diphosphate (ADP) receptor antagonists, such as *clopidogrel, ticlopidine*, and *prasugrel* are all prodrugs which require metabolic activation by the cytochrome P450 (CYP) enzyme system in order to exert their effects. These drugs selectively block the thrombolytic receptor P2Y12 on the platelet surface and prevent it from interacting with ADP. As a result, the binding of fibrinogen to its platelet receptor, the glycoprotein GP IIb/IIIa, is also prevented. ADP-receptor inhibition by these drugs is irreversible and lasts for the lifetime of the thrombocyte (approximately 7–10 days). Little data are available about the use of these drugs during pregnancy. Fourteen case reports describing the pregnancy outcomes of women who used clopidogrel during pregnancy have been published (Babic 2011, De Santis 2011, Duarte 2011, Myers 2011). In twelve (85%) of the 14 cases the infants were reported to be normal. Six of these normal infants were exposed to clopidogrel during the first trimester of pregnancy. A seventh infant whose mother was treated with clopidogrel from 6 weeks of pregnancy to delivery was born with patent foramen ovale, restrictive interventricular muscle communication and moderate mitral insufficiency (Santiago-Díaz 2009). In another case, fetal death occurred after maternal treatment with clopidogrel and coronary artery bypass graft surgery at 26 weeks of gestation (Shah 2004). Less clinical experience exists for ticlopidine. A normal infant was born to a woman who was treated with ticlopidine for 2 weeks prior to delivery (Sebastian 1998). Although no complications occurred at delivery, complete inhibition of platelet aggregation to ADP in the cord blood was observed. In another case report, a normal infant was born to a woman who was treated with ticlopidine throughout pregnancy and switched to heparin during the last 2 weeks (Ueno 2001). Similarly, no teratogenicity was observed in animal studies that utilized doses much higher than those used in humans (Watanabe 1980a, 1980b).

A case study reported increased bleeding tendency in a pregnant patient with coronary artery disease following mole resection on the forearm which was carried out one day prior to the planned delivery induction. Excessive bleeding occurred despite discontinuation of prophylactic therapy with clopidogrel and ASA seven days prior to the procedure, according to the recommendations. The author suggested that this case of heavy bleeding following a minor cosmetic intervention confirms the risk of serious bleeding complications, particularly spinal epidural hematomas, that can occur with the use of regional neuraxial anesthesia in patients managed with anticoagulant agents (Kuczkowski 2009). In another case in which clopidogrel was used during the entire pregnancy until 1 day prior to delivery there was hemorrhage after a caesarean section of the mother which necessitated a blood transfusion (Myers 2011).

Prasugrel is a third-generation thienopyridine that is more potent than clopidogrel. In animal experiments conducted by the manufacturer, prasugrel shows no evidence of teratogenicity at doses up to 40 times those typically used in humans. Only one case report on its use in human pregnancy is available in the literature. In this case, a normal infant was born to a woman who was treated with prasugrel throughout her entire pregnancy (Tello-Montoliu 2013). *Ticagrelor* is a cyclopentyltriazolopyrimidine that reversibly binds to the P2Y12 receptors. Ticagrelor is not a prodrug and, therefore, does not require metabolic activation in order to exert its effects. Ticagrelor has only been available on the market since January 2011, so there is no information about the use of this drug during pregnancy.

An additional strategy for inhibition of thrombocyte aggregation is the use of platelet glycoprotein (GP) IIb/IIIa antagonists, such as *abciximab*, *eptifibatide* and *tirofiban*. Binding to the GPIIb/IIIa receptor prevents fibrinogen, von Willebrand factor, vitronectin, and other molecules from binding to the receptor, thereby inhibiting thrombocyte aggregation. In contrast to the other medications of this group it is necessary to administer these drugs parenterally. Abciximab is the Fab-fragment of chimeric monoclonal antibodies which binds to GIIb/IIIa and to the vitronectin receptor on the surface of thrombocytes. In contrast to this eptifibatide and tirofiban are specific GPIIb/IIIa inhibitors. Abciximab was found not to significantly cross the term human placenta intact using an *in vitro* human placental lobule perfusion model (Miller 2003). Thus far no undesirable effects have been observed on the development of children whose mothers received an infusion of abciximab, eptifibatide or tirofiban for acute coronary intervention during pregnancy (Hajj-Chahine 2010, Al-Aqeedi 2008, Boztosun 2008, Sebastian 1998).

Due to its vasodilation effects, *dipyridamole* was originally used as a treatment for coronary disease. It is now licensed in combination with ASA in secondary prevention of ischemic strokes and transitory ischemic attacks (TIA). In addition to vasodilation, dipyridamole has antiplatelet activity. It has been used in combination with other anticoagulants to treat pregnant women with essential thrombocythemia to reduce the incidence of recurrent abortions and fetal growth restriction (Uzan et al. 1991). Congenital anomalies have been reported in infants born to mothers who were treated with dipyridamole during pregnancy, but the rate of anomalies reported in these studies is small and the pattern of anomalies is inconsistent (Chen 1982, Ibarra-Perez 1976, Tejani 1973). No increase in the frequency of congenital anomalies among infants of women who were treated with dipyridamole and ASA during the second and third trimesters of pregnancy has been observed in controlled trials (Uzan 1991, Wallenburg 1987, Beaufils 1985, 1986). Fetal wastage is high among women who are treated with dipyridamole during pregnancy, particularly when used in combination with warfarin (Sareli 1989). For low dose therapy with ASA see Section 2.1.2.

> **Recommendation.** In cases of intolerance with low dose ASA therapy, use of established inhibitors of thrombocyte aggregation, such as clopidogrel, is recommended. When one of the other above mentioned antithrombotics has been used during the first trimester, the termination of pregnancy or use of invasive diagnostics is not required. Ultrasound evaluation can be offered to confirm the normal development of the fetus. Precautions should be taken to minimize the risk for increased bleeding in both the mother and fetus prior to surgical interventions or prior to delivery.

2.9.7 Vitamin K antagonists

Pharmacology

Coumarin derivatives (4-hydroxycoumarin compounds) exert their anticoagulant activity indirectly by preventing vitamin K from acting as a cofactor in the hepatic synthesis of the vitamin K-dependent coagulation factors II, VII, IX and X (as well as the anticoagulants, proteins C and S). They are also called vitamin K antagonists (VKA). Anticoagulants with vitamin K antagonism include the coumarin derivatives *acenocoumarol, phenprocoumon, warfarin* and the indanediones, *fluindione* and *phenindione*. Most VKA are completely absorbed following oral administration and bound to albumin in the plasma by more than 95%. The elimination half-life is 24 hours for acencoumarol (including its metabolites), 36 hours for warfarin and 150 hours for phenprocoumon. The half-lives of the clotting factors range between 8–72 hours. Consequently, it takes several days for the inhibitory effect on the synthesis of the coagulation factors to result in reduced concentrations in the liver. Coumarin derivatives are metabolized in the liver and excreted by the kidneys. They are particularly susceptible to interactions with other drugs that are able to compete with them for plasma protein binding, alter their metabolism in the liver, or inhibit or stimulate synthesis of the clotting factors.

Coumarin embryopathy

VKAs readily cross the placental barrier and can reach the fetus. The teratogenic risk associated with the use of VKA during pregnancy continues to be of importance because maintaining long-term anticoagulation is essential in women with heart valve replacement. Substitution with LMWH in sufficient doses during the first trimester of pregnancy and prior to delivery improves fetal outcome but increases maternal morbidity and mortality (McLintock 2011, 2013, Abildgaard 2009, Vitale 1999). However, recent studies on the use of warfarin during pregnancy have shown that both maternal and fetal outcomes are greatly improved if low-dose warfarin (≤5 mg/d) is used throughout pregnancy and replaced with LMWH close to delivery (McLintock 2013, De Santo 2012, Malik 2012, Geelani 2005).

The embryotoxicity of VKA, particularly that of warfarin, is well-known. Warfarin has been found to produce a characteristic pattern of malformations in the children of women who took this drug during pregnancy. Common features of this pattern of malformations, collectively called coumarin embryopathy or fetal warfarin syndrome, include nasal hypoplasia, stippled epiphyses, and growth retardation (Hall 1980). In a review of 63 case reports of coumarin embryopathy published after 1955, van Driel (2002a) found that anomalies of the skeleton were the most predominant feature, occurring in 51 (81%) of the 63 cases. Midfacial hypoplasia, that included a small upward pointing nose with indentations between the tip of the nose and nares, depressed nasal bridge, defective development of the nasal septum, micrognathia, a prominent forehead, and a flattened appearance of the face, was described in 47 of the cases. Stippling in the epiphyseal regions (chondrodysplasia punctata) was described in 32 (51%) of the 63 cases, mostly along the axial skeleton, at the proximal femora and in the calcanei. Limb hypoplasia, primarily involving the distal digits, may be found in up to one-third of children with coumarin embryopathy (Pauli 1993). Other anomalies reported and summarized by van Driel (2002a) were CNS abnormalities, disturbances of eye and ear development, abnormal heart development, asplenia syndrome, kidney agenesis, cleft lip, jaw and palate and pulmonary hypoplasia. Minor physical anomalies reported were lowset or poorly developed ears, a high-arched palate, hypertelorism, antimongoloid palpebral fissures, and widely spaced nipples. Hepatopathy lasting up to 4 months of age in addition to features typical of coumarin embryopathy were described in a premature infant whose mother had been treated with phenprocoumon up until 24 weeks of pregnancy (Hetzel 2006). It is likely that the liver dysfunction observed in this infant resulted from a toxic effect of phenprocoumon on the fetus similar to that which occasionally occurs with the drug in adults.

Mechanisms of teratogenicity and fetotoxicity

Coumarin derivatives are thought to produce their teratogenic effects through inhibition of the synthesis of various vitamin K dependent proteins in the bones, cartilage and CNS. The classical features of coumarin embryopathy are phenotypically similar to those seen in X-linked recessive brachytelephalangic chondrodysplasia punctata (Conradi-Hunermann Syndrome) which is known to be caused by a mutation in the arylsulfatase E (ARSE) gene (Savarirayan 1999, Becker 1975). This gene mutation leads to a complete loss of functional ARSE. ARSE plays an important role in cartilage and bone development and its activity has been shown to be inhibited by warfarin *in vitro* (Savarirayan 1999, Franco 1995).

CNS abnormalities are thought to result from intracerebral hemorrhages and subsequent scarring, and are associated with exposure at any time during pregnancy, but mostly the second trimester of pregnancy. Of special concern are extensive cerebral hemorrhages during late pregnancy and during delivery (Oswal 2008, Simonazzi 2008, Hall 1980). One case report describes phenprocoumon poisoning in a woman who was admitted to the hospital at 38 weeks of pregnancy. She had an international normalized ratio (INR) that was not measurable (INR >10) and a phenprocoumon concentration that was twice the therapeutic levels of phenprocoumon. Sixteen days later and after treatment of the mother with prothrombin complex, antithrombin and oral vitamin K, a healthy girl was delivered by caesarean section without bleeding complications. The maternal coagulation parameters became normal 7 days after admission. In cord blood the level of phenprocoumon was 297 ng/mL (Hauck et al. 2011).

Frequency of malformations

In a review of all published case and cohort studies published between 1957 and 2002, coumarin embryopathy was observed in 23 (6%) of 394 live-born children whose mothers had been treated with a coumarin derivative during pregnancy; even when coumarin derivatives were used throughout the entire pregnancy (van Driel 2002a). A total of 17 studies with 979 pregnancies were analyzed in this review; 449 of the pregnancies were exposed to acenocoumarol, 327 to warfarin, and in 203 pregnancies the coumarin derivative was not specified. In a further case series, which included 71 pregnant women on warfarin therapy for artificial heart valves, four (6%) of the children had features of coumarin embryopathy (Cotrufo 2002). Here, as in other studies (Vitale 1999), a higher rate of poor pregnancy outcomes was observed when maternal doses of warfarin exceeded 5 mg/d. However, a case report on coumarin embryopathy with involvement of the optic nerve emphasized the low dose therapy in this case (Khan 2007).

The largest prospective cohort study to date, with 666 women who were treated during pregnancy with an oral anticoagulant, also reported a small risk for coumarin embryopathy (Schaefer et al. 2006). In this multicenter study, 226 pregnant women were treated with acenocoumarol, 280 with phenprocoumon, 99 with phenindione and 63 with warfarin. Four patients received two VKAs. The authors found a significantly increased risk for major malformations in the infants following maternal exposure to coumarin derivatives in the first trimester of pregnancy (odds ratio = 3.86, 95% confidence interval 1.86–8.00). However, the malformations that were observed were heterogeneous. Among the total of 356 live-born babies, there were only two (0.6%) coumarin embryopathies observed. In both of these cases the mother had been exposed to phenprocoumon during the critical period for coumarin embryopathy.

Critical period of susceptibility

Most publications state that the sensitive period for producing coumarin embryopathy is between 6–12 weeks of pregnancy without clearly
defining whether this is based on gestational or embryological age. A
critical review of all published reports, however, does not provide evidence for a highly sensitive period until week 8 after LMP (or week 6
postconception). Although there have been five cases published in the
literature in which maternal exposure to coumarins was reported to have
occurred prior to the 8th week after LMP, it is likely that the period of
pregnancy was calculated in weeks after conception (Hall 1989, Balde
1988) or causality was doubtful (Ruthnum 1987, Cox 1977) and/or additional contributing factors (such as open heart surgery during pregnancy)
were reported (Lapiedra 1986). Furthermore, the long half-lives of some
of the coumarins must be taken into account when considering the timing of embryonic and/or fetal exposure (Walfisch 2010). Warfarin, for
example, has a terminal half-life of 1 week. Therefore, discontinuation
of treatment or substitution with heparin at six weeks postconception to
avoid embryonic exposure may be too late.

Other adverse effects of coumarin therapy

Other adverse effects that have been associated with the use of coumarins during pregnancy include high rates of spontaneous abortion, stillbirth, preterm birth and low birth weight (Malik 2012, McLintock 2011,
Meister 2008, Schaefer 2006). The higher rate of infants with low birth
weight may be partially explained by the increased rate of prematurity;
however, Schaefer (2006) found reduced birth weight in full-term cou-
marin-exposed infants as well. It is possible that the underlying disease
of the mothers (e.g. defects of heart valves, embolism, various coagulopathies) contributed to the poor pregnancy outcomes in the coumarin-
exposed groups in these studies.

▶ **Mental development**

The long-term effects of prenatal exposure to coumarins were examined in a cohort of approximately 300 children aged 7.6 to 15.1 years
(van Driel 2001, 2002a, Wesseling 2000, 2001). Only two children in
the exposed cohort had features of coumarin embryopathy at the time
of birth. Both children were normally developed at the age of 9 and
13 years, respectively (van Driel 2002b). The average height and overall growth of the exposed children did not differ from a non-exposed
control group. None of the exposed children had abnormal neurological development. However, mild neurological deviations in the exposed
children were noted more frequently when the mother received treatment in the second or third trimester of pregnancy (Wesseling 2001).
The average IQ of the exposed children did not differ from the control
group significantly; however, 11 of the exposed children measured an IQ
<80 as opposed to three in the control group. These 11 children were all
exposed during the second and third trimesters of pregnancy and showed
no signs of dysmorphism. There were no differences between the two
groups in clinically relevant problem behavior, although less favorable
task-oriented and social-emotional behaviors were observed among the
exposed cohort (van Driel, 2001). Three other long-term studies with a
total of 72 children found no significant differences regarding physical
and mental development (Olthof 1994, Wong 1993, Chong 1984).

> **Recommendation.** Since VKAs are associated with a small, but increased, risk of embryopathy and other adverse effects, they are not recommended in the first trimester of pregnancy or prior to delivery. They are generally not recommended for use during pregnancy. Patients on VKA who are planning a pregnancy should preferably be placed on heparin (UH or LMWH) prior to pregnancy or, at the latest, prior to the 6th week after conception. This warrants adequate pregnancy testing. In high-risk patients with mechanical heart valves, an exception may be necessary because of the risk of valve thrombosis and failure or systemic thromboembolism. Here, oral anticoagulants throughout pregnancy until near term may be essential. The risk for coumarin embryopathy is small, particularly when therapy is discontinued prior to 6 weeks postconception or smaller doses (e.g. less than 5 mg/d for warfarin) are used. Therefore, interruption of a wanted pregnancy is not recommended if inadvertent exposure occurs in early pregnancy. Close follow-up by the obstetrician, including level II ultrasound, should be recommended in any case of VKA exposure during pregnancy.

2.9.8 Vitamin K

Vitamin K refers to a group of fat-soluble vitamins that are required for the synthesis of coagulation factors. Vitamin K_1 (*phytomenadione, phytonadione, phylloquinone*) is found in plants; vitamin K_2 (*menaquinone*) mostly occurs in animal products but is also synthesized from vitamin K_1 by various intestinal bacteria; vitamin K_3 (*menadione*) is a synthetic analog of vitamin K_1; and vitamin K_4 is the water-soluble form of menadione. High doses of vitamin K are used to reverse the anticoagulant effects of coumarins. Except in cases of malabsorption or in those who are undergoing treatment with antibiotics or anticonvulsants, there is no need for supplementation with vitamin K in pregnant women because usual dietary intake provides adequate amounts. The newborn infant is functionally deficient in vitamin K at birth. Breast-fed, but not formula-fed, newborns lack the intestinal bacteria that produce menaquinones. Furthermore, menaquinones are not stored in the newborn liver until 2–3 months of age when complementary foods are added to the diet. For these reasons, administration of vitamin K to the newborn is recommended to prevent Vitamin K Deficiency Bleeding (VKDB) in susceptible infants. The frequency of congenital anomalies did not appear to be increased among the infants of 28 women who received vitamin K_1, vitamin B_{12}, or liver extract during the first 4 lunar months of pregnancy in the Collaborative Perinatal Project (Heinonen 1977). Fourteen of these women received vitamin K_1. In a record linkage study, four out of five infants whose mothers were given prescriptions for vitamin K were reported to have major congenital anomalies (Rosa, cited in Briggs 2011). No adverse effects were observed among infants whose mothers were given prophylactic doses of vitamin K prior to delivery or among infants given fetal injections of vitamin K prior to delivery (Thorp 1995, Larsen 1978). No differences in intellectual development were observed at 2 years of age between children whose mothers had received prophylactic treatment with vitamin K prior to delivery and those whose mothers had not (Thorp 1997). No increased risk of childhood leukemia was found among the children of women who received vitamin K during pregnancy (Olsen 1994).

Vitamin K has been administered late during pregnancy for the prevention of intracranial hemorrhage in the newborn, but most studies have not shown a beneficial effect (Crowther 2010, Greer 2010, Choulika

Pregnancy

2.9 Anticoagulants, thrombocyte aggregation inhibitors, fibrinolytics and volume replacement agents

2004, Kazzi 1989). This is likely due to the limited amounts of vitamin K that are transferred from the mother to the fetus (Greer 2010).

Recommendation. Newborns should routinely receive 1–2 mg of vitamin K directly after birth. In those cases where the mother was treated with VKA (such as carbamazepine, phenobarbital, phenytoin, primidone, rifampin, or coumarin derivatives) parenteral administration directly after birth is advised, and the neonate should be given 1–2 mg vitamin K orally two to three times a week during the first 2 weeks after birth.

2.9.9   Fibrinolysis

Fibrinolytic drugs are used to dissolve thrombotic blocking. Fibrin, an end product of coagulation, is a polymer that is broken up into water-soluble parts by plasmin, a peptidase. These fibrin parts then dissolve along with the thrombus. Plasmin is formed from plasminogen, an endogenous glycoprotein, under the influence of endogenous activators like *urokinase* and *tissue-plasminogen activator*. Apart from these, exogenous substances such as *streptokinase* can enhance the formation of plasminogen. In the case of a hemorrhage as a result of fibrinoytic therapy, synthetic inhibitors like *tranexamic acid* and *p-aminomethyl-benzoic acid* (PAMBA) will have rapid hemostatic action.

Intrinsic fibrinolytics and derivatives

Urokinase is a thrombolytic enzyme predominantly formed in the kidney and excreted in the urine. The enzyme converts plasminogen into plasmin and promotes the dissolution of physiologically-occurring blood clots; for example, as in menstrual blood. Urokinase can be isolated from human kidney cell cultures or urine and can now also be produced by gene technology. Twelve case reports of normal infants born to women who were treated with urokinase during pregnancy, mostly after the first trimester, have been published (Murugappan 2006, Krishnamurthy 1999, La Valleur 1996, Glazier 1995, Kramer 1995, Turrentine 1995). Endogenous tissue plasminogen activator (t-PA) is a serine protease found in the endothelial cells that line the blood vessels. It can be produced using recombinant gene technology and is referred to as *rt-PA* or *alteplase*. Because of its large molecular size (527 amino acids) it is unlikely that transplacental passage occurs. There are more than 30 cases reported regarding the use of rt-PA during pregnancy (Li 2012, Akcay 2011, Holden 2011, Lonjaret 2011, Açar 2010, Biteker 2010, Ozer 2010, Kaya 2010, Bessereau 2007, Leonhardt 2006, Mehrkens 2006, Murugappan 2006, Bechtel 2005, Trukhacheva 2005, Goh 1999, Saviotti 1997, Baudo 1990). Most pregnancies that were treated with thrombolytic therapy with urokinase or alteplase were unremarkable. However, spontaneous abortions and premature deliveries occurred in some of the exposed pregnancies, which may be more related to the severity of the maternal disease than the treatment. So far, urokinase and alteplase have not been associated with an increased frequency of malformations in the children of women who are treated with these drugs during pregnancy. However, only about 23% of the exposures reported in these cases occurred in the first trimester of pregnancy. Very little data have been published regarding use of the recombinant t-PA variant, *tenecteplase*, during pregnancy. Several cases of successful thrombolysis with unremarkable pregnancy outcome have been reported (dos Santos 2012, Camacho Pulido 2008, Maegdefessel 2008, Bessereau 2007). Only two case reports describe maternal exposure to the recombinant analog, *reteplase*, during the 15th week of pregnancy in one case and in the 30th week of pregnancy in the other (Yap 2002, Rinaldi 1999). Normal infants were delivered in both cases. There is no information about the use of p-anisoylated plasminogen streptokinase activator complexes (*anistreplase*) during pregnancy.

> **Recommendation.** Urokinase and alteplase (rt-PA) should only be used during pregnancy in life-threatening circumstances. Reteplase, tenecteplase and anistreplase should only be used when it is therapeutically superior compared to other medications. Due to the danger of increased blood loss, special caution is needed when using fibrinolytics during the intrapartum period. Inadvertent use during the first trimester of pregnancy does not require the termination of pregnancy nor the use of invasive diagnostic procedures.

2.9.10   Streptokinase

Streptokinase is a plasminogen activator produced from β-hemolyzing streptococci of Group C. It is a protein, not an enzyme, and it combines with plasminogen to form the active complex that converts the free plasminogen to proteolysis plasmin. There are reports of around 200 patients who were treated with streptokinase during pregnancy, predominantly after the first trimester. No teratogenic or other adverse effects were observed in the infants (Srinivas 2012, Holden 2011, te Raa 2009, Nassar 2003, Anbarasan 2001, Henrich 2001, Turrentine 1995). No animal teratology studies of streptokinase have been published. For the use of streptokinase and other fibrinolytics, there have been discussions by some authors about an increased risk of spontaneous abortion and prematurity because of potential fibrinolysis of the fibrin layer between the chorionic villi and myometrium. The available data do not confirm this to date (Turrentine 1995). Only small amounts of streptokinase cross the placental barrier (Pfeifer 1970).

> **Recommendation.** It is acceptable to use streptokinase during pregnancy in life-threatening circumstances. Because of the danger of increased blood loss, it is advisable to exercise caution when fibrinolysis is performed during the perinatal phase. Treatment with streptokinase during the first trimester does not justify pregnancy interruption or the use of invasive diagnostic procedures. In cases of doubt or extreme maternal anxiety, a detailed ultrasound examination can be performed to confirm normal development of the fetus.

2.9.11   Antihemorrhagics

The body's own plasmin antagonists, such as α2-antiplasmin and α2-macroglobulin, are physiological inhibitors of fibrinolysis. The synthetic antifibrinolytics, *tranexamic acid* and *p-aminomethyl-benzoic acid*, are used therapeutically for treatment of coagulopathies with increased fibrinolytic activity, a malignant disease or following surgical interventions. A few case reports have been published regarding the use of tranexamic acid during pregnancy (e.g. Lindoff 1993, Walzman 1982) and all of the women in these cases were reported to have delivered normal live-born infants. Only one animal teratology study has been published and no substantial fetotoxic or teratogenic effects of tranexamic acid were found in the offspring in this study (Morita 1971). Successful pregnancy outcomes have been described after maternal treatment with cytostatic medications and tranexamic acid for promyelocytic leukemia (Carradice 2002). The concentration of tranexamic acid in umbilical cord blood was 70% of the maternal concentration (Kullander 1970). No information regarding the use of p-aminomethyl-benzoic acid during pregnancy has been published.

Aprotinin is a polypeptide that inhibits proteolytic enzymes such as chymotrypsin, trypsin, plasmin and plasminogen activators. As a foreign protein, it can induce sensitization. There is no information on its use during pregnancy.

Epsilon-aminocaproic acid is an inhibitor of fibrinolysis. The use of this agent is associated with an increased risk of thrombosis and embolism, with possible renal failure from thrombosis in glomerular capillary arteries. It was reported not to be teratogenic in rabbits (Howorka 1970). No information is available regarding its use in pregnant women.

Recommendation. The use of tranexamic acid, p-aminomethyl-benzoic acid, aprotinin, or epsilon-aminocaproic acid during pregnancy should be reserved for life-threatening situations. Inadvertent treatment during the first trimester does not justify termination of pregnancy or invasive diagnostic intervention. However, in some circumstances, ultrasound examination may be offered to confirm normal development of the fetus.

2.9.12   Other antihemorrhagics

Thrombopoietin-receptor agonists, such as *romiplostim* and *eltrombopag*, are used in the treatment of the autoimmune disease ITP (chronic idiopathic thrombocytopenic purpura). These compounds stimulate the thrombopoietin receptor to induce platelet production and reduce bleeding complications. These drugs are available for patients who cannot be treated with other therapies, such as immunoglobulins or corticosteroids, or surgery to remove the spleen.

Romiplostim is an Fc-Peptid-Fusion protein (peptibody) that is produced using recombinant DNA technology. It is injected subcutaneously once weekly. Romiplostim consists of a human IgG1-Fc-portion that has two single-chain subunits connected to a peptide containing two thrombopoetin-receptor-binding domains. It is known that IgG molecules are actively transported to the fetus via Fc-receptors beginning with the second trimester of pregnancy. It is possible that such a mechanism exists for romiplostim.

Eltrombopag is a small molecule that is administered orally. So far only one case report has been published describing a healthy, live-born infant with normal platelet count whose mother had been given both eltrombopag and romiplostim during the third trimester of pregnancy (Alkaabi 2012).

> **Recommendation.** Romiplostim and eltrombopag should only be used with urgent indications and after strict determination of benefit/risk analysis. Inadvertent treatment in the first trimester of pregnancy does not justify interruption of pregnancy or invasive diagnostic intervention. However, ultrasound examination is recommended to confirm normal development of the fetus.

2.9.13   Volume replacement substances and rheologics

▶ Dextrans

Dextrans are glucose polymers with molecular weights ranging between 1,000–40,000,000 daltons (Da). They are produced by lactic acid bacteria from solutions that contain saccharide, but also by the dental plaque-forming species, *Streptococcus mutans*. After fractionation there are several clinical products available: Dextran 40 (average molecular mass 40,000 Da), Dextran 60 (average molecular mass 60,000 Da) and Dextran 70 (average molecular mass 70,000 Da). Dextrans have an inhibitory effect on thrombocyte aggregation and coagulation factors and are used as volume expanders. The infusion of dextrans can lead to anaphylactic reactions in the mother which can also jeopardize the embryo. These anaphylactic reactions can be reduced by administering dextran 1 (or hapten-dextran which is a dextran fraction with a molecular mass of 1000 Da) immediately prior to the dextran infusion. Dextran 1 binds to the dextran-reactive antibodies thereby preventing the formation of large immune complexes and consequently an immune response. However there are reports about the use of dextrans during childbirth which led to anaphylactic shock and serious neonatal consequences despite dextran 1 prophylaxis (Barbier 1992, Berg 1991). Specific embryo- or fetotoxic effects have not been reported to date.

▶ Gelatin

Gelatin derivatives, such as *polygeline* and *modified fluid gelatin* (succinylated gelatin), are polypeptides used as plasma substitutes in the form of polymers with an average molecular mass of 30,000 to 35,000 Da. No specific embryotoxic or fetotoxic effects have been reported. As with the dextrans, anaphylactic reactions are possible after the use of gelatin.

▶ Hydroxyethyl starch

Hydroxyethyl starch (HES, HAES) is a high polymeric glucose compound that consists almost exclusively of amylopectin. The highly branched amylopectin starches are modified through the introduction of hydroxyethyl groups to the glucose subunits in order to limit degradation by alpha-amylase. Hetastarch products are grouped by their mean molecular weight which can range from 70,000 to 450,000 Da. These products differ by their substitution characteristics. HES is administered via infusion as a plasma volume expander. Anaphylactic reactions are rare. The effect of HES on coagulation is lower than for dextrans. A pruritus that is difficult to treat and lasts for weeks and months is a typical side effect which has been observed after the use of HES. No malformations

Pregnancy

2.9 Anticoagulants, thrombocyte aggregation inhibitors, fibrinolytics and volume replacement agents were observed among the infants of 25 women who were given HES early in pregnancy in association with paracentesis for ovarian hyperstimulation syndrome (Courtney 2005). The indication should be strict accordingly. Aside from precipitation in the placenta, no adverse effects were observed among newborn infants of women who were treated with HES prior to caesarean section delivery (Carvalho 2009, Siddik-Sayyid 2009, Davies 2006; Siddik 2000) or who received plasma volume expansion with HES during pregnancy for hypertensive disorders (Ganzevoort 2005, Heilmann 1991). Indications for HES should be strictly stipulated.

Recommendation. Dextrans, gelatins and hydroxyethyl starch are acceptable for pregnant women in critical situations when a therapeutic benefit is expected. The danger of anaphylactic reactions should be considered especially when dextran is used.

References

Abildgaard U, Sandset PM, Hammerstrøm J et al. Management of pregnant women with mechanical heart valve prosthesis: thromboprophylaxis with low molecular weight heparin. Thromb Res 2009; 124: 262–7.

Açar G, Simşek Z, Avci A et al. Right heart free-floating thrombus in a pregnant woman with massive pulmonary embolism: a case of 'emboli in transit'. J Cardiovasc Med 2010 Oct 16 [Epub ahead of print].

Akcay AB, Yuce M, Akcay M et al. Partial thrombus resolution with trofiban in a pregnant woman with mechanical prosthetic mitral valve thrombosis. Clin Appl Thromb Hemost 2011; 17: 476–9.

Al-Aqeedi RF, Al-Nabti AD. Drug-eluting stent implantation for acute myocardial infarction during pregnancy with use of glycoprotein IIb/IIIa inhibitor, aspirin and clopidogrel. J Invasive Cardiol 2008; 20: E146–9.

Alkaabi JK, Alkindi S, Riyami NA et al. Successful treatment of severe thrombocytopenia with romiplostim in a pregnant patient with systemic lupus erythematosus. Lupus 2012; 21: 1571–4.

Anbarasan C, Kumar VS, Latchumanadhas K et al. Successful thrombolysis of prosthetic mitral valve thrombosis in early pregnancy. J Heart Valve Dis 2001; 10: 393–5.

Andersen AS, Berthelsen JG, Bergholt T. Venous thromboembolism in pregnancy: prophylaxis and treatment with low molecular weight heparin. Acta Obstet Gynecol Scand 2010; 89: 15–21.

Andrew M, Mitchell L, Berry L et al. An anticoagulant dermatan sulfate proteoglycan circulates in the pregnant woman and her fetus. J Clin Invest 1992; 89: 321–6.

Babic Z, Gabric ID, Pintaric H. Successful primary percutaneous coronary intervention in the first trimester of pregnancy. Catheter Cardiovasc Interv 2011; 77: 522–5.

Badawy AM, Khiary M, Sherif LS et al. Low-molecular weight heparin in patients with recurrent early miscarriages of unknown aetiology. J Obstet Gynaecol 2008; 28: 280–4.

Bajoria R and Contractor SF. Transfer of heparin across the human perfused placental lobule. J Pharm Pharmacol 1992; 44: 952–9.

Balde MD, Breitbach GP, Wettstein A et al. Fallotsche Tetralogie nach Cumarineinnahme in der Frühschwangerschaft – eine Embryopathie? Geburtshilfe Frauenheilkd 1988; 48: 182–3.

Bar J, Cohen-Sacher B, Hod M et al. Low-molecular-weight heparin for thrombophilia in pregnant women. Int J Gyn Obstet 2000; 69: 209–13.

Barbier P, Jonville AP, Aufret E et al. Fetal risks with dextrans during delivery. Drug Saf 1992; 7: 71–3.

Bauder F, Beinder E, Arlettaz R et al. Intrauterine subdural hemorrhage in a preterm neonate possibly associated with maternal low-molecular weight heparin treatment. J Perinatol 2009; 29: 521–3.

Baudo F, Caimi TM, Redaelli R et al. Emergency treatment with recombinant tissue plasminogen activator of pulmonary embolism in a pregnant woman with antithrombin III deficiency. Am J Obstet Gynecol 1990; 163: 1274–5.

Bauersachs RM, Dudenhausen J, Faridi A et al. Risk stratification and heparin prophylaxis to prevent venous thromboembolism in pregnant women. Thromb Haemost 2007; 9: 1237–45.

Beaufils M, Uzan S, Donsimoni R, Colau JC. Prevention of pre-eclampsia by early antiplatelet therapy. Lancet 1985; 1: 840–2.

Beaufils M, Uzan S, Donsimoni R, Colau JC. Prospective controlled study of early antiplatelet therapy in prevention of preeclampsia. Adv Nephrol Necker Hosp 1986; 15: 87–94.

Bechtel JJ, Mountford MC, Ellinwood WE. Massive pulmonary embolism in pregnancy treated with catheter fragmentation and local thrombolysis. Obstet Gynecol 2005; 106: 1158–60.

Becker MH, Genieser NB, Feingold M. Chondrodysplasia punctata: is maternal warfarin therapy a factor? Am J Dis Child 1975; 129: 356–9.

Berg EM, Fasting S, Sellevold OP. Serious complications with dextran–70 despite hapten prophylaxis. Is it best avoided prior to delivery? Anaesthesia 1991; 46: 1033–5.

Bessereau J, Devignes O, Huon B et al. Case report of a successful pregnancy following thrombolysis for acute myocardial infarction. Arch Mal Coeur Vaiss 2007; 100: 955–8.

Biteker M, Duran NE, Ozkan M. Successful treatment of massive pulmonary embolism in a pregnant woman, with low-dose, slow infusion of tissue plasminogen activator. Turk Kardiyol Dern Ars 2010; 38: 32–4.

Boyle RK. Which heparin during the investigation of chest pain at term pregnancy? Emerg Med Australasia 2007; 19: 279–81.

Boztosun B, Olcay A, Avci A et al. Treatment of acute myocardial infarction in pregnancy with coronary artery balloon angioplasty and stenting: use of tirofiban and clopidogrel. Int J Cardiol 2008; 127: 413–6.

Briggs GG, Freeman RK, Yaffe SJ. Drugs in Pregnancy and Lactation: A Reference Guide to Fetal and Neonatal Risk, 9th edn. Philadelphia, Pa: Lippincott Williams & Wilkins, 2011.

Butwick AJ, Carvalho B. Neuraxial anesthesia in obstetric patients receiving anticoagulant and antithrombotic drugs. Int J Obstet Anesth 2010; 19: 193–201.

Camacho Pulido JA, Jiménez Sánchez JM, Montijano Vizcaíno A et al. Acute myocardial infarction in pregnancy of 39 week treated with fibrinolysis. An Med Interna 2008; 25: 31–2.

Carradice D, Austin N, Bayston K et al. Successful treatment of acute promyelocytic leukaemia during pregnancy. Clin Lab Haem 2002; 24: 307–11.

Carvalho B, Mercier FJ, Riley ET et al. Hetastarch co-loading is as effective as pre-loading for the prevention of hypotension following spinal anesthesia for cesarean delivery. Int J Obstet Anesth 2009; 18: 150–5.

Casele H, Haney EI, James A et al. Bone density changes in women who receive thromboprophylaxis in pregnancy. Am J Obstet Gynecol 2006; 195: 1109–13.

Chan WS, Anand S, Ginsberg JS. Anticoagulation of pregnant women with mechanical heart valves. A systematic review of the literature. Arch Intern Med 2000; 160: 191–6.

Chapman ML, Martinez-Borges AR, Mertz HL. Lepirudin for treatment of acute thrombosis during pregnancy. Obstet Gynecol 2008; 112: 432–3.

Chen WW, Chan CS, Lee PK et al. Pregnancy in patients with prosthetic heart valves: an experience with 45 pregnancies. Q J Med 1982; 51: 358–65.

Chong MK, Harvey D, de Swiet M. Follow-up study of children whose mothers were treated with warfarin during pregnancy. Br J Obstet Gynaecol 1984; 91: 1070–3.

Choulika S, Grabowski E, Holmes LB. Is antenatal vitamin K prophylaxis needed for pregnant women taking anticonvulsants? Am J Obstet Gynecol 2004; 190: 882–3.

Coppens M, Eikelboom JW, Gustafsson D et al. Translational success stories: development of direct thrombin inhibitors. Circ Res 2012; 111: 920–9.

Cotrufo M, de Feo M, de Santo LS et al. Risk of warfarin during pregnancy with mechanical valve prostheses. Obstet Gynecol 2002; 99: 35–40.

Courtney GG, Copeland JE, Racette N et al. Pregnancy outcome following use of hydroxyethyl starch (HES), human albumin (ALB) or no colloid infusion in women undergoing paracentesis for ovarian hyperstimulation syndrome (OHSS). Fertil Steril 2005; 84: S65.

Cox DR, Martin L, Hall BD. Asplenia syndrome after fetal exposure to warfarin. Lancet 1977; 26: 1134.

Crowther CA, Crosby DD, Henderson-Smart DJ. Vitamin K prior to preterm birth for preventing neonatal periventricular haemorrhage. Cochrane Database Syst Rev 2010; 1: CD000229.

Darki A, Kodali PP, McPheters JP et al. Hypereosinophilic syndrome with cardiac involvement in a pregnant patient with multiple sclerosis. Tex Heart Inst J 2011; 38: 163–5.

Davies P, French GWG. A randomised trial comparing 5 mL/kg and 10 mL/kg of pentastarch as a volume preload before spinal anaesthesia for elective caesarean section. Int J Obstet Anesth 2006; 15: 279–83.

Dempfle CE. Minor transplacental passage of fondaparinux in vivo. N Engl J Med 2004; 350: 1914–5.

Deruelle P, Coulon C. The use of low-molecular-weight heparins in pregnancy – how safe are they? Curr Opin Obstet Gynecol 2007; 19: 573–7.

De Santis M, de Luca C, Mappa I et al. Clopidogrel treatment during pregnancy: a case report and a review of literature. Intern Med 2011; 50: 1769–73.

De Santo LS, Romano G, Della Corte A et al. Mechanical aortic valve replacement in young women planning on pregnancy: Maternal and fetal outcomes under lows oral anticoagulation, a pilot observational study on a comprehensive pre-operative counseling protocol. J Am Coll Cardiol 2012: 59; 1110–5.

Dimitrakakis C, Papageorgiou P, Papageorgiou I et al. Absence of transplacental passage of the low molecular weight heparin enoxaparin. Haemostasis 2000; 30: 243–8.

Di Nisio M, Middeldorp S, Büller HR. Direct thrombin inhibitors. N Engl J Med 2005; 353: 1028–40. Erratum in: N Engl J Med 2005; 353: 2827.

Dizon-Townson D. Pregnancy-related venous thromboembolism. Clin Obstet Gynecol 2002; 45: 363–8.

dos Santos LF, Andrade C, Rodrigues B et al. Pregnancy and acute pulmonary embolism: a case report. Rev Port Cardiol 2012; 31: 389–94.

Duarte FP, O'Neill P, Centeno MJ. Myocardial infarction in the 31st week of pregnancy – case report. Rev Bras Anestesiol 2011; 61: 225–31.

Ebina Y, Hazama R, Nishimoto M et al. Resection of giant liver hemangioma in a pregnant woman with coagulopathy: case report and literature review. J Prenat Med 2011; 5: 93–6.

Ekbatani A, Asaro LR, Malinow AM. Anticoagulation in a parturient with heparin-induced thrombocytopenia. Int J Obstet Anesth 2010; 19: 82–7.

Fawzy M, Shokeir T, El-Tatongy M et al. Treatment options and pregnancy outcome in women with idiopathic recurrent miscarriage: a randomized placebo-controlled study. Arch Gynecol Obstet 2008; 278: 33–8.

Franco B, Meroni G, Parenti G et al. A cluster of sulfatase genes on Xp22.3: mutations in chondrodysplasia punctata (CDPX) and implications for warfarin embryopathy. Cell 1995; 81: 15–25.

Furlan A, Vianello F, Clementi M et al. Heparin-induced thrombocytopenia occurring in the first trimester of pregnancy: successful treatment with lepirudin. A case report. Haematologica 2006; 91: ECR40.

Ganzevoort W, Rep A, Bonsel GJ et al. A randomized trial of plasma volume expansion in hypertensive disorders of pregnancy: influence on the pulsatility indices of the fetal umbilical artery and middle cerebral artery. Am J Obstet Gynecol 2005; 192: 233–9.

Geelani MA, Singh S, Verma A et al. Anticoagulation in patients with mechanical valves during pregnancy. Asian Cardiovasc Thorac Ann 2005; 13: 30–3.

Gerhardt A, Scharf RE, Zotz RB. Successful use of danaparoid in two pregnant women with heart valve prosthesis and heparin-induced thrombocytopenia Type II (HIT). Clin Appl Thromb Hemost 2009; 15: 461–4.

Gnsberg JS, Hirsh J. Anticoagulants during pregnancy. Annu Rev Med 1989a; 40: 79–86.

Ginsberg JS, Hirsh J, Turner DC, et al. Risks to the fetus of anticoagulant therapy during pregnancy. Thromb Haemost, 1989b; 61: 197–203.

Glazier JJ, Eldin AM, Hirst JA et al. Primary angioplasty using a urokinase-coated hydrogel balloon in acute myocardial infarction during pregnancy. Cather Cardiovasc Diagn 1995; 36: 216–9.

Gogarten W, van Aken H, Büttner J et al. Rückenmarksnahe Regionalanästhesien und Thromboembolieprophylaxe/antithrombotische Medikation. 2., überarbeitete Empfehlungen der Deutschen Gesellschaft für Anästhesiologie und Intensivmedizin. Anästh Intensivmed 2007; 48: 109–24.

Goh KYC, Hsiang JNK, Zhu XL, Poon WS. Intraventricular recombinant tissue plasminogen activator for treatment of spontaneous intraventricular haemorrhage in pregnancy. J Clin Neurosci 1999; 6: 158–9.

Goland S, Elkayam U. Anticoagulation in pregnancy. Cardiol Clin 2012; 30: 395–405.

Greer FR. Vitamin K the basics – what's new? Early Hum Dev 2010; 86: 43–7.

Greer IA, Nelson-Piercy C. Low-molecular-weight heparins for thromboprophylaxis and treatment of venous thromboembolism in pregnancy: a systematic review of safety and efficacy. Blood 2005; 106: 401–7.

Greinacher A, Eckhardt T, Mussmann J et al. Pregnancy complicated by heparin associated thrombocytopenia: management by a prospectively in vitro selected heparinoid (Org 10172). Thromb Res 1993; 71: 123–6.

Hajj-Chahine J, Jayle C, Tomasi J et al. Successful surgical management of massive pulmonary embolism during the second trimester in a parturient with heparin-induced thrombocytopenia. Interact Cardiosvasc Throac Surg 2010; 11: 679–81.

Hall BD. Warfarin embryopathy and urinary tract anomalies: possible new association (letter). Am J Med Genet 1989; 34: 292–3.

Hall JG, Pauli RM, Wilson KM. Maternal and fetal sequelae of anticoagulation during pregnancy. Am J Med 1980; 68: 122–40.

Hanania G, Thomas D, Michel PL et al. Pregnancy and prosthetic heart valves: a French cooperative retrospective study of 155 cases. Eur Heart J 1994; 15: 1651–8.

Harenberg J, Jörg I, Bayerl C et al. Treatment of a woman with lupus pernio, thrombosis and cutaneous intolerance to heparins using lepirudin during pregnancy. Lupus 2005; 14: 411–2.

Harenberg J, Schneider D, Heilmann L, Wolf H. Lack of anti-factor Xa activity in umbilical cord vein samples after subcutaneous administration of heparin or low molecular mass heparin in pregnant women. Haemostasis 1993; 23: 314–20.

Hauck B, Zimmermann R, Ringwald J et al. Pregnancy outcome after maternal intoxication with phenprocoumon. Br J Clin Pharmacol 2011; 71: 139–40.

Heilmann L, Lorch E, Hojnacki B et al. Accumulation of two different hydroxyethyl starch preparations in the placenta after hemodilution in patients with fetal intrauterine growth retardation or pregnancy hypertension. Infusionstherapie 1991; 18: 236–43.

Heinonen OP, Slone D, Shapiro S. Birth Defects and Drugs in Pregnancy. Littleton, Mass: John Wright-PSG, 1977, p. 402.

Henrich W, Schmider A, Henrich M et al. Acute iliac vein thrombosis in pregnancy treated successfully by streptokinase lysis: a case report. J Perinat Med 2001; 29: 155–7.

Hetzel PG, Glanzmann R, Hasler PW et al. Coumarin embryopathy in an extremely low birth weight infant associated with neonatal hepatitis and ocular malformations. Eur J Pediatr 2006; 165: 358–60.

Holden EL, Ranu H, Sheth A et al. Thrombolysis for massive pulmonary embolism in pregnancy – a report of three cases and follow-up over a two year period. Thromb Res 2011; 127: 58–9.

Howorka E, Olasinski R, Wyrzykiewicz T. The effect of EACA administered to female rabbits during pregnancy on the fetuses. Patol Pol 1970; 21: 311–4.

Huhle G, Geberth M, Hoffmann U et al. Management of heparin-associated thrombocytopenia in pregnancy with subcutaneous r-hirudin. Gynecol Obstet Invest 2000; 49: 67–9.

Ibarra-Perez C, Arevalo-Toledo N, Alvarez-De La Cadena O et al. The course of pregnancy in patients with artificial heart valves. Am J Med 1976; 61: 504–12.

James AH, Brancazio LR, Gehrig TR et al. Low-molecular-weight heparin for thromboprophylaxis in pregnant women with mechanical heart valves. J Matern Fetal Neonatal Med 2006; 19: 543–9.

Kaya EB, Kocabas U, Aksoy H et al. Successful fibrinolytic treatment in a pregnant woman with acute mitral prosthetic valve thrombosis. Clin Cardiol 2010; 33: E101–3.

Kazzi NJ, Ilagan NB, Liang K-C, et al. Maternal administration of vitamin K does not improve the coagulation profile of preterm infants. Pediatrics 1989; 84: 1045–50.

Khan AO. Optic nerve dysfunction in a child following low-dose maternal warfarin exposure. Ophthalmic Genet 2007; 28: 183–4.

Kominiarek MA, Angelopoulos SM, Shapiro NL et al. Low-molecular-weight heparin in pregnancy: peripartum bleeding complications. J Perinatol 2007; 27: 329–34.

Kramer WB, Belfort M, Saade GR et al. Successful urokinase treatment of massive pulmonary embolism in pregnancy. Obstet Gynecol 1995; 86: 660–2.

Krishnamurthy P, Martin CB, Kay HH. Catheter-directed thrombolysis for thromboembolic disease during pregnancy: a viable option. J Matern Fetal Med 1999; 8: 24–7.

Kuczkowski KM. Clopidogrel and pregnancy: a situation pregnant with danger? Arch Gynecol Obstet 2009; 280: 693–4.

Kullander S, Nilsson IM. Human placental transfer of an antifibrinolytic agent (AMCA). Acta Obstet Gynecol Scand 1970; 49: 241–2.

Lagrange F, Vergnes C, Brun JL et al. Absence of placental transfer of pentasaccharide (Fondaparinux, Arixtra) in the dually perfused human cotyledon in vitro. Thromb Haemost 2002; 87: 831–5.

Lapiedra OJ, Bernal JM, Ninot S et al. Open heart surgery for thrombosis of a prosthetic mitral valve during pregnancy. Fetal hydrocephalus. J Cardiovasc Surg (Torino) 1986; 27: 217–20.

Larsen JF, Jacobsen B, Holm HH et al. Intrauterine injection of vitamin K before the delivery during anticoagulant therapy of the mother. Acta Obstet Gynecol Scand 1978; 57: 227–30.

La Valleur J, Molina E, Williams PP et al. Use of urokinase in pregnancy. Two success stories. Postgrad Med 1996; 99: 269–70, 272–3.

Lefkou E, Khamashta M, Hampson G et al. Review: Low-molecular-weight heparin induced osteoporosis and osteoporotic fractures: a myth or an existing entity? Lupus 2010; 19: 3–12.

Leonhardt G, Gaul C, Nietsch HH et al. Thrombolytic therapy in pregnancy. J Thromb Thrombolysis 2006; 21: 271–6.

Lepercq J, Conard J, Borel-Derlon A et al. Venous thromboembolism during pregnancy: a retrospective study of enoxaparin safety in 624 pregnancies. BJOG 2001; 108: 1134–40.

Li Y, Margraf J, Kluck B et al. Thrombolytic therapy for ischemic stroke secondary to paradoxical embolism in pregnancy: a case report and literature review. Neurologist 2012; 18: 44–8.

Lindqvist PG, Dahlback B. Bleeding complications associated with low molecular weight heparin prophylaxis during pregnancy. Thromb Haemost 2000; 84: 140–1.

Lindoff C, Rybo G, Astedt B. Treatment with tranexamic acid during pregnancy, and the risk of thrombo-embolic complications. Thromb Haemost 1993; 70: 238–40.

Lonjaret L, Lairez O, Galinier M, Minville V. Thrombolysis by recombinant tissue plasminogen activator during pregnancy: a case of massive pulmonary embolism. Am J Emerg Med 2011; 29: 694, e1–e2.

Maegdefessel L, Issa H, Scheler C et al. 27-year old pregnant woman with syncope and dyspnea after aortic alloplastic heart valve replacement 15 years ago. Internist (Berl) 2008; 49: 868–72.

Magnani HN. An analysis of clinical outcomes of 91 pregnancies in 83 women treated with danaparoid (Orgaran). Thromb Res 2010; 125: 297–302.

Malik HT, Sepehripour AH, Shipolini AR, McCormack DJ. Is there a suitable method of anticoagulation in pregnant patients with mechanical prosthetic heart valves? Interact Cardiovasc Thorac Surg 2012; 15: 484–8.

Maslovitz S, Many A, Landsberg JA et al. The safety of low-molecular-weight heparin therapy during labor. Obstet Gynecol Surv 2005; 60: 632–3.

Mätzsch T, Bergquist D, Bergquist A et al. No transplacental passage of standard heparin or an enzymatically depolymerized low molecular weight heparin. Blood Coagul Fibrinolysis 1991; 2: 273–8.

McLintock C. Anticoagulant therapy in pregnant women with mechanical prosthetic heart valves: no easy option. Thromb Res 2011; 127: S56–60.

McLintock C. Anticoagulant choices in pregnant women with mechanical heart valves: balancing maternal and fetal risks – the difference the dose makes. Thromb Res 2013; 131: S8–10.

McNamee K, Dawood F, Farquharson RG. Thrombophilia and early pregnancy loss. Best Pract Res Clin Obstet Gynaecol 2012; 26: 91–102.

Mehrkens JH, Steiger H-J, Strauss A, Winkler PA. Management of haemorrhagic type moyamoya disease with intraventricular haemorrhage during pregnancy. Acta Neurochir (Wien) 2006; 148: 685–9.

Mehta R, Golichowski A. Treatment of heparin induced thrombocytopenia and thrombosis during the first trimester of pregnancy. J Thromb Haemost 2004; 2: 1665–6.

Meister R, Schaefer C. Statistical methods for estimating the probability of spontaneous abortion in observational studies. Analyzing pregnancies exposed to coumarin derivatives. Reprod Toxicol 2008; 26: 31–35.

Miller RK, Mace K, Polliotti B et al. Marginal transfer of ReoPro™ (Abciximab) compared with immunoglobulin G (F105), inulin and water in the perfused human placenta in vitro. Placenta 2003; 24: 727–38.

Morita H, Tachizawa H, Okimoto T. Evaluation of the safety of tranexamic acid. 3. Teratogenic effects in mice and rats. Oyo Yakuri 1971; 5: 415–20.

Murugappan A, Coplin WM, Al-Sadat AN et al. Thrombolytic therapy of acute ischemic stroke during pregnancy. Neurology 2006; 66: 768–70.

Myers B, Westby J, Strong J. Prophylactic use of danaparoid in high-risk pregnancy with heparin-induced thrombocytopaenia-positive skin reaction. Blood Coagul Fibrinolysis 2003; 14: 485–7.

Myers GR, Hoffman MK, Marshall E. Clopidogrel use througout pregnancy in a patient with drug-eluting coronary stent. Obstet Gynecol 2011; 118: 432–3.

Nagler M, Haslauer M, Wuillemin WA. Fondaparinux – data on efficacy and safety in special situations. Thromb Res 2012; 129: 407–17.

Nassar AH, Abdallah ME, Moukarbel GV et al. Sequential use of thrombolytic agents for thrombosed mitral valve prosthesis during pregnancy. J Perinat Med 2003; 31: 257–60.

Nelson SM, Greer IA. Thromboembolic events in pregnancy: pharmacological prophylaxis and treatment. Expert Opin Pharmacother 2007; 8: 2917–31.

Olsen JH, Hertz H, Blinkenberg K, Verder H. Vitamin K regimens and incidence of childhood cancer in Denmark. BMJ 1994; 308: 895–6.

Olthof E, De Vries TW, Touwen BC et al. Late neurological, cognitive and behavioural sequelae of prenatal exposure to coumarins: a pilot study. Early Hum Dev 1994; 38: 97–109.

Oswal K, Agarwal A. Warfarin-induced fetal intracranial subdural hematoma. J Clin Ultrasound 2008; 36: 451–3.

Ozer O, Davutoglu V, Soydinc HE et al. Fibrinolytic therapy of prosthetic mitral valve thrombosis during pregnancy: three case reports and review of the literature. Clin Appl Thromb Hemost 2010; 16: 406–13.

Pauli RM, Haun JM. Intrauterine effects of coumarin derivatives. Dev Brain Dysfunct 1993; 6: 229–47.

Peeters LL, Hobbelen PM, Verkeste CM et al. Placental transfer of Org 10172, a low-molecular weight heparinoid, in the awake late-pregnant guinea pig. Thromb Res 1986; 44: 277–83.

Pfeifer GW. Distribution and placental transfer of 131-I streptokinase. Australas Ann Med 1970; 19: 17–8.

Pierangeli SS, Leader B, Barilaro G et al. Acquired and inherited thrombophilia disorders in pregnancy. Obstet Gynecol Clin North Am 2011; 38: 271–95.

Rinaldi JP, Yassine M, Aboujaoudé F et al. Successful thrombolysis on an aortic valve prosthesis by plasminogen tissue activator during pregnancy. Arch Mal Coeur Vaiss 1999; 92: 427–30.

Rowan JA, McLintock C, Taylor RS et al. Prophylactic and therapeutic enoxaparin during pregnancy: Indications, outcomes and monitoring. Aust N Z J Obstet Gynaecol 2003; 43: 123–8.

Ruthnum P, Tolmie JL. Atypical malformations in an infant exposed to warfarin during the first trimester of pregnancy. Teratology 1987; 36: 299–301.

Sanson BJ, Lensing AWA, Prins MH et al. Safety of low-molecular-weight heparin in pregnancy: a systematic review. Thromb Haemost 1999; 81: 668–72.

Santiago-Díaz P, Arrebola-Moreno AL, Ramírez-Hernández JA et al. Platelet antiaggregants in pregnancy. Rev Esp Cardiol 2009; 62: 1197–8.

Sareli P, England MJ, Berk MR. Maternal and fetal sequelae of anticoagulation during pregnancy in patients with mechanical heart valve prostheses. Am J Cardiol 1989; 63: 1462–5.

Savarirayan R. Common phenotype and etiology in warfarin embryopathy and X-linked chondrodysplasia punctata (CDPX) (letter). Pediatr Radiol 1999; 29: 322.

Saviotti M, Bongarzonddi A, Casazza F. Massive pulmonary embolism during the third trimester of pregnancy: effectiveness of alteplase therapy. G Ital Cardiol 1997; 27: 72–5.

Sbarouni E and Oakley CM. Outcome of pregnancy in women with valve prostheses. Br Heart J 1994; 71: 196–201.

Schaefer C, Hannemann D, Meister R et al. Vitamin K antagonists and pregnancy outcome. A multi-centre prospective study. Thromb Haemost 2006; 95: 949–57.

Schapkaitz E and Jacobson BF. Delayed hypersensitivity to low-molecular-weight heparin (LMWH) in pregnancy. S Afr Med J 2007; 97: 1255–7.

Schneider D, Heilmann L, Harenberg J. Placental transfer of low-molecular weight heparin. Geburtshilfe Frauenheilkd 1995; 55: 93–8.

Sebastian C, Scherlag M, Kugelmass A et al. Primary stent implantation for acute myocardial infarction during pregnancy: use of abciximab, ticlopidine, and aspirin. Cathet Cardiovasc Diagn 1998; 45: 275–9.

Serrano F, Nogueira I, Borges A, Branco J. Primary antiphospholipid syndrome: pregnancy outcome in a Portuguese population. Acta Reumatol Port 2009; 34: 492–7.

Shah P, Dzavik V, Cusimano RJ et al. Spontaneous dissection of the left main coronary artery. Can J Cardiol 2004; 20: 815–8.

Sharif S, Hay CR, Clayton-Smith J. Aplasia cutis congenita and low molecular weight heparin. BJOG 2005; 112: 256–8.

Siddik SM, Aouad MT, Kai GE et al. Hydroxyethylstarch 10% is superior to Ringer's solution for preloading before spinal anesthesia for Cesarean section. Can J Anaesth 2000; 47: 616–21.

Siddik-Sayyid SM, Nasr VG, Taha SK et al. A randomized trial comparing colloid preload to coload during spinal anesthesia for elective cesarean delivery. Anesth Analg 2009; 109: 1219–24.

Simonazzi G, Pilu G, Palareti G et al. Foetal cerebral hemispheric atrophy and porencephaly after intrauterine exposure to maternal warfarin for mechanical prosthetic heart valve. Prenat Diagn 2008; 28: 157–9.

Sørensen HT, Johnson SP, Larsen H et al. Birth outcomes in pregnant women treated with low-molecular-weight heparin. Acta Obstet Gynecol Scand 2000; 79: 655–9.

Srinivas BC, Moorthy N, Kuldeep A et al. Thrombolytic therapy in prosthetic valve thrombosis during early pregnancy. Indian Hedart J 2012; 64: 74–6.

Taniguchi S, Fkuda I, Watanabe K et al. Emergency pulmonary embolectomy during the second trimester of pregnancy: report of a case. Surg Today 2008; 38: 59–61.

Tanimura K, Ebina Y, Sonoyama A et al. Argatroban therapy for heparin-induced thrombocytopenia during pregnancy in a woman with hereditary antithrombin deficiency. J Obstet Gynaecol Res 2012; 38: 749–52.

Taylor S, Folkman J. Protamine is an inhibitor of angiogenesis. Nature 1982; 297: 307–12.

Tejani N. Anticoagulant therapy with cardiac valve prosthesis during pregnancy. Obstet Gynecol 1973; 42: 785–93.

Tello-Montoliu A, Seecheran NA, Angiolillo DJ. Successful pregnancy and delivery on prasugrel treatment: considerations for the use of dual antiplatelet therapy during pregnancy in clinical practice. J Thromb Thrombolysis 2013; 36: 348–51.

te Raa DG, Ribbert LSM, Snijder RJ et al. Treatment options in massive pulmonary embolism during pregnancy. A case-report and review of literature. Thromb Res 2009; 124: 1–5.

Thorp JA, Gaston L, Caspers DR, Pal ML Current concepts and controversies in the use of vitamin K. Drugs 1995; 49: 376–87.

Thorp JA, Yeast JD, Cohen GR et al. Does in-utero phenobarbital lower IQ? Follow up of the intracranial hemorrhage prevention trial. Am J Obstet Gynecol 1997; 176: S117.

Trukhacheva E, Scharff M, Gardner M, Lakkis N. Massive pulmonary embolism in pregnancy treated with tissue plasminogen activator. Obstet Gynecol 2005; 106: 1156–8.

Turrentine MA, Braems G, Ramirex MM. Use of thrombolytics for the treatment of thromboembolic disease during pregnancy. Obstet Gynecol Surv 1995; 50: 534–41.

Ueno M, Masuda H, Nakamura K et al. Antiplatelet therapy for a pregnant woman with a mechanical aortic valve: report of a case. Surg Today 2001; 31: 1002–4.

Uzan S, Beaufils M, Breart G et al. Prevention of fetal growth retardation with low-dose aspirin: findings of the EPREDA trial. Lancet 1991; 337: 1427–31.

van Driel D, Wesseling J, Sauer PJ et al. In utero exposure to coumarins and cognition at 8 to 14 years old. Pediatrics 2001; 107: 123–9.

Van Driel D, Wesseling J, Sauer PJ, et al. Teratogen update: Fetal effects after in utero exposure to coumarins overview of cases, follow-up findings, and pathogenesis. Teratology 2002a; 66: 127–40.

Van Driel D, Wesseling J, de Vries TW, et al. Coumarin embryopathy: long-term follow-up of two cases. Eur J Pediatr 2002b; 161: 231–2.

Vitale N, De Feo M, De Santo LS et al. Dose-dependent fetal complications of warfarin in pregnant women with mechanical heart valves. J Am Coll Cardiol 1999; 33: 1637–41.

Voke J, Keidan J, Pavord S et al. The management of antenatal venous thromboembolism in the UK and Ireland: a prospective multicentre observational survey. Br J Haematol 2007; 139: 545–58.

Walfisch A, Koren G. The "warfarin window" in pregnancy: the importance of half-life. J Obstet Gynaecol Can 2010; 32: 988–9.

Wallenburg HCS and Rotmans N. Prevention of recurrent idiopathic fetal growth retardation by low-dose aspirin and dipyridamole. Am J Obstet Gynecol 1987; 157: 1230–5.

Walzman M, Bonnar J. Effects of tranexamic acid on the coagulation and fibrinolytic systems in pregnancy complicated by placental bleeding. Arch Toxicol 1982; 5: 214–20.

Watanabe T, Aihara K, Ohura K, et al. Reproduction studies of ticlopidine hydrochloride. 2. Teratogenicity study in rats. Iyakuhin Kenkyu, 1980a; 11: 265–75.

Watanabe T, Ohura K, Tashiro K, et al. Reproduction studies of ticlopidine hydrochloride. 4. Teratogenicity study in rabbits. Iyakuhin Kenkyu, 1980b; 11: 287–93.

Wesseling J, van Driel D, Heymans HS et al. Behavioural outcome of school-age children after prenatal exposure to coumarins. Early Hum Dev 2000; 58: 213–24.

Wesseling J, van Driel D, Smrkovsky M et al. Neurological outcome in school-age children after in utero exposure to coumarins. Early Hum Dev 2001; 63: 83–95.

Winger EE, Reed JL. A retrospective analysis of fondaparinux versus enoxaparin treatment in women with infertility or pregnancy loss. Am J Reprod Immunol 2009; 62: 253–60.

Wittmaack FM, Greer FR, FitzSimmons J. Neonatal depression after a protamine sulfate injection. A case report. J Reprod Med 1994; 39: 655–6.

Wong V, Cheng CH, Chan KC. Fetal and neonatal outcome of exposure to anticoagulants during pregnancy. Am J Med Genet 1993; 45: 17–21.

Yap LB, Alp NJ, Forfar JC. Thrombolysis for acute massive pulmonary embolism during pregnancy. Int J Cardiol 2002; 82: 193–4.

Young SK, Al-Mondhiry HA, Vaida SJ et al. Successful use of argatroban during the third trimester of pregnancy: case report and review of the literature. Pharmacotherapy 2008; 28: 1531–6.

Epilepsy and antiepileptic medications

2.10

Christina Chambers and Christof Schaefer

2.10.1	Antiepileptic therapy	252
2.10.2	Antiepileptic and contraceptive drugs	253
2.10.3	Epilepsy and fertility	253
2.10.4	Frequency of seizures in pregnancy	254
2.10.5	Risk of malformations	254
2.10.6	Typical malformations and other anomalies	256
2.10.7	Pregnancy complications	256
2.10.8	Mental development dysfunction	257
2.10.9	"Damage mechanisms"	258
2.10.10	Folic acid and antiepileptic drugs	259
2.10.11	Vitamin K and antiepileptic drugs	259
2.10.12	Is epilepsy teratogenic?	260
2.10.13	Carbamazepine	260
2.10.14	Clobazam and clonazepam	263
2.10.15	Eslicarbazepine	264
2.10.16	Ethosuximide and other succinimides	264
2.10.17	Felbamate	265
2.10.18	Gabapentin	265
2.10.19	Lacosamide	266
2.10.20	Lamotrigine	267
2.10.21	Levetiracetam	268
2.10.22	Oxcarbazepine	269
2.10.23	Phenobarbital and primidone	270
2.10.24	Phenytoin	273
2.10.25	Pregabalin	274
2.10.26	Rufinamide	275
2.10.27	Sultiame	275
2.10.28	Tiagabine	275
2.10.29	Topiramate	276
2.10.30	Valnoctamide	277
2.10.31	Valproic acid	278
2.10.32	Vigabatrin	282
2.10.33	Zonisamide	283

Epilepsy affects 0.4–0.5% percent of pregnant women (Morrow 2003). About 80% of these women take at least one antiepileptic drug (AED) and are able to control their seizures (Kaaja 2003). In addition, antiepileptic drugs are also used to manage other conditions that afflict women of reproductive age, e.g. in psychiatry for manic-depressive symptoms, or in neurology for chronic pain. Children of mothers treated with antiepileptic drugs are, to a varying degree, subject to a higher risk of malformations, and sometimes also to mild facial dysmorphism, underdevelopment of the distal phalanges, intrauterine growth restriction, and functional developmental anomalies of the central nervous system (CNS). The latter was primarily noted for *valproic acid* (VPA) (Meador 2008). In general, the risk for the unborn is by far the greatest for VPA, while for *carbamazepine* the risk appears to be smaller than thought a few years ago. For the newer antiepileptic drugs extensive experience is only available for *lamotrigine*, which does not to date support an increased risk for malformations or other impairments of prenatally exposed offspring. Some concern has been raised for *topiramate* in terms of an increased risk for oral clefts and/or reduced birth weight. Epilepsy itself appears not to adversely affect prenatal development, the exception being the most severe forms with multiple grand-mal seizures.

CLASSIFICATION OF ANTIEPILEPTIC DRUGS

The following agents are older antiepileptic drugs: *carbamazepine, clobazam, clonazepam, ethosuximide, phenobarbital, phenytoin, sultiame* and *VPA*.

The newer antiepileptics include *eslicarbazepine, felbamate, gabapentin, lacosamide, lamotrigine, levetiracetam, oxcarbazepine, pregabalin, rufinamide, tiagabine, topiramate, vigabatrin,* and *zonisamide*.

2.10.1   Antiepileptic therapy

Recommendation.

- No woman who could become pregnant should receive antiepileptic medication without compelling reasons. In particular for non-epileptic neurologic or psychiatric indications the use of antiepileptic agents should be eschewed, the exception being the apparently well-tolerated lamotrigine.
- Because of teratogenic risks women should be advised about the use of appropriate contraception. The potential for a contraceptive medication to interact with the antiepileptic agent should be considered. Prior to discontinuing a contraceptive regimen, the anticonvulsive therapy should be optimized with consideration of embryotoxic properties.
- A woman suffering from epilepsy needs to know that the risk for major malformations increases two- to threefold when using antiepileptic medication.
- VPA should be avoided in women during the reproductive years. Exceptions being epilepsy that failed to respond to other treatments.
- Monotherapy is desirable, as the concomitant administration of several antiepileptic agents clearly increases the embryotoxic risk, although newer publications seem to suggest that VPA is the primary risk factor.
- Particularly during organogenesis, the medication dose should be kept as low as possible. If VPA has to be given, it should be distributed in 2–4 doses during the day.
- Determinations of levels of the free, unbound antiepileptic agent in the maternal blood should be performed once in each each trimester, and even more often, if antiepilectic drugs with a higher clearance are prescribed. Clearance increases during pregnancy especially with lamotrigine and levetiractam requiring a higher dose adjustment. To a lesser degree this applies also to oxcarbazepine, phenytoin, and carbamazepine.
- If, under antiepileptic therapy a child has been born with an anomaly that can reasonably be attributed to the drug, an alternative antiepileptic regimen should be considered as soon as possible prior to the next pregnancy. Because of their drug-specific pharmacologic susceptibility, mother and child have a higher risk of a recurrence in a subsequent pregnancy if the same antiepileptic agent is used. Empirically this recurrence risk has been estimated to be about 15% for VPA.
- If for several years no seizures have occurred, a woman should be assessed to determine if medication can be discontinued prior to a pregnancy. Approximately 50% of all epileptic patients can stop their medication at a given point (Morrow 2003).

- In cases of idiopathic, generalized seizures, lamotrigine is the best tolerated drug by the embryo/fetus, although VPA is more effective (Marson 2007). For focal epilepsy carbamazepine is as effective as VPA but poses lower risk.
- A stable medication setting should not be hastily altered or stopped during pregnancy.
- Neither a monotherapy, nor a combination therapy with several antileptic drugs are an indication for a pregnancy termination.
- Follow-up sonography should be offered to each pregnant woman treated with antiepileptic drugs, and each woman with epilepsy, treated or not.

2.10.2   Antiepileptic and contraceptive drugs

Certain antiepileptic drugs can lead to contraceptive failure. *Carbamazepine, phenobarbital, primidone, phenytoin, felbamate, oxcarbazepine* and *topiramate* are inducers of the hepatic cytochrome P450–3A4 enzyme system. This enzyme system is involved in the metabolism of estrogen and progestogen. The resulting increased metabolism of contraceptives can give rise to unwanted pregnancies (Dutton 2008). Thus it is not recommended to rely on hormonal therapy, including hormonal contraception, as even (as occasionally recommended) doubling the hormonal contraceptive dose will not guarantee prevention of pregnancy. An intrauterine device with local progestogen delivery would be preferable, or perhaps an intrauterine pessary, although somewhat less effective. Only if these methods cannot be tolerated, should a higher dose of hormonal contraception be considered, realizing the possible limitations of its reliability. In such cases, two daily doses of a low-dose monophasic formulation taken continuously for 3–9 months for each long-term cycle can be considered. Other recommendations aim for oral contraceptives with a higher dose to inhibit ovulation.

Effectiveness of hormonal contraceptives is not known to be impaired with the concomitant use of *benzodiazepines, ethosuximide, gabapentin, lamotrigine, levetiracetam, pregabalin, tiagabine, VPA, vigabatrin* and *zonisamide*.

However, estrogen-containing contraceptives can activate the degradation of lamotrigine, leading to an increased tendency for seizures without proper dosage adjustment, and, if appropriate dosing is initiated, after discontinuation of estrogen-containing contraceptives, there is potential for toxic side effects as the lamotrigine concentration increases (Dutton 2008).

In sensitive individuals, sex hormones can increase (estrogens) or decrease (progestogens) the disposition for seizures. This is of relevance in cycle-dependent seizures.

2.10.3   Epilepsy and fertility

Epilepsy and antiepileptic drugs can decrease fertility. Thus there is, at the moment, an unclarified association between temporal lobe epilepsy and VPA therapy on one side and polycystic ovary syndrome (PCOS) on the other side. PCOS may cause anovulatory infertility and is found in 10–25% of epileptic women, and at even higher rates in patients taking VPA, while its prevalence in the general population is 5–10%. Adiposity with hyperinsulinism or insulin resistance seems to play a part in PCOS. Thus antiepileptic medications that enhance weight gain, such as *VPA, carbamazepine, gabapentin* and *vigabatrin* need to be viewed critically.

2.10.4   Frequency of seizures in pregnancy

Seizures may occur more frequently during pregnancy because the dose of antiepileptic medication is inappropriately decreased (e.g. intentional reduction or discontinuation of medication to protect the child), sleep disturbances, and higher clearance (Fotopoulou 2009, López-Fraile 2009, Petrenaite 2009, Sabers 2009, Westin 2009). When antiepileptic drugs with higher clearance (*lamotrigine, carbamazepine, oxcarbazepine, levetiracetam, topiramate*) are dosed according to the patient's blood level, the risk of seizures does not appear to increase (e.g. Sabers 2009). Further, it has been shown that the risk for seizures during pregnancy is only about 10%, where patients experience no seizures during at least 9 months prior to the pregnancy (Harden 2009a).

2.10.5   Risk of malformations

Although well-established anticonvulsives belong to a class of medications that are among the most prescribed, and best investigated drugs with possible or proven teratogenicity, the determination of the individual risk of a patient remains a challenge (Tomson 2009).

The classic drugs *VPA, carbamazepine, phenobarbital*, and *phenytoin* are proven teratogens, yet the malformations seen in numerous studies differ markedly. There is agreement that the highest risk has been observed with VPA. The teratogenic risk of newer antiepileptics has not been defined in reliable studies that confirm their risk or safety. Only for *lamotrigine* are sufficient data on hand to assure good tolerance by the unborn.

Well over 100,000 women with epilepsy have been analyzed in major studies in previous years, and from established registries for epilepsy and pregnancy in Europe, EURAP (www.eurap.org) and UK Epilepsy and Pregnancy Register (Morrow 2006), in Australia (Vajda 2010b) and North America (http://aedpregnancyregistry.org/). Major malformations were seen in 1.2–11% when monotherapy was used (http://aedpregnancyregistry.org/; Meador 2008). When combination therapy with several antiepileptic agents is used, the risk is on average higher than with monotherapy (Mawer 2010, Harden 2009b, Meador 2008), and clearly greater than 10% in combination therapy that includes VPA. These values are up to four times higher than those seen in corresponding control groups of healthy pregnant women. A meta-analysis encompassing more than 65,000 pregnancies from 59 studies and epilepsy registries, found that 17.6% of infants born to women with epilepsy using monotherapy with VPA had malformations (95% CI 5.25–30.03) (Meador 2008). For carbamazepine, the rate of affected infants was 5.7% (95% CI 3.71–7.65). The malformation rates for both substances were significantly higher than for infants born to non-exposed mothers. The rates were not significantly increased for lamotrigine, phenobarbital, and phenytoin, while no analysis was conducted for other agents due to low numbers of exposed cases.

A study from England with 277 pregnant epileptic women (Mawer 2010) confirms the exceptionally high risk of VPA in mono- and combination therapies. While on average the major malformation rate of offspring of antiepileptic treated women was 6.6%, it was 11.3% when VPA was used alone and 16.7% when used in combination. Differentiating the daily dose above and below 1000 mg of monotherapy, the malformation rates were 16.0 and 7.1%, respectively; this difference was not significant due to the relatively low number of cases. Surprisingly, once the VPA–related cases had been excluded from the analysis, the authors found a malformation rate of only 3.0% for the cohort of pregnant women treated with all the other antileptic drugs. Carbamazepine was not found to have a significant elevation in risk for major malformations.

The North American Antiepileptic Drug Pregnancy Registry (http://aedpregnancyregistry.org/) as of the Spring 2012 newsletter (http://www2.massgeneral.org/aed/newsletter/Spring2012newsletter.pdf), currently contains data on over 7,000 pregnancies and indicates that the risk for major malformations was 2.0% for monotherapy with lamotrigine, 3.0% for carbamazepine, 2.9% for phenytoin, and 5.5% for phenobarbital. Here, too, VPA clearly had a higher risk with 9.3% of monotherapy exposed pregnancies resulting in a major malformation.

In contrast to other published results, Vajda (2010a) determined from the Australian Pregnancy Register of Antiepileptic Drugs in Pregnancy that combination therapies had a lower risk of malformation, and that the risk among polytherapy-treated pregnancies is, to a major degree, determined by the presence of VPA. According to their data, co-medication with lamotrigine can actually lower the risk of malformations in comparison to VPA given alone at the same dose. The authors discuss that lamotrigine enhances the elimination of VPA by degradation and glucuronidation. Accordingly, they challenge the general advice to use a monotherapy, especially when such treatment is not satisfactory. These results indicate that the avoidance of VPA is paramount.

Different malformation rates and relative risks in various studies can be explained by the methodological specifics of each study, the definition of (major) malformations, age of the child at the pediatric examination, as well as the composition of and malformation rates in the relevant control groups.

Two recent studies examined recurrence risk in women who took the same antiepileptic drug during two or more pregnancies. Using the Australian Register of Antiepileptic Drugs in Pregnancy, Vajda (2013b) evaluated 2637 births among 1243 women, and found that the rate of malformation in the subsequent pregnancy was 35.7% in women who had a malformed infant in the first pregnancy. In contrast, women who had a non-malformed infant in the first pregnancy had a malformation rate of 3.1% if they stayed on the same drug (odds ratio 17.6; 95% CI 4.5–68.7). The recurrence risk was highest in those who had a malformed infant and remained on VPA. In the second study using the United Kingdom Epilepsy and Pregnancy Register, Campbell (2013) evaluated 1534 pregnancies among 719 mothers who stayed on the same drug through two or more pregnancies, and found that those whose first child was malformed had a 16.8% risk of having a second child with a malformation, compared to a 9.8% rate among women whose first child did not have a malformation (relative risk 1.73, 95% CI 1.01–2.96). The recurrent risk rose to 50% in a third pregnancy if a mother had two previous malformed children while on the same drug. In this study, VPA and topiramate were associated with higher recurrence risks.

2.10.6   Typical malformations and other anomalies

It is not possible to map certain malformation patterns to individual antiepileptic drugs save for a few exceptions (Morrow 2003). There are malformations that are typical for VPA, such as neural tube defects, primarily lumbar spina bifida, and preaxial limb defects such as that of the radius. Specific developmental anomalies are described in the sections about the individual antiepileptic drugs.

The use of classical antiepileptic drugs primarily increases the risk of those anomalies that are also spontaneously more common (Tomson 2009). These include cardiac defects, cleft lip and palate (frequency each about 2%), neural tube defects (for VPA and *carbamazepine* 1–2%), anomalies of the urinary tract, especially hypospadias, skeletal anomalies such as club foot or hip dysplasia, and eye anomalies (ptosis, iris coloboma).

The term fetal anticonvulsant syndrome (FACS) has been applied to the constellation of minor malformations and other adverse effects that are similar across the carbamazepine, *phenytoin*, and *barbiturate embryopathies*. A syndrome refers to all symptoms beyond the major malformations, such as dysmorphism, growth restriction, microcephaly, and mental dysfunctions. The milder anomalies and dysmorphisms as well as functional deficits include:

- Midface hypoplasia (short nose, low and wide bridge of the nose or hypertelorism, epicanthus, long upper lip).
- Anomalies of the distal phalanges (small nails, short terminal phalanges of the fingers, finger-like thumb).
- Growth restriction.
- Microcephaly (especially with phenytoin and with antiepileptic combination therapy).
- Mental developmental dysfunctions, behavior problems, and suggestions of autism-like symptoms especially with VPA.

The detection of signs of dysmorphism is not always easy; it is based on subjective evaluation differences and sometimes requires a radiologic proof (Harvey 2003, Lu 2000).

Typically only some and not all malformations or dysmorphisms will be present. A recent small study has suggested that tooth enamel defects may be more common in children prenatally exposed to antiepileptic medications (Jacobsen 2013). In 38 children prenatally exposed to one or more anticonvulsant medications compared to 129 unexposed children in Denmark, 11% versus 4% had diffuse opacities, and numerous white opacities in the primary dentition, while 34% of exposed children versus 12% of unexposed had numerous white opacities in the permanent dentition.

Lymphocytes of the cord blood of offspring from mothers treated with antiepileptic drugs (primarily VPA and carbamazepine), demonstrated a significant increase of DNA damage as evidenced by presence of sister chromatid exchanges. Neither cytotoxic effects nor inhibition of cell-division kinetics were observed with these drugs (Witczak 2010).

2.10.7   Pregnancy complications

Pregnancy complications can be increased in women taking antiepileptic drugs; however, data are contradictory. In a comprehensive evidence-based analysis of more than 285 studies, Harden (2009a) con-cluded that there was no substantially higher risk (>2) for caesarean sections, no moderately increased risk (>1.5) for premature uterine contractions and delivery, but possibly a markedly higher risk for pre-mature uterine contractions and premature delivery for antiepileptic medication users who are also smokers. Data were considered insuf-ficient to estimate the risk for preeclampsia, pregnancy hypertension, and spontaneous abortion. Possibly there is a higher risk for an Apgar value of <7 at 1 minute and a likely increased risk for SGA (small for gestational age). In contrast, a Norwegian investigation with about 2,900 pregnancies with epilepsy found that women using antiepileptic drugs (1/3 of the cohort) displayed more frequently mild preeclampsia, premature delivery, and children with a birth weight <2,500 g, a head circumference below the 2.5 percentile, or lower Apgar scores. The authors also found that, independent of the specific antiepileptic ther-apy, intrauterine growth restriction and caesarean section were more common (Borthen 2009, Veiby 2009). A Swedish study saw a smaller head circumference primarily with carbamazepine, and to some degree also with VPA, but not with other antiepileptic drugs (Almgren 2009). Finally, a recent US study of 440 women with a seizure disorder were found to be no more likely to have a growth restricted infant or to expe-rience stillbirth, preterm delivery or preeclampsia than women without a seizure disorder (McPherson 2013).

2.10.8   Mental development dysfunction

CNS dysfunction is more common in children with midface hypopla-sia. Moore (2000) examined 57 children with a fetal anticonvulsant syndrome (FACS) and detected about 80% in behavior anomalies, speech impediments, and learning disorders; in 60%, two or more autistic features. Kjaer (2013) examined neurodevelopment in 4–5 year old children born to mothers with or without epilepsy, who did or did not use antiepileptic medications in pregnancy, using paren-tal questionnaires that were completed by 1,117 parents in Denmark. Behavioral problems as measured by the Strengths and Difficul-ties Questionnaire were more common in children born to mothers who took antiepileptic medication than either untreated epileptic mothers or non-epileptics. When comparing different antiepileptic medications, developmental problems were noted primarily after pre-natal exposure to VPA, and especially for autism spectrum disorders (Bromley 2010, 2013, Banach 2010, Meador 2009, Adab 2004, 2001). When evaluating the relative effects of prenatal antiepileptic exposure in children at 3 years of age, Meador (2011) found that all four of the commonly used anticonvulsants (VPA, carbamazepine, lamotrigine, or phenytoin) impair verbal versus non-verbal abilities. In a subse-quent analysis at 4.5 years of age, the deficits persisted for all four drugs; however, there was statistically significantly lower performance on mean IQ in VPA exposed relative to *carbamazepine, lamotrigine,* or *phenytoin* (Meador 2012). At the 6-year follow-up mark, findings persisted, with VPA exposed children doing less well on measures of verbal and memory ability compared to those exposed to other drugs, and in particular at high doses of VPA (Meador 2013). In that study, mean IQs were higher in children prenatally exposed to periconcep-tional folate supplements.

Pregnancy

2.10 Epilepsy and antiepileptic medications

2.10.9   "Damage mechanisms"

Different hypotheses have been proposed to explain the teratogenic effect of antiepileptic drugs; these are primarily derived from experimental studies. Thus a number of mechanisms can be invoked as possible explanation:

- *Carbamazepine, phenobarbital,* and *phenytoin* can interfere with the uptake of folic acid or alter its metabolism by stimulating the cytochrome-P450 enzyme system. VPA inhibits glutamate formyltransferase and also decreases the production of folinic acid. A genetically determined deficiency of methylentetrahydrolate reductase may possibly be of relevance.
- VPA inhibits the gene expression of histone deacetylase (HDAC). This enzyme participates in the control of the structure of nucleosomes. An HDAC deficiency results in a hyperacetylation of embryonal proteins particularly in the area of the caudal neural tube. Thus it represents a mechanism for the development of spina bifida that is independent of the folic acid pathway (Menegola 2006). Experiments also demonstrated an inhibition of HDAC by topiramate and the main metabolite of levetiracetam (Eyal 2004).
- VPA causes changes in gene expression that regulates cell growth (e.g. brain-derived growth factor (BDGF) and nerve growth factor (NGF)) and the corresponding receptors.
- A deficiency of the microsomal enzyme epoxide hydrolase in the mother and the embryo, leads to the accumulation of teratogenic epoxide metabolites in the presence of agents such as carbamazepine or phenytoin (Raymond 1995, Omtzigt 1993). These epoxide metabolites are produced by the enzyme monooxygenase that is linked to cytochrome-P450 and can bind to macromolecules. It can thus interfere with cell function and even lead to cell death (Wells 1997).
- Phenytoin decreases the mRNA expression of several growth factors (e.g. TGF-β, NT3 and WNT1) (Musselman 1994).
- Phenytoin inhibits the potassium channel resulting in hypoxia and a subsequnet reoxygenation (Danielsson 1997).
- Phenytoin has been implicated in the enhancement of gene expression of retinoic acid receptors in connection with a retinoic acid deficiency (Gelineau-van Waes 1999).
- VPA lowers the intracellular pH, for example in the limb buds (cited in Dean 2002).

Clinical observations of familial accumulation of typical anomalies after use of antiepileptic drugs and results of gene sequence analyses, suggest that a genetic disposition is required for the teratogenic effect of damaging medications. An interplay of external (medication-related) and genetic factors was first discussed about 25 years ago in relation to a dizygotic pair of twins that had been exposed to phenytoin. One twin was healthy, while the other demonstrated the typical phenytoin anomalies although the intrauterine environment was the same (Phelan 1982). Individual genetic patterns of metabolism can also explain the differences seen in a trizygotic triplet pregnancy, where the mother took phenytoin and phenobarbital. The three children displayed various degrees of intrauterine growth restriction as well as hypoplasia of the midface and the distal phalanges. One member of the triplet set also had a cleft lip and palate and another craniosynostosis (Bustamante 1978).

2.10.10   Folic acid and antiepileptic drugs

While a high dose of folic acid supplementation is recommended when folic acid antagonists are used in pregnancy, the proof of effective protection against the embryotoxic and teratogenic effects of antiepileptic medications, has not been demonstrated (Jentink 2010a, Hernández-Diaz 2000). A study conducted at the National Health Services Maternity Hospitals in Liverpool and Manchester, UK (Mawer 2010), and the UK Registry for Epilepsy and Pregnancy (Pittschieler 2008), also did not find a protective effect of a higher folic acid dose when compared to a standard dose. Generally, folic acid prophylaxis is recommended for all women when planning a pregnancy and during the first trimester. US recommendations, in a country with food fortification, are 0.4 mg/day (Chapter 2.18). The general recommendation for epileptic patients who want to conceive, is that they be treated with folic acid supplements at a dose of 0.8 mg/day from before conception until the end of organogenesis (gestational week 10). The absence of any additional effectiveness of higher doses argues against greater supplementation. Additionally, it needs to be considered that folic acid enhances the drug metabolism of the hepatic hydroxylases so that the concentration of antiepileptic medication could be lowered in the mother. Provided nutritional balance is present, this and the lack of proof for additional benefit argue against the continuation of folic acid intake past the first trimester in epileptic women.

2.10.11   Vitamin K and antiepileptic drugs

Independent of the maternal medication, newborns and especially premature infants exhibit a deficiency of vitamin K that needs to be substituted right after birth to prevent bleeding problems. In addition, *carbamazepine, ethosuximide, oxcarbazepine, phenytoin, phenobarbital, primidone, topiramate, vigabatrin* and *zonisamide* belong to a group of medications that induce enzymes leading to a decrease in vitamin K-dependent clotting factors. The prothrombin precursor PIVKAII (protein induced by vitamin K absence or antagonist II) represents an indirect marker and can be elevated in the newborn (Howe 1999).

It has often been recommended that when a mother uses drugs that counteract vitamin K, she should be given vitamin K1 during the last 4 weeks of gestation, initially 10 mg/day, and in the last 2 weeks 20 mg/day. The effectiveness of this regimen remains controversial (Harden 2009c, Hey 1999).

Kaaja (2002) did not find a higher rate of bleeding complications in 667 newborns whose mothers had taken antiepileptic drugs (among them 463 caramazepine, 212 phenytoin and 44 phenobartital), in comparison with 1,324 children of healthy mothers. The mothers had not been given vitamin K during pregnancy, but all children received 1 mg vitamin K1 (preferably intramuscularly) at birth. In another study of about 200 children of mothers with antiepileptic therapy who had not received vitamin K prophylaxis during pregnancy, no increase in a bleeding tendency was apparent in the newborns exposed to antiepileptic drugs compared with the control infants (Choulika 2004).

Vitamin K is absorbed orally as well as parenterally, but just after delivery the oral route may be unreliable, so that an IM injection of

Pregnancy

2.10 Epilepsy and antiepileptic medications

0.5–1.0 mg vitamin K1 is recommended. This therapy appears to be superior to the oral administration, particularly for the prevention of late bleeding problems (after two weeks) (American Academy of Pediatrics 2003). If oral prophylaxis is chosen, it needs to be ascertained that the newborn actually swallows the dose.

2.10.12   Is epilepsy teratogenic?

According to the current state of knowledge, observed malformations in newborns are the result of antiepileptic therapy and not the epilepsy itself. However, this distinction is difficult to demonstrate conclusively, as only in minor forms of epilepsy can treatment be foregone. Some authors observed higher rates of malformation when mothers suffered a grand mal seizure during the first trimester (Lindhout 1992). Mastroiacovo (1998) described in a very small cohort a significantly increased risk of malformation when epilepsy was not treated (4/31 = 13%). Most other investigations did not find teratogenic effects, either with untreated epilepsy or with grand mal seizures during pregnancy. No distinguishing link has been illustrated between the duration of the antiepileptic treatment prior to pregnancy and the pregnancy outcome (Dansky 1991). An analysis of the Belfast UK Epilepsy and Pregnancy Registry detected a 3.5% rate of major congenital malformations in 239 pregnancies of mothers whose epilepsy had not been treated, while the rate on average was 3.7% for those treated with monotherapy ($n = 2598$) and 6.0% for those treated with polytherapy ($n = 770$) (Morrow 2006).

Fried (2004) evaluated 10 studies in a meta-analysis covering 400 pregnancies of mothers whose epilepsy was not treated. They did not detect a teratogenic effect of epilepsy itself, but indicated that untreated epilepsy tends to occur in women with a less severe form of the disease, and with a lower frequency of seizures. Data from the Finnish Birth Registry were evaluated by Artama (2005) which showed 26 malformations in 939 pregnancies corresponding to a unsuspicious malformation rate of 2.8%. Holmes (2000) examined 57 children of mothers who reported a history of epilepsy but were not treated nor suffered seizures during pregnancy. These children showed no impairment of intellectual development and no dysmorphism of face and fingers that are often seen after anticonvulsive therapy in pregnancy. Adab (2004), however, reported that verbal IQ was significantly more often lower (<70), where more than five generalized tonic-clonic seizures had occured during pregnancy, irrespective of any antiepileptic treatment.

2.10.13   Carbamazepine

Carbamazepine has structural similarities to tricyclic antidepressant medications and is used for grand mal seizures, focal and complex focal seizures, as a phasic prophylactic and mood stabilizer, and for trigeminal neuralgia. As with other antiepileptic agents, the anticonvulsive effect of carbamazepine is explained by its membrane-stabilizing ability.

Carbamazepine is well absorbed after oral administration, binds readily to proteins, and has a plasma half-life of 1–2 days. In the fetus, 50–80% of the maternal concentration is attained. The ratio of concentration to dose of carbamazepine decreases down to 40% during the third trimester and can necessitate a dose increase for adjustment (Sabers 2009).

The effectiveness of oral contraceptives can be reduced by the marked induction of the cytochrome P450 enzyme (Chapter 2.10.2).

Typical malformations

Like other classic antiepileptic drugs, carbamazepine has a teratogenic effect not only in animals but also in humans. However, according to currently available studies, the malformation rate is judged to be only slightly increased (Harden 2009b). A specific carbamazepine syndrome had been postulated towards the end of the 1980s and included epicanthus, upward slanting eyes, short nose, elongated philtrum, hypoplasia of the distal phalanges, microcephaly, and developmental delay (Jones 1989). Other investigators could not confirm the specificity of these anomalies or failed to find an accumulation of hypoplasias of the distal phalanges. Typical for carbamazepine, though less frequently seen compared with VPA, is the risk for neural tube defects. Meningomyelocele (spina bifida) has been estimated to occur 2.6 times more frequently (95% CI 1.2–5.3) with carbamazepine monotherapy compared to those not exposed to any antiepileptic drug (Jentink 2010b). This association was confirmed in a case-control study from the U.S. National Birth Defects Prevention Study, where the adjusted odds ratio for NTD's was 5.0 (95% CI 1.9–12.7) (Werler 2011). Other malformations that had been reported to be increased include cleft palate, anomalies of heart and limbs, hip problems, inguinal hernia, and hypospadias (Harden 2009b, Ornoy 1996). Vajda (2013a), using the Australian Register of Antiepileptic Drugs in Pregnancy, found a statistically significant association between carbamazepine and renal anomalies.

However, a 2010 review of eight cohort studies as well as the European birth defects monitoring program (EUROCAT) did not find clear-cut evidence for additional specific malformations other than spina bifida (Jentink 2010b) although power was limited for more rare defects.

Frequency of malformations

According to a meta-analysis encompassing 1,255 exposed pregnant women, the rate major malformation rate is doubled with carbamazepine from about 2 to 5% (Matalon 2002). However, the Belfast UK Epilepsy and Pregnancy Register revealed only a 2.2% rate of major malformations when carbamazine was used as monotherapy in 900 pregnancies (Morrow 2006). Also, a Finnish study did not see a significantly increased risk of major malformations, when more than 900 pregnant women were studied who were primarily exposed to carbamazepine monotherapy (Artama 2005). Kaaja (2003) compared 740 children who had been exposed prenatally to antiepileptic drugs with 239 children whose mother had a history of epilepsy, but were not treated during their pregnancy. A significantly increased risk for major malformations was found, only when carbamazepine was used in combination but not as monotherapy.

A meta-analysis looking at 59 studies and epilepsy registries covering more than 65,000 pregnancies in epileptic mothers, indicated a malformation rate of 5.7% (95% CI 3.71–7.65) for monotherapy with carbamazepine (Meador 2008), a rate significantly higher than that seen in non-exposed mothers. In the North American Antiepileptic Drug in Pregnancy Registry, a 3.0% rate of major malformations was reported in 1,033 first-trimester carbamazepine monotherapy exposed compared

Pregnancy

2.10 Epilepsy and antiepileptic medications

to 1.1% in a healthy control group (http://www2.massgeneral.org/aed/newsletter/Spring2012newsletter.pdf). A review of cohort studies calculated the risk for major malformations in carbamazepine exposed pregnancies to be 3.3% (Jentink 2010b). In an analysis of 1,402 prospectively identified monotherapy carbamazepine exposed pregnancies in the EURAP Epilepsy and Pregnancy Registry, a dose response relationship was seen – with a malformation rate at 1 year of age of 3.4% for infants whose mothers took <400 mg/day, a rate of 5.3% for mothers on doses between 400 and 1,000 mg/day, and a rate of 8.7% for doses at or above 1000 mg/day (Tomson 2011).

Other somatic anomalies

Holmes (2001) and a pediatrician trained in dymorphologic disorders checked 316 newborns whose mothers had been treated with antiepileptic medications. They looked for one or more of the following characteristics: major malformations, microcephaly, growth restriction, facial dysmorphism, and finger hypoplasia. Results were compared with two control groups: 98 children whose mother had a history of epilepsy, but were not treated during pregnancy, and 508 children of healthy mothers. The rate of anomalies was significantly higher when a combination treatment was used with more than one antiepileptic drug. The result was not significantly different when carabamazepine was utilized as a monotherapy with 8/58 anomalies (14%).

Dean (2002) compared 149 prenatally exposed children with 38 (older) siblings whose mothers had not yet taken antiepileptic drugs during their pregnancy. Monotherapy with carbamazepine resulted in a higher, but not statistically significant risk for major malformations (11 versus 5%). However, the frequency of facial dysmorphism was significantly higher in the group exposed to carbamazepine as compared to their non-exposed siblings (60 versus 25%).

Diav-Citrin (2001) found that birth weight was reduced on average by 250 g when they evaluated the data of 210 carbamazepine-exposed pregnant women. A Swedish group noted a decreased head circumference, especially with carbamazepine, and to a smaller degree with VPA, but not with other antiepileptic drugs (Almgren 2009). A case report describes a boy who displayed symptoms of a cholestatic hepatitis for 5 weeks after birth, and whose mother had been treated with a monotherapy of carbamazepine during pregnancy and lactation (Frey 2002). With regard to vitamin K deficiency in the newborn see Section 2.10.11.

Functional disturbances

Dean (2002) observed significant effects regarding a delay in postnatal development, anomalies in behavior, and other abnormalities in later childhood (visual disturbances, otitis media, and joint problems). While the results of this study should be viewed with caution because of limitations in case numbers and methodology, the high number of affected children is of concern. Ornoy (1996) noted an impairment of cognitive development, especially in children who also displayed facial dysmorphism. In contrast, Gaily (2004) did not see a reduction in verbal and nonverbal IQ in 86 children after monotherapy with carbamazepine when compared to a nonexposed control group. Harden (2009b) came to a similar conclusion in their review.

A study with 309 children at the age of 3 years also found no significant medication effect in the carbamazepine subgroup with regard to IQ values (Meador 2009). In a sub-segment of this study, extent and quality of cognitive originality at the age of 3 were not negatively impacted when compared to VPA (McVearry 2009). Another investigation with 210 children noted a higher rate of developmental delay with carbamazepine (20.4%), in contrast to lamotrigine (2.9%) and controls (4.5%) (Cummings 2011). This effect was clearly less pronounced than with the valproate group (39.6%).

Recommendation. The contradictory, and to some degree negative, results regarding the overall risk of malformations with carbamazepine should not obscure the repeatedly observed risk of specific anomalies such as spina bifida, or lead to the false conclusion that teratogenicity is absent. If epilepsy requiring treatment and control has been achieved with carbamazepine, the medication can and should be continued in pregnancy. Monotherapy should be the aim. The level of medication has to be checked on a regular basis. The daily dose should be as low as therapeutically possible. In addition, liver and kidney function as well as hematological parameters need to be monitored in the pregnant patient. When treatment is continued until birth, it is possible that the newborn may be affected; thus clinical symptoms should be looked for during the first days of life. Treatment with carbamazepine during the first trimester does not justify a risk-based termination (Chapter 1.15). As an additional precaution a follow-up sonography should be offered.

Regarding the extended folic acid prophylaxis when planning a pregnancy see Section 2.10.10, and with regard to vitamin K prophylaxis of the newborn see Section 2.10.11.

Carbamazepine should be replaced by other medications for psychiatric and non-epileptic indications.

2.10.14   Clobazam and clonazepam

The benzodiazepines, *clobazam* and *clonazepam*, have been approved as antiepileptic medications, clobazam also as an anxiolytic. Few data are available about the application of clobazam in pregnancy. Thus experience with other benzodiazepines has to be referred to (Chapter 2.11). A meta-analysis of the use of benzodiazepines in the first trimester showed no problems when data from cohort studies were analyzed. However, analysis of all data from case-control studies displayed a higher rate of major malformations, specifically isolated oral clefts (Dolovich 1998). An update of this meta-analysis (Enato 2011) of cohort studies encompassing more than 3,000 pregnant women, failed to show a higher risk of malformations. Primarily, the drugs evaluated were *alprazolam*, *chlordiazepoxide*, *diazepam*, and *oxazepam*. The doubling of risk for oral clefts as suggested by case-control studies indicates that for 1,000 embryos and fetuses exposed during the first trimester, one extra oral cleft is to be expected.

With regard to clonazepam, experiences have been published for about 300 pregnant women mostly during the first trimester (Lin 2004, Vajda 2003, Weinstock 2001, Ornoy 1998). Observed anomalies such as tetralogy of Fallot, microcephaly, and various forms of dysmorphism do not indicate a specific pattern, nor is their frequency alarming. An

Pregnancy

2.10 Epilepsy and antiepileptic medications

observation not confirmed by others describes a paralytic ileus during the third trimester, when long-term therapy with clonazepam had been conducted (Haeusler 1995). The symptoms of the newborn improved shortly after birth. The North American Antiepileptic Drug in Pregnancy Registry reported two major malformations in 64 first trimester clonazepam monotherapy exposed (3.1%) in comparison to 1.1% in a healthy control group (http://www2.massgeneral.org/aed/newsletter/Spring2012newsletter.pdf).

Available data do not suggest an appreciable teratogenic potential. In the newborn, similar adjustment problems have to be expected as with diazepam, where treatment has been long-term and until birth. On the one hand neonatal respiratory depression is possible, on the other hand, after long-term exposure, the newborn may exhibit restlessness, tremor, muscular hypertonicity, vomiting and diarrhea. Seizures are possible in the neonatal period, and a floppy infant syndrome may last months with muscle weakness, lethargy, disturbances in temperature regulation, and sucking weakness.

> **Recommendation.** If there is an indication for clonazepam, treatment may also be conducted during the first trimester. If a long-term therapy has been instituted, especially during the last trimester, the newborn should be observed for possible symptoms at least for two days. The same holds for a high dose during labor that may lead to a respiratory depression. Treatment with clobazam or clonazepam does not justify a risk-based termination (Chapter 1.15).

2.10.15   Eslicarbazepine

Eslicarbazepine, the main metabolite of eslicarbazepine acetate, is a carboxamide derivative like *carbamazepine* and *oxcarbazepine*. It is used for the management of focal seizures. There are not sufficient experiences about its application in pregnancy; no case reports of human teratogenicity have been reported.

> **Recommendation.** Eslicarbazepine cannot be recommended due to a lack of experience. As with other antiepileptic drugs a higher risk of malformation cannot be excluded. The (unintended) application during the first trimester is not a justification for a risk-based termination (Chapter 1.15). A follow-up sonography should be offered to confirm the normal development of the fetus.

2.10.16   Ethosuximide and other succinimides

Ethosuximide is exclusively effective for absence seizures (petit mal). Only a small fraction of it is bound by plasma proteins.

Few reports address the use of ethosuximide in pregnancy. Typical patterns of malformation were not observed in the offspring of 57 treated women (Lindhout 1992). Another case collection of 18 women exposed during the first trimester did not show evidence of malformations (Rosa 1995, cited by Briggs 2011). While available reports do not allow for a differentiated risk assessment, a significant risk potential does not appear to be present. The higher tendency of neonatal bleeding problems due to vitamin K antagonism is discussed in Section 2.10.11.

Experiences with the *succinimides*, *mesuximide* and *phensuximide* are insufficient regarding pregnancy.

> **Recommendation.** If ethosuximide is indicated for petit mal seizures, it may be continued during pregnancy. Mesuximide and phensuximide are less well examined and thus not recommended. Monotherapy should be aimed for. The medication level needs to be monitored on a regular basis. The daily dose should be as low as therapeutically possible. When treatment continues until birth, it is possible that the newborn may be affected. Thus the neonate should be monitored clinically for the first few days. During pregnancy, follow-up sonography should be offered to ascertain the normal development of the fetus.
> Regarding extended folic acid prophylaxis when planning a pregnancy see Section 2.10.10, and regarding vitamin K prophylaxis of the newborn see Section 2.10.11.

2.10.17   Felbamate

Felbamate is used for the management of the Lennox-Gastaut syndrome during childhood. The manufacturer has reported seven exposed pregnancies leading to the birth of four normal children, two terminations, and one miscarriage.

> **Recommendation.** Felbamate cannot be recommended due to the lack of sufficient experience. As is the case with other antiepileptic drugs, especially combination drugs, a higher risk of malformation cannot be excluded. An (unintended) exposure during the first trimester does not justify a risk-based termination (Chapter 1.15). A follow-up sonography should be offered to ascertain the normal development of the fetus.

2.10.18   Gabapentin

Gabapentin is primarily used to treat focal epilepsy and for neuropathic pain. It circulates freely in the blood stream, unbound by proteins. There are several dozen cases available from a prescription study (Wilton 2002) and from the Australian Registry for Epilepsy and Pregnancy. All these prospectively and retrospectively collected reports contain four major malformations: one child with holoprosencephaly and cyclopia (Rosa 1995), another with atresia of the external auditory canal (cited by Briggs 2011; both in combination with other anticonvulsants). The third child had hypospadias after combination therapy with VPA, and the fourth unilateral renal atresia after combination therapy with phenobarbital. The manufacturer's Gabapentin Pregnancy Registry reported on 39 gabapentin-exposed women with 48 pregnancy outcomes including previous pregnancies. Of these, 17 pregnancies were exposed to monotherapy at the time of conception, and one resulted in a child with unilateral renal agenesis. The other malformed infant (hypospadias) occurred in a pregnancy also exposed to VPA (Montouris 2003). The Belfast UK

Pregnancy

2.10 Epilepsy and antiepileptic medications

Epilepsy and Pregnancy Registry data reported one major malformation among 31 pregnancies treated with gabapentin monotherapy (3.2%) (Morrow 2006). Chambers (2005) reported 13 prenatally exposed newborns; two of these (one with monotherapy) showed facial dysmorphism similar to that seen with classic antiepileptic medications. The Danish Medical Birth Register study identified 59 gabapentin exposed pregnancies and one malformed infant for a rate of 1.7% (Molgaard-Nielsen 2011). Fujii (2013) reported on 223 pregnancies exposed to gabapentin as an anticonvulsant, or for treatment of pain or psychiatric indications, and found no evidence of an excess of major birth defects.

The North American Antiepileptic Drug in Pregnancy Registry has reported one major malformation in 145 pregnancies (0.7%) treated in the first trimester with gabapentin monotherapy in comparison to 1.1% in a healthy control group (http://www2.massgeneral.org/aed/newsletter/Spring2012newsletter.pdf).

Tomson (2009) suggest in their review of 250 pregnancies treated with gabapentin monotherapy that no specific pattern of major malformations, nor an accumulation of smaller anomalies or dysmorphism is evident. It has been reported that gabapentin was successfully used for hyperemesis gravidarum in seven pregnant women (Guttuso 2010). Two of the children were found to have anomalies (hydronephrosis, tethered spinal cord). Case numbers and uneven methodology of the data currently available are insufficient to confirm or exclude a risk. Animal experiments do not provide evidence that gabapentin is teratogenic.

> **Recommendation.** According to available clinical data and results from animal experiments, it appears that the teratogenic risk of gabapentin is not higher, but perhaps even lower, when compared to classic antiepileptic medications. It may be used to treat epilepsy in pregnancy recognizing that a teratogenic risk has not been fully excluded. The combination with VPA is to be avoided. In the situation of non-epileptic indications, the appropriate medication for the specific indication should be prefered, such as pain medication, antiemetics, or psychopharmaceuticals. The use of gabapentin during the first trimester does not justify a risk-based termination (Chapter 1.15). Follow-up sonography should be offered to ascertain the normal development of the fetus.

2.10.19   Lacosamide

Lacosamide is an adjunct medication for focal seizures. Teratogenicity was not observed in animal experiments. A small case series with seven prospectively, and two retrospectively documented pregnancies with lacosamide, disclosed fetuses and children with anomalies (two cases of mild hydronephrosis, hemangioma, cryptorchidism) and normal appearing newborns (Hoeltzenbein 2011).

> **Recommendation.** Lacosamide cannot be recommended in view of the lack of experience. Treatment in the first trimester does not justify a risk-based termination (Chapter 1.15). As with other antiepileptic drugs, when used in combination with therapy, a higher risk of malformation has to be expected. A follow-up sonography should be offered.

2.10.20   Lamotrigine

Lamotrigine is administered in patients with partial and secondary generalized tonic-clonic seizures as well as to prevent recurrences in patients with bipolar psychiatric disorders. Chemically, lamotrigine is a phenyltriazine that inhibits dihydrolfolic acid reductase. Nevertheless, it does not appear to act as a folic acid antagonist in adults. Protein binding of lamotrigine is about 58% and thus clearly lower than with classic anticonvulsants.

In contrast to VPA, lamotrigine has not been reported to impact menstrual cyclicity and fertility in a significant way. When women with polycystic ovary syndrome (PCOS) are switched from VPA to lamotrigine, their symptoms improve (for a review of gender-specific pharmacology see Schmitz 2003, Isojärvi 1998). A slight impairment of the activity of oral contraceptives is possible as enzyme activity is stimulated (Section 2.10.2). Estrogenic contraceptives can enhance the metabolism of lamotrigine and thus increase the potential for seizures. Also, when contraceptives are discontinued, rising lamotrigine concentrations can lead to toxic side effects (Dutton 2008), and/or an ensuing pregnancy may be exposed to unintentionally high lamotrigine concentrations.

Clearance of lamotrigine is markedly increased during pregnancy, especially during the second trimester with a maximum rise of 264%. To avoid a higher tendency for seizures, monthly determinations of serum levels are necessary to direct dose adjustments (Fotopoulou 2009, Sabers 2009). The gestational increases in medication dose can lead to toxic symptoms after delivery, if the dose is not adjusted quickly. Both during pregnancy and when taking oral contraceptives, the pharmacokinetics of lamotrigine appears to be influenced by enzyme induction involving the 2-N-glucuronide pathway (Ohman 2008).

Toxicology

Case series and pregnancy registries involving several thousand pregnancies describing outcomes following lamotrigine monotherapy, have not shown clear evidence of teratogenic effects (GlaxoSmithKline 2010, Hunt 2009, Dolk 2008 – updated 2010, Vajda 2010a, Mølgaard-Nielsen 2011). The Lamotrigine Pregnancy Registry conducted by the manufacturer contains 1,558 prospectively captured pregnant women treated with monotherapy during the first trimester. The Registry's final report showed a major malformation rate of 2.2% for monotherapy (95% CI 1.6–31.0), while the rate was 10.7% when lamotrigine was used in combination with VPA (Cunnington 2011).

The Belfast UK Epilepsy and Pregnancy Register noted a 2.4% rate of major malformations in 1,229 pregnancies after monotherapy; these included one cleft lip and palate defect (Hunt 2009). It cannot be excluded that the Belfast UK and manufacturer's Registries may have overlapping data. The Belfast data revealed a significantly higher risk of malformations of 5.4% when the dose exceeded 200 mg/day (Morrow 2006). The same pattern was also seen in 1,280 monotherapy lamotrigine exposed pregnancies in the EURAP Registry, with a rate of 2.0% malformed at follow-up to 1 year of age at a prenatal dose <300 mg/day, whereas the rate was 4.5% for doses at or above 300 mg (Tomson 2011). This dose relationship could not be confirmed by the data of the manufacturer or the Australian Epilepsy Registry (Vajda 2010a).

The 2012 newsletter of the North American Antiepileptic Drug in Pregnancy Registry indicated that the malformation rate with monotherapy was 2.0% in 1,562 pregnancies, compared to 1.1% in the unexposed (http://www2.massgeneral.org/aed/newsletter/Spring2012newsletter.pdf). However, this same Registry has suggested that there is an excess of isolated oral clefts with lamotrigine monotherapy, with seven affected infants in 1,562 exposed (0.44%), estimated to be six fold higher than the general population risk (Holmes 2008, 2012). This observation was not confirmed in other studies: the rate of oral clefts was 0.1% in 1,151 exposed in the UK and Ireland Registers, 0.1% of 1,558 exposed in the manufacturer's Lamotrigine Pregnancy Registry, 0.2% in 1,280 exposed in the EURAP Registry, and 0.1% of 1,019 exposed in the Denmark population based study (Cunnington 2011, Tomson 2011, Mølgaard-Nielsen 2011, Hunt 2009). Nonetheless, a sufficiently powered case-control study is needed to confirm or refute the suggested association.

In summary, there is no clear evidence of an increased risk overall or a risk of specific patterns of major malformations for lamotrigine.

An investigation with 210 children noted no higher rate of developmental delay in young children with prenatal lamotrigine exposure (2.9%) compared to controls (4.5%) (Cummings 2011). In addition, a study from the Australian Pregnancy Register (Nadebaum 2011) found no difference in mean language scores of children exposed to lamotrigine monotherapy compared to the normal range.

Animal experiments have not demonstrated evidence for teratogenicity.

Recommendation. Lamotrigine is currently the antiepileptic medication with the largest amount of data that appear not to be concerning. If applicable, it should be preferred when a pregnancy is planned, as neither animal experiments nor appreciable clinical data suggest teratogenicity when used in monotherapy. Especially if VPA therapy is conducted, a change to lamotrigine is to be aimed for prior to pregnancy. A follow-up sonography can be offered to ascertain the normal development of the fetus. The significant increase of the lamotrigine clearance during pregnancy requires monthly determination of serum levels with corresponding dose adjustments, and after delivery, an appropriate lowering of the dose. Lamotrigine can also be used in the interval to prevent recurrences in pregnant patients with bipolar disease.

2.10.21   Levetiracetam

Levetiracetam is used for focal and generalized epilepsy. With a steady dose, its level decreases during pregnancy to 40–50%, apparently due to increased renal excretion (López-Fraile 2009, Westin 2008, Tomson 2007). Thus monitoring of its levels and corresponding dose adjustment are indicated during pregnancy; after birth, these changes need to be reversed again.

The UK and Ireland Epilepsy and Pregnancy Registers found two major malformations in 304 pregnancies managed by monotherapy (0.7%), while the rate in 367 polytherapy exposed pregnancies was 5.6% – highest in combination with VPA or carbamazepine (Mawhinney 2013). The North American Antiepileptic Drug in Pregnancy Registry noted 11 major malformations in 450 pregnancies (2.4%) with monotherapy compared to 1.1% in the healthy control group (http://www2.massgeneral.org/aed/newsletter/Spring2012newsletter.pdf).

Overall there are more than 250 analyzed pregnancies from a number of case series and registries including a report of about 95 pregnancies from the manufacturer's registry (Bronstein 2007), that were summarized in two reviews (Longo 2009, Tomson 2009). Most of the patients were treated with antiepileptic combination therapy. Observed malformations did not indicate a specific risk in terms of frequency and extent of malformations; defects were seen primarily with combination therapies. In the UK Epilepsy and Pregnancy Registry cohorts, 51 young children were evaluated for developmental delay and compared to 97 general population children. Similarly, in the Danish Medical Birth Register, among 58 levetiracetam exposed pregnancies, no malformations were noted (Mølgaard-Nielsen 2011).

Relative to neurodevelopmental outcomes, no significant differences were found in the proportion who fell below the average range on the standard developmental quotient (8%) compared to controls (Shallcross 2011).

Animal experiments with rats and rabbits have shown minor limb deformities.

> **Recommendation.** If epilepsy necessitates therapy and is well managed with levetiracetam, the medication may be continued in pregnancy, if the current residual uncertainty about its teratogenic risk is acceptable. A combination with VPA needs to be avoided. Treatment in the first trimester is not a justification for a risk-based termination (Chapter 1.15). A follow-up sonography should be offered to ascertain a normal development of the fetus.

2.10.22   Oxcarbazepine

Oxcarbazepine is used for focal epilepsy. While a structural derivative of carbamazepine it is not degradated like carbamazepine via (embryo-) toxic epoxide metabolites, but is reduced to the pharmacologically active monohydroxy derivatives (MHD) and carbamazepine-10, 11trans-dihydrodiol (DHD). Only about 40% of oxcarbazepine is bound to protein. Under steady-state conditions plasma contains mostly the active MHD (Mazzucchelli 2006). Induction of enzymes may lead to oral contraceptive failure. Thus hormonal contraceptives should not be used as primary methods of contraception when taking this drug (Section 2.10.2). The concentration/dose ratio decreases to nearly 40% in the third trimester (Sabers 2009, Christensen 2006) necessitating a dose adjustment during pregnancy as well as after delivery.

Levels in the umbilical cord are similar to those in maternal blood.

Toxicology

Kaaja (2003) found one major malformation in an investigation that included nine children who had been exposed prenatally to oxcarbazepine. This result (1/9 = 11%) was thought to be a significant elevation when compared to the controls with 239 children whose mothers had a history of epilepsy, but were not treated. Another study from Finland describes one urogenital defect among 99 pregnancies treated with monotherapy (Artama 2005). Some of these 99 pregnancies may have already been reported by Kaaja (2003).

Meischenguiser (2004) observed only one major malformation among 55 newborns (20 with combination therapy, 35 with monotherapy), namely a heart defect, in combination therapy with phenobarbital. All children in the monotherapy group were healthy. These 55 case reports

Pregnancy

2.10 Epilepsy and antiepileptic medications

apparently contained 42 children also described by Rabinowicz (2002). Sabers (2004) detected two heart defects in 37 pregnancies (one of them in combination therapy with *lamotrigine*). A review by Montouris (2005) calculated a malformation frequency of 2.4% (6/248) with monotherapy using oxcarbazepine. There were no malformations reported in a smaller case series by Eisenschenk (2006).

Tomson (2009) analyzed about 300 pregnancies from case series and registries, and found four major malformations with mono-therapy. A recent study from Denmark did not detect an increase in malformations when looking at 393 prenatally exposed children (Mølgaard-Nielsen 2011). The North American Antiepileptic Drug in Pregnancy Registry reported four major malformations in 182 first trimester oxcarbazepine monotherapy exposed (2.2%), compared to 1.1% in an unexposed comparison group (http://www2.massgeneral. org/aed/newsletter/Spring2012newsletter.pdf).

Another observation was the low birth rate, when one partner was treated with oxcarbazepine (Artama 2006).

In animal studies oxcarbazepine has teratogenic effects. Cranio-facial, cardiovascular, and skeletal changes were observed in rats at doses (adjusted to body surface) that correspond to human therapeutic levels.

Recommendation. If epilepsy requires treatment and is well managed with oxcarbazepine, treatment may be continued with the medication, if the current uncertainty about the teratogenic risk is acceptable. Combination with VPA must be avoided. Oxcarbazepine treatment in the first trimester does not justify a risk-based termination (Chapter 1.15). A follow-up sonography should be offered to ascertain the normal development of the fetus.

Regarding the extended folic acid prophylaxis when planning a pregnancy, see Section 2.10.10, and regarding vitamin K prophylaxis of the newborn, see Section 2.10.11.

2.10.23   Phenobarbital and primidone

Among the barbiturates, primarily *phenobarbital* and *primidone* have been used in the management of epilepsy. Primidone is converted to the anticonvulsant metabolites phenobarbital and phenylethylmalonamide. *Barbexaclone* is a compound of phenobarbital and levopropylhexedrine, a psychostimulant that lessens the sedative effect of the barbiturate.

Phenobarbitol and primidone have been successfully administered in focal epilepsy and grand mal seizures. Phenobarbital has been utilized as a sedative and anticonvulsive for more than 100 years (Hauptmann 1912), which provides extensive experience in pregnancy. Oral pheno-barbital is well absorbed. In blood about 50% is bound to protein. During pregnancy the free, unbound portion of the medication drops notably. The kidneys excrete about 25% unchanged, and 75% after oxidation and metabolization. The half-life is about 2–6 days.

Regarding the inhibition of oral contraceptives see Section 2.10.2.

Phenobarbital reaches the fetus rapidly and stimulates fetal liver enzymes especially during the perinatal period. This also holds for the glu-curonidating enzymes that are responsible for the excretion of bilirubin.

Typical malformations

Heinonen (1977) did not detect evidence of teratogenicity in 1,415 pregnant women who had been treated with phenobarbital during the first trimester. In contrast, they found a slightly increased risk for cardiovascular defects with other barbiturates. Jones (1992) diagnosed facial dysmorphism in seven of 46 newborns who had been prenatally exposed. Dysmorphism is also known with other antiepileptic medications and includes epicanthus, hypertelorism, flat nasal bridge, and an upturned nasal tip. Eleven of these children exhibited hypoplastic fingernails and three of 16 showed a delay in development. Already during the 1970s, reports appeared describing intrauterine and postnatal delays in growth when phenobarbital had been used in pregnancy. In contrast to long-term antiepileptic use, single dose applications of barbiturates (other than phenobarbital) for example, in the context of anesthesia, are unlikely to be teratogenic.

Frequency of major malformations

Samrén (1999) did not find that higher rates of malformation occurred with monotherapy of phenobarbital (5/172 = 3%) or primidone (1/151 = 1%). Two other studies reported a 5% malformation rate with phenobarbital monotherapy (Canger 1999, Kaneko 1999). Holmes (2004) examined the North American Antiepileptic Drug in Pregnancy Registry noted 11 major malformations in 199 first trimester phenobarbital monotherapy exposed pregancies (5.5%) compared to 1.1% in 442 unexposed (http://www2.massgeneral.org/aed/newsletter/Spring2012newsletter.pdf). The authors discussed the frequently neglected issue that in poor countries no alternatives are available to the inexpensive phenobarbital, and undesirable side effects have to be accepted or remain unnoted. Some investigators point out that caffeine in combination with phenobarbital additionally increases the malformation risk (Samrén 1999). A review with a meta-analysis that incorporated 59 studies calculated a malformation risk of 4.9% after monotherapy. This value was not significantly increased compared to non-exposed control groups (Meador 2008). Harden (2009b) summarized in their review that phenobarbital may possibly increase the risk of heart defects. Furthermore, Tomson (2011) have demonstrated that in 217 monotherapy exposed pregnancies, the rate of major malformations at 1 year of age was 5.4% in infants born to women who took <150 mg/day, while the rate was 13.7% in infants born to mothers on higher doses.

Other developmental anomalies

Holmes (2001) and a pediatrician trained in dymorphologic disorders checked 316 newborns whose mothers had been treated with antiepileptic medications looking for one or more of the following characteristics: major malformations, microcephaly, growth restriction, facial dysmorphism, and finger hypoplasia. Results were compared with two control groups: 98 children whose mothers had a history of epilepsy but did not receive treatment during pregnancy, and 508 children of healthy mothers. A significantly increased proportion of children (17/64 = 27%) whose mothers had received phenobarbital monotherapy displayed at least one of the above named developmental anomalies. Dean (2002) compared 149 prenatally exposed children with 38 (older) siblings whose mothers had not yet taken antiepileptic drugs during their pregnancy. An increase in the rate of major malformations was noted for monotherapy with phenobarbital, but did not reach statistical

Pregnancy

2.10 Epilepsy and antiepileptic medications

significance (10% versus 5%). Facial dysmorphism (21%) and delays in development (10%) were not more common than in the untreated control group.

Withdrawal symptoms were observed in newborns whose mothers took 60–300 mg/day during the last months of pregnancy. Hyper-irritability and tremor may appear delayed 3–14 days after birth. Clinical symptoms were reported to be more common in the subset of 23 infants with higher serum levels of phenobarbital postpartum (Zuppa 2011).

Also noted was that phenobarbital may disrupt the metabolism of ste-roids, vitamin D and vitamin K, leading to hypocalcemia, clotting and bleeding disorders in the newborn (Section 2.10.11). The comparison of treatment with phenobarbital in the third trimester versus placebo to prevent intracranial hemorrhage in 436 preterm infants did not show a benefit from the treatment, but in a follow-up at 18–22 months corrected age the treatment was also not associated with impairments in neuro-logic development (Shankaran 2002).

Numerous single cases and results of epidemiologic studies (Adams 2004, van der Pol 1991) suggest that after antiepileptic treatment with phenobarbital delays in mental development, notably in speech develop-ment, are more common than in healthy controls. Koch (1999) reeval-uated 116 children at the age of 11–18 years. They found a significantly reduced intelligence quotient (IQ), when combination therapy with phe-nobarbital and primidone had been used during pregnancy. The IQ was lower with an increasing dose of primidone. The result was independent of socio-economic status. Nevertheless, an impact of maternal IQ cannot be excluded. In a review of the prenatal influence of antiepileptic med-ications, Harden (2009b) indicate that a negative effect upon cognitive function is possible.

One case of sirenomelia in a still born from a mother who was on phenobarbital (0.1 g/day), and carbamazepine (0.4 g/day) during the first four months of her pregnancy, followed by only phenobarbital (0.1 g/day) until delivery was reported from a hospital in Craiova, Romania (Tica 2013).

Recommendation. In summary, the risk of malformations with an antiepileptic monotherapy of phenobarbital does not exceed the background risk by twofold or more. An impact upon the mental development cannot be excluded. Primidone should be assessed similar to phenobarbital. If a new treatment is started, phe-nobarbital and primidone are not drugs of choice for women in their reproductive years. However, if treatment for epilepsy is required and the condition is well man-aged with these medications, they may be continued during pregnancy as long as their risks are being considered. The aim should be monotherapy. The medication level needs to be regularly monitored. The daily dose should be effective, yet kept as low as possible. When therapy continues until birth, effects on the newborn are possible. Therefore the newborn needs to be observed for clinical symptoms during the first days of life. A high dose during labor can lead to respiratory depres-sion in the neonate. Treatment with barbiturates during the first trimester does not justify a risk-based termination (Chapter 1.15). A follow-up sonography should be offered to ascertain the normal development of the fetus.

Regarding the extended folic acid prophylaxis when planning a pregnancy, see Section 2.10.10, and regarding vitamin K prophylaxis of the newborn, see Section 2.10.11.

2.10.24   Phenytoin

Phenytoin and *mephenytoin* are hydantoins and have been used as antiepileptic treatments since 1938. They have a marked anticonvulsive potency and are effective in grand mal seizure, focal epilepsy, and also in the case of status epilepticus without showing sedative-hypnotic properties. On occasion phenytoin has been used for eclampsia (Friedman 1993). Phenytoin is inactivated in the liver by hydroxylation and its major metabolite is excreted by the kidneys. The half-life varies between 20 and 50 hours. Phenytoin is accumulated in fatty tissue. Its plasma concentration is lowered during pregnancy. During the last trimester, this process is in part compensated by an increase in the unbound fraction of the drug. The decreased plasma concentration has been viewed as a cause for a higher tendency for seizures in pregnancy. If necessary, the level of the unbound phenytoin fraction should be determined in the plasma. The interference with the effectiveness of oral contraceptives is discussed in Section 2.10.2. Fosphenytoin is a water-soluble that is administered intravenously to deliver phenytoin.

Typical malformations

Phenytoin's teratogenic potential was discovered in 1964 (Janz 1964), although it has not been replicated in all studies (Samrén 1999). Most commonly noted malformations include heart defects, cleft lip/palate, and urogenital anomalies. Early on, the typical malformations were labeled "fetal hydantoin syndrome" (Sections 2.10.5 and 2.10.6).

Frequency of major malformations

Kaaja (2003) examined prenatally exposed children and controls whose mothers had a history of epilepsy but were not treated. They found a malformation rate for phenytoin that was not significantly elevated at 2% (3/124). The Belfast UK Epilepsy and Pregnancy Registry showed that phenytoin in monotherapy could be linked to major malformations in 3.7% of 82 pregnancies (Morrow 2006). The North American Antiepileptic Drug in Pregnancy Registry noted 12 major malformations in 416 first-trimester phenytoin monotherapy exposed pregnancies (2.9%) compared to 1.1% in healthy controls (http://www2.massgeneral.org/aed/newsletter/Spring2012newsletter.pdf).

Other developmental anomalies

Dean (2002) compared 149 prenatally exposed children with 38 (older) siblings whose mothers had not taken antiepileptic drugs during pregnancy. An increase in the rate of major malformations was noted for phenytoin monotherapy (16% versus 5%), also facial dysmorphism was more common (52% versus 25%), but only the difference in postnatal developmental delay was statistically significant (33% versus 11%). The results of this study have to be viewed with some reservation, one reason being the small numbers of cases. On the other hand, the high number of affected children is of concern.

Holmes (2001) and a pediatrician trained in dymorphologic disorders checked 316 newborn whose mothers had been treated with antiepileptic medications looking for one or more of the following characteristics: major malformations, microcephaly, growth restriction, facial dysmorphism, and finger hypoplasia. Results were compared with two control groups: 98 children whose mothers had a history of epilepsy but did not receive treatment during pregnancy, and 508 children of healthy mothers. A significantly increased proportion of children (18/87 = 21%) whose mothers had received monotherapy with phenytoin displayed at least one of the above named developmental anomalies.

Limitations of cognitive development have been observed more often than expected in offspring after phenytoin exposure (Scolnik 1994, Vanoverloop 1992, Hättig 1987). Facial dysmorphism may suggest an increased risk for effects on cognitive performance (Orup 2000). Koch (1999) have reexamined 116 children at the ages of 11 to 18 and detected a significantly lower IQ, when combination therapy with phenytoin and primidone had been used during pregnancy. The result was independent of socio-economic status, but an influence of the maternal IQ cannot be excluded. A later review about prenatal influence of antiepileptics confirmed that a negative impact upon cognitive development is possible (Harden 2009b). One publication suggested conflicts in the development of the gender-specific identity of exposed offspring; however, other authors have not confirmed this (Dessens 1999).

Newborns that have been exposed to phenytoin can develop clotting problems due to vitamin K deficiency (Section 2.10.11).

Some publications address a possible risk of a transplacental carcinogenesis due to phenytoin: 12 prenatally exposed children were presented who had neuroectodermal tumors, six of them neuroblastomas (review in Briggs 2011). The case numbers are too small to prove a connection.

Recommendation. In summary, the risk of major malformations with antiepileptic monotherapy of phenytoin does not exceed more than twofold that of the background risk. An impact upon mental development cannot be excluded. Phenytoin is not an antiepileptic drug of choice when women in the reproductive years are started on therapy; it is, however, acceptable to continue its use during a pregnancy, if treatment for epilepsy is required and the condition well managed, as long as its risk is being considered. The aim should be a monotherapy. The medication dose needs to be monitored on a regular basis. The daily dose should be effective, yet kept as low as possible. When therapy continues until birth, effects on the newborn are possible. Therefore the newborn needs to be observed for clinical symptoms during the first days of life. A treatment with phenytoin during the first trimester does not justify a risk-based termination (Chapter 1.15). A follow-up sonography should be offered to ascertain the normal development of the fetus.

Regarding the extended folic acid prophylaxis when planning a pregnancy, see Section 2.10.10, and regarding vitamin K prophylaxis of the newborn, see Section 2.10.11.

2.10.25   Pregabalin

Pregabalin is used for the treatment of partial seizures with or without generalization and for neuronal pain. It is thought that its analgesic effect is mediated by a selective link to sub-units of voltage-gated calcium channels at the ends of the primarily afferent nocireceptors of the spinal cord. Further, pregabalin modulates the calcium influx at the nerve endings, resulting in a decreased release of stimulatory transmitting factors and a dampening of hyper excitation. An interaction with hormonal contraceptives could not be shown. In animal studies, skeletal anomalies were seen in rats and rabbits and neural tube effects in rats. In fetal rats, developmental problems were apparent already at plasma concentrations corresponding to the twofold therapeutic level in humans. Insufficient data are available about teratogenic effects in humans.

> **Recommendation.** With a lack of relevant experience pregabalin cannot be recommended in pregnancy. As with other antiepileptic medications, especially combination drugs, an increased risk of malformation cannot be excluded. An (unintended) exposure during the first trimester does not justify a risk-based termination (Chapter 1.15). A follow-up sonography should be offered to ascertain the normal development of the fetus.

2.10.26 Rufinamide

Rufinamide is a carboxamide derivative like carbamazepine and oxcarbazepine. It is used for seizure disorders in the context of the Lennox-Gastaut syndrome. Rufinamide induces the hepatic CYY3A4 enzyme activity and thereby reduces the effectiveness of oral contraceptives resulting potentially in an unwanted pregnancy. There is insufficient experience about its use in pregnancy.

> **Recommendation.** With a lack of relevant experience rufinamide cannot be recommended in pregnancy. As with other antiepileptic medications, especially combination drugs, an increased risk of malformation cannot be excluded. An (unintended) exposure during the first trimester does not justify a risk-based termination (Chapter 1.15). A follow-up sonography should be offered to ascertain the normal development of the fetus.

2.10.27 Sultiame

Sultiame is primarily used to treat focal epilepsy in children up to puberty. A greater than 30-year-old case collection describes 11 pregnant women, three of them suffering a miscarriage. It did not report on malformations. These data are insufficient to assess a risk for its use in pregnancy.

> **Recommendation.** With a lack of relevant experience sultiame cannot be recommended in pregnancy. As with other antiepileptic medications, especially combination drugs, an increased risk of malformation cannot be excluded. An (unintended) exposure during the first trimester does not justify a risk-based termination (Chapter 1.15). A follow-up sonography should be offered to ascertain the normal development of the fetus.

2.10.28 Tiagabine

Tiagabine acts as a selective reuptake inhibitor of gamma aminobutyric acid (GABA), an inhibitory neurotransmitter. Thus the increase of the level of extracellular GABA results in anticonvulsant activity. It is used to treat focal epilepsy. Most of it (96%) is bound by proteins. In a study by Leppik (1999) 22 patients exposed to tiagabine during pregnancy were identified; nine of which were delivered and among these, one breech delivered neonate with a hip dislocation was noted. Two additional exposed children from the Austrialian registry did not display malformations (Vajda 2003). In animal experiments rats developed facial and other anomalies when high doses (100 mg/kg/d) were administered.

> **Recommendation.** With a lack of relevant experience tiagabine cannot be recommended in pregnancy. As with other antiepileptic medications, especially combination drugs, an increased risk of malformation cannot be excluded. An (unintended) exposure during the first trimester does not justify a risk-based termination (Chapter 1.15). A follow-up sonography should be offered to ascertain the normal development of the fetus.

2.10.29   Topiramate

Topiramate is used to treat focal and generalized epilepsy. Only about 15% is bound to proteins. Enzyme induction in the liver leads to hormonal contraceptives failure. Thus non-hormonal contraceptives should be used as the primary choice to prevent pregnancy (Section 2.10.2). Due to increased glomerular filtration and enzymatic induction, the concentration/dose ratio of topiramate decreases until the third trimester by about 30–40% on average (Ohman 2009, Westin 2009). Thus blood level determinations are needed during pregnancy with appropriate dose adjustments, and subsequently, a downward dose correction after birth.

A population-based study in Denmark noted five major malformations in 108 topiramate exposed live births (4.6%) compared to 2.4% among unexposed in the entire cohort (Mølgaard-Nielsen 2011). Similar rates have been reported by the UK and Ireland Registers (Hunt 2008, Morrow 2006), the Australian Register (Vajda 2013a), a US claims database (Green 2012), and the North American Antiepileptic Drug in Pregnancy Registry which noted 15 major malformations in 359 first trimester topiramate monotherapy exposed pregnancies (4.2%) compared to 1.1% in healthy controls (http://www2.massgeneral.org/aed/newsletter/Spring2012newsletter.pdf).

However, the North American Registry has suggested that there may be an increased risk specifically for oral clefts, with five of these specific defects identified among the 15 malformed (Hernández-Díaz 2012). The UK Register also suggested, based on small numbers, that the rate of oral clefts was approximately 11 times the background rate (Hunt 2008). However, this and other registry studies are too limited in the number of topiramate monotherapy exposures to adequately address this question. An analysis of pooled data from two US multi-site case-control studies identified seven malformed infants with oral clefts, and prenatally exposed to topiramate which translated to a significantly elevated odds ratio of 5.4 (95% CI 1.5–20.1) compared to non-malformed controls (Margulis 2012).

Topiramate exposure has also been suggested to be associated with hypospadias in data from the Australia Register (Vajda 2011, 2013a), although the findings are based on a small number of the exposed and affected.

A case report describes a child with thumb aplasia on the right hand and thumb hypoplasia on the other hand, syndactyly of the second and third toes, and hypoplasia of the right orbicular muscle (Vila Ceren 2005). Another case report presents two siblings, both of them suffering a seizure after birth. The authors suggest that this was triggered by hypocalcaemia caused by an adrenal hypofunction due to topiramate (Gorman 2007).

A meta-analysis covering more than 400 analyzed pregnancies exposed to monotherapy does not provide clear evidence of either teratogenicity or safety (Day 2011).

Twenty-one percent of the newborns in the North American Registry whose mothers had used topiramate were small for gestational age on birth weight in comparison to 4.9% among unexposed, while there was no increase in preterm delivery (Hernández-Díaz 2010). This finding was also reported in another small study of 52 pregnancies (Ornoy 2008).

One small study of neurodevelopment in nine preschool age children prenatally exposed to topiramate compared to 18 unexposed children, suggested the exposed children did significantly worse that the comparison children, especially in cognitive functioning, but numbers were too small to draw definitive conclusions (Rihtman 2012).

Topiramate has teratogenic properties in animal models; at only 20% of the dose used therapeutically in humans (based on body surface) mice were noted to develop craniofacial defects; rats and rabbits displayed limb reduction defects.

> **Recommendation.** If epilepsy requires treatment and is well managed with topiramate, treatment may be continued with the medication, if the current uncertainty about the teratogenic risk is acceptable. Combination with VPA must be avoided. Topiramate treatment in the first trimester does not justify a risk-based termination (Chapter 1.15). A follow-up sonography should be offered to ascertain the normal development of the fetus.

Regarding the extended folic acid prophylaxis when planning a pregnancy, see Section 2.10.10, and regarding vitamin K prophylaxis of the newborn, see Section 2.10.11.

2.10.30   Valnoctamide

Valnoctamide is a structural isomer of valpromide, a derivative of the teratogenic VPA. In experimental studies, valnoctamide is reported to have a similar anticonvulsive effect as VPA; it has been applied to treat bipolar disorders in clinical studies. It is not metabolized to a free acid like VPA that is considered to have teratogenic potential, and thus it has been speculated that it may be safer. Animal experiments would suggest this, but human experience is lacking.

> **Recommendation.** With a lack of relevant experience, valnoctamide cannot be recommended. A treatment during the first trimester does not justify a risk-based termination (Chapter 1.15). As with other antiepileptic medications, especially combination drugs, an increased risk of malformation cannot be excluded. A follow-up sonography should be offered to ascertain the normal development of the fetus.

Pregnancy

2.10 Epilepsy and antiepileptic medications

2.10.31   Valproic acid

Valproic acid (VPA) (sodium valproate, 2-propylpentanoic acid) is a relatively newer drug of the classic antiepileptics that is used for various forms of epilepsy. Its anticonvulsant effectiveness was discovered in 1963. The therapeutic effect appears to be caused by an increase in the level of the inhibitory neurotransmitter GABA. VPA is also used in other neurological and psychiatric indications, such as bipolar disorder.

Oral VPA is well absorbed and 95% of it is bound to plasma proteins. Being lipophilic, VPA easily crosses the blood–brain barrier and the placenta.

At the end of a pregnancy, VPA is metabolized more by the liver, while less of it is bound in the plasma. Both effects could balance each other, so that the active available agent remains about stable (Nau 1981).

VPA blood levels in the umbilical cord are at birth 1.7 times higher than the maternal levels (Nau 1981). Newborns excrete VPA more slowly as their liver enzymes are not yet mature. Thus the half-life in newborns may be prolonged from 8–15 to 15–60 hours. VPA may possibly increase irregularities of the menstrual cycle, and has been linked to the polycystic ovary syndrome (PCOS) that is accompanied by infertility and increased testosterone levels (Isojärvi 1993). A negative impact on the effectiveness of oral contraceptives by the induction of enzyme has not been reported.

Typical malformations

In the 1980s a fetal valproate syndrome was defined that included dysmorphic facial features, such as epicanthus, thin arched eye brows, flat nasal bridge, short, upturned nose, flat philtrum, thin upper lip, as well as thin, overlapping fingers and toes, and hyperconvex nails (Kozma 2001). More important than single features is the clustering of typical anomalies which may become attenuated with time, making some features harder to recognize as the child grows older. In addition, trigonocephaly (an abnormal skull shape due to premature closure of the frontal suture) has been noted. This craniosynostosis may require surgical correction during the first months of life to prevent a negative impact upon cognitive development. Numerous case reports describe neural tube defects (Robert 1982) and other malformations such as preaxial limb deformities (Cole 2009, Rodriguez-Pinilla 2000, Sharony 1993, Robert 1992) that may include missing or double thumbs, radial aplasia, anomalies of ribs or vertebrae, heart defects, hypospadias (Rodriguez-Pinilla 2008), porencephaly, and other brain anomalies (Arpino 2000). Rodriguez-Pinilla (2000) calculated that the risk for missing or hypoplastic limb defects was about six times higher than in controls; accordingly, 0.4% of exposed children are affected.

A meta-analysis from pooled data looking at VPA and various malformations by Jentink (2010c) concluded that there was statistically significant evidence of associations between VPA exposure and spina bifida, atrial septal defect, cleft palate, hypospadias, polydactyly, and craniosynostosis. Similar significant associations were found by Vajda (2013a) except in relation to cleft palate and hypospadias, and by Werler (2011) in relation to neural tube defects, oral clefts, and hypospadias. Typically for VPA, there is primarily an up to 20-fold increased risk for spina bifida and other neural tube defects if the mother received treatment between the 17th and 28th day after conception (Dansky 1991). This indicates that about 1–2% of exposed children will be affected. Table 2.10.1 summarizes the most important anomalies linked with VPA.

Table 2.10.1 Congenital anomalies linked to prenatal treatment with VPA

Organ system	Anomaly
Neural tube	Spina bifida, anencephaly
Heart	Ventricular septal defect, atrial septal defect, aortic stenosis, ductus arteriosus apertus, *anomaly of right pulmonary artery*
Extremities	Radial ray deficiency, polydactyly, cleft hand, overlapping toes, camptodactyly *hypoplasia of ulna or tibia, missing fingers, oligodactyly*
Urogenital tract	Hypospadia, *renal hypoplasia, hydronephrosis, duplication of renal collecting system*
CNS	*Hydranencephaly, porencephaly, arachnoidal cysts, cerebral atrophy, partial agenesis of corpus callosum, septum pellucidum aplasia, lissencephaly, Dandy Walker anomaly*
Eyes	*Bilateral cataract, optical nerve hypoplasia, anomaly of lacrimal duct, microphthalmia, bilateral iris defect, corneal cloudiness*
Respiratory system	*Tracheomalacia, lung hypoplasia, extensive laryngeal hypoplasia, abnormal lobe formation of right lung*
Abdominal wall	*Omphalocele*
Skin	Capillary hemangiomas, *aplasia cutis of scalp*

Rare anomalies in italics; according to Kini 2006.

Frequency of major malformations

For monotherapy with VPA the overall malformation rate has been reported to be as high as 18% (Vajda 2010b), and thus is at least two-fold and up to more than four-fold higher than that of untreated pregnant women not suffering from epilepsy. The majority of investigations have demonstrated that the rate of malformation due to monotherapy VPA is significantly higher than monotherapy with any other antiepileptic medication (Vajda 2010b, Veiby 2009, Diav-Citrin 2008, Morrow 2006, Artama 2005, Wyszynski 2005, Alsdorf 2004, Wide 2004, Kaaja 2003, Mastroiacovo 1998, Samrén 1999, http://www2.massgeneral.org/aed/newsletter/Spring2012newsletter.pdf).

Thousands of VPA-exposed pregnancies have been summarized in some reviews and meta-analyses (e.g. Harden 2009b, Tomson 2009, Meador 2008).

One meta-analysis that included 59 studies and epilepsy registries with more than 65,000 pregnancies of epileptic women, determined a malformation rate of 17.6% (95% CI 5.25–30.03) for VPA monotherapy (Meador 2008). In comparison, for *carbamazepine* the rate was 5.7% (95% CI; 3.71–7.65). Both are significantly higher than the rate for non-exposed mothers. Rates were not significantly elevated for *lamotrigine, phenobarbital* and *phenytoin*, while for all the other antiepileptics case numbers were too low to determine the rate.

An assessment of eight cohort studies described 14 types of malformations that were significantly more common with VPA (Jentink 2010c). These 14 types were analyzed using data from European malformation registries to see if there was a link with maternal VPA therapy. Results indicated significantly higher risks for the following malformations after adjustment for other factors (odds ratios are provided): Spina bifida 12.7; atrial septum defect 2.5; cleft palate 5.2; hypospadias 4.8; polydactyly 2.2; craniosynostosis 6.8.

Two recent studies from the Australian and UK Registers have demonstrated that the risk for malformations is increased in women who have one child with a malformation, and stay on the same anticonvulsant in a subsequent pregnancy. This was especially true for VPA exposed pregnancies (Campbell 2013, Vajda 2013b).

Dose-response relation

Some studies have examined the risk of malformation in relation to the VPA dose. A significantly higher risk was seen when more than 1000 mg/day was administered or serum levels exceeded 70 µg/mL (Kaneko 1999, Samrén 1999, 1997, Mawhinney 2012). A study from Israel noted a rate of 21.9% malformations when the daily dose was 1000 mg or higher (including combination therapy) in comparison to 1.3% for <1000 mg/day (Diav-Citrin 2008). Similarly, Tomson (2011) in 1,010 monotherapy VPA pregnancies involved in the EURAP Registry, found the rate of major malformations was 5.6% at doses <700 mg/day, 10.4% at doses between 700 and 1500 mg/day, and 24.2% at doses at or above 1500 mg/day. Morrow (2006) found a higher risk of 9.1% major malformations when doses of >1000 mg VPA were used in monotherapy in comparison to lower dosing. However, the difference was not statistically significant. An especially marked increase in the risk for neural tube defects, heart malformations, cleft palate, and hypospadias was noted by Vajda (2005) when the daily dose exceeded 1,400 mg/day. They discuss different pathways of metabolism according to dose, resulting possibly in different teratogenic pathways. In a later publication, Vajda (2013a) further refined the association between higher doses of VPA and specific defects, suggesting that risk for spina bifida and hypospadias are specifically related to dose. However, some investigators have not found a threshold for dose or serum concentration (Kaaja 2003). Jentink (2010d) cautioned against underestimating the malformation risk when low doses of VPA are given during pregnancy, especially when compared to other antiepileptic agents.

Other abnormalities

Dean (2002) compared 149 prenatally exposed children with 38 (older) siblings whose mothers had not taken antiepileptic remedies during their pregnancy. For VPA monotherapy a significantly higher risk was seen for facial dysmorphism (70% versus 25%). Also diseases of childhood were more commonly noted, such as visual impairment, otitis media and joint problems. While the results of this study need to be looked at with some reservation, the high prevalence of affected children, both exposed and controls, is noteworthy. Authors of another study caution against an overestimation of facial dysmorphism (Kini 2006). They noted dysmorphism was most commonly linked with VPA, but also reported that 45% of children of untreated epileptic mothers displayed corresponding features.

Neonatal abnormalities

Fetal hypoxia with low Apgar values, microcephaly and diminished postnatal growth have been observed with VPA. A Swedish study found especially for carbamazepine, but to a lesser degree also for VPA, a decreased head circumference in contrast to all other antiepileptic drugs (Almgren 2009). Necrosis of liver cells has been reported in some children after maternal VPA therapy (Legius 1987), also bleeding due to fibrinogen deficiency and disrupted thrombocytic function (Bavoux 1994), and hypoglycemia of the newborn (Ebbesen 1998).

Mental development anomalies

Koch (1996) indicated that hyperexcitability and other neurologic abnormalities during the course of childhood correlate with the umbilical VPA concentration at birth. Some authors suggest an impairment of cognitive development (Ornoy 1996), especially in children with facial dysmorphism. Numerous publications of the past decade reported deficits in mental development, behavior problems such as attention deficit and hyperactivity, as well as autism-like symptoms (see below) when VPA was used.

An investigation of 57 children with an antiepileptic syndrome, of which 46 had been exposed to VPA, showed that 80% displayed delays in speech development, learning difficulties, and abnormal behavior. In 60% at least two autistic features could be found. Four children were diagnosed as having autism and another two children were diagnosed as having Asperger's syndrome (Moore 2000). Another study with 40 children of mothers who had used antiepileptic monotherapy detected a majority of anomalies in the VPA group. Gaily (2004) noted in 13 children who had been exposed to a VPA monotherapy, or combination therapy, that the verbal IQ was decreased, a finding not apparent in the 86 children who had been exposed to carbamazepine monotherapy. In contrast, another study showed that the type of maternal epilepsy and the occurrence of generalized tonic-clonic seizure during pregnancy, had no effect on the intelligence of children. Adab (2001) conducted a study that included 70 schoolchildren with prenatal exposure to VPA, and found that this group needed significantly more educational intervention. A follow-up examination showed a negative impact upon speech development (verbal IQ) in those children whose mother's dose had exceeded 800 mg/day. Dysmorphism was linked to a lower verbal IQ (<79): 55% of children with medium to severe dysmorphism had a verbal IQ of <79 compared to 22% with slight or no dysmorphism. Other antiepileptics did not reveal significant results, but five or more generalized tonic-clonic seizures during pregnancy correlated significantly with a lower verbal IQ, independent of the antiepileptic medication (Adab 2004). Eriksson (2005) detected a lower IQ in 13 children exposed to VPA than in non-exposed children, or children whose mothers had taken carbamazepine. In a review by Banach (2010), it was noted that more recent studies, such as one encompassing 42 VPA-exposed children (Bromley 2010), confirmed the higher risk with VPA in regard to different developmental parameters in two-year-olds in contrast to other antiepileptics, untreated epilepsies, and healthy control mothers. Twenty-nine percent of VPA-exposed children were found below the average on total development score, which as a proportion is 3.5 times higher than that seen in children of healthy mothers. In particular, daily doses of >900 mg increased the risk. Seizures during pregnancy had no negative impact on developmental score. Another study with 309 children evaluated at the age of 3 also noted significantly lower IQs in 53 VPA-exposed children, and predominantly in those where daily doses exceeded 1,000 mg. In contrast to children prenatally exposed to carbamazepine, lamotrigine, and phenytoin, children exposed to VPA displayed no correlation with maternal IQ values (Meador 2009). In a subgroup in this study, prenatally VPA-exposed children showed lower scores on cognitive originality at the age of three, in contrast to carbamazepine- and lamotrigine-exposed children (McVearry 2009).

Pregnancy

2.10 Epilepsy and antiepileptic medications

In a case study in 1994, Christianson (1994) linked autism spectrum disorders (ASD) to intrauterine VPA exposure. They presented two pairs of siblings: three of the children demonstrated global development disorders with speech impediments and dysmorphism, one of these children had also been diagnosed as having infantile austism; the fourth child showed mild dysmorphism and a reduced IQ, primarily verbal. Williams (2001) subsequently reported on six children with fetal valproate syndrome (FVS), cognitive deficits, and evidence of autistic symptoms. In an updated nested case-control study by Christensen (2013) in Denmark, 5,437 individuals with autism spectrum disorder were identified, and the estimated absolute risk of autism in the sample was 1.58%. Among the 432 children with prenatal exposure to VPA, the risk was 4.15% (adjusted hazard ratio 1.7, 95% CI 0.9–3.2).

The hypothesis of a link between VPA and autism is supported by observations that VPA is able to modify the expression of HoxA1 in the embryo, and allelic variants of the HoxA1 gene have been found in people with autism. Other teratogenic factors too, such as prenatal exposure to rubella infection, misoprostol, alcohol abuse, and thalidomide have been suspected to have the potential to induce autism-like symptoms. In the case of thalidomide, autistic symptoms were noted more frequently if the exposure had occurred during the time of neural tube closure (Stromland 1994). Neuropathologic studies have been reported about a human who had been exposed prenatally to VPA and also, in the context on animal experiments, about rats who had been exposed to VPA *in utero*. In both situations a lesion of the nuclei of the cranial nerves was identified in the brain stem, and also cerebellar anomalies with a decreased number of Purkinje cells (Arndt 2005, Rodier 1997). Other investigators have demonstrated severe alterations of serotonergic nerves in rats treated with VPA. Disruption of these nerves can also be observed in autistic patients (Miyazaki 2005).

> **Recommendation.** VPA is more toxic during pregnancy than any other antiepileptic medication based on current knowledge. It increases the risk of malformation by a factor of 2 to 4, and in addition, adversely affects mental development. If a VPA-affected child has been born, the risk of having another VPA-affected child has been empirically estimated to be about 50%. VPA should be strictly avoided during the reproductive years, the latest at the planning of a pregnancy; it can only be used in situations where other treatments for epilepsy have failed. If no alternative to VPA is available (such as lamotrigine, or even carbamazepine) monotherapy is to be preferred. The daily dose should be below 1000 mg and be distributed over 3–4 single doses. Plasma levels need to be monitored on a regular basis and should not exceed 70 µg/mL, if possible. With regard to the extended folic acid prophylaxis when planning a pregnancy see Section 2.10.10. Treatment with VPA does not justify a risk-based termination (Chapter 1.15). A follow-up sonography should be offered to ascertain the normal development of the fetus.

2.10.32   Vigabatrin

Vigabatrin is now only used in exceptional cases when all other antiepileptics (for focal epilepsy and West syndrome in childhood) have failed. It inhibits the GABA aminotransferase irreversibly, resulting in an increase in the level of the inhibitory neurotransmitter GABA in the central nervous system. Thereby abnormal discharges that trigger seizures will be suppressed. Although the half-life is only 4–8 hours, its inhibitory effect lasts 3–5 days. In plasma, vigabatrin is not bound to proteins. Vigabatrin can irreversibly reduce the visual field of a patient. Animal experiments suggest neuropathologic changes with the formation of microvacuoles at various locations within the CNS.

Vigabatrin crosses the placenta (Tran 1998). About 400 pregnancies have been documented in several case series (Morrell 1996, Case collection of the manufacturer), revealing a conspicuous rate of congenital anomalies: 18% in Morrell's study (1996), and 57 of 239 live births in the registry of the manufacturer that contained 331 pregnancies in total. The registry contains both, prospectively and retrospectively collected cases with mono- and combination therapy; thus these data do not allow a risk analysis. A typical malformation pattern has not been recognized. Two reports mention diaphragmatic hernia (Kramer 1992) and hypospadias (Lindhout 1994), albeit in combination therapy with carbamazepine. Among twelve pregnancies of the Australian Epilepsy Registry no malformations were reported (Vajda 2013a). In a small number of children who had follow-up examinations evidence of visual damage was not evident (Lawthom 2009, Sorri 2005).

Recommendation. Vigabatrin cannot be recommended due to its general side effects. Its use in the first trimester does not justify a risk-based termination (Chapter 1.15). As with other antiepileptic drugs, especially when used in combination, a higher malformation rate cannot be excluded. A follow-up sonography should be offered to ascertain the normal development of the fetus.

Regarding the extended folic acid prophylaxis when planning a pregnancy, see Section 2.10.10, and regarding vitamin K prophylaxis of the newborn, see Section 2.10.11.

2.10.33   Zonisamide

Zonisamide is primarily administered in the treatment of focal epilepsy. In a case series with 26 pregnancies no anomalies were noted in the offspring, among them four children who had been exposed to monotherapy (Kondo 1996). When mothers had been treated with a combination therapy (VPA and/or phenytoin), one child was found to have an atrial septum defect, another anencephaly, and five other children were healthy (Oles 2008, Ohtahara 2007, Kawada 2002). The North American Antiepileptic Drug in Pregnancy Registry has followed 90 first trimester zonisamide monotherapy exposed pregnancies, and identified no major malformations (0%) compared to 1.1% in an unexposed control group (http://www2.massgeneral.org/aed/newsletter/Spring2012newsletter.pdf).

Recommendation. Zonisamide cannot be recommended due a lack of experience in pregancy. Its use in the first trimester does not justify a risk-based termination (Chapter 1.15). As with other antiepileptic drugs, especially when used in combination, a higher malformation rate cannot be excluded. A follow-up sonography should be offered to ascertain the normal development of the fetus.

References

Adab N, Jacoby A, Smith D et al. Additional educational needs in children born to mothers with epilepsy. J Neurol Neurosurg Psychiatry 2001; 70: 15–21.

Adab N, Kini U, Vinten J et al. The longer term outcome of children born to mothers with epilepsy. J Neurol Neurosurg Psychiatry 2004; 75: 1575–83.

Adams J, Holmes LB, Janulewicz P. The adverse effect profile of neurobehavioral teratogens: phenobarbital. Birth Defects Res A 2004; 70: 280.

Almgren M, Källén B, Lavebratt C. Population-based study of antiepileptic drug exposure in utero – influence on head circumference in newborns. Seizure 2009; 18: 672–5.

Alsdorf RM, Wyszynski DF, Holmes LB et al. Evidence of increased birth defects in the offspring of women exposed to valproate during pregnancy: findings from the AED pregnancy registry. Birth Defects Res A 2004; 70: 245.

American Academy of Pediatrics. Committee on Fetus and Newborn: Controversies concerning vitamin K and the newborn. Pediatrics 2003; 112: 191–2.

Arndt TL, Stodgell CJ, Rodier PM. The teratology of autism. Int J Dev Neurosci 2005; 23: 189–99.

Arpino C, Brescianini S, Robert E et al. Teratogenic effects of antiepileptic drugs: use of an international database on malformations and drug exposure (MADRE). Epilepsia 2000; 41: 1436–43.

Artama M, Auvinen A, Raudaskoski T et al. Antiepileptic drug use of women with epilepsy and congenital malformations in offspring. Neurology 2005; 64: 1874–8.

Artama M, Isojarvi JI, Auvinen A. Antiepileptic drug use and birth rate in patients with epilepsy – a population-based cohort study in Finland. Hum Reprod 2006; 21: 2290–5.

Banach R, Boskovic R, Einarson T et al. Long-term developmental outcome of children of women with epilepsy, unexposed or exposed prenatally to antiepileptic drugs: a meta-analysis of cohort studies. Drug Saf 2010; 33: 73–9.

Bavoux F, Fournier-Perhilou AI, Wood C et al. Neonatal fibrinogen depletion caused by sodium valproate [letter]. Ann Pharmacother 1994; 28: 1307.

Borthen I, Eide MG, Veiby G et al. Complications during pregnancy in women with epilepsy: population-based cohort study. BJOG 2009; 116: 1736–42.

Briggs GG, Freeman RK, Yaffe SJ. *Drugs in Pregnancy and Lactation*. 9th edn. Baltimore: Williams & Wilkins 2011.

Bromley RL, Mawer GE, Briggs M et al. Liverpool and Manchester Neurodevelopment Group: The prevalence of neurodevelopmental disorders in children prenatally exposed to antiepileptic drugs. J Neurol Neurosurg Psychiatry 2013; 84: 637–43.

Bromley RL, Mawer G, Love J et al. Liverpool and Manchester Neurodevelopment Group (LMNDG): Early cognitive development in children born to women with epilepsy: a prospective report. Epilepsia 2010; 51: 2058–65.

Bronstein KS, Leppik I, Montouris G et al. Keppra® Pregnancy Registry. Epilepsia 2007; 48: 325.

Bustamante SA, Stumpff LC. Fetal hydantoin syndrome in triplets: A unique experiment of nature. Am J Dis Child 1978; 132: 978–9.

Campbell E, Devenney E, Morrow J et al. Recurrence risk of congenital malformations in infants exposed to antiepileptic drugs in utero. Epilepsia 2013; 54:165–71.

Canger R, Battino D, Canevini MP et al. Malformations in offspring of women with epilepsy: a prospective study. Epilepsia 1999; 40: 1231–6.

Chambers CD, Kao KK, Felix RJ et al. Pregnancy outcome in infants prenatally exposed to newer anticonvulsants {Abstract}. Birth Defects Res A 2005; 73: 316.

Choulika S, Grabowski E, Holmes LB. Is antenatal vitamin K prophylaxis needed for pregnant women taking anticonvulsants? Am J Obstet Gynecol 2004; 190: 882–3.

Christianson AL, Chesler N, Kromberg JG. Fetal valproate syndrome: clinical and neurodevelopmental features in two sibling pairs. Dev Med Child Neurol 1994; 36: 361–9.

Christensen J, Sabers A, Sidenius P. Oxcarbazepine concentrations during pregnancy: a retrospective study in patients with epilepsy. Neurology 2006; 67: 1497–9.

Christensen J, Grønborg TK, Sørensen MJ et al. Prenatal valproate exposure and risk of autism spectrum disorders and childhood autism. JAMA 2013; 309: 1696–703.

Cole RL, van Ross ER, Clayton-Smith J. Fibular aplasia in a child exposed to sodium valproate in pregnancy. Clin Dysmorphol 2009; 18: 37–9.

Cummings C, Stewart M, Stevenson M et al. Neurodevelopment of children exposed in utero to lamotrigine, sodium valproate and carbamazepine. Arch Dis Child 2011 Jul; 96: 643–7.

Cunnington MC, Weil JG, Messenheimer JA et al. Final results from 18 years of the International Lamotrigine Pregnancy Registry. Neurology 2011; 76: 1817–23.

Danielsson BR, Azarbayjani F, Skold AC et al. Initiation of phenytoin teratogenesis: pharmacologically induced embryonic bradycardia and arrhythmia resulting in hypoxia and possible free radical damage at reoxygenation. Teratology 1997; 56: 271–81.

Dansky LV, Finnell RH. Parental epilepsy, anticonvulsant drugs and reproductive outcome: epidemiologic and experimental findings spanning three decades: 2. Human studies. Reprod Toxicol 1991; 5: 301–35.

Day W, Yee S, Peterson C et al. Assessment of the teratogenic risk in fetuses exposed to topiramate in utero [Abstract]. Birth Defects Research A 2011; 91: 356.

Dean JCS, Hailey H, Moore SJ et al. Long-term health and neurodevelopment in children exposed to antiepileptic drugs before birth. J Med Genet 2002; 39: 251–9.

Dessens AB, Cohen-Kettenis PT, Mellenbergh GJ et al. Prenatal exposure to anticonvulsants and psychosexual development. Arch Sex Behav 1999; 28: 31–44.

Diav-Citrin O, Shechtman S, Arnon J et al. Is carbamazepine teratogenic? A prospective controlled study of 210 pregnancies. Neurology 2001; 57: 321–4.

Diav-Citrin O, Shechtman S, Bar-Oz B et al. Pregnancy outcome after in utero exposure to valproate: evidence of dose relationship in teratogenic effect. CNS Drugs 2008; 22: 325–34.

Dolk H, Jentink J, Loane M et al. Does lamotrigine use in pregnancy increase orofacial cleft risk relative to other malformations? Neurology 2008; 71: 714–22.

Dolovich LR, Addis A, Régis Vaillancourt JM et al. Benzodiazepine use in pregnancy and major malformation or oral cleft: meta-analysis of cohort and case-control studies. BMJ 1998; 317: 838–43.

Dutton C, Foldvary-Schaefer N. Contraception in women with epilepsy: pharmacokinetic interactions, contraceptive options, and management. Int Rev Neurobiol 2008; 83: 113–34.

Ebbesen F, Jergensen AM, Hoseth E et al. Neonatal hypoglycaemia after exposure in utero to valproate. Pediatr Res 1998; 44: 439.

Eisenschenk S. Treatment with oxcarbazepine during pregnancy. Neurologist 2006; 12: 249–54.

Enato E, Moretti M, Koren G. The fetal safety of benzodiazepines: an updated meta-analysis. J Obstet Gynaecol Can 2011; 33: 46–8.

Eriksson K, Viinikainen K, Mönkkönen A et al. Children exposed to valproate in utero – population-based evaluation of risks and confounding factors for long-term neurocognitive development. Epilepsy Res 2005; 65: 189–200.

Eyal S, Yagen B, Sobol E et al. The activity of antiepileptic drugs as histone deacetylase inhibitors. Epilepsia 2004; 45: 737–44.

Fujii H, Goel A, Bernard N et al. Pregnancy outcomes following gabapentin use: results of a prospective comparative cohort study. Neurology 2013; 80: 1565–70.

Fotopoulou C, Kretz R, Bauer S et al. Prospectively assessed changes in lamotrigine-concentration in women with epilepsy during pregnancy, lactation and the neonatal period. Epilepsy Res 2009; 85: 60–4.

Frey B, Braegger CP, Ghelfi D. Neonatal cholestatic hepatitis from carbamazepine exposure during pregnancy and breast feeding. Ann Pharmacother 2002; 36: 644–7.

Fried S, Kozer E, Nulman I et al. Malformation rates in children of women with untreated epilepsy: a meta-analysis. Drug Saf 2004; 27: 197–202.

Friedman SA, Lim HK, Baker CA et al. Phenytoin versus magnesium sulfate in pre-eclampsia: a pilot study. Am J Perinatol 1993; 10: 233–8.

Gaily E, Kantola-Sorsa E, Hiileesma V et al. Normal intelligence in children with prenatal exposure to carbamazepine. Neurology 2004; 62: 28–32.

Gelineau-van Waes J, Bennett GD, Finnell RH. Phenytoin-induced alterations in craniofacial gene expression. Teratology 1999; 59: 23–34.

GlaxoSmithKline. Lamotrigine pregnancy registry. Final report, 1 September 1992 through 31 March 2010; issued July 2010. http://pregnancyregistry.gsk.com/documents/lam_spring_2010_final_report.pdf.

Gorman MP, Soul JS. Neonatal hypocalcemic seizures in siblings exposed to topiramate in utero. Pediatr Neurol 2007; 36: 274–6.

Green MW, Seeger JD, Peterson C et al. Utilization of topiramate during pregnancy and risk of birth defects. Headache 2012; 52: 1070–84.

Guttuso T Jr, Robinson LK, Amankwah KS. Gabapentin use in hyperemesis gravidarum: a pilot study. Early Hum Dev 2010; 86: 65–6.

Haeusler MCH, Hoellwarth ME, Holzer P. Paralytic ileus in a fetus-neonate after maternal intake of benzodiazepine. Prenat Diagn 1995; 15: 1165–7.

Harden CL, Hopp J, Ting TY et al. American Academy of Neurology; American Epilepsy Society. Management issues for women with epilepsy – focus on pregnancy (an evidence-based review): I. Obstetrical complications and change in seizure frequency: Report of the Quality Standards Subcommittee and Therapeutics and Technology Assessment Subcommittee of the American Academy of Neurology and the American Epilepsy Society, Review. Epilepsia 2009a; 50: 1229–36.

Harden CL, Meador KJ, Pennell PB et al. Academy of Neurology; Epilepsy Society: Management issues for women with epilepsy – focus on pregnancy (an evidence-based review): II. Teratogenesis and perinatal outcomes: Report of the Quality Standards Subcommittee and Therapeutics and Technology Subcommittee of the American Academy of Neurology and the American Epilepsy Society, Review. Epilepsia 2009b; 50: 1237–46.

Harden CL, Pennell PB, Koppel BS et al. Management issues for women with epilepsy – focus on pregnancy (an evidence-based review): III. Vitamin K, folic acid, blood levels, and breast-feeding: Report of the Quality Standards Subcommittee and Therapeutics and Technology Assessment Subcommittee of the American Academy of Neurology and the Epilepsy Society, Review. Epilepsia 2009c; 50: 1247–55.

Harvey EA, Coull BA, Holmes LB. Anticonvulsant teratogenesis 5: observer bias in a cohort study. Birth Defects Res A 2003; 67: 452–6.

Hättig H, Steinhausen H-C. Children of epileptic parents: a prospective development study. In: Rauh H, Steinhausen H-C (eds). *Psychobiology and Early Development*. Amsterdam: Elsevier 1987, pp. 155–69.

Hauptmann A. Luminal bei Epilepsie. Münch Med Wochenschr 1912; 59: 1907–8.

Heinonen OP, Slone D, Shapiro S. *Birth Defects and Drugs in Pregnancy*. Littleton/USA: Publishing Sciences Group 1977.

Hernández-Díaz S, Mittendorf R, Holmes LB. Comparative Safety of Topiramate during pregnancy {Abstract}. Birth Defects Res A 2010; 88: 408.

Hernández-Díaz S, Smith CR, Shen A et al. Comparative safety of antiepileptic drugs during pregnancy. Neurology 2012; 78: 1692–9.

Hernández-Díaz S, Werler MM, Walker AM et al. Folic acid antagonists and the risk of birth defects. N Engl J Med 2000; 343: 1608–14.

Hey E. Effect of maternal anticonvulsant treatment on neonatal blood coagulation. Arch Dis Child Fetal Neonatal Ed 1999; 81: F208–10.

Holmes LB, Baldwin EJ, Smith CR et al. Increased frequency of isolated cleft palate in infants exposed to lamotrigine during pregnancy. Neurology 2008; 70: 2152–8.

Holmes LB, Harvey EA, Coull BA et al. The teratogenicity of anticonvulsant drugs. N Engl J Med 2001; 344: 1132–8.

Holmes LB, Hernandez-Diaz S. Newer anticonvulsants: lamotrigine, topiramate and gabapentin. Birth Defects Res A Clin Mol Teratol 2012 Aug; 94: 599–606.

Holmes LB, Rosenberger PB, Harvey EA et al. Intelligence and physical features of children of women with epilepsy. Teratology 2000; 61: 196–202.

Holmes LB, Wyszynski DF, Lieberman E. The AED (Antiepileptic Drug) Pregnancy Registry. A 6-year experience. Arch Neurol 2004; 61: 673–8.

Hoeltzenbein M, Supcun-Ritzler S, Langthaler M et al. Lacosamide during pregnancy: Experience of the Berlin Institute for Clinical Teratology and Drug Risk Assessment in Pregnancy. Reprod Toxicol 2011; 31: 259.

Howe AM, Oakes DJ, Woodman PDC et al. Prothrombin and PIVKA-II levels in cord blood from newborns exposed to anticonvulsants during pregnancy. Epilepsia 1999; 40: 980–4.

Hunt SJ, Craig JJ, Morrow JI. Increased frequency of isolated cleft palate in infants exposed to lamotrigine during pregnancy. Neurology 2009; 72: 1108.

Hunt S, Russell A, Smithson WH et al. Topiramate in pregnancy. Preliminary experience from the UK Epilepsy and Pregnancy Register. Neurology 2008; 71: 272–6.

Isojärvi JI, Laatikainen TJ, Pakarinen AJ et al. Polycystic ovaries and hyperandrogenism in women taking valproate for epilepsy. N Engl J Med 1993; 329: 1383–8.

Isojärvi JIT, Rättya J, Myllylä VV. Valproate, lamotrigine, and insulin-mediated risks in women with epilepsy. Ann Neurol 1998; 43: 446–51.

Jacobsen PE, Henriksen TB, Haubek D et al. Developmental enamel defects in children prenatally exposed to antiepileptic drugs. PLoS One 2013; 8: e58213.

Janz D, Fuchs V. Are anti-epileptic drugs harmful when given during pregnancy? German Med Monogr 1964; 9: 20–3.

Jentink J, Bakker MK, Nijenhuis CM et al. Does folic acid use decrease the risk for spina bifida after in utero exposure to valproic acid? Pharmacoepidemiol Drug Saf 2010a; 19: 803–7.

Jentink J, Dolk H, Loane MA et al. EUROCAT Antiepileptic Study Working Group: Intra-uterine exposure to carbamazepine and specific congenital malformations: systematic review and case-control study. BMJ 2010b; 341: c6581.

Jentink J, Loane MA, Dolk H et al. EUROCAT Antiepileptic Study Working Group: Valproic acid monotherapy in pregnancy and major congenital malformations. N Engl J Med 2010c; 362: 2185–93, Review.

Jentink J, Wang H, de Jong-van den Berg LT. Valproic acid use in pregnancy and congenital malformations. New Engl J Med 2010d; 363: 1771–2.

Jones KL, Johnson KA, Chambers CC. Pregnancy outcome in women treated with pheno-barbital monotherapy. Teratology 1992; 45: 452.

Jones KL, Lacro RV, Johnson KA et al. Pattern of malformations in the children of women treated with carbamazepine during pregnancy. N Engl J Med 1989; 320: 1661–6.

Kaaja E, Kaaja R, Hiilesmaa V. Major malformations in offspring of women with epilepsy. Neurology 2003; 60: 575–9.

Kaaja E, Kaaja R, Matila R et al. Enzyme-inducing antiepileptic drugs in pregnancy and the risk of bleeding in the neonate. Neurology 2002; 58: 549–53.

Kaneko S, Battino D, Andermann E et al. Congenital malformations due to antiepileptic drugs. Epilep Res 1999; 33: 145–58.

Kawada K, Itoh S, Kusaka T et al. Pharmacokinetics of zonisamide in perinatal period. Brain Develop 2002; 24: 95–7.

Kini U. Fetal valproate syndrome: a review. Paed Perinat Drug Ther 2006; 7: 123–30.

Kini U, Adab N, Vinten J et al. Liverpool and Manchester Neurodevelopmental Study Group: Dysmorphic features: an important clue to the diagnosis and severity of fetal anticonvulsant syndromes. Arch Dis Child Fetal Neonatal Ed 2006; 91: F90–5.

Kjaer D, Christensen J, Bech BH et al. Preschool behavioral problems in children prenatally exposed to antiepileptic drugs – a follow-up study. Epilepsy Behav 2013 Nov; 29: 407–11.

Koch S, Jäger-Roman E, Losche G et al. Antiepileptic drug treatment in pregnancy: drug side effects in the neonate and neurological outcome. Acta Paediatr 1996; 85: 739–46.

Koch S, Titze K, Zimmermann RB et al. Long-term neuropsychological consequences of maternal epilepsy and anticonvulsant treatment during pregnancy for school-age children and adolescents. Epilepsia 1999; 40: 1237–43.

Kondo T, Kaneko S, Amano Y et al. Preliminary report on teratogenic effects of zonisamide in the offspring of treated women with epilepsy. Epilepsia 1996; 37: 1242–4.

Kozma C. Valproic acid embryopathy: report of two siblings with further expansion of the phenotypic abnormalities and a review of the literature. Am J Med Genet 2001; 98: 168–75.

Kramer G. Vigabatrin: Wirksamkeit und Verträglichkeit bei Epilepsien im Erwachsenenal-ter. Akt Neurol 1992; 19: 28–40.

Lawthom C, Smith PE, Wild JM. In utero exposure to vigabatrin: no indication of visual field loss. Epilepsia 2009; 50: 318–21.

Legius E, Jaeken J, Eggermont E et al. Sodium valproate, pregnancy, and infantile fatal liver failure. Lancet 1987; 2: 1518–9.

Leppik IE, Gram L, Deaton R et al. Safety of tiagabine: summary of 53 trials. Epilepsy Res 1999; 33: 235–46.

Lin AE, Peller AJ, Westgate M-N et al. Clonazepam use in pregnancy and the risk of malfor-mations. Birth Defects Res A 2004; 70: 534–6.

Lindhout D, Omtzigt JGC. Pregnancy and the risk of teratogenicity. Epilepsia 1992; 33: 41–8.

Lindhout D, Omtzigt JGC. Teratogenic effects of antiepileptic drugs: Implication for the management of epilepsy in women of childbearing age. Epilepsia 1994; 35: 19–28.

Longo B, Forinash AB, Murphy JA. Levetiracetam use in pregnancy. Ann Pharmacother 2009; 43: 1692–5.

López-Fraile IP, Cid AO, Juste AO et al. Levetiracetam plasma level monitoring during pregnancy, delivery, and postpartum: clinical and outcome implications. Epilepsy Behav 2009; 15: 372–5.

Lu MCK, Sammel MD, Cleveland RH et al. Digit effects produced by prenatal exposure to antiepileptic drugs. Teratology 2000; 61: 277–83.

Margulis AV, Mitchell AA, Gilboa SM et al. Use of topiramate in pregnancy and risk of oral clefts. Am J Obstet Gynecol 2012; 207: 405.

Marson AG, Al-Kharusi AM, Alwaidh M et al. SANAD Study group: The SANAD study of effectiveness of valproate, lamotrigine, or topiramate for generalised and unclassifiable epilepsy: an unblinded randomised controlled trial. Lancet 2007; 369: 1016–26.

Mastroiacovo P et al. Epilepsy and anticonvulsants during pregnancy. ENTIS study, preliminary results. Vortrag anlässlich der 9. ENTIS-Jahreskonferenz 1998.

Matalon S, Schechtman S, Goldzweig G et al. The teratogenic effect of carbamazepine: a meta-analysis of 1,255 exposures. Reprod Toxicol 2002; 16: 9–17.

Mawer G, Briggs M, Baker GA et al. Liverpool & Manchester Neurodevelopment Group: Pregnancy with epilepsy: obstetric and neonatal outcome of a controlled study. Seizure 2010; 19: 112–9.

Mawhinney E, Campbell J, Craig J et al. Valporate and the risk for congenital malformations: Is formulation and dosage regime important? Seizure 2012; 21: 215–8.

Mawhinney E, Craig J, Morrow J et al. Levetiracetam in pregnancy: results from the UK and Ireland epilepsy and preganancy registers. Neurology 2013; 80: 400–5.

Mazzucchelli I, Onat FY, Ozkara C et al. Changes in the disposition of oxcarbazepine and its metabolites during pregnancy and the puerperium. Epilepsia 2006; 47: 504–9.

McPherson JA, Harper LM, Odibo AO et al. Maternal seizure disorder and risk of adverse pregnancy outcomes. Am J Obstet Gynecol 2013 May; 208: 378, e1–5.

McVearry KM, Gaillard WD, van Meter J et al. A prospective study of cognitive fluency and originality in children exposed in utero to carbamazepine, lamotrigine, or valproate monotherapy. Epilepsy Behav 2009; 16: 609–16.

Meador KJ, Baker GA, Browning N et al. NEAD Study Group: Cognitive function at 3 years of age after fetal exposure to antiepileptic drugs. N Engl J Med 2009; 360: 1597–605.

Meador KJ, Baker GA, Browning N et al. Relationship of child IQ to parental IQ and education in children with fetal antiepileptic drug exposure. Epilepsy Behav 2011; 21: 147–52.

Meador KJ, Baker GA, Browning N et al. Effects of fetal antiepileptic drug exposure: outcomes at age 4.5 years. Neurology 2012 Apr 17; 78: 1207–14.

Meador KJ, Baker GA, Browning N et al. Fetal antiepileptic drug exposure and cognitive outcomes at age 6 years (NEAD study): a prospective observational study. Lancet Neurol 2013; 12: 244–52.

Meador KJ, Reynolds MW, Crean S et al. Pregnancy outcomes in women with epilepsy: a systematic review and meta-analysis of published pregnancy registries and cohorts. Epilepsy Res 2008; 81: 1–13.

Menegola E, Di Renzo F, Broccia ML et al. Inhibition of histone deacetylase as a new mechanism of teratogenesis. Birth Defects Res C Embryo Today 2006; 78: 345–53.

Meischenguiser R, D'Giano CH, Ferraro SM. Oxcarbazepine in pregnancy: clinical experience in Argentina. Epilepsy Behav 2004; 5: 163–7.

Miyazaki K, Narita N, Narita M. Maternal administration of thalidomide or valproic acid causes abnormal serotonergic neurons in the offspring: implication for pathogenesis of autism. Int J Dev Neurosci 2005; 23: 287–97.

Mølgaard-Nielsen D, Hviid A. Newer-generation antiepileptic drugs and the risk of major birth defects. JAMA 2011; 305: 1996–2002.

Montouris G. Gabapentin exposure in human pregnancy: results from the Gabapentin Pregnancy Registry. Epilepsy Behav 2003; 4: 310–7.

Montouris G. Safety of the newer antiepileptic drug oxcarbazepine during pregnancy. Curr Med Res Opin 2005; 21: 693–701.

Moore SJ, Turnpenny P, Quinn A et al. A clinical study of 57 children with fetal anticonvulsant syndrome. J Med Genet 2000; 37: 489–97.

Morrell MJ. The new antiepileptic drugs and women, efficacy, reproductive health, pregnancy, and fetal outcome. Epilepsia 1996; 37: S34–S44.

Morrow JI, Craig JI. Anti-epileptic drugs in pregnancy: current safety and other issues. Expert Opinion Pharmacother 2003; 4: 445–56.

Morrow JI, Russell A, Gutherie E et al. Malformation risk of anti-epileptic drugs in pregnancy: a prospective study from the UK epilepsy and pregnancy register. J Neurol Neurosurg Psychiatry 2006; 77: 193–8.

Musselman AC, Bennett GD, Greer KA et al. Preliminary evidence of phenytoin-induced alteration in embryonic gene expression in a mouse model. Reprod Toxicol 1994; 8: 383–95.

Nadebaum C, Anderson VA, Vajda F et al. Language skills of school-aged children prenatally exposed to antiepilptic drugs. Neurology 2011; 76: 719–26.

Nau H, Rating D, Koch S et al. Valproic acid and its metabolites: placental transfer, neonatal pharmacokinetics, transfer via mother's milk and clinical status in neonates of epileptic mother's. J Pharmacol Exp Ther 1981; 219: 768–77.

Ohman I, Luef G, Tomson T. Effects of pregnancy and contraception on lamotrigine disposition: new insights through analysis of lamotrigine metabolites. Seizure 2008; 17: 199–202.

Ohman I, Sabers A, de Flon P et al. Pharmacokinetics of topiramate during pregnancy. Epilepsy Res 2009; 87: 124–9.

Ohtahara S, Yamatogi Y. Erratum to "Safety of zonisamide therapy: prospective follow-up survey". Seizure 2007; 16: 87–93.

Oles KS; Bell WL. Zonisamide concentrations during pregnancy. Ann Pharmacother 2008; 42: 1139–41.

Omtzigt JGC, Los JF, Meijer JWA et al. The 10,11-epoxide-10,11-diol pathway of carbamazepine in early pregnancy in maternal serum, urine, and amniotic fluid: effect of dose, co-medication, and relation to outcome of pregnancy. Ther Drug Monit 1993; 15: 1–10.

Ornoy A, Arnon J, Shechtman S et al. Is benzodiazepine use during pregnancy really teratogenic? Reprod Toxicol 1998; 12: 511–5.

Ornoy A, Cohen E. Outcome of children born to epileptic mothers treated with carbamazepine during pregnancy. Arch Dis Child 1996; 75: 517–20.

Ornoy A, Zvi N, Arnon J et al. The outcome of pregnancy following topiramate treatment: A study on 52 pregnancies. Reprod Toxicol 2008; 25: 388–9.

Orup Jr HI, Coull BA, Adams J et al. Changes in cranio-facial features in children exposed to antiepileptic drugs in utero {Abstract}. Teratology 2000; 61: 448.

Petrenaite V, Sabers A, Hansen-Schwartz J. Seizure deterioration in women treated with oxcarbazepine during pregnancy. Epilepsy Res 2009; 84: 245–9.

Phelan MC, Pellock JM, Nance WE. Discordant expression of fetal hydantoin syndrome in heteropaternal dizygotic twins. N Engl J Med 1982; 307: 99–101.

Pittschieler S, Brezinka C, Jahn B et al. Spontaneous abortion and the prophylactic effect of folic acid supplementation in epileptic women undergoing antiepileptic therapy. J Neurol 2008; 255: 1926–31.

Rabinowicz A, Meischenguiser R, Ferraro SM et al. Single center, 7-year experience of oxcarbazepine exposure during pregnancy. Epilepsia 2002; 43: 208–9.

Raymond GV, Buehler BA, Finell RH et al. Anticonvulsant teratogenesis: 3. Possible metabolic basis. Teratology 1995; 51: 55–6.

Rihtman T, Parush S, Ornoy A. Preliminary findings of the developmental effects of in utero exoposure to topiramate. Reprod Toxicol 2012; 34: 308–11.

Robert E, Guibaud P. Maternal valproic acid and congenital neural tube defects. Lancet 1982; 2: 937.

Robert E, Jouk PS. Preaxial limb defects after valproic acid exposure during pregnancy. In: Mastroiacovo P, Källén B, Castilla E (eds.) Proceedings of the First International Meeting of the Genetic and Reproductive Epidemiology Research Society (GRERS). Rome: Ghedini Editore 1992; 101–5.

Rodier PM, Ingram JL, Tisdale B et al. Linking etiologies in humans and animal models: studies of autism. Reprod Toxicol 1997; 11: 417–22.

Rodriguez-Pinilla E, Arroyo I, Fondevilla J et al. Prenatal exposure to valproic acid during pregnancy and limb deficiencies: a case-control study. Am J Med Genet 2000; 90: 376–81.

Rodriguez-Pinilla E, Mejías C, Prieto-Merino D et al. Risk of hypospadias in newborn infants exposed to valproic acid during the first trimester of pregnancy: a case-control study in Spain. Drug Saf 2008; 31: 537–43.

Rosa F. Holoprosencephaly and antiepileptic exposures. Teratology 1995; 51: 230.

Sabers A, Dam M, A-Rogvi-Hansen B et al. Epilepsy and pregnancy: lamotrigine as main drug used. Acta Neurol Scand 2004; 109: 9–13.

Sabers A, Petrenaite V. Seizure frequency in pregnant women treated with lamotrigine monotherapy. Epilepsia 2009; 50: 2163–6.

Samrén EB, van Duijn CM, Koch S et al. Maternal use of antiepileptic drugs and the risk of major congenital malformations: a joint European prospective study of human teratogenesis associated with maternal epilepsy. Epilepsia 1997; 38: 981–90.

Samrén EB, van Duijn CM, Lieve Christiaens GCM et al. Antiepileptic drug regimens and major congenital abnormalities in the offspring. Ann Neurol 1999; 46: 739–46.

Schmitz B. Lamotrigin bei Frauen mit Epilepsie. Nervenarzt 2003; 74: 833–40.

Scolnik D, Nulman I, Rovet J et al. Neurodevelopment of children exposed in utero to phenytoin and carbamazepine monotherapy. JAMA 1994; 271: 767–70.

Shallcross R, Bromley RL, Irwin B et al. Child development following in utero exposure: levetiracetam vs sodium valproate. Neurology 2011; 76: 383–9.

Shankaran S, Paille L, Wright L et al. Neurodevelopmental outcome of premature infants after antenatal phenobarbital exposure. Am J Obstet Gynecol 2002; 187: 171–7.

Sharony R, Garber A, Viskochil D et al. Preaxial ray reduction defects as part of valproic acid-embryofetopathy. Prenat Diagn 1993; 13: 909–18.

Sorri I, Herrgård E, Viinikainen K et al. Ophthalmologic and neurologic findings in two children exposed to vigabatrin in utero. Epilepsy Res 2005; 65: 117–20.

Stromland K, Nordin V, Miller M et al. Autism in thalidomide embryopathy: a population study. Dev Med Child Neurol 1994; 36: 351–6.

Tica OS, Tica AA, Brailoiu CG et al. Sirenomelia after phenobarbital and carbamazepine therapy in pregnancy. Birth Defects Res A Clin Mol Teratol 2013; 97: 425–8.

Tomson T, Battino D. Teratogenic effects of antiepileptic medications. Neurol Clin 2009; 27: 993–1002.

Tomson T, Battino D, Bonizzoni E et al. Does-dependent risk of malformations with antiepileptic drugs: an analysis of data from the EURAP epilepsy and pregnancy registry. Lancet Neurol 2011; 10: 609–17.

Tomson T, Palm R, Källén K et al. Pharmacokinetics of levetiracetam during pregnancy, delivery, in the neonatal period, and lactation. Epilepsia 2007; 48: 1111–6.

Tran A, O'Mahoney T, Rey E et al. Vigabatrin: placental transfer in vivo and excretion into breast milk of the enantiomers. Br J Clin Pharmacol 1998; 45: 409–11.

Vajda FJ, Eadie MJ. Maternal valproate dosage and foetal malformations. Acta Neurol Scand 2005; 112: 137–42.

Vajda FJ, Graham JE, Hitchcock AA et al. Is lamotrigine a significant human teratogen? Observations from the Australian Pregnancy Register. Seizure 2010a; 19: 558–61.

Vajda FK. Graham J, Hitchcock AA et al. Foetal malformations after exposure to antiepileptic drugs in utero assessed at birth and 12 months later: observations from the Australian pregnancy register. Acta Neurol Scand 2011; 124: 9–12.

Vajda FJ, Hitchcock AA, Graham J et al. The teratogenic risk of antiepileptic drug polytherapy. Epilepsia 2010b; 51: 805–10.

Vajda FJ, O'Brien TJ, Hitchcock A et al. The Australian registry of anti-epileptic drugs in pregnancy: experience after 30 months. J Clin Neurosci 2003; 10: 543–9.

Vajda, FJ, O'Brien TJ, Graham J et al. Associations between particular types of fetal malformation and antiepileptic drug exposure in utero. Acta neurologica Scandinavica 2013a; 128: 228–34.

Vajda, FJ, O'Brien TJ, Lander CM et al. Teratogenesis in repeated pregnancies in antiepileptic drug-treated women. Epilepsia 2013b; 54: 181–6.

van der Pol MC, Hadders-Algra M, Huisjes HJ et al. Antiepileptic medication in pregnancy: late effects on the children's central nervous system development. Am J Obstet Gynecol 1991; 164: 121–8.

Vanoverloop D, Schnell RR, Harvey EA et al. The effects of prenatal exposure to phenytoin and other anticonvulsants on intellectual function at 4 to 8 years of age. Neurotoxicol Teratol 1992; 14: 329–35.

Veiby G, Daltveit AK, Engelsen BA et al. Pregnancy, delivery, and outcome for the child in maternal epilepsy. Epilepsia 2009; 50: 2130–9.

Vila Ceren C, Demestre Guasch X, Raspall Torrent F et al. Topiramate and pregnancy. Neonate with bone anomalies. An Pediatr (Barc) 2005; 63: 363–5.

Weinstock L, Cohen LS, Bailey JW et al. Obstetrical and neonatal outcome following clonazepam use during pregnancy: a case series. Psychother Psychosom 2001; 70:158–62.

Wells PG, Kim PM, Nicol CJ et al. Reactive intermediates. In: Kavlock RJ, Daston GP (eds.), Drug Toxicity in Embryonic Development. Vol. 1. Handbook of Experimental Pharmacology. Heidelberg: Springer 1997: 451–516.

Werler MM, Ahrens KA, Bosco JL et al. Use of antiepileptic medications in pregnancy in relation to risks of birth defects. Ann Epidemiol 2011; 21: 842–50.

Westin AA, Nakken KO, Johannessen SI et al. Serum concentration/dose ratio of topiramate during pregnancy. Epilepsia 2009; 50: 480–5.

Westin AA, Reimers A, Helde G et al. Serum concentration/dose ratio of levetiracetam before, during and after pregnancy. Seizure 2008; 17: 192–8.

Wide K, Windbladh B, Källén B. Major malformations in infants exposed to antiepileptic drugs in utero with emphasis on carbamazepine and valproic acid: a nation-wide population-based register study. Acta Paediatr 2004; 93: 174–6.

Williams G, King J, Cunningham M et al. Fetal valproate syndrome and autism: additional evidence of an association. Dev Med Child Neurol 2001; 43: 202–6.

Wilton LV, Shakir S. A postmarketing surveillance study of gabapentin as add-on therapy for 3.100 patients in England. Epilepsia 2002; 43: 983–92.

Witczak M, Kociszewska I, Wilczyński J et al. Evaluation of chromosome aberrations, sister chromatid exchange and micronuclei in cultured cord-blood lymphocytes of newborns of women treated for epilepsy during pregnancy. Mutat Res 2010; 701: 111–7.

Wyszynski D, Nambisan M, Surve T et al. Antiepileptic Drug Pregnancy Registry: Increased risk of major malformations in offspring exposed to valproate during pregnancy. Neurology 2005; 64; 961–5.

Zuppa AA, Carducci C, Scorrano A et al. Infants born to mothers under phenobarbital treatment: correlation between serum levels and clinical features of neonates. Eur J Obstet Gynecol Reprod Biol 2011; 159: 53–6.

Pregnancy

2.10 Epilepsy and antiepileptic medications

Psychotropic drugs

2.11

Katherine L. Wisner and
Christof Schaefer

2.11.1	Psychiatric disorder during pregnancy	294
2.11.2	Antidepressant treatment	294
2.11.3	Selective serotonin-reuptake-inhibitors (SSRI)	295
2.11.4	Tri- and tetracyclic antidepressants	302
2.11.5	Individual antidepressants	303
2.11.6	Antipsychotic treatment	313
2.11.7	Individual antipsychotic drugs	316
2.11.8	Lithium and other anti-manic agents	322
2.11.9	Anxiolytics, hypnotics, sedatives in general	324
2.11.10	Benzodiazepines	325
2.11.11	Zaleplon, zolpidem and zopiclone	327
2.11.12	Other anxiolytics and hypnotics	328
2.11.13	Psychoanaleptics	328
2.11.14	Anti-Parkinson drugs and restless legs syndrome	329

Women of childbearing age are often affected with depressive, psychotic or other psychiatric disorders, which require medication during pregnancy. Psychopharmaceuticals during pregnancy constitute both a potential risk to the developing fetus as well as a possible benefit through improvement of the disease state. According to the current knowledge there is no strong teratogen among the classical psychopharmaceuticals. The risk for Ebstein's anomaly with the mood stabilizer *lithium* has been confirmed but was overestimated. However, many drugs used in psychiatry are insufficiently tested with respect to their effects on the fetus. *Valproic acid* should be avoided during pregnancy due to its established physical and neurobehavioral teratogenicity, and it is not a drug of first choice for the management of women of childbearing age. This chapter provides a detailed overview on SSRI and the other antidepressants, on antipsychotics, mood stabilizers, anxiolytics, hypnotics and, among others, on restless leg treatment.

Drugs During Pregnancy and Lactation. **http://dx.doi.org/10.1016/B978-0-12-408078-2.00012-3**
Copyright © 2015 Elsevier B.V. All rights reserved.

2.11.1   Psychiatric disorder during pregnancy

Like other serious medical disorders, psychiatric illnesses adversely impact the course and outcome of pregnancy. Characterized by physiological and circadian rhythm dysregulation, maternal psychiatric disorders create an adverse milieu for the growing fetus. Stress has a prominent role in the pathogenesis of psychiatric and general medical disorders, particularly early adverse events such as child physical or sexual abuse. Extensive research has demonstrated the effects of negative emotional states, such as anxiety and depression, and stress during pregnancy on birth outcomes and fetal/infant development (Dunkel Schetter 2012). High levels of maternal life stress are significantly associated with an increased risk of offspring congenital malformations, mental disorders, and eye, ear, respiratory, digestive, skin, musculoskeletal, and genitourinary diseases (Tegethoff 2011). In a population-based case control study, high maternal stress levels were associated with an increased risk of cleft palate, cleft lip, transposition of the great arteries, and tetralogy of Fallot, after adjustment for multiple potential confounding variables (Carmichael 2007). A meta-analytic study of women with high depressive symptom levels or major depressive disorders (Grote 2010a) found that newborns were at increased risk for preterm birth and small for gestational age status. The concept of fetal programming, the observation that characteristics of the fetal milieu predispose individuals to diseases over the life course, has intensified the importance of optimizing pregnancy health. Antenatal depression was an independent risk factor for offspring depression at 18 years of age, independent of post-birth maternal depression (Pearson 2013). The authors concluded with the intriguing point that treating maternal depression antenatally could prevent offspring depression in early adulthood.

Exposure to medications during pregnancy constitutes both a potential risk to the developing fetus as well as a possible benefit through improvement of the disease state. The possibility that prenatal psychopharmacologic treatment may prevent adverse outcomes during human pregnancy is less commonly considered than the possibility of harm. The art of medicine is exemplified by balancing the risks and benefits of medication with the woman's illness management during pregnancy. Most women prefer a collaborative stance with the physician, who provides information and support, while the woman applies her values to the components of the decision making process and derives a choice (Patel 2011).

In the following sections, the impact of psychotropic drug classes, individual agents and the impact of the diseases they are used to treat are reviewed.

2.11.2   Antidepressant treatment

The frequency of reported antidepressant use at any time during pregnancy increased from 2.5% in 1998 to 8.1% in 2005 in the USA (Alwan 2011). A sharp decrease in frequency of use occurred by the third month after conception. The rate of antidepressant use after the first trimester of pregnancy was about 2%.

Recommendation.

- A primary factor for the choice of an antidepressant during pregnancy is the woman's treatment history. The drug to which she has responded, or ideally, remitted (recovered fully to functional status prior to depressive episode), with an acceptable side effect burden deserves first consideration. The rationale for selecting a drug for which the patient's response and side effect burden is not known should be justified carefully.
- Non-pharmacological approaches with an evidence base for the treatment of major depression during pregnancy include psychotherapy (Spinelli 1997), bright morning light therapy (Wirz-Justice 2011), acupuncture (Manber 2010) and transcranial magnetic stimulation (Kim 2011).
- As a group, selective SSRI antidepressants are the most frequently used drugs for the pharmacological treatment of major depressive disorder due to their low toxicity, particularly in overdose situations. SSRI are among the most comprehensively studied group of medications taken by pregnant women.
- The serotonin-norepinephrine reuptake inhibitors (SNRI) have been included with the group of SSRI medications as well as separately for pregnancy exposure studies.
- Tricyclic antidepressants (TCA) are less well studied than SSRI; however, they are useful for women who are not responsive to SSRI or have prohibitive side effects. All antidepressants have similar efficacy for depression.
- One advantage to TCA is that the serum levels are associated with likelihood of response, which is useful in evaluating treatment refractory patients. Serum level monitoring is also an advantage in the rapidly changing pharmacokinetic milieu induced by the dynamic state of pregnancy, which often require dosage change to maintain efficacy (Stika 2001).
- Bupropion, a dopamine-norepinephrine reuptake inhibitor, has been studied in pregnancy and is also FDA-indicated as an adjunct to behavioral treatment for smoking cessation.
- Optimize the dose of a single drug before considering additional drug treatments.
- Always inquire about alcohol, cigarettes and other drug use, environmental exposures, as well as over the counter and prescribed medication intake, and record them in the patient's medical chart prior to writing any prescriptions.
- A reduction or discontinuation of an antidepressant medication before the birth to reduce the fetal load at birth is theoretically appealing, no clear advantages for the newborn has been demonstrated to offset potential risk for maternal recurrence (Warburton et al. 2010).
- Information about the impact of drugs in pregnancy is constantly evolving. A free resource for updates is the US National Library of Medicine (http://toxnet.nlm.nih.gov/) for DART (Developmental and Reproductive Toxicology Database).

2.11.3   Selective serotonin-reuptake-inhibitors (SSRI)

Among the SSRIs are *fluoxetine, sertraline, paroxetine, citalopram, escitalopram* (the active isomer of citalopram), and *fluvoxamine*. They are heterogeneous chemically and structurally unrelated to tricyclic antidepressants. They selectively inhibit the reuptake of serotonin from the synaptic cleft. The SSRI have considerably lower anticholinergic effect than tricyclics.

Pregnancy

2.11 Psychotropic drugs

All SSRIs cross the placenta. The concentration relationship between cord blood and maternal plasma is between 0.3 and 0.9. Citalopram is transferred the most, followed by fluoxetine. The lowest transfer is found with sertraline, followed by paroxetine (Rampono 2009, Hendrick 2003).

Clinical and preclinical data demonstrate the substantial impact of SSRI exposure on neural plasticity and brain development (Pawluski 2012). Prior to functioning as a neurotransmitter, serotonin (5-hydroxytryptamine = 5-HT) functions in the embryo to regulate migration of the neural crest cells, the growth of the axons and the synaptic communication system. Results of animal studies show that elevated serotonin levels are associated with neuroanatomical abnormalities with a decreased number of β-adrenergic and serotonin receptors as well as abnormal serotonin receptor binding in the central nervous system (CNS). In cell cultures, 5-HT or the 5-HT transporter is involved in the development of the heart and that fluoxetine impairs the differentiation of the cardiomyocytes (Kusakawa 2008, Sari 2003). However, these studies are not performed in the context of the maternal disease state of major depression, and whether SSRIs could protect against the impact of maternal disease in offspring in the short- and long-term is an important research question (Pawluski 2012).

Maternal treatment

Pregnancy brings dramatic physiological changes associated with the potential for loss of drug efficacy, or alternatively an increase in toxicity, across pregnancy. Freeman (2008) reported non-significant group changes in sertraline bioavailability across pregnancy in nine women, although serum levels were lowest in the third trimester. Sit (2008) found that the level/dose ratios for sertraline decreased by a mean of 60% between 20 weeks and delivery and were similar to those in early pregnancy by 4–6 weeks postpartum. The level/dose ratios of fluoxetine and norfluoxetine decreased by 50% in the third trimester and were similar to those observed in early pregnancy by 12 weeks postpartum (Sit 2010). For paroxetine, P450 2D6 genotyping has been applied to study paroxetine plasma levels during pregnancy in 74 Dutch women (Ververs 2009). Women who were extensive or ultrarapid metabolizers for 2D6 showed steadily decreasing paroxetine concentrations during the course of pregnancy, which was associated with increasing depression scores. In contrast, plasma paroxetine concentrations of women who were intermediate or poor metabolizers increased during pregnancy. However, the impact of these changes on clinical care, and the relationship of alterations in serum levels to depressive symptom relapse (or side effects), and, in response, dose escalation (or reduction) has not been systematically elucidated.

SSRI have been evaluated for association with postpartum hemorrhage due to their effects on platelet serotonin. Salkeld (2008) found that SSRI did not confer increased risk of hemorrhage at the time of delivery compared with non-SSRI antidepressants. In contrast, Palmsten and colleagues reported that exposure to serotonin and non-serotonin reuptake inhibitors near delivery was associated with an elevated risk of one excess case for every 80 to 100 women, and commented about the possibility of residual confounding (Palmsten 2013a).

Congenital malformations

Because of the prevalence of depression and anxiety disorders in women of childbearing age, the SSRIs are among the medications with the most comprehensive data to guide use during pregnancy. Most studies have not found an elevated total rate of malformations associated with SSRIs as a grouped exposure (Malm 2011, Nordeng 2011, Reis 2010, survey in Ellfolk 2010, Wichman 2009, Einarson 2008, Oberlander 2008, Alwan 2007, Davis 2007, Louik 2007, Hallberg 2005). However, associations between specific malformations and SSRI exposure during the first trimester have been reported (Pedersen 2009, Alwan 2007, Louik 2007). The only consistently reported malformation is cardiac defects – particularly septum defects (Colvin 2011, Kornum 2010, Merlob 2009, Pedersen 2009, Diav-Citrin 2008, Oberlander 2008, Källén 2007).

Two large-scale, North American case-controls have been published. Alwan (2007) analyzed data from 9,622 infants with birth defects and 4,092 control infants from the National Birth Defects Prevention Study. No significant associations between SSRI use during early pregnancy and congenital heart defects or most other categories or subcategories of birth defects were observed. Maternal SSRI use was associated with anencephaly (214 infants, nine exposed; adjusted OR, 2.4; 95% CI 1.1 to 5.1), craniosynostosis (432 infants, 24 exposed; adjusted OR, 2.5; 95% CI 1.5 to 4.0), and omphalocele (181 infants, 11 exposed; adjusted OR, 2.8; 95% CI 1.3 to 5.7). These associations between SSRI use and birth defects resulted in small absolute risks. Outcome data were collected by maternal interview after birth which also presents the possibility of recall bias when a negative birth outcome occurs. Louik (2007) did not confirm the association between overall use of SSRIs and craniosynostosis, omphalocele, or heart defects. The only significant association in common was specifically between sertraline use and omphalocele (OR, 5.7; 95% CI 1.6 to 20.7), which was based on only three subjects. They did not find significantly increased risks of congenital heart defects associated with overall use of SSRIs or of non-SSRI antidepressants. However, they did find a doubling of the risk of septal defects associated with sertraline exposure (OR, 2.0), based on 13 exposed subjects, and a tripling of the risk of right ventricular outflow tract obstruction defects associated with paroxetine use (OR, 3.3), based on six exposed subjects.

In the Pedersen (2009) study, filled prescriptions for SSRIs were not associated with major malformations overall but were associated with septal heart defects (OR 1.99, 95% CI 1.13 to 3.53). For individual SSRIs, the odds ratio for septal heart defects was 3.25 (1.21 to 8.75) for sertraline, 2.52 (1.04 to 6.10) for citalopram, and not significant for fluoxetine. Redemptions for more than one type of SSRI were associated with septal heart defects (4.70, 1.74 to 12.7). The absolute increase in the prevalence of malformations was low – for example, the prevalence of septal heart defects was 0.5% among unexposed children, 0.9% among children whose mothers were prescribed any SSRI, and 2.1% among children whose mothers filled prescriptions for more than one type of SSRI. One interpretation of these data is that the mothers who were prescribed SSRI, and particularly those who were prescribed more than one SSRI, have more severe underlying psychiatric disorders which bring additional confounding factors that remain unmeasured.

Grigoriadis (2013) conducted a meta-analysis to determine whether antenatal antidepressant exposure was associated with congenital malformations, cardiovascular defects, septal heart defects (ventral septal defects and atrial septal defects), and ventral septal defects only. Nineteen studies were included. Antidepressant exposure was not associated with most congenital malformations or major malformations. However, an increased risk for cardiovascular malformations (RR = 1.36; 95% CI 1.08–1.71; $p = 0.008$) and septal heart defects (RR = 1.40; 95% CI 1.10–1.77; $p = 0.005$) was observed. The RR for ventral septal defects was similar to septal defects, although not significant (RR = 1.54; 95% CI 0.71–3.33; p = 0.274). Pooled effects were significant for paroxetine and cardiovascular malformations (RR = 1.43; 95% CI 1.08–1.88; p = 0.012). The authors concluded that antidepressants do not appear to be associated with an increased risk of most congenital malformations, but statistical significance was found for cardiovascular malformations. Given that the RRs are marginal, they may be the result of uncontrolled confounders. Although the RRs were statistically significant, none reached clinically significant levels.

An intriguing design (Jimenez-Solem 2012) was used to evaluate the relationship between SSRI use and cardiac malformations. From 848,786 women in the Danish Medical Birth Registry, 4,183 filled a prescription for an SSRI for the period covering the first trimester and 806 women discontinued their medication prior to and during pregnancy. The risks for cardiac malformations were similar for SSRI exposed (adjusted OR 2.01, 95% CI 1.60 to 2.53) and SSRI paused (non-exposed) pregnancies (adjusted OR = 1.85, 95% CI 1.07 to 3.20; p = 0.94). The authors found similar increased risks of specific congenital malformations of the heart for the individual SSRIs and no association with dosage was observed. They concluded that the association between SSRI use and congenital malformations of the heart may be confounded by indication (Källén 2012). Methodological issues inherent in studies based on prescription databases also complicate interpretation of this literature.

Preterm birth, intrauterine growth retardation

Women with major depression (MDD = major depressive disorder) during pregnancy have higher rates of small for gestational age infants and preterm delivery. MDD or clinically significant depressive symptoms were associated with an increase in the relative risks for preterm birth by 39%, for low birth weight by 49%, and for intrauterine growth restriction by 45% (Grote 2010b). Adverse pregnancy outcomes have also been reported for depressed women treated with antidepressants. Meta-analyses have shown that SSRI-treated women have a 2- to 3-fold greater risk for preterm birth as well as a higher rate of low birth weight infants compared to women unexposed to SSRI (Lattimore 2005, Källén 2004). Preterm birth rates were similar in women exposed continuously to MDD (no SSRI) or to SSRI (23% and 21%, respectively) compared to women with neither exposure (6%; Wisner 2009).

Consideration of the impact of antenatal SSRI and MDD exposures on fetal and infant growth is important because epidemiologic studies have demonstrated that infants born either small or large for gestational age have higher rates of chronic illnesses such as diabetes and cardiovascular disease as adults (Harder 2007, Barker 1989). Maternal depression was associated with slower rates of fetal body and head growth, while in SSRI-treated pregnant women only delayed head growth was observed (El Marroun 2012). In a prospective study, no significant impact of *in utero* exposure to MDD or SSRI on infant weight, length or head circumference through 12 months was reported (Wisner 2013). In an Australian investigation of the association between prenatal SSRI prescription dispensing and overweight in offspring at 4–5 years of age (Grzeskowiak 2012), female offspring of exposed mothers were less likely to be overweight compared with female offspring of mothers with an untreated psychiatric illness and female offspring of unexposed mothers. No association with overweight was observed among male offspring. Differentiating between the contribution of MDD or depressive symptoms and that of antidepressant treatment on growth presents a clinical challenge.

The risk of preeclampsia was studied in a population-based health-care utilization database of nearly 70,000 pregnancies in women with depression (Palmsten 2012). The risk of preeclampsia in unmedicated women with depression was similar to the risk in women without depression (2.3%). Compared to women with untreated depression, women treated with SSRI, SNRI, and TCA monotherapy had adjusted relative risks of 1.22 (95% CI 0.97, 1.54), 1.95 (95% CI 1.25, 3.03), and 3.23 (95% CI 1.87, 5.59), respectively. Although the risk of preeclampsia is higher in treated women, this group of women also may have more severe underlying depressive disorder.

Neonatal adaptation disorders

Neonatal adaptation difficulties in the offspring of pregnant SSRI-treated women include central nervous, gastrointestinal, and respiratory system signs that result from serontonergic overstimulation or alternatively withdrawal (Moses-Kolko 2005, Zeskind 2004, Laine 2003). Neonatal signs include restlessness, rigidity, jitteriness, feeding difficulty, respiratory distress, frequent startle reactions and longer REM phases as well as a less variability in behavioral patterns (Moses-Kolko 2005). The signs begin in the first days of life and continue in the typical infant for less than 2 weeks, and for a month in very rare cases (Laine 2003). Sanz (2005) described 93 spontaneous reports of newborns with signs associated with SSRI to the international WHO Drug Monitoring Centre in Uppsala (Sweden). Of these 93 cases of neonatal adaptation syndrome, 64 were associated with paroxetine, and 13 had seizures. Paroxetine is generally the SSRI most frequently implicated, followed by fluoxetine (Moses-Kolko 2005). In addition to the receptor-specific differences between the SSRI, the short half-life of paroxetine may account for withdrawal symptoms. Inter-individual differences are also possibly caused by genetic polymorphism of the metabolizing enzymes and the 5-HT transporter activity (Hilli 2009, Oberlander 2008).

In addition to the mild neonatal adaptation syndrome, late gestational SSRI exposure has been associated with an increased risk for persistent pulmonary hypertension of the newborn (PPHN). Chambers (2006) reported an increased risk from the baseline frequency of 1–2 per 1,000 to 6–12 per 1,000 newborns. Källén (2008) used the Swedish Medical Birth Register to explore the association between SSRI use and PPHN. Potential confounders were evaluated and included: older maternal age, parity, maternal BMI, and maternal smoking. Adjusting for these variables and year of birth, an association between maternal use of SSRI and PPHN in births after 34 completed weeks was identified with a risk ratio of 2.4 (95% CI 1.2–4.3) for women who reported the drug use in early pregnancy. For the subgroup of the women who had prescriptions for SSRI later in pregnancy, the risk estimate was 3.6 (95% CI 1.2–8.3).

Kieler (2012) evaluated a Scandinavian population-based cohort study to examine the risk for PPHN with SSRI exposure after gestational week 33. They reported an absolute risk of 3 per 1,000 live-born infants compared with the background incidence of 1.2 per 1000 (aOR 2.1, 95% CI 1.5–3.0). The risk associated with individual agents similar. Other researchers could not confirm an association of SSRI exposure with PPHN (Wilson 2011, Andrade 2009, Wichman 2009). Maternal depression, obesity, smoking and surgical delivery are also risk factors for PPHN, and confounding factors associated with depression remain a concern in interpreting these data (Occhiogrosso 2012). Doppler ultrasound measures of the right pulmonary artery at 36 weeks gestation

Pregnancy

2.11 Psychotropic drugs

was used to evaluate SSRI- and non-exposed fetuses and no significant difference was found. However, in the subset of SSRI-exposed infants with transient neonatal respiratory difficulties, fetal right pulmonary artery flow was increased but it was not associated with PPHN (Lim 2012).

A recent meta-analysis (Grigoriadis 2014) on PPHN covering seven studies concluded that the risk was increased for infants exposed to SSRIs in late pregnancy (OR 2.50; 1.32–4.73), independent of the potential moderator variables examined. Although the statistical association was significant, clinically the absolute risk of PPHN of the newborn remained low.

Increased bleeding in newborns after fetal exposure to SSRI was reported (Mhanna 1997) and two case reports associated paroxetine treatment in late pregnancy with functional thrombocyte disturbance, which was associated with subarachnoidal or ventricular bleeding and seizures in mature newborns (Duijvestijn 2003, Salvia-Roiges 2003). However, a study of 27 full-term babies and their mothers found neither laboratory chemical nor clinical indications of thrombocyte function disturbances (Maayan-Metzger 2006).

In a small study of 52 newborns, an extended QT interval was observed compared to non-exposed children (409 vs. 392 milliseconds) (Dubnov-Raz 2008). In case reports, necrotizing enterocolitis in newborns was also reported in association with prenatal SSRI or venlafaxine exposure, including in term infants (Treichel 2009).

Salisbury (2011) examined potential effects of major depression with and without SSRI treatment on newborn neurobehavior in a prospective study. Women were seen at an outpatient research center twice during pregnancy at 26–28 and 36–38 weeks. Three exposure groups were studied: control ($n = 56$), major depression ($n = 20$) or major depression plus SSRI exposure ($n = 36$). Infants were assessed on a single occasion within 3 weeks of birth with the NICU Network Neurobehavioral Assessment Scale (NNNS). Full-term infants exposed to depression+SSRI had a lower gestational age than the controls or depression-exposed infants and (controlling for gestational age) lower quality of movement and more CNS stress signs. In contrast, depression-exposed infants had the highest quality of movement scores, while having lower attention scores than controls and depression + SSRI-exposed infants. Depression + SSRI-exposed infants have a different neurobehavioral profile than depression-exposed infants in the first 3 weeks after delivery. Both groups may have different neurobehavioral profiles with increasing age from birth.

Long-term development

Although animal studies have revealed adverse effects of fetal SSRI exposure on developmental outcomes (Ansorge 2008), human investigations have found no impact on either cognitive development or behavior. However, motor skill deficits have been reported in infants (Gentile 2011). Compared with offspring of mothers with depression, SSRI-exposed infants scored lower on the psychomotor index of the Bayley Scales of Infant Development – Second Edition (BSID-II) and the motor quality factor of the BSID-II Behavioral Rating Scale (Casper 2003), although their neurological examinations were normal. Longer duration of prenatal exposure increased the risk for lower psychomotor functioning in infants (Casper 2011). Delayed motor milestones were also described (by parental report) in a large ($n=415$) Danish National Birth Cohort (Pedersen 2010) in infants exposed prenatally to SSRI compared to infants exposed to maternal depression or antidepressants. However, these infants were still within the normal range of development and the differences in motor skill achievement were not significant at 19 months of age. Hanley (2013) also found that 10-month-old infants ($n = 31$) with prenatal SSRI exposure had lower gross motor functioning and social–emotional and adaptive behavior on the Bayley Scales of Infant Development (Third Edition) than non-exposed infants after controlling for prenatal and postpartum maternal depressed mood, smoking and alcohol use during pregnancy.

In contrast, Johnson (2012) studied 6-month-old infants and found no significant differences on the Infant Neurological International Battery between those exposed *in utero* to antidepressants compared to no psychotropic drug exposure controls. A comparison between children exposed prenatally to SSRIs and children in two control groups (209 tricyclic antidepressants, 185 non-drug exposed) also showed no significant differences between exposed and unexposed infants in rates of developmental delay or other neurological disorder in either the tricyclic antidepressant or SSRI groups (Simon 2002). Oberlander (2010) found that prenatal exposure to both maternal depressed mood and SSRI antidepressants were associated with increased internalizing behavior during early childhood, whereas current maternal depression increased risk for externalizing behavior. Increased child anxiety and depression symptoms were predicted by higher third-trimester maternal anxiety only in children with SLC6A4 two short S alleles. In contrast, increased aggression and externalizing behaviors were predicted by third-trimester maternal anxiety only in children with two copies of the L allele.

A significant association between dispensing of an SSRI prescription and autism spectrum disorder was observed (Croen 2011). However, the number of women exposed to SSRIs was low, and the proportion of children with autism statistically attributable to prenatal SSRI exposure was 2.1% for exposure during the year before delivery, and 2.3% for exposure during the first trimester. A history of maternal depression (adjusted odds ratio 1.49, 95% CI 1.08–2.08) was associated with an increased risk of autism spectrum disorders in offspring (Rai 2013). In the subsample with available data on drugs, this association was confined to women reporting antidepressant use during pregnancy (3.34, 1.50 to 7.47, $p = 0.003$), irrespective of whether SSRIs or other drugs were used. All associations were higher in cases of autism without intellectual disability. Antidepressant use during pregnancy explained 0.6% of the cases of autism spectrum disorder. Sørensen (2013) identified 668,468 Danish children and their parents in the Civil Registration System. Children exposed prenatally to antidepressants (ascertained by prescription filling) had an adjusted hazard ratio of 1.5 (95% CI 1.2–1.9) for autism spectrum disorder compared with unexposed children. Restricting the analysis to children of women with a diagnosis of affective disorder, the adjusted hazard ratio was 1.2 (95% CI 0.7–2.1), and the risk was further reduced when exposed children were compared with their unexposed siblings (adjusted hazard ratio 1.1; 95% CI 0.5–2.3). The authors concluded that there was no significant association between prenatal exposure to antidepressant medication and autism spectrum disorders in offspring after controlling for important confounding factors. In another study Danish investigators linked information on maternal use of SSRIs before and during pregnancy, autism spectrum disorders diagnosed in the offspring, and a range of confounders. The use of SSRIs during pregnancy was not associated with a significantly increased risk of autism spectrum disorders (adjusted rate ratio, 1.20; 95% CI 0.90–1.61; Hviid 2013).

Pregnancy

2.11 Psychotropic drugs

2.11.4   Tri- and tetracyclic antidepressants

A meta-analysis of the efficacy and tolerability of selective serotonin reuptake inhibitors (SSRIs) against tricyclic antidepressants (TCAs) (Anderson 2000) showed that the overall efficacy between the TCAs and SSRIs was comparable; however, SSRIs were not as effective in treating inpatients and amitriptyline was more effective than SSRI comparators. SSRIs had a modest advantage in terms of tolerability against most TCAs. The SSRIs are dramatically less toxic in overdose situations than the TCAs, due to lower cardiac toxicity.

TCA block the reuptake of the neurotransmitters (i.e. noradrenaline and serotonin) in the adrenergic neurons. The prototype of the TCA is imipramine. Similar medications are *clomipramine*, *dibenzepin* and *lofepramine*. Specific drugs have stimulating effects in some patients, such as with *desipramine* (metabolite of *imipramine*), *nortriptyline* (metabolite of *amitriptyline*; and *trimipramine* (chemically similar to imipramine). Other drugs typically have sedative effects, such as amitriptyline, *dosulepine*, *doxepin* and the chemically related *opipramol*, which has characteristics of both antidepressants and antipsychotics.

Maprotiline and *mianserin* belong to the group of tetracyclic antidepressants. Maprotiline primarily inhibits the synaptic reuptake of noradrenaline. In contrast to maprotiline and the tricyclic antidepressants, mianserin has minimal anticholinergic effects. *Ketanserin*, related to mianserin, was used for the treatment of preeclampsia and for tocolysis without any fetotoxic effects (Steyn 1998, Bolte 1997).

Maternal treatment and pregnancy complications

An advantage of the use of TCA during pregnancy is the availability of meaningful serum levels to assess dose adequacy across the changing milieu of pregnancy (Stika 2001). Oral dosages are likely to change as pregnancy progresses, particularly in the third trimester, to a mean of 1.6 times the nonpregnant dose to achieve a similar serum level (Wisner 1993). Less anticholinergic secondary amine drugs, such as nortriptyline and desipramine, are typically preferred to minimize side effects such as constipation, which is common in the later stages of pregnancy.

Simon (2002) reported that TCA exposure was not associated with any significant difference in perinatal outcomes. Reis (2010) reported an association between antidepressant treatment and prepregnancy diabetes and chronic hypertension, and also with pregnancy complications including induced delivery, caesarean birth, preterm birth, neonatal complications (particularly the sub group exposed to TCA) and PPHN. However, the contributors to these outcomes may be from the drug, the underlying depressive disorder and its sequelae or both.

Congenital malformations

In the 1970s and 1980s malformations such as anomalies of the limbs, heart, polydactyly and hypospadias were associated with tricyclic antidepressant exposure. However, increased rates of congenital malformations were not replicated in a total of approximately 1,000 pregnancies (Davis 2007, Pearson 2007, Simon 2002, McElhatton 1996). Reis (2010) found a slightly elevated risk of cardiac septum defects on the basis of Swedish health databases, which include about 1,600 pregnant women who reported taking or were prescribed TCA in the first trimester. The majority (about 75%) were treated with clomipramine.

Neonatal adaptation disorders

Neonatal symptoms such as jitteriness, excitability, respiratory distress syndrome and, sporadically, seizures were observed in newborns exposed in utero to TCA (Davis 2007, Källén 2004, Bromiker 1994, Schimmell 1991). Källén (2004) reported a higher risk for neonatal adaptation problems with TCA than with the SSRIs. The study included nearly 1,000 pregnant women with over a third of the women taking clomipramine ($n = 353$). This and other studies (e.g. Ericson 1999) have also observed a higher birth weight after tricyclic exposure than with SSRIs.

Long-term development

Nulman (1997) studied the children of 80 mothers who had received a TCA, 55 preschool children whose mothers had received fluoxetine, and 84 children not exposed to any agent known to affect the fetus adversely. The mean (±SD) global IQ scores were 118 ± 17 in the children of mothers who received a TCA, 117 ± 17 in those whose mothers received fluoxetine, and 115 ± 14 in those in the control group. Language scores were similar in all three groups. The results were similar in children exposed to a TCA or fluoxetine during the first trimester and those exposed throughout pregnancy. There were no significant differences in temperament, mood, arousability, activity level, distractibility, or behavior problems in the three groups of children. A later prospective study, by the same group of authors, also found no developmental problems in children (15 to 71 months) whose mothers had taken TCA throughout pregnancy (46 mother–child pairs, of which 36 were in the 1997 study). However, the duration of the maternal depression negatively affected the IQ and the frequency of maternal depressive episodes impacted speech development (Nulman 2002).

2.11.5   Individual antidepressants

In this section, information about individual agents is presented when available. For additional experience with antidepressants during pregnancy, effects on neonatal adjustment and Recommendation, see Sections 2.11.2, 2.11.3 and 2.11.4.

The majority of studies on TCA were conducted with the class rather than individual agents.

Myles (2013) performed a meta-analysis to evaluate the strength of the association between individual SSRIs and major, minor, and cardiac malformations among infants born to women taking these medications. *Fluoxetine* (OR 1.14, 95% CI 1.01–1.30) and *paroxetine* (OR 1.29, 95% CI 1.11–1.49) were associated with increased risk of major malformations. Paroxetine was associated with an increased risk for cardiac malformations (OR 1.44, 95% CI 1.12–1.86). *Sertraline* and *citalopram* were not significantly associated with congenital malformations. The authors emphasize the importance of data for individual medications within the SSRI class, and that confounding by indication is a concern in that different medications may be used for psychiatric disorders of different type and severity.

▶ **Agomelatine**

Agomelatine is a melatonergic MT1/MT2-agonist and 5-HT2C-antagonist that induces a phase advance of sleep, body temperature decline and

Pregnancy

2.11 Psychotropic drugs

the onset of melatonin release. The drug is not widely available and its efficacy has been debated. No data in human pregnancy are available.

▶ Amitriptyline

Amitriptyline is a TCA that is frequently used for its sedative effect; however, it has substantial anticholinergicity, which may increase the constipation and orthostatic hypotension experienced by women in the latter months of pregnancy. There is no evidence of teratogenic effects (Reis 2010, McElhatton 1996).

▶ Atomoxetine

Atomoxetine , an SNRI, is a non-stimulant drug used for the treatment of attention deficit/hyperactivity disorder. Atomoxetine is metabolized through P450 2D6. No human pregnancy data are available.

▶ Bupropion

Bupropion, also called *amfebutamone*, is an atypical antidepressant that inhibits the reuptake of noradrenaline and, to a lesser extent, dopamine. It is also indicated for use in smoking cessation. In the manufacturer's register of over 700 pregnant women treated in the first trimester (data on file; GlaxoSmithKline), no increased risk for malformations or any specific pattern of malformations was reported. Cole (2007b) evaluated the rate of congenital and cardiovascular malformations after first trimester exposure to bupropion (1,213 infants) compared with other antidepressant exposure (4,743 infants) and to bupropion exposure outside the first trimester (1,049 infants). The prevalence of malformations did not significantly differ across groups. Similarly, a study of 136 women exposed to bupropion during the first trimester resulted in no malformations and infants had a mean gestational age of 40 weeks (Chun-Fai-Chan 2005).

In contrast, Alwan (2010) conducted a retrospective case-control study of 6,853 infants with major heart defects compared to 5,869 control infants. Mothers of infants with left outflow tract defects were more likely to have reported taking bupropion during the first trimester than mothers of control infants (aOR 2.6; 95% CI 1.2–5.7; $p = 0.01$); however, the magnitude of the individual risk was considered low.

Smokers who used either bupropion or nicotine replacement therapy were more likely to stop or reduce smoking and were at decreased risk for giving birth prematurely or having an infant with low birth weight compared to pregnant smokers (Bérard 2007b).

A case report of fetal arrhythmia at 32 weeks gestation was associated with maternal treatment with bupropion (100 mg/day) from 30 weeks. The arrhythmia improved after discontinuation of bupropion (Leventhal 2010). It is important to note that case reports do not establish causality.

Figueroa (2010) found that exposure to bupropion during pregnancy (OR = 3.63, $p = 0.02$), especially during the second trimester (OR = 14.66, $p < 0.001$), was associated with increased risk of attention deficit hyperactivity disorder in offspring while exposure to SSRI was not (OR = 0.91, $p = 0.74$).

► **Citalopram**

Similar to other SSRIs, increased rates of malformations have not been consistently reported for *citalopram*. In the retrospective cohort study by Malm (2011), which did not indicate increased risk for malformations for SSRI as a class, analysis of individual drugs showed that citalopram use was associated with neural tube defects (aOR 2.46, 95% CI 1.20–5.07). However, fetal alcohol spectrum disorders were 10 times more common in the SSRI exposed offspring than in unexposed offspring and alcohol exposure has an established association with neural tube defects. Mothers who purchased prescriptions for SSRI were also 20 times more likely to have purchased another psychotropic drug.

Pregnant women who were taking citalopram and contacted the Canadian Teratogen Information Center ($n = 125$) were matched to a disease-matched group of women and a nonteratogen exposure group (Sivojelezova 2005). After birth, women were contacted to report pregnancy outcomes. Seventy-one (54%) women continued to take the drug throughout pregnancy. Fetal survival rates, mean birth weights, and duration of pregnancy were not statistically different among the three groups. Of 108 live-born infants whose mothers were exposed to citalopram in the first trimester, there was one (0.9%) male infant born with a major malformation. There was a relative risk of 4.2 (95% CI 1.71–10.26) in neonates exposed to citalopram in late pregnancy to be admitted to special-care nurseries as compared with the unexposed infants.

Six of 19 congenital defects out of 94 citalopram exposed pregnancies reported to the FDA involved the eye and were discussed by the authors in context with retinal and optic nerve changes in the rodents treated with citalopram (Tabacova 2004). Voluntary reporting to any adverse reporting system, such as the FDA, has an important function of generating hypotheses about relationships between drugs and adverse events. However, they are limited by identifying spurious associations and over-estimating the magnitude of associations.

► **Clomipramine**

*Clomipramine,*a TCA, is a unique antidepressant agent in that it has substantial serotonergic effects and was the first drug indicated for the treatment of obsessive compulsive disorder. The substantial serotonergic and anticholinergic side effects have relegated clomipramine to a second line drug for most patients.

The ratios of umbilical cord to maternal serum concentration at delivery of clomipramine and desmethylclomipramine were 0.60 ± 0.50 and 0.80 ± 0.60, respectively. Obstetrical complications, such as preterm delivery and gestational hypertension, were increased compared to the national average (Loughhead 2006b).

Ten infants exposed to clomipramine in utero were evaluated for neonatal withdrawal symptoms at 12, 24 and 48 h after birth (ter Horst 2012). Symptoms included short duration of sleep after feeding, poor feeding, mild to severe tremors, hyperactive Moro reflex and tachypnea, tachycardia and cyanosis. The drug's half-life in newborns was 42 ± 16 hours; however, the correlation of withdrawal symptoms and plasma concentration was weak.

Pregnancy

2.11 Psychotropic drugs

▶ Desipramine

Desipramine, an SNRI, is an active metabolite of the prototype TCA imipramine. It has a stimulating effect in some patients.

▶ Doxepin

Doxepin is a TCA that is often used for its sedative properties.

▶ Duloxetine

Duloxetine, an SNRI, is indicated for treatment of depression and anxiety disorders, neuropathic pain, diabetic peripheral neuropathy, musculoskeletal pain, fibromyalgia and, in some countries, stress incontinence. The manufacturer's database for the reporting of adverse events and the FDA Adverse Events Reporting System (AERS) through 2011 were reviewed (Hoog 2013). The databases provided voluntary reporting data from women who had been treated with duloxetine during pregnancy. In the manufacturer's data, 233 prospectively reported cases were available. The rates of miscarriages, congenital anomalies, ectopic pregnancy and stillbirth were similar to historic control rates in the general population. For the AERS database analysis, there was no disproportionate elevation of adverse pregnancy outcomes including congenital anomalies, miscarriage, ectopic pregnancy and stillbirth in patients treated with duloxetine compared to historical data from patients exposed to other antidepressants.

▶ Escitalopram

Escitalopram is the S(+)enantiomer of racemic citalopram. Like *citalopram*, escitalopram is a well-tolerated antidepressant for treatment of depression and anxiety disorders. Klieger-Grossmann (2012) analyzed pregnancy outcomes in women exposed to escitalopram ($n = 212$), other antidepressants ($n = 212$) and nonteratogenic drug exposures ($n = 212$). No depressed comparison group was included. Among the escitalopram exposures were 172 (81%) live births, 32 (15%) miscarriages, six (2.8%) therapeutic abortions, three stillbirths (1.7%), and three major malformations (1.7%). Escitalopram was not associated with an increased risk for major malformations but an increase in the risk for categorical low birth weight (<2,500 g), lower mean birth weight (escitalopram, $3,198 \pm 594$ g; other antidepressants, $3,470 \pm 540$; nonteratogen controls 3470 ± 540 g $p<0.001$).

▶ Fluoxetine

Fluoxetine is an SSRI with stimulating action in some patients. This agent was the first SSRI medication approved by the FDA for marketing in 1987. Fluoxetine is used to treat depression, obsessive-compulsive and panic disorders, bulimia and premenstrual dysphoric disorder. Riggin (2013) performed a systematic review of the literature for women who were exposed to fluoxetine during the first trimester and compared outcomes with those of unexposed control subjects. The odds ratio for major malformations associated with maternal fluoxetine use in cohort studies was 1.12 (95% CI 0.98–1.28). For cardiac malformations the overall odds ratio was 1.6 (95% CI 1.31–1.95). In contrast, two case-control studies assessing cardiac malformations yielded a combined odds ratio of 0.63 (95% CI 0.39–1.03). A register-based retrospective nation-wide cohort study, using the Danish Medical Birth Registry observed that risks of congenital malformations of the heart were similar for pregnancies exposed to an SSRI throughout the first trimester, adjusted OR 2.01 (95% CI 1.60–2.53), and for pregnancies with paused SSRI treatment during pregnancy, adjusted OR 1.85 (95% CI 1.07–3.20), p value for difference: 0.94. The authors found similar increased risks of specific congenital malformations of the heart for the individual SSRIs. The authors concluded that the apparent association between SSRI use and congenital malformations of the heart may be due to residual confounding (Jimenez-Solem 2012).

▶ Fluvoxamine

Fluvoxamine is an SSRI which is used for obsessive compulsive disorder and other anxiety disorders. It is used infrequently compared to other SSRIs (Sivojelezova 2004). Women with fluvoxamine exposure during pregnancy were matched (on age, time of first call to the teratogen information service, and smoking/drinking habits) to a disease-control group of women with depression and SSRI use in pregnancy. Data from 92 women showed that fetal survival rates, birth weight, and rates of major malformations did not differ statistically between both groups. In the fluvoxamine group, two (4.7%) major malformations compared to two (4.3%) in the disease-control group were observed. These preliminary results suggest that the use of fluvoxamine during pregnancy is not associated with an increased risk of major malformations above the baseline risk.

▶ Imipramine

Imipramine is the prototype TCA and is discussed under combined TCA exposures.

▶ Maprotiline

Maprotiline is a tetracyclic antidepressant. It is a strong norepinephrine reuptake inhibitor with only weak effects on serotonin and dopamine reuptake. In approximately 100 exposed pregnancies included in grouped data with other antidepressants, no preliminary indication of teratogenic effects was observed (Reis 2010, McElhatton 1996).

▶ Mianserin

Mianserin is a tetracyclic antidepressant that is structurally similar to mirtazapine. No pregnancy exposure data for human pregnancy was located.

Pregnancy

2.11 Psychotropic drugs

▶ **Mirtazapine**

Mirtazapine is a tetracyclic antidepressant with noradrenergic and specific serotonergic antidepressant effects that is used for the treatment of depression. It is also used as an anxiolytic, hypnotic, antiemetic and appetite stimulant. Its antiemetic action has been efficacious for women with hyperemesis gravidarum. Djulus (2006) analyzed information from teratogen information sites with disease-matched pregnant women with depression taking other antidepressants and pregnant women exposed to nonteratogens. For 104 pregnancies, there were 77 live births, one stillbirth, 20 miscarriages, six therapeutic abortions, and two major malformations in the mirtazapine group. The differences among the three groups were in the rate of miscarriage, which was higher in both antidepressant groups (19% in the mirtazapine group and 17% in the other antidepressant group) than in the nonteratogen group (11%), but none of the differences were statistically significant. The rate of preterm births (prior to 37 weeks' gestation) was also higher in the mirtazapine group (10%) and in the other antidepressant group (7%) than in the nonteratogen group (2%). The difference was statistically significant between the mirtazapine group and the nonteratogen group ($p = 0.04$).

Mirtazapine was effective in the treatment of 11 pregnant women with hyperemesis gravidarum due to its action to block 5-HT^3 receptors which helps prevent nausea and vomiting in addition to its antianxiety, antidepressant effects as well as improving sleep continuity and increasing appetite (Guclu 2005, Rohde 2003, Saks 2001).

▶ **Moclobemide**

Moclobemide reversibly and selectively inhibits the enzyme monoamine oxidase (MAO), which oxidatively inactivates the transmitter substances in the adrenergic system (noradrenalin and adrenalin). MAO inhibitor substances are structurally related to amphetamines and are used primarily for treatment-refractory depression. MAO inhibitors can increase the risk for gestational hypertension and reduce placental perfusion with negative effects on fetal development. In addition, they can negate tocolysis with betamimetics and interact with the narcotics during childbirth. Normal development was documented in four children who were exposed during the entire pregnancy and while breastfeeding (Taylor 2008). A single case report of moclobemide in pregnancy also described a healthy pregnancy with normal development of the infant through 14 months (Rybakowski 2001).

▶ **Nortriptyline**

Nortriptyline is a TCA and the main active metabolite of amitriptyline. It is a drug of choice among TCA, and serum levels are available to direct dosing in conjunction with clinical assessment.

Maternal and umbilical cord sera were collected at delivery from ten women taking nortriptyline (Loughhead 2006b). The placental passage ratios of nortriptyline and its active metabolite, *cis*-10-hydroxynortriptyline, were 0.68 ± 0.40 and 1.40 ± 2.40, respectively, which are higher than those reported in placenta perfusion studies.

► **Opipramol**

Opipramol is a TCA; no data specific to this drug were located.

► **Phenelzine**

Phenelzine irreversibly blocks monoamine oxidase (MAO), and the effect persists for at least 14–21 days after discontinuation. This drug is used for patients who do not respond to other agents. While taking phenelzine, dietary intake of *tyramine* must be limited to avoid a hypertensive crisis. Few reports of its use during pregnancy have been published, and drug interactions during labor and delivery must be carefully considered (Gracious 1997).

► **Paroxetine**

Paroxetine is the SSRI that has been most consistently related to malformations, specifically cardiac malformations; however, several studies have demonstrated positive associations that become non-significant after adjustment for confounding variables. Louik (2007) did not find significant associations between overall use of SSRI and birth defects; however, they did find a tripling of the risk of right ventricular outflow tract obstruction defects associated with paroxetine use (OR, 3.3), based on six exposed subjects. Among 66 comparisons in the Louik (2007) study, two had lower confidence bounds that exceeded 1.0: paroxetine's association with neural-tube defects and clubfoot (four and 10 exposed subjects, respectively).

To examine the association between paroxetine and cardiovascular defects, Einarson (2008) used teratology information services around the world, to evaluate two exposure cohorts: (1) prospectively ascertained, unpublished cases of infants exposed to paroxetine in the first trimester of pregnancy versus unexposed infants ($n = 1,174$), and (2) outcomes of infants exposed to paroxetine ($n = 2,061$) derived from publications in which all SSRI were included. For the first cohort, the rates of cardiac defects in the paroxetine group and in the unexposed group were both 0.7%. The rate in the second cohort was 1.5%. Because the incidence in more than 3,000 infants was well within the population incidence of about 1%, the authors concluded that paroxetine was not associated with an increased risk of cardiovascular defects following use in early pregnancy.

Diav-Citrin (2008) conducted a multicenter, prospective, controlled study to assess the rate of major congenital anomalies after first-trimester exposure to paroxetine compared to non-teratogens. They studied 410 paroxetine first-trimester exposed pregnancies and 1,467 controls. There was a higher rate of major anomalies, primarily cardiovascular malformations, in the paroxetine exposed group compared to controls. However, following adjustment for confounders, the OR for paroxetine was no longer significant, and the authors commented that the diversity of cardiovascular anomalies did not support a common underlying mechanism of teratogenicity.

Bakker (2010) studied 678 cases with isolated heart defects and 615 controls. The first trimester exposure rate was 1.5% for cases and 1.0% for controls. After excluding mothers who used paroxetine outside the first trimester, or who had used another SSRI, they found no significantly increased risk for heart defects overall , but did find a significantly increased risk for atrium septum defects (three exposed cases; OR, 5.7; 95% CI 1.4–23.7).

The only study to evaluate dosage of paroxetine (Bérard 2007a) was an analysis of medication databases that included all pregnancies in Quebec. Two nested case-control studies were used to compare the prevalence of paroxetine use in the first trimester of pregnancy to the prevalence of other antidepressant exposures during the same time period. Cases were defined as major malformations or cardiac malformations diagnosed in the first year of life; controls were defined as no major or minor malformations. Multivariate logistic regression techniques were used to analyze data. Among the 1,403 women meeting inclusion criteria, 101 infants with major congenital malformations were identified, 24 of whom had cardiac malformations. Adjusting for possible confounders, the use of paroxetine or other SSRI during the first trimester did not increase the risk of congenital cardiac malformations compared with the use of non-SSRI antidepressants. A dose-response relationship was observed in that women exposed to >25 mg/day of paroxetine during the first trimester of pregnancy were at increased risk of having an infant with major congenital malformations (aOR = 2.23, 95% CI = 1.19, 4.17) or major cardiac malformations (AOR = 3.07, 95% CI = 1.00, 9.42). Women on higher doses of medication are also more likely to have greater severity of the underlying illness and its sequelae.

Two meta-analyses also found significant increases in risks for heart malformations. Wurst (2010) reported combined cardiac defects (prevalence odds ratio, 1.46; 95% CI 1.17–1.82) and aggregated congenital defects (1.24; 95% CI 1.08–1.43) with first trimester paroxetine use. Bar-Oz (2007) found that first-trimester paroxetine exposure was associated with a significant increase in the risk for cardiac malformation (OR, 1.72; 95% CI 1.22–2.42). They also reported that women using antidepressants in pregnancy had a 30% higher rate of ultrasound procedures, which would increase identification of anomalies. Infants of women who received SSRI underwent approximately twice as many echocardiograms in the first year of life compared with children of women who were unexposed. Significantly more women receiving paroxetine used the drug for anxiety or panic than women receiving other SSRI (OR, 4.11; 95% CI 2.39–7.08). The authors concluded that a detection bias was a possible contributor to the apparent increased rate of cardiovascular malformation of children exposed *in utero* to paroxetine.

Cole (2007a) studied mono- or mono/polytherapy exposure to paroxetine and other antidepressants. For paroxetine, there were 815 infants born to 791 women exposed as monotherapy and 1,020 infants born to 989 women exposed as mono- or polytherapy. AORs for all congenital malformations associated with paroxetine were 1.89 (95% CI 1.20–2.98) for monotherapy and 1.76 (95% CI 1.18–2.64) for mono- or polytherapy. AORs for cardiovascular malformations associated with paroxetine were not signficant: 1.46 (95% CI 0.74–2.88) for monotherapy and 1.68 (95% CI 0.95–2.97) for mono- or polytherapy. The authors concluded that their results suggest the possibility of a modestly increased occurrence of congenital malformations following first trimester exposure to paroxetine compared to other antidepressants.

To summarize, paroxetine has received the most attention among SSRI due to reports of a slightly elevated risk for cardiac malformations in some, but not all studies. Confounding factors and greater vigilance for defects are also possible interpretations of positive studies. Neonatal adjustment disorders may be more marked with paroxetine than with other SSRI (Moses-Kolko 2005). Unless paroxetine is the most favorable drug for the individual woman's psychiatric care, other SSRI are preferred for treatment during pregnancy.

▶ **Reboxetine**

Reboxetine is an SNRI, the effectiveness of which has been questioned and the tolerability of which has been judged critically (Eyding 2010). Individual case reports and around 40 pregnancies in two studies are available (Reis 2010, Lennestål 2007), which are not sufficient for a differentiated risk assessment.

▶ **Sertraline**

Sertraline is among the SSRI of first choice for treatment during pregnancy due to its tolerability and minimal interactions with other medications.

In the North American case-control study by Louik (2007), the only significant association in common with that of the parallel study by Alwan (2007) was between *sertraline* use and *omphalocele* (OR, 5.7; 95% CI, 1.6–20.7), which was based on only three affected subjects. Among 66 comparisons (Louik 2007), two had lower confidence bounds that exceeded 1.0: sertraline's association with anal atresia and limb-reduction defects (three exposed subjects for each defect). These were previously unreported associations, and the authors recommended cautious interpretation. They commented that due to the absence of pre-existing hypotheses and multiple comparisons for birth defects, distinguishing random variation from true elevations in risk is difficult and further study is necessary. They cautioned that these estimates should not be interpreted as strong evidence of increased risks.

In the Pedersen (2009) study, filled prescriptions for sertraline were associated with septal heart defects, with six of 352 exposed children (OR 3.25, 1.21–8.75) which are not supported by the majority of other studies.

▶ **Tranylcypromine**

Tranylcypromine is an irreversible inhibitor of monoamine oxidase (MAO), which oxidatively inactivates the transmitter substances in the adrenergic system (epinephrine and norepinephrine). Tranylcypromine is only used for women who do not respond to other medications. MAOs are structurally related to amphetamines and can exacerbate hypertension during pregnancy and potentially reduce placental perfusion. When taking tranylcypromine, dietary intake of tyramine must be limited to avoid a hypertensive crisis. Little information about tranylcypromine use during pregnancy is available, and drug interactions during labor and delivery must be carefully considered (Gracious 1997).

Two cases of multiple fetal anomalies associated with high-dose tranylcypromine therapy and other medications (100 mg/day, *pimozide* 1 mg/day and *diazepam* 5–10 mg/day) have been reported (Kennedy 2001). The first case resulted in a stillbirth at 31 weeks. Postmortem examination revealed hypertelorism, an atrioventricular septal defect, single coronary ostium, right pulmonary isomerism and multiple placental infarcts. In the second case, the patient presented with a 19 week fetus with a malformed head and a fetal echocardiogram revealed atrioventricular septal defect. She delivered surgically at 38 weeks; the infant had a normal female karyotype but had hypertelorism, low-set overfolded ears, cleft palate, micrognathia, distal phalangeal hypoplasia, agenesis of the corpus callosum and atrioventricular septal defect.

Trazodone

Trazodone has prominent sedative effects and is often prescribed in low doses as a hypnotic agent. Einarson (2003) studied 147 pregnant women from five centers who had been exposed to trazodone ($n = 58$) or *nefazodone* ($n = 89$) during the first trimester. The comparison groups were women who took other antidepressant drugs ($n = 147$) or nonteratogenic drugs ($n = 147$). Of the 121 live births in the trazodone/nefazodone group, two (1.6%) had major malformations. The results suggest that these drugs do not increase the rates of major malformations above the baseline rate.

Trimipramine

Trimipramine is a TCA with sedative effects. No data specific to this agent were located.

Venlafaxine

Venlafaxine is an SNRI. Data from the National Birth Defects Prevention Study, a population-based, case-control study in the United States, was used to evaluate the relationship between venlafaxine and birth defects (Polen 2013). Among the 27,045 participants who met inclusion criteria, 0.17% of mothers with normal infants and 0.40% of mothers of infants with birth defects reported use of venlafaxine from 1 month preconception through the third month of pregnancy. Statistically significant associations were found for anencephaly, atrial septal defect (ASD) secundum or ASD not otherwise specified, coarctation of the aorta, cleft palate, and gastroschisis. The data suggested associations between periconceptional use of venlafaxine and some birth defects. However, sample sizes were small, confidence intervals were wide, and multiple comparisons were made. Results from a prospective controlled study of 71 women exposed to venlafaxine compared to nonteratogen exposures (Di Gianantonio 2006) suggested that the use of venlafaxine does not increase the rate of adverse pregnancy outcomes.

Palmsten found that the risk for preeclampsia was higher among women receiving venlafaxine 1.57 (95% CI 1.29–1.91) (Palmsten 2013b).

Fluid obtained during amniocentesis was analyzed and the ratio of venlafaxine concentrations of amniotic fluid to maternal serum were higher for three cases of venlafaxine, which averaged 172% (SD = 91%), than for SSRI ($n = 22$), which averaged 11.6% (SD = 9.9%) (Loughhead 2006a).

Boucher (2009) measured cord and maternal drug concentrations at birth and in neonates on day 3. Median cord/maternal distribution ratio was 0.72 for venlafaxine and 1.08 for the *O*-desmethyl metabolite.

Neonatal abstinence scores were significantly higher in exposed than non-exposed infants on day 1. Mild behavioral symptoms in the early perinatal period were transient. Rampono (2009) correlated neonatal clinical signs over time with serum concentrations of venlafaxine and its active metabolite in the neonatal period in seven subjects. Median maternal venlafaxine dose was 75 mg/day (37.5–300 mg/day). Five neonates presented with multiple clinical signs including tachypnea and respiratory distress. Respiratory distress was present within the first hours after birth, with other symptoms appearing subsequently. The elimination half-life, calculated for three neonates, ranged between 12 and 15 hours for venlafaxine and between 10 and 37 hours for O-desmethylvenlafaxine. Neonatal clinical signs emerged as drug concentrations declined which suggests discontinuation as the etiology.

Because venlafaxine has a relatively short half-life and higher incidence of abrupt discontinuation syndrome in adults, the rate of poor neonatal adaptation associated with venlafaxine in late pregnancy was evaluated (Tanaka 2007). Infants exposed to venlafaxine were compared to those exposed to paroxetine and to those with no exposure to antidepressants. From 83 subjects, five of 36 (13.8%) in the venlafaxine group, two of 23 (8.7%) in the paroxetine group, and none of the 24 in the non-exposed group had poor neonatal adaptation.

Three case reports describe seizures in newborns as possible withdrawal symptoms, but epileptiform changes by EEG were documented in only one (Hoppenbrouwers 2010). The mother was a 28-year-old multigravida who was treated with venlafaxine 75 mg daily during pregnancy. She smoked 8 to 10 cigarettes daily. At 18 hours of age, the infant was admitted to the NICU. The serum concentrations of venlafaxine and its active metabolite were below the sensitivity of the assay. At the age of 1 month the infant showed normal growth and neurodevelopment.

The development of four groups of children with the following maternal prenatal treatment were compared: venlafaxine, SSRI, untreated depressed women, and non-depressed healthy women. Children exposed to venlafaxine, SSRI, and maternal depression during fetal life had similar intelligence quotients (IQs; 105, 105, and 108, respectively), which were significantly lower than children of non-depressed mothers (112). The authors concluded that factors other than antidepressant exposure during pregnancy predicted children's intellect and behavior (Nulman 2012).

2.11.6   Antipsychotic treatment

Among the classic antipsychotics, also called typical antipsychotics or first generation neuroleptics, are the phenothiazines (*chlorpromazine, fluphenazine, levomepromazine, perazine, perphenazine, promethazine, prothipendyl, thioridazine,* and *zuclopenthixol*), the thioxanthenes (*chlorprothixene* and *flupentixol*), and the butyrophenones (*haloperidol, benperidol, bromperidol, droperidol, melperone, pimozide* and *pipamperone* as well as the structurally related *fluspirilene*). Atypical antipsychotics (second generation antipsychotics) include *amisulpride, aripiprazole, asenapine, clozapine, iloperidone, lurasidone, olanzapine, paliperidone, quetiapine, risperidone, sertindole, sulpiride* and *ziprasidone*.

Antipsychotic drugs block dopamine-2 receptors and reduce symptoms such as hallucinations and delusions. The atypical agents are associated with

Pregnancy

2.11 Psychotropic drugs

fewer extrapyramidal side effects such as tardive dyskinesia, tremor, rigidity, akathisia, bradykinesia, and dystonia compared to the first generation antipsychotics. However, side effects of the atypicals include somnolence, dry mouth, akathisia, and elevated hepatic enzymes. Although hyperprolactinemia is primarily associated with typical antipsychotics, the atypical drug risperidone is also likely to induce hyperprolactinemia. Standard clinical practice does not include serum level monitoring for antipsychotic drugs.

The metabolic side effects of atypical antipsychotics are prominent. Weight gain, elevated lipids, and metabolic syndrome frequently occur with atypical antipsychotic therapy, particularly olanzapine (Lieberman 2005). Overweight and obese women are at increased risk of multiple pregnancy complications, including gestational diabetes, hypertension, preeclampsia, surgical delivery, and postpartum weight retention (ACOG 2013). Infants of overweight or obese pregnant women have increased risk of stillbirth, congenital anomalies, preterm birth, macrosomia with birth injury, intrapartum anesthesia difficulties, and childhood obesity. Use of an atypical antipsychotic agent should be accompanied by close monitoring of gestational weight gain and glucose tolerance throughout pregnancy (Sit 2013).

According to a population-based Swedish cohort study, women who used antipsychotics during pregnancy had increased risk for gestational diabetes (Bodén 2012a). Two groups of women who filled prescriptions for an antipsychotic during pregnancy were compared to women not exposed to antipsychotics. The groups included women with prescriptions for: (1) olanzapine and/or clozapine, the most obesogenic and diabetogenic antipsychotics ($n = 169$), (2) other antipsychotics ($n = 338$), or (3) no antipsychotics ($n = 357,696$). Exposure to other antipsychotics was associated with an increased risk of gestational diabetes (aOR, 1.77; 95% CI 1.04–3.03). The risk increase with olanzapine and/or clozapine was of similar magnitude but was not statistically significant (aOR, 1.94; 95% CI 0.97–3.91).

Pregnancy is associated with dramatically altered physiology. Although no data about the need for dose adjustments in pregnancy are available, the clinical status of the pregnant woman should be monitored for sustained efficacy. Changes in liver metabolism with pregnancy may contribute to decreased serum levels of risperidone, aripiprazole, and iloperidone, which are metabolized by CYP2D6, and possibly quetiapine, metabolized by CYP3A4; conversely, these changes may lead to increased serum levels of clozapine and olanzapine, which are principally metabolized by CYP1A2 (Robakis 2013).

The reproductive risks of atypical antipsychotics have received less research attention than antidepressants. According to a Swedish study, pregnant women who received either typical or atypical drugs had increased risks for preterm birth, low birthweight, and major malformations compared to the general population. The malformations (mainly atrial and ventricular septal defects) affected only infants with exposure to first generation antipsychotics (Reis 2008). The rates of preterm birth were similar among patients who received typical or atypical agents. Although genetic liability and gene-environment interactions contribute to these outcomes, maternal risk factors, substance abuse, nutritional status, and biological and behavioral sequelae of severe mental illness are likely to be the major determinants of reproductive adversity in this group of women.

Another study found that infants of mothers who received typical antipsychotic drugs weighed less than infants of mothers who received atypical or non-antipsychotic drugs (Newham 2008). Significantly more large-for-gestational age babies were born to mothers who received atypical agents (20%) compared to mothers who received typical agents (2%), or non-antipsychotics (3%).

The largest cohort study on second-generation antipsychotic agents (SGAs) is based on data from the German national teratology service (Habermann 2013). The pregnancies of 561 women exposed to SGAs (study cohort) were prospectively followed and compared to 284 pregnant women exposed to first-generation antipsychotic agents (FGAs) and to 1,122 pregnant women using drugs known as not harmful to the unborn. Major malformation rates of SGA exposed were higher compared to non-teratogen exposed controls (aOR 2.17; 95% CI 1.20–3.91), possibly reflecting a detection bias concerning atrial and ventricular septal defects. Postnatal disorders occurred significantly more often in infants prenatally exposed to SGAs (15.6%) and FGAs (21.6%) compared to 4.2% for non-teratogens cohort II. Cumulative incidences of elective terminations of pregnancy were significantly higher in both the SGA (17%) and FGA (21%) compared to non-teratogen exposed (3%), whereas the rates of spontaneous abortions did not differ. The numbers of stillbirths and neonatal deaths were within the reference range. Preterm birth and low birth weight were more common in infants exposed to FGAs. The authors concluded that their findings did not reveal a major teratogenic risk for SGAs.

Infants born to pregnant women treated with antipsychotics may exhibit extrapyramidal and other symptoms including agitation, increased or decreased muscle tone, tremor, sleepiness, respiratory difficulties, and feeding problems. Infants prenatally exposed to antipsychotics showed significantly lower neuromotor development scores than those with no psychotropic exposure (Johnson et al. 2012). The neuromotor scores were also significantly associated with maternal psychiatric history, including depression, psychosis, and overall severity/chronicity, which again illustrates the difficulty separating the impact of medication from the underlying psychotic disorder.

Recommendation.

- A risk benefit model for decision making has been published (Wisner 2007). A primary factor in the choice of an antipsychotic drug during pregnancy is the woman's treatment history. The drug to which she has responded with an acceptable side effect burden deserves first consideration.
- Optimize the dose of a single drug before considering additional drug treatments.
- First generation antipsychotics also have anti-nauseant effects, which may reduce morning sickness.
- The Clinical Antipsychotic Trials in Intervention Effectiveness (CATIE) study (Lieberman 2005) of 1,493 patients with schizophrenia, demonstrated that the efficacy of the typical agent perphenazine was similar to that of quetiapine, risperidone, and ziprasidone. Olanzapine was the most effective agent but was associated with greater weight gain and increases in measures of glucose and lipid metabolism.
- With atypical antispychotics, particularly clozapine and olanzapine, weight gain, hyperglycemia and glucose intolerance have been observed in pregnant women.
- Always inquire about alcohol, cigarettes and other drug use, environmental exposures, as well as over the counter and prescribed medication intake, and record them in the patient's medical chart prior to writing any prescriptions.

Pregnancy

2.11 Psychotropic drugs

- Central nervous, gastrointestinal and respiratory adaptation disturbances have been described in newborns exposed in utero to antipsychotic drugs. The adaptation disturbances are usually limited; however, some infants had extrapyramidal symptoms and other symptoms that continued for weeks to months.
- Classic antipsychotics, such as butyrophenones and phenothiazine/thioxanthenes, may reduce fertility via increasing prolactin.
- With the exception of amisulpride, sulpiride and risperidone, atypical antipsychotics do not increase prolactin concentrations. Hyperprolactinemia carries the risk of undesired pregnancy if there is a change from first generation to second generation antipsychotics and the prolactin lowering of fertility ceases (McKenna 2004).
- Information about the impact of drugs in pregnancy is constantly evolving. A free resource for updates is the US National Library of Medicine (http://toxnet.nlm.nih.gov/) for DART (Developmental and Reproductive Toxicology Database).

2.11.7   Individual antipsychotic drugs

▶ Amisulpride

Amisulpride is an atypical antipsychotic. Because of the risk for hyperprolactinemia, conception may be compromised in women who desire a pregnancy. No information about exposure to this agent in human pregnancy is available.

▶ Aripiprazole

Aripiprazole is an atypical antipsychotic used to treat schizophrenia, bipolar disorder and treatment refractory depression (in combination with an antidepressant). It is characterized by mixed dopaminergic agonism (in regions of reduced dopaminergic activity) and antagonism. Aripiprazole is associated with reduction in prolactin levels, and interference with breastfeeding has been reported (Mendhekar 2006) after a normal pregnancy. There are cohort studies (Lutz 2010) and case reports on around 100 pregnancies (Habermann 2013, Gentile 2010), with no indication of specific teratogenicity in this limited literature.

▶ Asenapine

Asenapine is an atypical antipsychotic drug for the treatment of schizophrenia and mania. No data on its use in pregnancy are available.

▶ Benperidol

Benperidol is the butyrophenone with the highest neuroleptic potency and substantial side effects (extrapyramidal-motor symptoms). Its use is reserved for treatment-resistant patients.

▶ Bromperidol

Bromperidol is a butyrophenone structurally related to haloperidol; no human pregnancy data are available.

► Chlorpromazine

Chlorpromazine is the prototype phenothiazine which, in the 1970s, was also used to treat nausea in pregnant women at doses lower than for antipsychotic treatment. Slone (1977) evaluated first-trimester chlorpromazine exposure in 142 women and found no evidence of increased risk of birth defects, perinatal mortality, abnormal birth-weight, or abnormal IQ score at 4 years of age. Kris (1961, 1965) studied 52 children who had been exposed to chlorpromazine during fetal life (50–150 mg/day) through ages 2–4 years. No increased risk for physical or developmental problems was observed. A record review found that outcomes for 52 women who received chlorpromazine (Sobel 1960) were similar to a control group of untreated women who delivered at the same psychiatric hospital; however, the infants of three women who were treated with high doses (500–600 mg/day) exhibited respiratory distress and died.

Jaundice, hypotonicity, lethargy and extrapyramidal syndromes have been described in infants exposed *in utero* to chlorpromazine.

► Chlorprothixene

Chlorprothixene is among the thioxanthenes. It is a low potency neuroleptic used for sedation. Minimal information is available with respect to human pregnancy (Reis 2008); however, there is no indication of an increased risk of malformations with the phenothiazines and thioxanthenes.

► Clozapine

Clozapine was the first atypical antipsychotic available. Due to the risk of agranulocytosis and myocarditis as well as seizures, clozapine is prescribed for treatment-refractory patients. Regular white cell count monitoring is required. To date there are no reports of agranulocytosis in exposed newborns.

There have been no indications of increased malformations from approximately 400 pregnancies published to date (Habermann 2013, Gentile 2010, Reis 2008, McKenna 2005). Multiple case reports and a Swedish study (Bodén 2012a) describe a doubling of the risk for gestational diabetes in women treated with clozapine (or olanzapine) compared to untreated women. A case report describes reduced fetal heart-rate variability at the end of the pregnancy (Yogev 2002). Sedation of the newborn, jitteriness, or other withdrawal symptoms as well as seizures and floppy-infant symptoms have been described (Gentile 2010).

► Droperidol

Droperidol is a butyrophenone that is used for postoperative nausea and vomiting and as an antipsychotic. It has been evaluated in two studies with a total of more than 100 pregnant women, who received the medication for nausea. There was no indication of birth defects (Turcotte 2001, Nageotte 1996).

Pregnancy

2.11 Psychotropic drugs

▶ Flupentixol

Flupentixol is among the thioxanthenes and is frequently used as a depot medication. There are published results on flupentixol for about 100 pregnancies (Reis 2008), which give no indication of an increased risk for malformations.

The concentration of the active drug flupentixol in umbilical cord serum was lower than that in maternal serum with a ratio of 0.24 (Kirk 1980).

▶ Fluphenazine

Fluphenazine is a phenothiazine and is among the classic antipsychotic drugs. There are published reports on fluphenazine for about 200 pregnancies (Gentile 2010), which, as is the case for the other phenothiazines, gives no indication of an increased risk of malformations.

▶ Fluspirilene

Fluspirilene is a diphenylbutylpiperidine with characteristics similar to those of butyrophenones. There are about 40 prospectively analyzed pregnancies (Diav-Citrin 2005), in which no indication of increased risk for birth defects was found.

▶ Haloperidol

Haloperidol is the most important representative of the butyrophenones and is the best studied in pregnancy. It has a high antipsychotic potency with minimal sedative effects. Due to the substantial occurrence of extrapyramidal symptoms, *biperiden* is frequently given in addition. Although case reports of limb reduction anomalies associated with haloperidol exposure were published, later case series and prospective studies did not confirm an increase in birth defects. In an evaluation of haloperidol for the treatment of hyperemesis gravidarum, 100 women and their offspring were studied (Van Vaes 1969). No adverse effects were noted on birth weight, duration of pregnancy, or fetal or neonatal mortality, and no malformations were observed. Data are available on a total of over 400 pregnant women, treated primarily in the first trimester or throughout pregnancy, as well as from retrospective case-control studies (Gentile 2010, Reis 2008, Diav-Citrin 2005).

▶ Iloperidone

Iloperidone is a new atypical antipsychotic used to treat schizophrenia. No data about its use in pregnancy are available.

▶ Levomepromazine

Levomepromazine is a phenothiazine with low potency and marked sedative and hypotensive side effects. There are around 50 published results on pregnancies with levomepromazine (Reis 2008), which, as is the case with the other phenothiazines, gave no indication of an increased risk of malformations.

▶ **Lurasidone**

Lurasidone is a newer atypical antipsychotic used to treat schizophrenia and depressive episodes associated with bipolar disorder. No data are currently available for the use of this drug during pregnancy.

▶ **Melperone**

Melperone is one of the butyrophenones. It is a low-potency neuroleptic that is used for sedation and sleep promotion. It has more limited extrapyramidal side effects than haloperidol. Few data are available in pregnancy.

▶ **Olanzapine**

Olanzapine is a second generation antipsychotic with sedating effects. It is used for the treatment of both schizophrenia and bipolar disorder. No increased risk for birth defects has been observed in the majority of studies covering more than 400 pregnancies in total (Habermann 2013, Gentile 2010, Reis 2008, McKenna 2005, Levinson 2003, Mendhekar 2002, Biswas 2001, Malek-Ahmadi 2001, Nagy 2001, Neumann 2001, Goldstein 2000, Kirchheiner 2000). Brunner (2013) analyzed prospective post-marketing reproductive data from a worldwide safety database maintained by the manufacturer. In a sample of 610 mothers, 9.8% had preterm births, 8% had other perinatal conditions and 4.4% had congenital anomalies. These rates were consistent with outcomes in the general population.

The metabolic side effects of olanzapine are prominent. Weight gain and elevated lipids frequently occur with olanzapine therapy (Lieberman 2005). Metabolic disorders, obesity, and gestational diabetes also contribute to the risk of malformations. Babu (2010) reported that olanzapine exposure was associated with higher birth weight compared with use of other psychotropic medications, and the difference was not explained by dose, duration of exposure, gestational age, maternal age, or infant sex.

Sedation and persistent jaundice in an infant were associated with maternal olanzapine intake during pregnancy (Goldstein 2000). Seizures occurred in the neonatal period in three retrospectively recorded children whose mothers were treated with olanzapine until the birth (Goldstein 2000; unpublished data, C.S.). A plasma level of olanzapine obtained from a neonate was about a third (11 ng/mL) of the maternal level (range 25–34 ng/mL); delivery and development of the infant through 6 months were normal (Aichhorn 2008).

▶ **Paliperidone**

Paliperidone is an atypical antipsychotic and an active metabolite of *risperidone*.

▶ **Perazine**

Perazine is a phenothiazine and a moderately potent antipsychotic agent. With the phenothiazines in general, there is no indication of an elevated risk for malformations.

▶ Perphenazine

Perphenazine is among the phenothiazines and was the first generation antipsychotic selected for the Clinical Antipsychotic Trials in Intervention Effectiveness (CATIE) study (Lieberman 2005) which showed that the efficacy of perphenazine was similar to that of *quetiapine, risperidone,* and *ziprasidone.* There are published results on about 100 perphenazine exposures in pregnancy (Reis 2008), which, as with other phenothiazines, gave no indication of an increased risk of malformations.

▶ Pimozide

Pimozide is a rarely used butyrophenone. There are only a few documented pregnancies available which do not indicate an increased risk for birth defects but are not sufficient for a differentiated risk assessment (Gentile 2010).

▶ Pipamperone

Pipamperone is a butyrophenone and a low-potency neuroleptic with sedating action. It is structurally related to haloperidol.

▶ Promethazine

Promethazine is a phenothiazine and a low-potency neuroleptic with sedating action. During pregnancy promethazine is used for its antiemetic action. There are published results on several hundred pregnancies with promethazine (e.g. Bartfai 2008, Diav-Citrin 2003). In an intriguing design for toxicity analysis, Petik (2008) looked at women who attempted suicide by promethazine overdose in the first trimester and found no increased risk for birth defects or preterm birth. There was also no difference in birth weight between exposed children and their siblings. Mean intelligence quotient was not reduced and the rate of behavioral problems was not increased in the exposed children.

▶ Prothipendyl

Prothipendyl is structurally related to the phenothiazines.

▶ Quetiapine

Quetiapine is an atypical antipsychotic used in the treatment of schizophrenia and bipolar disorder as well as an augmentation for treatment refractory depression (in combination with an antidepressant). Studies and case series with a total of about 400 pregnancies have been published and 150 pregnancies have been documented by the manufacturer. No increased risk for birth defects has been reported (Habermann 2013, survey in Gentile 2010, Reis 2008, McKenna 2005, Taylor 2003, Tényi 2002).

► **Risperidone**

Risperidone is an atypical antipsychotic. A comprehensive review of the Benefit Risk Management Worldwide Safety database for case reports of risperidone exposure during pregnancy indicated that exposure does not appear to increase the risk of spontaneous abortions or structural malformations compared to the general population (Coppola 2007). Extrapyramidal effects in neonates were observed following maternal exposure to risperidone during the third trimester.

► **Sertindole**

Sertindole is an atypical antipsychotic for which insufficient data on use in pregnancy are available.

► **Sulpiride**

Sulpiride, structurally related to *amisulpride,* is an atypical, low-potency antipsychotic for which insufficient information about use in pregnancy is available.

► **Thioridazine**

Thioridazine is a phenothiazine and moderately potent antipsychotic. In lower doses it is also used for sedation. There are published results on thioridazine for more than 50 pregnancies (Reis 2008), which, as is the case with the other phenothiazines, show no increased risk of malformations.

► **Ziprasidone**

Ziprasidone is an atypical antipsychotic. There are reports of about 50 pregnancies (e.g. Habermann 2013) which have not shown an increased risk for defects. A single case of cleft palate associated with ziprasidone use in pregnancy was reported (Peitl 2010).

► **Zotepine**

Zotepine is among the phenothiazines but is characterized as an atypical neuroleptic. There are only a few case reports on zotepine which, as is the case with the other phenothiazines, do not give any indication of an increased rate of malformations.

► **Zuclopenthixol**

Zuclopenthixol is among the thioxanthenes. There are published results on zuclopenthixol in about 75 pregnancies (Reis 2008). There has been no indication of an increased rate of malformations with thioxanthenes

Pregnancy

2.11 Psychotropic drugs

(Vladimir 2013). A depot preparation of zuclopenthixol was used to treat a woman in two successive pregnancies which resulted in two normal female offspring who developed normally through ages of 6 months and of 3.5 years.

2.11.8   Lithium and other anti-manic agents

▶ **Lithium**

The course of bipolar disorder across pregnancy was clarified by Bergink (2012) who found that all women with a history of episodes limited to the postpartum period remained stable throughout pregnancy without pharmacotherapy, while 24.4% of women with chronic bipolar disorder relapsed during pregnancy despite drug treatment. This work suggests that women with chronic bipolar symptomatology are candidates for continued pharmacotherapy during pregnancy. Viguera (2000) and colleagues demonstrated that discontinuation of pharmacotherapy resulted in relapse in 52% of pregnant bipolar women.

Lithium remains the primary drug for acute and maintenance treatment for bipolar disorder (Yonkers 2004). Dosing is guided by serum levels, but the difference between the therapeutic and toxic concentrations is narrow. Following oral administration, lithium is well-absorbed and excreted in the urine essentially unchanged. During pregnancy, lithium clearance through the kidneys is increased by 50–100%. Lithium treatment during pregnancy is challenging because progressively increasing clearance necessitates higher doses and frequent level monitoring to sustain therapeutic serum levels. Dehydration increases the serum concentrations and women with hyperemesis, poor fluid intake, or treatment with diuretics or non-steroidal anti-inflammatory agents can develop toxic levels rapidly. Lithium crosses the placenta and reaches a concentration in the fetus that is similar to that of the maternal serum. Lithium may cause fetal polyuria which increases the risk for polyhydramnios (Yonkers 2004, Ang 1990).

Lithium clearance declines rapidly after birth; therefore, the dose must be discontinued 24–48 hours before a scheduled induction or caesarean delivery or stopped with the onset of labor. This strategy reduces the neonatal concentrations at birth as well as the risk for complications related to lithium treatment. Adequate hydration during labor and delivery is imperative. After delivery, the pre-conception dose can be used because the pregnancy-related increase in renal clearance resolves quickly (Newport 2005).

In the 1970s, first-trimester lithium exposure was associated with cardiac malformations, particularly Ebstein's anomaly (a downward displacement of the tricuspid valve). The Lithium Baby Register was established in Denmark and expanded internationally to collect data on the outcomes of lithium-exposed fetuses. When it was closed in 1979, there were reports on 225 children; 25 (11%) had malformations, 18 of which were in the heart and large blood vessels. Other anomalies were reported in the external ear, brain, ureters, and endocrine system (Kozma 2005). However, clinicians are less likely to contact a Registry to report a normal pregnancy outcome than an abnormal one. Subsequent prospective cohort and retrospective case-control studies showed more favorable outcomes than described in the Registry (Diav-Citrin 2006, Kozma 2005, Cohen 1994, Jacobson 1992, Zalzstein 1990). The risk of Ebstein's anomaly, which occurs spontaneously in one of every 20,000 children, increases to about 1 in 1,000 lithium-exposed fetuses; that is, it occurs about 20 times more frequently with lithium therapy than in the general population (Shepard 2002). However, some investigators have questioned whether lithium is teratogenic due to methodological difficulties with the available studies (Yacobi 2008). Referral for detailed fetal cardiac evaluation is appropriate to assess for malformations (Benoit 2004).

Several investigators (Gentile 2012, Han 2012) recommend supplementation with folic acid for lithium-treated women (ideally prior to conception) in order to reduce the risk for neural tube defects (Gentile 2012). Additionally, one randomized trial demonstrated reduction in affective morbidity for patients who were supplemented with 0.3 to 0.4 mg/day of folic acid (Coppen 1986), after confirming that vitamin B12 levels were adequate (Blencowe 2010). The American Academy of Neurology recommends routine supplementation of folic acid of at least 0.4 mg/day for women of childbearing potential who take antiepileptic drugs (www.aan.com), and similar dosing has been advocated for women treated with lithium.

Lithium-exposed neonates are at risk for large-for-gestational age status, hypotonia, feeding difficulties, depressed reflexes, cyanosis, apnea, bradycardia, hypothyroidism, and diabetes insipidus. The neonatal symptoms are usually transient and are linked with higher maternal serum concentrations at delivery (>0.64 mEq/L) (Newport 2005).

In newborns lithium has been associated with breathing disorders and cardiac difficulties (persistent fetal circulation, atrial flutter, and pathological pulmonary vascular resistance) in individual cases. Transient diabetes insipidus (necessitating treatment with antidiuretic hormone) (Pinelli 2002), seizures, and hypothyroidism have also been described (Malzacher 2003, Zegers 2003, Frassetto 2002, Llewellyn 1998). These adverse effects resolve within a few weeks after birth. In newborns with marked hypothyroidism and congenital goiter, thyroid supplementation for several weeks has been reported (Frassetto 2002). Floppy infant syndrome with lethargy, poor sucking, tachypnea, tachycardia, cyanosis, temperature regulation disorders, and muscular hypotonicity may occur. The later development of such children was normal (Kozma 2005).

The development of 67 children from the Lithium Baby Registry was compared to that of their non-exposed siblings at 5 years of age or greater. Parental report of developmental abnormalities did not differ (Schou 1976). Growth, neurological, cognitive, and behavioral development of children exposed to lithium in utero were normal in 15 children studied at 3–15 years of age. Developmental milestones were normal in infants exposed prenatally to lithium (van der Lugt 2012).

Recommendation.

- The lowest lithium level that is efficacious with manageable side effects can be used as the level to target with dose adjustments as pregnancy progresses and renal clearance increases.
- Consider folate supplementation in women of childbearing age; half of pregnancies are unplanned and early pregnancy supplementation is optimal.

Pregnancy

2.11 Psychotropic drugs

- After exposure to lithium in the early first trimester a detailed ultrasound examination or a fetal echocardiogram can be offered to evaluate fetal cardiac development.
- The frequency of dosing should be increased to avoid large, rapid increases in lithium serum level due to few higher dose administrations, unless compliance will be reduced.
- If fluid loss through emesis, dehydration, or diuretic use occurs, reduce or discontinue lithium temporarily and check serum levels frequently to reduce the risk for toxicity.
- Renal function impairment, such as may occur with preeclampsia, results in increased serum lithium levels and dose adjustment or discontinuation must be considered.
- Always inquire about alcohol, cigarette, and other drug use, environmental exposures, and over the counter and prescribed medication intake; record them in the patient's medical chart prior to writing any prescriptions.
- Lithium clearance declines rapidly after birth and the dose must be discontinued 24–48 hours before a scheduled induction or caesarean delivery or with the onset of labor.
- Restart lithium at the pre-pregnancy dose after the mother is medically stable.
- Due to immature renal elimination, particularly in the first few days of life, the baby should be monitored for toxic signs.
- Information about the impact of lithium in pregnancy is constantly evolving. A free resource is the US National Library of Medicine (http://toxnet.nlm.nih.gov/) for DART (Developmental and Reproductive Toxicity).

Women with bipolar disorder are at higher risk than the general population for adverse outcomes independent of drug treatment (Bodén 2012b). Bodén and colleagues compared pregnant women who had bipolar disorder and had filled a prescription for lithium, antipsychotics, or anticonvulsants ($n = 320$) to untreated women with bipolar disorder ($n = 554$) and to non-bipolar women ($n = 331\ 263$). Both untreated (OR 1.57, 95% CI 1.30–1.90) and treated (OR 2.12, 1.68–2.67) bipolar women had higher rates of labor induction or planned caesarean delivery than the general population. The risk of preterm birth in both treated and untreated women was increased by 50%. Untreated women (OR 1.68, 1.07–2.62) and treated women (OR 1.26, 0.67–2.37) had a higher risk for the birth of a microcephalic infant. Similar trends were observed for risks of infants being small for gestational age, weight, and length. Infants of untreated (OR1.51, 1.04–2.43) and treated women (OR 1.18, 0.64–2.16) had increased risk for neonatal hypoglycemia.

▶ Antiepileptics

Antiepileptic drugs, such as *lamotrigine, valproic acid, carbamazepine* and *oxcarbazepine* are also prescribed as mood stabilizers for women with bipolar disorder. Because valproic acid in particular has significant physical and neurodevelopmental teratogenic potential, it should be avoided in women of childbearing potential unless other agents are ineffective. Lamotrigine is the antiepileptic drug of choice for use in pregnancy, and guidelines are available (Clark 2013). For more information on antiepileptic drugs, see Chapter 2.10.

2.11.9   Anxiolytics, hypnotics, sedatives in general

Anxiolytics are used in the treatment of anxiety and these drugs minimize the influence of negative emotions on physiological activation. Many agents are used as hypnotics to treat sleep disorders; however, sleep disturbances have many different etiologies and behavioral treatments are effective in many cases. Chronic medication treatment with some agents risks dependency.

2.11.10   Benzodiazepines

Pharmacology

Benzodiazepine derivatives are used as anxiolytics, hypnotics and antiepileptics (Chapter 2.10). The half-lives of benzodiazepines are impacted by the biologic activity of the metabolites which are formed in the liver via oxidation. The very short-acting benzodiazepines (half-life <6 hours) are used for induction of anesthesia and as hypnotics. They include *brotizolam, flurazepam, midazolam* and *triazolam*.

The short-acting benzodiazepines (half-life 6–24 hours) are available as sedatives and hypnotics. These include *alprazolam, bromazepam, clotiazepam, flunitrazepam, loprazolam, lorazepam, lormetazepam, metaclazepam, nitrazepam, oxazepam* and *temazepam*.

Long-acting benzodiazepines (half-life >24 hours to several days) are primarily prescribed as sedatives, anxiolytics and antiepileptics. They include *chlordiazepoxide, clobazam, and* clonazepam. *Diazepam* is quickly absorbed after oral administration and is primarily transported in the blood bound to the plasma protein. In the liver, hydroxylation and metabolism to the active desmethyldiazepam occurs, which is excreted via the kidneys after glucuronidation. The half-life is 1–2 days. Diazepam crosses the placenta. The concentration in cord blood is up to three times higher than in the maternal blood. In the newborn, the half-life is considerably prolonged due to the limited clearance.

Risk of malformations

Most studies have been done more than a decade ago; however, a recent review drew a similar conclusion to older studies that little evidence for major malformations associated with benzodiazepines exists (Bellantuono 2013).

The most experience is with *diazepam*. In connection with benzodiazepine therapy in the first trimester, heart malformations, lip and palate clefts, inguinal hernias and other, complex, malformations were described (McElhatton 1994). Bonnot (2001) found no evidence of increased risk with benzodiazepines for malformations. However, they did find an association between anal atresia and *lorazepam*.

Two case-control studies with around 400 pregnant women exposed to *chlordiazepoxide* (Czeizel 2004), as well as 10 patients with *alprazolam*, about 100 with *clonazepam* (Chapter 2.10), 18 with *medazepam*, 18 with *nitrazepam* and 13 with *tofisopam*, there was also no indication of any birth defects (Lin 2004, Eros 2002).

A small number of case studies from the Hungarian malformation register on overdoses by women during suicidal attempts with alprazolam (Gidai 2008c), chlordiazepoxide (Gidai 2008b), diazepam (Gidai 2008a) and nitrazepam, Gidai (2010) reported malformations in offspring. However, the number of cases is small and the anomalies observed are heterogeneous; which makes drawing conclusions from these data difficult.

Pregnancy

2.11 Psychotropic drugs

Laegreid (1989) described eight children whose mothers abused prescription drugs throughout the entire pregnancy with at least 30 mg diazepam or at least 75 mg oxazepam daily. All of the children had facial dysmorphia, and some also had microcephaly as well as postpartum toxic symptoms (apnea) and withdrawal symptoms. Later, varied distinctive mental retardation, attention disorders and hyperkinesis were observed. These case presentations were criticized because the kind and scope of the exposure was not sufficiently certain and, in one case, Zellweger syndrome could not be ruled out. In follow-up examinations, an improvement in the symptoms of the 18-month-old children was observed (Laegreid 1992).

In a meta-analysis by Dolovich (1998), the collected data of cohort studies with pregnant women who were treated with benzodiazepines showed no increased risk for anomalies. However, conclusion of an analysis of the available retrospective case-control studies revealed an increased risk for major malformations or for isolated oral clefts after treatment with benzodiazepines (Dolovich 1998). An update of the 1998 Dolovich meta-analysis, which incorporated cohort studies with a total of more than 4,000 pregnant women (Enato 2011), did not reveal any increased risk of malformations (OR 1.07; 95% CI 0.91–1.25). Alprazolam, chlordiazepoxide, diazepam and oxazepam were the primary substances recorded. In this updated meta-analysis, two additional large cohort studies with a total of 3,000 pregnant women exposed in the first trimester (Oberlander 2008, Wikner 2007a) were included. Wikner (2007a) stressed that women who take benzodiazepines tend to smoke more frequently, take other psychotropic medications and have less education. These factors should be considered as potential confounding variables for the outcome of the pregnancy, including the occurrence of oral clefts. The doubling of the frequency of oral clefts would mean that, based on a background risk of 8.5/10,000, one additional oral cleft could be expected in every 1,000 fetuses exposed in the first trimester.

Postnatal adaptation disorders

When benzodiazepines have been given in high doses during birth or when diazepam or other benzodiazepines have been taken regularly over a longer period of time, including the last trimester, a risk of adaptational problems in newborns has been verified. After high doses over the short-term (as with therapy for eclampsia), the newborn must be observed for respiratory depression. Following longer-term continuous exposure during pregnancy, withdrawal signs such as restlessness, tremor, muscular hypotonicity, vomiting and diarrhea occur. Seizures may occur in the neonatal phase and floppy-infant syndrome with muscular flaccidity, lethargy, disturbances of temperature regulation and weak sucking are possible and may continue for weeks or months. Due to the accumulation in fetuses, even low doses of diazepam (<10 mg) can, in individual cases, lead to clinical signs in the newborn (Peinemann 2001).

The newborn metabolizes benzodiazepines significantly more slowly than an adult, which results in a half-life of up to 80 hours for diazepam compared to 8 hours in toddlers. The long-term effects of prenatal exposure on later development of the child have not been systematically assessed. Benzodiazepines can compete with bilirubin for albumin binding and, theoretically, may increase neonatal icterus.

Recommendation.

- Benzodiazepines are the drugs of choice for the brief treatment of acute anxiety symptoms and, in certain cases, sleep disturbances during pregnancy.
- For sleep disorders requiring continuous medication, the antidepressants trazodone or amitriptyline are preferable.
- After exhausting all the non-medicinal options for treatment and medicinal alternatives (such as antidepressants), benzodiazepines should only be prescribed for as short a period as clinically feasible.
- Ongoing therapy in the last trimester, for example, as supplementary medication to inhibit contractions at the time of delivery should be followed by close observation for neonatal complications in the first few days of life.
- Depending on the half-life of the benzodiazepine, the possibility of a dose reduction should be discussed with the mother before the expected date of birth.

2.11.11 Zaleplon, zolpidem and zopiclone

Eszopiclone, zaleplon, zolpidem and *zopiclone* are hypnotics with agonistic action on benzodiazepine receptors. They are not chemically related to the benzodiazepines. The epidemiological data available do not indicate an increased risk for birth defects.

Using insurance data, a Taiwanese study identified 2,497 women who used zolpidem during pregnancy and compared them with a control group. At least 535 were exposed in the first trimester. They found minimally increased risks for intrauterine growth retardation and prematurity, but not for selected CNS malformations (Wang 2010). In a study of the Swedish birth register, no indications of an increased risk for birth defects using benzodiazepines or benzodiazepine agonists in the first trimester were found. In this sample, 61 women had been prescribed zolpidem (Wikner 2007b). The authors emphasized that women who take benzodiazepine agonists more frequently smoke, take other psychotropic drugs, and have less education. These factors should be considered as potential confounding factors that impact outcome. In another study, no major malformations were observed in 17 children who were exposed to zolpidem during the first trimester (Juric 2009).

A further publication on the Swedish data on zaleplon, zolpidem and zopiclone with more than 1,300 pregnant women exposed in the first trimester revealed no increased overall rate of malformations, with only one association with non-atresial intestinal malformations, based on four children (Wikner 2011). The authors discussed this finding as a possible chance result of multiple comparisons.

Two small prospective studies with a total of 70 pregnant women treated in the first trimester with zopiclone, did not find any indications of birth defects (Stephens 2008, Diav-Citrin 1999).

There is no experience during pregnancy on *eszopiclone*, the S-enantiomer of zopiclone

Recommendation. Benzodiazepine agonists may be briefly prescribed during pregnancy. The most data are available for zolpidem. After use in the third trimester or until birth, adaptation disorders of the newborn may occur with these agents.

Pregnancy

2.11 Psychotropic drugs

2.11.12 Other anxiolytics and hypnotics

Until the introduction of benzodiazepines, barbituric acid derivatives were the most important hypnotics. Since then, barbiturates are rarely used for this purpose. Today, *phenobarbital* (*phenobarbitone*) is occasionally prescribed. Experience on barbiturates during pregnancy has been collected primarily from the treatment of epilepsy (Chapter 2.10). With brief use for anesthesia, barbiturates have not been shown to be related to birth defects. If given during labor, barbiturates can cause respiratory depression in the newborn.

Buspirone is an anxiolytic psychoactive drug of the azapirone class. It is not chemically or pharmacologically related to the benzodiazepines, barbiturates, or other sedative/anxiolytic drugs. It is rarely used for anxiety and restless states. There are individual case reports which have not, to date, revealed any specific teratogenicity.

Chloral hydrate has been used for over 100 years and is, thereby, the oldest hypnotic still in use. After absorption, chloral hydrate is quickly converted to the metabolite, *trichlor ethanol*, which is also hypnotically active, and to some extent, metabolized to *trichloroacetic acid*. In one study, chromosomal changes were observed (Sora 1987). There are only few data on its use during pregnancy, which do not indicate an increased risk of malformations (Heinonen 1977).

Clomethiazole is used for acute withdrawal symptoms after chronic alcohol abuse.

Diphenhydramine: See Chapter 2.4 on the use of H_1 antihistamines during pregnancy.

Doxylamine: See Chapter 2.4 on the use of H_1 antihistamines during pregnancy.

Hydroxyzine is an antihistamine with sedative, antiemetic, and anxiolytic properties. Available studies, covering a total of around 240 pregnancies, do not indicate developmental toxicity (Diav-Citrin 2003, Einarson 1997).

Melperone has no relevance as a hypnotic.

Meprobamate is one of the oldest tranquilizers but since the introduction of benzodiazepines, it no longer has any therapeutic significance. In a study of 400 women who had received meprobamate in the first trimester, the rate of congenital heart defects was increased (Milkovich 1974). This observation was not replicated in other studies.

Recommendation.

- Regular use anxiolytics at the end of pregnancy can cause adaptation disorders in the newborn.
- For sleep disorders requiring medication, sedating antihistamines, trazodone, amitriptyline, and, if necessary benzodiazepines or zolpidem are preferable to these agents.

2.11.13 Psychoanaleptics

Psychoanaleptics are psychostimulators which enhance the activity of the CNS. The methylxanthines *caffeine* and *theobromine* (Chapter 2.21) belong to the group of psychoanaleptics.

The most frequently used analeptics are derivatives of *phenylethyl-amine*. The prototype of this group is amphetamine (Chapter 2.21). These drugs are related to the sympathomimetics, enhance mental performance, and repeated use can lead to addiction. Drugs such as *amfetaminil*, *fenethylline*, and *methylphenidate* belong to this group, as well as *modafinil* and *sodium oxybate* used for narcolepsy with cataplexy, and *pemoline*, an oxazolidine, used for attention deficit disorder.

Pottegård (2014) evaluated the rate of major malformations following first-trimester exposure to methylphenidate in Denmark. Exposure was defined as redeeming at least one prescription for methylphenidate within a time window defined as 14 days before conception to the end of the first trimester. Propensity score matching was used to match each exposed subject to 10 unexposed subjects on maternal age, smoking status, body mass index, education, calendar year of completion of pregnancy, and use of antipsychotics, antidepressants, anxiolytics, and nonsteroidal anti-inflammatory drugs. The sample included 222 exposed and 2,220 unexposed pregnancies. No statistically significant increase in major malformations (point prevalence ratio = 0.8; 95% CI 0.3–1.8) or cardiac malformations (point prevalence ratio = 0.9; 95% CI 0.2–3.0) was observed. Wajnberg (2011) found no differences compared to a control group in gestational age and birth weight or the rate of miscarriage. With increasing use into adulthood for attention deficit disorder, more exposures in pregnancy are likely to occur.

There is one published case report on modafinil exposure during pregnancy which was followed by the birth of a healthy child (Williams 2008).

> **Recommendation.** If stimulants are used during pregnancy, the expected benefit which outweighs the risk should be documented. The most data are available for methylphenidate.

2.11.14   Anti-Parkinson drugs and restless legs syndrome

During pregnancy, anti-Parkinson drugs play a role for restless legs syndrome (RLS). This syndrome is related to parity, and its symptoms may worsen during pregnancy. Treatment with levodopa or dopamine agonists is the first-line therapy for RLS; however, there are limited data on treatment in pregnancy.

Amantadine enhances the dopamine activity and is used as an anti-Parkinson drug. In addition, it is effective as a virustatic against influenza-A viruses. In humans, malformations have been identified in case series and individual case reports, which comprised more than 150 pregnancies with exposure at different times (Greer 2010).

In total, about 60 case reports on *levodopa* (L-dopa) in combination with *benserazide* or *carbidopa* do not indicate any prenatal toxicity (e.g. Dostal 2013).

There is a case series with 12 pregnant women on *pramipexol*, which provides no indication of teratogenic effects. There are only individual cases for *ropinirole* and *rotigotine* (e.g. Dostal 2013).

Dostal (2013) conducted the first prospective case series on RLS treatment during pregnancy. It is based on data from the German national teratology service and includes a detailed literature review. The investigation includes levodopa (with either benserazide or carbidopa), pramipexole,

Pregnancy

2.11 Psychotropic drugs

rotigotine, and ropinirole in 59 pregnancies and their outcomes. For specific treatments, the numbers of exposed pregnancies/live-born children/spontaneous abortions/induced abortions/minor malformations were as follows: levodopa only: 38/29/3/7/3; pramipexole only: 12/9/3/0/0; rotigotine only: 2/2/0/0/0; ropinirole only: 3/2/0/1/0; levodopa combined with pramipexole: 3/3/0/0/0; levodopa combined with ropinirole: 1/1/0/0/0. The number of live-born children with levodopa only included one pair of twins. No major birth defects were found with any of these treatments; however, three infants exposed to levodopa had minor anomalies. The authors concluded that this small prospective case series showed no evidence of increased risk above baseline for major malformations or other adverse outcomes for levodopa and pramipexole. If necessary, levodopa treatment may be considered as an alternative to cabergoline, which has substantially more data for use in pregnancy.

Medications other than the dopamine-agonist-acting ergotamine derivatives, which are used as medication for Parkinson's Disease, include *bromocriptine, cabergoline, α-dihydroergocryptine, lisuride* and *pergolide*. Some of these drugs are used by women in reproductive age for prolactinomas and associated fertility disorders (Chapter 2.15).

Additional anti-Parkinson drugs, which are used for treatment of extrapyramidal symptoms induced by antipsychotics are: *biperiden, benzatropine, bornaprine, budipin, metixen, piribedil, pridinol, procyclidine, tetrabenazine*; for hyperkinetic movement disorders *tiapride* and *trihexyphenidyl* as well as the monoaminoxidase-B-inhibitors (MAO-B-inhibitors) *selegiline* and *rasagiline*. With the exception of the older ergotamine derivatives, there is minimal experience with most of these drugs during pregnancy.

> **Recommendation.** Treatment with anti-Parkinson drugs may be necessary during pregnancy; for example, in the context of therapy for a prolactinoma with ergotamine-derivatives or for extrapyramidal side-effects of an antipsychotic treatment.With marked restless-legs symptoms, cabergoline or levodopa are reasonable choices.

References

ACOG. Obesity in pregnancy. http://www.acog.org/Resources_And_Publications/Committee_Opinions/Committee_on_Obstetric_Practice/Obesity_in_Pregnancy, 2013.

Aichhorn W, Yazdi K, Kralovec K et al. Olanzapine plasma concentration in a newborn. J Psychopharmacol 2008; 22: 923–4.

Alwan S, Reefhuis J, Botto LD et al. Maternal use of bupropion and risk for congenital heart defects. Am J Obstet Gynecol 2010; 203: 52–6.

Alwan S, Reefhuis J, Rasmussen SA et al. National Birth Defects Prevention Study: Use of selective serotonin-reuptake inhibitors in pregnancy and the risk of birth defects. N Engl J Med 2007; 356: 2684–92.

Alwan S, Reefhuis J, Rasmussen SA et al. National Birth Defects Prevention Study: Patterns of antidepressant medication use among pregnant women in a United States population. J Clin Pharmacol 2011; 51: 264–70.

Anderson IM. Selective serotonin reuptake inhibitors versus tricyclic antidepressants: a meta-analysis of efficacy and tolerability. J Affect Disord 2000; 58: 19–36.

Andrade SE, McPhillips H, Loren D et al. Antidepressant medication use and risk of persistent pulmonary hypertension of the newborn. Pharmacoepidemiol Drug Saf 2009; 18: 246–52.

Ang MS, Thorp JA, Parisi VM. Maternal lithium therapy and polyhydramnios. Obstet Gynecol 1990; 76: 517–9.

Ansorge MS, Morelli E, Gingrich JA. Inhibition of serotonin but not norepinephrine transport during development produces delayed, persistent perturbations of emotional behaviors in mice. J Neurosci 2008; 28: 199–207.

Babu GN, Desai G, Tippeswamy H, Chandra PS. Birth weight and use of olanzapine in pregnancy: a prospective comparative study. J Clin Psychopharmacol 2010; 30: 331–2.

Bakker MK, Kerstjens-Frederikse WS, Buys CH et al. First-trimester use of paroxetine and congenital heart defects: a population-based case-control study. Birth Defects Res A Clin Mol Teratol 2010; 88: 94–100.

Barker DJ, Osmond C, Golding J et al. Growth in utero, blood pressure in childhood and adult life, and mortality from cardiovascular disease. BMJ 1989; 298: 564–7.

Bar-Oz B, Einarson T, Einarson A et al. Paroxetine and congenital malformations: meta-analysis and consideration of potential confounding factors. Clin Ther 2007; 29: 918–26.

Bartfai Z, Kocsis J, Puho EH et al. A population-based case-control teratologic study of promethazine use during pregnancy. Reprod Toxicol 2008; 25: 276–85.

Bellantuono C, Tofani S, Di Sciascio G, Santone G. Benzodiazepine exposure in pregnancy and risk of major malformations: a critical overview. 2013; 35: 3–8.

Benoit R. Does lithium exposure warrant referral for fetal echocardiogram? Am J Obstet Gynecol 2004; 191: S127.

Bérard A, Ramos E, Rey E et al. First trimester exposure to paroxetine and risk of cardiac malformations in infants: the importance of dosage. Birth Defects Res B Dev Reprod Toxicol 2007a; 80: 18–27.

Bérard A , Rey E, Oraichi D. Effect of smoking cessation interventions during pregnancy on the newborn. Pharmacoepidemiol Drug Saf 2007b; 16: S133.

Bergink V, Bouvy PF, Vervoort JS et al. Prevention of postpartum psychosis and mania in women at high risk. Am J Psychiatry 2012; 169: 609–15.

Biswas PN, Wilton LV, Pearce GL et al. The pharmacovigilance of olanzapine: results of a post-marketing surveillance study on 8858 patients in England. J Psychopharmacology 2001; 15: 265–71.

Blencowe H, Cousens S, Modell B et al. Folic acid to reduce neonatal mortality from neural tube disorders. Int J Epidemiol 2010; 39: i110–21.

Bodén R, Lundgren M, Brandt L et al. Antipsychotics during pregnancy: relation to fetal and maternal metabolic effects. Arch Gen Psychiat 2012a; 69: 715–21.

Bodén R, Lundgren M, Brandt L et al. Risks of adverse pregnancy and birth outcomes in women treated or not treated with mood stabilisers for bipolar disorder: population based cohort study. BMJ 2012b; 345: e7085.

Bolte AC, van Eyck J, Bruinse HW et al. Ketanserin versus dihydralazine in the management of early-onset pre-eclampsia: maternal and neonatal outcome. Am J Obstet Gynecol 1997; 176: 15.

Bonnot O, Vollset SE, Godet PF et al. Maternal exposure to lorazepam and anal atresia in newborns: results from a hypothesis-generating study of benzodiazepines and malformations. J Clin Psychopharmacol 2001; 21: 456–8.

Boucher N, Koren G, Beaulac-Baillargeon L. Maternal use of venlafaxine near term: correlation between neonatal effects and plasma concentrations. Ther Drug Monit 2009; 31: 404–9.

Bromiker R, Kaplan M. Apparent intrauterine fetal withdrawal from clomipramine hydrochloride. JAMA 1994; 272: 1722–3.

Brunner E, Falk DM, Jones M et al. Olanzapine in pregnancy and breastfeeding: a review of data from global safety surveillance. BMC Pharmacol Toxicol 2013; 14: 38.

Carmichael SL, Shaw GM, Yang W et al. Maternal stressful life events and risks of birth defects. Epidemiology 2007; 18: 356–61.

Casper RC, Fleisher BE, Lee-Ancajas JC et al. Follow-up of children of depressed mothers exposed or not exposed to antidepressant drugs during pregnancy. J Pediatr 2003; 142: 402–8.

Casper RC, Gilles AA, Fleisher BE et al. Length of prenatal exposure to selective serotonin reuptake inhibitor (SSRI) antidepressants: effects on neonatal adaptation and psychomotor development. Psychopharmacology 2011; 217: 211–9.

Chambers CD, Hernandez-Diaz S, van Marter LJ et al. Selective serotonin-reuptake inhibitors and risk of persistent pulmonary hypertension of the newborn. N Engl J Med 2006; 354: 579–87.

Chun-Fai-Chan B, Koren G, Fayez I et al. Pregnancy outcome of women exposed to bupropion during pregnancy: a prospective comparative study. Am J Obstet Gynecol 2005; 192: 932–6.

Clark CT, Klein AM, Perel JM et al. Lamotrigine dosing for pregnant patients with bipolar disorder. 2013; 170: 1240–7.

Cohen LS, Friedman JM, Jefferson JW et al. A reevaluation of risk of in utero exposure to lithium. JAMA 1994; 271: 146–50.

Cole JA , Ephross SA, Cosmatos IS, Walker AM. Paroxetine in the first trimester and the prevalence of congenital malformations. Pharmacoepidemiol Drug Saf 2007a; 16: 1075–85.

Cole JA, Modell JG, Haight BR et al. Bupropion in pregnancy and the prevalence of congenital malformations. Pharmacoepidemiol Drug Saf 2007b; 16: 474–84.

Colvin L, Slack-Smith L, Stanley FJ et al. Dispensing patterns and pregnancy outcomes for women dispensed selective serotonin reuptake inhibitors in pregnancy. Birth Defects Res A Clin Mol Teratol 2011; 91: 142–52.

Coppen S. Chaudhry and C. Swade. Folic acid enhances lithium prophylaxis. J Affect Dis 1986; 10: 9–13.

Coppola D. Evaluating the postmarketing experience of risperidone use during pregnancy: pregnancy and neonatal outcomes. Drug Saf 2007; 30: 247–64.

Croen LA, Grether JK, Yoshida CK et al. Antidepressant use during pregnancy and childhood autism spectrum disorders. Arch Gen Psychiatry 2011; 68: 1104–12.

Czeizel AE, Rockenbauer M, Sørensen HAT et al. A population-based case-control study of oral chlordiazepoxide during pregnancy and risk of congenital abnormalities. Neurotoxicol Teratol 2004; 26: 593–8.

Davis RL, Rubanowice D, McPhillips H et al. HMO Research Network Center for Education, Research in Therapeutics: Risks of congenital malformations and perinatal events among infants exposed to antidepressant medications during pregnancy. Pharmacoepidemiol Drug Saf 2007; 16: 1086–94.

Di Gianantonio E. Venlafaxine in pregnancy: A prospective controlled study. Reprod Toxicol 2006; 22: 269.

Diav-Citrin O, Okotore B, Lucarelli K et al. Pregnancy outcome following first-trimester exposure to zopiclone: a prospective controlled cohort study. Am J Perinatol 1999; 16: 157–60.

Diav-Citrin O, Shechtman S, Aharonovich A et al. Pregnancy outcome after gestational exposure to loratadine or other antihistamines: a prospective controlled cohort study. J Allergy Clin Immunol 2003; 111: 1239–43.

Diav-Citrin O, Shechtman S, Ornoy S et al. The safety of haloperidol and penfluridol in pregnancy: a multicenter, prospective, controlled study. J Clin Psychiatry 2005; 66: 317–22.

Diav-Citrin O, Shechtman S, Weinbaum D et al. Paroxetine and fluoxetine in pregnancy: a prospective, multi-center, controlled, observational study. Br J Clin Pharmacol 2008; 65: 695–705.

Diav-Citrin O. Pregnancy outcome after in-utero exposure to lithium: a prospective controlled cohort study. Birth Defects Res A Clin Mol Teratol 2006; 76: 424.

Djulus J, Koren G, Einarson TR et al. Exposure to mirtazapine during pregnancy: a prospective comparative study of birth outcomes. J Clin Psychiatry 2006; 67: 1280–4.

Dolovich LR, Addis A, Regis Vaillancourt et al. Benzodiazepine use in pregnancy and major malformations or oral cleft: meta-analysis of cohort and case-control studies. BMJ 1998; 317: 839–43.

Dostal M, Weber-Schoendorfer C, Sobesky J, Schaefer C. Pregnancy outcome following use of levodopa, pramipexole, ropinirole and rotigotine for restless legs syndrome during pregnancy: a case series. Eur J Neurol 2013; 20: 1241–6.

Dubnov-Raz G, Juurlink DN, Fogelman R et al. Antenatal use of selective serotonin-reuptake inhibitors and QT interval prolongation in newborns. Pediatrics 2008; 122: e710–5.

Duijvestijn YCM, Kalmeijer MD, Passier ALM et al. Neonatal intraventricular haemorrhage associated with maternal use of paroxetine. Br J Clin Pharmacol 2003; 56: 581–2.

Dunkel Schetter C, Tanner L. Anxiety, depression and stress in pregnancy: implications for mothers, children, research, and practice. Curr Opin Psychiatry 2012; 20: 141–8.

Einarson A, Bailey B, Jung G et al. Prospective controlled study of hydroxyzine and cetirizine in pregnancy. Ann Allergy Asthma Immunol 1997; 78: 183–6.

Einarson A, Bonari L, Voyer-Lavigne S et al. A multicentre prospective controlled study to determine the safety of trazodone and nefazodone use during pregnancy. Can J Psychiatry 2003; 48: 106–10.

Einarson A, Pistelli A, de Santis M et al. Evaluation of the risk of congenital cardiovascular defects associated with use of paroxetine during pregnancy. Am J Psychiatry 2008; 165: 749–52.

El Marroun H, Jaddoe VW, Hudziak JJ et al. Maternal use of selective serotonin reuptake inhibitors, fetal growth, and risk of adverse birth outcomes. Arch Gen Psychiatry 2012; 69: 706–14.

Ellfolk M, Malm H. Risks associated with in utero and lactation exposure to selective serotonin reuptake inhibitors (SSRIs). Reprod Toxicol 2010; 30: 249–60.

Enato E, Moretti M, Koren G. The fetal safety of benzodiazepines: an updated meta-analysis. J Obstet Gynaecol Can 2011; 33: 46–8.

Ericson A, Källén B, Wiholm BE. Delivery outcome after the use of antidepressants in early pregnancy. Eur J Clin Pharmacol 1999; 55: 503–8.

Eros E, Czeizel AE, Rockenbauer M et al. A population-based case-control teratologic study of nitrazepam, medazepam, tofisopam, alprazolam and clonazepam treatment during pregnancy. European J Obstet Gynecol Reprod Biol 2002; 101: 147–54.

Eyding D, Lelgemann M, Grouven U et al. Reboxetine for acute treatment of major depression: systematic review and meta-analysis of published and unpublished placebo and selective serotonin reuptake inhibitor controlled trials. BMJ 2010; 341: c4737.

Figueroa R. Use of antidepressants during pregnancy and risk of attention-deficit/hyperactivity disorder in the offspring. J Dev Behav Pediatr 2010; 31: 641–8.

Frassetto F, Martel FT, Barjhoux CE et al. Goiter in a newborn exposed to lithium in utero. Ann Pharmacother 2002; 36: 1745–8.

Freeman MP Nolan PE Jr, Davis MF et al. Pharmacokinetics of sertraline across pregnancy and postpartum. J Clin Psychopharmacol 2008; 28: 646–53.

Gentile S. Antipsychotic therapy during early and late pregnancy. A systematic review. Schizophr Bull 2010; 36: 518–544.

Gentile S. Lithium in pregnancy: the need to treat, the duty to ensure safety. Expert Opinion on Drug Safety 2012; 11: 425–37.

Gentile S, Galbally M. Prenatal exposure to antidepressant medications and neurodevelopmental outcomes: a systematic review. J Affect Disord 2011; 128: 1–9.

Gidai J, Acs N, Banhidy F et al. No association found between use of very large doses of diazepam by 112 pregnant women for a suicide attempt and congenital abnormalities in their offspring. Toxicol Ind Health 2008a; 24: 29–39.

Gidai J, Acs N, Bánhidy F et al. A study of the teratogenic and fetotoxic effects of large doses of chlordiazepoxide used for self-poisoning by 35 pregnant women. Toxicol Ind Health 2008b; 24: 41–51.

Gidai J, Acs N, Banhidy F et al. An evaluation of data for 10 children born to mothers who attempted suicide by taking large doses of alprazolam during pregnancy. Toxicol Ind Health 2008c; 24: 53 60.

Gidai J, Acs N, Bánhidy F et al. Congenital abnormalities in children of 43 pregnant women who attempted suicide with large doses of nitrazepam. Pharmacoepidemiol Drug Saf 2010; 19: 175–82.

Goldstein DJ, Corbin LA, Fung MC. Olanzapine-exposed pregnancies and lactation: early experience. J Clin Psychopharmacol 2000; 20: 399–403.

Gracious BL, Wisner KL. Phenelzine use throughout pregnancy and the puerperium: case report, review of the literature, and management recommendations. Depress Anxiety 1997; 6: 124–8.

Greer LG, Sheffield JS, Rogers VL et al. Maternal and neonatal outcomes after antepartum treatment of influenza with antiviral medications. Obstet Gynecol 2010; 115: 711–716.

Grigoriadis S, VonderPorten EH, Mamisashvili L, Antidepressant exposure during pregnancy and congenital malformations: is there an associatioin? A systematic review and meta-analysis of the best evidence. J Clin Psychiat 2013; 74: e293–308.

Grigoriadis S, Vonderporten EH, Mamisashvili L et al. Prenatal exposure to antidepressants and persistent pulmonary hypertension of the newborn: systematic review and meta-analysis. BMJ 2014; 358: f6932.

Grote NK, Bridge JA, Gavin AR et al. A meta-analysis of depression during pregnancy and the risk of preterm birth, low birth weight, and intrauterine growth restriction. Arch Gen Phychiatry 2010a; 67: 1012–24.

Grote V, Vik T, von Kries R et al. Maternal postnatal depression and child growth: a European cohort study. BMC Pediatr 2010b; 10: 14.

Grzeskowiak LE, Gilbert AL, Morrison JL. Prenatal exposure to selective serotonin reuptake inhibitors and risk of childhood overweight. J Dev Orig Health Dis 2012; 3: 253–61.

Guclu S, Gol M, Dogan E et al. Mirtazapine use in resistant hyperemesis gravidarum: report of three cases and review of the literature. Arch Gynecol Obstet 2005; 272: 298–300.

Habermann F, Fritzsche J, Fuhlbrück F et al. Atypical antipsychotic drugs and pregnancy outcome: A prospective cohort study. J Clin Psychopharmacol 2013; 33: 453–62.

Pregnancy

2.11 Psychotropic drugs

Hallberg P, Sjöblom V. The use of selective serotonin reuptake inhibitors during pregnancy and breastfeeding: a review and clinical aspects. J Clin Pharmacol 2005; 25: 59–73.

Han M, Neves AL, Serrano M et al. Effects of alcohol, lithium, and homocysteine on non-muscle myosin-II in the mouse placenta and human trophoblasts. Am J Obstet Gynecol 2012; 207: 140, e7–19.

Hanley GE, Brain U, Oberlander TF. Infant developmental outcomes following prenatal exposure to antidepressants, and maternal depressed mood and positive affect. Early Hum Dev 2013; 89: 519–24.

Harder T, Rodekamp E, Schellong K et al. Birth weight and subsequent risk of type 2 diabetes: a meta-analysis. Am J Epidemiol 2007; 165: 849–57.

Heinonen OP, Slone D, Dick LM et al. Birth Defects and Drugs in Pregnancy. Littleton/USA: Publishing Sciences Group, 1977.

Hendrick V, Stow ZN, Altshuler LL. Placental passage of antidepressant medications. Am J Psychiatry 2003; 160: 993–6.

Hilli J, Heikkinen T, Rontu R et al. MAO-A and COMT genotypes as possible regulators of perinatal serotonergic symptoms after in utero exposure to SSRIs. Eur Neuropsychopharmacol 2009; 19: 363–70.

Hoog SL, Cheng Y, Elpers J, Dowsett SA. Duloxetine and pregnancy outcomes: safety surveillance findings. Int J Med Sci 2013; 10: 413–9.

Hoppenbrouwers CJ, Bosma J, Wennink HJ et al. Neonatal seizures on EEG after in utero exposure to venlafaxine. Br J Clin Pharmacol 2010; 70: 454–6.

Hviid A, Melbye M, Pasternak B. Use of selective serotonin reuptake inhibitors during pregnancy and risk of autism. N Engl J Med 2013; 369: 2406–15.

Jacobson SJ, Jones K, Johnson K et al. Prospective multicentre study of pregnancy outcome after lithium exposure during first trimester. Lancet 1992; 339: 530–3.

Jimenez-Solem E, Andersen JT, Petersen M et al. Exposure to selective serotonin reuptake inhibitors and the risk of congenital malformations: a nationwide cohort study. BMJ Open 2012; 2: e001148.

Johnson KC, LaPrairie JL, Brennan PA et al. Prenatal antipsychotic exposure and neuromotor performance during infancy. Arch Gen Psychiatry 2012; 69: 787–94.

Juric S, Newport DJ, Ritchie JC et al. Zolpidem (Ambien) in pregnancy: placental passage and outcome. Arch Womens Ment Health 2009; 12: 441–6.

Källén B. Neonate characteristics after maternal use of antidepressants in late pregnancy. Arch Pediatr Adolesc Med 2004; 158: 312–6.

Källén B. The problem of confounding in studies of the effects of maternal drug user on pregnancy outcome. Obstet Gynecol Int 2012: 148616.

Källén B, Olausson PO. Maternal use of selective serotonin re-uptake inhibitors and persistent pulmonary hypertension of the newborn. Pharmacoepidemiol Drug Saf 2008; 17: 801–6.

Källén B, Otterblad Olausson P. Maternal use of selective serotonin re-uptake inhibitors in early pregnancy and infant congenital malformations. Birth Defects Res A 2007; 79: 301–8.

Kennedy DS, Evans M, Wand I, Webster WF. Fetal abnormalities with high-dose tranylcypromine in two consecutive pregnancies {Abstract}. Teratology 2001; 64: 324.

Kieler H, Artama M, Engeland A et al. Selective serotonin reuptake inhibitors during pregnancy and risk of persistent pulmonary hypertension in the newborn: population based cohort study from the five Nordic countries. BMJ 2012; 344: d8012.

Kim DR, Epperson N, Paré E et al. An open label pilot study of transcranial magnetic stimulation for pregnant women with major depressive disorder. J Women's Health 2011; 20: 255–61.

Kirchheiner J, Berghöfer A, Bolk-Weischedel D. Healthy outcome under olanzapine – treatment in a pregnant woman. Pharmacopsychiatry 2000; 33: 78–80.

Kirk L, Jorgensen A. Concentrations of Cis(Z)-flupentixol in maternal serum, amniotic fluid, umbilical cord serum, and milk. Psychopharmacology 1980; 72: 107–8.

Klieger-Grossmann C, Weitzner B, Panchaud A et al. Pregnancy outcomes following use of escitalopram: a prospective comparative cohort study. J Clin Pharmacol 2012; 52: 766–70.

Kornum JB, Nielsen RB, Pedersen L et al. Use of selective serotonin-reuptake inhibitors during early pregnancy and risk of congenital malformations: updated analysis. Clin Epidemiol 2010; 2: 29–36.

Kozma C. Neonatal toxicity and transient neurodevelopmental deficits following prenatal exposure to lithium: Another clinical report and a review of the literature. Am J Med Genet 2005; 132A: 441–4.

Kris EB. Children born to mothers maintained on pharmacotherapy during pregnancy and postpartum. Recent Adv Biol Psychiatr 1961; 4: 180–7.

Kris EB. Children of mothers maintained on pharmacotherapy during pregnancy and postpartum. Curr Ther Res 1965; 7: 785–9.

Kusakawa S, Yamauchi J, Miyamoto Y et al. Estimation of embryotoxic effect of fluoxetine using embryonic stem cell differentiation system. Life Sci 2008; 83: 871–7.

Laegreid L, Hagberg G, Lundberg A. Neurodevelopment in late infancy after prenatal exposure to benzodiazepines – a prospective study. Neuropediatrics 1992; 23: 60–7.

Laegreid L, Olegard R, Walstrom J et al. Teratogenic effects of benzodiazepine use during pregnancy. J Pediatr 1989; 114: 126–31.

Laine KL, Heikkinen T, Ekblad U et al. Effects of exposure to selective serotonin reuptake inhibitors during pregnancy on serotonergic symptoms in newborns and cord blood monoamine and prolactin concentrations. Arch Gen Psychiatry 2003; 60: 720–6.

Lattimore KA, Donn SM, Kaciroti N et al. Selective serotonin reuptake inhibitor (SSRI) use during pregnancy and effects on the fetus and newborn: a meta-analysis. J Perinatol, 2005; 25: 595–604.

Lennestål R, Källén B. Delivery outcome in relation to maternal use of some recently introduced antidepressants. J Clin Psychopharmacol 2007; 27: 607–13.

Leventhal K, Byatt N, Lundquist R. Fetal cardiac arrhythmia during bupropion use. Acta Obstet Gynecol Scand 2010; 89: 980–1.

Levinson AJ, Zipursky RB. Antipsychotics and the treatment of women with psychosis. In Steiner M, Koren G (eds) Handbook of Female Psychopharmacology. London: Dunitz 2003, p. 63.

Lieberman JA, Stroup TS, McEvoy JP et al. Effectiveness of antipsychotic drugs in patients with chronic schizophrenia. N Engl J Med 2005; 353: 1209–23.

Lim K, Sanders A, Brain U et al. Third trimester fetal pulmonary artery Doppler blood flow velocity characteristics following prenatal selective serotonin reuptake inhibitor (SSRI) exposure. Early Hum Dev 2012; 88: 609–15.

Lin AE, Peller AJ, Westgate MN et al. Clonazepam use in pregnancy and the risk of malformations. Birth Defects Res A 2004; 70: 534–6.

Llewellyn A, Stowe ZN, Strader JR. The use of lithium and management of women with bipolar disorder during pregnancy and lactation. J Clin Psychiatry 1998; 59: 57–64.

Loughhead AM, Fisher AD, Newport DJ et al. Antidepressants in amniotic fluid: another route of fetal exposure. Am J Psychiatry 2006a; 163: 145–7.

Loughhead AM, Stowe ZN, Newport DJ et al. Placental passage of tricyclic antidepressants. Biol Psychiatry 2006b; 59: 287–90.

Louik C, Lin AE, Werler MM et al. First-trimester use of selective serotonin-reuptake inhibitors and the risk of birth defects. N Engl J Med 2007; 356: 2675–83.

Lutz UC Hiemke C, Wiatr G et al. Aripiprazole in pregnancy and lactation: A case report. J Clin Psychopharmacol 2010; 30: 204–5.

Maayan-Metzger A, Kuint J, Lubetsky A et al. Maternal selective serotonin reuptake inhibitor intake does not seem to affect neonatal platelet function tests. Acta Haematol 2006; 115: 157–61.

Malek-Ahmadi P. Olanzapine in pregnancy. Ann Pharmacother 2001; 35: 1294–5.

Malm H, Artama M, Gissler M et al. Selective serotonin reuptake inhibitors and risk for major congenital anomalies. Obstet Gynecol 2011; 118: 111–20.

Malzacher A, Engler H, Drack G et al. Lethargy in a newborn: lithium toxicity or lab error? J Perinat Med 2003; 31: 340–2.

Manber R, Schnyer RN, Lyell D et al. Acupuncture for depression during pregnancy: a randomized controlled trial. Obstet Gynecol 2010; 115: 511–20.

McElhatton PR, Garbis HM, Eléfant E et al. The outcome of pregnancy in 689 women exposed to therapeutic doses of antidepressants. A collaborative study of the European Network of Teratology Information Services (ENTIS). Reprod Toxicol 1996; 10: 285–94.

McElhatton PR. The effects of benzodiazepine use during pregnancy and lactation. Reprod Toxicol 1994; 8: 461–75.

McKenna K, Einarson A, Levinson A et al. Significant changes in antipsychotic drug use during pregnancy. Vet Human Toxicol 2004; 46: 44–6.

McKenna K, Koren G, Tetelbaum M et al. Pregnancy outcome of women using atypical antipsychotic drugs: a prospective comparative study. J Clin Psychiatry 2005; 66: 444–9.

Mendhekar DN, Sunder KR, Andrade C. Aripiprazole use in a pregnant schizoaffective woman. Bipolar Disord 2006; 8: 299–300.

Mendhekar DN, War L, Sharma JB et al. Olanzapine and pregnancy. Pharmacopsychiatry 2002; 35: 122–3.

Merlob P, Birk E, Sirota L et al. Are selective serotonin reuptake inhibitors cardiac teratogens? Echocardiographic screening of newborns with persistent heart murmur. Birth Defects Res A Clin Mol Teratol 2009; 85: 837–41.

Mhanna MJ, Bennett JB, Izatt SD. Potential fluoxetine chloride (Prozac) toxicity in a newborn. Pediatrics 1997; 100: 158–9.

Milkovich L, van den Berg BJ. Effects of prenatal meprobamate and chlordiazepoxide hydrochloride on human embryonic and fetal development. N Engl J Med 1974; 291: 1268–71.

Morrell MJ. Folic acid and epilepsy. Epilepsy Curr 2002; 2: 31–4.

Moses-Kolko EL, Bogen D, Perel J et al. Neonatal signs after late in utero exposure to serotonin reuptake inhibitors. JAMA 2005; 293: 2372–83.

Myles N. Systematic meta-analysis of individual selective serotonin reuptake inhibitor medications and congenital malformations. Aust NZ J Psychiatry 2013; 47: 1002–12.

Nageotte MP, Briggs GG, Towers CV et al. Droperidol and diphenhydramine in the management of hyperemesis gravidarum. Am J Obstet Gynecol 1996; 174: 1801–5.

Nagy A, Tenyi T, Lenard K et al. Olanzapine and pregnancy. Orv Hetil 2001; 142: 137–8.

Neumann NU, Frasch K. Olanzapin und Schwangerschaft. Nervenarzt 2001; 72: 876–8.

Newham JJ, Thomas SH, MacRitchie K et al. Birth weight of infants after maternal exposure to typical and atypical antipsychotics: prospective comparison study. Br J Psychiatry 2008; 192: 333–7.

Newport DJ, Viguera AC, Beach AJ et al. Lithium placental passage and obstetrical outcome: Implications for clinical management during late pregnancy. Am J Psychiatry 2005; 162: 2162–70.

Nordeng H, Gelder M, Spigset O et al. Antidepressant exposure, maternal depression and pregnancy outcome – results from the Norwegian mother and child cohort study {Abstract}. Reprod Toxicol 2011; 31: 263.

Nulman I, Koren G, Rovet J et al. Neurodevelopment of children following prenatal exposure to venlafaxine, selective serotonin reuptake inhibitors, or untreated maternal depression. Am J Psychiatry 2012; 169: 1165–74.

Nulman I, Rovet J, Stewart DE et al. Child development following exposure to tricyclic antidepressants or fluoxetine throughout fetal life: a prospective, controlled study. Am J Psychiatry 2002; 159: 1889–95.

Nulman I, Rovet J, Stewart DE et al. Neurodevelopment of children exposed in utero to antidepressant drugs. N Engl J Med 1997; 336: 258–62.

Oberlander TF, Papsdorf M, Brain UM et al. Prenatal effects of selective serotonin reuptake inhibitor antidepressants, serotonin transporter promoter genotype (SLC6A4), and maternal mood on child behavior at 3 years of age. Arch Pediatr Adolesc Med 2010; 164: 444–51.

Oberlander TF, Warburton W, Misri S et al. Major congenital malformations following prenatal exposure to serotonin reuptake inhibitors and benzodiazepines using population-based health data. Birth Defects Res B Dev Reprod Toxicol 2008; 83: 68–76.

Occhiogrosso M, Omran SS, Altemus M. Persistent pulmonary hypertension of the newborn and selective serotonin reuptake inhibitors: lessons from clinical and translational studies. Am J Psychiat 2012; 169: 134–40.

Palmsten K , Hernández-Díaz S, Huybrechts KF. Use of antidepressants near delivery and risk of postpartum haemorrhage: cohort study of low income women in the United States. BMJ 2013a; 347: f4877.

Palmsten K, Huybrechts KF, Michels KB et al. Antidepressant use and risk for preeclampsia. Epidemiology 2013b; 24: 682–91.

Palmsten K, Setoguchi S Margulis AV et al. Elevated risk of preeclampsia in pregnant women with depression: depression or antidepressants? Am J Epidemiol 2012; 175: 988–97.

Patel SR, Wisner KL. Decision making for depression treatment during pregnancy and the postpartum period. Depress Anxiety 2011; 28: 589–95.

Pawluski JL. Perinatal selective serotonin reuptake inhibitor exposure: impact on brain development and neural plasticity. Neuroendocrinology 2012; 95: 39–46.

Pearson KH, Nonacs RM, Viguera AC et al. Birth outcomes following prenatal exposure to antidepressants. J Clin Psychiatry 2007; 68: 1284–9.

Pearson RM, Evans J, Kounali D et al. Maternal depression during pregnancy and the postnatal period: risks and possible mechanisms for offspring depression at age 18 years. JAMA Psychiatry 2013; 70: 1312–9.

Pedersen LH, Henriksen TB, Olsen J. Fetal exposure to antidepressants and normal milestone development at 6 and 19 months of age. Pediatrics 2010; 125: e600–8.

Pedersen LH, Henriksen TB, Vestergaard M et al. Selective serotonin reuptake inhibitors in pregnancy and congenital malformations: population based cohort study. BMJ 2009; 339: b3569.

Peinemann F, Daldrup T. Severe and prolonged sedation in five neonates due to persistence of active diazepam metabolites. Eur J Pediatr 2001; 160: 378–81.

Peitl RV. Ziprasidone as a possible cause of cleft palate in a newborn. Psychiatria Danubina, 2010; 22: 117–9.

Petik D, Acs N, Bánhidy F et al. A study of the potential teratogenic effect of large doses of promethazine used for a suicide attempt by 32 pregnant women. Toxicol Ind Health 2008; 24: 87–96.

Pinelli JM, Symington AJ, Cunningham KA et al. Case report and review of the perinatal implications of maternal lithium use. Am J Obstet Gynecol 2002; 187: 245–9.

Polen KN, Rasmussen SA, Riehle-Colarusso T, Reefhuis J. Association between reported venlafaxine use in early pregnancy and birth defects, national birth defects prevention study, 1997–2007. National Birth Defects Prevention Study. Birth Defects Res A Clin Mol Teratol 2013; 97: 28–35.

Pottegård A, Hallas J, Andersen JT et al. First-trimester exposure to methylphenidate: a population-based cohort study. J Clin Psychiatry 2014; 75: e88–93.

Rai D, Lee BK, Dalman C et al. Parental depression, maternal antidepressant use during pregnancy, and risk of autism spectrum disorders: population based case-control study. BMJ 2013; 346: f2059.

Rampono J, Simmer K, Ilett KF et al. Placental transfer of SSRI and SNRI antidepressants and effects on the neonate. Pharmacopsychiatry 2009; 42: 95–100.

Reis M, Källén B. Delivery outcome after maternal use of antidepressant drugs in pregnancy: an update using Swedish data. Psychol Med 2010; 40: 1723–33.

Reis M, Källén B. Maternal use of antipsychotics in early pregnancy and delivery outcome. J Clin Psychopharmacol 2008; 28: 279–88.

Riggin L, Frankel Z, Moretti M et al. The fetal safety of fluoxetine: a systematic review and meta-analysis. J Obstet Gynaecol Can 2013; 35: 362–9. Erratum appears in J Obstet Gynaecol Can 2013; 35: 691.

Robakis T, Williams KE. Atypical antipsychotics during pregnancy: Make decisions based on available evidence, individualized risk/benefit analysis. Curr Psychiat 2013; 12: 12–8.

Rohde A, Dembinski J, Dorn C. Mirtazapine (Remergil) for treatment resistant hyperemesis gravidarum: rescue of a twin pregnancy. Arch Gynecol Obstet 2003; 268: 219–21.

Rybakowski JK. Moclobemidc in pregnancy. Pharmacopsychiatry 2001; 34: 82–3.

Saks BR. Mirtazapine: treatment of depression, anxiety, and hyperemesis gravidarum in the pregnant patient. A report of 7 cases. Arch Womens Ment Health 2001; 3: 165–70.

Salisbury AL, Wisner KL, Pearlstein T et al. Newborn neurobehavioral patterns are differentially related to prenatal maternal major depressive disorder and serotonin reuptake inhibitor treatment. Depress Anxiety 2011; 28: 1008–19.

Salkeld E, Ferris LE, Juurlink DN. The risk of postpartum hemorrhage with selective serotonin reuptake inhibitors and other antidepressants. J Clin Psychopharmacol 2008; 28: 230–4.

Salvia-Roiges GL, Gonce-Mellgren A, Esque-Ruiz MT et al. Neonatal convulsions and subarachnoidal hemorrhage after in utero exposure to paroxetine. Rev Neurol 2003; 36: 724–6.

Sanz EJ, De-las-Cuevas C, Kiuru A et al. Selective serotonin reuptake inhibitors in pregnant women and neonatal withdrawal syndrome: a database analysis. Lancet 2005; 365: 482–7.

Sari Y, Zhou FC. Serotonin and its transporter on proliferation of fetal heart cells. Int J Dev Neurosci 2003; 21: 417–24.

Schimmell MS, Katz EZ, Shaag Y et al. Toxic neonatal effects following maternal clomipramine therapy. J Toxicol Clin Toxicol 1991; 29: 479–84.

Schou M. What happened later to the lithium babies? Arch Psychiar Scand 1976; 54: 193–7.

Shepard TH, Brent RL, Friedman JM et al. Update on new developments in the study of human teratogens. Teratology 2002; 65: 153–61.

Simon GE, Cunningham ML, Davis RL. Outcomes of prenatal antidepressant exposure. Am J Psychiatry 2002; 159: 2055–61.

Sit D, Luther J, Dills JLJ et al. Abnormal screening for gestational diabetes, maternal mood disorder, and preterm birth. Bipolar Dis 2013; DOI: 10.1111/bdi.12129.

Sit D, Perel JM, Luther JF et al. Disposition of chiral and racemic fluoxetine and norfluoxetine across childbearing. J Clin Psychopharmacol 2010; 30: 381–6.

2.11 Psychotropic drugs

Pregnancy

Sit DK, Perel JM, Helsen JC et al. Changes in antidepressant metabolism and dosing across pregnancy and early postpartum. J Clin Psychiatry 2008; 69: 652–8.

Sivojelezova A. Fluvoxamine (LUVOX™) use in pregnancy. Clin Pharmacol Ther 2004; 75: 25.

Sivojelezova A, Shuhaiber S, Sarkissian L et al. Citalopram use in pregnancy: prospective comparative evaluation of pregnancy and fetal outcome. Am J Obstet Gynecol 2005; 193: 2004–9.

Slone D, Siskind V, Heinonen OP. Antenatal exposure to the phenothiazines in relatin to congenital malformations, parinatal mortality rate, birth weight and intelligence quotient score. Am J Obsetr Gynecol 1977; 128: 486–8.

Sobel DE. Fetal damage due to ECT, insulin coma, chlorpromaine, or reserpine. Arch Gen psych 1960; 2: 606–11.

Sora S, Agostini Carbone ML. Chloral hydrate, methylmercury hydroxide and ethidium bromide affect chromosome segregation during meiosis of Saccharomyces cerevisiae. Mutat Res 1987; 190: 13–7.

Sørensen MJ, Grønborg TK, Christensen J et al. Antidepressant exposure in pregnancy and risk of autism spectrum disorders Clin Epidemiol 2013; 5: 449–59.

Spinelli MG. Interpersonal psychotherapy for depressed antepartum women: a pilot study. Am J Psychiatry 1997; 154: 1028–30.

Stephens S, Wilson G, Gilfillan C et al. Preliminary data on therapeutic exposure to zopiclone during pregnancy. Reprod Toxicol 2008; 26: 73–74.

Steyn DW, Odendaal HJ. The effect of oral ketanserin on fetal heart rate parameters. J Matern Fetal Investig 1998; 8: 126–9.

Stika C, Frederiksen M. Drug therapy in pregnant and nursing women. In Principles of Clinical Pharmacology. Atkinson AJ Jr, Daniels CE, Dedrick R, Grudzinskas CV, eds. San Diego: Academic Press, 2001; pp. 227–91.

Tabacova SA, McCloskey CA, Fisher JE. Adverse developmental events reported to FDA in association with maternal citalopram treatment in pregnancy. Birth Defects Res A 2004; 70: 361.

Tanaka T, Choi J, Nomura Y et al. The incidence of poor neonatal adaptation syndrome following exposure to venlafaxine in late pregnancy. Birth Defects Res A Clin Mol Teratol 2007; 79: 446.

Taylor T, Kennedy D. Safety of moclobemide in pregnancy and lactation, four case reports. Birth Defects Res A Clin Mol Teratol 2008; 82: 413.

Taylor TM, O'Toole MS, Ohlsen RI et al. Safety of quetiapine during pregnancy. Am J Psychiatry 2003; 160: 588–9.

Tegethoff M, Greene N, Olsen J et al. Stress during pregnancy and offspring pediatric disease: A National Cohort Study. Health Perspect 2011; 119: 1647–52.

Tényi T, Trixler M, Keresztes Z. Quetiapine and pregnancy. Am J Psychiatry 2002; 159: 674.

ter Horst PG, van der Linde S, Smit JP et al. Clomipramine concentration and withdrawal symptoms in 10 neonates. Br J Clin Pharmacol 2012; 73: 295–302.

Treichel M, Schwendener Scholl K, Kessler U et al. Is there a correlation between venlafaxine therapy during pregnancy and a higher incidence of necrotizing enterocolitis? World J Pediatr 2009; 5: 65–7.

Turcotte V, Ferreira E, Duperron L. Utilité du dropéridol et de la diphenhydramine dans l'hyperemesis gravidarum. J Soc Obstet Gynaecol Can 2001; 23: 133–9.

van der Lugt NM, van de Maat JS, van Kamp IL et al. Fetal, neonatal and developmental outcomes of lithium-exposed pregnancies. 2012; 88: 375–8.

Van Vaes A, van de Velde E. Safety evaluation of haloperidol in the treatment of hyperemesis gravidarum. J Clin Pharmacol 1969; 9: 224–7.

Ververs FF, Voorbij HA, Zwarts P et al. Effect of cytochrome P450 2D6 genotype on maternal paroxetine plasma concentrations during pregnancy. Clin Pharmacokinet 2009; 48: 677–83.

Viguera AC, Nonacs R, Cohen LS et al. Risk of recurrence of bipolar disorder in pregnant and nonpregnant women after discontinuing lithium maintenance. Am J Psychiatry 2000; 157: 179–84.

Vladimir J, Dragan M, Ružić et al. Zuclopenthixol decanoate in pregnancy: successful outcomes in two consecutive offsprings of the same mother. Vojnosanitetski Pregled: Military Medical & Pharmaceutical Journal of Serbia & Montenegro 2013; 70: 526–9.

Wajnberg R, Diav-Citrin O, Shechtman S et al. Pregnancy outcome after in-utero exposure to methylphenidate: A prospective comparative cohort study (abstract). Reprod Toxicol 2011; 31: 267.

Wang LH, Lin HC, Lin CC et al. Increased risk of adverse pregnancy outcomes in women receiving zolpidem during pregnancy. Clin Pharmacol Ther 2010; 88: 369–74.

Warburton W, Hertzman C, Oberlander TF. A register study of the impact of stopping third trimester selective serotonin reuptake inhibitor exposure on neonatal health. Acta Psychiatr Scand 2010; 121: 471–9.

Wichman CL, Moore KM, Lang TR et al. Congenital heart disease associated with selective serotonin reuptake inhibitor use during pregnancy. Mayo Clin Proc 2009; 84: 23–7.

Wikner BN, Källén B. Are hypnotic benzodiazepine receptor agonists teratogenic in humans? J Clin Psychopharmacol 2011; 31: 356–9.

Wikner BN, Stiller CO, Bergman U et al. Use of benzodiazepines and benzodiazepine receptor agonists during pregnancy: neonatal outcome and congenital malformations. Pharmacoepidemiol Drug Saf 2007a; 16: 1203–10.

Wikner BN, Stiller CO, Källén B et al. Use of benzodiazepines and benzodiazepine receptor agonists during pregnancy: maternal characteristics. Pharmacoepidemiol Drug Saf 2007b; 16: 988–94.

Williams SF, Alvarez JR, Pedro HF et al. Glutaric aciduria type II and narcolepsy in pregnancy. Obstet Gynecol 2008; 111: 522–4.

Wilson KL, Zelig CM, Harvey JP et al. Persistent pulmonary hypertension of the newborn is associated with mode of delivery and not with maternal use of selective serotonin reuptake inhibitors. Am J Perinatol 2011; 28: 19–24.

Wirz-Justice A, Bader A, Frisch U et al. A randomized, double-blind, placebo-controlled study of light therapy for antepartum depression. J Clin Psychiatry 2011; 72: 986–93.

Wisner KL, Bogen DL, Sit D et al. Does fetal exposure to SSRIs or maternal depression impact infant growth? Am J Psych 2013; 170: 485–93.

Wisner KL, Perel JM, Wheeler SB. Tricyclic dose requirements across pregnancy. Am J Psychiat 1993; 150: 1541–2.

Wisner KL, Sit DK, Hanusa BH et al. Major depression and antidepressant treatment: impact on pregnancy and neonatal outcomes. Am J Psychiatry 2009; 166: 557–66.

Wisner KL, Sit DK, Moses EL. Antipsychotic treatment during pregnancy: A model for decision making. Adv Schizophr Clin Psychiatry 2007; 3: 48–55.

Wurst KE, Poole C, Ephross SA et al. First trimester paroxetine use and the prevalence of congenital, specifically cardiac, defects: a meta-analysis of epidemiological studies. Birth Defects Res A Clin Mol Teratol 2010; 88: 159–70.

Yacobi S, Ornoy A. Is lithium a real teratogen? What can we conclude from the prospective versus retrospective studies? Isr J Psychiatry Relat Sci 2008; 45: 95–106.

Yogev Y, Ben-Haroush A, Kaplan B. Maternal clozapine treatment and decreased fetal heart rate variability. Int J Gynecol Obstet 2002; 79: 259–60.

Yonkers KA, Wisner KL, Stowe Z et al. Management of bipolar disorder during pregnancy and the postpartum period. Am J Psychiatry 2004; 161: 608–20.

Zalzstein E, Koren G, Einarson T et al. A case-control study on the association between first trimester exposure to lithium and Ebstein's anomaly. Am J Cardiol 1990, 65: 817–8.

Zegers B, Andriessen P. Maternal lithium therapy and neonatal morbidity. Eur J Pediatr 2003; 162: 348–9.

Zeskind PS, Stephens LE. Maternal selective serotonin reuptake inhibitor use during pregnancy and newborn neurobehavior. Pediatrics 2004; 113: 368–75.

Pregnancy

2.11 Psychotropic drugs

Immunosuppression, rheumatic diseases, multiple sclerosis, and Wilson's disease 2.12

Corinna Weber-Schöndorfer

2.12.1	Azathioprine/6-mercaptopurine	341
2.12.2	Selective immunosuppressants	342
2.12.3	Biologics	345
2.12.4	Multiple sclerosis	352
2.12.5	Interferons	354
2.12.6	Other immunostimulatory drugs	356
2.12.7	Transplantation	358
2.12.8	Drugs for rheumatic diseases	358
2.12.9	Drugs for Wilson's disease	363

Immunomodulators include immunosuppressive and immunostimulatory agents. Within the group of immunosuppressants (Sections 2.12.1–2.12.3) a differentiation is made between glucocorticoids, conventional synthetic disease-modifying drugs and biologics. The immunostimulatory drugs (Sections 2.12.5–2.12.6) basically include the cytokines, interferons, glatiramer and colony stimulating factors.

2.12.1   Azathioprine/6-mercaptopurine

Azathioprine (AZA) is an antimetabolite which is 80% metabolized to *6-mercaptopurine* (6-MP). 6-MP in turn, is changed into the active metabolite 6-thioguaninenucleotide (6-TGN). Approximately 47% of orally given AZA is absorbed, whereas 6-MP is, on average, only 16% absorbed. The placental transfer is limited (Hutson 2011); however, 6-TGN was found in similar concentrations in the erythrocytes of three mothers and their healthy newborns (de Boer 2006). Jharap and colleagues prospectively analyzed thiopurine metabolism before, during, and after pregnancy in 30 mother–child pairs (31 infants). During pregnancy, maternal 6-TGN decreased, while 6-methylmercaptopurine (6-MMP) increased. Fetal 6-TGN concentrations correlated positively with maternal 6-TGN levels. Jharap (2014) discussed whether the maternally derived metabolites, and not the parent drug, cross the placental barrier.

Experience from nearly 40 studies, case series or reports, with a total of more than 2,000 pregnant women – of whom half had taken AZA during the entire pregnancy – have not revealed teratogenic risks (e.g. Ban 2014, Casanova 2013, Goldstein 2007, Armenti, 2005, Moskovitz 2004,

Polifka 2002). Only a Swedish study (Cleary 2009) found a weak association between AZA and atrial or ventricular septal defects (adjusted OR 3.18; 95%–CI 1.45 to 6.04), whereas the total malformation risk was not significantly increased. The authors question the causality with the medication and consider this an incidental result due to multiple testing. The latter study was included in a recently published meta-analysis (Akbari 2013) which did not find a significantly increased risk for malformation.

Lower birth weight and a higher rate of prematurity (Akbari 2013) have occasionally been observed after long-term AZA therapy; however, these adverse outcomes might well be a consequence of maternal illness and disease activity. While with pregnant transplant recipients on AZA, an association between maternal leukopenia and impaired neonatal hematopoiesis has occasionally been observed (e.g. Davison 1985), two studies with pregnant women treated with lower AZA doses because of autoimmune diseases, found no effect on the infant's immune system (Biggioggero 2007, Motta 2007).

There are limited and conflicting data on long-term neurodevelopment of children exposed *in utero* to AZA (e.g. Gayed 2013, Marder 2013).

Paternal exposure: A meta-analysis covering three studies on male patients with inflammatory bowel disease treated with AZA, did not find an increased risk for congenital malformations (Akbari 2013). This is in line with an observational prospective cohort study on 115 expecting fathers who were treated with AZA because of various treatment indications (Hoeltzenbein 2012b), and with the findings of Viktil (2012), who reported on, among others, about 124 pregnancies fathered by men on AZA treatment.

> **Recommendation.** AZA/6-MP is one of the best studied drugs amongst immunosuppressants. A teratogenic potential in humans has not been recognized. It may be prescribed during pregnancy. A detailed ultrasound examination may be offered to confirm normal fetal development.

2.12.2   Selective immunosuppressants

▶ Cyclosporine

The calcineurin inhibitor, *ciclosporine* or *cyclosporine A* (CyA) is among the well-studied immunosuppressants. CyA was first approved for use in organ transplant patients and is, meanwhile, also used for severe courses of some autoimmune diseases. Some 30–64% of the maternal concentration of the substance can reach the fetus.

Experience of a large number of case reports and series, and from the transplantation registries (Armenti 2005, Bar 2001, Lamarque 1997) have not revealed teratogenic risk. Intrauterine growth retardation, a higher rate of caesarean deliveries, prematurity and increased maternal complications, such as, for instance, hypertension and preeclampsia have been described (Paziana 2013); however, these adverse outcomes might well be a consequence of maternal illness. In two case series, no effects on the infant immune system were found in children of mothers with autoimmune diseases and immunosuppressive therapy during pregnancy (Biggioggero 2007, Motta 2007). This is in line with the findings of earlier studies (e.g. Rieder 1997). A hepatoblastoma in a 2-year-old child is the only case described of a malignancy after continuous maternal treatment (Roll 1997).

In a cohort study, in which 39 intrauterine CyA-exposed children were compared with non-exposed children with respect to possible long-term effects, no differences in intelligence, visual motor abilities and behavior could be determined (Nulman 2010).

> **Recommendation.** Among immunosuppressants cyclosporine is one of the best studied drugs. A teratogenic potential in humans has not been recognized. It may be prescribed during pregnancy. A detailed ultrasound examination may be offered to confirm normal fetal development.

► Mycophenolate (MMF)

The selective immunosuppressants *mycophenolate mofetil* and *mycophenolic acid* are used after organ transplants, for rheumatoid arthritis and for systemic lupus erythematosus (SLE). Mycophenolate mofetil is quickly absorbed after oral intake and rapidly changed into its active metabolite, mycophenolic acid. The metabolite has a mean half-life of 12–16 hours and it appears to cross the placenta (Tjeertes 2007).

MMF is the most recently recognized human teratogen. The specific pattern of birth defects consists of malformations of the ear, in particular, microtia and atresia of the external ear, cleft lip, and other malformations such as tracheal-esophageal atresia (Anderka 2009) or heart defects (Lin 2011).

The experiences with pregnancy are based on transplantation registries (Termini 2011, Coscia 2009), the manufacturer's (Roche) database (77 pregnancies) and retrospective case reports, which describe 20 children or fetuses with a distinct pattern of malformations (e.g. Anderka 2009). Some of these pregnancies were also recorded by the Roche database or the transplantation registry. In a study by the European Network of Teratology Information Services (ENTIS), 57 prospectively ascertained pregnancies with maternal MMF treatment were evaluated: a spontaneous abortion risk of about 45% and an increased risk for major birth defects of 26% were observed, of which at least four fetuses/infants had a clinical phenotype consistent with mycophenolate embryopathy (Hoeltzenbein 2012a).

Paternal exposure: An evaluation of the National Transplantation Pregnancy Registry could identify 152 male transplant recipients with MMF therapy who fathered 205 pregnancies. There was neither an increased rate of major birth defects nor a distinct pattern of anomalies (Jones 2013).

> **Recommendation.** Mycophenolate is teratogenic. When planning a pregnancy, MMF should be replaced by another immunosuppressant. It should be avoided during the pregnancy if possible (Section 2.12.7, Transplantation). An accidental exposure during pregnancy does not, however, justify a risk-grounded termination of pregnancy, but a detailed ultrasound examination should be carried out (Chapter 1.15).

► Tacrolimus

Tacrolimus (FK-506) is a macrolide obtained from Streptomyces, which is used orally as an immunosuppressant after organ transplantation

Pregnancy

2.12 Immunosuppression, rheumatic diseases, multiple sclerosis, and Wilson's disease

or locally for skin diseases (Chapter 2.17). It crosses the placenta with *in utero* exposure being approximately 71% of maternal blood concentrations. Its pharmacokinetic is altered during pregnancy. Due to decreased albumin level during pregnancy unbound tacrolimus concentration increases (e.g. Hebert 2013).

The experience in pregnancy rests on retrospective case reports (e.g. Alsuwaida 2011, Costa, 2011), case series and studies (e.g. Christopher 2006, Garcia-Donaire 2005, Jain 2004), including a small prospective study with 49 children of 37 mothers with liver transplants (Jain 2003), and on the National Transplantation Registry established in 1991 by the drug manufacturers (Armenti 2005). Altogether, more than 250 pregnancies with tacrolimus have been documented, from which no teratogenic risk can be deduced. The malformations observed up to now do not occur frequently, and there is no recognizable pattern.

As with therapy with other immunosuppressants, preeclampsia, premature births, lower birth weights and caesarean sections have been observed more frequently; however, these adverse outcomes might well be a consequence of maternal disease. Gestational diabetes appears to occur more frequently with tacrolimus, and newborns with decreased kidney function and hyperkalemia have been described frequently (e.g. Kainz 2000). A case of anuria which continued for 36 hours was the gravest finding (Jain 1997).

> **Recommendation.** As yet, no teratogenic potential has been recognized for humans. Systemic use of tacrolimus during pregnancy is acceptable in well-grounded cases (Section 2.12.7). A detailed ultrasound examination should be offered to confirm normal fetal development. After tacrolimus exposure in late pregnancy, the newborn's kidney function and potassium levels should be checked as a precaution.

▶ Further selective immunosuppressants

Everolimus is a derivative of *sirolimus* and is used in transplant patients, and in higher doses, as an antineoplastic drug. There are only a few documented case reports on its use during pregnancy, all with favorable outcome (Margoles 2014, Veroux, 2011, Carta 2012).

Sirolimus inhibits the T-cell proliferation via another mechanism in comparison with cyclosporine or tacrolimus. More than 10 case reports give no indications of any teratogenicity (e.g. Framarino dei 2011, Chu 2008, Sifontis 2006, Armenti 2005).

Paternal exposure: There is evidence that sirolimus can lead to oligospermia, which was reversible in some patients after ceasing the therapy (Zuber 2008, Deutsch 2007).

There is no documented experience for the selective calcineurin inhibitor *pimecrolimus* during pregnancy. After dermal use, no relevant systemic concentrations are expected, and thus effects on the expected child appear unlikely (Chapter 2.17).

> **Recommendation.** Due to insufficient data, everolimus and sirolimus therapy are reserved for refractory situations (Section 2.12.7). *Pimecrolimus* should be avoided. After systemic therapy, a detailed ultrasound examination should be offered to confirm the normal development of the fetus.

2.12.3   Biologics

Biologics used for medical treatment are genetically engineered proteins which can activate or suppress the body's target function in order to act as a therapeutic. Among others, *monoclonal antibodies* are biologics. The therapeutically used ones carry the ending -mab. *Mabs* are used for different treatment indications. As well as this chapter, they can be found in "Antiasthmatics and cough medications" (see Chapter 2.3), "Anticoagulants, thrombocyte aggregation inhibitors, fibrinolytics and volume replacement agents" (see Chapter 2.9) and "Antineoplastic drugs" (see Chapter 2.13). Biologics for immunomodulation are described below. Recommendations are only given, if sufficient experience is available. All other agents are dealt with together and no recommendations are given.

The substances reviewed below are not only very expensive, but can also have severe adverse effects, such as serious infections or anaphylaxis. For more details please refer to the product labeling or to a standard pharmacology book.

▶ **Adalimumab**

Adalimumab (ADA), a fully human monoclonal IgG1-antibody and *tumor necrosis factor α-(TNF α-) blocker* with a half-life of 14 days, is used in severe forms of rheumatoid arthritis, ankylosing spondylitis, psoriasis, psoriasis-arthritis or Crohn's disease, as a rule after failure of established immunosuppressants.

In total, approximately 270 pregnancies (abstracts included) exposed during the first trimester are published in case reports (e.g. Dessinioti 2011), case series (e.g. Bortlik 2013, Schnitzler 2011, Weber-Schoendorfer 2011), a small study on 83 anti-TNF-α-exposed pregnancies of which 23 were adalimumab exposed (Diav-Citrin 2014), and a study currently conducted by the North American Teratology Centers (OTIS, Organization of Teratology Information Specialists) for which an interim report on 161 pregnancies is available (Johnson 2011). Even though malformations were described in a few pregnancies, there is no distinct pattern.

The high molecular weight of 148,000 Da makes placental transfer during embryogenesis unlikely. Nevertheless, through an active process, there is an increasing transfer of the monoclonal antibody by the mature placenta after the twentieth week of pregnancy. Because TNF-α plays an important role in the development of the fetal immune system, there are theoretical concerns about its use, especially in the late second and third trimester. Thirty-five pregnancy courses to date on continuous adalimumab therapy, or on treatment in the second half of the pregnancy, have shown that therapeutic concentrations can be reached in the newborn (Bortlik 2013, Mahadevan 2013, Fritzsche 2012). Zelinkova (2013) determined the cord blood concentrations in 13 pregnancies in which ADA therapy already ended before gestational week 30. In only 5 out of 13 samples ADA was detected in cord blood. The median ratio of infant's ADA drug level to mother's was 179% (range 98–293%) (Mahadevan 2013).

The experience with a longer follow-up period after therapy in late pregnancy is considerably sparser (e.g. Coburn 2006, Mishkin 2006, Vesga 2005). Up to now, there is only one case reporting adverse effects on the infant immune system after maternal TNF-inhibitor therapy. Cheent (2010) reported on a boy born healthy, whose mother was treated

Pregnancy

2.12 Immunosuppression, rheumatic diseases, multiple sclerosis, and Wilson's disease

for Crohn's disease throughout pregnancy with infliximab. At the age of 3 months, he received a BCG live vaccine, which led to a disseminated BCG infection and ultimately to the child's death. On the contrary, a recently published case report of a 3-month-old preterm infant with chicken pox who fully recovered is reassuring (Johnsson, 2013). His mother received ADA until gestational week 34 and went into labor 2 days later.

Paternal exposure: Six pregnancies fathered by men on adalimumab with apparent favorable pregnancy outcome were reported by Viktil (2012).

> **Recommendation.** ADA does not need to be stopped when planning a pregnancy. However, treatment in the second/third trimester should be reserved for well-grounded indications. Discontinuation of therapy is mostly recommended by gestational week 30. A detailed ultrasound examination may be offered to confirm normal fetal development. With treatment in the second half of pregnancy, the pregnant woman and the fetus should be closely and sonographically monitored. As a matter of precaution, children who were exposed to ADA in later pregnancy should not be immunized with a live vaccine before 6 months of life.

▶ Certolizumab pegol

Certolizumab pegol (CZP) is a pegylated (polyethylene glycol) antigen-binding fragment (Fab) of a recombinant humanized anti-TNF-α monoclonal antibody, which is approved for severe courses of rheumatoid arthritis (in some countries only together with MTX) and by the FDA also for Crohn's disease. Its half-life is 14 days. The molecular structure of CTZ is different from infliximab (IFX) and ADA. It lacks an Fc portion which among others is necessary for an active transport across the placenta.

Experience during the first trimester is limited to less than 20 published pregnancies which did not indicate a teratogenic risk as yet (e.g. review by Marchioni 2013). In addition, 59 pregnancies were reported from clinical trial reports and 82 from spontaneous post-marketing reports. According to an analysis by the manufacturer, no particular fetal risks have been reported; however, data quality does not seem to be high (Clowse 2013).

CZP has a low placental transfer which was shown by Mahadevan (2013). Ten mothers of 12 infants (including twins) had received their last CZP dose in median 19 days before delivery. The median ratio of cord blood to maternal drug concentration was 3.9% (range 1.5–24%). The mechanism of transfer is not yet known.

> **Recommendation.** Although teratogenicity is not suspected, experience with CZP during organogenesis is still insufficient. A detailed ultrasound examination should be offered after exposure during the 1st trimester. As placental transfer of CZP is low, therapy may be continued until delivery if necessary.

▶ Etanercept

Etanercept is approved for treatment of moderately severe to severe courses of rheumatoid arthritis, with or without methotrexate, as well as for psoriasis-arthritis, plaque-psoriasis, Bechterew's disease (ankylosing spondylitis) and juvenile idiopathic arthritis, following insufficient response to the usual basic therapeutics. It is a functionally soluble TNF-α-inhibitor, a fusion protein, consisting of a portion of the human TNF-receptor and the Fc domain of human IgG1, which among others, leads to a placental transfer. It has a half-life of about 70 hours.

Meanwhile, published experience covers more than 300 pregnancies. However, most data come from abstracts (e.g. Hultzsch 2011), posters (Johnson 2008), case descriptions (e.g. Scioscia 2011, Roux 2007), case series (e.g. Rump 2010) or registries (Viktil 2012, Verstappen 2011). Most of the children described here were exposed in the first trimester and born healthy.

Preliminary results of an OTIS study of 139 pregnancies exposed in the first trimester were published as poster (Johnson 2008). A higher number of malformations than expected was observed, but the malformations were heterogeneous. Confounders such as co-medication, e.g. methotrexate, have not been considered in the preliminary findings. A small cohort study on 83 anti-TNF-α-exposed pregnancies among them 25 with etanercept, did not find an increased malformation risk (Diav-Citrin 2014). An evaluation of the British Society for Rheumatology Biologics Register included 71 prospectively recorded pregnancies with anti-TNF therapy, among them 48 with etanercept, nine with infliximab and 14 with adalimumab, and revealed a 27% miscarriage rate. Even if only pregnancies without MTX as a co-medication were considered, the miscarriage rate remained high. However, the total number of pregnancies evaluated was small, the group of drugs was heterogeneous and the results have not been confirmed by other studies up to now (Verstappen 2011). Furthermore, since TNF-α can play an important role in causing spontaneous abortions, the TNF-α inhibitors adalimumab or etanercept were used in patients with IVF treatment or recurrent miscarriage (Winger 2009, 2008). Thereby, no negative effects on the pregnancy were observed. This also argues against an increased spontaneous abortion rate after etanercept therapy.

A report (Carter 2006) on a child with VACTERL syndrome (V: vertebral defects; A: anal atresia; C: cardiac anomalies; T: tracheal-esophageal fistula; E: esophageal atresia; R: radial and renal problems; L: limb anomalies) following continuous intrauterine exposure has led to discussion. However, there are no further comparable observations after etanercept treatment. Also the analysis of the FDA data base (Carter 2009) was unable to turn up any additional children with a VACTERL syndrome among the 22 retrospectively recorded pregnancies with anomalies. However, the authors assessed isolated malformations, such as septal heart defects as part of the VACTERL syndrome. Furthermore, this publication has grave methodological shortcomings in that, for instance, the respective exposure periods were not mentioned.

With continuous treatment, etanercept crosses the placenta in limited amounts as indicated through simultaneous measurements in the mother's blood and the cord blood. In the cord blood 1/30 (Murashima 2009) and 1/14 (Berthelsen 2010) of the maternal concentration was found. The experience of use in later pregnancy is very limited, with fewer than 20 cases, but does not indicate any negative effects on the newborn (e.g. Umeda 2010).

Paternal exposure: Forty pregnancies fathered by men on etanercept with mostly favorable outcomes were reported (Viktil 2012). Among those was one child with a septal heart defect and penoscrotal malformation.

Pregnancy

2.12 Immunosuppression, rheumatic diseases, multiple sclerosis, and Wilson's disease

Recommendation. Etanercept is not considered a teratogen; however, experience during pregnancy is still insufficient. Substitution of treatment should be considered when planning a pregnancy. After accidental treatment during the pregnancy, etanercept should be replaced, if at all possible. There is no indication for a risk-grounded pregnancy termination. However, a detailed ultrasound examination should be offered (Chapter 1.15). Although placental transfer is low, treatment after the first trimester should be reserved for well-grounded individual cases.

▶ Infliximab

Infliximab (IFX) is a TNF-α inhibitor and full IgG1-antibody which is approved for severe cases of rheumatoid arthritis, together with methotrexate, for pronounced psoriasis and psoriasis-arthritis, ankylosing spondylitis as well as for chronic inflammatory bowel disease. It has an average terminal half-life of about 9 days, and is still detectable to some extent in the serum after 12 weeks, and in steady-state, is infused every 6 to 8 weeks.

The approximately 500 pregnancy courses after treatment in the first trimester come from registries (Snoeckx 2008, Katz 2004), case series (e.g. Bortlik 2013, Schnitzler 2011), case reports (e.g. Chaparro 2011) and a small prospective cohort study among which were 35 infliximab exposed pregnancies (Diav-Citrin 2014). Up to now, there are no larger controlled studies. No teratogenicity has been observed as yet.

The high molecular weight of 144,200 Da makes placental transfer during embryogenesis unlikely. Nevertheless, through an active process, there is an increasing transfer of the monoclonal antibody by the mature placenta after the twentieth week of pregnancy. Because TNF-α plays an important role in the development of the fetal immune system, there are theoretical concerns about its use, especially in the late second and the third trimester. The few publications to date on continuous therapy or on treatment in the second half of the pregnancy, have shown that therapeutic concentrations can be reached in the newborn (Bortlik 2013, Mahadevan 2013). Zelinkova (2013) determined the cord blood concentrations in 18 cases. In most of these cases, IFX therapy ended before gestational week 30. The mean IFX cord levels were significantly lower when the treatment had been stopped 10 weeks or more before delivery. The median ratio of infant's IFX drug level to mother's was 160% (range 87–400%) (Mahadevan 2013). In one infant, a slow postpartum clearance was documented with measurable levels up to 6 months of age. This argues for an increased half-life in fetuses, neonates and young infants. Antibodies against IFX, which about 60% of the patients in treatment develop, were not observed in this child at the age of 6 months (Vasiliauskas 2006). There is currently only one case reporting adverse effects of the infant immune system after maternal IFX. As has been noted previously, Cheent (2010) reported on a boy born healthy, whose mother was treated for Crohn's disease throughout pregnancy with IFX. At the age of 3 months, he received a BCG live vaccine, which led to a disseminated BCG infection and ultimately to the child's death. However, a recently published case report of a 3-month-old preterm infant with chicken pox who fully recovered is reassuring (Johnsson 2013). His mother had received ADA until gestational week 34 and went into labor 2 days later.

Paternal exposure: In two small case series/case reports, changes of form and motility of the sperm were described after the father's infliximab therapy (Mahadevan 2005, Montagna 2005). However, a comparative analysis of semen samples of 26 men on TNF-antagonists and healthy volunteers, showed no significant impairment in the patients with inactive disease receiving long-term TNF-inhibitors (Villiger 2010). Saougou reported about 14 healthy children fathered by men on infliximab therapy (Saougou 2013).

> **Recommendation.** IFX does not need to be stopped when planning a pregnancy. However, treatment in the second/third trimester should be reserved for well-grounded indications. Discontinuation of therapy is mostly recommended by gestational week 30. A detailed ultrasound examination may be offered to confirm normal fetal development. With treatment in the second half of pregnancy, the pregnant woman and the fetus should be closely and sonographically monitored. As a matter of precaution, children who were exposed to IFX in the late pregnancy should not be immunized with a live vaccine before the sixth month of life.

▶ Natalizumab

Natalizumab is an alpha-4 integrin inhibitor, which is used for severe relapsing remitting multiple sclerosis, and in some countries also for Crohn's disease. After temporary removal from the market due to progressive multifocal leukoencephalopathy (PML), it was again approved in the USA and following that also, for the first time, in Europe. The risk of PML increases with the duration of therapy.

Apart from one infant with hexadactyly, there were no malformations recorded among the 29 live-born children from a small study of 35 prospectively recorded pregnancies (Hellwig 2011). Also, three additional children, of whom two were exposed throughout the pregnancy, were healthy (Fagius 2014, Hoevenaren 2011). The manufacturer reported on 222 prospectively recorded pregnancies, including five pairs of twins, from which there were 186 live-born children, 26 spontaneous abortions and 10 terminations. The results, which have thus far only been published as an abstract, report "isolated" malformations without giving any details (Cristiano 2011). Four cases published on natalizumab therapy in later pregnancy report about healthy children (Schneider, 2013, Bayas 2011, Hoevenaren 2011). However, in two children the chemotaxis rate of neonatal T lymphocytes were analyzed and found to be impaired at the age of 2 weeks and restored at 2 months (Schneider 2013). The clinical relevance of this finding remains unclear.

> **Recommendation.** Although teratogenicity is not currently suspected, experience with natalizumab during organogenesis is still insufficient. A detailed ultrasound examination should be offered after exposure during the 1st trimester. As effects on lymphocytes in newborns and various changes in the differential blood count in treated patients have been shown, a differential blood count in the neonate may be recommended after exposure in late pregnancy as a matter of precaution. If possible, therapy with natalizumab should not be undertaken during pregnancy.

Pregnancy

2.12 Immunosuppression, rheumatic diseases, multiple sclerosis, and Wilson's disease

▶ **Additional Mabs and other biologics**

Abatacept is used, together with methotrexate, for treatment of rheumatoid arthritis. It is a fusion protein from the extracellular domain of human cytotoxic T-lymphocytes-antigen-4 (CTLA-4), which is bound to the Fc portion of human immunoglobulin G1 (IgG1). Abatacept interferes with the activation of T-lymphocytes and thus should be able to limit an excessive immune response or inflammation. It has a half-life of more than 13 days and must be infused intravenously. In animal experiments no teratogenicity was observed. Studies on rats showed placental transfer. During the pre-marketing phase of the medication, there were 10 pregnancies, of which the majority were terminated or ended with a spontaneous abortion (Ojeda-Uribe 2013, Pham 2009). One healthy child was reported (Ojeda-Uribe 2013, Pham 2009) with the last abatacept infusion at 2.5 gestational weeks.

Aflibercept is a recombinant fusion protein which specifically inhibits the vascular endothelial growth factor-A and also binds to the placental growth factor. It is administered into the vitreous. As it is newly marketed, there are no reports on its use during pregnancy. For drugs in ophthalmology see also Chapter 2.17.

Alemtuzumab is a humanized monoclonal IgG_{1k}-antibody which has now been approved for multiple sclerosis (Section 2.12.4). There are no data for its use in pregnancy.

Anakinra is an interleukin (IL)-1 receptor antagonist, which is approved for treatment of rheumatoid arthritis in combination with methotrexate. A placental transfer of 1–3% in Rhesus monkeys was measured. To date, three healthy children after intrauterine anakinra exposure have been reported (Fischer-Betz 2011, Berger 2009).

Basiliximab which blocks the IL-2 receptors on the surface of activated T-lymphocytes is used, together with other immunosuppressants, as a prophylaxis against rejection during and after kidney transplantation. There is no experience on its use during pregnancy.

Belatacept was approved by the EMA and FDA in 2011. It is a selective co-stimulatory blocker of T-cell activation, and intended to be used for the prophylaxis of renal transplant rejection in combination with glucocorticoids and mycophenolate. The chemical structure is similar to abatacept. There are no data for its use in pregnancy.

Belimumab was approved by the FDA and EMA in 2011 as therapy for SLE, except for severe courses with kidney or CNS involvement. It inhibits B-cell activating factor. Studies in cynomolgus monkeys did not find an increased malformation rate. Umbilical cord blood concentrations of belimumab were about one-quarter of maternal blood concentrations, suggesting that this drug crosses the placenta in late pregnancy (Auyeung-Kim 2009). Human pregnancy data are limited to pregnancies which occurred during clinical trials. Of 83 pregnancies with known outcomes, 42% were live births among which were three infants with birth defects. One was a chromosomal translocation also found in the mother; no details are given on the other two malformations (Peart 2014).

Bevacizumab, a humanized IgG1antibody, is an angiogenesis inhibitor which binds the vascular endothelial growth factor and thereby prevents the production of new vessels. Therefore, it is used with some cancers in combination with cytostatics (doses between 5 and 15 mg/kg IV every 2 or 3 weeks) and off-label in ophthalmology for moist macular degeneration, for choroidal neovascularization (e.g. intravitreal injection of 1.25 mg) and also, to some extent, with macular edema. There are at least seven publications available that describe 10 healthy children after intravitreal injection during pregnancy, one preterm infant with prematurity related problems after emergency C-section because of maternal preeclampsia, and three early spontaneous abortions (e.g. Sullivan, 2014, Gomez 2012, Introini 2012, Tarantola 2010). Among the 11 live-births, seven were exposed in the first trimester, one in the second, one in the third, another both in the second and third, and the 11th child throughout pregnancy. Two cases with systemic use of bevacizumab presented by Cross (2012), suggest that interference with vascular endothelial growth factor signaling is sufficient to induce a preeclampsia-like syndrome in nonpregnant patients. Although bevacizumab has a high molecular weight of 149,000 Da, a transfer from the vitreous body into the circulation has been found. It seems to be equally effective as ranibizumab, but persists longer in the systemic circulation after an intravitreal injection (Rosenfeld 2011). For drugs in ophthalmology, see also Chapter 2.17.

Canakinumab, a fully human monoclonal antibody against interleukin-1β, is approved as an orphan drug for the rare, inherited CAPS-Syndrome (cryopyrin-associated periodic syndrome). There are no published data on its use during pregnancy as yet.

Daclizumab binds to the interleukin-2 receptor and is used in transplantation medicine. There are no human data. Recently, it has been tested in relapsing remitting multiple sclerosis.

Eculizumab, an orphan drug, has been approved for treatment of paroxysmal nocturnal hemoglobinuria (PNH) – a rare acquired severe illness of the blood-producing stem cells. Intravascular hemolysis with consequent anemia, and a high incidence of venous and arterial thrombotic events and other complications of PNH, led to high maternal, fetal morbidity and mortality during pregnancy. As a starting point with the multiple symptoms, eculizumab can reduce the intravascular hemolysis by binding the humanized type IgG 2/4 to the C5 protein of the complementary system and blocking the terminal activation. Up to now, at least nine cases with eculizumab exposure throughout pregnancy because of PNH have been published, in which the children were healthy (e.g. Danilov 2010, Kelly 2010, Marasca 2010). Eculizumab has also been approved for atypical hemolytic-uremic syndrome. One pregnancy with successful therapy beginning in week 26 and delivery of a full-term healthy baby has been reported (Ardissino 2013). There is an anecdotal report about therapy of preeclampsia with eculizumab. Trace levels of eculizumab were found in the cord blood samples (Burwick 2013).

Golimumab is an IgG1-antibody and TNF-α-blocker with a terminal half-life of 12 ± 3 days, which can be used together with methotrexate for rheumatoid arthritis, psoriasis-arthritis or Bechterew's disease after failure of the usual immunosuppressants. There are no human data on its use during pregnancy. Experiments with macaque monkeys suggest high placental transfer in later pregnancy (Arsenescu 2011).

Inolimomab is an anti-interleukin-2 receptor monoclonal antibody for corticosteroid-refractory acute graft-versus-host disease. There are no human data on its use in pregnancy.

Muromonab-CD3 is used for treatment of acute rejection reactions after organ transplants. There is no experience during pregnancy.

Ranibizumab, approved for neovascular eye diseases and diabetic macular edema, is the fragment of a Mab and, thereby, has a molecular weight of only 48,000 Da. The maximum serum concentrations after intravitreal injections, reported by the manufacturer lie between 0.79 and 2.90 ng/mL. There is one case report with a successful therapy in the third trimester of pregnancy and a healthy child (Sarhianaki 2012). For drugs in ophthalmology, see also Chapter 2.17.

Rilonacept, a fusion protein, which binds to IL-1 β and thus blocks its action, has been approved as an orphan drug for the treatment of CAPS since 2011 by the FDA. There is no experience on its use in pregnancy.

Tocilizumab, an IL-6-receptor antibody, has been available since 2010 for treatment of moderately severe (juvenile) rheumatoid arthritis. Experience of its use in pregnancy is limited to 31 pregnancies reported in an abstract (Rubbert-Roth 2010). Outcomes included 13 elective terminations, seven spontaneous abortions and 11 live-born infants, of which 10 were healthy. One died shortly postpartum from complications following placenta previa.

Ustekinumab is an IL-12 and IL-23 inhibitor, which is approved for moderate to severe plaque psoriasis for patients with failed other immunosuppressive therapy. Across clinical studies, about 26 pregnancies with early pregnancy exposure and known outcomes have been recognized from which no specific risk can be drawn so far (Fotiadou 2012). Independently, one spontaneous abortion (Fotiadou 2012) and one healthy full-term infant (Andrulonis 2012) have been reported.

2.12.4   Multiple sclerosis

Multiple sclerosis is an autoimmune disease of the central nervous system. The clinical course, severity, disability and symptoms vary from patient to patient. Multiple sclerosis typically presents in women between the ages of 20 and 40 years, which means that they are often affected in their reproductive age. The three major forms are relapsing remitting multiple sclerosis, which represents the most frequent form (85%) at disease onset, the primary progressive multiple sclerosis and the secondary progressive form. The higher objectives of treating multiple sclerosis are to prevent relapses and delay disability progression; however, treating relapses and improving multiple sclerosis-related symptoms such as depression and bladder disturbances are other indications for a medicinal drug treatment.

Relapse therapy is carried out with a cortisone preparation, mostly prednisone/prednisolone or *methylprednisolone* (Chapter 2.15) administered IV over 3 to 5 days. *Plasmapheresis* is considered as an individual treatment decision in patients with severe and otherwise not properly responding relapses. The disease-modifying drugs are intended to minimize the severity and frequency of the relapses as well as the extent of the disability progression.

According to neurological recommendations for nonpregnant patients (Wiendl 2008), first line treatments for relapsing remitting multiple sclerosis are the disease-modifying drugs *interferon β-1a*, *interferon β-1b* (Section 2.12.5) and *glatiramer acetate* (Section 2.12.6). Azathioprine (AZA) (Section 2.12.1) seems to be less efficient than the other disease-modifying drugs. The monoclonal antibody *natalizumab* (Section 2.12.3) has shown promising results, but may have serious adverse effects such as progressive multifocal leukoencephalopathy or liver injury. Therefore, it should only be considered for escalation therapy. The latter also refers to the cancer drugs *mitoxantrone* (Chapter 2.13) and *cyclophosphamide* (Chapter 2.13). Intravenous *immunoglobulins* are considered reserve drugs in the majority of countries.

Some new oral drugs have recently been marketed: *Fingolimod* reduces the relapse rate under certain circumstances slightly better compared to interferon β-1a, but not the disability progression (AkdÄ 2011). Severe side-effects might further limit its use, among others deadly infections, brady-cardia and atrioventricular block. Fingolimod is a sphingosine 1-phosphate receptor modulator that prevents lymphocytes from leaving lymph nodes and entering the peripheral bloodstream (Lu 2014a). The FDA has approved *dimethyl fumarate* (Chapter 2.7) for relapse reduction in multiple sclerosis in 2013; however, results on disability progression have been inconsistent. This drug has been on the market for psoriasis in some countries. The mode of action in multiple sclerosis has not been clearly determined as yet. The newly marketed *teriflunomide*, a metabolite of *leflunomide* (Section 2.12.8), is a selective immunosuppressant with anti-inflammatory properties.

The immunosuppressive monoclonal antibody *alemtuzumab* (Section 2.12.3) formerly approved for chronic lymphocytic leukemia (Chapter 2.13) was withdrawn by the marketing authorization holder for commer-cial reasons, after it had been shown to be effective in relapsing remitting multiple sclerosis and relaunched with a lower dose suitable for multiple sclerosis therapy at higher prices.

There are some immunosuppressive drugs licensed for other diseases which are occasionally used in the treatment of multiple sclerosis such as *rituximab* (Chapter 2.13) and *mycophenolate* (Section 2.12.2). *Laqui-nimod*, which belongs to the quinolones, has shown low-level evidence for use as a disease-modifying therapy for multiple sclerosis as yet (He 2013). *Laquinimod* is currently being assessed for licensing by the EMA. As *statins* (Chapter 2.5) have anti-inflammatory and immunomodulatory properties in addition to lipid-lowering effects, they have been tested in the treatment of multiple sclerosis as well. However, there is no convinc-ing evidence to support the addition of statins to interferon therapy in multiple sclerosis (e.g. Kamm 2012).

Fampridine or *dalfampridine* are orally available potassium blockers and approved to improve walking range, although there is still uncer-tainty concerning its lasting effectiveness. *Nabiximols (Tetrahydrocan-nabinol/Cannabidiol)* is used for the reduction of spasticity in multiple sclerosis.

Cladribine (Chapter 2.13), licensed for hairy cell leukemia was not approved for multiple sclerosis by the FDA. *Ocrelizumab, pegylated interferon β-1a*, and *daclizumab* are currently in phase 3 trials.

▶ Pregnancy and multiple sclerosis

In general, there is nothing that argues against pregnancy in a woman with multiple sclerosis. Pregnancy complications in women with mul-tiple sclerosis do not seem to be more frequent in comparison with the general population (e.g. Jalkanen 2010). In advanced pregnancy, above all, in the last trimester, the relapse rate declines considerably. Different explanations for this phenomenon have been discussed. Recent research suggests that not only endogenous changes of the maternal immune system during pregnancy are responsible, but also fetal antigens which directly interact with the maternal immune system (Patas 2013). In the first 3 months postpartum relapses occur more frequently. Most studies found this independent of whether the mother breastfeeds or not. How-ever, in one small study (Hellwig 2012), after exclusive breastfeeding some beneficial effects on postpartum relapse rate were observed. Only after 6 months does the risk of relapse again corresponds to that before pregnancy. A relapse can be treated as usual at all stages of the pregnancy, and also while breastfeeding, with high doses of methylprednisolone/ prednisolone.

▶ **Prenatal toxicity of multiple sclerosis medication**

The disease modifying medications of choice consist of *interferon-β* (Section 2.12.5) and *glatiramer acetate* (Section 2.12.6). There is sufficient experience with continuous *azathioprine* (Section 2.12.1) treatment from other diseases. Also, after treatment with *immunoglobulins*, no negative effects have been observed up to now. The use of other basic therapeutics should, however, be very carefully weighed. *Mycophenolate* (Section 2.12.2) has proven to be teratogenic in humans, and should best be avoided in women of reproductive age if possible. It is recommended to change therapy with *cyclophosphamide* (Chapter 2.13) and *mitoxantrone* (Chapter 2.13) prior to conception. For more details on these drugs see the corresponding chapters.

The manufacturer reported on 69 pregnancies with known outcomes after maternal *fingolimod* treatment. In eight of these pregnancies, fingolimod was discontinued at least 6 weeks before conception, resulting in seven healthy children and one pregnancy which was electively terminated. The outcome of the remainder was 28 live births, nine spontaneous abortions and 24 elective abortions, on which there were no details except for one with a Tetralogy of Fallot. In two of the newborns malformations were observed, a unilateral bowing of the tibia and an acrania (Karlsson 2014). Data are too sparse for a well-grounded risk assessment. However, these results together with the findings from animal experience, suggest teratogenicity and the long half-life warrant caution. Medication should best be avoided during pregnancy.

From clinical studies pregnancy outcomes for 25 *dimethyl fumarate* recipients are available resulting in 15 healthy live births, three spontaneous abortions and seven elective terminations (Gold 2013).

There is no experience on use in pregnancy for *teriflunomide, laquinimod*, and *fampridine/dalfampridine*.

For all other drugs see the corresponding chapters as cited above.

Paternal exposure: A study examining birth outcomes of pregnancies fathered by men with multiple sclerosis did not find an association between paternal multiple sclerosis and multiple sclerosis-related clinical factors with birth outcomes (Lu 2014b).

> **Recommendation.** A decision concerning continuing disease-modifying therapy during pregnancy should be undertaken jointly between neurologists and obstetricians. As the disease activity of multiple sclerosis often declines during the second and third trimester, it might be possible to pause treatment with DMD. After delivery it is mostly recommended to start therapy with disease-modifying drugs right away. The disease-modifying drugs of choice are interferons β and glatiramer. A relapse can be treated at all stages of the pregnancy with the usual high doses of methylprednisolone/prednisolone.

2.12.5   Interferons

Interferons (IFN) are naturally occurring protein-like macromolecules with antiviral activity. They are present in all tissues, even in the embryo and fetus. Four classes of interferons, α, β, γ und τ are distinguished. IFN-α is important for the physiological maintenance of the pregnancy. IFN-α and -γ are of significance for ovarian function. The role of interferons in cell growth and differentiation is not yet clear. Most of the interferons on the market today are produced with gene technology.

Some of the side-effects of interferon therapy can be fever, leukopenia, hypotension, fatigue and anorexia. It is conceivable that a fever could lead to undesirable fetal side-effects. With almost all of the preparations produced with gene technology, an increased absorption rate (abortion rate) has been observed in animal experiments using doses many times higher than the human therapeutic dose.

▶ Interferon-α and peginterferon-α

Interferon-α_{2a} and *interferon-α_{2b}* are used for chronic hepatitis B or C and some malignant diseases, and have a half-life of 4 to 7 hours. With pegylated IFN-α, this is a conjugate of IFN-α with polyethylene glycol, from which a longer half-life of 50–130 hours with *peginterferon-α_{2a}*, and 30.7 hours with *peginterferon-α_{2b}* result. The first is indicated for hepatitis C or B, the latter only for hepatitis C. Treatment for hepatitis C can be given as monotherapy or together with ribavirin (Chapter 2.6). *Interferon-α_{n3}* is used for the treatment of genital warts (Chapter 2.17).

Most of the available experience on IFN-α therapy during pregnancy is on essential thrombocythemia (ET) and, in addition, chronic myeloid leukemia as well as other hematological diseases. Complications of ET include a high risk for spontaneous abortion and thrombohemorrhagic events. Melillo (2009) found a higher live birth rate among pregnant women with ET on IFN therapy than on low-dose ASS therapy (Chapter 2.1). Tefferi and Passamonti (2009) considered IFN-α as first choice therapy during pregnancy to be justified only for high risk patients (for therapy of ET see also hydroxyurea and anagrelide (Chapter 2.13). In more than 50 case reports on the use of IFN-α for ET (e.g. review by Yazdani 2012), at least eight on hepatitis C (e.g. Seror 2009), around 15 on chronic myeloid leukemia (e.g. Regierer 2006, Mubarak 2002) and some with additional indications, have shown no teratogenic or fetotoxic effects with mostly continuous therapy. The complications observed were mostly caused by the underlying maternal disease.

No specific malformation risk from pegylated interferons has been described up to now.

Recommendation. Interferons-α and peginterferons-α may be used in all phases of pregnancy for appropriate indications after a benefit-risk assessment. A detailed ultrasound examination may be offered after exposure in the first trimester to confirm normal fetal development.

▶ Interferon-β

Human *interferon-β* can be used for severe, uncontrollable viral illnesses. Although concrete experience during pregnancy is limited, the assumption is that there is no teratogenic risk, due to the high molecular weight and the good experience with other interferons.

Interferon-β_{1a} (preparation for i.m. and s.c. applications available) and *interferon-β_{1b}* (s.c.) are approved for relapsing forms of multiple sclerosis. Results of some 250 prospectively recorded pregnancies from case series and smaller studies (e.g. review by Lu 2012b), as well as an analysis of 425 prospectively recorded pregnancies with s.c. IFN-β_{1a} exposure from the database of Merck Serono (Sandberg-Wollheim 2011) have been published. Likewise, no increased risks were recorded in the company registry on i.m. interferon-β_{1a} based on 302 exposed pregnancies (Tomczyk 2012). The quality of the publications is quite variable (Lu 2012a, 2012b, Auyeung-Kim 2009). For instance, in the study from Merck Serono, information on the exposure time is available only for 187/425 pregnancies. Summing up, no teratogenic risk and no increased risk of spontaneous abortion can be deduced from the studies so far.

On several occasions, a lower mean birth weight in comparison to control groups was described. This has been discussed as an effect of the disease, particularly of the disease activity. However, some authors attribute this to the IFN-β medication. The experience mostly refers to pregnant women with exposure during the first trimester.

> **Recommendation.** Interferon-β_{1a} and interferon-β_{1b} may be administered before and during pregnancy. Since the disease activity of multiple sclerosis declines over the course of the pregnancy, especially in the third trimester, interrupting treatment might be warranted. If continuous therapy is necessary, it is acceptable throughout pregnancy. A detailed ultrasound examination may be offered after exposure in the first trimester to confirm normal fetal development.

▶ Interferon-γ

Interferon-γ_{1b} is used to reduce infection in patients with septic granulomatosis and with marble bone disease. In animal experiments, an increased rate of abortion (monkeys) at approximately 100 times the human dose was described (manufacturer's package leaflet information for Imukin®). We are unaware of any published experience on its use in humans during pregnancy.

2.12.6   Other immunostimulatory drugs

▶ Glatiramer

Glatiramer acetate (GA) is used for treatment of relapsing remitting multiple sclerosis. It is also approved for patients with a clinically isolated multiple sclerosis-typical syndrome, where a first attack has not yet been confirmed as multiple sclerosis.

It consists of synthetic polypeptides, which contain the four naturally occurring amino acids glutamine acid, lysine, alanine and tyrosine. Within the subcutaneous tissue, the major part of a dosage is rapidly split into smaller fragments. Therefore, administration has to be strictly subcutaneous. The way it works is not yet fully understood.

According to the manufacturer's information (Teva Pharmaceutical Industries, Ltd, Petah Tikva, Israel), experimental animal studies with rats and rabbits using 18- to 36-fold human therapeutic doses did not reveal negative effects on prenatal growth. Thirty pregnancies were registered during the trial phase and 215 after marketing approval. Thereby, no particular fetal risks have been reported (Coyle 2003).

Studies and case series of different quality have analyzed approximately 100 pregnancies on GA with mostly favorable outcomes (overview by Lu 2012b). A minority of the women were treated throughout pregnancy.

One of the studies, a prospective cohort study, reported on 31 fetuses – the majority of them exposed in the first trimester – among which there were two with malformations (AV-canal, club foot) (Weber-Schoendorfer 2009). No malformations were reported in another prospective study based on 16 live-born infants with intrauterine GA exposure (Giannini 2012), and in an observational retrospective cohort study among others, including seven GA-exposed pregnancies (Lu 2012a).

> **Recommendation.** Glatiramer does not need to be stopped when planning a pregnancy. If it seems advisable not to interrupt treatment due to the individual course of the disease, continuing the therapy during the pregnancy seems acceptable. Detailed ultrasound examination should be offered to confirm the normal development of the fetus.

▶ Granulocyte colony-stimulating factor (G-CSF)

Granulocyte colony-stimulating factor (G-CSF) is normally present during pregnancy. Recombinant G-CSFs are, for example, *filgrastim*, *lenograstim*, *nartograstim* and *pegfilgrastim*. There are data indicating transplacental transfer of, for example, filgastrim. There are different treatment indications for G-CSF. It can be given to enhance the number and function of mature neutrophils in neutropenic patients. It has been administered in order to stimulate neonatal granulopoiesis. Some studies indicate that G-CSF is a promising treatment in women with unexplained recurrent miscarriage. Furthermore, it is an accompanying therapy in patients with hematological malignancies receiving chemotherapy. Preparation for hematopoietic stem cell donation is another treatment indication. The experiences of more than 150 exposed pregnancies have not shown an increased risk, neither for the pregnant mother nor for the fetus. However, experience during the first trimester is still limited (review by Pessach 2013).

> **Recommendation.** For relevant treatment indications, G-CSF, e.g. filgrastim, as the best studied drug of this group, can be administered during pregnancy.

▶ Further immunostimulants

Plerixafor is used (together with G-CSF) for an improved mobilization of hematopoietic stem cells in peripheral blood as preparation for an autolog stem cell transplantation. According to the manufacturer, in animal experiments a teratogenic potential was determined. There is no experience on its use in pregnant patients. *Palivizumab* is a monoclonal antibody, which is used for the prevention of severe respiratory syncytial virus (RSV) illnesses in premature infants.

See also Chapter 2.13 for immunostimulatory drugs used in cancer therapy such as BCG immunotherapy; Chapter 2.19 for herbal immunostimulants such as *Echinacea purpurea* and Chapter 2.17 for substances used in dermatology such as *imiquimode*.

Pregnancy

2.12 Immunosuppression, rheumatic diseases, multiple sclerosis, and Wilson's disease

> **Recommendation.** Plerixafor should not be used during pregnancy, if possible. An incidental exposure during pregnancy does not, however, justify a risk-grounded termination, but a detailed ultrasound examination should be carried out (Chapter 1.15).

2.12.7   Transplantation

Pregnancies in organ transplant patients are relatively common. However, obstetric complications occur more frequently than in pregnancies of the general population. Even if most of the transplant recipients' pregnancies are successful, a higher proportion of preeclampsia, hypertension, low-birth weight babies, C-sections and preterm deliveries has been observed. A higher spontaneous abortion rate is inconsistently described. Interestingly, the increased risk for preeclampsia already existed in pregnancies during the years before transplantation. Complication rates seem to depend on the kind of organ transplant, the time difference between transplantation and conception, the underlying disease and overall, the stability of the graft (e.g. Blume 2013, Brosens 2013, Kim 2008).

A lot of medicinal drugs are available for the prophylaxis of organ transplant rejection: *azathioprine* (Section 2.12.1), *cyclosporine* (Section 2.12.2), and the teratogenic *mycophenolate, everolimus, tacrolimus* and *sirolimus* (Section 2.12.2), *basiliximab* and *belatacept* (Section 2.12.3), and *corticoids* (Chapter 2.15). *Muromonab-CD3* (OKT3) (Section 2.12.3) is indicated for acute rejection reaction, as are *antithymocyte globulins*.

Azathioprine and cyclosporine are the best studied for use in pregnancy. Mycophenolate should be avoided in pregnancy, if possible. There is no experience in pregnancy with *gusperimus*, a guanidine derivate, and with *mizoribine*, both used in the treatment of renal graft rejection. The latter is also licensed for glomerulonephritis, lupus nephritis and rheumatoid arthritis. For details regarding the use of the other drugs in pregnancy see the corresponding chapters.

Paternal exposure: The course and outcome of almost 800 pregnancies fathered by solid-organ transplant recipients is comparable to the normal population, according to the data of the American Pregnancy Registry (Coscia 2009). A Chinese working group also describes no increased malformation risk in the offspring of more than 200 male renal transplant recipients (Xu 2008).

> **Recommendation.** As stability of the graft is most important for an uncomplicated and successful pregnancy, medication for prophylaxis of transplant rejection should usually not be changed *during* a pregnancy.

2.12.8   Drugs for rheumatic diseases

The range of rheumatic diseases is varied and includes (mentioning just some important ones that frequently occur in younger women): rheumatoid arthritis, ankylosing spondylitis, SLE, psoriasis-arthritis and vasculitis. The basic pharmacological therapy for rheumatic diseases involves the use of so-called disease modifying antirheumatic drugs (DMARD) or basic therapeutics. Among the conventional DMARDs are the long-used substances, *sulfasalazine, chloroquine* or *hydroxychloroquine, methotrexate* (MTX) in low doses, *leflunomide* (Section 2.12.8), as well as *cyclophosphamide* (Chapter 2.13) for highly active inflammatory processes. *Gold* preparations and *D-penicillamine* (Section 2.12.9) have declined in significance. *Azathioprine* (Section 2.12.1) and *cyclosporine* (Section 2.12.2) are only used occasionally.

In patients with rheumatoid arthritis failing to respond to the conventional synthetic DMARDs or when poor prognostic factors are present, therapy with biological DMARDs should be started. In this instance, TNF-α-blockers *adalimumab, etanercept* and *infliximab* (Section 2.12.3) should be mentioned. As further biologics for the therapy of rheumatic diseases, the monoclonal antibodies *certolizumab pegol, golimumab, tocilizumab* (Section 2.12.3), and *rituximab* (Chapter 2.13) can be considered as well as *abatacept* and *anakinra* (Section 2.12.3). *Tofacitinib* for therapy of rheumatoid arthritis has recently been approved by the FDA as well as in Japan and Russia, but not as yet by the EMA. The Task Force of The European League Against Rheumatism (EULAR) is convinced of its efficacy, and recommends it after one or two biological treatments have failed (EULAR: The European League Against Rheumatism, 2013). There is no human data on the use of the tyrosinkinase inhibitor tofacitinib during pregnancy. The teratogenic *mycophenolate* (Section 2.12.2) is also used for some rheumatic diseases.

Rapidly acting inflammation inhibitors are non-steroidal antirheumatics (NSAR) or COX-2 inhibitors (Chapter 2.1) as well as glucocorticoids (Chapter 2.15), which are often prescribed in combination with DMARDs, especially at the beginning of therapy.

Since some rheumatic diseases, e.g. SLE or an antiphospholipid syndrome, can pose particular risks for a pregnancy, caring for a pregnant woman should be undertaken jointly between rheumatology and gynecology centers. With *SLE*, among other matters, such as maternal involvement of the kidney, it must be clarified whether and how frequently fetal echocardiography should be carried out – especially when anti-SSA/Ro and SSB/La antibodies (with or without SLE) are present. The aim is to diagnose cardiac conduction disorders at an early stage in order to prevent the development of a heart block or to better handle their complications.

▶ Sulfasalazine

Sulfasalazine or *salazosulfapyridine* is a poorly absorbed sulfonamide that is metabolized in the intestine to sulfapyridine and *5-aminosalicylic acid (5-ASA)*. Most of the experience with this drug during pregnancy is in connection with the treatment of inflammatory bowel diseases (Chapter 2.5). A meta-analysis of seven studies (Rahimi 2008) found no statistically significant risk of malformations among 642 pregnancies exposed to ASA-substances, in comparison to a control group with 1,158 pregnant women. Furthermore, a study by Viktil (2012) with antirheumatic drugs in pregnancy did not find an increased adverse outcome after sulfasalazine exposure. A Swedish study on the use of 5-ASA drugs in early pregnancy analyzed an increased risk for cardiovascular defects, mainly septal heart defects. Results were also statistically significant for the 1,342 sulfasalazine exposed pregnancies (OR 1.68; 95% CI 1.13–2.50) (Kallen 2014). However, the study has several methodological shortcomings, such as multiple testing among others. A recent study from UK included 551 women with 5-ASA exposure during the first trimester, which neither found an overall increased malformation risk, nor an increased risk for heart defects (adjusted OR 0.66; 95% CI 0.18–2.48) (Ban 2014).

Paternal exposure: Sulfasalazine can lead to a reversible reduction of the number and motility of the sperm (e.g. Toovey 1981, Toth 1979).

Recommendation. Sulfasalazine may be used in all phases of pregnancy.

▶ Low dose methotrexate (MTX)

Outside of pregnancy, low-dose *methotrexate* (*MTX*) is a first line therapeutic for rheumatoid arthritis (EULAR: The European League Against Rheumatism, 2013), and is also used for a variety of other autoimmune or inflammatory diseases. MTX, as a folic acid analog, belongs to the anti-metabolites. It competitively inhibits the enzyme dihydrofolate reductase and has a half-life of 12 to 24 hours. About 5 to 35% of the substance is stored for many months in the liver cells and erythrocytes as a polygluta-mate derivative. The therapeutic dosage in low-dose therapy is between 7.5 and 25 mg/weekly. MTX is also used for malignancies, non-surgical treatment of ectopic pregnancy, and elective termination of pregnancy – however, in other dosages Chapter 2.13).

MTX is a teratogen with a (variable) pattern of malformations. The typical pattern of anomalies consists of skull, limb and other skeletal defects, some minor craniofacial abnormalities and growth restriction (Feldkamp 1993). Holoprosencephaly and malformations of the urogenital tract (e.g. Corona-Rivera 2010) as well as cardiac defects (Piggott 2011) have been discussed as possible expansions of the phenotype.

Most MTX embryopathies have been observed after a failed attempt of termination (with or without *misoprostol*) (Chapter 2.13). Among published case reports involving at least 38 MTX-exposed fetuses/infants with birth defects, two infants were described with an MTX phenotype after a typical low-dose therapy (Martin 2013, Buckley 1997). However, in the study by Martin, a genetic syndrome was not thoroughly ruled out. By contrast, there are case reports (e.g. Angelucci 2010, Ostensen 2000) and case series with healthy children (e.g. Chakravarty 2003). A prospective French study reported on 28 low-dose MTX-exposed pregnancies including 19 live births without major birth defects (Lewden 2004).

In an international prospective observational cohort study, 188 post-conception and 136 pre-conception MTX-exposed pregnancies were compared with a disease-matched and a non-autoimmune group. In the post-conception cohort, the cumulative incidence of spontaneous abortion was 42.5% – exceeding both comparison groups. Furthermore, there was an elevated risk for major birth defects of 6.6%, but none of the malformations was consistent with the typical MTX-embryopathy. No adverse effects were noted in the pre-conception cohort (Weber-Schoendorfer 2014). According to international recommendations low-dose MTX therapy should be discontinued at least 3 months before conception (Visser 2009). The results of the study do not confirm the necessity of this advice.

Paternal exposure: An evaluation of about 20 pregnancies and a case series with 42 pregnancies fathered by men on MTX, showed an overall favorable outcome (Beghin 2011). This was confirmed by the results of a prospective cohort study, involving 113 pregnancies fathered by men who were treated with low-dose MTX around conception or longer. Neither the spontaneous abortion risk, nor the rate of major birth defects, or the gestational age at delivery and birth weights differed between the exposed and controls (Weber-Schoendorfer 2013).

Recommendation. MTX is a teratogen which should not be used during pregnancy. However, the specific MTX embryopathy, which has been linked to higher dosages, has only rarely been observed after maternal low-dose treatment. Adverse pregnancy outcomes seem to be dose and exposure time dependent. Inadvertent low-dose MTX exposure during early pregnancy was shown to increase the spontaneous abortion rate and also slightly, the rate of major birth defects. This does not justify a risk-grounded termination of pregnancy (Chapter 1.15), but the treatment should be stopped immediately and a level II ultrasound should be offered to examine fetal development. A 3-month MTX free interval prior to conception may not be necessary after paternal treatment. In cases of inevitable paternal MTX therapy it seems tolerable not to postpone family planning.

▶ Chloroquine and hydroxychloroquine

Hydroxychloroquine and *chloroquine* are given, for instance for SLE. Both belong to the group of 4-aminochinolines and have similar pharmacological characteristics, whereby, hydroxychloroquine is somewhat more potent, so that 400 mg of hydroxychloroquine sulfate approximately corresponds to 500 mg of chloroquine phosphate. Both substances cross the placenta (Law 2008). For chloroquine and malaria, see Chapter 2.6.

Among the children of more than 600 pregnant women with rheumatic diseases, who were recorded in various studies and case series (Cooper 2014, Diav-Citrin 2013, Costedoat-Chalumeau 2003), and who were mostly exposed to hydroxychloroquine, no appreciably elevated risk of malformations was observed. In one of these studies, among the 117 children exposed *in utero*, neither visual, acoustic, nor other developmental deficits were found at the age of 2 (Costedoat-Chalumeau 2003). The authors explored this question to scrutinize the applicability of animal experimental results and the causal connection between one case description (Hart 1964), and chloroquine intake. In this publication, seven pregnancies of a mother with SLE were described, of which three healthy children were not exposed *in utero* to chloroquine. One exposed pregnancy ended in a spontaneous abortion. Of the three exposed live-born children, one had a Wilms tumor which was surgically removed at the age of four, and the other two showed a severe cochleovestibular paresis.

Since ocular side-effects, among them retinopathies and corneal changes, are known side-effects of chloroquine/hydroxychloroquine therapy, some studies have pursued the question of whether these side-effects also occur in children after intrauterine exposure. Klinger (2001) examined 21 children ophthalmologically, and Cimaz (2004) examined six children by funduscopy and electroretinogram. Both found no anomalies. Renault (2009) carried out an electroretinogram with 21 children exposed prenatally and tested the visually evoked potentials. In six of the children – among them three preterm infants – pathological results were found. Their comparison group was comprised of historic control children from 1996. Their method was rightly criticized (Ingster-Moati 2010).

Occasionally, an increased rate of spontaneous abortion, a higher rate of preterm deliveries and lower birth weights have been reported with antirheumatic chloroquine/hydroxychloroquine therapy. However, this seems to be attributable to the mother's underlying disease. For this and other reasons, most authors expressly recommend continuation of the therapy for SLE during the entire pregnancy, because the risk of an exacerbation of the disease with consequences for the mother, the pregnancy and the fetus, is greater than the residual risk from the maternal

Pregnancy

2.12 Immunosuppression, rheumatic diseases, multiple sclerosis, and Wilson's disease

medication. In a case-control study, Izmirly (2010) compared 50 newborns with neonatal lupus with 151 control children with respect to the frequency of maternal hydroxychloroquine medication during pregnancy. The mothers in both groups had anti-SSA/Ro- and SSB/La-antibodies. Significantly more healthy children were exposed *in utero* to hydroxychloroquine ($p = 0.002$; OR 0.28; 95%-CI 0.12 to 0.63).

> **Recommendation.** An antirheumatic therapy with hydroxychloroquine or chloroquine can be continued, or even begun during pregnancy. Following use in the first trimester, a detailed ultrasound examination may be offered. Up to now, there are no sufficient grounds for routine ophthalmological examination in the first or second year of life after continuous intrauterine hydroxychloroquine/chloroquine exposure.

▶ Leflunomide

Leflunomide is approved for treatment of rheumatoid arthritis and in some countries also for psoriasis-arthritis. It is a pyrimidine synthesis inhibitor, which is quickly metabolized into an active component. In humans, this inhibits the enzyme dihydroorotate dehydrogenease, whereby there is a reduced proliferation of autoimmune active T-lymphocytes. The half-life is 2 weeks.

In animal experiments, leflunomide was teratogenic in serum concentrations, which correspond to the therapeutic values in humans. Skeletal malformations, anophthalmia or microphthalmia and hydrocephalus have been described. However, at these serum concentrations maternal toxicity appeared, so that the teratogenic character of the damage has been discussed controversially. The drug safety information leaflet specifies a concentration of <0.02 mg/l as safe, which is more than 100-fold lower than the blood concentrations which are characterized in rats and rabbits as "no-effect level", meaning that this implies a wide safety range. Because of the warnings in the package leaflet, many pregnant women terminate the pregnancy.

The experience in humans rests on case reports or case series (e.g. Heine 2008, De Santis 2005), on data from the company registries and two North American prospective studies with 45 and 64 exposed pregnant women, respectively (Cassina 2012, Chambers 2010). However, neither a significant increase in the frequency of malformations, nor a distinct pattern of malformations has been shown in the live-born children. The malformation rate in the study by Chambers (2010), in which >95% of pregnant women had received a "washing out" therapy with colestyramine, was also not significantly higher than in the two comparison groups (pregnant women with rheumatoid arthritis, but without leflunomide and healthy pregnant women). There are only few case reports with an unfavorable outcome (e.g. Neville 2007). In the latter, causality is debatable.

> **Recommendation.** Up to now, there is no support for the teratogenicity of leflunomide in humans. Due to the still limited experience, leflunomide should not be used during pregnancy. However, incidental intake in early pregnancy does not justify a risk-grounded termination of the pregnancy (Chapter 1.15). Nevertheless, the therapy should be changed and a "wash-out" therapy with *colestyramine* or *activated charcoal* should be carried out as recommended by the manufacturer. It is advisable to determine the concentration of the substance before and after the "wash out" procedure, and to carry out a detailed ultrasound examination.

▶ Gold preparations

Gold preparations such as *sodium aurothiomalate* (gold sodium thiomalate) with a half-life of 225 to 250 days are old basic therapeutics, which are used primarily with rheumatoid arthritis. In humans, in contrast to animal experiments, no teratogenic potential has been discovered. The placental transfer of gold compounds into the fetal liver and kidneys is documented. Case reports and case collections, among them, on 119 pregnant women treated with gold in the first trimester and, to some extent, beyond that because of bronchial asthma (in Japan), showed no increased risks for fetal malformations or other adverse effects in the newborn (Miyamoto 1974).

> **Recommendation.** Although teratogenicity is not suspected as yet, experience with gold compounds during pregnancy is still insufficient. Gold therapy seems acceptable during pregnancy; however, a detailed ultrasound examination should be offered to confirm the normal development of the fetus.

2.12.9   Drugs for Wilson's disease

Wilson's disease is an autosomal-recessive disturbance of the hepatic copper metabolism, which leads to a toxic accumulation of copper, primarily in the liver and the brain. Once the diagnosis has been made, treatment needs to be life-long, including a pregnancy and the lactation period. The European Association for the Study of the Liver stated, "There is a lack of high-quality evidence to estimate the relative treatment effects of the available drugs in Wilson's disease" (European Association for the Study of the Liver 2012). The main available drugs are *D-penicillamine, trientine, zinc, tetrathiomolybdate* and *dimercaprol* (synonyms: *2,3-dimercaptopropanol* or *British Anti-Lewisite*). The latter is considered to be obsolete. The current standard therapy consists of either one of the two chelating agents D-penicillamine and trientine, or of zinc for maintenance treatment whereas tetrathiomolybdate remains an experimental therapy. Controlled studies on the effectiveness of Vitamin E as an adjunct are lacking to date (European Association for the Study of the Liver 2012).

▶ D-Penicillamine

The chelating agent *D-penicillamine* is currrently mainly used in Wilson's disease by promoting the urinary excretion of copper. In addition, D-penicillamine has some antiphlogistic characteristics and induces metallothionein. Due to its effect as a pyridoxine antimetabolite, supplemental pyridoxine should be provided (European Association for the Study of the Liver 2012).

Six cases with congenital cutis laxa partly combined with inguinal hernias and with other serious malformations have been published (Pinter 2004, Rosa 1986). Maternal drug treatment indication varied from cystinuria to rheumatoid arthritis and Wilson's disease. A cleft lip and palate, also observed with high doses in animal experiments, was observed in one case report (Martinez-Frias 1998). Among other

Pregnancy

2.12 Immunosuppression, rheumatic diseases, multiple sclerosis, and Wilson's disease

possibilities, a zinc deficiency caused by penicillamine as the cause of the malformations has been discussed. A case report from Israel (Hanukoglu 2008) describes transient, hypothyroid struma (goiter) in two siblings whose mother had taken penicillamine for Wilson's disease during both pregnancies. Subclinical hypothyroidism has also been found among children with Wilson's disease who had been treated with penicillamine.

By contrast, there are more than 150 published, mostly unremarkable, courses of pregnancy (e.g. European Association for the Study of the Liver 2012, Sinha 2004).

Summarizing the experience to date, there is at most only a minimal teratogenic risk to humans.

▶ Trientine

Trientine (triethylene tetramine dihydrochloride or trien) was introduced in 1969. It not only acts as a chelating agent and promotes urinary copper excretion, but also inhibits intestinal copper absorption through metallothionein induction. Trientine is an effective treatment for Wilson's disease. It is mostly prescribed in patients who are intolerant of penicillamine (European Association for the Study of the Liver 2012).

Among more than 20 pregnancies with trientine treatment, there was no indication of specific anomalies in the mothers or the newborns (author's own observations 2013, Devesa 1995, Walshe 1986). A mild iron deficiency is frequently observed as a side-effect of treatment.

▶ Zinc salts

Zinc preparations with sufficiently high zinc content inhibit intestinal copper absorption and induce enterocyte metallothionein. Zinc is ideal as a maintenance therapy for a decopperized patient. As an initial therapy, it is considered primarily for asymptomatic patients. It may also be considered as first-line therapy in neurological patients (European Association for the Study of the Liver 2012).

A small prospective study evaluated 26 pregnancies with continuous zinc therapy for Wilson's disease. Among the 26 live-born children, one had a heart malformation and another microcephaly. A teratogenic effect cannot be deduced from this (Brewer 2000). Malik reported on four successful pregnancies with healthy babies after intrauterine zinc exposure (Malik 2013).

> **Recommendation.** The copper status should be optimized prior to pregnancy. Treatment needs to be continued during pregnancy and lactation. Depending on the copper status, all three agents seem to be acceptable during pregnancy. With penicillamine the benefits of continuation outweigh the potential minimal elevated malformation risk. A control of the neonate's thyroid status may be recommended after long-term exposure with penicillamine. When planning a pregnancy and if clinically possible, zinc is the preferred treatment option. In any case, a detailed ultrasound examination should be offered to confirm the normal development of the fetus.

References

Akbari M, Shah S, Velayos FS et al. Systematic review and meta-analysis on the effects of thiopurines on birth outcomes from female and male patients with inflammatory bowel disease. Inflamm. Bowel Dis 2013; 19: 15–22.

AkdÄ (2011). Gilenya (Fingolimod). www.akdae.de/Arzneimitteltherapie/NA/ Archiv/2011021-Gilenya.pdf (accessed 12-9-2013).

Alsuwaida A. Successful management of systemic lupus erythematosus nephritis flare-up during pregnancy with tacrolimus. Mod Rheumatol 2011; 21: 73–5.

Anderka MT, Lin AE, Abuelo DN et al. Reviewing the evidence for mycophenolate mofetil as a new teratogen: case report and review of the literature. Am J Med Genet A 2009; 149A: 1241–8.

Andrulonis R, Ferris LK. Treatment of severe psoriasis with ustekinumab during pregnancy. J Drugs Dermatol 2012; 11: 1240.

Angelucci E, Cesarini M, Vernia P. Inadvertent conception during concomitant treatment with infliximab and methotrexate in a patient with Crohn's disease: is the game worth the candle? Inflamm Bowel Dis 2010; 16: 1641–2.

Ardissino G, Wally OM, Maria BG et al. Eculizumab for atypical hemolytic uremic syndrome in pregnancy. Obstet Gynecol 2013; 122: 487–9.

Armenti VT, Radomski JS, Moritz MJ et al. Report from the National Transplantation Pregnancy Registry (NTPR): outcomes of pregnancy after transplantation. Clin Transpl 2005; 69–83.

Arsenescu R, Arsenescu V, de Villiers WJ. TNF-alpha and the development of the neonatal immune system: implications for inhibitor use in pregnancy. Am J Gastroenterol 2011; 106: 559–62.

Auyeung-Kim DJ, Devalaraja MN, Migone TS et al. Developmental and peri-postnatal study in cynomolgus monkeys with belimumab, a monoclonal antibody directed against B-lymphocyte stimulator. Reprod Toxicol 2009; 28: 443–55.

Ban L, Tata LJ, Fiaschi L et al. Limited risks of major congenital anomalies in children of mothers with IBD and effects of medications. Gastroenterology 2014; 146: 76–84.

Bar OB, Hackman R, Einarson T et al. Pregnancy outcome after cyclosporine therapy during pregnancy: a meta-analysis. Transplantation 2001; 71: 1051–5.

Bayas A, Penzien J, Hellwig K. Accidental natalizumab administration to the third trimester of pregnancy in an adolescent patient with multiple sclerosis. Acta Neurol Scand 2011; 124: 290–2.

Beghin D, Cournot MP, Vauzelle C et al. Paternal exposure to methotrexate and pregnancy outcomes. J Rheumatol 2011; 38: 628–32.

Berger CT, Recher M, Steiner U et al. A patient's wish: anakinra in pregnancy. Ann Rheum Dis 2009; 68: 1794–5.

Berthelsen BG, Fjeldsoe-Nielsen H, Nielsen CT et al. Etanercept concentrations in maternal serum, umbilical cord serum, breast milk and child serum during breastfeeding. Rheumatology (Oxford) 2010; 49: 2225–7.

Biggioggero M, Borghi MO, Gerosa M et al. Immune function in children born to mothers with autoimmune diseases and exposed in utero to immunosuppressants. Lupus 2007; 16: 651–6.

Blume C, Sensoy A, Gross MM et al. A comparison of the outcome of pregnancies after liver and kidney transplantation. Transplantation 2013; 95: 222–7.

Bortlik M, Machkova N, Duricova D et al. Pregnancy and newborn outcome of mothers with inflammatory bowel diseases exposed to anti-TNF-alpha therapy during pregnancy: three-center study. Scand J Gastroenterol 2013; 48: 951–8.

Brewer GJ, Johnson VD, Dick RD et al. Treatment of Wilson's disease with zinc. XVII: Treatment during pregnancy. Hepatology 2000; 31: 364–70.

Brosens I, Pijnenborg R, Benagiano G. Risk of obstetrical complications in organ transplant recipient pregnancies. Transplantation 2013; 96: 227–33.

Buckley LM, Bullaboy CA, Leichtman L et al. Multiple congenital anomalies associated with weekly low-dose methotrexate treatment of the mother. Arthritis Rheum 1997; 40: 971–3.

Burwick RM, Feinberg BB. Eculizumab for the treatment of preeclampsia/HELLP syndrome. Placenta 2013; 34: 201–3.

Carta P, Caroti L, Zanazzi M. Pregnancy in a kidney transplant patient treated with everolimus. Am J Kidney Dis 2012; 60: 329

Carter JD, Ladhani A, Ricca LR et al. A safety assessment of tumor necrosis factor antagonists during pregnancy: a review of the Food and Drug Administration database. J Rheumatol 2009; 36: 635–41.

Carter JD, Valeriano J, Vasey FB. Tumor necrosis factor-alpha inhibition and VATER association: a causal relationship. J Rheumatol 2006; 33: 1014–7.

Casanova MJ, Chaparro M, Domenech E et al. Safety of thiopurines and anti-TNF-alpha drugs during pregnancy in patients with inflammatory bowel disease. Am J Gastroenterol 2013; 108: 433–40.

Cassina M, Johnson DL, Robinson LK et al. Pregnancy outcome in women exposed to leflunomide before or during pregnancy. Arthritis Rheum 2012; 64: 2085–94.

Chakravarty EF, Sanchez-Yamamoto D, Bush TM. The use of disease modifying antirheumatic drugs in women with rheumatoid arthritis of childbearing age: a survey of practice patterns and pregnancy outcomes. J Rheumatol 2003; 30: 241–6.

Chambers CD, Johnson DL, Robinson LK et al. Birth outcomes in women who have taken leflunomide during pregnancy. Arthritis Rheum 2010; 62: 1494–503.

Chaparro M, Gisbert JP. Successful use of infliximab for perianal Crohn's disease in pregnancy. Inflamm Bowel Dis 2011; 17: 868–9.

Cheent K, Nolan J, Shariq S et al. Case Report: Fatal case of disseminated BCG infection in an infant born to a mother taking infliximab for Crohn's disease. J Crohns Colitis 2010; 4: 603–5.

Christopher V, Al-Chalabi T, Richardson PD et al. Pregnancy outcome after liver transplantation: a single-center experience of 71 pregnancies in 45 recipients. Liver Transpl 2006; 12: 1138–43.

Chu SH, Liu KL, Chiang YJ et al. Sirolimus used during pregnancy in a living related renal transplant recipient: a case report. Transplant Proc 2008; 40: 2446–8.

Cimaz R, Brucato A, Meregalli E et al. Electroretinograms of children born from mothers treated with hydroxychloroquine (HCQ) during pregnancy and breast-feeding {Abstract}. Lupus 2004; 13: 755.

Cleary BJ, Kallen B. Early pregnancy azathioprine use and pregnancy outcomes. Birth Defects Res A Clin Mol Teratol 2009; 85: 647–54.

Clowse M, Wolf D, Förger F et al. Outcomes of Pregnancy in Subjects Exposed to Certolizumab {Poster}. Ann Rheum Dis 2013; 72: A431.

Coburn LA, Wise PE, Schwartz DA. The successful use of adalimumab to treat active Crohn's disease of an ileoanal pouch during pregnancy. Dig Dis Sci 2006; 51: 2045–7.

Cooper WO, Cheetham TC, Li DK et al. Brief report: risk of adverse fetal outcomes associated with immunosuppressive medications for chronic immune-mediated diseases in pregnancy. Arthritis Rheumatol 2014; 66: 444–50.

Corona-Rivera JR, Rea-Rosas A, Santana-Ramirez A et al. Holoprosencephaly and genitourinary anomalies in fetal methotrexate syndrome. Am J Med Genet A 2010; 152A: 1741–6.

Coscia LA, Constantinescu S, Moritz MJ et al. Report from the National Transplantation Pregnancy Registry (NTPR): outcomes of pregnancy after transplantation. Clin Transpl 2009: 103–22.

Costa ML, Surita FG, Passini R et al. Pregnancy outcome in female liver transplant recipients. Transplant Proc 2011; 43: 1337–9.

Costedoat-Chalumeau N, Amoura Z, Duhaut P et al. Safety of hydroxychloroquine in pregnant patients with connective tissue diseases: a study of one hundred thirty-three cases compared with a control group. Arthritis Rheum 2003; 48: 3207–11.

Coyle PK, Johnson K, Pardo L et al. Pregnancy outcomes in patients with multiple sclerosis treated with glatiramer acetate (copaxone). J Neurol Neurosurg Psychiatry 2003; 74: 443.

Cristiano L, Bozic C, Bloomgren G. Preliminary evaluation of pregnancy outcomes from the Tysabri (Natalizumab) pregnancy exposure register. Mult Scler 2011; 17: S457.

Cross SN, Ratner E, Rutherford TJ et al. Bevacizumab-mediated interference with VEGF signaling is sufficient to induce a preeclampsia-like syndrome in nonpregnant women. Rev Obstet Gynecol 2012; 5: 2–8.

Danilov AV, Brodsky RA, Craigo S et al. Managing a pregnant patient with paroxysmal nocturnal hemoglobinuria in the era of eculizumab. Leuk Res 2010; 34: 566–71.

Davison JM, Dellagrammatikas H, Parkin JM. Maternal azathioprine therapy and depressed haemopoiesis in the babies of renal allograft patients. Br J Obstet Gynaecol 1985; 92: 233–9.

de Boer NK, Jarbandhan SV, de Graaf F et al. Azathioprine use during pregnancy: unexpected intrauterine exposure to metabolites. Am J Gastroenterol 2006; 101: 1390–2.

De Santis M, Straface G, Cavaliere A et al. Paternal and maternal exposure to leflunomide: pregnancy and neonatal outcome. Ann Rheum Dis 2005; 64: 1096–7.

Dessinioti C, Stefanaki I, Stratigos AJ et al. Pregnancy during adalimumab use for psoriasis. J Eur Acad Dermatol Venereol 2011; 25: 738–9.

Deutsch MA, Kaczmarek I, Huber S et al. Sirolimus-associated infertility: case report and literature review of possible mechanisms. Am J Transplant 2007; 7: 2414–21.

Devesa R, Alvarez A, de las Heras G et al. Wilson's disease treated with trientine during pregnancy. J Pediatr Gastroenterol Nutr 1995; 20: 102–3.

Diav-Citrin O, Blyakhman S, Shechtman S et al. Pregnancy outcome following in utero exposure to hydroxychloroquine: A prospective comparative observational study. Reprod Toxicol 2013; 39: 58–62.

Diav-Citrin O, Otcheretianski-Volodarsky A, Shechtman S et al. Pregnancy outcome following gestational exposure to TNF-alpha-inhibitors: A prospective, comparative, observational study. Reprod Toxicol 2014; 43: 78–84.

EULAR: The European League Against Rheumatism. EULAR Issues Updated Rheumatoid Arthritis (RA) Management Recommendations. http://www.eular.org/myUploadData/files/EULAR%20RA%20recommendations%20FINAL.pdf (accessed 1-9-2013).

European Association for the Study of the Liver. EASL Clinical Practice Guidelines: Wilson's disease. J Hepatol 2012; 56: 671–85.

Fagius J, Burman J. Normal outcome of pregnancy with ongoing treatment with natalizumab. Acta Neurol Scand 2014; 129(6): e27–9.

Feldkamp M, Carey JC. Clinical teratology counseling and consultation case report: low dose methotrexate exposure in the early weeks of pregnancy. Teratology 1993; 47: 533–9.

Fischer-Betz R, Specker C, Schneider M. Successful outcome of two pregnancies in patients with adult-onset Still's disease treated with IL-1 receptor antagonist (anakinra). Clin Exp Rheumatol 2011; 29: 1021–3.

Fotiadou C, Lazaridou E, Sotiriou E, Ioannides D. Spontaneous abortion during ustekinumab therapy. I Dermatol Case Rep 2012; 6: 105–7.

Framarino dei MM, Corona LE, De Luca L et al. Successful pregnancy in a living-related kidney transplant recipient who received sirolimus throughout the whole gestation. Transplantation 2011; 91: e69–71

Fritzsche J, Pilch A, Mury D et al. Infliximab and adalimumab use during breastfeeding. J Clin Gastroenterol 2012; 46: 718–9.

Garcia-Donaire JA, Acevedo M, Gutierrez MJ et al. Tacrolimus as basic immunosuppression in pregnancy after renal transplantation. A single-center experience. Transplant Proc 2005; 37: 3754–5.

Gayed M, Leone F, Toescu V et al. Long-term outcomes of children born to mothers with SLE (oral Abstract). Rheumatology (Oxford) 2013; 52: 126.

Giannini M, Portaccio E, Ghezzi A et al. Pregnancy and fetal outcomes after Glatiramer Acetate exposure in patients with multiple sclerosis: a prospective observational multicentric study. BMC Neurol 2012; 12: 124.

Gold R, Phillips T, Havrdova E et al. BG-12 (Dimethyl Fumarate) and Pregnancy: Preclinical and Clinical Data from the Clinical Development Program (Poster P02.129) 2013.

Goldstein LH, Dolinsky G, Greenberg R et al. Pregnancy outcome of women exposed to azathioprine during pregnancy. Birth Defects Res A Clin Mol Teratol 2007; 79: 696–701.

Gomez Ledesma I, de Santiago Rodriguez MA, Follana Neira I et al. Neovascular membrane and pregnancy. Treatment with bevacizumab. Arch Soc Esp Oftalmol 2012; 87: 297–300.

Hanukoglu A, Curiel B, Berkowitz D et al. Hypothyroidism and dyshormonogenesis induced by D-penicillamine in children with Wilson's disease and healthy infants born to a mother with Wilson's disease. J Pediatr 2008; 153: 864–6.

Hart CW, Naunton RF. The ototoxicity of chloroquine phosphate. Arch Otolaryngol 1964; 80: 407–12.

He D, Han K, Gao X et al. Laquinimod for multiple sclerosis. Cochrane Database Syst Rev 2013; 8: CD010475.

Hebert MF, Zheng S, Hays K et al. Interpreting tacrolimus concentrations during pregnancy and postpartum. Transplantation 2013; 95: 908–15.

Heine K, Poets CF. A pair of twins born after maternal exposure to leflunomide. J Perinatol 2008; 28: 841–2.

Hellwig K, Haghikia A, Gold R. Pregnancy and natalizumab: results of an observational study in 35 accidental pregnancies during natalizumab treatment. Mult Scler 2011; 17: 958–63.

Hellwig K, Haghikia A, Rockhoff M et al. Multiple sclerosis and pregnancy: experience from a nationwide database in Germany. Ther Adv Neurol Disord 2012; 5: 247–53.

Hoeltzenbein M, Elefant E, Vial T et al. Teratogenicity of mycophenolate confirmed in a prospective study of the European Network of Teratology Information Services. Am J Med Genet A 2012a; 158A: 588–96.

Hoeltzenbein M, Weber-Schoendorfer C, Borisch C et al. Pregnancy outcome after paternal exposure to azathioprine/6-mercaptopurine. Reprod Toxicol 2012b; 34: 364–9.

Hoevenaren IA, de Vries LC, Rijnders RJ et al. Delivery of healthy babies after natalizumab use for multiple sclerosis: a report of two cases. Acta Neurol Scand 2011; 123: 430–3.

HultzschS, Weber-Schoendorfer C, Schaefer C. Pregnancy outcomes after exposure to etanercept {Abstract}. Reprod Toxicol 2011; 31: 260.

Hutson JR, Lubetsky A, Walfisch A et al. The transfer of 6-mercaptopurine in the dually perfused human placenta. Reprod Toxicol 2011; 32: 349–53.

Ingster-Moati I, Albuisson E. Visual neurophysiological dysfunction in infants exposed to hydroxychloroquine in utero. Acta Paediatr 2010; 99: 4–5.

Introini U, Casalino G, Cardani A et al. Intravitreal bevacizumab for a subfoveal myopic choroidal neovascularization in the first trimester of pregnancy. J Ocul Pharmacol Ther 2012; 28: 553–5.

Izmirly PM, Kim MY, Llanos C et al. Evaluation of the risk of anti-SSA/Ro-SSB/La antibody-associated cardiac manifestations of neonatal lupus in fetuses of mothers with systemic lupus erythematosus exposed to hydroxychloroquine. Ann Rheum Dis 2010; 69: 1827–30.

Jain A, Venkataramanan R, Fung JJ et al. Pregnancy after liver transplantation under tacrolimus. Transplantation 1997; 64: 559–65.

Jain AB, Reyes J, Marcos A et al. Pregnancy after liver transplantation with tacrolimus immunosuppression: a single center's experience update at 13 years. Transplantation 2003; 76: 827–32.

Jain AB, Shapiro R, Scantlebury VP et al. Pregnancy after kidney and kidney-pancreas transplantation under tacrolimus: a single center's experience. Transplantation 2004; 77: 897–902.

Jalkanen A, Alanen A, Airas L. Pregnancy outcome in women with multiple sclerosis: results from a prospective nationwide study in Finland. Mult Scler 2010; 16: 950–5.

Jharap B, de Boer NK, Stokkers P et al. Intrauterine exposure and pharmacology of conventional thiopurine therapy in pregnant patients with inflammatory bowel disease. Gut 2014; 63: 451–7.

Johnson DL, Jones KL, Chambers CD. Pregnancy outcomes in women exposed to etanercept: The OTIS autoimmune diseases in pregnancy project {Poster}. http://www.pregnancystudies.org/wp-content/uploads/Etanercept_in_Pregnancy_Oct_2008.pdf (accessed 12-9-2013).

Johnson D, Luo Y, Jones K et al. Pregnancy outcomes in women exposed to adalimumab: an update on the autoimmune diseases in pregnancy project. Arthritis & Rheumatism 2011; 63: S730–S731.

Johnsson A, Avlund S, Grosen A et al. Chicken pox infection in a three months old infant exposed in utero to Adalimumab. J Crohns Colitis 2013; 7: e116–7.

Jones A, Clary MJ, McDermott E et al. Outcomes of pregnancies fathered by solid-organ transplant recipients exposed to mycophenolic acid products. Prog Transplant 2013; 23: 153–7.

Kainz A, Harabacz I, Cowlrick IS et al. Review of the course and outcome of 100 pregnancies in 84 women treated with tacrolimus. Transplantation 2000; 70: 1718–21.

Kallen B. Maternal use of 5-aminosalicylates in early pregnancy and congenital malformation risk in the offspring. Scand J Gastroenterol 2014; 49: 442–8.

Kamm CP, El-Koussy M, Humpert S et al. Atorvastatin added to interferon beta for relapsing multiple sclerosis: a randomized controlled trial. J Neurol 2012; 259: 2401–13.

Karlsson G, Francis G, Koren G et al. Pregnancy outcomes in the clinical development program of fingolimod in multiple sclerosis. Neurology 2014; 82: 674–80.

Katz JA, Antoni C, Keenan GF et al. Outcome of pregnancy in women receiving infliximab for the treatment of Crohn's disease and rheumatoid arthritis. Am J Gastroenterol 2004; 99: 2385–92.

Kelly R, Arnold L, Richards S et al. The management of pregnancy in paroxysmal nocturnal haemoglobinuria on long term eculizumab. Br J Haematol 2010; 149: 446–50.

Kim HW, Seok HJ, Kim TH et al. The experience of pregnancy after renal transplantation: pregnancies even within postoperative 1 year may be tolerable. Transplantation 2008; 85: 1412–9.

Klinger G, Morad Y, Westall CA et al. Ocular toxicity and antenatal exposure to chloroquine or hydroxychloroquine for rheumatic diseases. Lancet 2001; 358: 813–4.

Lamarque V, Leleu MF, Monka C et al. Analysis of 629 pregnancy outcomes in transplant recipients treated with Sandimmun. Transplant Proc 1997; 29: 2480.

Law I, Ilett KF, Hackett LP et al. Transfer of chloroquine and desethylchloroquine across the placenta and into milk in Melanesian mothers. Br J Clin Pharmacol 2008; 65: 674–9.

Lewden B, Vial T, Elefant E et al. Low dose methotrexate in the first trimester of pregnancy: results of a French collaborative study. J Rheumatol 2004; 31: 2360–5.

Lin AE, Singh KE, Strauss A et al. An additional patient with mycophenolate mofetil embryopathy: cardiac and facial analyses. Am J Med Genet A 2011; 155A: 748–56.

Lu E, Dahlgren L, Sadovnick A et al. Perinatal outcomes in women with multiple sclerosis exposed to disease-modifying drugs. Mult Scler 2012a; 18: 460–7.

Lu E, Wang BW, Guimond C et al. Disease-modifying drugs for multiple sclerosis in pregnancy: a systematic review. Neurology 2012b; 79: 1130–5.

Lu E, Wang BW, Alwan S et al. A review of safety-related pregnancy data surrounding the oral disease-modifying drugs for multiple sclerosis. CNS Drugs 2014a; 28: 89–94.

Lu E, Zhu F, Zhao Y et al. Birth outcomes of pregnancies fathered by men with multiple sclerosis. Mult Scler 2014b [Epub ahead of print].

Mahadevan U, Terdiman JP, Aron J et al. Infliximab and semen quality in men with inflammatory bowel disease. Inflamm Bowel Dis 2005; 11: 395–9.

Mahadevan U, Wolf DC, Dubinsky M et al. Placental transfer of anti-tumor necrosis factor agents in pregnant patients with inflammatory bowel disease. Clin Gastroenterol Hepatol 2013; 11: 286–92.

Malik A, Khawaja A, Sheikh L. Wilson's disease in pregnancy: case series and review of literature. BMC Res Notes 2013; 6: 421.

Marasca R, Coluccio V, Santachiara R et al. Pregnancy in PNH: another eculizumab baby. Br J Haematol 2010; 150: 707–8.

Marchioni RM, Lichtenstein GR. Tumor necrosis factor-alpha inhibitor therapy and fetal risk: a systematic literature review. World J Gastroenterol 2013; 19: 2591–602.

Marder W, Ganser MA, Romero V et al. In utero azathioprine exposure and increased utilization of special educational services in children born to mothers with systemic lupus erythematosus. Arthritis Care Res (Hoboken) 2013; 65: 759–66.

Margoles HR, Gomez-Lobo V, Veis JH et al. Successful maternal and fetal outcome in a kidney transplant patient with everolimus exposure throughout pregnancy: a case report. Transplant Proc 2014; 46: 281–3.

Marder MC, Barbero P, Groisman B et al. Methotrexate embryopathy after exposure to low weekly doses in early pregnancy. Reprod Toxicol 2013; 43: 26–9.

Martinez-Frias ML, Rodriguez-Pinilla E et al. Prenatal exposure to penicillamine and oral clefts: case report. Am J Med Genet 1998; 76: 274–5.

Melillo L, Tieghi A, Candoni A et al. Outcome of 122 pregnancies in essential thrombocythemia patients: A report from the Italian registry. Am J Hematol 2009; 84: 636–40.

Mishkin DS, Van DW, Becker JM et al. Successful use of adalimumab (Humira) for Crohn's disease in pregnancy. Inflamm Bowel Dis 2006; 12: 827–8.

Miyamoto T, Miyaji S, Horiuchi Y et al. Gold therapy in bronchial asthma with special emphasis upon blood level of gold and its teratogenicity (author's transl). Nihon Naika Gakkai Zasshi 1974; 63: 1190–7.

Montagna GL, Malesci D, Buono R et al. Asthenoazoospermia in patients receiving anti-tumour necrosis factor {alpha} agents. Ann Rheum Dis 2005; 64: 1667.

Moskovitz DN, Bodian C, Chapman ML et al. The effect on the fetus of medications used to treat pregnant inflammatory bowel-disease patients. Am J Gastroenterol 2004; 99: 656–61.

Motta M, Ciardelli L, Marconi M et al. Immune system development in infants born to mothers with autoimmune disease, exposed in utero to immunosuppressive agents. Am J Perinatol 2007; 24: 441–7.

Mubarak AA, Kakil IR, Awidi A et al. Normal outcome of pregnancy in chronic myeloid leukemia treated with interferon-alpha in 1st trimester: report of 3 cases and review of the literature. Am J Hematol 2002; 69: 115–8.

Murashima A, Watanabe N, Ozawa N et al. Etanercept during pregnancy and lactation in a patient with rheumatoid arthritis: drug levels in maternal serum, cord blood, breast milk and the infant's serum. Ann Rheum Dis 2009; 68: 1793–4.

Neville CE, McNally J. Maternal exposure to leflunomide associated with blindness and cerebral palsy. Rheumatology (Oxford) 2007; 46: 1506.

Nulman I, Sgro M, Barrera M et al. Long-term neurodevelopment of children exposed in utero to ciclosporin after maternal renal transplant. Paediatr Drugs 2010; 12: 113–22.

Ojeda-Uribe M, Afif N, Dahan E et al. Exposure to abatacept or rituximab in the first trimester of pregnancy in three women with autoimmune diseases. Clin Rheumatol 2013; 32: 695–700.

Ostensen M, Hartmann H, Salvesen K. Low dose weekly methotrexate in early pregnancy. A case series and review of the literature. J Rheumatol 2000; 27: 1872–5.

Patas K, Engler JB, Friese MA et al. Pregnancy and multiple sclerosis: feto-maternal immune cross talk and its implications for disease activity. J Reprod Immunol 2013; 97: 140–6.

Paziana K, Del MM, Cardonick E et al. Ciclosporin use during pregnancy. Drug Saf 2013; 36: 279–94.

Peart E, Clowse ME. Systemic lupus erythematosus and pregnancy outcomes: an update and review of the literature. Curr Opin Rheumatol 2014; 26: 118–23.

Pessach I, Shimoni A, Nagler A. Granulocyte-colony stimulating factor for hematopoietic stem cell donation from healthy female donors during pregnancy and lactation: what do we know? Hum Reprod Update 2013; 19: 259–67.

Pham T, Claudepierre P, Constantin A et al. Abatacept therapy and safety management. Joint Bone Spine 2009; 76: S3–55

Piggott KD, Sorbello A, Riddle E et al. Congenital cardiac defects: a possible association of aminopterin syndrome and in utero methotrexate exposure? Pediatr Cardiol 2011; 32: 518–20.

Pinter R, Hogge WA, McPherson E. Infant with severe penicillamine embryopathy born to a woman with Wilson disease. Am J Med Genet A 2004; 128A: 294–8.

Polifka JE, Friedman JM. Teratogen update: azathioprine and 6-mercaptopurine. Teratology 2002; 65: 240–61.

Rahimi R, Nikfar S, Rezaie A et al. Pregnancy outcome in women with inflammatory bowel disease following exposure to 5-aminosalicylic acid drugs: a meta-analysis. Reprod Toxicol 2008; 25: 271–5.

Regierer AC, Schulz CO, Kuehnhardt D et al. Interferon-alpha therapy for chronic myeloid leukemia during pregnancy. Am J Hematol 2006; 81: 149–50.

Renault F, Flores-Guevara R, Renaud C et al. Visual neurophysiological dysfunction in infants exposed to hydroxychloroquine in utero. Acta Paediatr 2009; 98: 1500–3.

Rieder MJ, McLean JL, Morrison C et al. Long-term follow-up of children with in utero exposure to immunosuppressives [abstract]. Teratology 1997; 55: 37.

Roll C, Luboldt HJ, Winter A et al. Hepatoblastoma in a 2-year-old child of a liver-transplanted mother. Lancet 1997; 349: 103.

Rosa FW. Teratogen update: penicillamine. Teratology 1986; 33: 127–31.

Rosenfeld PJ. Bevacizumab versus ranibizumab for AMD. N Engl J Med 2011; 364: 1966–7.

Roux CH, Brocq O, Breuil V et al. Pregnancy in rheumatology patients exposed to anti-tumour necrosis factor (TNF)-alpha therapy. Rheumatology (Oxford) 2007; 46: 695–8.

Rubbert-Roth A, Goupille PM, Moosavi S et al. First experiences with pregnancies in RA patients (pts) receiving tocilizumab (TCZ) therapy {abstract}. Arthritis Rheum 2010; 62: 384.

Rump JA, Schonborn H. Conception and course of eight pregnancies in five women on TNF blocker etanercept treatment. Z Rheumatol 2010; 69: 903–9.

Sandberg-Wollheim M, Alteri E, Moraga MS et al. Pregnancy outcomes in multiple sclerosis following subcutaneous interferon beta-1a therapy. Mult Scler 2011; 17: 423–30.

Saougou I, Markatseli TE, Papagoras C et al. Fertility in male patients with seronegative spondyloarthropathies treated with infliximab. Joint Bone Spine 2013; 80: 34–7.

Sarhianaki A, Katsimpris A, Petropoulos IK et al. Intravitreal administration of ranibizumab for idiopathic choroidal neovascularization in a pregnant woman. Klin Monbl Augenheilkd 2012; 229: 451–3.

Schneider H, Weber CE, Hellwig K et al. Natalizumab treatment during pregnancy – effects on the neonatal immune system. Acta Neurol Scand 2013; 127: e1–4.

Schnitzler F, Fidder H, Ferrante M et al. Outcome of pregnancy in women with inflammatory bowel disease treated with antitumor necrosis factor therapy. Inflamm Bowel Dis 2011; 17: 1846–54.

Scioscia C, Scioscia M, Anelli MG et al. Intentional etanercept use during pregnancy for maintenance of remission in rheumatoid arthritis. Clin Exp Rheumatol 2011; 29: 93–5.

Seror J, Sentilhes L, Lefebvre-Lacoeuille C et al. Interferon-alpha for treatment of essential thrombocythemia during pregnancy: case report and review of the literature. Fetal Diagn Ther 2009; 25: 136–40.

Sifontis NM, Coscia LA, Constantinescu S et al. Pregnancy outcomes in solid organ transplant recipients with exposure to mycophenolate mofetil or sirolimus. Transplantation 2006; 82: 1698–702.

Sinha S, Taly AB, Prashanth LK et al. Successful pregnancies and abortions in symptomatic and asymptomatic Wilson's disease. J Neurol Sci 2004; 217: 37–40.

Snoeckx Y, Keenan G, Sanders M et al. Pregnancy outcomes in women taking infliximab: the infliximab safety database [abstract]. Arthritis Rheum 2008; 58: S426.

Sullivan L, Kelly SP, Glenn A et al. Intravitreal bevacizumab injection in unrecognised early pregnancy. Eye (Lond) 2014: doi: 10.1038/eye.2013.311 [Epub ahead of print].

Tarantola RM, Folk JC, Boldt HC et al. Intravitreal bevacizumab during pregnancy. Retina 2010; 30: 1405–11.

Tefferi A, Passamonti F. Essential thrombocythemia and pregnancy: Observations from recent studies and management recommendations. Am J Hematol 2009; 84: 629–30.

Termini S, Helms M, Coscia L et al. National Transplantation Pregnancy Registry (NTPR): The Use of an Internal Control Group to Identify a Specific Pattern of Malformation (Workshop Abstracts). Birth Defects Res A Clin Mol Teratol 2011; 91: 387.

Tjeertes IF, Bastiaans DE, van Ganzewinkel CJ et al. Neonatal anemia and hydrops fetalis after maternal mycophenolate mofetil use. J Perinatol 2007; 27: 62–4.

Tomczyk S, Richmann S, Wallace K et al. Pregnancy outcomes from the AVONEX (Interferon Beta-1a) pregnancy exposure Registry (Poster P06.191). 64th Annual Meeting of the American Academy of Neurology (April 21–28, 2012 New Orleans, Louisiana).

Toovey S, Hudson E, Hendry WF et al. Sulphasalazine and male infertility: reversibility and possible mechanism. Gut 1981; 22: 445–51.

Toth A. Male infertility due to sulphasalazine. Lancet 1979; 2: 904.

Umeda N, Ito S, Hayashi T et al. A patient with rheumatoid arthritis who had a normal delivery under etanercept treatment. Intern Med 2010; 49: 187–9.

Vasiliauskas EA, Church JA, Silverman N et al. Case report: evidence for transplacental transfer of maternally administered infliximab to the newborn. Clin Gastroenterol Hepatol 2006; 4: 1255–8.

Veroux M, Corona D, Veroux P. Pregnancy under everolimus-based immunosuppression. Transpl Int 2011; 24: e115–7.

Verstappen SM, King Y, Watson KD et al. Anti-TNF therapies and pregnancy: outcome of 130 pregnancies in the British Society for Rheumatology Biologics Register. Ann Rheum Dis 2011; 70: 823–6.

Vesga L, Terdiman JP, Mahadevan U. Adalimumab use in pregnancy. Gut 2005; 54: 890.

Viktil KK, Engeland A, Furu K. Outcomes after anti-rheumatic drug use before and during pregnancy: a cohort study among 150,000 pregnant women and expectant fathers. Scand J Rheumatol 2012; 41: 196–201.

Villiger PM, Caliezi G, Cottin V et al. Effects of TNF antagonists on sperm characteristics in patients with spondyloarthritis. Ann Rheum Dis 2010; 69: 1842–4.

Visser K, Katchamart W, Loza E et al. Multinational evidence-based recommendations for the use of methotrexate in rheumatic disorders with a focus on rheumatoid arthritis: integrating systematic literature research and expert opinion of a broad international panel of rheumatologists in the 3E Initiative. Ann Rheum Dis 2009; 68: 1086–93.

Walshe JM. The management of pregnancy in Wilson's disease treated with trientine. QJ Med 1986; 58: 81–7.

Weber-Schoendorfer C, Chambers C, Wacker E et al. Pregnancy outcome after methotrexate treatment for rheumatic disease prior to or during early pregnancy: a prospective multi-center cohort study. Arthritis Rheumatol 2014; 66: 1101–10.

Weber-Schoendorfer C, Fritzsche J, Schaefer C. Pregnancy outcomes in women exposed to adalimumab or infliximab: The experience of the Berlin Institute for Clinical Teratology and Drug Risk Assessment in Pregnancy (Abstract). Reproductive Toxicology 2011; 31: 267–8.

Weber-Schoendorfer C, Hoeltzenbein M, Wacker E et al. No evidence for an increased risk of adverse pregnancy outcome after paternal low-dose methotrexate (MTX): an observational cohort study. Rheumatology (Oxford) 2013; 53: 757–63.

Weber-Schoendorfer C, Schaefer C. Multiple sclerosis, immunomodulators, and pregnancy outcome: a prospective observational study. Mult Scler 2009; 15: 1037–42.

Wiendl H, Toyka KV, Rieckmann P et al. Basic and escalating immunomodulatory treatments in multiple sclerosis: current therapeutic recommendations. J Neurol 2008; 255: 1449–63.

Winger EE, Reed JL. Treatment with tumor necrosis factor inhibitors and intravenous immunoglobulin improves live birth rates in women with recurrent spontaneous abortion. Am J Reprod Immunol 2008; 60: 8–16.

Winger EE, Reed JL, Ashoush S et al. Treatment with adalimumab (Humira) and intravenous immunoglobulin improves pregnancy rates in women undergoing IVF. Am J Reprod Immunol 2009; 61: 113–20.

Xu LG, Jin LM, Zhu XF et al. A report of 212 male renal transplant recipients who fathered 216 offspring after transplantation. Transplantation 2008; 86: 1480–1.

Yazdani BP, Matok I, Garcia BF et al. A systematic review of the fetal safety of interferon alpha. Reprod Toxicol 2012; 33: 265–8.

Zelinkova Z, van der Ent C, Bruin KF et al. Effects of discontinuing anti-tumor necrosis factor therapy during pregnancy on the course of inflammatory bowel disease and neonatal exposure. Clin Gastroenterol Hepatol 2013; 11: 318–21.

Zuber J, Anglicheau D, Elie C et al. Sirolimus may reduce fertility in male renal transplant recipients. Am J Transplant 2008; 8: 1471–9.

Antineoplastic drugs

Jan M. Friedman and
Corinna Weber-Schöndorfer

2.13

2.13.1	Malignancy and pregnancy	374
2.13.2	Breast cancer	376
2.13.3	Vinca alkaloids and analogs	377
2.13.4	Podophyllotoxin derivatives	377
2.13.5	Nitrosourea alkylators	378
2.13.6	Nitrogen mustard analog alkylators	378
2.13.7	Other alkylating agents	379
2.13.8	Cytotoxic anthracycline antibiotics	380
2.13.9	Other cytotoxic antibiotics	381
2.13.10	Folate antagonists	382
2.13.11	Purine antagonists	383
2.13.12	Pyrimidine antagonists	383
2.13.13	Taxanes and other cytostatic agents	385
2.13.14	Monoclonal antibodies	385
2.13.15	Platin compounds	386
2.13.16	Thalidomide and its analogs	387
2.13.17	Tyrosine kinase inhibitors	388
2.13.18	Antineoplastic drugs with endocrine effects	389
2.13.19	Other antineoplastic agents	390

Malignant disease is rare in pregnancy and requires expert interdisciplinary medical and psychosocial support. To give a pregnant woman the best chance for survival, cancer is often treated in the same way that it would be if the woman were not pregnant. Antineoplastic therapy in the first trimester is of greatest concern with respect to possible teratogenic effects, but only a few antineoplastic treatments (*thalidomide, methotrexate, cyclophosphamide, tretinoin* and possibly *cytarabine*) have been implicated in producing embryopathies. A few other treatments, most notably *anthracyclines* and *trastuzumab*, are associated with toxic fetal effects later in pregnancy. Most of the information available on other treatments is reassuring, but the supporting data are usually quite limited.

Drugs During Pregnancy and Lactation. **http://dx.doi.org/10.1016/B978-0-12-408078-2.00014-7**

Clinical estimation of fetal risks associated with maternal cancer therapy in pregnancy needs to be very careful and critical and should include an appropriate statement of uncertainty.

Black Box Warning

The data available to assess the risks, and especially the safety, of the embryo or fetus for maternal cancer chemotherapy during pregnancy are very limited. Almost all available human data come from case reports and clinical series (NTP 2013, Selig 2012). There are serious methodological and statistical limitations in trying to generalize from such data (NTP 2013), and, as a result, the absence of an observed effect in case reports and most clinical series cannot provide much reassurance. On the other hand, the occurrence of a birth defect in a child after maternal treatment during pregnancy does not necessarily imply a causal relationship between the treatment and the birth defect, even if no other cause of the child's problems is apparent. Maternal therapy for cancer often involves administration of several medications simultaneously, and the tumor itself may produce substances that can affect fetal development. In such circumstances, it is difficult to distinguish the effects of one exposure from another or from a particular combination of exposures.

Case reports and clinical series may be useful in recognizing major teratogenic effects, especially if they frequently produce patterns of malformations that are extremely uncommon in other circumstances. However, even if a causal relationship can be established, case reports are not able to provide quantitative estimates of risk, and risk estimates obtained from clinical series are usually very crude. Although much of the information included in this chapter is reassuring, the supporting data are usually quite limited, and clinical application needs to be very careful, very critical, and include a healthy dose of skepticism.

The intent of cancer chemotherapy is to kill or inhibit the growth of rapidly dividing cells, and embryos and fetuses are composed largely of rapidly dividing cells. In addition, normal prenatal development depends on proper functioning of the same signaling and regulatory pathways that cancer chemotherapy may be designed to disrupt. There is almost always at least a theoretical potential for maternal cancer chemotherapy during pregnancy to damage the embryo or fetus. In the absence of adequate data on the outcome of exposed human pregnancies, one must assume that some degree of teratogenic risk exists, especially with first-trimester exposure. Avoiding chemotherapy in the mother during pregnancy is usually the safest option for the embryo or fetus in the short-term, but doing so may reduce or even preclude effective treatment of the mother's malignancy. Thus, decisions about treating cancer in a pregnant woman always need to be individualized and often are difficult.

2.13.1   Malignancy and pregnancy

Currently available evidence indicates that previous chemotherapy for cancer does not measurably increase the rate of spontaneous abortion or stillbirths in subsequent pregnancies (Falconer 2002). Similarly, malformations, genetic defects, and chromosomal anomalies do not appear to be more frequent than expected among the children of cancer survivors who were previously treated with chemotherapy (Green 2009). Some kinds of cancer chemotherapy may reduce subsequent fertility, depending on the drugs administered, their dose, and the duration of therapy, as well as on the age of the patient at the time of treatment (Ben-Aharon 2010).

Generally, radiotherapy much earlier in life does not cause permanent infertility in either men or women. Neither does it increase the risk of birth defects or genetic disease in children born of subsequent pregnancies. An exception may be prior irradiation of the ovaries and/or uterus, which has been associated with an elevated risk of infertility or premature menopause. One study has also shown increased rates of premature births, growth retardation, and stillbirths and perinatal deaths among infants of women who had previously received such therapy (Signorello 2010). Tissue damage after irradiation of the uterus was suspected as the cause, especially if the radiotherapy took place before menarche.

Malignant illness during pregnancy is rare, occurring in 0.2–1 per 1000 pregnancies. Breast cancer, lymphomas, melanomas and ovarian cancer are seen most often (Lee 2012, Cardonick 2010b). There is no clear evidence that pregnancy itself influences the prognosis for a cancer.

If malignant disease is diagnosed in the first trimester, many couples choose to terminate the pregnancy, owing to the potential teratogenic risk of the expected therapy. There is, therefore, the least experience with maternal treatment early in pregnancy, but it is clear from documented cases that chemotherapy does not usually lead to major fetal malformations that are apparent at birth (Selig 2012). Moreover, intellectual development does not usually seem to be impaired, although available studies are very limited in terms of the number of patients and range of chemotherapeutic treatments included (Amant 2012b, Nulman 2001).

Only a few antineoplastic medications (for example, *anthracyclines* or *trastuzumab*) have been reported to produce specific adverse fetal pharmacologic effects. Multiple agent chemotherapy in the second or third trimester may lead to growth retardation or transient bone marrow depression with fetal anemia, leucopenia or thrombocytopenia, but intrauterine death appears to be infrequent. Premature delivery of a pregnant woman who has cancer may be undertaken once fetal lung maturity has been achieved in order to have a "free hand" to provide maternal treatment without exposing the fetus to potentially toxic substances.

Recommendation. Generally speaking, following antineoplastic therapy, a waiting period of 2 years for the woman and 6 months for the man before conceiving is recommended. However, if a pregnancy occurs sooner, there is no evidence that the risk to the fetus is measurably increased by the previous treatment. If there is a prior history of cancer chemotherapy or radiotherapy – especially irradiation of the abdomen and pelvis, but also the skull or spine – the course of the pregnancy should be carefully monitored.

Malignant illnesses during pregnancy are rare and require expert interdisciplinary medical and psychosocial support. The decision of the couple about antineoplastic therapy during pregnancy should be made together with the healthcare team after consideration of available information about the individual risks to both the mother and the fetus. Every malignant illness during pregnancy requires individualized counseling and treatment.

As a rule, neoplasms in pregnant women are treated in the same way that they would be if the patient were not pregnant to give her the best chance for survival (Backes 2011, Brewer 2011, Azim 2010). Therefore, in contrast to other chapters, few therapy recommendations will be given in this section from an embryotoxicological perspective. Pregnant women who have cancer should be offered serial detailed ultrasound examinations to monitor fetal development. Maternal chemotherapy after 35 weeks gestation is generally not recommended because both the mother and fetus are thought to benefit from a few weeks of recovery prior to delivery (Amant 2012a, Azim 2011, Cardonick 2010a).

Pregnancy

2.13 Antineoplastic drugs

Antineoplastic therapy in the first trimester, which may occur before the pregnancy is recognized, is of greatest concern with respect to possible teratogenic effects, but such treatment may or may not be associated with teratogenic risk that is great enough to justify consideration of pregnancy termination (Chapter 1.15). Again, management should be individualized by the healthcare team in consultation with the woman and her family.

2.13.2   Breast cancer

Breast cancer is one of the most frequently diagnosed malignancies in pregnancy. Breast cancer in pregnancy is increasing because the incidence of breast cancer increases with age, and older women are becoming pregnant more often in industrialized nations. However, the increase in breast cancer during pregnancy appears to be greater than expected as a result of increased maternal age alone (Lee 2012).

Large population-based registry studies (Johansson 2011, 2013) and series including 100 or more women who received various chemotherapeutic regimens for breast cancer have been reported (Amant 2013, Loibl 2012b, Cardonick 2010a), and the results of these and many smaller clinical studies have recently been reviewed (NTP 2013, Azim 2012, Cardonick 2010a, McGrath 2011). In general, these studies show similar, or only slightly worse, survival for women who are treated for breast cancer during pregnancy when other prognostic factors are taken into consideration.

Most of the reported experience is with treatment after the first trimester of pregnancy. Breast cancer chemotherapy generally seems to be well tolerated by the fetus in the second and third trimesters, at least in terms of serious adverse outcomes that are apparent in infancy, if premature delivery can be avoided (Abdel-Hady 2012, Loibl 2012a) (see the individual medications detailed below). Treatment with *trastuzumab* is an apparent exception – there is a substantial risk of fetal renal dysfunction with trastuzumab therapy during the second half of pregnancy (see discussion below). Surgical treatment of breast cancer can undertaken at any point in pregnancy, with maternal risks that are similar to those in nonpregnant women and fetal risks that are similar to those associated with other kinds of surgery (Colfry 2013, Amant 2012b).

Recommendation. Treatment of breast cancer in a pregnant woman should be individualized, taking into account the nature of the patient's disease, the stage of her pregnancy, her general state of health, and the multitude of personal, family, and social issues raised by the situation. In general, however, optimal treatment of the malignancy requires therapy in accordance with established protocols for the stage of the cancer in nonpregnant women (Amant 2012b, Loibl 2012b, Azim 2011, Sukumvanich 2011). Surgery, including sentinel-lymph node localization (Chapter 2.20), can be carried out in the first trimester or later in pregnancy with maternal and fetal risks that are considered to be acceptable. Chemotherapy can be used, if necessary, but should generally not begin until after the first trimester of pregnancy to limit teratogenic risk to the fetus. Chemotherapy cycles should be timed so that the birth does not take place in the period of blood count depression, if possible. Trastuzumab treatment and radiation therapy usually should be postponed until after delivery.

2.13.3   Vinca alkaloids and analogs

Vinca alkaloids are cytotoxic agents that disrupt microtubule formation. They have many effects on cellular activities, including inhibition
of mitotic spindle formation and mitotic arrest. *Vinblastine* and *vincristine* are natural alkaloids, while *vindesine, vinorelbine* and *vinflunine* are
semisynthetic derivatives.

At least 16 infants have been reported whose mothers were treated
with *vinblastine*, usually in combination with other cytotoxic agents,
during the first trimester of pregnancy (NTP 2013, Selig 2012). In most
cases, the child appeared normal at birth, although instances of cleft lip
and palate, foot malformations, hydrocephalus, thumb anomaly, and
atrial septal defect have been described (NTP 2013, Selig 2012, Dilek
2006, Mulvihill 1987, Thomas 1976, Garrett 1974). More than 50 children
whose mothers received cancer chemotherapy that included vinblastine
during the second or third trimester of pregnancy have been reported
(NTP 2013, Selig 2012). Most of these infants appeared normal at birth,
but fetal growth retardation and transient anemia have been described.

At least 57 infants without congenital anomalies and at least seven children with malformations have been reported after maternal vincristine
therapy during the first trimester of pregnancy (NTP 2013, Selig 2012).
Two of the children had cleft lip and palate, but the malformations were
different in all of the others. In each of these cases, the mother was also
treated with other chemotherapeutic agents. More than 160 apparently
normal children have been reported after maternal vincristine treatment
later in pregnancy (NTP 2013, Selig 2012), but premature delivery, fetal
growth retardation and neonatal bone marrow suppression have also
been observed (NTP 2013, Fernandez 1989, Avilés 1988, Pizzuto 1980,
Doney 1979).

Three of 10 children born to women who were treated with vinorelbine and other chemotherapeutic drugs during the first trimester were
reported to have malformations (Selig 2012) – one child with atrial septal
defect (Thomas 1976), one with hydrocephalus (Mulvihill 1987), and one
with cleft palate and tracheoesophageal fistula (Abellar 2009). At least
16 infants, most of whom appeared to be healthy, have been reported
after maternal treatment with vinorelbine later in pregnancy (NTP 2013,
Selig 2012).

One normal infant whose mother was treated with vindesine during the
third trimester of pregnancy has been reported (Fassas 1984). There is, as
yet, no reported experience with vinflunine treatment during pregnancy.

2.13.4   Podophyllotoxin derivatives

Etoposide and *teniposide* are semisynthetic alkaloids that inhibit DNA
synthesis by blocking topoisomerase.

Reports describe five apparently healthy children whose mothers were
treated with etoposide and other cancer chemotherapeutic agents during
the first trimester of pregnancy and more than 40 infants whose mothers were treated with etoposide in combination with other drugs later in
pregnancy (NTP 2013, Selig 2012, Brudie 2011, Benjapibal 2010, Avilés
1991). Most of these children appeared normal, but transient neonatal
anemia, pancytopenia or hair loss was sometimes seen (Hsu 1995, Murray
1994, Buller 1992, Raffles 1989). A premature infant, whose mother was
treated with etoposide, *bleomycin* and *cisplatin* in the 26th/27th week of

pregnancy developed cerebral atrophy (Elit 1999). The glandular hypospadias observed in a boy whose mother was treated after the 21st week of gestation with etoposide, bleomycin, and cisplatin (Ghaemmaghami 2009) was unrelated to the treatment, which occurred after formation of the penile urethra was completed.

Only three reports of infants born after maternal treatment with teniposide during pregnancy are available (Selig 2012, Lambert 1991, Lowenthal 1982); all involved combination therapy in the second or third trimester of pregnancy. Two of the children appeared normal; the outcome in the third case was said to be "adverse" but was not described further.

2.13.5   Nitrosourea alkylators

A child with microphthalmia was born to a woman who was treated with *carmustine* (BCNU), *dacarbazine, cisplatin*, and *tamoxifen* during the first and second trimesters of pregnancy (Li 2007). Two other women who were treated with the same combination of drugs beginning at the 23rd week of gestation have been reported. One had a child with atrial septal defect, strabismus and a nevus (Selig 2012), and the other woman had a healthy child (DiPaola 1997).

Only two infants have been reported whose mothers were treated with *lomustine* (CCNU) during the first trimester of pregnancy, and both had cleft lip and palate (Selig 2012, Mulvihill 1987). The therapy also included other anticancer agents in both cases.

One normal infant whose mother was treated with *nimustine* during the second half of pregnancy has been reported (Ishida 2009). No information is available on the outcomes of pregnancies in which the mother was treated with *bendamustine*.

2.13.6   Nitrogen mustard analog alkylators

Chlorambucil blocks the initiation of DNA replication. There are at least eight reports on its use in the first trimester of pregnancy (NTP 2013, Selig 2012). In two cases, the fetus was found to have unilateral renal agenesis. Chlorambucil was the only drug used to treat one of these mothers (Shotton 1963); the other woman had also been treated with prednisone for autoimmune disease (Steege 1980). A woman with severe dermatosclerosis who had been treated with chlorambucil during the first trimester of pregnancy had an infant with multiple cardiovascular malformations who died on the third day of life (Thompson 1983). In another case, the fetus had retinal defects (Rugh 1965). Few cases have been described in which the mother was treated with chlorambucil beginning later in pregnancy, but all of the infants were reported to be normal (NTP 2013).

An extremely rare but characteristic pattern of malformations has been reported in at least 12 children whose mothers were treated with *cyclophosphamide* during the first trimester of pregnancy (NTP 2013). The most frequently described features of this cyclophosphamide embryopathy included growth retardation, developmental delay, microcephaly and major malformations of the distal limbs in association with minor anomalies of the ears, nose, jaw and midface (Lazalde 2012, Leyder 2011, Paskulin 2005, Paladini 2004, Vaux 2003, Enns 1999). The frequency of this embryopathy among infants whose mothers were treated with cyclophosamide during the first trimester of pregnancy is unknown, but most infants born to women who are treated with cyclophosphamide early in pregnancy appear normal at birth (NTP 2013, Selig 2012). Maternal treatment with cyclophosphamide later in pregnancy has not been associated with an increased risk of fetal malformations, although oligohydramnios, premature delivery and neonatal bone marrow suppression are unusually frequent (NTP 2013, Selig 2012).

Ifosfamid and *trofosfamid* are structurally similar to cyclophosphamide. Ten infants whose mothers were treated with ifosfamid in combination with other cancer chemotherapeutic agents during pregnancy have been reported (NTP 2013), but only one of these women was treated during the first trimester (Shufaro 2002). None of the infants had major malformations. However, nine of these children were born prematurely, and oligohydramnios and fetal growth retardation were frequent.

Siepermann (2012) reported a child whose mother was treated with *trofosfamid, etoposide* and *idarubicin* during the second half of pregnancy. The baby was born without malformations and showed normal neurological development to age 2 years.

There are only three reports of maternal melphalan treatment in the first trimester of pregnancy, resulting in two miscarriages and one early therapeutic abortion (Zemlickis 1992, Jochimsen 1981). A mother who was treated in the first trimester with *bendamustine* gave birth to a healthy child (Schardein 2000). There is no experience in pregnancy with *estramustine*.

2.13.7   Other alkylating agents

Busulfan exerts its alkylating effect specifically on the bone marrow and is, therefore, used in preparation for bone marrow transplantation. At least 49 pregnancies, among them at least 31 with use during the first trimester, have been reported (NTP 2013, Selig 2012, Briggs 2011). At least six of these children or fetuses had malformations, but they differed in each case.

Malformations have been reported in two of 9 children born to women who were treated with *dacarbazine* during the first trimester of pregnancy (NTP 2013, Selig 2012). One child had microphtalmia with associated visual impairment (Li 2007), and another had metacarpal agenesis and hypoplasia of the thumb (Dilek 2006). Most infants born to women treated with dacarbazine later in pregnancy appear healthy at birth, although premature delivery and fetal growth retardation are frequent (NTP 2013, Selig 2012).

Four infants whose mothers were treated with *mechlorethamine* (*nitrogen mustard*) and other cytotoxic agents during the first trimester of pregnancy had major congenital anomalies, including oligodactyly in two cases (Thomas 1982, Garrett 1974) hydrocephalus in one (Zemlickis 1992), and renal hypoplasia in another (Mennuti 1975). At least a dozen infants without major birth defects have also been described following maternal mechlorethamine therapy in the first trimester, and a similar number have been reported following maternal exposure that did not begin before the second or third trimester (NTP 2013, Selig 2012).

Five of 15 infants born to women who were treated with *procarbazine* during the first trimester of pregnancy were reported to have major malformations (NTP 2013, Selig 2012). Four of these infants are described in the previous paragraph because their mothers were also treated with

Pregnancy

2.13 Antineoplastic drugs

mechlorethamine (Zemlickis 1992, Thomas 1982, Mennuti 1975, Garrett 1974). Another infant with cleft lip and palate has been described whose mother was not treated with mechlorethamine but who did receive other chemotherapeutic agents as well as *probarbazine* early in pregnancy (Mulvihill 1987).

Three apparently normal infants born to women who were treated with *temozolomide* during the second or third trimester of pregnancy have been reported (McGrane 2012, Bodner-Adler 2006, Ducray 2006). There is no reported experience with *thiophosphamide* or *treosulfan* treatment during pregnancy.

2.13.8   Cytotoxic anthracycline antibiotics

Anthracyclines, a class that includes *doxorubicin (adriamycin)*, *daunorubicin*, *epirubicin* and *idarubicin*, intercalate and damage DNA, inhibit topoisomerase II, and interfere with DNA and RNA synthesis. Anthracylcines are widely used in combination chemotherapy of a variety of malignant neoplasms.

First-trimester treatment with doxorubicin, usually in combination with other cancer chemotherapeutic drugs, has been described in more than 50 pregnancies (NTP 2013, Selig 2012). No congenital anomalies were seen in most of these infants, but four had digital and other skeletal malformations (Dilek 2006, Paskulin 2005, Thomas 1982, Ebert 1997), one had imperforate anus (Murray 1994), and another was reported to have microcephaly and hydrocephalus (Kim 1996).

Clinical series and case reports describe about 400 infants whose mothers were treated with doxorubicin, usually in combination with other chemotherapeutic agents, during the second or third trimester of pregnancy (NTP 2013, Selig 2012). Most of these children are reported to be healthy – few birth defects have been observed, but premature delivery, fetal growth retardation or myelosuppression may occur (NTP 2013, Cardonick 2010a, Hahn 2006). Because cardiotoxicity is a well-recognized adverse effect of daunorubicin treatment in children (Lipshultz 2006), fetal echocardiography and serial ultrasonography have been recommended for pregnancies in which the mother is treated with an anthracycline (Meyer-Wittkopf 2001).

There are reports of at least 13 pregnant women who were treated with daunorubicin during the first trimester of pregnancy (NTP 2013, Selig 2012). No malformations were observed in most of these infants, but one had polydactyly (Selig 2012), and another had multiple congenital anomalies, although daunorubicin is unlikely to have been responsible in this case (Artlich 1994). Experience with maternal treatment during the second or third trimester of pregnancy is much more extensive, and few birth defects have been reported among these infants (NTP 2013, Selig 2012, Germann 2004). However, fetal death or stillbirth has been described repeatedly after daunorubicin treatment in pregnancy (NTP 2013, Germann 2004), and one stillborn infant had diffuse myocardial necrosis (Schaison 1979), a finding that is of particular concern because cardiotoxicity is a well-recognized adverse effect of daunorubicin treatment in children (Lipshultz 2006). Transient myelosuppression has also been observed repeatedly among infants whose mothers were treated with daunorubicin late in pregnancy (NTP 2013).

More than 70 infants have been described whose mothers were treated with epirubicin and other cancer chemotherapeutic agents during pregnancy; almost all of these exposures occurred after completion of the first trimester (NTP 2013, Peccatori 2009, Mir 2008). There is one report of malformations in a fetus exposed to epirubicin, cyclophosphamide and 5-fluorouracil during the first trimester of pregnancy (Leyder 2011), but the pattern of skeletal and other anomalies resembles cyclophosphamide embryopathy (see Section 2.13.6). A normal outcome has been reported in four other pregnancies in which the mother was treated with epirubicin during the first trimester (Andreadis 2004, Avilés 1991). There are few congenital anomalies among the infants whose mothers were treated later in pregnancy, but many instances of premature delivery and occasional stillbirths and fetal deaths have been reported (NTP, 2013). Neonatal anemia and leukopenia have also been observed (Giacalone 1999, Cuvier 1997).

Only 19 infants whose mothers were treated with idarubicin and other cancer chemotherapeutic agents during pregnancy have been described, all with exposure during the second or third trimester (NTP 2013). Malformations were only seen in one child (Niedermeier 2005), but this infant and three others had evidence of prenatal or postnatal cardiac dysfunction that later resolved (Baumgärtner 2009, Siu 2002, Achtari 2000). This is of particular concern because cardiotoxicity is known to occur in some children who are treated with anthracyclines (Lipshultz 2006). Oligohydramnios, fetal growth retardation, fetal death, and premature delivery have been repeatedly reported in the pregnancies of women who were treated with combination chemotherapy that included idarubicin during the second or third trimester (NTP 2013).

Mitoxantrone is not a classic anthracycline but a related substance. No malformations were observed among 15 infants whose mothers received mitoxantrone and other cancer chemotherapeutic agents (NTP 2013, Selig 2012), but none of these treatments occurred during the first trimester. Three children whose mothers had been treated during pregnancy with *cytosine* and mitoxantrone for acute leukemia showed good long-term development (Avilés 2001). Mitoxantrone is also used as a second-line therapy in multiple sclerosis, but the published experience with this treatment in pregnancy is very limited (Houtchens 2013, Lu 2012). One report describes a woman with multiple sclerosis who was treated with mitoxantrone until the 30th week of gestation and subsequently developed oligohydramnios and fetal growth retardation; the infant had no malformations (de Santis 2007).

2.13.9   Other cytotoxic antibiotics

Bleomycin is a cytotoxic glycopeptide antibiotic, which is generally used in combination with other chemotherapeutic agents. Malformations (metacarpal agenesis and phalangeal hypoplasia of the thumb) were reported in one of 24 infants of women who were treated with bleomycin and other cytotoxic drugs during the first trimester of pregnancy (NTP 2013, Selig 2012, Dilek 2006). In one other case, the fetus was found to have toxic degenerative changes of the kidney and liver on pregnancy termination (Peres 2001). At least 80 infants whose mothers were treated with bleomycin during the second or third trimester of pregnancy have been reported (NTP 2013, Selig 2012). Most of these children had no congenital anomalies, but one infant had cerebral atrophy (Elit 1999), and another, who was born at 27 weeks gestation, had bilateral hearing loss (Raffles 1989). Many of these infants were delivered prematurely or were small for gestational age (NTP 2013).

Pregnancy

2.13 Antineoplastic drugs

No malformations were observed among 16 children whose mothers had been treated with *dactinomycin* (*actinomycin D*) during the second or third trimester of pregnancy, but premature delivery was very frequent (NTP 2013, Selig 2012). No information on the use of mitomycin during pregnancy is available.

2.13.10   Folate antagonists

▶ **Aminopterin**

As early as the 1950s, a characteristic pattern of malformations was described among children born following failed abortion attempts with *aminopterin* (Thiersch 1952). Typical features of this aminopterin embryopathy, which has been reported in more than a dozen children, include short stature, craniosynostosis, hydrocephalus, abnormal ears, wide-spaced eyes, small jaw, and cleft palate (Hyoun 2012, Warkany 1978).

▶ **High-dose methotrexate**

Methotrexate (also called *amethopterin*) is a methyl derivative of aminopterin and has replaced it in therapy. Methotrexate is used for a wide range of indications. Here we limit ourselves to experience with methotrexate in weekly doses of 10 mg or more, and often several times more (for low-dose methotrexate, see Chapter 2.12). Such doses are often used in combination with other antineoplastic agents for the treatment of cancer but may also be used for medical termination of ectopic or unwanted pregnancy or for treatment of severe immunopathic disease.

More than 25 children have been reported with a characteristic recurrent pattern of malformations following maternal treatment with 10 mg/week or more of methotrexate early in pregnancy (Hyoun 2012, Feldkamp 1993). Typical features of this methotrexate embryopathy include growth deficiency, abnormal head shape, craniosynostosis, wide-spaced eyes, abnormal ears, and skeletal defects. Intellectual disability may also occur. The pattern of anomalies is strikingly similar to the aminopterin embryopathy described above. The critical exposure period for classical methotrexate embryopathy appears to be 6–8 weeks after conception (Hyoun 2012, Feldkamp 1993), although a susceptibility to conotruncal heart defects may occur with maternal methotrexate treatment a little earlier in pregnancy (Hyoun 2012). Not surprisingly, methotrexate treatment early in pregnancy is also associated with miscarriage (Donnenfeld 1994, Kozlowski 1990).

Most infants born to women treated with methotrexate in doses above 10 mg/week in pregnancy appear normal (NTP 2013, Hyoun 2012, Selig 2012). The risk of methotrexate embryopathy is probably greater with higher dose treatment during the critical period of pregnancy, but apparently normal infants have been born to women treated with 150–1000 mg of methotrexate during the first trimester (Selig 2012). Prenatal diagnosis of major malformations associated with methotrexate embryopathy is sometimes possible by ultrasound examination in the second or third trimester (Usta 2007, Goffman 2006, Seidahmed 2006).

In the second and third trimesters of pregnancy, maternal treatment with high doses of methotrexate has been associated with fetal growth retardation, myelosuppression, premature delivery, and fetal death (NTP 2013).

▶ **Pemetrexed**

No pregnancies have been reported in which the mother was treated with the antimetabolite *pemetrexed*.

2.13.11   Purine antagonists

6-Mercaptopurine (6-MP) is a purine analog that inhibits nucleic acid synthesis (see Chapter 2.12 for discussion of *azathioprine*, a pro-drug of 6-mercaptopurine). At least 52 infants have been reported whose mothers were treated with 6-mercaptopurine, usually in combination with other medications for cancer or inflammatory bowel disease, during the first trimester of pregnancy (NTP 2013, Selig 2012, Polifka 2002). In most cases, the baby appeared normal at birth, but two children had multiple congenital anomalies. One had severe intrauterine growth retardation, cleft palate, bilateral microphthalmia and corneal opacity, hypoplastic thyroid and ovaries, and poorly developed external genitalia (Diamond 1960). The other child had pulmonary hypoplasia and dysplasia and malformations of the urinary bladder and urethra (Nørgård 2003). Other case reports describe an infant with polydactyly (Mulvihill 1987), one with hydrocephalus (Francella 2003), and a child with a notched uvula and auditory processing defect whose brother had a submucous cleft palate, bifid uvula, and partial meatal stenosis (Tegay 2002).

No major malformations have been observed among 41 children whose mothers were treated with 6-mercaptopurine during the second or third trimester of pregnancy (NTP 2013, Selig 2012), although preterm delivery, fetal growth retardation and transient myelosuppression are often seen (NTP 2013, Polifka 2002).

Thioguanine is a purine analog that inhibits DNA and RNA synthesis and causes cell death. Multiple skeletal malformations were observed in two case reports in which the mother was treated with thioguanine and *cytarabine* during the first trimester of pregnancy (Artlich 1994, Schafer 1981). No malformations were observed in at least seven other infants whose mothers had been treated with thioguanine during the first trimester (De Boer 2005, Schardein 2000). The frequency of congenital anomalies among infants born to women who were treated with thioguine later in pregnancy appears to be low, although prematurity and low birth weight are common (NTP 2013, Selig 2012).

No malformations were seen in the infant of woman who was treated during the first trimester of pregnancy with *cladribine* (Alothman 1994). Fetal growth retardation, transient neonatal cardiomyopathy and transient cerebral ventriculomegaly were observed in a premature infant whose mother was treated with *fludarabine* and other antineoplastic agents, including an *anthracycline*, during the second and third trimesters of pregnancy (Baumgärtner 2009). Fetal death occurred in another case after similar treatment (Paşa 2009). There have been no reports on the use of *nelarabine* or *clofarabine* during pregnancy.

2.13.12   Pyrimidine antagonists

The pyrimidine antagonist, *cytarabine* (also called *cytosine arabinoside*), is used to treat leukemia or non-Hodgkin lymphoma. The existence of

Pregnancy

2.13 Antineoplastic drugs

a cytarabine embryopathy has been suggested by the occurrence of an unusual pattern of limb malformations in four children whose mothers were treated with cytarabine early in pregnancy and by the observation of similar malformations in experimental teratology studies in laboratory animals (Vaux 2003). These four children had oligodactyly, ectrodactyly, or longitudinal hemimelia (Ebert 1997, Artlich 1994, Schafer 1981, Wagner 1980); one child also had bilateral microtia and another also had craniosynostosis. In addition, published case reports and clinical series describe at least 24 infants without malformations whose mothers were treated with cytarabine, usually in combination with other cancer chemotherapeutic agents, early in pregnancy (NTP 2013, Selig 2012).

More than 100 infants have been reported whose mothers were treated with cytarabine, usually in combination with other antineoplastic agents, in the second and third trimesters of pregnancy (NTP 2013, Selig 2012). Congenital anomalies are infrequent among these children and do not appear to be related to the maternal treatment. Premature delivery is common, and transient myelosuppression has been described repeatedly in infants whose mothers were treated with cytarabine late in pregnancy (NTP 2013). Fetal death also appears to be relatively frequent after treatment of pregnant women with cancer chemotherapy that includes cytarabine (NTP 2013).

5-Fluorouracil (5-FU) is a pyrimidine analog that interferes with DNA and RNA synthesis. At least five fetuses or infants with major malformations have been reported after treatment of the mother with 5-fluorouracil during the first trimester of pregnancy. In one case, a causal relationship is unlikely because the malformations probably developed before the treatment began (Stephens 1980); the malformations were not described in a second case (Rosa, cited in Briggs 2011). One child whose mother was treated with 5-flurouracil and methotrexate from gestational week 7.5 through gestational week 28 and also had radiation therapy during the second trimester had microcephaly and associated minor anomalies (Bawle 1998). In two other cases, a mother who was treated with 5-fluorouracil during the first trimester of pregnancy had a fetus or infant with distal limb malformations and other anomalies (microcephaly, cerebral ventriculomegaly, prenatal onset growth retardation and bicuspid aortic valve in one instance and micrognathia in the other) (Leyder 2011, Paskulin 2005). Although these malformations have been attributed to concurrent therapy with *cyclophosphamide*, this interpretation may not be correct – skeletal malformations have also been produced by 5-fluorouracil treatment of pregnant rodents or rabbits in experimental studies (Kuwagata 1998, Naya 1997, DeSesso 1994). In at least nine other cases, maternal systemic treatment with 5-fluorouracil during the first trimester of pregnancy was followed by the delivery of an apparently normal infant (NTP 2013).

No malformations were observed in eight infants whose mothers were treated during the first trimester of pregnancy or two infants whose mothers were treated in periconceptinal period with topical 5-fluorouracil applied to the vulva or vagina (Van Le 1991, Kopelman 1990, Odom 1990) (see Chapter 2.17).

Congenital anomalies did not appear to be unusually frequent among more than 160 infants whose mothers were treated with 5-fluorouracil during the second or third trimesters of pregnancy (NTP 2013, Selig 2012).

Congenital anomalies were not noted in three infants whose mothers were treated with *gemcitabine* during the second or third trimester of pregnancy (Cardonick 2010b, Gurumurthy 2009, Kim 2008). All three children were delivered prematurely, and two of them had neonatal anemia.

An apparently normal infant was born to a woman who had been treated with *capecitabine* and *oxaliplatin* during the first trimester of pregnancy (Cardonick 2010b). No information has been reported on pregnancies in women who were treated with *azacitidine*.

2.13.13   Taxanes and other cytostatic agents

▶ **Taxanes**

Taxanes inhibit cell division by interfering with microtubule function.

Paclitaxel is an alkaloid produced by yew trees. Growth retardation but no malformations occurred in an infant whose mother was treated with paclitaxel and *carboplatin* during the first trimester of pregnancy (Cardonick 2012). At least 40 infants whose mothers were treated with paclitaxel during the second or third trimester, usually in combination with other antineoplastic agents, have been reported (NTP 2013, Selig 2012). Two of these children were noted to have anomalies – one infant had pyloric stenosis (Cardonick 2010a, 2012) and the other was a twin with Tourette syndrome, dyslexia, and Asperger syndrome whose co-twin was normal (Cardonick 2012). Two of the pregnancies were complicated by oligohydramnios (Shieh 2011, Bader 2007), but one of the mothers was concurrently treated with *trastuzumab*, which has been strongly associated with the development of oligohydramnios (Zagouri 2013).

Docetaxel is a structural analog of paclitaxel. There are three case reports on its use in combination with other chemotherapeutic agents during the first trimester of pregnancy; none of these infants was noted to have birth defects (Massey Skatulla 2012, Kim 2008, Ibrahim 2006). At least 20 infants whose mothers were treated with docetaxel in combination with other antineoplastic drugs during the second or third trimesters of pregnancy have been reported (NTP 2013). Most of the infants were normal, but the woman mentioned in the previous paragraph who was treated with paclitaxel beginning in the second trimester of pregnancy and subsequently gave birth to an infant with pyloric stenosis was also treated with docetaxal late in the pregnancy (Cardonick 2010a, 2012).

▶ **Other cytostatics**

Bortezomib is a proteasome-inhibitor that has been used to treat multiple myeloma and other tumors. *Trabectedin* inhibits cellular proliferation by blocking DNA excision repair. There is no reported experience with either bortezomib or trabectedin therapy during pregnancy.

2.13.14   Monoclonal antibodies

Antibodies directed to various tumor antigens are used to treat a variety of malignancies. Because maternally-produced isoantibodies and autoantibodies are well-recognized causes of fetal damage in conditions like Rh hemolytic disease (Eder 2006) and congenital heart block (Krishnan 2012), the administration of anti-tumor antibodies to pregnant women has been a cause of concern. This is exacerbated because therapeutic antibodies, once administered, often remain in the mother's circulation for months, because antibodies are actively transported across the placenta in later pregnancy, and because animal teratology studies, which are routinely used to assess the safety of new medications, may not be useful for many therapeutic antibodies because of their species specificity.

Trastuzumab is a "humanized" mouse IgG-antibody against epidermal growth factor receptor-2 (also called HER2). Trastuzumab therapy is used in the treatment of breast cancer, gastric cancer and other cancers that overexpress the HER2 gene. No malformations were reported among 12 infants whose mothers were treated with trastuzumab during the first trimester of pregnancy, but reduced amounts of amniotic fluid were observed in most of at least 16 pregnancies in which treatment occurred during the second or third trimester (NTP 2013, Zagouri 2013, Selig 2012). The infants born of these pregnancies often had neonatal renal dysfunction or neonatal respiratory distress, and four of them died within the first few months of life (Beale 2009, Warraich 2009, Weber-Schöndorfer 2008, Witzel 2008).

Rituximab is a chimeric mouse-human IgG-antibody directed against CD20, a protein expressed on the surface of B-lymphocytes. Rituximab is used to treat non-Hodgkin's lymphomas and chronic lymphocytic leukemia as well as rheumatoid arthritis and other immunopathic diseases. One infant whose mother was treated with rituximab in the first trimester of pregnancy (NTP 2013) was reported to have a major congenital anomaly – a ventricular septal defect (Chakravarty 2011). This report also includes a pregnancy that was terminated in which the fetus was found to have trisomy 13; the mother had been treated at some point with rituximab, but when the treatment occurred with respect to conception of the affected fetus is not stated. Another woman is reported to have had twins, one of whom had a club foot, but the nature and timing of her treatment are not described (Chakravarty 2011). This report also includes 88 live-born infants whose mothers were treated with rituximab sometime before delivery, and usually before conception, who are said to have had healthy infants. It is impossible to determine from these data, which were obtained from the manufacturer's routine postmarketing surveillance, how many of the pregnancies were actually exposed to rituximab (Chakravarty 2011). There are also several reports of transient myelosuppression involving B-lymphocytes, granulocytes, or red blood cells in various combinations after maternal rituximab treatment during or before pregnancy (NTP 2013, Gall 2010, Decker 2006).

There is no reported experience with pregnancy outcomes after maternal treatment with *alemtuzumab, cetuximab, catumaxomab, ibritumomab-tiuxetan, ofatumumab* or *panitumumab* during pregnancy. For *bevacizumab*, see Chapter 2.12.

2.13.15   Platin compounds

Cisplatin, carboplatin, and *oxaliplatin* crosslink DNA and also act as alkylating agents. These drugs are used to treat a variety of solid tumors, often in combination with other cancer chemotherapeutic agents.

A woman who was treated with cisplatin, *cyclophosphamide* and *doxorubicin* in the first trimester of pregnancy had a child with blepharophimosis, microcephaly and enlarged cerebral ventricles (Kim 1996). In another case, a woman who was treated with *carmustine, dacarbazine*, and *tamoxifen* in the first trimester of pregnancy had a child with microphthalmia and visual impairment (Li 2007). At least four other cases have been reported in which a child without congenital anomalies was born after maternal ciplatin treatment during the first trimester (NTP 2013, Selig 2012).

More than 100 infants whose mothers were treated with cisplatin, usually in combination with other anticancer drugs, during the second or third trimester of pregnancy have been described (NTP 2013, Selig 2012). Most of these children were born without apparent malformations, although one had cerebral atrophy and vetriculomegaly (Elit 1999). Many of the infants were born prematurely, and transient neonatal bone marrow suppression has been repeatedly reported (NTP 2013).

Gastroschisis was observed in a spontaneously aborted fetus whose mother was treated with carboplatin alone during the second trimester of pregnancy (Cardonick 2010b), but it seems likely that the malformation developed before the treatment in this case. Sixteen other women who were treated with carboplatin during the second trimester of pregnancy are reported to have had infants without birth defects (NTP 2013, Selig 2012). No experience with first-trimester treatment has been described.

Four infants have been reported whose mothers were treated with oxaliplatin during the first trimester of pregnancy (NTP 2013). One of these babies, whose mother was also treated with *vinorelbine* and *irinotecan*, was born with cleft lip, cleft palate, and esophageal atresia with tracheoesophageal fistula (Abellar 2009). One of two infants born after maternal oxaliplatin treatment in the second and third trimesters of pregnancy had congenital hypothyroidism (Kanate 2009). No congenital anomalies were reported in any of the other children whose mothers were treated with oxaliplatin during pregnancy.

2.13.16   Thalidomide and its analogs

Although thalidomide was removed from the market throughout the world in 1961–62 after recognition that it had caused severe malformations in an estimated 10,000 children, it was reintroduced for the treatment of leprosy and has subsequently been used as an immunomodulatory drug in conditions like systemic lupus erythematosus and graft-versus host disease. More recently, thalidomide has been used to treat multiple myeloma, myelodysplasia and other neoplasms (Xu 2013). *Lenalidomide* and *pomalidomide* are structural analogs of thalidomide and are also used for the treatment of multiple myeloma and other neoplastic conditions (Saini 2013). Special precautions have been put into place to avoid prescribing thalidomide and its analogs to women who are, or may become, pregnant during treatment (BfArM 2013, Celgene REMS Program 2013).

A characteristic embryopathy occurs frequently among the children of women who have been treated with thalidomide between 34 and 50 days after the beginning of the mother's last menstrual period (Miller 1999, Smithells 1992). Typical features of thalidomide embryopathy have been described in children of women who took as little as one 50 mg capsule during this time. Limb reduction defects are the most characteristic feature: the upper limbs are usually involved in a symmetrical fashion, and the preaxial bones, especially the thumb, are most often affected. In the lower limbs, which are less frequently involved, long bone deficiency or absence, club feet, and supernumary toes are most often seen. People with thalidomide embryopathy may also have microtia, ocular abnormalities, cardoivascular malformations, and neurodevelopmental disorders.

There is no reported experience with lenalidomide or pomalidomide treatment in human pregnancies, but their chemical similarity to thalidomide raises serious concern that they also can produce serious birth defects. Treatment of pregnant macaques with lenalidomide in doses similar to or greater than those used in humans causes limb and other malformations in the offspring (Amin 2009).

2.13.17   Tyrosine kinase inhibitors

About 100 infants whose mothers were treated with the tyrosine kinase inhibitor *imatinib* for chronic myelogenous leukemia or gastrointestinal stromal tumor during the first trimester of pregnancy have been described (NTP 2013, Selig 2012, Ali 2009, Pye 2008). The exact number of exposed pregnancies, and the number of infants with birth defects are unclear because some of the cases are probably reported more than once. In addition, many of the cases were not identified until after the outcome of the pregnancy was known, so that the reported experience is likely to be biased toward abnormal outcomes. Malformations observed among the children of women who were treated with imatinib early in pregnancy include omphalocele (3 cases), congenital heart defects (3 cases), hypospadias (3 cases), unilateral renal agenesis (2 cases), and hemivertebrae (2 cases). Babies with hydrocephalus, craniosynostosis or meningocele have also been noted. Five of the infants had multiple congenital anomalies, including a fetus with warfarin embryopathy whose mother was also treated with warfarin (Pye 2008). Most of the infants whose mothers were treated with imatinib early in pregnancy appeared normal at birth.

Very little experience is available with use of other tyrosine kinase inhibitors in pregnancy. A pregnant woman who conceived while on imatinib therapy was switched to *dasatinib* therapy at about 3 weeks gestation, and at 16 weeks was found to have fetal hydrops (Berveiller 2012). The pregnancy was terminated, and no cause for the hydrops was found on fetal autopsy. Apparently normal infants have been born to four other women who were treated with dasantinib during the first trimester of pregnancy (Conchon 2010, Kroll 2010, Cortes 2008).

An apparently healthy infant was born to a woman who received *nilotinib* therapy in the first trimester of pregnancy (Conchon 2009).

Gefitinib is an epidermal growth factor receptor inhibitor that is used to treat non-small cell lung cancer. One case has described a healthy infant whose mother was treated with gefitinib during the third trimester of pregnancy (Lee 2011).

A healthy child without congenital anomalies was born to a woman who was treated with *erlotinib* monotherapy for the first 8 weeks of pregnancy (Zambelli 2007). In another case in which erotinib treatment was continued throughout pregnancy, oligohydramnios and fetal growth retardation occurred in the third trimester, but no malformations were present in the infant (Rivas 2012). A healthy infant was also delivered to a woman who was treated with erlotinib for a short time during the third trimester of pregnancy (Lee 2011).

No congenital anomalies and normal development in infancy were observed in a child whose mother was treated with *lapatinib* during the first and second trimesters of pregnancy (Kelly 2006). No information about women who were treated with *sorafenib* or *sunitinib* during pregnancy has been reported.

2.13.18 Antineoplastic drugs with endocrine effects

The estrogen antagonist *tamoxifen* is used to treat breast cancer. A summary of the outcomes of pregnancies in women who had been treated with tamoxifen include spontaneous adverse experience reports submitted to the manufacturer, as well as previously published cases and series (Braems 2011). Most infants born to women treated with tamoxifen in pregnancy appear normal at birth, but congenital anomalies were described in 15 live-born infants, two stillbirths and six fetuses from pregnancies that had been terminated (NTP 2013, Braems 2011). The anomalies observed after maternal treatment in the first trimester included genital ambiguity in female infants (Braems 2011, Tewari 1997), Goldenhar syndrome (Cullins 1994), Pierre-Robinson sequence (Berger 2008), idiopathic chylothorax (Braems 2011), microphthalmus and severe far-sightedness (Li 2007), and two cases in which "fetal defects" were not further described (Braems 2011). In two other instances, malformations were reported after maternal tamoxifen treatment later in pregnancy, and a vaginal adenoma was observed in a 2.5-year-old girl after maternal treatment late in pregnancy (Braems 2011). Several other birth defects occurred after tamoxifen treatment at an unknown time during pregnancy. The congenital anomalies varied from cases to case, but minor genital anomalies were noted in female infants in two instances (Braems 2011). Many of the cases were not identified until after the outcome of the pregnancy was known, so the reported experience is likely to be biased toward abnormal outcomes and the total number of exposed pregnancies is unknown.

There is no experience during pregnancy with the estrogen antagonists *toremifene* and *fulvestrant*.

The aromatase inhibitors, *letrozole*, *anastrozole*, and *exemestane*, are used in the therapy of hormone-dependent breast cancer and also in the treatment of infertility. The frequency of congenital anomalies among 514 infants born to women in whom ovulation had been induced with letrozole was no higher than expected in a retrospective cohort study performed through five fertility centers (Tulandi 2006). Similarly, no congenital anomalies were observed among 112 infants whose mothers had conceived after ovulation induced with letrozole in a partially overlapping clinical series (Forman 2007). These findings are inconsistent with an earlier report from one of these centers that higher frequencies of "locomotor malformations" and cardiac anomalies occurred among infants born to women whose ovulation had been induced with letrozole (Biljan 2005). Two (6.6%) of 30 infants born to women whose ovulation had been induced with letrozole had major congenital anomalies in another series (Badawy 2009). None of these studies provides any information about the effects of maternal letrozole treatment during embryogenesis.

There are no reports of infant outcomes following treatment of women with *anastrozole* or *exemestane* during pregnancy. No congenital anomalies were observed among 11 infants born to women whose ovulation had been induced with anastrozole (Badawy 2009).

Goserelin is an LHRH agonist that is used for the treatment of hormone-responsive breast cancer. Apparently normal female infants were born to two women who were treated with goserelin throughout the first trimester of pregnancy (Ishizuka 2013, Jiménez-Gordo 2000). Another woman who was treated with goserelin during the first and second trimester of pregnancy developed severe oligohydramnios, and her baby died of pulmonary hypoplasia shortly after delivery (Warraich 2009). This woman also received *trastuzumab* treatment, which is strongly associated with the development of oligohydramnios (Zagouri 2013; Section 2.13.14).

Pregnancy

2.13 Antineoplastic drugs

Mitotane, which suppresses and is cytotoxic to adrenal cortex, is used to treat adrenal carcinoma. No malformations have been observed in one embryo, one fetus or three infants whose mothers were treated with mitotane early in pregnancy (Tripto-Shkolnik 2013, Kojori 2011, Gerl 1992, Leiba 1989, Luton 1973). Histological abnormalities of the adrenal anlage were seen in an embryo that was therapeutically aborted because the mother became pregnant while being treated with mitotane (Leiba 1989).

The progestins, *medroxyprogesterone acetate* and *megestrol acetate*, are used at high doses to treat endometrial cancer and metastastic breast cancer. Virilization of the genitalia of female infants whose mothers were treated with other synthetic progestins during pregnancy has been repeatedly reported (Schardein 1980, 2000) and has been described at least twice after maternal medroxyprogesterone acetate treatment during prenancy (Burstein 1964, Eichner 1963). There have also been occasional reports of hypospadias in boys whose mothers were treated during pregnancy with synthetic progestins (Schardein 1980, 2000). This has been reported three times after maternal medroxyprogesterone acetate treatment (Harlap 1975, Aarskog 1970, Goldman 1967) and once after high-dose therapy with megestrol acetate (Farrar 1997). See Chapter 2.15 which discusses the effects of lower dose medroxyprogesterone acetate treatment for other indications.

2.13.19   Other antineoplastic agents

Hydroxycarbamide (also called *hydroxyurea*) is an antimetabolite that interferes with DNA synthesis and repair. Hydroxycarbamide is used in the treatment of melanoma, chronic myeloid leukemia, and a variety of solid tumors. Other uses include therapy for essential thrombocythemia, polycythemia vera and sickle cell disease. Much of the reported experience with hydroxycarbamide treatment during pregnancy has been for these non-neoplastic conditions.

An infant with vertebral anomalies, ambiguous genitalia and growth retardation was born to a woman with a familial chronic myeloproliferative syndrome that was treated with hydroxycarbamide early in pregnancy (Pérez-Encinas 1994). More than two dozen other apparently normal infants have been described whose mothers were treated with hydroxycarbamide during the first trimester of pregnancy (NTP 2013, Selig 2012). Among a similar number of infants born after maternal hydroxycarbamide treatment later in pregnancy, one had pyloric stenosis (Heartin 2004) and two others had congenital anomalies that developed during the first trimester and therefore cannot be attributed to the maternal treatment (Ault 2006, Choudhary 2006).

Tretinoin (all-trans-retinoic acid, ATRA) is used orally in the treatment of acute myelocytic or promyelocytic leukemia. Systemic tretinoin therapy in the first trimester of pregnancy is assumed to have teratogenic potential because isotretinoin, a stereoisomer of tretinoin, is strongly teratogenic when taken at therapeutic doses early in human pregnancy (Lammer 1985, see also Chapter 2.17), because retinoic acid plays an important role in normal embryogenesis (Rhinn 2012), and because teratogenic effects have been observed in pregnant monkeys, rabbits, and rodents treated systemically with tretinoin in doses similar to or greater than those used to treat leukemia in humans (Kochhar 1997). Only two infants whose mothers were treated with tretinoin during the first trimester of pregnancy have been described (NTP 2013, Simone 1995); neither was reported to have malformations. About 30 infants whose mothers were treated with tretinoin later in pregnancy, usually in combination with other chemotherapeutic agents, have been reported (NTP 2013, Yang 2009, Valappil 2007). One infant had bilateral renal agenesis, which must have occurred before the treatment began (Sham 1996), and another infant had a transient cardiomyopathy that was attributed to maternal *idarubicin* therapy (Siu 2002). Two others had cardiac arrhythmias in infancy (Terada 1997, Harrison 1994). No congenital anomalies were described in any of the other children.

Bexarotene is a synthetic retinoid that is used to treat cutaneous T-cell lymphoma. No reports of infants whose mothers were treated with bexarotene during pregnancy are available, but such treatment during the first trimester may be associated with a high risk of malformations because baxarotene is a retinoid.

Arsenic trioxide is used intravenously for the treatment of acute promyelocytic leukemia. Although there is no reported experience with this treatment in human pregnancy, the toxicity of arsenic in adults (Miller 2002) and the embryotoxic and teratogenic activity that has been demonstrated in experimental animal studies (DeSesso 2001) raise concern about damage to the embryo or fetus with maternal arsenic trioxide treatment in human pregnancy. See also Chapter 2.22.2.

An infant with cleft lip and palate, esophageal atresia, and tracheoesophageal fistula was born to a woman who was treated throughout pregnancy with *oxaliplatin, vinorelbine* and the topoisomerase inhibitor, *irinotecan* (Abellar 2009). No malformations were observed in two other children whose mothers were treated with irinotecan during the second half of pregnancy (Cirillo 2012, Taylor 2009). No information is available on the effects of topotecan treatment in human pregnancy.

Asparaginase is a bacterial enzyme that reduces the availability of asparagine, an amino acid that is necessary for the growth of some tumor cells. Asparaginase is used in combination with other chemotherapeutics to treat acute leukemia or lymphoma. A woman who was treated with asparaginase during the first trimester of pregnancy had a stillborn baby with polydacyly (Selig 2012). No major malformations were observed in at least 18 other infants whose mothers were treated with asparaginase during pregnancy; only one of these women was treated during the first trimester (NTP 2013, Selig 2012). *Pegaspargase* is asparaginase conjugated with polyethylene glycol. There is no reported experience with pegaspargase treatment in pregnancy.

An apparently normal child was born to a woman who was treated with amsacrine during the first trimester of pregnancy (Blatt 1980). No congenital anomalies were seen in an infant whose mother was treated with amasacrine and other drugs during the third trimester, but transient neonatal myelosuppression occurred (Udink ten Cate 2009).

High-dose *celecoxib* is used to reduce the number of intestinal polyps in familial adenomatous polyposis. (For lower doses of celecoxib as an anti-inflammatory agent in pregnancy, see Chapter 2.1.) No reports of maternal high-dose celecoxib use during pregnancy are available, but a significant association with the mother receiving a prescription for celecoxib during pregnancy was observed in a case-control study of 4705 spontaneous abortions (Nakhai-Pour 2011). This drug inhibits prostaglandin synthesis, and treatment of a woman late in pregnancy would be expected to produce premature closure of the fetal ductus arteriosus and consequent changes in neonatal cardiovascular function, as occurs with other drugs of this class.

There is no reported experience with use of the following substances in pregnancy: *aldesleukin, methyl-(5-amino-4-oxo-pentanoate) (methyl aminolevulinate), miltefosine, pentostatin, porfimer sodium, temoporfin,* or *temsirolimus.* For *everolimus,* see Chapter 2.12.

References

Aarskog D. Clinical and cytogenetic studies in hypospadias. Acta Paediatr Scand 1970; 203: 7–62.

Abdel-Hady el-S, Hemida RA, Gamal A et al. Cancer during pregnancy: perinatal outcome after in utero exposure to chemotherapy. Arch Gynecol Obstet 2012; 286: 283–6.

Abellar RG, Pepperell JR, Greco D et al. Effects of chemotherapy during pregnancy on the placenta. Pediatr Dev Pathol 2009; 12: 35–41.

Achtari C, Hohlfeld P. Cardiotoxic transplacental effect of idarubicin administered during the second trimester of pregnancy. Am J Obstet Gynecol 2000; 183: 511–2.

Ali R, Ozkalemkas F, Kimya Y et al. Imatinib use during pregnancy and breast feeding: a case report and review of the literature. Arch Gynecol Obstet 2009; 280: 169–75.

Alothman A, Sparling TG. Managing hairy cell leukemia in pregnancy. Ann Intern Med 1994; 120: 1048–9.

Amant F, Loibl S, Neven P, Van Calsteren K. Breast cancer in pregnancy. Lancet 2012a; 379: 570–9.

Amant F, Van Calsteren K, Halaska MJ et al. Long-term cognitive and cardiac outcomes after prenatal exposure to chemotherapy in children aged 18 months or older: an observational study. Lancet Oncol 2012b; 13: 256–64.

Amant F, von Minckwitz G, Han SN et al. Prognosis of Women With Primary Breast Cancer Diagnosed During Pregnancy: Results From an International Collaborative Study. J Clin Oncol 2013; 31: 2532–9.

Amin RP, Fuchs A, Christian MS et al. An embryo-fetal developmental toxicity study of lenalidomide in cynomolgus monkeys. Birth Defects Res A Clin Mol Teratol 2009; 85: 435.

Andreadis C, Charalampidou M, Diamantopoulos N et al. Combined chemotherapy and radiotherapy during conception and first two trimesters of gestation in a woman with metastatic breast cancer. Gynecol Oncol 2004; 95: 252–5.

Artlich A, Möller J, Tschakaloff A et al. Teratogenic effects in a case of maternal treatment for acute myelocytic leukaemia – neonatal and infantile course. Eur J Pediatr 1994; 153: 488–1.

Ault P, Kantarjian H, O'Brien S et al. Pregnancy among patients with chronic myeloid leukemia treated with imatinib. J Clin Oncol 2006; 24: 1204–8.

Avilés A, Diaz Maqueo JC, Talavera A et al. Growth and development of children of mothers treated with chemotherapy during pregnancy: current status of 43 children. Am J Hematol 1991; 36: 243–8.

Avilés A, Neri N. Hematological malignancies and pregnancy: a final report of 84 children who received chemotherapy in utero. Clin Lymphoma 2001; 2: 173–7.

Avilés A, Niz J. Long-term follow-up of children born to mothers with acute leukemia during pregnancy. Med Pediatr Oncol 1988; 16: 3–6.

Azim HA Jr, Del Mastro L, Scarfone G, Peccatori FA. Treatment of breast cancer during pregnancy: regimen selection, pregnancy monitoring and more. Breast 2011; 20: 1–6.

Azim HA Jr, Pavlidis N, Peccatori FA. Treatment of the pregnant mother with cancer: a systematic review on the use of cytotoxic, endocrine, targeted agents and immunotherapy during pregnancy. Part II: Hematological tumors. Cancer Treat Rev 2010; 36: 110–21.

Azim HA Jr, Santoro L, Russell-Edu W et al. Prognosis of pregnancy-associated breast cancer: a meta-analysis of 30 studies. Cancer Treat Rev 2012; 38: 834–42.

Backes CH, Moorehead PA, Nelin LD. Cancer in pregnancy: fetal and neonatal outcomes. Clin Obstet Gynecol 2011; 54: 574–90.

Badawy A, Shokeir T, Allam AF et al. Pregnancy outcome after ovulation induction with aromatase inhibitors or clomiphene citrate in unexplained infertility. Acta Obstet Gynecol Scand 2009; 88: 187–91.

Bader AA, Schlembach D, Tamussino KF et al. Anhydramnios associated with administration of trastuzumab and paclitaxel for metastatic breast cancer during pregnancy. Lancet Oncol 2007; 8: 79–81.

Baumgärtner AK, Oberhoffer R, Jacobs VR et al. Reversible foetal cerebral ventriculomegaly and cardiomyopathy under chemotherapy for maternal AML. Onkologie 2009; 32: 40–3.

Bawle EV, Conard JV, Weiss L. Adult and two children with fetal methotrexate syndrome. Teratology 1998; 57: 51–5.

Beale JM, Tuohy J, McDowell SJ. Herceptin (trastuzumab) therapy in a twin pregnancy with associated oligohydramnios. Am J Obstet Gynecol 2009; 201: e13–4.

Ben-Aharon I, Gafter-Gvili A, Leibovici L et al. Pharmacological interventions for fertility preservation during chemotherapy: a systematic review and meta-analysis. Breast Cancer Res Treat 2010; 122: 803–11.

Benjapibal M, Chaopotong P, Leelaphatanadit C et al. Ruptured ovarian endodermal sinus tumor diagnosed during pregnancy: case report and review of the literature. J Obstet Gynaecol Res 2010; 36: 1137–41.

Berger JC, Clericuzio CL. Pierre Robin sequence associated with first trimester fetal tamoxifen exposure. Am J Med Genet A 2008; 146A: 2141–4.

Berveiller P, Andreoli A, Mir O et al. A dramatic fetal outcome following transplacental transfer of dasatinib. Anticancer Drugs 2012; 23: 754–7.

Biljan MM, Hemmings R, Brassard N. The outcome of 150 babies following the treatment with letrozole or letrozole and gonadotropins. Fertil Steril 2005; 84: S95 (abstract O-231).

Blatt J, Mulvihill JJ, Ziegler JL et al. Pregnancy outcome following cancer chemotherapy. Am J Med 1980; 69: 828–32.

Bodner-Adler B, Bodner K, Zeisler H. Primitive neuroectodermal tumor (PNET) of the brain diagnosed during pregnancy. Anticancer Res 2006; 26: 2499–501.

Braems G, Denys H, De Wever O et al. Use of tamoxifen before and during pregnancy. Oncologist 2011; 16: 1547–51.

Brewer M, Kueck A, Runowicz CD. Chemotherapy in pregnancy. Clin Obstet Gynecol 2011; 54: 602–18.

Briggs GG, Freeman RK, Yaffe SJ. Drugs in Pregnancy and Lactation, 9th edn, Baltimore: Williams & Wilkins 2011.

Brudie LA, Ahmad S, Radi MJ, Finkler NJ. Metastatic choriocarcinoma in a viable intrauterine pregnancy treated with EMA-CO in the third trimester: a case report. J Reprod Med 2011; 56: 359–63.

Buller RE, Darrow V, Manetta A et al. Conservative surgical management of dysgerminoma concomitant with pregnancy. Obstet Gynecol 1992; 79: 887–890.

BfArM. Bundesinstitut für Arzneimittel und Medizinprodukte, 2013: Bekanntmachung zur Arzneimittelverschreibungsverordnung (AMVV) thalidomide/lenalidomide/pomalidomide Available online at http://www.bfarm.de/EN/Home/home_node.html.

Burstein R, Wasserman HC. The effect of Provera on the fetus. Obstet Gynecol 1964; 23: 931–4.

Cardonick E, Bhat A, Gilmandyar D, Somer R. Maternal and fetal outcomes of taxane chemotherapy in breast and ovarian cancer during pregnancy: case series and review of the literature. Ann Oncol 2012; 23: 3016–23.

Cardonick E, Dougherty R, Grana G et al. Breast cancer during pregnancy: maternal and fetal outcomes. Cancer J 2010a; 16: 76–82.

Cardonick E, Usmani A, Ghaffar S. Perinatal outcomes of a pregnancy complicated by cancer, including neonatal follow-up after in utero exposure to chemotherapy: results of an international registry. Am J Clin Oncol 2010b; 33: 221–8.

Celgene REMS Program. 2013; Available online at www.celgeneriskmanagement.com/REMS-Portal/rems/portal/REMSPortal.portal.

Chakravarty EF, Murray ER, Kelman A et al. Pregnancy outcomes after maternal exposure to rituximab. Blood 2011; 117: 1499–506.

Choudhary DR, Mishra P, Kumar R et al. Pregnancy on imatinib: fatal outcome with meningocele. Ann Oncol 2006; 17: 178–9.

Cirillo M, Musola M, Cassandrini PA et al. Irinotecan during pregnancy in metastatic colon cancer. Tumori 2012; 98: 155e-7e.

Colfry AJ III. Miscellaneous syndromes and their management: occult breast cancer, breast cancer in pregnancy, male breast cancer, surgery in stage IV disease. Surg Clin North Am 2013; 93:519–31.

Conchon M, Sanabani SS, Bendit I et al. Two successful pregnancies in a woman with chronic myeloid leukemia exposed to nilotinib during the first trimester of her second pregnancy: case study. J Hematol Oncol 2009; 2: 42.

Conchon M, Sanabani SS, Serpa M et al. Successful pregnancy and delivery in a patient with chronic myeloid leukemia while on dasatinib therapy. Adv Hematol 2010; 2010: 136252.

Cortes J, O'Brien S, Ault P et al. Pregnancy outcomes among patients with chronic myeloid leukemia treated with dasatinib [Abstract]. Blood 2008; 112: 3230.

Cullins SL, Pridjian G, Sutherland CM. Goldenhar's syndrome associated with tamoxifen given to the mother during gestation (letter). JAMA 1994; 271: 1905–6.

Pregnancy

2.13 Antineoplastic drugs

Cuvier C, Espie M, Extra JM, Marty M. Vinorelbine in pregnancy. Eur J Cancer 1997; 33: 168–9.

De Boer NK, van Elburg RM, Wilhelm AJ et al. 6-Thioguanine for Crohn's disease during pregnancy: thiopurine metabolite measurements in both mother and child. Scand J Gastroenterol 2005; 40: 1374–7.

De Santis M, Straface G, Cavaliere AF et al. The first case of mitoxantrone exposure in early pregnancy. Neurotoxicology 2007; 28: 696–7.

Decker M, Rothermundt C, Holländer G et al. Rituximab plus CHOP for treatment of diffuse large B-cell lymphoma during second trimester of pregnancy. Lancet Oncol 2006; 7: 693–4. Erratum in: Lancet Oncol 2006; 7: 706.

DeSesso JM, Scialli AR, Goeringer GC. Developmental toxicity of 5-fluorouracil and amelioration by folate analogs in the New Zealand white rabbit embryo. Teratology 1994; 49: 369.

DeSesso JM. Teratogen update: inorganic arsenic. Teratology 2001; 64: 170–3.

Diamond I, Anderson MM, McCreadie SR. Transplacental transmission of busulfan (myleran) in a mother with leukemia. Production of fetal malformation and cytomegaly. Pediatrics 1960; 25: 85–90.

Dilek I, Topcu N, Demir C et al. Hematological malignancy and pregnancy: a single-institution experience of 21 cases. Clin Lab Haematol 2006; 28: 170–6.

DiPaola RS, Goodin S, Ratzell M et al. Chemotherapy for metastatic melanoma during pregnancy. Gynecol Oncol 1997; 66: 526–30.

Doney KC, Kraemer KG, Shepard TH. Combination chemotherapy for acute myelocytic leukemia during pregnancy: three case reports. Cancer Treat Rep 1979; 63: 369–71.

Donnenfeld AE, Pasuszak A, Noah J et al. Methotrexate exposure prior to and during pregnancy. Teratology 1994; 49: 79–81.

Ducray F, Colin P, Cartalat-Carel S et al. Management of malignant gliomas diagnosed during pregnancy. Rev Neurol (Paris) 2006; 162: 322–9.

Ebert U, Loffler H, Kirch W. Cytotoxic therapy and pregnancy. Pharmacol Ther 1997; 74: 207–20.

Eder AF. Update on HDFN: new information on long-standing controversies. Immunohematology 2006; 22: 188–95.

Eichner E. The clinical uses of Provest. Int J Fertil 1963; 8: 673–80.

Elit L, Bocking A, Kenyon C et al. An endodermal sinus tumor diagnosed in pregnancy: case report and review of the literature. Gynecol Oncol 1999; 72: 123–7.

Enns GM, Roeder E, Chan RT et al. Apparent cyclophosphamide (Cytoxan) embryopathy: a distinct phenotype? Am J Med Genet 1999; 86: 237–41.

Falconer AD, Fernis P. Pregnancy outcomes following treatment of cancer. J Obstet Gynaec 2002; 22: 43–4.

Farrar DJ, Aromin I, Uvin SC et al. Hypospadias associated with the use of high dose megestrol acetate in an HIV infected woman. Genitourin Med 1997; 73: 226.

Fassas A, Kartalis G, Klearchou N et al. Chemotherapy for acute leukemia during pregnancy. Five case reports. Nouv Rev Fr Hematol 1984; 26: 19–24.

Feldkamp M, Carey JC. Clinical teratology counseling and consultation case report: low dose methotrexate exposure in the early weeks of pregnancy. Teratology 1993; 47: 533–9.

Fernandez H, Diallo A, Baume D, Papiernik E. Anhydramnios and cessation of fetal growth in a pregnant mother with polychemotherapy during the second trimester. Prenat Diagn 1989; 9: 681–2.

Forman R, Gill S, Moretti M et al. Fetal safety of letrozole and clomiphene citrate for ovulation induction. J Obstet Gynaecol Can 2007; 29: 668–71.

Francella A, Dyan A, Bodian C et al. The safety of 6-mercatopurine for childbearing patients with inflammatory bowel disease: a retrospective cohort study. Gastroenterology 2003; 124: 9–17.

Gall B, Yee A, Berry B et al. Rituximab for management of refractory pregnancy-associated immune thrombocytopenic purpura. J Obstet Gynaecol Can 2010; 32: 1167–71.

Garrett MJ. Teratogenic effects of combination chemotherapy. Ann Intern Med 1974; 80: 667.

Gerl H, Benecke R, Knappe G et al. Pregnancy and partus in Cushing's disease treated with o,p'-DDD. Acta Endocrinol (Copenh) 1992; 126: 133.

Germann N, Goffinet F, Goldwasser F. Anthracyclines during pregnancy: embryo-fetal outcome in 160 patients. Ann Oncol 2004; 15: 146–50.

Ghaemmaghami F, Abbasi F, Abadi AG. A favorable maternal and neonatal outcome following chemotherapy with etoposide, bleomycin, and cisplatin for management of grade 3 immature teratoma of the ovary. J Gynecol Oncol 2009; 20: 257–9.

Giacalone PL, Laffargue F, Benos P. Chemotherapy for breast carcinoma during pregnancy: A French national survey. Cancer 1999; 86: 2266–72.

Goffman D, Cole DS, Bobby P, Garry DJ. Failed methotrexate termination of pregnancy: a case report. J Perinatol 2006; 26: 645–57.

Goldman AS, Bongiovanni AM. Induced genital anomalies. Ann NY Acad Sci 1967; 142: 755–67.

Green DM, Sklar CA, Boice JD Jr et al. Ovarian failure and reproductive outcomes after childhood cancer treatment: results from the Childhood Cancer Survivor Study. J Clin Oncol 2009; 27: 2374–81.

Gurumurthy M, Koh P, Singh R et al. Metastatic non-small-cell lung cancer and the use of gemcitabine during pregnancy. J Perinatol 2009; 29: 63–5.

Hahn KM, Johnson PH, Gordon N et al. Treatment of pregnant breast cancer patients and outcomes of children exposed to chemotherapy in utero. Cancer 2006; 107: 1219–26.

Harlap S, Prywes R, Davies AM. Birth defects and oestrogens and progesterones in pregnancy. Lancet 1975; 1: 682–3.

Harrison P, Chipping P, Fothergill GA. Successful use of all-trans retinoic acid in acute promyelocytic leukaemia presenting during the second trimester of pregnancy. Br J Haematol 1994; 86: 681–2.

Heartin E, Walkinshaw S, Clark RE. Successful outcome of pregnancy in chronic myeloid leukaemia treated with imatinib. Leuk Lymphoma 2004; 45: 1307–8.

Houtchens MK, Kolb CM. Multiple sclerosis and pregnancy: therapeutic considerations. J Neurol 2013; 260: 1202–14.

Hsu K-F, Chang Ch-H, Chou Ch-Y. Sinusoidal fetal heart rate pattern during chemotherapy in a pregnant woman with acute myelogenous leukemia. J Formos Med Assoc 1995; 94: 562–5.

Hyoun SC, Običan SG, Scialli AR. Teratogen update: methotrexate. Birth Defects Res A Clin Mol Teratol 2012; 94: 187–207.

Ibrahim N, Saadeddin A, Al Sabbagh T. TAC chemotherapy during the first trimester of pregnancy – the first case report. J Oncol Phram Pract 2006; 12: 25.

Ishida I, Yamaguchi Y, Tanemura A et al. Stage III melanoma treated with chemotherapy after surgery during the second trimester of pregnancy. Arch Dermatol 2009; 145: 346–8.

Ishizuka S, Satou S. A case of delivery of healthy infant in breast cancer patient incidentally treated with goserelin acetate and tamoxifen during pregnancy. Breast Cancer 2013 May 1 (Epub ahead of print).

Jiménez-Gordo AM, Espinosa E, Zamora P et al. Pregnancy in a breast cancer patient treated with a LHRH analogue at ablative doses. Breast 2000; 9: 110–2.

Jochimsen PR, Spaight ME, Urdaneta LF. Pregnancy during adjuvant chemotherapy for breast cancer. JAMA 1981; 245: 1660–1.

Johansson AL, Andersson TM, Hsieh CC et al. Increased mortality in women with breast cancer detected during pregnancy and different periods postpartum. Cancer Epidemiol Biomarkers Prev 2011; 20: 1865–72.

Johansson AL, Andersson TM, Hsieh CC et al. Stage at diagnosis and mortality in women with pregnancy-associated breast cancer (PABC). Breast Cancer Res Treat 2013; 139: 183–92.

Kanate AS, Auber ML, Higa GM. Priorities and uncertainties of administering chemotherapy in a pregnant woman with newly diagnosed colorectal cancer. J Oncol Pharm Pract 2009; 15: 5–8.

Kelly H, Graham M, Humes E et al. Delivery of a healthy baby after first-trimester maternal exposure to lapatinib. Clin Breast Cancer 2006; 7: 339–41.

Kim JH, Kim HS, Sung CW et al. Docetaxel, gemcitabine, and cisplatin administered for non-small cell lung cancer during the first and second trimester of an unrecognized pregnancy. Lung Cancer 2008; 59: 270–3.

Kim WY, Wehbe TW, Akerley W. A woman with a balanced autosomal translocation who received chemotherapy while pregnant. Med Health R I 1996; 79: 396–9.

Kochhar DM, Christian MS. Tretinoin: a review of the nonclinical developmental toxicology experience. J Am Acad Dermatol 1997; 36: S47–59.

Kojori F, Cronin CM, Salamon E et al. Normal adrenal function in an infant following a pregnancy complicated by maternal adrenal cortical carcinoma and mitotane exposure. J Pediatr Endocrinol Metab 2011; 24: 203–4.

Kopelman JN, Miyazawa K. Inadvertent 5-fluorouracil treatment in early pregnancy: a report of three cases. Reprod Toxicol 1990; 4: 233–5.

Kozlowski RD, Steinbrunner JV, MacKenzie AH et al. Outcome of first-trimester exposure to low-dose methotrexate in eight patients with rheumatic disease. Am J Med 1990; 88: 589–92.

Pregnancy

2.13 Antineoplastic drugs

Krishnan A, Pike JI, Donofrio MT. Prenatal evaluation and management of fetuses exposed to Anti-SSA/Ro antibodies. Pediatr Cardiol 2012; 33: 1245–52.

Kroll T, Ames MB, Pruett JA et al. Successful management of pregnancy occurring in a patient with chronic myeloid leukemia on dasatinib. Leuk Lymphoma 2010; 51: 1751–3.

Kuwagata M, Takashima H, Nagao T. A comparison of the in vivo and in vitro response of rat embryos to 5-fluorouracil. J Vet Med Sci 1998; 60: 93–9.

Lambert J, Wijermans PW, Dekker GA et al. Chemotherapy in non-Hodgkin's lymphoma during pregnancy. Neth J Med 1991; 38: 80–85.

Lammer EJ, Chen DT, Hoar RM et al. Retinoic acid embryopathy. N Engl J Med 1985; 313: 837–41.

Lazalde B, Grijalva-Flores J, Guerrero-Romero F. Klippel-Feil syndrome in a boy exposed inadvertently to cyclophosphamide during pregnancy: a case report. Birth Defects Res A Clin Mol Teratol 2012; 94: 249–52.

Lee CH, Liam CK, Pang YK et al. Successful pregnancy with epidermal growth factor receptor tyrosine kinase inhibitor treatment of metastatic lung adenocarcinoma presenting with respiratory failure. Lung Cancer 2011; 74: 349–51.

Lee YY, Roberts CL, Dobbins T et al. Incidence and outcomes of pregnancy-associated cancer in Australia, 1994–2008: a population-based linkage study. BJOG 2012; 119: 1572–82.

Leiba S, Weinstein R, Shindel B et al. The protracted effect of o,p′-DDD in Cushing's disease and its impact on adrenal morphogenesis of young human embryo. Ann Endocrinol (Paris) 1989; 50: 49–53.

Leyder M, Laubach M, Breugelmans M et al. Specific congenital malformations after exposure to cyclophosphamide, epirubicin and 5-fluorouracil during the first trimester of pregnancy. Gynecol Obstet Invest 2011; 71: 141–4.

Li RH, Tam WH, Ng PC et al. Microphthalmos associated with Dartmouth combination chemotherapy in pregnancy: a case report. J Reprod Med 2007; 52: 575–6.

Lipshultz SE. Exposure to anthracyclines during childhood causes cardiac injury. Semin Oncol 2006; 33: S8–14.

Loibl S, Han SN, Amant F. Being pregnant and diagnosed with breast cancer. Breast Care (Basel) 2012a; 7: 204–9.

Loibl S, Han SN, von Minckwitz G et al. Treatment of breast cancer during pregnancy: an observational study. Lancet Oncol 2012b; 13: 887–96.

Lowenthal RM, Funnell CF, Hope DM et al. Normal infant after combination chemotherapy including teniposide for Burkitt's lymphoma in pregnancy. Med Pediatr Oncol 1982; 10: 165–9.

Lu E, Wang BW, Guimond C et al. Disease-modifying drugs for multiple sclerosis in pregnancy: a systematic review. Neurology 2012; 79: 1130–5.

Luton JP, Remy JM, Valcke JC et al. Recovery or remission of Cushing's disease following long term administration of op′DDD in seventeen patients (author's translation). Ann Endocrinol (Paris) 1973; 34: 351–76.

Massey Skatulla L, Loibl S, Schauf B, Muller T. Pre-eclampsia following chemotherapy for breast cancer during pregnancy: case report and review of the literature. Arch Gynecol Obstet 2012; 286: 89–92.

McGrane J, Bedford T, Kelly S. Successful pregnancy and delivery after concomitant temozolomide and radiotherapy treatment of glioblastoma multiforme. Clin Oncol (R Coll Radiol) 2012; 24: 311.

McGrath SE, Ring A. Chemotherapy for breast cancer in pregnancy: evidence and guidance for oncologists. Ther Adv Med Oncol 2011; 3: 73–83.

Mennuti MT, Shepard TH, Mellman WJ. Fetal renal malformation following treatment of Hodgkin's disease during pregnancy. Obstet Gynecol 1975; 46: 194–6.

Meyer-Wittkopf M, Barth H, Emons G, Schmidt S. Fetal cardiac effects of doxorubicin therapy for carcinoma of the breast during pregnancy: case report and review of the literature. Ultrasound Obstet Gynecol 2001; 18: 62–6.

Miller MT, Strömland K. Teratogen update: thalidomide: a review, with a focus on ocular findings and new potential uses. Teratology 1999; 60: 306–21.

Miller WH Jr, Schipper HM, Lee JS et al. Mechanisms of action of arsenic trioxide. Cancer Res 2002; 62: 3893–903.

Mir O, Berveiller P, Rouzier R et al. Chemotherapy for breast cancer during pregnancy: is epirubicin safe? Ann Oncol 2008; 19: 1814–5.

Mulvihill JJ, McKeen EA, Rosner F et al. Pregnancy outcome in cancer patients: experience in a large cooperative group. Cancer 1987; 60: 1143–50.

Murray NA, Acolet D, Deane M et al. Fetal marrow suppression after maternal chemotherapy for leukaemia. Arch Dis Child 1994; 71: F209–10.

Nakhai-Pour HR, Broy P, Sheehy O, Bérard A. Use of nonaspirin nonsteroidal antiinflammatory drugs during pregnancy and the risk of spontaneous abortion. CMAJ 2011; 183: 1713–20.

NTP (National Toxicology Program): NTP Monograph on Developmental Effects and Pregnancy Outcomes Associated with Cancer Chemotherapy Use during Pregnancy; May 2013. Available online at http://ntp.niehs.nih.gov/ntp/ohat/cancer_chemo_preg/chemopregnancy_monofinal_508.pdf.

Naya M, Yasuda M. Effects of glutathione and related compounds on teratogenicity of 5-fluorouracil or cadmium hydrochloride in mice. Cong Anom 1997; 37: 337–44.

Niedermeier DM, Frei-Lahr DA, Hall PD. Treatment of acute myeloid leukemia during the second and third trimesters of pregnancy. Pharmacotherapy 2005; 25: 1134–40.

Nørgård B, Pedersen L, Fonager K et al. Azathioprine, mercaptopurine and birth outcome: a population-based cohort study. Aliment Pharmacol Ther 2003; 17: 827–34.

Nulman I, Laslo D, Fried S et al. Neurodevelopment of children exposed in utero to treatment of maternal malignancy. Br J Cancer 2001; 85: 1611–8.

Odom LD, Plouffe l, Butler WJ. 5-Fluorouracil exposure during the period of conception: report on two cases. Am J Obstet Gynecol 1990; 163: 76–7.

Paladini D, Vassallo M, D'Armiento MR et al. Prenatal detection of multiple fetal anomalies following inadvertent exposure to cyclophosphamide in the first trimester of pregnancy. Birth Defects Res A Clin Mol Teratol 2004; 7: 99–100.

Paşa S, Altintaş A, Çil T, Ayyildiz O. Fetal loss in a patient with acute myeloblastic leukemia associated with FLAG-IDA regime. Int J Hematol Oncol 2009; 19: 110–2.

Paskulin GA, Gazzola Zen PR, de Camargo Pinto LL et al. Combined chemotherapy and teratogenicity. Birth Defects Res A Clin Mol Teratol 2005; 73: 634–7.

Peccatori FA, Azim HA Jr, Scarfone G et al. Weekly epirubicin in the treatment of gestational breast cancer (GBC). Breast Cancer Res Treat 2009; 115: 591–4.

Peres RM, Sanseverino MTV, Guimararaes JLM et al. Assessment of fetal risk associated with exposure to cancer chemotherapy during pregnancy: a multicenter study. Braz J Med Biol Res 2001; 34: 1551–9.

Pérez-Encinas M, Bello JL, Pérez-Crespo S et al. Familial myeloproliferative syndrome. Am J Hematol 1994; 46: 225–9.

Pizzuto J, Aviles A, Noriega L et al. Treatment of acute leukemia during pregnancy: presentation of nine cases. Cancer Treat Rep 1980; 64: 679–83.

Polifka JE, Friedman JM. Teratogen uptake: azathioprine and 6-mercaptopurine. Teratology 2002; 65: 240–61.

Pye SM, Cortes J, Ault P et al. The effects of imatinib on pregnancy outcome. Blood 2008; 111: 5505–8.

Raffles A, Williams J, Costeloe K et al. Transplacental effects of maternal cancer chemotherapy. Case Report. Br J Obstet Gynaecol 1989; 96: 1099–100.

Rhinn M, Dollé P. Retinoic acid signalling during development. Development 2012; 139: 843–58.

Rivas G, Llinas N, Bonilla C et al. Use of erlotinib throughout pregnancy: A case-report of a patient with metastatic lung adenocarcinoma. Lung Cancer 2012; 77: 469–72.

Rugh R, Skaredoff L. Radiation and radiomimetic chlorambucil and the fetal retina. Arch Ophthalmol 1965; 74: 382–93.

Saini N, Mahindra A. Novel immunomodulatory compounds in multiple myeloma. Expert Opin Investig Drugs 2013; 22: 207–15.

Schafer AI. Teratogenic effects of antileukemic chemotherapy. Arch Intern Med 1981; 14: 514–5.

Schaison G, Jacquillat C, Auclerc G, Weil M. Fetal risk of cancer chemotherapy. Bull Cancer 1979; 66: 165–70.

Schardein JL. Chemically Induced Birth Defects, 3rd edn, New York: Marcel Dekker 2000.

Schardein JL. Congenital abnormalities and hormones during pregnancy: a clinical review. Teratology 1980; 22: 251–70.

Seidahmed MZ, Shaheed MM, Abdulbasit OB et al. A case of methotrexate embryopathy with holoprosencephaly, expanding the phenotype. Birth Defects Res A 2006; 76: 138–42.

Selig BP, Furr JR, Huey RW et al. Cancer chemotherapeutic agents as human teratogens. Birth Defects Res A Clin Mol Teratol 2012; 94: 626–50.

Sham RL. All-trans retinoic acid-induced labor in a pregnant patient with acute promyelocytic leukemia. Am J Hematol 1996; 53: 145.

Pregnancy

2.13 Antineoplastic drugs

Shieh MP, Mehta RS. Oligohydramnios associated with administration of weekly paclitaxel for triple-negative breast cancer during pregnancy. Ann Oncol 2011; 22: 2151–2.

Shotton D, Monie IW. Possible teratogenic effect of chlorambucil on a human fetus. JAMA 1963; 186: 74–5.

Shufaro Y, Uzieli B, Pappo O, Abramov Y. Pregnancy and delivery in a patient with metastatic embryonal sarcoma of the liver. Obstet Gynecol 2002; 99: 951–3.

Siepermann M, Koscielniak E, Dantonello T et al. Oral low-dose chemotherapy: Successful treatment of an alveolar rhabdomyosarcoma during pregnancy. Pediatr Blood Cancer 2012; 58: 104–6.

Signorello LB, Mulvihill JJ, Green DM et al. Stillbirth and neonatal death in relation to radiation exposure before conception: a retrospective cohort study. Lancet 2010; 376: 624–30.

Simone MD, Stasi R, Venditti A et al. All-trans retinoic acid (ATRA) administration during pregnancy in relapsed acute promyelocytic leukemia. Leukemia 1995; 9: 1412–3.

Siu BL, Alonzo MR, Vargo TA et al. Transient dilated cardiomyopathy in a newborn exposed to idarubicin and all-trans-retinoic acid (ATRA) early in the second trimester of pregnancy. Int J Gynecol Cancer 2002; 12: 399–402.

Smithells RW, Newman CGH. Recognition of thalidomide defects. J Med Genet 1992; 29: 716–723.

Steege JF, Caldwell DS. Renal agenesis after first trimester exposure to chlorambucil. South Med J 1980; 73: 1414–5.

Stephens TD, Golbus MS, Miller TR et al. Multiple congenital anomalies in a fetus exposed to 5-fluorouracil during the first trimester. Am J Obstet Gynecol 1980; 137: 747–9.

Sukumvanich P. Review of current treatment options for pregnancy-associated breast cancer. Clin Obstet Gynecol 2011; 54: 164–72.

Taylor J, Amanze A, di Federico E et al. Irinotecan use during pregnancy. Obstet Gynecol 2009; 114: 451–2.

Tegay DH, Tepper R, Willner JP. 6-Mercaptopurine teratogenicity. Postgrad Med J 2002; 78: 572.

Terada Y, Shindo T, Endoh A et al. Fetal arrhythmia during treatment of pregnancy-associated acute promyelocytic leukemia with all-trans retinoic acid and favorable outcome. Leukemia 1997; 11: 454–5.

Tewari K, Bonebrake RG, Asrat T et al. Ambiguous genitalia in infant exposed to tamoxifen in utero. Lancet 1997; 350: 183.

Thiersch JB. Therapeutic abortion with a folic acid antagonist, 4-amino pteroylglutamic acid (4-amino PGA) administered by the oral route. Am J Obst Gynec 1952; 63: 1298–304.

Thomas L, Andes WA. Fetal anomaly associated with successful chemotherapy for Hodgkin's disease during the first trimester of pregnancy. Clin Res 1982; 30: 424A.

Thomas PR, Peckham MJ. The investigation and management of Hodgkin's disease in the pregnant patient. Cancer 1976; 38: 1443–1451.

Thompson J, Conklin KA. Anesthetic management of a pregnant patient with scleroderma. Anesthesiology 1983; 59: 69–71.

Tripto-Shkolnik L, Blumenfeld Z, Bronshtein M et al. Pregnancy in a patient with adrenal carcinoma treated with mitotane: a case report and review of literature. J Clin Endocrinol Metab 2013; 98: 443–7.

Tulandi T, Martin J, Al-Fadhli R et al. Congenital malformation among 911 newborns conceived after infertility treatment with letrozole or clomiphene citrate. Fertil Steril 2006; 85: 1761–5.

Udink ten Cate FE, ten Hove CH, Nix WM et al. Transient neonatal myelosuppression after fetal exposure to maternal chemotherapy. Case report and review of the literature. Neonatology 2009; 95: 80–5.

Usta IM, Nassar AH, Yunis KA, Abu-Musa AA. Methotrexate embryopathy after therapy for misdiagnosed ectopic pregnancy. Int J Gynaecol Obstet 2007; 99: 253–5.

Valappil S, Kurkar M, Howell R. Outcome of pregnancy in women treated with all-trans retinoic acid; a case report and review of literature. Hematology 2007; 12: 415–8.

Van Le L, Pizzuti DJ, Greenberg M, Reid R. Accidental use of low-dose 5-fluorouracil in pregnancy. J Reprod Med 1991; 36: 872–4.

Vaux KK, Kahole NCO, Jones KL. Cyclophosphamide, methotrexate and cytarabine embryopathy: Is apoptosis the common pathway? Birth Defects Res A 2003; 67: 403–8.

Wagner VM, Hill JS, Weaver D et al. Congenital abnormalities in baby born to cytarabine treated mother. Lancet 1980; 2: 98–9.

Warkany J. Aminopterin and methotrexate: folic acid deficiency. Teratology 1978; 17: 353–7.

Warraich Q, Smith N. Herceptin therapy in pregnancy: continuation of pregnancy in the presence of anhydramnios. J Obstet Gynaecol 2009; 29: 147–8.

Weber-Schöndorfer C, Schaefer C. Trastuzumb exposure during pregnancy. Reprod Toxicol 2008; 25: 390–1.

Witzel ID, Müller V, Harps E et al. Trastuzumab in pregnancy associated with poor fetal outcome. Ann Oncol 2008; 19: 191–2.

Xu M, Hou Y, Sheng L, Peng J. Therapeutic effects of thalidomide in hematologic disorders: a review. Front Med 2013; 7: 290–300.

Yang D, Hladnik L. Treatment of acute promyelocytic leukemia during pregnancy. Pharmacotherapy 2009; 29: 709–24.

Zagouri F, Sergentanis TN, Chrysikos D et al. Trastuzumab administration during pregnancy: a systematic review and meta-analysis. Breast Cancer Res Treat 2013; 137: 349–57.

Zambelli A, Prada GA, Fregoni V et al. Erlotinib administration for advanced non-small cell lung cancer during the first 2 months of unrecognized pregnancy. Lung Cancer 2008; 60: 455–7.

Zemlickis D, Lishner M, Degendorfer P et al. Fetal outcome after in utero exposure to cancer chemotherapy. Arch Intern Med 1992; 152: 573–6.

Uterine contraction agents, tocolytics, vaginal therapeutics and local contraceptives

2.14

Gerard H.A. Visser and Angela Kayser

2.14.1	Prostaglandins	401
2.14.2	Oxytocin	403
2.14.3	Ergot alkaloids	404
2.14.4	Tocolytics in general	405
2.14.5	β_2-Sympathomimetics	406
2.14.6	Calcium antagonists	407
2.14.7	Magnesium sulfate	407
2.14.8	Oxytocin receptor antagonists	408
2.14.9	Prostaglandin antagonists	408
2.14.10	Other tocolytics	409
2.14.11	Vaginal therapeutics	409
2.14.12	Spermicide contraceptives	410
2.14.13	Intrauterine devices	410

Uterine contraction agents and tocolytics are among the most frequently used drugs in obstetrics. The former are generally effective but carry the risk of uterine overstimulation and fetal asphyxia in cases of labor induction or augmentation. They should be titrated carefully and the fetal condition should be monitored continuously. Other indications include induction of abortion and prevention/treatment of post-partum hemorrhage.

Tocolytic drugs are only moderately effective, and their use has not been unequivocally associated with an improved neonatal outcome. Therefore, agents with the highest safety profile should be given when considering using these drugs.

2.14.1   Prostaglandins

Pharmacology and toxicology

Prostaglandins (PG) have a large number of biologic and reproductive functions. Of practical significance during pregnancy are the prostaglandins designated as PGE_2, $PGF_{2\alpha}$ and PGI_2 (*prostacyclin*).

Prostaglandins are synthesized from *arachidonic acid* by the enzyme phospholipase A_2. The half-life of naturally occurring prostaglandins, such as those produced in the uterus is only a few minutes. The kidneys, liver, intestinal tract, and lungs contain enzymes that quickly destroy prostaglandins and limit their activity. The synthesis of prostaglandins in the genital tract is influenced by the hormones estradiol, progesterone and by catecholamines.

PGE_2 causes so-called ripening of the cervix, characterized by connective tissue changes that facilitate softening, effacement, and dilatation of the cervix during uterine contractions. $PGF_{2\alpha}$ promotes contractions. PGI_2 is an arteriolar dilator. Deficiency of prostacyclin is associated with hypertensive disorders of pregnancy.

In practice, the following uses of prostaglandins can be distinguished:

- Preparation for labor induction by ripening the cervix with *dineprostone*, a PGE_2 analog, applied in the form of intravaginal suppositories or as a gel intracervically, or with *misoprostol* (a PGE_2 analog) applied.
- Induction intravaginally of labor or enhancement of contractions with dinoprostone, applied as intravaginal suppositories, as vaginal inserts, or as a gel intracervically or extra-amniotically.
- Treatment of post-partum uterine atony with *dinoprostol* or *sulprostone* application intravenously or into the myometrium, or transcervically into the uterus, or misoprostol rectally or orally.
- Induction of abortion with dinoprostone (PGE_2) as an intracervical gel, with sulprostone cervically or in the myometrium, with dinoprostone extra-amniotically, and with *gemeprost*, intravaginally or misoprostol intravaginally or orally.
- Sub-involution of the uterus after birth can be treated with *oxytocin* or ergotamine derivatives like *methylergometrine*.

With all contraction stimulants, overstimulation of the myometrium can occur. Because myometrial contractions are associated with a decrease in perfusion of the uterine vessels, a potential adverse effect of these agents is embryonic or fetal hypoxia. A disruption type malformation due to reduced perfusion and, in extreme cases, fetal death might be the consequences (Bond 1994). Misoprostol is a complementary drug for medical termination of pregnancy up to 63 days of gestation; where this is permitted under national law and where culturally acceptable, and for induction of labor (Stuart 2008). Failed abortion attempts with misoprostol have been associated with the occurrence of Moebius sequence (cranial nerve defects and limb defects) in the offspring. Other malformations, such as cranial bone defects, omphalocele, and gastroschisis, have also been observed. In these abortion attempts, misoprostol was used orally, often combined with vaginal administration as well. The most common total dose was 800 µg, with a range from 200 to 16,000 µg (four tablets daily for 20 days). All cases were exposed in the first trimester, most commonly in the second month (Orioli 2000, Gonzalez 1998, Hofmeyr 1998, Castilla 1994, Schüler 1992). In a retrospective Brazilian case-control study it was found that nearly half of the 94 women with a child with Moebius sequence had used misoprostol orally or vaginally (Pastuszak 1998).

A 200 µg dose of misoprostol has been associated with increased uterine artery resistance indices by Doppler ultrasound, suggesting that perfusion reduction could underlie the disruption-type malformations (Yip 2000).

In a relatively small prospective controlled study in 86 women, on the contrary, no adverse effects on pregnancy or neonates were observed (Schüler 1999). The same held for a French collaborative study of 125 pregnancies exposed to misoprostol (Bellemin 1999).

However, a systematic review and meta-analysis, including 4,899 cases of congenital anomalies and 5,742 controls, concluded that misoprostol is associated with an increased risk of Moebius sequence (OR = 25; 95%

CI 11–58), and terminal transverse limb defects (OR = 12; 95% CI 5–29) (Da Silva Dal Pizzol 2006). In a subsequent study of 118 pregnancies, these authors found a doubling of the incidence of congenital malformations as compared to non-exposed infants not exposed to misoprostol at early gestation (Da Silva Dal Pizzol 2008).

In summary, an increased teratogenic risk after (accidental) exposure to misoprostol may exist. Amongst women with an offspring with Moebius syndrome, the likelihood of exposure to misoprostol in the first trimester is high; however, the absolute risk is probably low following misoprostol exposure in the first trimester of pregnancy (Goldberg 2001).

Misoprostol given either orally or rectally in a dose of up to 800 μg is increasingly used in low-income settings to prevent post-partum hemorrhage. It is cheap, stable and can be easily distributed at community level. However, current evidence has not shown a reduction in maternal mortality, with maternal pyrexia as a side-effect (Hofmeyr 2013). Oxytocin infusion as a first-line therapy has been shown to be more effective in preventing post-partum hemorrhage (Mousa 2014). Off-label use of misoprostol for this indication may be the first choice in a low resource setting, but there remains a need for large randomized trials to further elucidate the relative effectiveness and risks of various dosages (Hofmeyr 2013).

Misoprostol is also increasingly used for the induction of an abortion or labor, and in the post-partum period, due to its simple oral administration and favorable costs. Titrating the misoprostol dose on the basis of the frequency and intensity of uterine contractions is frequently applied, particularly in developing countries. For labor induction after rupture of the membranes, it is the most effective drug that can be applied without an increased risk for infection. Overstimulation and pathologic fetal heart rate patterns in individual cases, however, are a reason to warn against indiscriminate use of misoprostol (Wing 2006). Misoprostol should not be used in term pregnancies with a uterine scar from a previous caesarean section or from major uterine surgery (ACOG 2006).

Misoprostol is not approved for any indication in pregnancy, and administration of misoprostol for cervical ripening and/or labor induction currently is considered off-label (Wing 2006).

> **Recommendation.** Prostaglandins may be used for cervical ripening and induction of labor. When pregnancy continues after a failed abortion attempt with prostaglandins, it is advisable to perform detailed ultrasound scanning (at 12–14 and 18–20 weeks) to verify morphologic development of the fetus on the grounds of possible embryotoxicity. Misoprostol is not approved for any indication in pregnancy.

2.14.2   Oxytocin

Pharmacology and toxicology

Oxytocin is an octapeptide produced in the hypothalamus, stored in the posterior pituitary, and from there released into the blood. Inactivation occurs via a specific oxytocinase in the liver, spleen, and ovaries. During pregnancy, oxytocin is inactivated by another enzyme produced by the placenta, a cystinaminopeptidase. Oxytocin has a plasma half-life of about 10 minutes.

The sites of oxytocin action are the uterine muscle and the myoepithelial cells surrounding the milk-producing units of the breast. The conditions for the action of oxytocin on a pregnant uterus are complex and controlled by several factors. Among these factors are decreases in estrogen and progesterone concentrations in the blood, with a reduction in the α- and β-adrenergic activity in the uterine muscles. During pregnancy the concentration of oxytocin in the blood is slightly elevated, but towards the end of pregnancy both the concentration and the number of oxytocin receptors in the myometrium increase significantly. During the course of labor, a three- to four-fold increase in the plasma concentration of oxytocin is observed.

Because of its structural similarity to vasopressin, oxytocin has antidiuretic hormone activity, promoting the reabsorption of salt-free fluid in the distal renal tubules. High doses of oxytocin (>40 mU/min) given with electrolyte-free solutions can lead to water intoxication, with cramps, coma and, rarely, death. Reduction of fluid intake and monitoring of electrolytes can eliminate the risk of water intoxication.

The oxytocin analog *pitocin* is used in low doses intravenously as a standard treatment for the induction or augmentation of labor. As with all contraction stimulants, overstimulation of the myometrium can occur. In that case, oxytocin increases the basal tone in the uterus, leading to a decrease in uteroplacental perfusion, with the possibility of fetal hypoxia and even fetal death occurring.

A second risk from overstimulation is uterine rupture, particularly in the presence of a scarred uterus; this may lead to fetal death and substantial maternal blood loss, shock, loss of the uterus, and even maternal death. Uterine rupture, except when an emergency caesarean delivery can be performed, will inevitably lead to the death of the child. Oxytocin should be applied with extreme caution for induction or augmentation of labor, and only in combination with careful monitoring of maternal uterine contractions and the fetal heart rate (i.e. electronic fetal heart rate monitoring, cardiotocography).

Oxytocin, either given intravenously or intramuscularly is the agent of first choice for routine primary prevention of post-partum hemorrhage. The long acting oxytocin derivate *carbetocin* has been developed to reduce post-partum hemorrhage following a caesarean delivery. A recent Cochrane review has indicated that this agent significantly reduced the need for therapeutic uterotonics as compared to oxytocin (RR 0.62. 95% CI 0.44–0.88), without reducing the overall incidence of post-partum hemorrhage. It is also associated with less blood loss, as compared to syntometrine in the prevention of post-partum hemorrhage in women having a vaginal delivery (Su 2012).

> **Recommendation.** Oxytocin (pitocin) may be used when indicated for induction or augmentation of labor. It should be applied extremely carefully, and only in combination with monitoring of uterine activity and fetal heart rate.

2.14.3   Ergot alkaloids

Pharmacology and toxicology

Ergot alkaloids (ergotamine derivatives; see also Chapter 2.1.7) are used to increase the strength of uterine contraction to limit post-partum bleeding and promote post-partum involution. Because ergot-associated contractions are tonic rather than rhythmic, these agents cannot be used during labor. Tonic contraction of the uterus during labor could result in fetal hypoxia and even death. The use of these agents is associated with a slight risk of acute coronary syndrome or myocardial infarction, especially in hypertensive women, but the combined risk is relatively low (<1 per 10,000) (Bateman 2013). It is also associated with an increased risk for manual removal of a retained placenta. For primary prevention of post-partum hemorrhage, oxytocin is generally considered an agent of first choice.

Pharmacologic agents in this group include ergometrine and methyler-gometrine (methylergonovine).

> **Recommendation.** Ergot alkaloids are used only after birth for post-partum uterine hypotonia. They are contraindicated during pregnancy. Accidental use during the first trimester does not automatically require termination of pregnancy. Detailed ultrasound scanning can exclude morphologic developmental disorders. For other ergotamine derivatives, see Chapters 2.1.14.

2.14.4   Tocolytics in general

Tocolytic agents can stop uterine contractions and temporarily delay delivery. Critical analyses have demonstrated that most tocolytics are effective for prolongation of pregnancy for only 48–72 hours (Haas 2009, 2012). This period allows for transport of the pregnant woman to a peri-natal center, and for administration of glucocorticoids for lung matura-tion (Haas 2009, Higby 1999, Katz 1999). No protocol of (long-term) tocolysis has unequivocally contributed to improvement in neonatal outcome (Haas 2009, 2012). When prescribing tocolytics, strict guide-lines must be observed and tocolytics should generally not be given for more than 48 hours. There is no evidence that maintenance therapy with intravenous or oral tocolytic drugs, given after a period of acute preterm contractions, will prolong gestational age (Roos 2013, Dodd 2012).

Tocolytic drugs are usually given to prolong gestation during the preterm period. However, they may also be given during term labor, as acute tocolysis, to stop contractions in case of spontaneous or induced tachysystole (i.e. too many contractions), and/or to stop contractions when arranging a caesarean delivery (de Heus 2008a). In one random-ized controlled trial it has been found that the condition at birth of these infants was indeed better after acute intra-partum tocolysis (Briozzo 2007). Both oxytocin antagonists and β-adrenergic agents have been shown to be effective in this regard (de Heus 2008b).

Among the most common agents used, as tocolytics are calcium antag-onists, β-adrenergic agents, oxytocin antagonists, prostaglandin antago-nists, and magnesium sulfate. Magnesium sulfate has been shown not to be effective as a tocolytics drug, but may be used as a neuro-protective agent. The tocolytic action and side effects of the other four agents is schemati-cally shown in Table 2.14.1 (Haas 2012, 2009, RCOG 2011). The drugs of first choice are the calcium channel antagonists and oxytocin antagonist (RCOG 2011). Prostaglandin antagonists have the highest probability of postponing delivery, and have only few maternal side effects, but may have negative effects on the fetus when given after 32 weeks.

Pregnancy

2.14 Uterine contraction agents, tocolytics, vaginal therapeutics and local contraceptives

Table 2.14.1 The action and side effects of the four tocolytic agents schematically (according to Haas 2012, 2009, RCOG 2011)

Treatment	Tocolytic drug	Side effects	Tocolytic effects
1	Indomethacin	++++	++++
2	β-Agonists	+++	++
3	Calcium channel blockers	++	++
4	Oxytocin antagonists	+	++

2.14.5   β₂-Sympathomimetics

Pharmacology and toxicology

β-Adrenergic agents have long been the most widely used contracting inhibitors (tocolytics), but are applied less frequently because of their pronounced side effects (de Heus 2009, Papatsonis 2003, Goldenberg 2002) and the short-acting effect (maximum of 48 hours) on the uterine musculature due to development of tachyphylaxis (Schiff 1993). *Ritodrine* and *fenoterol* are the most frequently used inhibitors of uterine contractions. *Clenbuterol, salbutamol, terbutaline*, and the less selective *isoxsuprine* are also used for tocolysis.

Maternal cardiovascular side effects, such as palpitations and pulmonary edema, are serious complications from intravenous application. In a prospective series of 175 cases, serious adverse drug reactions occurred in three cases (1.7%), and mild adverse drug reactions (ADRs) in 2.3% of cases (de Heus 2009). Side effects requiring a change of medication is 23 times higher compared to *atosiban* (Haas 2012).

A suspected cardioprotective effect of verapamil led for a time to the combining of both pharmaceutical agents (Weidinger 1973), until reports appeared of pulmonary edema following this combination (Grospietsch 1981). The effectiveness of oral treatment with these agents has not been demonstrated. Oral administration may not produce blood levels adequate to maintain tocolysis, and effectiveness is limited by tachyphylaxis (Schiff 1993). Maybe the only current and remaining indication for β-sympathomimetic agents is in its use during term labor to stop excessive contractions and improve the fetal condition (de Heus 2008a, 2008b, Briozzo 2007). These agents and oxytocin antagonists are the only agents that have been shown to reduce contractions acutely and significantly in these circumstances.

The use of fenoterol and other β-sympathomimetics, especially when combined with corticosteroids to enhance fetal lung maturity, can result in impaired carbohydrate tolerance, sometimes leading to an abrupt increase in insulin need in insulin-dependent diabetics. As in their mothers, β-sympathomimetics can cause fetal and neonatal cardiovascular side effects, as well as impaired carbohydrate tolerance in the neonate.

Transient alterations in neonatal behavior and hyperkinetic behavior have been observed (Thayer 1997).

> **Recommendation.** Use of tocolytics like β₂-sympathomimetics is difficult to justify at this time. Maternal, fetal, and neonatal cardiovascular side effects and impaired carbohydrate tolerance can occur. The only current potential role for these agents is acute tocolysis during term labor in cases of excessive contractions.

2.14.6   Calcium antagonists

Pharmacology and toxicology

Calcium antagonists, such as *nifedipine* or *nicardipine*, are used for tocolysis. The oral use of slow-release preparations is considered an advantage over intravenous treatment schedules. Several studies have demonstrated that these agents are well tolerated and effective compared with other tocolytics, such as β_2-sympathomimetics (Haas 2012, Papatsonis 2000, 1997, El-Sayed 1998, Jannet 1997). However, severe adverse and mild drug reactions occur in total in about 2% of cases (de Heus 2009). Myocardial infarction and serious dyspnea with lung edema have been reported during tocolysis with calcium antagonists (Oei 2006, van Geijn 2005). Combined administration of calcium antagonists and magnesium may seriously potentiate the activity of magnesium, inducing hypotension and neuromuscular blockade, and thus endangering the mother and fetus.

> **Recommendation.** Tocolysis with calcium antagonists is acceptable when clearly indicated and following a normal course of pregnancy. Caution is required regarding its use simultaneously with magnesium sulfate.

2.14.7   Magnesium sulfate

Pharmacology and toxicology

Magnesium sulfate, although not actually an antihypertensive, has proved valuable in the treatment of preeclampsia. Magnesium sulfate is the drug of choice for the prevention and treatment of seizures in eclampsia. Intravenous administration of the drug as an initial loading dose of 4–6 g, followed by an infusion of 2–3.5 g/h, was found not to be harmful. A significantly lower risk of repeated convulsions in eclampsia has been reported.

Magnesium sulfate also acts to inhibit contractions, but is not very effective as a tocolytic (Crowther 2002). Although it is still being used in the USA for tocolysis, there are better alternatives, such as *atosiban* or *nifedipine*. Grimes and colleagues have presented convincing arguments that intravenous magnesium sulfate tocolysis should be stopped (Grimes 2006). Recently, it has been shown that magnesium sulfate acts as a neuroprotective agent when given during preterm labor. Six randomized controlled trials have shown that magnesium sulfate results in a 30% lower incidence of cerebral palsy, and in a 40% lower incidence of motor dysfunction without affecting perinatal mortality or other neurological impairments or disabilities in the first years of life (Doyle 2012, Conde-Agudelo 2009). When given before 28 weeks the number needed to treat to prevent one case of moderate to severe cerebral palsy is about 30 (before 32 weeks, $n = 63$). An intravenous loading dose of 4 g with 1–2 g/h maintenance of 12 to 24 hours has been suggested, although clear dose-response studies are still lacking. Therefore, there is an indication to use magnesium sulfate during preterm labor, not to stop preterm contractions, but as a neuroprotective agent. Treatment should be restricted to gestational ages below 32 weeks.

Magnesium, when used in higher doses or when kidney function is limited, can cause marked muscle hypotonia in both mother and newborn.

In extreme cases, especially when a calcium antagonist such as nifedipine enhances its effect, a dangerous drop in maternal blood pressure can occur, which may result in fetal hypoxia.

> **Recommendation.** Magnesium sulfate can be used for appropriate indications such as preeclampsia and eclampsia. It is the drug of choice for treatment of seizures in eclampsia. Its use as a tocolytic is questionable, but it is recommended as a neuroprotective drug in case of preterm labor before 32 weeks of gestation.

2.14.8   Oxytocin receptor antagonists

Pharmacology and toxicology

Atosiban is a new intravenously used compound registered for tocolysis. Global availability, however, is limited due to cost. Atosiban competes with oxytocin for binding to oxytocin receptors in the myometrium, thus preventing the increase of free calcium in the cell. In a worldwide double-blind randomized trial of atosiban versus β-agonists (Worldwide Atosiban versus β-agonists Study Group 2001), both compounds resulted in similar rates of delivery within 48 hours and 7 days after the start of therapy. Atosiban, though, resulted in far fewer and particularly, less severe maternal side effects, and as a consequence substantially less discontinuations of therapy (Wing 2006). Atosiban is considered a safe drug in comparison with calcium antagonists and β-mimetics. Also, in a prospective study severe ADRs were absent in 576 treated women, while mild ADRs occurred in only 0.2% (de Heus 2009). Adverse drug reactions were significantly lower as compared to betamimetics or calcium-channel blocking agents. According to the Royal College of Obstetricians and Gynaecologists (Greentop) guidelines, both oxytocin antagonists and calcium-channel blockers should be considered as a first choice (RCOG 2011). However, given its favorable side-effect profile, oxytocin antagonists should be the first choice for women at increased risk, such as in multiple gestations and in preexisting maternal cardiovascular disease and diabetes.

> **Recommendation.** Atosiban appears to be safe when used properly, and can be considered for tocolysis during the preterm period and for reduction of excessive (induced) contractions at term.

2.14.9   Prostaglandin antagonists

Pharmacology and toxicology

Prostaglandin synthetase inhibitors such as *indomethacin* and *sulindac* are used as an adjunct in tocolysis (Higby 1999). These agents can produce premature closure of the ductus arteriosus and impairment of renal function, with subsequent oligohydramnios. In short-term tocolysis (maximum 48 hours) before the thirty-second week of pregnancy this is seldom problematic, although the magnitude of the risks is still a subject of debate (for further detail, see also Chapter 2.1).

> **Recommendation.** Additional use of prostaglandin synthetase inhibitor in tocolysis is controversial, and should be reserved for treatment before 32 weeks of gestation.

2.14.10   Other tocolytics

Nitroglycerin administered as a patch or intravenously, has not been shown to be an effective tocolytic agent when compared to β-sympatho-mimetics. Ethyl alcohol has been used in the past for tocolysis, for its presumed inhibition of oxytocin release by the posterior pituitary gland. To be effective, substantial maternal serum levels are needed! The harmful effects of alcohol on the development of the child are well known, and thus alcohol is an obsolete tocolytic (see Chapter 2.21.1).

> **Recommendation.** Alcohol is contraindicated.

2.14.11   Vaginal therapeutics

Pharmacology and toxicology

In women with bacterial vaginosis, the normal vaginal flora is characterized by high concentrations of *Gardnerella vaginalis* and anaerobic bacteria, and a decrease in *Lactobacillus* species. This condition is present in about 20% of pregnancies. Bacterial vaginosis in pregnancy has been associated with adverse outcomes of pregnancy, such as preterm labor, preterm birth, preterm premature rupture of the outer membranes (PPROM), chorioamnionitis, and low birth weight of the infant and maternal infection, especially in women with at least one other factor known to be associated with preterm delivery – in particular, cervical incompetence (Leitich 2007).

Currently, treatment of bacterial vaginosis during pregnancy has not been proven unequivocally to be efficient in reducing the risk of preterm birth or PPROM. In a recent Cochrane review it was concluded that antibiotic treatment can eradicate bacterial vaginosis in pregnancy, however without significantly reducing the overall risk of (recurrent) preterm birth (Brocklehurst 2013). These results are not encouraging. However, in two trials (only) in women with an abnormal vaginal flora (Nugent score <6) a reduction in preterm labor was found, and similarly in two trials, it was found that early clindamycin may reduce miscarriage. Overall there was no clear difference between oral and vaginal treatment, nor between *metronidazole* and *clindamycin*. Despite the presence of 21 trials of good quality, there remain many uncertainties regarding the treatment of bacterial vaginosis. The use of the Nugent score to identify an abnormal vaginal flora may identify women that will benefit from treatment, but further trials are needed.

For local therapy of vaginal candida infection, see Chapter 2.6. Antimycotics of first choice for local therapy of vaginal candidiasis are *nystatin*, *clotrimazole*, and *miconazole*.

Vaginal douching with *povidone iodine* solutions increases maternal serum iodine levels and transiently alters maternal and fetal thyroid function (from week 12 of gestation). Therefore, its use should be avoided during pregnancy (see Chapter 2.17.2).

To date, there is no indication that vaginally administered estrogens or disinfectants, such as *dequalium*, *hexetidine*, and *policresulenum*, have a teratogenic effect. However, it is good therapeutic practice to avoid obsolete and controversial agents.

> **Recommendation.** When treatment of bacterial vaginosis is indicated, oral antibiotics are the first choice (see details in Chapter 2.6). Vaginal administration of metronidazole or other antibiotics appears to be less effective.

2.14.12   Spermicide contraceptives

The "over-the-counter" (OTC) available spermicides, sold as cream, gel, tablets or foam, contain *nonoxinol-9*. This form of contraception had always been considered harmless. However, in one study of more than 700 children born to mothers who became pregnant in spite of the use of vaginal contraceptives, a slight increase in rate of malformations was observed (Jick 1981). A meta-analysis did not confirm this finding (Einarson 1990). Several publications suggest that by damaging the vaginal mucosa and disturbing the vaginal flora, the use of these spermicides may facilitate HIV infection (Rosenstein 1998, Stafford 1998).

> **Recommendation.** Conception using vaginal spermicidals containing nonoxinol-9 has not been associated with an identifiable risk of birth defects.

2.14.13   Intrauterine devices

In women who use a copper IUD as a contraceptive, the copper concentration in the fallopian tubes is elevated, but copper and ceruloplasmin levels in the serum are not changed (Wollen 1994). A number of reports suggest that pregnancy in association with copper IUDs, results in an increased rate of spontaneous abortions and preterm birth in the group in which the IUD remained in the uterus, compared with the group in which the IUD was removed or expelled. No increase in the rate of birth defects was documented. This is also to be expected with *levonorgestrel*-containing "intrauterine systems."

> **Recommendation.** From the embryotoxicity point of view, an IUD remaining *in utero* is no indication for termination of pregnancy or invasive diagnostic procedures. However, increased spontaneous abortion has been reported with retained IUDs.

References

ACOG. Committee Opinion No. 342. Induction of labor for vaginal birth after cesarean delivery. Obstet Gynaecol 2006; 108: 465–7.

Bateman BT, Huybrechts KF, Hernandez-Diaz S et al. Methyergonovine maleate and the risk of myocardial ischemia and infarction. Am J Obstet Gynecol 2013; 209: 459.e1–459.e13.

Bellemin B, Carlier P, Vial T et al. Misoprostol exposure during pregnancy: a French collaborative study. Presentation at the 10th Annual Conference of the European Network of Teratology Information Services (ENTIS), Madrid, 1999.

Bond GR, Van Zee A. Overdosage of misoprostol in pregnancy. Am J Obstet Gynecol 1994; 71: 561–2.

Briozzo L, Matinez A, Nozar M et al. Tocolysis and delayed delivery versus emergency delivery in cases of non-reassuring fetal status during labor. J Obstet Gynaecol Res 2007; 33: 266–73.

Brocklehurst P, Gordon A, Heatly E et al. Antibiotics for treating bacterial vaginosis in pregnancy. Cochrane Database Syst Rev 2013; CD000262.pub4.

Castilla EE, Orioli IM. Teratogenicity of misoprostol: data from the Latin-American collaborative study of congenital malformations (ECLAMC). Am J Med Genet 1994; 51: 161–2.

Conde-Agudelo A, Romero R. Antenatal magnesium sulfate for the prevention of cerebral palsy in preterm infants less than 34 weeks' gestation: a systematic review and meta-analysis. Am J Obstet Gynecol 2009; 200: 595–609.

Crowther CA, Hiller JE, Doyle LW. Magnesium sulphate for preventing preterm birth in threatened preterm labour. Cochrane Database Syst Rev 2002: CD001060.

Da Silva dal Pizzol T, Pozzobon Knop F, Serrate Mengue S. Prenatal exposure to misoprostol and congenital anomalies: systematic review and meta-analysis. Reproduct Toxicol 2006; 22: 666–71.

Da Silva Dal Pizzol T, Vieira Sanseverino MT, Mengue SS. Exposure to misoprostol and hormones during pregnancy and risk of congenital anomalies. Cad Saude Publica 2008; 24: 1447–53.

de Heus R, Mulder EJH, Derks JB et al. Acute tocolysis for uterine reduction in term labour; a review. Obstet Gynecol Surv 2008a; 63: 383–8.

de Heus R, Mulder EJH, Derks JB et al. A prospective randomized trial of acute tocolysis in term labour with atosiban or ritodrine. Eur J Obstet Gynecol Reprod Biol 2008b; 139: 139–45.

de Heus R, Mol BW, Erwich JJHM, et al. Adverse drug reactions to tocolytic treatment for preterm labour: a prospective cohort study. BMJ 2009; 338; b744.

Dodd JM, Crowther CA, Middleton P. Oral betamimetics for maintenance therapy after threatened preterm labour. Cochrane Database Syst Rev 2012; 12: CD003927.

Doyle LW. Antenatal magnesium sulfate and neuroprotection. Curr Opin Pediatr 2012; 24: 54–9.

Einarson TR, Koren G, Mattice D et al. Maternal spermicide use and adverse reproductive outcome: a meta-analysis. Am J Obstet Gynecol 1990; 162: 655–60.

El-Sayed Y, Holbrook RH Jr, Gibson R et al. Diltiazem for maintenance tocolysis of preterm labor: comparison to nifedipine in a randomized trial. J Matern Fetal Med 1998; 7: 217–21.

Goldberg AB, Greenberg MB, Darney PD. Misoprostol and pregnancy. N Engl J Med 2001; 344: 38–47.

Goldenberg RL. The management of preterm labor. Obstet Gynecol 2002; 100: 1020–37.

Gonzalez CH, Marques-Dias MJ, Kim CA et al. Congenital abnormalities in Brazilian children associated with misoprostol misuse in first trimester of pregnancy. Lancet 1998; 351: 1624–7.

Grimes DA, Nanda K. Magnesium sulfate tocolysis: time to quit. Obstet Gynecol 2006; 108: 986–9.

Grospietsch G, Fenske M, Kühn W. Pathophysiologie der Lungenödementstehung bei der tokolytischen Therapie mit Fenoterol. Arch Gynäkol 1981; 232: 504–12.

Haas DM, Caldwel DM, Kirkpatrick P et al. BMJ 2012; 345: e6226.

Haas DM, Imperiale TF, Kirkpatrick PR et al. Tocolytic therapy: a meta-analysis and decision analysis. Obstet Gynecol 2009; 113: 585–94.

Higby K, Suiter CR. A risk-benefit assessment of therapies for premature labour. Drug Saf 1999; 21: 35–56.

Hofmeyr GJ, Milos D, Nikodem VC et al. Limb reduction anomaly after failed misoprostol abortion. S Afr Med J 1998: 88; 566–7.

Hofmeyr GJ, Gulmezoglu AM, Novikova N et al. Post-partum misoprostol for preventing maternal mortality and morbidity. Cochrane Database Syst Rev 2013; 7: CD008982.

Jannet D, Abankwa A, Guyard B et al. Nicardipine versus salbutamol in the treatment of premature labor. A prospective randomized study. Eur J Obstet Gynecol Reprod Biol 1997; 73: 11–6.

Jick H, Walker AM, Rothman KJ et al. Vaginal spermicides and congenital disorders. J Am Med Assoc 1981; 245: 1329–32.

Katz VL, Farmer RM. Controversies in tocolytic therapy. Clin Obstet Gynecol 1999; 42: 802–19.

Leitich H, Kiss H. Asymptomatic bacterial vaginosis and intermediate flora as risk factors for adverse pregnancy outcome. Best Pract Res Clin Obstet Gynecol 2007; 21: 375–90.

Mousa HA, Blum J, Abou El Senoun G et al. Treatment of primary post-partum hemorrhage. Cochrane Database Syst Rev 2014; 1: CD003249.

Oei SG. Calcium channel blockers for tocolysis: a review of their role and safety following reports of serious adverse events. Eur J Obstet Gynecol 2006; 126: 137–45.

Orioli IM, Castilla EE. Epidemiological assessment of misoprostol teratogenicity. Br J Obstet Gynaecol 2000; 107: 519–23.

Papatsonis DN, Kok JH, van Geijn HP et al. Neonatal effects of nifedipine and ritodrine for preterm labor. Obstet Gynecol 2000; 95: 477–81.

Papatsonis DN, van Geijn HP, Ader HJ et al. Nifedipine and ritodrine in the management of preterm labor: a randomized multicenter trial. Obstet Gynecol 1997; 90: 230–34.

Papatsonis DN, van Geijn HP, Bleker OP et al. Hemodynamic and metabolic effects after nifedipine and ritodrine tocolysis. Int J Gynaecol Obstet 2003; 82: 5–10.

Pastuszak AL, Schüler L, Speck-Martins CE et al. Use of misoprostol during pregnancy and Möbius' syndrome in infants. N Engl J Med 1998; 338: 1881–5.

RCOG Green-top guideline 1B. Tocolysis for women in preterm labour. RCOG 2011.

Roos C, Spaanderman ME, Schuit E et al. Effect of maintenance tocolysis with nifedipine in threatened preterm labour on perinatal outcome: a randomised controlled trial. JAMA 2013; 309: 41–7.

Rosenstein IJ, Stafford MK, Kitchen VS et al. Effect on normal vaginal flora of three intra-vaginal microbiocidal agents potentially active against human immunodeficiency virus type 1. J Infect Dis 1998; 177: 1386–90.

Schiff E, Sivan E, Terry S et al. Currently recommended oral regimens for ritodrine tocolysis result in extremely low plasma levels. Am J Obstet Gynecol 1993; 169: 1059–64.

Schüler L, Ashton PW, Sanseverino MT. Teratogenicity of misoprostol. Lancet 1992; 339: 437.

Schüler L, Pastuszak A, Sanseverino MTV et al. Pregnancy outcome after exposure to miso-prostol in Brazil: a prospective, controlled study. Reprod Toxicol 1999; 13: 147–51.

Stafford MK, Ward H, Flanagan A et al. Safety study of nonoxynol-9 as a vaginal microbi-cide: evidence of adverse effects. J Acquir Immune Defic Syndr Hum Retrovirol 1998; 17: 327–31.

Stuart MC, Kouimtzi M, Hill SR eds. WHO Model of Essential Medicines 2008, WHO Geneva.

Su LL, Chong YS, Samuel M. Carbetocin for preventing post-partum haemorrhage. Cochrane Database Syst Rev 2012; 2: CD005457.

Thayer JS, Hupp SC. In utero exposure to terbutaline. Effects on infant behavior and mater-nal self esteem. J Obstet Gynecol Neonatal Nurs 1997; 27: 691–700.

van Geijn HP, Lenglet JE, Bolte AC. Nifedipine trials: effectiveness and safety aspects. Br J Obstet Gynaecol 2005; 112: 79–83.

Weidinger H, Wiest H. Die Behandlung des Spätabortes und der drohenden Frühgeburt mit Thll65a in Kombination mit Isoptin. Z Geburtsh Perinatol 1973; 177: 233–7.

Wing DA, Gaffaney CA. Vaginal misoprostol administration for cervical ripening and labor induction. Clin Obstet Gynecol 2006; 49: 627–41.

Wollen A, Sandvei R, Skare A et al. The localization and concentration of copper in the fallopian tube in women with or without an intrauterine contraceptive device. Acta Obstet Gynecol Scand 1994; 73: 195–9.

Worldwide Atosiban versus Beta-agonists Study Group. Effectiveness and safety of the oxytocin antagonist atosiban versus beta-adrenergic agonists in the treatment of preterm labour. Br J Obstet Gynaecol 2001; 108: 133–42.

Yip SK, Tse AOK, Haines CJ et al. Misoprostol's effect on uterine arterial blood flow and fetal heart rate in early pregnancy. Obstet Gynecol 2000; 95: 232–5.

Hormones

Asher Ornoy and Corinna Weber-Schöndorfer

2.15

2.15.1	Hypothalamic releasing hormones	414
2.15.2	Anterior pituitary hormones	415
2.15.3	Prolactin antagonists/dopamine agonists	416
2.15.4	Posterior pituitary hormones	417
2.15.5	Thyroid function and iodine supply during pregnancy	417
2.15.6	Hypothyroidism, triiodothyronine (T3) and thyroxin (T4)	418
2.15.7	Hyperthyroidism and thyrostatics	419
2.15.8	Glucocorticoids	423
2.15.9	Diabetes mellitus and pregnancy	426
2.15.10	Insulin	428
2.15.11	Oral antidiabetics (OAD)	430
2.15.12	Estrogens	434
2.15.13	Gestagens	435
2.15.14	Duogynon®	437
2.15.15	Diethylstilbestrol	437
2.15.16	Androgens and anabolics	438
2.15.17	Cyproterone and danazol	439
2.15.18	Mifepristone (RU486)	440
2.15.19	Clomiphene	440
2.15.20	Erythropoietin	441

Hormones are the body's own messenger substances which carry out specific regulating functions in the cells of their respective effector organs and thereby control physiologic processes. Their regulation takes place on three levels, the hypothalamic level (primary releasing function), the stimulator level in the pituitary gland, and the glandular level in the respective organs. The secretion of the hormones is controlled via feedback mechanisms among the three levels or via the blood levels of the substance they are regulating (e.g. insulin and glucose, glucagon and glucose, calcium and parathyroid hormone).

Drugs During Pregnancy and Lactation. http://dx.doi.org/10.1016/B978-0-12-408078-2.00016-0

When a mother is treated with hormones, there may also be effects on the fetus at the various levels of these regulatory mechanisms. Drugs affecting the maternal endocrine system might also affect the fetal system. Maternal endocrine diseases (e.g. diabetes, hyper- or hypothyroidism) might have negative effects on the embryo and fetus often not related to the fetal hormones (e.g. diabetic embryopathy and fetopathy).

The classical hormones, antihormones and maternal disease of the endocrine system discussed in this chapter are distinguished from local tissue factors or mediators, which also include, among other substances, the prostaglandins (Chapter 2.14) and leukotrienes.

2.15.1   Hypothalamic releasing hormones

Hypothalamic releasing hormones (e.g. gonadotropin releasing hormone, GnRH) can cross the placenta due to their relatively low molecular size. They are used today as diagnostics for endometriosis, uterine myomas, in reproductive medicine, and for some hormone-dependent malignant illnesses. GnRH agonists are also used to prevent premature menopause in younger patients with malignancies after chemotherapy, though their effectiveness and safety are controversial (Blumenfeld 2008).

The following are used as diagnostics:

- With the synthetic substance, *protirelin*, which is equivalent to the natural hypothalamic thyrotropin-releasing hormone (TRH) test is carried out.
- With the help of *corticorelin*, the corticotropic function of the anterior pituitary can be examined (i.e. when pituitary tumors are suspected).
- *Somatorelin*, a synthetic analog of the growth hormone-releasing hormone (GHRH) is used as a diagnostic where there is suspicion of growth hormone deficiency.
- *Gonadorelin* is the physiologic GnRH, which releases LH and FSH from the pituitary and is used both as a diagnostic and as a medication (i.e. for substitution treatment of a GnRH-insufficiency). The gonadorelin analog, *triptorelin*, is used in the course of assisted reproduction as well as in women with endometriosis and with uterine myomas.
- *Leuprorelin* (a GnRH analog), and *goserelin*, luteinizing hormone-releasing hormone (LHRH) agonist are approved for endometriosis, uterine myomas and breast cancer.
- The GnRH analogs, *buserelin* and *nafarelin*, are used for the treatment of endometriosis and in assisted reproduction.

Among more than 340 pregnant women accidentally treated with GnRH analogs in the first trimester, there was neither an increase in birth defects or miscarriages, nor an inhibitory effect on intrauterine growth (survey in Cahill 1998). In a study comprising only six children, developmental problems such as attention deficits disorder, motor and language disturbances, were diagnosed in four children. One child also had epilepsy. The authors attributed this to a possible developmental toxic effect of the GnRH analogs (Lahat 1999). These findings were not corroborated by other studies.

The GnRH antagonists, *cetrorelix* and *ganirelix* are intended to prevent a premature increase of the luteinizing hormone (LH) and, thereby, premature ovulation in the context of assisted reproduction. A comparison of the effects on pregnancy between the GnRH antagonist, ganirelix, and the analog, buserelin, on the triggering of ovulation, showed no differences between the two groups of 1,000 women each, with respect to the live birth rate and the frequency of congenital malformations (Bonduelle 2010). The clinical experiences with the accidental administration of GnRH antagonists with an already existing pregnancy are insufficient for a risk assessment. However, up to now, there have been no suspicions of damage to the embryo.

Naturally occurring *somatostatin* as well as the similarly structured synthetically manufactured somatostatin and *octreotide,* a synthetic octapeptide derivative of somatostatin, inhibit the release of both the somatotropin (STH) and thyroid stimulating hormone (TSH). Thus, somatostatin occupies a special position among the hypothalamic hormones. Therapeutically, somatostatin analogs are used as hemostatics, with carcinoids and for reducing the effects of growth hormone in acromegaly.

The treatment of pregnant women with octreotide was reported in more than 15 cases, without observation of any side effects. Most women were treated for acromegaly, and at least seven patients received the drug throughout pregnancy. The somatostatin analogs cross the placenta. No effects on the children exposed *in utero* have been reported as yet. One girl was examined regularly until she was six, with laboratory, neurological and clinical testing (Maffei 2010). *Lanreotide,* an analog of somatostatin, has been used since 2005 as a therapy for acromegaly.

> **Recommendation.** There is scarcely any indication for the use of hypothalamic releasing hormones (agonists) or for GnRH-antagonists during pregnancy. The therapy for acromegaly is an exception for which there is currently no general recommendation but also no contraindication for use in pregnancy.

2.15.2   Anterior pituitary hormones

The hormones produced in the anterior pituitary gland stimulate or regulate the body's endocrine glands. The release of pituitary hormones is controlled by hypothalamic releasing hormones. Pituitary hormones do not cross the placenta due to their high molecular weight. Therefore, a direct effect on the fetus is not to be expected. The following hormones are among the pituitary hormones.

ACTH, the adrenocorticotropic hormone, stimulates the synthesis of the glucocorticoids and mineralocorticoids in the adrenal cortex. *Tetracosactid,* a synthetically produced preparation mimicking ACTH is available to treat West's syndrome ("infantile epileptic encephalopathy").

Gonadotropins, the follicle-stimulating hormone (FSH) and the LH as well as human chorionic gonadotropin, produced in the placenta during pregnancy and similar to LH. *Urofollitrophin, chorionic gonadotropin, chorionic gonadotropin alfa, corifollitropin alfa, follitropin alfa, follitropin beta, lutropin alfa* and *menotropin* (HMG) are the medications available which mimic the action of natural hormones. Indications for hormone treatment are: induction of ovulation and maintenance of the corpus luteum.

The stimulation of ovulation with gonadotropins can lead to multiple pregnancies with 5–6% of the cases resulting in triplets. Two publications described one complex malformation and four neuroblastoma cases in the first year of life after gonadotropin stimulation (Mandel 1994, Litwin 1991). These findings were not confirmed by other studies, nor were other risks for the course of pregnancy described. Hence, there is no appreciable indication of damage when pituitary hormones are accidentally administered during pregnancy.

Pregnancy

2.15 Hormones

Somatotropin or growth hormone (GH; a structurally and function-ally similar hormone to somatotropin) is produced by the placenta in increasing quantities as the pregnancy progresses. It is also termed human placental lactogen (HPL) or, less often, human chorianic soma-tomammotropin (HCS). Functionally, it has similarities to prolactin (see below). Medications with gene technologically produced STH are avail-able for the treatment of dwarfism. *Mecasermin*, a human insulin-like growth factor-1 (IGF-1), produced with gene technology and, thereby, a somatotropin agonist, is indicated for growth disturbances with a severe lack of IGF-1.

Pegvisomant is a somatotropin receptor antagonist, which is used for acromegaly and for which several case reports are available. One such example is a case described by Brian (2007), of a woman who was treated during pregnancy with 15 mg per day of pegvisomant and gave birth to a healthy child. The pegvisomant concentration in the cord blood was just at the detectable limit and the baby's hormone levels were within the normal range.

Naturally occurring TSH stimulates the synthesis of the thyroid gland hormones. The medication known as *thyrotropin alfa* is used to detect the remains of the thyroid after a thyroidectomy.

Recommendation. There is scarcely any indication for giving anterior pituitary hormones or their antagonists during pregnancy. The therapy for acromegaly is an exception for which there is currently no general recommendation.

2.15.3   Prolactin antagonists/dopamine agonists

Infertility resulting from hyperprolactinemia hypogonadism (galactorrhea-amenorrhea syndrome) or a prolactinoma is usually reversible after treat-ment with centrally acting dopamine agonists. Should ophthalmological problems associated with macroprolactinomas, for example, arise in the course of the pregnancy, it is recommended to resume therapy.

Bromocriptine, an ergot alkaloid derivative, is used for hyperprolac-tinemia (Chapter 4.11.3) and, in higher doses, for Parkinson's disease (Chapter 2.11.14). A study of 2,587 pregnancies in which bromocriptine was given during the first weeks of pregnancy, gave no indication of tera-togenic effects (Krupp 1987). Since most women stopped the therapy after discovering the pregnancy, the result confirms, at the same time, the harm-lessness for the developing fetus of a continuing hyperprolactinemia.

Cabergoline, a synthetic ergot alkaloid with a longer-lasting effective-ness is given for the same indications as bromocriptine but has a higher effectiveness and a more positive side-effect profile. In about 500 pregnan-cies there was no indication of teratogenic effects (i.e. Lebbe 2010, Ono 2010), even when treatment was continuous in some cases or had to be resumed in the course of the pregnancy (i.e. Laloi-Michelin 2007, de Turris 2003). Up to now, there has been no indication of postnatal developmen-tal disturbances (Lebbe 2010). A pediatrician has examined the children at regular intervals, in some cases up to the age of six (Ono 2010).

Lisuride was used in a small retrospective study of 27 pregnancies to 17 hyperprolactinemic women. Most of them were treated with lisuride and there were 22 normal children, four induced abortions and one spontaneous abortion, possibly demonstrating that lisuride does not negatively affect pregnancies (Ventz 1996).

Metergoline can probably be evaluated similarly to the other prolactin antagonists.

Experiences with the selective dopamine-D2-receptor agonist, *quinagolide*, which is not among the ergot alkaloids, are available for 10 pregnancies with healthy children. In four cases, therapy was needed throughout pregnancy (Morange 1996). An additional 159 pregnancies collected by the manufacturer, where the mothers were treated for an average of 37 days of their pregnancy, had no indication of developmental toxic effects (cited in Webster 1996).

> **Recommendation.** Bromocriptine and cabergoline are the dopamine agonists of choice for hyperprolactinemia. After conception they should be stopped if it is therapeutically possible. This also applies to lisuride, metergoline and quinagolide for which a differentiated risk analysis is not yet possible due to limited experience in these products.

2.15.4   Posterior pituitary hormones

Oxytocin (Chapter 2.14) and *vasopressin* (adiuretin) are secreted from the neurohypophysis, the posterior lobe of the pituitary. Structurally, these octapeptide hormones are similar to the hypothalamic hormones.

Vasopressin, or the antidiuretic hormone (ADH), is the natural representative of synthetic analogs, *desmopressin* and *terlipressin*. Desmopressin is used for treatment of already existing *diabetes insipidus* or diagnosed during pregnancy. It is also approved parenterally as an antihemorrhagic drug to increase factor VIII coagulation activity with hemophilia A and the von Willebrand-Jürgens disease. Case reports on more than 50 pregnancies found no specific risk (Sánchez-Luceros 2007, Siristatidis 2004, Ray 1998). There is no experience available in pregnancy for terlipressin, which is approved as an emergency medication for esophageal varices bleeding and which, in animal experiments, acts as an abortifacient.

Tolvaptan is a selective vasopressin-V2-receptor antagonist, which is used for hyponatremia resulting from inadequate ADH secretion. There are no reports on its use during pregnancy.

> **Recommendation.** Oxytocin can be used in obstetrics for inducing and strengthening contractions. Desmopressin may be used as a substitution for ADH deficiency during pregnancy and, if urgently indicated, also as an antihemorrhagic agent.

2.15.5   Thyroid function and iodine supply during pregnancy

Hormonal changes and the altered metabolic needs during pregnancy are accompanied by a physiological adaptation of the thyroid function. This is an important prerequisite for normal embryonic and fetal development as well as for an uncomplicated pregnancy.

The fetal thyroid begins to function at the end of the third month of pregnancy. Before that, the placenta and embryo are exclusively dependent on the thyroid hormone supply via the mother.

Pregnancy

2.15 Hormones

During pregnancy, the mother's need for iodine increases. Both the maternal as well as the fetal thyroid function are dependent on a sufficient iodine supply. In regions where iodine is in short supply, sufficient iodine should be assured even before a pregnancy.

The daily iodine requirement during pregnancy is 260 μg. In many countries, the intake of iodine is frequently insufficient. Since a supply through iodized salt, iodized foods and sea fish appears to be unreliable, 200–300 μg of iodine should be substituted with tablets throughout the entire pregnancy. Giving iodine can also be undertaken with an elevated thyroid peroxidase auto-antibody titer of the thyroid (TPO-AK), because autoimmune thyroiditis of the Hashimoto type is neither induced nor worsened by this.

2.15.6 Hypothyroidism, triiodothyronine (T3) and thyroxin (T4)

Hypothyroidism can be a cause of infertility and, if untreated, may lead to increased complications during pregnancy, e.g. to more spontaneous abortions, hypertension of pregnancy, placenta previa or placenta abruptio (Gärtner 2009). In populations with a sufficient iodine supply, chronic thyroiditis is the most common cause of thyroid hypoactivity. Also thyroid antibodies, without manifest hypothyroidism, increase the risk of spontaneous abortions (Gärtner 2009) and premature births (Negro 2006). This was also confirmed by the results of a meta-analysis (Thangaratinam 2011). Levothyroxine seems to lower this risk. Depending on the severity and duration of (untreated) hypothyroidism during pregnancy, there may be impairment of neuropsychological development of the child. This is known, in particular in connection with iodine deficiency (Berbel 2009). Pop (2003) studied the developmental outcome of 63 children born to mothers with low free thyroxin (fT4) during pregnancy compared to 62 children born to euthyroid mothers and found on the Bayley developmental scales an average reduction of 10 points on the mental scales, and of 8 points on the motor scales in the first and second year of life. Similarly, Li (2010) found delayed development at 25–30 months of age in offspring of women with subclinical hypothyroidism, hypothyroxinemia or elevated levels of thyroid peroxidase antibodies. In a study from The Netherlands (Henrichs 2010) maternal hypothyroxinemia was found to be a significant risk factor in the offspring for language and cognitive delay at 30 months.

Haddow (1999) came to similar conclusions in a study on 60 seven to nine-year-old children. Many authors recommend screening for thyroid function disturbances, including thyroid antibody determinations before or, at least, after confirmation of a pregnancy.

The active thyroid hormones are the L-forms of *triiodothyronine* (T3) and *thyroxin* (T4), which are only metabolically active in a free, non-protein bound form. T3 is the biologically effective hormone, which takes effect relatively quickly and has a shorter period of effectiveness, while T4 can be seen as a less effective prohormone, which is deionized as needed to T3. The placenta needs thyroid hormones for its development. It deionates T4 to T3 (reverses T3), and T3 to T2. The placenta only allows limited passage of thyroid hormones. However, with fetal thyroid gland agenesis, there is a quantitative transfer (of maternal thyroxin) due to the high concentration gradient.

Levothyroxine and *liothyronine* or combination preparations are the medications available as substitution therapy. Teratogenic or feto-toxic effects are not to be expected with the usual doses that restore physiological relationships. During pregnancy, the need for thyroid hormone increases so that hypothyroid women must adapt the dose accordingly.

There are indications that selenium (i.e. selenase) can lower the thyroid peroxidase autoantibody (TPO-AB) titer when there is a selenium deficiency (Toulis 2010). The thyroid is rich in this essential trace element, which is a component of glutathione peroxidase and deiodase which deiodates T4 to the active hormone triiodothyronine (T3). With immune thyroiditis, selenium can be given in a dose of about 200 µg/ daily, together with thyroxin. In a prospective, placebo-controlled study of 151 pregnant women with elevated TP-AK, of whom half were in the intervention group, a decline in the frequency of maternal postpartum thyroid function disturbances and postpartum hypothyroidism was observed (Negro 2007). However, it is not clear whether this also has positive effects on the course of the pregnancy (e.g. the frequency of preeclampsia) and the outcome of pregnancy (e.g. the rate of prematurity; Reid 2010).

Recommendation. Pregnant women with healthy thyroids should also take iodine prophylactically. Hypothyroidism must, as a rule, be treated with levothyroxine. At the beginning of a pregnancy (from the fifth week of pregnancy), the T4 dose should be increased by about 30%, by 25–50 µg at the beginning of the pregnancy. In the second trimester, a further dose increase is needed to an approximately 40–50% higher dose compared to the pre-pregnancy dose. The TSH values allow for monitoring the therapeutic adaptation. Women with chronic thyroiditis without hypothyroidism should receive thyroxin during pregnancy. Further studies are needed to judge whether selenium is a good therapeutic option for a pregnant woman with TPO-AB.

2.15.7 Hyperthyroidism and thyrostatics

Untreated manifested hyperthyroidism is a risk for the mother and the fetus. Fetal growth retardation, preeclampsia, prematurity, and intrauterine death or stillbirths have been described. With Grave's disease, as well as Hashimoto thyroiditis, which, as a rule, lead to hypothyroidism, the thyroid gland auto-antibodies should be determined at the beginning of the pregnancy and early in the third trimester. High values, especially of TSH-R immunoglobulin (TSI) are an indication of how these antibodies can be transferred transplacentally. Observations of how frequently transient hyperthyroidism in the fetus or the newborn can occur in this way, lie between 1 and 10.3% (Rosenfeld 2009). Selenium supplementation in pregnant women with thyroiditis, if possible several months before a planned pregnancy, should be considered as this may reduce the level of the thyroid antibodies that are able to reach the fetus (Toulis 2010).

Hyperthyroidism in pregnant women is usually treated with thyrostatics. With severe thyrotoxicosis in the mother, operative treatment may be indicated during pregnancy.

Radioactive iodine therapy (Chapter 2.20) is contraindicated. Among the thyrostatics are propylthiouracil, carbimazol and its active metabolite, thiamazol (or methimazol). All of these substances can reach the fetus.

Thyrostatic treatment is the therapy of choice for hyperthyroid pregnant women.

Thyroid function, i.e. the levels of free thyroxine (FT4) and anti-TSH receptor antibodies should be routinely monitored in pregnancy to reduce the possibility of fetal thyroid dysfunction (Chan 2007). Today, carefully adjusted thyrostatic therapy scarcely ever leads to a serious congenital goiter in the newborn (Diav-Citrin 2002). During pregnancy, therapy with thyrostatics should be kept at the lowest possible dose, involve clinical findings such as the mother's heart beat frequency, as monitoring parameters, and should not be combined with thyroxin.

Hyperthyroidism may adversely affect pregnancy outcome. Mitsuda (1992) observed reduced birth weight in 6.5% of neonates of 230 pregnancies of mothers with Grave's disease and thyroid dysfunction in 16.5% of the neonates. There were apparently no other problems in the neonates. Other investigators also reported reduced birth weight, increased prematurity and abnormal thyroid functions in the neonates (Ramprasad 2012).

▶ **Propylthiouracil (PTU)**

Propylthiouracil (PTU), which came on the market more than 60 years ago, is more commonly used in the USA than in Europe. It is estimated that 100,000 people were treated with PTU in 2008 in the USA. The rare sudden acute liver toxicity has limited the recommendation as the drug of first choice for pregnant women. Over the last 20 years, 22 cases of serious liver toxicity after PTU in adults, of which nine died and five had liver transplants, have been reported to the Food and Drug Administration (FDA 2009). Presumably, the actual number is higher because 16 PTU-caused liver transplants have been carried out alone in the past 17 years in the USA (Rivkees 2010). Bahn (2009) found an increased rate of hepatotoxicity of PTU in children below 17 years compared to adults, and no such increase after metimazole treatment.

In a recent review on the use of PTU and hepatic toxicity, Glinoer (2012) recommend that PTU was not used in children and should be reduced in its use in adults. However, they do recommend its use during pregnancy.

Recommendations of the drug of choice in pregnancy are supported by the lack of teratogenicity (i.e. Rosenfeld 2009, Diav-Citrin 2002). A newer case-control study found an association between PTU and *situs inversus*, but the authors have doubts about a connection (Clementi 2010). The FDA MedWatch data bank analysis from 1970 to 2008 revealed nine malformations among 15 PTU cases reported, but without a specific malformation pattern (Tabacova 2010). The transplacental transfer of the various thyrostatics is very similar, so that with all of them, fetal/newborn hypothyroidism and goiter may occur (Bliddal 2011, Corral 2010). The observed frequency for neonatal elevated TSH values after intrauterine PTU exposure lies between 9.5% (of which a good half of them also had a concurrent goiter; Rosenfeld 2009) and 21% (Momotani 1997). Under clinical conditions, the hyperthyroidism is not always detectable at the recommended pediatric check-up of these infants between 7–10 days of age. As a rule, normalization of the thyroid values occurs in the first month of life.

► **Thiamazole (methimazole) and carbimazole**

Carbimazole and *thiamazole* or *methimazole* have been on the market as long as PTU. Only five cases of severe liver toxicity in adults have been reported to the Food and Drug Administration (2009). Of these, three died (i.e. fewer than after PTU use). In order to be able to compare this side effect of the two substances, figures on the frequency of methimazole use would also be needed.

Carbimazole and thiamazole (methimazole) can lead to a rare embryopathy, the skin defect (aplasia cutis), particularly in the area of the head covered by hair, choanal atresia, esophageal atresia, tracheo-esophageal fistulas and other malformations of the gastrointestinal tract (Ono 2009) and includes discrete facial dysmorphism, growth retardation, and mental as well as motor delay (i.e. Foulds 2005, Barbero 2004, Karg 2004, Ferraris 2003, Karlsson 2002, Clementi 1999). In some 20 to 30 case reports, malformation or a combination of them, that fit with the phenotype mentioned, have been described: at least 15 children had an aplasia cutis (i.e. Abe 2010) and in at least 13 cases, a choanal atresia (i.e. Kannan 2008). In some children, both malformations occurred. Also the FDA MedWatch data bank analysis between 1970 and 2008 revealed that, among the 32 reported pregnancies during methimazole treatment, many malformations showed the familiar pattern, consisting of scalp defects, facial dysmorphias and choanal atresia (Tabacova 2010).

In a prospective multicenter case control study of 204 methimazole-exposed pregnancies, eight children were malformed demonstrating no increased risk of malformations. However, among the eight malformed children, one had a choanal atresia and another had an esophageal atresia (di Gianantonio 2001). In a case control study by Barbero (2008), an association with intrauterine methimazole exposure was found in 10 of 61 children (16.4%) with choanal atresia, while in the control group of healthy children, only 2/183 (1.1%) had been exposed to methimazole *in utero*. Another study (Clementi 2010), which divided 18,131 children with malformations into 52 groups and analyzed medication intake in the first trimester with respect to an association with the intake of thyrostatics, found a statistically significant connection between carbimazole/methimazole exposure and omphaloccles as well as choanal atresias. It may be assumed that unilateral choanal atresia after methimazole exposure occurs more frequently than has been reported to date, because this is not always diagnosed shortly after birth.

To summarize, the total rate of malformations after methimazole exposure does not seem to be increased; however, methimazole, with an estimated frequency of 1/1,000–1/10,000 exposed fetuses, can lead to the above-mentioned malformation syndrome (Cooper 2002, Diav-Citrin 2002). Two smaller studies found no effects on the physical and intellectual development of children exposed *in utero* (Eisenstein 1992, Messer 1990). Transplacental transfer of the various thyrostatics is similar, so that fetal/neonatal hypothyroidism and goiter may occur with all of them (Bliddal 2011). According to an earlier study, about 14% the newborns are affected (Momotani 1997).

► **Sodium perchlorate and others**

Sodium perchlorate is only rarely indicated for excessive iodine intake. During pregnancy it can impair the iodine transfer to the fetus and lead to a hypothyroid goiter.

> **Recommendation.** Manifest hyperthyroidism should be treated during pregnancy with thyrostatics, whereby a dose as low as therapeutically possible should be chosen; a combination with thyroxin is contraindicated. Due to the lack of teratogenicity, PTU is seen in many places as the drug of choice in pregnancy. Since an embryopathy after carbimazole, thiamazole/methimazole seldom occurs and the very rare severe liver toxicity is more frequently observed in PTU-treated patients than after carbimazole/thiamazole, these risks have to be weighed up against each other. At least in the first trimester, PTU is preferable. On the other hand, a woman who was already stably adapted to (low doses) of carbimazole/thiamazole (methimazole) should not change the treatment. Therapy with thiamazole (methimazole) and carbimazole in the first trimester warrants a second trimester detailed ultrasound diagnostic examination.

Both fetal hypothyroidism (as a consequence of the medication) and fetal hyperthyroidism (through the transfer of maternal auto-antibodies) have been described. Therefore, the thyroid of the fetus should be examined sonographically and monitoring of the thyroid function in the newborn, as well as on days 10–14 postpartum are recommended.

▶ Parathyroid hormone (PTH)

Parathyroid hormone (PTH), is secreted by the parathyroid glands as a polypeptide containing 84 amino acids with a molecular weight of 9.4 kiloDaltons. The 1-34 amino acid is the active part of PTH. It acts to increase the concentration of calcium (Ca^{2+}) in the blood, by increasing bone resorption; hence, causing the release of calcium and phosphate. The latter is lost in the kidney because of decreased reabsorption from the proximal tubule in the kidney. PTH increases calcium and magnesium absorption from the gut by increasing the activation of vitamin D as it increases 1 alpha hydroxylase activity producing its active metabolite 1,25-dihydroxy D (calcitriol). PTH opposes the action of calcitonin, a hormone produced by the parafollicular cells (C cells) of the thyroid gland, which acts to decrease calcium concentration. Severe *hypomagnesemia* or *hypercalcemia* and increased *calcitriol* inhibit PTH secretion. PTH increases the concentration of calcium in the blood by acting upon the parathyroid hormone 1 receptor (PTH and PTHrp), which are found in high levels in bone and kidney, and in the central nervous system, pancreas, testis, and placenta (Kovacs 2001). Being a protein, it has a short half-life of about 4 minutes. PTH, as well as vitamin D, regulates fetal placental calcium and phosphate homeostasis and are important players in fetal bone mineralization (Young 2012, Simmonds 2010) partially by regulating the genes involved in calcium transfer in the placenta and increasing its transfer through the placenta. There is a tight relationship between PTH and vitamin D (see also Chapter 2.18.9). Due to its high molecular weight, PTH is not supposed to cross the placenta. Hence, hyperparathyroidism in pregnancy is not reported to harm fetal development. On the other hand, the resulting hypercalcemia might affect the fetus. PTH treatment in pregnancy is not contraindicated.

> **Recommendation.** There is no need for treatment with PTH as the cases of hyperparathyroidism are treated with calcitriol and calcium with continuous monitoring of blood calcium. If treatment in pregnancy is indicated, it can be given with appropriate monitoring of maternal blood calcium levels. In the rare cases of hyperparathyroidism in pregnancy (i.e. adenoma of the parathyroids) there were no reports of fetal damage.

2.15.8   Glucocorticoids

Pharmacology

The adrenal cortex synthesizes two different groups of hormones: the glucocorticoids and mineralocorticoids, which, among other things, regulate the carbohydrate and mineral metabolism. During pregnancy, changes in the hormone balance of the adrenal cortex occur. From about the third month on, the concentration of cortisol in the serum rises and excretion increases until the end of the pregnancy.

Therapeutically, glucocorticoids are of high clinical importance and used extensively. A difference is made between the non-halogenated and the halogenated corticoids. The exclusively locally, dermally or inhalatively used derivatives are discussed in other sections (see Chapters 2.3.2). *Cortisol* and *prednisolone*, but not *betamethasone* and *dexamethasone*, are enzymatically inactivated in the placenta. Perinatally, only 10% of the maternal concentration of prednisone and prednisolone are found in the fetal blood. With betamethasone it is 30% and with dexamethasone nearly 100%.

Primary indications for glucocorticoid treatment

Glucocorticoids are effective in therapy for allergic, inflammatory and proliferative diseases. Thereby, unphysiologically high doses are used. Furthermore, they are used in substitution therapy for adrenal cortex failure and for the induction of fetal lung maturation.

In Table 2.15.1, the doses of the various glucocorticoids, whose effectiveness correspond to 10 mg prednisolone, are summarized.

Substitution therapy during pregnancy is seldom indicated, i.e. with Addison's disease giving *fludrocortisone* together with hydrocortisone.

Table 2.15.1 Effectiveness comparison of the various glucocorticoids

10 mg prednisolone corresponds to	Halogenate, fluoridated	Characteristics
Betamethasone	1.5 mg +	Mineral corticoids: There is almost no effect. Duration of effectiveness 36–54 hours
Budesonide		Oral bioavailability only 9–13% (Crohn's patients. Effective primarily locally in the GI tract
Cloprednol	5 mg +	
Deflazacort	12 mg	
Dexamethasone	1.5 mg +	No mineral corticoid effect. Duration of effect > 36 hours
Fluocortolone	10 mg +	Cushing threshold dose: 20 mg/day
Hydrocortisone	40 mg	Cushing threshold dose: 0–40 mg/daily. Clear mineral corticoid effect. Biological half-life 8–12 hours
Methylprednisolone	8 mg	No mineral corticoid effect. Duration of effect 12–36 hours
Prednisone	10 mg	Minimal mineral corticoid effect. Duration of effect 18–36 hours
Triamcinolone	8 mg +	Lesser mineral corticoid effect than prednisolone

Pregnancy

2.15 Hormones

The required doses of mineralocorticoids and glucocorticoids help to achieve physiological relationships and do not cause any side effects in either the mother or the exposed fetus.

Long-term treatment with high therapeutic doses for allergic, inflammatory or proliferative illnesses may lead to severe maternal side effects such as Cushing-like symptoms and osteoporosis. When it is stopped, adrenal cortex failure may occur. Should treatment of the fetus be necessary, *dexamethasone*, in particular, is preferable due to the better placental transfer. By contrast, the fluorinated corticoids are not appropriate for long-term systemic therapy of the mother.

Teratogenic effects

The largest experience with systemically used glucocorticoids is available for *prednisone* and *prednisolone*, the biologically active form of prednisone, particularly in the first trimester. In animal experiments, glucocorticoids have a teratogenic effect. They may cause a cleft palate, particularly in mice. On the question of clefts of the lip and palate in human beings, retrospective studies have not been able to completely rule out a slightly elevated risk (Carmichael 2007, Pradat 2003, Rodriguez-Pinilla 1998). A meta-analysis of all the cohort and case-control studies published so far has revealed a significantly increased risk for cleft formation (odds-ratio 3.4) with a total malformation rate that is not elevated (Park-Wyllie 2000). A prospective controlled study of 311 mothers exposed in the first trimester found neither an increase in the total risk of malformations nor a single case of cleft lip and palate (Gur 2004). Hardy (2005) also did not observe any association between oral steroid medication and the formation of clefts. Moreover, in a recent study from Denmark by Bay Bjorn (2012) of 1,449 pregnant women who used corticosteroids in the first trimester of pregnancy, there was only one case of oral cleft (0.08%) and the rate of major anomalies was similar to that of a control group of 83,043 "control" pregnancies of women not treated with glucocorticosteroids.

To summarize, a small risk of cleft palate with or without lip involvement cannot be ruled out if there is treatment with high doses of glucocorticoids in the sensitive phase between the eighth and eleventh weeks of pregnancy. A safe dose cannot be specified, but with low doses (i.e. 10–15 mg of prednisolone/daily) the individual risk seems to be negligible.

Fetotoxic effects

With high dose glucocorticoid maternal treatment, there may be intrauterine growth retardation, premature birth as well as transient hypoglycemia, hypotension and electrolyte disturbances in the newborn, depending on the duration of therapy, the dose and the indication. It seldom comes – as in the following unusual case – to severe neonatal adrenal insufficiency that appeared 3 hours after the birth of an otherwise healthy, full-term boy, who had no infection. After hydrocortisone substitution therapy, the newborn recovered without consequences. In the preceding 4 weeks, his mother had received 32 mg/daily of methyl prednisolone orally and 100 mg of hydrocortisone rectally due to an exacerbated Crohn's disease (Homar 2008).

Long-term effects

Miller (2004) studied body weight, the baseline concentration of cortisol, and cortisol values after stress induction due to immunizations up to the age of 4 months or longer. No differences were observed between children with longer prednisolone exposure and those of healthy mothers.

Induction of lung maturity

Pregnant women have been treated for decades for threatened premature births with dexamethasone or betamethasone, in order to promote the maturation of the newborn's lungs and prevent respiratory distress syndrome (RDS). The survival rate of a premature baby increases as a result of this therapy and brain hemorrhage occurs less frequently. The common clinical practice in the late 1990s was that after the initial administration, corticoids were repeated weekly, as long as the birth did not take place. This procedure was changed, as there were indications of an increased risk for infantile cerebral palsy and later behavioral anomalies, and one-time administration was recommended. In recent years, a large number of studies have been published, which have examined betamethasone versus dexamethasone and a one- versus two-time cycle with respect to effectiveness and neonatal side effects or possible long-term effects on the child.

Today, many European countries recommend a one-time betamethasone cycle (i.e. 12 mg betamethasone, i.m. and after 24 hours, a repetition with 12 mg) for pregnant women with threatening or medically indicated premature births (singletons and multiple births) between the twenty-fourth (from achieving viability) to the thirty-fourth week of pregnancy. After the thirty-fourth week of pregnancy, medical support for lung maturation is not necessary as a rule (Porto 2011). The more extensive recommendations of the World Association of Perinatal Medicine Prematurity Working Group (SAPM) are similar.

For the time being, the recommendation for a one-time betamethasone cycle is being adhered to. However, newer study results indicate a more favorable effect on neonatal morbidity with a two-time cycle (Miracle 2008). The chief argument for maintaining the one-time cycle is the lack of convincing studies on long-term effects on the child's behavior.

Repeated antenatal administration of corticosteroids has led to more serious negative effects on birth weight, body length and head circumference than one-time administration (Rodriguez-Pinilla 2006). Studies, which compared premature infants (<34 weeks), with one- versus two-time glucocorticoid exposures, with respect to neonatal mortality and morbidity, found no differences in mortality between the two groups. With neonatal morbidity, however, particularly as far as respiratory function is concerned, those premature infants with a two-time prepartum glucocorticoid cycle fared better (McEvoy 2010, Garite 2009).

Animal experimental studies and experiences from clinical studies of prematures suggest that betamethasone affects the neurophysiologic development of fetuses and newborns less than dexamethasone (Lee 2006). Contrary to individual reports, newborn sepsis does not occur frequently after the induction of lung maturation with glucocorticoids. A higher body-mass index of the mother before the pregnancy (BMI ≥25) had no significant influence on the morbidity of prematures when prenatal corticoids were given (Hashima 2010).

Long-term effects

Betamethasone
A Dutch study compared premature infants (born at less than 32 weeks of pregnancy) of 171 mothers who had received betamethasone (in a dose which is currently recommended) with those of 818 mothers who were not treated with glucocorticoids. At the age of 19 years, 84 of those exposed *in utero* were still able to be compared with 328 "controls": the low death rate in the betamethasone group (22% versus 35%) was not

associated in the survivors with a higher metabolic risk. However, the glomerular filtration rate in the exposed group was slightly reduced, but without clinical relevance (Finken 2008).

In a randomized study with 142 prematures from Helsinki, it was observed that repeated intrauterine betamethasone administration did not influence the temperament of the small child. However, when there was more than 24 hours between the second cycle and birth, these children were significantly more impulsive at age 2. The "Early Child Behavior" questionnaire, which was filled out by the parents, served as a basis for the analysis. Independent of the frequency of the administration of betamethasone, the birth weight was correlated with the temperament. Lighter prematures displayed less emotional control and motor activity as well as greater shyness at 2 years of age (corrected age) (Pesonen 2009).

Two hundred and fifty-nine Finnish prematures, among them 120 with two-time and 139 with only one-time betamethasone treatment (the so-called placebo group) were examined at 2 years of age by neuropsychologists, pediatricians or neuro-pediatricians in accordance with strict standardized measures. The groups did not differ in their physical or neurological development (Peltoniemi 2009).

Recommendation.

- Substitution with corticoids should be continued during pregnancy whenever needed.
- The induction of lung maturation with a threatening premature birth is currently carried out with a one-time betamethasone cycle between the twenty-fourth (achievement of viability) and the thirty-fourth week of pregnancy. In individual cases, a second cycle follows after the twenty-eighth week of pregnancy has passed.
- A systemic, antiallergic, antiinflammatory or immunosuppressive treatment of the mother with glucocorticoids may also be carried out for relevant indications. Prednisone and prednisolone are the drugs of choice for this.
- With the rarely necessary higher dose treatment over many weeks, fetal growth should be observed sonographically. If this therapy continues until birth, adrenal insufficiency in the newborn must be considered and treated if it occurs.
- Emergency treatments are obviously not subject to any dosage limitations.

Treatment of the mother with high doses of glucocorticoids during weeks 8–11 of pregnancy may warrant an ultrsonographic evaluation of the fetal face for the detection of clefting of the lip and palate (CL/CLP).

2.15.9   Diabetes mellitus and pregnancy

Diabetes mellitus (DM) is the collective term for heterogeneous disturbances of metabolism, the principal symptom of which is chronic hyperglycemia. Primarily, three types are differentiated. While type 1 is caused by insufficient secretion of insulin, type 2 and gestational diabetes (GDM) are characterized by disturbed insulin action. Type 1 or type 2 diabetes, can also be a major factor in infertility for men and women. GDM usually develops in the second half of pregnancy. The rate of pre-gestational diabetes (PGDM) and GDM are rising steadily in parallel with the striking rise in type 2 diabetes among adults. The rate of PGDM among pregnant women is now about 0.5%, and almost 40% of these women suffer from type 2 diabetes (Kinsley 2007). Maternal type 1 as well as type 2 diabetes pre-existing or starting at the beginning of a pregnancy (PGDM), recognizable by an elevated HbA1c-value, is correlated with an increased rate of malformations. HbA1c, as the "blood sugar memory", marks the metabolic situation of the patient for the duration of the survival time of the erythrocytes (120 days). The higher the HbA1c, the higher the risk of malformations and other pregnancy complications. The rate of congenital malformations in the offspring of PGD mothers, is about 5–10% in direct correlation with the severity of diabetes, being higher with poorer control of the disease (Reece 2012, Allen 2007).

The malformations associated with maternal diabetes include, in particular, heart defects, neural tube and brain anomalies, skeletal anomalies including caudal regression syndrome, omphalocels, malformations of the urinary tract and bile duct atresia with anomalies of the spleen. Frequently there are multiple malformations. It is difficult to define a threshold value beneath which an increased rate of malformations would not be expected. Overweight women without known diabetes mellitus are also at higher risk of having a child with neural tube defects. With a preconceptional HbA1c <7.5%, however, the risk for malformations in the baby is likely only modestly increased (Allen 2007).

Depending on the periconceptional metabolic adaptation, the rate of miscarriage is increased. Perinatal mortality and the premature birth rate are significantly above average. Neonatal morbidity is characterized by macrosomic newborns with insufficiently mature organs, underdevelopment and postpartum metabolic disturbances, in particular of hypoglycemia and sometimes hypocalcemia. With good control of diabetes, birth weight is normalized. In severe diabetes with nephropathy, birth weight might be below normal. In all newborns of diabetic mothers, hypoglycemia must be ruled out. The rate of caesarean deliveries and shoulder dystocia with vaginal births is increased in macrosomic children. Similarly, uteroplacental problems, hypertension of pregnancy also occurs more frequently. The vast majority of diabetes type 2 or GDM develops on the basis of a metabolic syndrome. In the beginning, there is insulin resistance of the insulin-dependent tissues so that an elevated insulin concentration is necessary for utilization of glucose in the tissues. Through hyperinsulinemia, the feeling of hunger is increased, which, in turn, leads to an increased intake of food, further obesity, etc. – a vicious circle. Effective weight reduction in these patients leads to lowered insulin concentrations and to an increased sensibility and density of insulin receptors. Weight reduction to a body mass index of (BMI) <27 kg/m^2 should be achieved before a planned pregnancy! (On the risk of existing obesity for the pregnancy see Chapter 2.5.15.)

Good metabolic adjustment with euglycemia is the goal of therapy during pregnancy, because diabetic fetopathy is mainly due to hyperglycemia in the mother, which also leads to hyperglycemia in the fetus. This reacts with increased fetal insulin production, which leads to β-cell-hypertrophy/-hyperplasia. Fetal hyperinsulinemia also promotes the development of RDS through the creation of hyaline membranes and impairment of the surfactant production in the fetal pneumocytes resulting in hyaline membrane disease.

Hypoglycemia is a relatively common complication during strict control of diabetes. If not severe enough to harm the mother, it apparently does not harm the developing embryo and fetus. Episodes of hypoglycemia, sometimes severe, usually occur in the first trimester of pregnancy (Evers 2002).

Pregnancy

2.15 Hormones

Children of diabetic mothers with insufficient diabetic control during pregnancy (mostly from unrecognized or insufficiently treated GDM) have a high risk of developing "metabolic syndrome" later in life. This is characterized by overweight and/or obesity, hypertension, cardiovascular disease and type 2 diabetes. Overweight and GDM are rapidly increasing in children and adults in industrialized countries. After a pregnancy with GDM, the maternal risk to develop diabetes mellitus type 2 increases. An attempt should be made to lower that risk with weight reduction, dietary and life style changes.

► Neurodevelopmental outcome

Children born to mothers with PGDM or GDM are at increased risk of having slight gross and fine motor deficits. They also have an increased rate of learning difficulties and attention deficit hyperactivity disorder (ADHD), as observed by several investigators in preschool and school-aged children. Their cognitive abilities are normal (Ornoy 1998, 1999).

The results of the international HAPO study (The Hyperglycemia and Adverse Pregnancy Outcome Study, Coustan 2010) have been published. This sought to find the blood glucose threshold values for an unfavorable course of pregnancy. Twenty-five thousand women from four continents took part in this study. The goal was to create standards with a predictive value for the diagnosis of GDM. The following recommendations were suggested for the diagnosis of GDM: when more than one of the following criteria of an oral glucose tolerance test (OGTT with 75 g glucose over 2 hours) was achieved or exceeded, fasting blood sugar, at the beginning of the glucose load, ≥92 mg/dL (5.1 mmol/L) 1-hour post glucose intake plasma glucose value ≥180 mg/dL (10 mmol/L); 2-hours plasma glucose value ≥153 mg/dL (8.5 mmol/L) (Coustan 2010). These guidelines are generally implemented in many countries as international guidelines.

> **Recommendation.** With diabetes mellitus, exact maintenance of euglycemia is the most important prerequisite for an uncomplicated course of pre- and postnatal development of the child and minimal maternal morbidity. Ideally, this goal should be achieved prior to pregnancy. LGA babies (large for gestational age), as a result of insufficient therapy, are the chief danger, however, SGA babies (small for gestational age) as a result of too strict blood sugar and episodes of hypoglycemia, are also described, especially in women with nephropathy. Hence, fetal growth should be monitored periodically. Every pregnant diabetic woman should be cared for professionally in an interdisciplinary way.

2.15.10   Insulin

The endocrine part of the pancreas produces and secretes insulin, glucagon and somatostatins. Of clinical importance is, above all, the disturbance of insulin production. Glucagon is important for the reverse regulation in hypoglycemia.

During pregnancy, the insulin sensitivity changes: during the eighth to twelfth week, there is increased insulin sensitivity with a higher risk of hypoglycemia, while in the second half of the pregnancy, insulin sensitivity declines. Thus, insulin therapy must constantly be adapted to the changing requirements of the altered glucose metabolism in pregnancy.

Immediately after birth, the original insulin sensitivity returns to normal. Hence, GDM disappears.

Human insulin, by contrast to oral antidiabetics, does not cross the placenta. Better blood sugar control and advantages for the newborn's condition can be achieved if an intensified insulin dose regime with at least three daily injections of short-acting insulin pre-prandially, perhaps complemented by a long-acting insulin dose at night, are given or when an insulin pump is used. Should this not be possible with women with type 2 diabetes, or GDM, a conventional intensified therapy, i.e. separates administration of basal and prandial insulin or even mixed insulin with a sufficient proportion of short-acting insulin, may be worth considering.

Extensive experience with human insulin substitution therapy in pregnant diabetics gives no indication of embryotoxic or teratogenic effects. This also applies to high doses of insulin, which are often necessary in the third trimester, due to high insulin resistance as a result of overweight and obesity in pregnant women with type 2 diabetes, Thus, human insulin, for which 25 years of good experience are available world-wide, is the drug of first choice for pregnant women.

For many years, there have been insulin analogs: short-acting insulin lispro, insulin aspart and insulin glulisin as well as the long-acting insulin glargine and insulin detemir. The requirements of insulin analogs, in addition to good glycemic control, are that they may not cross the placenta, cause scarcely any production of antibodies and have only minimal IGF-I activity, a parameter for the promotion of retinopathy. Insulin lispro and insulin aspart reach peak plasma concentrations double so high in half the time of regular insulin and can, therefore, be injected immediately before eating.

Insulin lispro has been quite well studied in nearly 1,000 pregnancies, largely in retrospective or smaller prospective studies (i.e. Durnwald 2008, Scherbaum 2002). However, there are currently no (i.e. Wyatt 2005, Garg 2003, Masson 2003) controls available. No increased rate of congenital malformations has been observed (i.e. Lapolla 2008, Wyatt 2005). Achievement of glucose control with insulin lispro is comparable to that with human insulin. Aggravation of diabetic retinopathy with insulin lispro has not been observed as yet, but has also not been sufficiently studied (i.e. Loukovaara 2003, Persson 2002, Buchbinder 2000). The production of insulin antibodies with insulin lispro and human insulin treatment is equally low.

The experience with insulin aspart is more comprehensive insofar as there are not only small studies with different designs, but also a European randomized multicenter study of 322 pregnant diabetics, who received either insulin aspart or human insulin while maintaining basal substitution with long-acting or delayed-acting insulin. There were no significant differences in the rate of hypoglycemia, the levels of HbA1c and the progression of retinopathy (Mathiesen 2007). There was a slight tendency in the aspart group to fewer spontaneous abortions and premature births. In addition, insulin aspart was associated in 157 pregnant women with lower postprandial glucose blood levels and fewer episodes of hypoglycemia compared to 165 pregnant women treated with human insulin (Kinsley, 2007) The rate of malformations, perinatal mortality and the state of the newborns were similar (Hod 2008, Kinsley 2007). In a subgroup of 97 women, comparative measurements of specific insulin aspart or human insulin antibodies in the mother and in the cord blood were undertaken. Furthermore, in both cohorts, there was a search for the relevant crossreactive antibodies in the mothers and in the cord

Pregnancy

2.15 Hormones

blood and a correlation between the concentration of these antibodies in the mother and in the cord blood was determined. Significant differences between insulin aspart and human insulin were not observed (McCance 2008). Similar results were found in a small study of Pettitt (2007). Insulin aspart is specifically approved for pregnancy.

There is no experience available on insulin *glulisin* (Lambert 2013).

Even though a range of small studies or retrospective case series on the tolerance for insulin *glargine* during pregnancy, involving a total of around 650 pregnant women, is available, the experience is not sufficient. Frequently, these are retrospective case series without controls (i.e. Henderson 2009); the designs of the (small) comparative studies are very different. A case-control study of 64 pregnant women (20 with type 1 diabetes and 44 with GDM), among whom half had injected insulin glargine or intermediately-acting human insulin in the third trimester, showed no significant differences with respect to neonatal complications, macrosomia and hypoglycemia (Price 2007). A small prospective cohort study (Negrato 2010) on 56 treated women as well as a study with 52 pregnant women (Fang 2009) treated with insulin glargine came to similar conclusions that there is no difference between insulin glargine and NPH insulin regarding pregnancy outcome. A recent prospective study on 46 women treated with insulin glargine compared to insulin detemir did not find any difference regarding glycemic control and pregnancy outcome (Callesen 2013). A meta-analysis of 331 pregnant women treated with insulin clargine compared with 371 pregnant women treated with NPH insulin also did not find any difference in pregnancy outcomes (Pollex 2011). No study has been able to rebut the previous indications that retinopathy can worsen when insulin glargine is given during pregnancy (Gallen 2008).

Experience with the insulin *detemir* is limited. There are retrospective case series with 10 pregnant women who had type 1 diabetes mellitus, after continuous insulin detemir therapy, from which neither a special risk nor greater safety of the therapy during pregnancy could be deduced (Lapolla 2009). The recent prospective study by Callesen (2013) on 67 women treated during pregnancy with insulin detemir described no difference from treatment with insulin glargine.

> **Recommendation.** Type 1 diabetes mellitus must be well controlled with insulin before pregnancy. Human insulin is the drug of choice. A woman who is in good control with insulin lispro or insulin aspart must not be changed during pregnancy. Long-acting analogs, however, should be stopped and substituted. Pregnant women with type 2 diabetes or GDM, who cannot be adequately treated with diet, should be put on human insulin. Also, with blood sugar levels at a critical threshold and fetal macrosomia, insulin therapy should be instigated. In pregnant women who already required insulin, the need can greatly increase. For therapy control, ultrasound biometry of the growing fetus should also be used. Since glucocorticoids and tocolytics limit the carbohydrate tolerance of the mother, particularly careful metabolic controls are advisable when these medications are being given.

2.15.11   Oral antidiabetics (OAD)

Oral antidiabetics (OAD) are not hormones and do not work in the way that insulin does: they are not substitutes. They are primarily used for the treatment of type 2 diabetes. Evidence-based end-point related positive effectiveness proofs on the diabetes-specific late complications are available for insulin, metformin and sulfonylurea preparations. Oral antidiabetics are also often used in pregnancy, especially for the treatment of GDM together with diet.

The following OADs can be differentiated:

- Sulfonylurea derivatives stimulate the cells in the pancreas that still have the ability to function: among these are *glibenclamide, gliclazide, glimepiride* and *gliquidone.*
- Metformin is on the market as the only biguanide. It decreases the glucose synthesis in the liver, leads to a delayed glucose resorption from the intestines and to increased glucose uptake in the muscular system.
- Inhibitors of the alpha-glucosidases, such as *acarbose* and *miglitol,* limit the carbohydrate resorption in the intestine.
- Glinides, such as *nateglinide* and *repaglinide* are postprandial glucose regulators, which lead to short-term increase in insulin secretion.
- Incretin mimetics, such as *vildagliptin, sitagliptin* and *saxagliptin,* like the hormones secreted in the intestine, are intended to increase the insulin secretion as required when eating. With diabetes, less incretin is produced than in healthy people. Sitagliptin blocks the normally rapid enzymatic breakdown of incretins.
- Glitazones, such as *pioglitazone* and *rosiglitazone,* as so-called insulin sensitizers, are intended to improve the sensitivity of the peripheral cells for insulin.
- *Exenatide* and *liraglutide* are glucagon-like peptides (GLP-1)-receptor antagonists, which may only be used subcutaneously and only in combination with some other oral antidiabetics. In animal research, both were developmentally toxic. The transplacental transfer of exenatide was only minimal in a placenta model (Hiles 2003). There is no experience available during pregnancy.

▶ Glibenclamide

In a placenta model *in vitro, glibenclamide* (=*glyburide*) was only minimally transferred to the fetus (Koren 2001) and in animal experiments it was not teratogenic. In humans as well, no teratogenicity has been described. The increased rate of congenital malformations observed in some older studies is certainly to be seen as a consequence of insufficiently treated type 2 diabetes. Newer case reports and a retrospective analysis of 379 pregnancies with pre-existing diabetes, did not observe any increased risk of congenital malformations: 93/379 were treated continuously with glibenclamide or metformin. Two hundred and forty-nine were switched over from OAD to insulin and 37 were treated with insulin after the failure of diet alone (Ekpebegh 2007). However, these experiences do not permit a differentiated risk assessment.

Studies on glibenclamide in the second/third trimester (e.g. in the treatment of GDM) are considerably more numerous. Randomized studies found no differences in the course of pregnancy and the condition of the newborn between the women treated with human insulin and many hundreds treated with glibenclamide. Differences in the number of hypoglycemic children and the average birth weight were also not significant (Lain 2009, Jacobson 2005, Langer 2000, 2005, Kremer 2004). Jacobson (2005) observed preeclampsia with glibenclamide significantly more frequently. Three newer meta-analyses, which, to some extent, use these same studies, determined no differences in the comparison between

Pregnancy

2.15 Hormones

glibenclamide and insulin in the treatment of GDM. Moretti (2008) analyzed nine studies with a total of 754 women exposed to glibenclamide and 637 women treated with insulin. However, this involved some retrospective and some prospective studies. For three, only the abstract was readily available and only seven gave information about the final macrosomia/birth weight. Further, in some of these studies, the women had to be switched to human insulin because of insufficient blood sugar control. Nicholson (2009) and Dhulkotia (2010) analyzed randomized studies on OAD versus human insulin. The publication of Langer (2005), with 404 pregnant women, represents the largest and most significant study. Half of the pregnant women were treated with glibenclamide and the other half with insulin. There were no differences in the pregnancy outcome between these groups. However, all these results are apparently not sufficient to question recommendations for insulin therapy with GDM.

▶ **Metformin**

Metformin, by contrast to *glibenclamide,* does not stimulate insulin secretion and does not cause hypoglycemia. With overweight diabetics, giving an agent that leads to increased insulin sensitivity and to a lower need for insulin makes more sense than giving glibenclamide.

Although metformin is only approved for diabetes mellitus type 2, it is also used for GDM and for women with polycystic ovary syndrome (PCOS) in the context of fertility treatment. Many studies (i.e. Vanky 2010) and a meta-analysis on the basis of eight smaller retrospective and prospective studies of exposure in the first trimester, did not find any increased risk of congenital malformation. However, the quality of the data may be questioned if, in the meta-analysis (Gilbert 2006), only five malformations in 496 metformin-exposed pregnancies (1.0%) were reported – a value which lies below the basic risk – while in the disease-matched control group, 7.5% malformations were observed.

Two newer studies examine the effectiveness of metformin by comparison to human insulin for GDM. 100 pregnant women, who continuously received metformin, were compared with 100 pregnant women who were treated exclusively with human insulin (Balani 2009). Women, who needed insulin in addition to metformin for blood glucose control, were described separately. The pregnant women in the metformin group showed a lower weight gain and generally scored better on some of the baby's outcome parameters. An Australian study with 363 pregnant women who had developed GDM and were treated with metformin (46.3% needed insulin in addition), found no significant differences to the insulin-treated comparison group (Rowan 2008).

There have been discussions on whether metformin lowers the increased rate of spontaneous abortion with PCOS and contributes to the prevention of GDM. Vanky (2010) carried out a randomized, placebo controlled, double blind study on 257 pregnant women with PCOS, who received metformin ($n = 135$) or a placebo ($n = 138$) until birth. Metformin was unable to lower neither the prevalence of preeclampsia nor the rate of prematurity or the frequency of GDM (17.6% in the metformin and 16.9% in the placebo group). Ghazeeri (2012) summarized the data on the effects of Metformin on PCOS. They found that women with PCOS are at increased risk to developing GDM, hypertension of pregnancy, preeclampsia and preterm birth. Metformin improved pregnancy rates and the outcome of their pregnancies without any recognizable damage to the embryo and fetus.

In some studies a lowering of the rate of spontaneous abortions with metformin in women with PCOS could be shown (Sohrabvand 2009, Palomba 2005, Jakubowicz 2002). How long metformin should be given for "stabilization of the pregnancy" with PCOS, and which pregnant women profit from, is controversial. To date, there is no clear documentation that giving it beyond the sixth to eighth week of pregnancy leads to better results.

Rosiglitazone

Other antidiabetics

Some individual case descriptions (Choi 2006, Holmes 2006, Kalyoncu 2005, Yaris 2004) and a case series with eight women who were treated for PCOS with *rosiglitazone* until the twelfth week of pregnancy (Haddad 2008), do not permit a differentiated risk assessment despite babies born healthy. Rosiglitazone was removed from the market in 2010 because of cardiovascular side-effects (i.e. heart attack).

Pioglitazone

Pioglitazone was not teratogenic in animal studies and there is no experience available on use during pregnancy. A retrospective study reported on nine patients with therapy-resistant PCOS and a desire to have a baby. The children were healthy (Ota 2008). Several countries advise against the use of pioglitazone-containing medications because both the French and also the US boards for the evaluation of medicines (i.e. FDA) had determined an increased incidence of bladder cancer with their use.

There are three case reports on healthy children (born) after *repaglinide* therapy in early pregnancy (Mollar-Puchades 2007, Napoli 2006).

> **Recommendation.** A type 2 mother diabetic should also be switched to insulin when planning a pregnancy, although continued therapy with oral antidiabetics may also be considered. In any case, the use of any oral antidiabetic drug does not justify a risk-grounded termination of the pregnancy. A detailed second trimester ultrasound study is indicated for pregnant women with type 2 diabetes as well as follow up on the fetal growth. Should there be important grounds in individual cases against insulin therapy, metformin would be the most likely OAD to be considered.

Glucagon

Glucagon is a 29 amino acids polypeptide hormone of high molecular weight (3,483 Dalton), secreted by the alpha cells in the pancreatic islets. Its effects oppose those of insulin as it raises blood glucose levels by increasing glycogenolysis and gluconeogenesis. It may be used in an injectable form to rapidly raise blood glucose levels in case of severe hypoglycemia in type 1 diabetic patients treated with insulin, especially if the patient is unconscious (Ringholm 2013, Rayburn 1987). It acts by activation of phosphorylase A that releases glucose-1-phosphate from glycogen. The levels of blood glucagon are increased in the third trimester

Pregnancy

2.15 Hormones

of pregnancy in women with GDM (Grigorakis 2000). It is unknown whether this increase has any relation to the development of GDM or is a reflection of increased insulin insensitivity.

Women with type 1 diabetes treated with insulin often develop severe hypoglycemia especially during the first trimester of pregnancy (Ringholm 2013). These hypoglycemic episodes might endanger the mother as well as the developing embryo and fetus. The rate of such episodes can be reduced by insulin pumps and by educating the pregnant women, preferably before pregnancy. Such interventions carried out on 104 of 212 pregnancies were found to reduce the incidence of severe hypoglycemia by 36% without increasing the levels of HbA1c. Many of the women in both cohorts were treated for their hypoglycemia with glucagon without any increase in the rate of major congenital anomalies. Only two of the 2012 children born had major congenital anomalies (Ringholm 2013). It is, however, difficult to draw firm conclusions from this study because of its small size and the fact that this was not the main purpose of their study.

There seems to be no specific studies on the safety of glucagon during pregnancy. Due to its high molecular weight glucagon is not expected to cross the placental barrier. Indeed, several studies have demonstrated that there seems to be no passage through the human placenta (Spellacy 1976, Johnston 1972).

> **Recommendation.** Glucagon may be given during pregnancy at any phase whenever severe hypoglycemia is diagnosed and intravenous glucose is not recommended. There seems to be no transfer through the placenta to the fetus.

2.15.12   Estrogens

Estrogens (Oestrogens) are a pharmacologically heterogeneous group of hormones which have a stimulating action on the growth of the uterus, the fallopian tubes and, in particular, the endometrium. In addition, estrogens produce thickening of the vaginal epithelium and an increase in cervical secretions and cause a widening of the cervical canal. Therapeutically, estrogens are used today for hormonal contraception, for symptoms of post-menopausal estrogen deficiency, in the context of a hypogonadotropic amenorrhea and for treatment of malignancies (Chapter 2.13) as well as for local administration with certain forms of hair loss.

Among the available substances are conjugated estrogens, *estradiol* and its derivatives *ethinyl estradiol* (component of most of the estrogen-containing (contraceptive) "pills"), *estradiol valerate* and *estriol*.

▶ **Experiences**

The relatively low-dosed preparations for hormonal contraception (combination preparations of estrogen and gestagen) and preparations for treatment of amenorrhea are quite well studied due to their frequent accidental use in early pregnancy. According to the current state of our knowledge, they do not pose any appreciable risk of malformations (Nørgaard 2009, Ahn 2008, Jellesen 2008, Wogelius 2006, Raman-Wilms 1995), not even for disturbances of gender differentiation, when treatment took place during the sensitive period after the eighth week of pregnancy. These studies were able to refute the association between urinary tract anomalies and taking of oral contraceptives (Li 1995) as well as that of cardiac malformations, which were described in some case reports in the 1970s.

Effects of intrauterine exposure to estrogens on possible later fertility problems are not, as yet, confirmed. In a review, all the previous studies on disturbances of male reproduction due to intrauterine estrogen action were analyzed. Here, the medication of the mother, physiologically elevated estrogen levels (i.e. in twin pregnancies), vegetarian (soy) diets (soy contains non-steroid phytoestrogens; see also West 2005) and environmental contaminants with an estrogen-like action (organochloride binding such as PCB or dioxins; Chapter 2.23) were considered. In any case, a certain association was recognized with testicular cancer, but not with hypospadias, undescended testicles or sperm count (Storgaard 2006).

Recommendation. During pregnancy there is no indication for treatment with estrogens. The (accidental) use of oral contraceptives in early pregnancy does not require either a risk-grounded termination of the pregnancy or additional diagnostics (Chapter 1.15). This also applies to the low-dosed preparations commonly used today and treatment of amenorrhea with ethinyl estradiol and norethisterone acetate. The accidental administration of high dosed preparations for other indications also does not justify a risk-grounded termination of the pregnancy. However, a detailed ultrasound examination should then be offered.

2.15.13   Gestagens

Among the gestagens are the naturally occurring progesterone, which is also increasingly produced by the placenta during pregnancy, and a range of synthetic agents, which bind to the progesterone receptors and create a secretory transformation on the proliferated endometrium. In addition, progesterone leads to a decrease in the readiness of the uterine musculature to contract, to narrowing of the cervical canal and to the development and maturation of the milk duct system of the breast. The synthetic gestagens have, to some degree, very variable biological effects.

The following substances are available as medications: *chlormadinon*, a gestagen with antiandrogenic characteristics, *desogestrel*, a progestagen, *dienogest*, which also has antiandrogenic characteristics, *drospirenon* with mild antiandrogenic and mild antimineral corticoids, *dydrogesterone, etonogestrel, gestodene, hydroxyprogesterone caproate, levonorgestrel*, (Synonym: *d-norgestrel, medrogestone, medroxyprogesterone, norelgestromin, norethisterone* and *norgestimate*.

The gestagen, megestrol, and, to some extent also medroxyprogesterone, are used exclusively as antineoplastic medications (Chapter 2.13.18).

▶ **Experiences**

For more than 40 years, progesterone as well as its partially or completely synthesized derivatives (e.g. hydroxyprogesterone), have been used to treat threatened miscarriage. This is largely outdated even though it is repeatedly discussed controversially. Progesterone is considered, at best, with repeated threatening spontaneous abortion and the absence of other more obvious causes. Also being discussed is whether progesterone can lower the rate of prematurity. In some studies, positive effects were

Pregnancy

2.15 Hormones

determined (Barros 2010, Fonseca 2007, Coomarasamy 2006), in others they were not (Briery 2011, Berghella 2010). A randomized placebo controlled double-blind study of 500 pregnant women (Norman 2009) found no positive progesterone effect with premature twins. The analysis of previously available studies also showed that progesterone cannot prevent premature births in twin pregnancies (Norman 2009).

The relatively low dosed gestagen preparations for hormonal contraception, including emergency contraception ("the morning-after pill") and products for treating amenorrhea are fairly well studied due to their frequent (accidental) use during pregnancy. They pose no appreciable risk for genital or extra-genital malformations according to the current state of knowledge (Nørgaard 2009, Ahn 2008, Jellesen 2008, Wogelius 2006, Martinez-Frias 1998, Raman-Wilms 1995, Källén 1991), not even for gender differentiation disturbances if treatment was in the sensitive period after the eighth week of pregnancy. A connection between urinary tract anomalies or heart malformations and the intake of oral contraceptives, which was suggested by case reports from the 1970s, has been refuted (Li 1995).

Emergency contraception (EC) today is carried out as a pure gestagen therapy with 1.5 mg levonorgestrel or with the new progesterone receptor modulator ulipristal. Safety, tolerance and side-effects of levonorgestrel have such a positive profile, that in some countries a prescription-free purchase is possible. With this therapy, ovulation is prevented and no abortion is induced. Embryotoxic effects in case of an intact pregnancy have not been described as yet (Zhang 2009, American Academy of Pediatrics 2005).

The second-generation antiprogestin, ulipristal acetate (30 mg in a single dose), has been studied for use as EC and has been found to be highly effective and well-tolerated (Fine 2010, Glasier 2010, Creinin 2006). It has been marketed for use as EC in Europe since 2009; it was approved by the FDA in 2010 (see overview Trussell 2013). There is not enough experience available on ulipristal to make a risk assessment of developmental disorders at this time.

Negative effects of this intrauterine exposure on fertility in adulthood have not been observed up to now. Development into adolescence seems age-appropriate, according to large long-term studies, i.e. on depot preparations with medroxyprogesterone ("three-month shot") (Pardthaisong 1992).

When 19-norgestagenes, with their androgenizing potential, are repeatedly taken in significantly higher doses than the contraceptive doses common today, a transient enlargement of the clitoris could occur (survey in Briggs 2011).

Recommendation. During pregnancy there is no undisputed indication for therapy with gestagens. Nevertheless, neither the outdated therapy for miscarriage prophylaxis nor contraceptives accidentally taken in early pregnancy require a risk-grounded termination of pregnancy or additional diagnostics (Chapter 1.15). This applies to the one or multiphase preparations in the low doses common today, emergency contraception with levonorgestrel and treatment of amenorrhea with norethisterone acetate and ethinyl estradiol. After failed emergency contraception with ulipristal, a detailed, second trimester ultrasound study can be considered.

Similarly, the (accidental) administration of high-dose preparations for other indications does not justify a risk-grounded termination of the pregnancy. In such a case, the organ development of the fetus can be studied by a detailed ultrasound examination.

2.15.14   Duogynon®

Duogynon® was offered as a dragee (0.02 mg ethinyl estradiol plus 10 mg norethisterone acetate) until 1973 and as an injection (3 mg estradiol benzoate plus 50 mg progesterone) until 1978. There were also oral preparations with estradiol benzoate and progesterone. Duogynon was offered both as a pregnancy test and for treatment of secondary amenorrhea – an indication that has meanwhile long been outdated. The removal of the preparation from the market, which followed, is not tantamount to proof of an increased risk of malformations.

The ingredients of duogynon continue to be available as medications up to today. Ethinyl estradiol and the gestagen, norethisterone acetate, are components of various contraceptive pills. However, norethisterone acetate is significantly lower dosed in the products available today – rather than 10 mg, only in the range of 1 mg. Estradiol with 1–2 mg is contained in preparations for hormone substitution therapy. Progesterone is largely prescribed in significantly higher doses of between 100 and 600 mg daily as prophylaxis against spontaneous abortion and is taken for many weeks by pregnant women. This treatment is only controversial with respect to its effectiveness but not because of possible teratogenicity.

According to the current state of scientific knowledge, there is no serious indication of teratogenic effects for any of the above-mentioned four ingredients. Multiple studies have been carried out on this topic and have not been able to confirm a connection between the earlier use of duogynon or comparable preparations and an increase in malformations. The hypothesis of a causal connection rests largely on individual case reports in which intake of the medication was documented in connection with a malformation. However, malformations occur "spontaneously", independently of any intake of medication, or at random in 3 to 4% of children. In most cases, the cause is unknown. If, then, taking medication in early pregnancy is remembered, it seems reasonable to assume a causal connection. In this way, a connection with the malformation can be postulated with practically every medication due to the coincidental concurrence (of the two events). However, such a suspicion has only been confirmed with a few medications. The hormonal preparations discussed here are not among them.

Since the substances contained in duogynon continue to be used up to the current world-wide, an accumulation of malformations must be registered. Proven is a masculinization of female fetuses with long-term norethisterone therapy from the 10th week of pregnancy due to the androgenic effect of this gestagen. An enlargement of the clitoris, for instance, could also result.

2.15.15   Diethylstilbestrol

Diethylstilbestrol (DES) is a synthetic non-steroidal estrogenic drug that causes cancer in animal tests. Up to 1971 it was prescribed – mostly in the USA – for therapy against threatened abortions, premature birth and other pregnancy complications. The discovery of increased rates of vaginal clear-cell adenocarcinoma in adolescence, among daughters whose mothers had received DES during pregnancy, caused an international sensation (Herbst 1975). This is the only proven example in human beings of prenatally caused cancer ("transplacental carcinogenesis"). The risk for this illness, which is otherwise rare among young women, is given

Pregnancy

2.15 Hormones

as up to 0.14%. Other cancer risks such as, for instance, breast cancer, cannot be clearly proven (Hatch 1998). A Dutch study followed 12,091 formerly DES-exposed daughters from 1992 to 2008 to examine the incidence of cancers (average age at registration, 29 years). The risk for all kinds of cancers together were within the usual range, however, there was an increased risk for adenocarcinoma of the vagina and cervix at advanced ages, while melanomas occurred more frequently at younger ages (Verloop 2010).

In addition, a least 25% of the young women exposed in utero during the first trimester showed anomalies of the vagina, uterus or fallopian tubes (Mittendorf 1995). Furthermore, there were indications of an increased risk for premature births and other pregnancy complications among the women formerly exposed in utero (Papiernik 2005). Also, an increased incidence of depression was discussed in one study (O'Reilly 2010). With male offspring, there was apparently an elevated risk for cryptorchidism, testicular hypoplasia and abnormal semen cell morphology (Mittendorf 1995). Palmer (2009), in a cohort study, also found slightly elevated risks for cryptorchidism, cysts of the epididymis and testicular infections.

Experimental results indicate that epigenetic changes can be caused by DES, which can be passed on to the next generation (transgenerational effect). Among the offspring of those exposed in utero to DES, higher risks of hypospadias (Storgaard 2006, Palmer 2005, Klip 2002), ovarian cancer and leukemia in infancy have been discussed (Chantrain 2009, Titus-Ernstoff 2008). Furthermore, there are studies, which provide support of a slightly elevated risk of malformations among offspring of those exposed in utero to DES Titus-Ernstoff 2010), such as, for instance, esophageal atresias and/or tracheo-esophageal fistulas (Felix 2007). Treatment with diethylstilbestrol has long been obsolete. It was used in Central Europe until 1978, although, by contrast to the USA, on a significantly lesser scale. (Centers for Disease Control and Prevention 2006).

2.15.16 Androgens and anabolics

There are no indications for using androgens or anabolics, such as, for instance, nandrolone or metenolone during pregnancy. Only testosterone is available for substitution therapy. Tibolone is quickly metabolized to metabolites with estrogen-, gestagen- and androgen-like activity and is approved for treatment of estrogen deficiency symptoms in postmenopausal women. However, it is also used as an anabolic. In connection with strength sports and body building, "black market" imported preparations, which can also contain androgens or anabolics without the corresponding declaration, are frequently used. Occasionally they are also "accidentally" continued during a pregnancy.

The practical experience on prenatal tolerance for androgens and anabolics is insufficient for a differentiated risk assessment – also with respect to an androgenizing effect.

> **Recommendation.** Androgens and anabolics are absolutely contraindicated during pregnancy. However, accidental use does not require a risk based termination of the pregnancy (Chapter 1.15). Particularly with repeated use, development of the organs should be monitored with a detailed ultrasound examination.

2.15.17   Cyproterone and danazol

Cyproterone acetate is a most frequently prescribed antiandrogen, which also has gestagen characteristics during reproductive years. Diane-35, and other similar preparations, contain 2 mg of cyproterone acetate and 0.035 mg of ethinyl estradiol and are no longer approved just as contraceptives but only when there is an existing androgenization symptom (e.g. with serious acne). The use of Diane-35 has been limited in many countries since 1995, because of a suspicion of liver tumors. There are also reports of thromboembolic adverse drug reactions associated with cyproterone/ethinylestradiol (Wooltorton 2003) especially in first users.

Mono preparations with considerably higher doses of cyproterone acetate (tablets 10–50 mg; injection 300 mg) are available for other indications.

The antiandrogenic effect of cyproterone acetate can theoretically lead to feminization of male fetuses. Yet even in the case of accidental continuation of treatment using 2 mg daily into the sensitive phase beyond the eighth week of pregnancy, no feminization was observed. Thirteen pregnant women with male fetuses, who had taken 2 mg/daily during (virtually) the entire genital development phase and other pregnant women, who had even used 25–100 mg cyproterone daily were registered by the manufacturer (Bye 1986). The live-born boys were normally developed. Also, with a late miscarriage, there was no developmental disturbance determined. Similarly, additional case reports or case series on the intake of 2 mg/daily do not indicate any teratogenic effects in humans (i.e. Tews 1988, Bergh 1987). However, the scope of experiences is insufficient for a differentiated definitive risk assessment.

Danazol is a synthetic ethisterone derivative, a modified progestogen, also known as 17-alpha-ethinyl testosterone which reversibly inhibits the synthesis and/or the release of hypophyseal gonadotropins LH and FSH (follicle-stimulating hormone) and has a weak androgenic effect. Danazol is approved in Europe (Switzerland) and the USA. There it was approved as the first drug to specifically treat endometriosis in the early 1970s and further for therapy of hereditary angioneurotic edema and fibrocystic mastopathy. It has also been tried for other indications such as contraception. Danazol crosses the placenta. Several publications on over 100 women exposed in pregnancy revealed an apparently considerable risk of masculinization of female fetuses, when they continued to be treated with 200 mg or more daily after the eighth week of pregnancy (when the androgen receptors begin to function). With normal internal genitalia, over 50% of the girls exposed prenatally had an enlargement of the clitoris or a fully developed female pseudohermaphroditism. In the later development, there were no further anomalies such as, for instance, virilization or disturbed sexual behavior (survey in Briggs 2011). An increased rate of spontaneous abortions associated with danazol could also have been caused by endometriosis as the basic illness.

> **Recommendation.** Cyproterone and danazol are absolutely contraindicated during pregnancy. Accidental use, however, does not justify a risk-grounded termination of pregnancy (Chapter 1.15). A detailed ultrasound study should be offered.

2.15.18   Mifepristone (RU486)

Pharmacology

Mifepristone is a progesterone and glucocorticoid antagonist that was approved as an abortifacient in many countries. A dose of 600 mg is required for the termination of early pregnancy. In combination with a prostaglandin preparation, 200 mg are just as effective (Peyron 1993).

Among the pharmacologic effects of mifepristone are a lowering of LH secretion, more rapid corpus luteum regression and increased contractility of the uterine muscles. Effects on the placental production of progesterone, chorionic gonadotropin (hGG) and human placental lactogen have also been observed.

The effectiveness of mifepristone for birth control as an "interceptive" medication (by contrast to a contraceptive, it is effective only after conception), as a contraceptive and for emergency contraception, as well as for ending ectopic pregnancies, but the preparation has not caught on due to insufficient success. Mifepristone crosses the placenta.

Toxicology

Results of animal experiments are contradictory with respect to teratogenicity. In a human case series with 70 pregnancies, carried to term after termination attempts with *mifepristone*, various malformations, among them four children with club foot (Sitruk-Ware1998) were observed. A specific teratogenic effect cannot be clearly deduced from this publication and from other case descriptions which mostly comprise healthy newborns (Pons 1991, Lim 1990). The fact that mifepristone is frequently given together with the teratogenic misoprostol (Chapter 2.14) complicates the risk-assessment of mifepristone. Generally speaking, however, a failed attempt at a medicinal termination of pregnancy, can pose a risk to fetal development.

In 4,673 pregnancies following a mifepristone induced abortion, no increased rate of complications was found compared to a similarly sized control group (Zhu 2009).

Recommendation. Should a pregnancy be continued after the accidental use of mifepristone, confirmation of normal organ development should be confirmed with a detailed ultrasound diagnosis. A risk grounded termination of the pregnancy following a failed medicinal abortion attempt, is not necessarily indicated (Chapter 1.15).

2.15.19   Clomiphene

The estrogen antagonist *clomiphene*, has been used for a considerable time for treating absent ovulation without hyperprolactinemia. An overdose, particularly in combination with HCG (human chorionic gonadotropin) can lead to overstimulation of the ovaries. Among the undesirable side effects are increased rates of pregnancies with multiples and enlargement of the ovaries. Apparently, the effect is based on competitive inhibition of the estrogen receptors in the pituitary and hypothalamus, which leads to increased LH secretion.

The discussion of whether, clomiphene causes neural tube defects (van Loon 1992) or other malformations (Reefhuis 2011), continues. A case report describes a vitreous body anomaly in a baby whose mother had taken clomiphene until the sixth week of pregnancy (Bishai 1999).

In Japan, 1,034 pregnancies induced by clomiphene were observed over a period of 5 years. Of the 935 live-born children, 2.3% had malformations, a rate that was not higher compared to a control group (Kurachi 1983). However, whether treatment with clomiphene took place only before the beginning of a pregnancy or afterwards, was not differentiated. The manufacturer's collection of cases showed 58 malformations among 2,379 clomiphene-treated patients (2.4%). Among 158 women who had also taken clomiphene after conception, there were malformations in eight children (5.1%). A study with data from a malformation register found an increased incidence for craniosynostosis in 20 pregnant women who had taken clomiphene before or during the pregnancy (Reefhuis 2002). A further, similarly designed work with an unknown number of cases, determined a significantly more frequent penoscrotal hypospadias after clomiphene (Meijer 2005). By contrast, no increased risk of hypospadias was determined in a Danish case-control study (Sørensen 2005).

Among 911 newborns from pregnancies induced through clomiphene or *letrozole*, there were no differences in the rate of malformations. In the letrozole group, cardiac malformations were underrepresented (Tulandi 2006). An increased individual risk cannot be documented with the currently available study results.

Recommendation. Clomiphene may be prescribed for the induction of ovulation if the patient is informed of the still-not-entirely-rebutted risk of a slight increase in congenital anomalies and if she also accepts the significantly higher occurrence of a multiple embryos pregnancy. An existing pregnancy must be ruled out before the start of treatment.

2.15.20 Erythropoietin

The erythropoietin derivatives manufactured with gene technology *epoetin alfa, epoetin beta, epoetin delta, epoetin theta, epoetin zeta* and *darbepoetin alfa* are designated as recombinant human erythropoietin. All of them have a comparable biological effect to the body's own erythropoietins, that is, the stimulation of erythropoiesis. A supplementary therapeutic use for the new derivatives, epoetin delta, theta and zeta has not been determined

Erythropoietins are used for pronounced anemia, i.e. with chronic kidney diseases and after kidney transplants, but also in cancer and HIV therapy as well as with thalassemia and with therapy-resistant anemia during pregnancy. Whether the serious maternal hypertension and worsening of the pregnant woman's kidney function described in four pregnancies can be attributed to treatment with erythropoietin, could not be conclusively determined (Briggs 2011).

Recombinant human erythropoietin has a high molecular weight of 23,000 Dalton and does not cross the placenta (Dorado 1974). It has been shown in numerous reports and case series to be well tolerated during pregnancy (Krafft 2009). There is no appreciable risk for the embryo/fetus. Erythropoietin is used with good success and tolerance in newborns and also in premature infants (Brown 2009).

Pregnancy

2.15 Hormones

There is less experience with darbepoetin alfa during pregnancy than with epoetin. However, up to now, negative effects have not been described (Ghosh 2007, Sobiło-Jarek 2006, Goshorn 2005).

Recommendation. Epoetin alfa or epoetin beta may be given during pregnancy for appropriate indications. If possible, the other epoetins and darbepoetin alfa should not be used due to limited experience.

References

Abe M, Syuto T, Yokoyama Y et al. Aplasia cutis congenita after methimazole exposure in utero successfully treated with basic fibroblast growth factor. Int J Dermatol 2010; 49: 334–5.

Ahn HK, Choi JS, Han JY et al. Pregnancy outcome after exposure to oral contraceptives during the periconceptional period. Hum Exp Toxicol 2008; 27: 307–13.

Allen VM, Armson BA, Wilson RD et al. Teratogenicity associated with pre-existing and gestational diabetes. J Obstet Gynecol Can 2007; 29: 927–44.

American Academy of Pediatrics Committee on Adolescence. Emergency contraception. Pediatrics 2005; 116: 1026–35.

Bahn RS, Burch HS, Cooper DS et al. The role of propylthiouracil in the management of Graves' disease in adults: report of a meeting jointly sponsored by the American Thyroid Association and the Food and Drug Administration. Thyroid 2009; 19: 673–4.

Balani J, Hyer SL, Rodin DA et al. Pregnancy outcomes in women with gestational diabetes treated with metformin or insulin: a case-control study. Diabet Med 2009; 26: 798–802.

Barbero P, Ricagni C, Mercado G et al. Choanal atresia associated with prenatal methimazole exposure: three new patients. Am J Med Gen 2004; 129: 83–6.

Barbero P, Valdez R, Rodriguez H et al. Choanal atresia associated with maternal hyperthyroidism treated with methimazole: a case-control study. Am J Med Genet A 2008; 146A: 2390–5.

Barros FC, Bhutta ZA, Batra M et al. GAPPS Review Group. Global report on preterm birth and stillbirth (3 of 7): evidence for effectiveness of interventions. BMC Pregnancy Childbirth 2010; 10: S3.

Bay Bjorn AM, Ehrenstein V, Holmager Hundborg H et al. Use of corticosteroids in early pregnancy is not associated with risk of oral clefts and other congenital malformations in offspring. Am J Ther 2012 [Epub ahead of print].

Berbel P, Mestre JL, Santamarfa A et al. Delayed neurobehavioral development in children born to pregnant women with mild hypothyroxinemia during the first month of gestation: the importance of early iodine supplementation. Thyroid 2009; 19: 511–9.

Bergh T, Bakos O. Exposure to antiandrogen during pregnancy: case report. BMJ (Clin Res Ed) 1987; 294: 677–8.

Berghella V, Figueroa D, Szychowski JM et al. Vaginal Ultrasound Trial Consortium: 17-alpha-hydroxyprogesterone caproate for the prevention of preterm birth in women with prior preterm birth and a short cervical length. Am J Obstet Gynecol 2010; 202: 351, e1–6.

Bishai R, Arbour L, Lyons C et al. Intrauterine exposure to clomiphene and neonatal persistent hyperplastic primary vitreous. Teratology 1999; 60: 143–5.

Bliddal S, Rasmussen ÅK, Sundberg K et al. Graves' disease in two pregnancies complicated by fetal goitrous hypothyroidism: successful in utero treatment with levothyroxine. Thyroid 2011; 21: 75–81.

Blumenfeld Z, Avivi I, Eckman A et al. Gonadotropin-releasing hormone agonist decreases chemotherapy-induced gonadotoxicity and premature ovarian failure in young female patients with Hodgkin lymphoma. Fertil Steril 2008; 89: 166–73.

Bonduelle M, Oberyé J, Mannaerts B et al. Large prospective, pregnancy and infant follow-up trial assures the health of 1000 fetuses conceived after treatment with the GnRH antagonist ganirelix during controlled ovarian stimulation. Hum Reprod 2010; 25: 1433–40.

Brian SR, Bidlingmaier M, Wajnrajch MP et al. Treatment of acromegaly with pegvisomant during pregnancy: maternal and fetal effects. J Clin Endocrinol Metab 2007; 92: 3374–7.

Briery CM, Veillon EW, Klauser CK et al. Women with preterm premature rupture of the membranes do not benefit from weekly progesterone. Am J Obstet Gynecol 2011; 204: 54, e1–5.

Briggs GG, Freeman RK, Jaffe SJ. Drugs in Pregnancy and Lactation. 9th edn. Baltimore: Williams & Wilkins 2011.

Brown MS, Eichorst D, Lala-Black B et al. Higher cumulative doses of erythropoietin and developmental outcomes in preterm infants. Pediatrics 2009; 124: e681–7.

Buchbinder A, Miodovnik M, McElvy S et al. Is insulin lispro associated with the development or progression of diabetic retinopathy during pregnancy? Am J Obstet Gynecol 2000; 183: 1162–5.

Bye P. Comments on "Conception during Diane' therapy – a successful outcome". Br J Dermatol 1986; 114: 516.

Cahill DJ. Risks of GnRH agonist administration in early pregnancy in ovulation induction. In: Filiconi M, Flamigni C (eds.) Risk of GnRH Agonist Administration in Early Pregnancy in Ovulation Induction. Update 98. New York: Parthenon Publishing Group 1998, pp. 97–105.

Callesen NF, Damm J, Mathiesen JM et al. Treatment with the long-acting insulin analogues detemir or glargine during pregnancy in women with type 1 diabetes: comparison of glycemic control and pregnancy outcome. J Matern Fetal Med 2013; 26: 588–92.

Carmichael SL, Shaw GM, Ma C et al. National Birth Defects Prevention Study. Maternal corticosteroid use and orofacial clefts. Am J Obstet Gynecol 2007; 197(6): 585, e1–7; discussion 683–4, e1–7.

Centers for Disease Control and Prevention (CDC) 2006. Diethylstilbestrol (DES) available at www.cdc.gov/DES/

Chan GV, Mandel SJ. Therapy insight: management of Graves disease during pregnancy. Nat Clin Pract Endocrinol Metab 2007; 470–8.

Chantrain CF, Sauvage D, Brichard B et al. Neonatal acute myeloid leukemia in an infant whose mother was exposed to diethylstilboestrol in utero. Pediatr Blood Cancer 2009; 53: 220–2.

Choi JS, Han JY, Ahn HK et al. Exposure to rosiglitazone and fluoxetine in the first trimester of pregnancy. Diabetes Care 2006; 29: 2176.

Clementi M, di Gianantonio E, Cassina M et al. SAFE-Med Study Group: Treatment of hyperthyroidism in pregnancy and birth defects. J Clin Endocrinol Metab 2010; 95: E337–41.

Clementi M, di Gianantonio E, Pelo E et al. Methimazole embryopathy: delineation of the phenotype. Am J Med Genet 1999; 83: 43–6.

Coomarasamy A, Thangaratinam S, Gee H et al. Progesterone for the prevention of preterm birth: a critical evaluation of evidence. Eur J Obstet Gynecol Reprod Biol 2006; 129: 111–8.

Cooper DS, Mandel S. Author's response: severe embryopathy and exposure to methimazole in early pregnancy. J Clin Endocrinol Metab 2002; 87: 948–9.

Coustan DR, Lowe LP, Metzger BE et al. International Association of Diabetes and Pregnancy Study Groups: The Hyperglycemia and Adverse Pregnancy Outcome (HAPO) study: paving the way for new diagnostic criteria for gestational diabetes mellitus. Am J Obstet Gynecol 2010; 202: 654, e1–6.

Corral E, Reascos M, Preiss Y et al. Treatment of fetal goitrous hypothyroidism: value of direct intramuscular L-thyroxine therapy. Prenat Diagn 2010; 30: 899–901.

Creinin MD, Schlaff W, Archer DF et al. Progesterone receptor modulator for emergency contraception: a randomized controlled trial. Obstet Gynecol 2006; 108: 1089–97.

De Turris P, Venuti L, Zuppa AA. Long-term treatment with cabergoline in pregnancy and neonatal outcome: report of a clinical case. Pediatr Med Chir 2003; 25: 178–80.

Dhulkotia JS, Ola B, Fraser R et al. Oral hypoglycemic agents versus insulin in management of gestational diabetes: a systematic review and metaanalysis. Am J Obstet Gynecol 2010; 203: 457, e1–9.

Diav-Citrin O, Ornoy A. Teratogen update: Antithyroid drugs – methimazole, carbimazole and propylthiouracil. Teratology 2002; 65: 38–44.

Di Gianantonio E, Schaefer C, Mastroiacovo PP et al. Adverse effects of prenatal methimazole exposure. Teratology 2001; 64: 262–6.

Dorado M, Espada J, Langton AA et al. molecular weight estimation of human erythropoietin by SDS – polyacrylamide gel electrophoresis. Biochemical Med 1974: 10: 1–7.

Durnwald CP, Landon MB. A comparison of lispro and regular insulin for the management of type 1 and type 2 diabetes in pregnancy. J Matern Fetal Neonatal Med 2008; 21: 309–13.

Pregnancy

2.15 Hormones

Eisenstein Z, Weiss M, Katz Y et al. Intellectual capacity of subjects exposed to methimazole or propylthiouracil in utero. Eur J Pediatr 1992; 151: 558–9.

Ekpebegh CO, Coetzee EJ, van der Merwe L et al. A 10-year retrospective analysis of pregnancy outcome in pregestational Type 2 diabetes: comparison of insulin and oral glucose-lowering agents. Diabet Med 2007; 24: 253–8.

Evers IM, Ter Braak EWMT, De Valk HW et al. Risk indicators predictive for severe hypoglycemia during the first trimester of type 1 diabetic pregnancy. Diabetes Care 2002; 25: 554–9.

Fang YM, MacKeen D, Egan JF et al. Insulin glargine compared with Neutral Protamine Hagedorn insulin in the treatment of pregnant diabetics. J Matern Fetal Neonatal Med 2009; 22: 249–53.

Felix JF, Steegers-Theunissen RP, de Walle HE et al. Esophageal atresia and tracheoesophageal fistula in children of women exposed to diethylstilbestrol in utero. Am J Obstet Gynecol 2007; 197: 38, e1–5.

Ferraris S, Valenzise M, Lerone M et al. Malformations following methimazole exposure in utero: an open issue. Birth Defects Res A 2003; 67: 989–92.

Fine P, Mathé H, Ginde S et al. Ulipristal acetate taken 48–120 hours after intercourse for emergency contraception. Obstet Gynecol 2010; 115: 257–63.

Finken MJ, Keijzer-Veen MG, Dekker FW et al. Dutch POPS-19 Collaborative Study Group: Antenatal glucocorticoid treatment is not associated with long-term metabolic risks in individuals born before 32 weeks of gestation. Arch Dis Child Fetal Neonatal Ed 2008; 93: F442–7.

Fonseca EB, Celik E, Parra M et al. Fetal Medicine Foundation Second Trimester Screening Group: Progesterone and the risk of preterm birth among women with a short cervix. N Engl J Med 2007; 357: 462–9.

Food and Drug Administration (FDA). Information for Healthcare Professionals – Propylthiouracil-Induced Liver Failure. 06.04.2009 Available at www.fda.gov/Drugs/DrugSafety/PostmarketDrugSafetyInformationforPatientsandProviders/DrugSafetyInformationforHeathcareProfessionals/ucm162701.htm

Foulds N, Walpole I, Elmslie F et al. Carbimazole embryopathy: an emerging phenotype. Am J Med Gen 2005; 132: 130–5.

Gärtner R. Thyroid diseases in pregnancy. Curr Opin Obstet Gynecol 2009; 21: 501–7.

Gallen IW, Jaap A, Roland JM et al. Survey of glargine use in 115 pregnant women with Type 1 diabetes. Diabet Med 2008; 25: 165–9.

Garg SK, Frias JP, Anil S et al. Insulin lispro therapy in pregnancies complicated by type 1 diabetes: glycemic control and maternal and fetal outcomes. Endocr Pract 2003; 9: 187–93.

Garite TJ, Kurtzman J, Maurel K et al. Obstetric Collaborative Research Network: Impact of a "rescue course" of antenatal corticosteroids: a multicenter randomized placebo-controlled trial. Am J Obstet Gynecol 2009; 200: 248, e1–9.

Ghazieeri GS, Nassar AH, Younes Z et al. Pregnancy outcomes and the effects of metformin treatment in women with polycystic ovary syndrome; an overview. Acta Obst Gynecol Scand 2012; 91:58–78.

Ghosh A, Ayers KJ. Darbepoetin alfa for treatment of anaemia in a case of chronic renal failure during pregnancy – case report. Clin Exp Obstet Gynecol 2007; 34: 193–4.

Gilbert C, Valois M, Koren G. Pregnancy outcome after first-trimester exposure to metformin: a meta-analysis. Fertil Steril 2006; 86: 658–63.

Glasier AF, Cameron ST, Fine PM et al. Ulipristal acetate versus levonorgestrel for emergency contraception: a randomised non-inferiority trial and meta-analysis. Lancet 2010; 375: 555–62.

Glinoer D, Cooper DS. The propylthiouracil dilemma. Curr Opi Endcrinol Diabetes Obes 2012; 19: 402–7.

Goshorn J, Youell TD. Darbepoetin alfa treatment for post-renal transplantation anemia during pregnancy. Am J Kidney Dis 2005; 46: 81–6.

Grigorakis SI, Alevizaki M, Beis C et al. Hormonal parameters in gestational diabetes mellitus during the third trimester: high glucagon levels. Gynecol Obstet Invest 2000; 49: 106–9.

Gur C, Diav-Citrin O, Shechtman S et al. Pregnancy outcome after first trimester exposure to corticosteroids: a prospective controlled study. Reprod Toxicol 2004; 18: 93–101.

Haddad GF, Jodicke C, Thomas MA et al. Case series of rosiglitazone used during the first trimester of pregnancy. Reprod Toxicol 2008; 26: 183–4.

Haddow JE et al. Maternal thyroid deficiency during pregnancy and subsequent neuropsychological development of the child. N Engl J Med 1999; 341: 549–55.

HAPO Study Cooperative Research Group. Hyperglycaemia and Adverse Pregnancy Outcome (HAPO) Study. associations with maternal body mass index. BJOG 2010; 117: 575–84.

Hardy JR, Leaderer BP, Holford TR et al. Asthma medication in pregnancy and risk of orofacial clefts: A cohort study of 81,975 mother-baby pairs from United Kingdom's general practice research database {Abstract}. Birth Defects Res A 2005; 73: 300.

Hashima JN, Lai Y, Wapner RJ et al. Eunice Kennedy Shriver National Institute of Child Health and Human Development Maternal-Fetal Medicine Units Network: The effect of maternal body mass index on neonatal outcome in women receiving a single course of antenatal corticosteroids. Am J Obstet Gynecol 2010; 202: 263, e1–5.

Hatch EE, Palmer JR, Titus-Ernstoff L et al. Cancer risk in women exposed to diethylstilbestrol in utero. JAMA 1998; 280: 630–4.

Henderson CE, Machupalli S, Marcano-Vasquez H et al. A retrospective review of glargine use in pregnancy. J Reprod Med 2009; 54: 208–10.

Henrichs J, Bongers-Schokking JJ, Schenk JJ et al. Maternal thyroid function during early pregnancy and cognitive functioning in early childhood: the generation R study. J Clin Endocrinol Metab 2010; 95: 4227–34.

Herbst AL, Poskanzer DC, Robboy SJ et al. Prenatal exposure to stilbestrol. N Engl J Med 1975; 292: 334–9.

Hiles RA, Bawdon RE, Petrella Em. Ex vivo human placental transfer of the peptides pramlintide and exenatide (synthetic exendin-4). Hum Exp Toxicol 2003; 22: 623–8.

Hod M, Damm P, Kaaja R et al. Insulin Aspart Pregnancy Study Group: Fetal and perinatal outcomes in type I diabetes pregnancy: a randomized study comparing insulin aspart with human insulin in 322 subjects. Am J Obstet Gynecol 2008; 198: 186, e1–7.

Holmes HJ, Casey BM, Bawdon RE. Placental transfer of rosiglitazone in the ex vivo human perfusion model. Am J Obstet Gynecol 2006; 195: 1715–9.

Homar V, Grosek S, Battelino T. High-dose methylprednisolone in a pregnant woman with Crohn's disease and adrenal suppression in her newborn. Neonatology 2008; 94: 306–9.

Jacobson GF, Ramos GA, Ching JY et al. Comparison of glyburide and insulin for the management of gestational diabetes in a large managed care organization. Am J Obstet Gynecol 2005; 193: 118–24.

Jakubowicz DJ, Iuorno MJ, Jakubowicz S et al. Effects of metformin on early pregnancy loss in the polycystic ovary syndrome. J Clin Endocrinol Metab 2002; 87: 524–9.

Jellesen R, Strandberg-Larsen K, Jørgensen T et al. Maternal use of oral contraceptives and risk of fetal death. Paediatr Perinat Epidemiol 2008; 22: 334–40.

Johnston DI, Bloom SR, Greene KR, Beard RW. Failure of the human placenta to transfer pancreatic glucagon. Biol Neonate 1972; 21: 375–80.

Kalyoncu NI, Yaris F, Ulku C et al. A case of rosiglitazone exposure in the second trimester of pregnancy. Reprod Toxicol 2005; 19: 563–4.

Källén B, Mastroiacovo P, Lancaster PA et al. Oral contraceptives in the etiology of isolated hypospadias. Contraception 1991; 44: 173–82.

Kannan L, Mishra S, Agarwal R et al. Carbimazole embryopathy – bilateral choanal atresia and patent vitello intestinal duct: a case report and review of literature. Birth Defects Res A Clin Mol Teratol 2008; 82: 649–51.

Karg E, Bereg E, Gaspar L et al. Aplasia cutis congenita after methimazole exposure in utero. Pediatr Dermatol 2004; 21: 491–4.

Karlsson FA, Axelsson O, Melhus H. Severe embryopathy and exposure to methimazole in early pregnancy. J Clin Endocrinol Metab 2002; 87: 946–51.

Kinsley B. Achieving better outcomes in pregnancies complicated by type 1 and type 2 diabetes. Clin Ther 2007; 29: s153–8.

Klip H, Werloop J, van Gool JD et al. Hypospadias in sons of women exposed to diethylstilbestrol in utero: a cohort study. Lancet 2002; 359: 1102–7.

Koren G. Glyburide and fetal safety; transplacental pharmacokinetic considerations. Reprod Toxicol 2001; 15: 227–9.

Kovacs CS, Chafe LL, Fudge JN et al. PTH regulates fetal blood calcium and mineralization independently of PTHrP. Endocrinilogy 2001; 142: 4983–93.

Krafft A, Bencaiova G, Breymann C. Selective use of recombinant human erythropoietin in pregnant patients with severe anemia or nonresponsive to iron sucrose alone. Fetal Diagn Ther 2009; 25: 239–45.

Kremer CJ, Duff P. Glyburide for the treatment of gestational diabetes. Am J Obstet Gynecol 2004; 190: 1438–9.

Krupp P, Monka C. Bromocriptine in pregnancy: Safety aspects. Klin Wochenschr 1987; 65: 823–7.

Pregnancy

2.15 Hormones

Kurachi K, Aono T, Minigawa J et al. Congenital malformations of newborn infants after clomiphen-induced ovulation. Fertil Steril 1983; 40: 187–9.

Lahat E, Raziel A, Friedler S et al. Long-term follow-up of children born after inadvertent administration of a gonadotrophin-releasing hormone agonist in early pregnancy. Human Reproduction 1999; 14: 2656–60.

Lain KY, Garabedian MJ, Daftary A et al. Neonatal adiposity following maternal treatment of gestational diabetes with glyburide compared with insulin. Am J Obstet Gynecol 2009; 200: 501, e1–6.

Laloi-Michelin M, Ciraru-Vigneron N, Meas T. Cabergoline treatment of pregnant women with macroprolactinomas. Int J Gynaecol Obstet 2007; 99: 61–2.

Lambert K, Holt RI. The use of insulin analogues in pregnqancy. Diabetes Obes Metab 2013; 15: 888–900.

Langer O, Conway DL, Berkus MD et al. A comparison of glyburide and insulin in women with gestational diabetes mellitus. N Engl J Med 2000; 343: 1134–8.

Langer O, Yogev Y, Xenakis EMJ et al. Insulin and glyburide therapy: dosage, severity level of gestational diabetes, and pregnancy outcome. Am J Obstet Gynecol 2005; 192: 134–9.

Lapolla A, Dalfrà MG, Spezia R et al. Outcome of pregnancy in type 1 diabetic patients treated with insulin lispro or regular insulin: an Italian experience. Acta Diabetol 2008; 45: 61–6.

Lapolla A, di Cianni G, Bruttomesso D et al. Use of insulin detemir in pregnancy: a report on 10 Type 1 diabetic women. Diabet Med 2009; 26: 1181–2.

Lee BH, Stoll BJ, McDonald SA et al. National Institute of Child Health and Human Development Neonatal Research Network: Adverse neonatal outcomes associated with antenatal dexamethasone versus antenatal betamethasone. Pediatrics 2006; 117: 1503–10.

Lebbe M, Hubinont C, Bernard P et al. Outcome of 100 pregnancies initiated under treatment with cabergoline in hyperprolactinaemic women. Clin Endocrinol (Oxf) 2010; 73: 236–42.

Li DK, Daling JR, Mueller BA et al. Oral contraceptive use after conception in relation to the risk of congenital urinary tract anomalies. Teratology 1995; 51: 30–6.

Li Y, Shan Z, Teng W et al. Abnormalities of maternal thyroid function during pregnancy affect neuropsychological development of their children at 25–30 months. Clin Endocrinol 2010; 72: 825–9.

Lim BH, Lees DA, Bjornsson S et al. Normal development after exposure to mifepristone in early pregnancy. Lancet 1990; 336: 257–8.

Litwin A, Amodai I, Fisch B et al. Limb-body wall complex with complete absence of external genitalia after in vitro fertilization. Fertil Steril 1991; 55: 634–6.

Loukovaara S, Immonen I, Teramo KA et al. Progression of retinopathy during pregnancy in type 1 diabetic women treated with insulin lispro. Diabetes Care 2003; 26: 1193–8.

Maffei P, Tamagno G, Nardelli GB et al. Effects of octreotide exposure during pregnancy in acromegaly. Clin Endocrinol (Oxf) 2010; 72(5): 668–77. Erratum in: Clin Endocrinol (Oxf) 2010; 72: 856.

Mandel M, Toren A, Rechavi G et al. Hormonal treatment in pregnancy: a possible risk factor for neuroblastoma. Med Pediatr Oncol 1994; 23: 133–5.

Martinez-Frias ML, Rodriguez-Pinilla E, Bermejo E et al. Prenatal exposure to sex hormones: a case-control study. Teratology 1998; 57: 8–12.

Masson EA, Patmore JE, Brash PD et al. Pregnancy outcome in type 1 diabetes mellitus treated with insulin lispro (Humalog). Diab Med 2003; 20: 46–50.

Mathiesen E, Kinsley B, Amiel S et al. on behalf of the Insulin Aspart Pregnancy Study Group: Maternal glycemic control and hypoglycemia in type 1 diabetic pregnancy. Diabetes Care 2007; 30: 771–6.

McCance DR, Damm P, Mathiesen ER et al. Evaluation of insulin antibodies and placental transfer of insulin aspart in pregnant women with type 1 diabetes mellitus. Diabetologia 2008; 51: 2141–3.

McEvoy C, Schilling D, Peters D et al. Respiratory compliance in preterm infants after a single rescue course of antenatal steroids: a randomized controlled trial. Am J Obstet Gynecol 2010; 202: 544, e1–9.

Meijer WM, de Jong-van den Berg, van den Berg MD et al. Clomiphene and hypospadias: the necessity to investigate on a detailed level {Abstract}. Reprod Toxicol 2005; 20: 472–3.

Messer PM, Hauffa BP, Olbricht T. Antithyroid drug treatment of Graves' disease in pregnancy: long-term effects on somatic growth, intellectual development and thyroid function of the offspring. Acta Endocrinol (Copenh) 1990; 123: 311–6.

Miller NM, Williamson C, Fisk NM et al. Infant cortisol response after prolonged antenatal prednisolone treatment. BJOG 2004; 111: 1471–4.

Miracle X, Di Renzo GC, Stark A et al. Coordinators of World Association of Perinatal Medicine Prematurity Working Group: Guideline for the use of antenatal corticosteroids for fetal maturation. J Perinat Med 2008; 36: 191–6.

Mitsuda N, Tamaki H, Amino N et al. Risk factors for developmental disorders in infants born to women with Graves disease. Obstet Gynecol 1992; 80: 359–64.

Mittendorf R: Teratogen update: carcinogenesis and teratogenesis associated with exposure to diethylstilbestrol (DES) in utero. Teratology 1995; 51: 435–45.

Mollar-Puchades MA, Martin-Cortes A, Perez-Calvo A et al. Use of repaglinide on a pregnant woman during embryogenesis. Diabetes Obes Metab 2007; 9: 146–7.

Momotani N, Noh JY, Ishikawa N et al. Effects of propylthiouracil and methimazole on fetal thyroid status in mothers with Graves' hyperthyroidism. J Clin Endocrinol Metab 1997; 82: 3633–6.

Morange I, Barlier A, Pellegrini I et al. Prolactinomas resistant to bromocriptine: long-term efficacy of quinagolide and outcome of pregnancy. Europ J Endocrinol 1996; 135: 413–20.

Moretti ME, Rezvani M, Koren G. Safety of glyburide for gestational diabetes: a meta-analysis of pregnancy outcomes. Ann Pharmacother 2008; 42: 483–90.

Napoli A, Ciampa F, Colatrella A et al. Use of repaglinide during the first weeks of pregnancy in two type 2 diabetic women. Diabetes Care 2006; 29: 2326–7.

Negrato CA, Rafacho A, Negrato G et al. Glargine versus NPH insulin therapy in pregnancies complicated by diabetes: an observational cohort study. Diabetes Res Clin Pract 2010; 89: 46–51.

Negro R, Formoso G, Mangieri T et al. Levothyroxine treatment in euthyroid pregnant women with autoimmune thyroid disease: effects on obstetrical complications. J Clin Endocrinol Metab 2006; 91: 2587–91.

Negro R, Greco G, Mangieri T et al. The influence of selenium supplementation on post-partum thyroid status in pregnant women with thyroid peroxidase autoantibodies. J Clin Endocrinol Metab 2007; 92: 1263–8.

Nicholson W, Bolen S, Witkop CT et al. Benefits and risks of oral diabetes agents compared with insulin in women with gestational diabetes: a systematic review. Obstet Gynecol 2009; 113: 193–205.

Nørgaard M, Wogelius P, Pedersen L et al. Maternal use of oral contraceptives during early pregnancy and risk of hypospadias in male offspring. Urology 2009; 74: 583–7.

Norman JE, Mackenzie F, Owen P et al. Progesterone for the prevention of preterm birth in twin pregnancy (STOPPIT): a randomised, double-blind, placebo-controlled study and meta-analysis. Lancet 2009; 373: 2034–40.

Ono K, Kikuchi A, Takikawa KM et al. Hernia of the umbilical cord and associated ileal prolapse through a patent omphalomesenteric duct: prenatal ultrasound and MRI findings. Fetal Diagn Ther 2009; 25: 72–5.

Ono M, Miki N, Amano K et al. Individualized high-dose cabergoline therapy for hyperprolactinemic infertility in women with micro- and macroprolactinomas. J Clin Endocrinol Metab 2010; 95: 2672–9.

Ornoy A, Ratzon N, Greenbaum C et al. Neurobehavior of children born to diabetic mothers at early school age. Arch Dis Child 1998; 79: F94–9.

Ornoy A. Wolf A, Ratzon N et al. Neurodevelopmental impact of diabetic alterations on early school-age children born to mothers with Gestational Diabetes. Arch Dis Child 1999; 81: F10–14.

O'Reilly EJ, Mirzaei F, Forman MR et al. Diethylstilbestrol exposure in utero and depression in women. Am J Epidemiol 2010; 171: 876–82.

Ota H, Goto T, Yoshioka T et al. Successful pregnancies treated with pioglitazone in infertile patients with polycystic ovary syndrome. Fertil Steril 2008; 90: 709–13.

Palmer JR, Herbst AL, Noller KL et al. Urogenital abnormalities in men exposed to diethylstilbestrol in utero: a cohort study. Environ Health 2009; 8: 37.

Palmer JR, Wise LA, Robboy SJ et al. Hypospadias in sons of women exposed to diethylstilbestrol in utero. Epidemiology 2005; 16: 583–6.

Palomba S, Orio F, Falbo A et al. Prospective parallel randomized, double-blind, double-dummy controlled clinical trial comparing clomiphene citrate and metformin as the first-line treatment for ovulation induction in nonobese anovulatory women with polycystic ovary syndrome. J Clin Endocrinol Metab 2005; 90: 4068–74.

Papiernik E, Pons JC, Hessabi M. Obstetrical outcome in 454 women exposed to diethylstilbestrol during their fetal life: a case-control analysis. J Gynecol Obstet Biol Reprod (Paris) 2005; 34: 33–40.

Pardthaisong T, Yenchit C, Gray R. The long-term growth and development of children exposed to Depo-Provera during pregnancy and lactation. Contraception 1992; 45: 313–24.

Park-Wyllie L, Mazzotta P, Pastuszak A et al. Birth defects after maternal exposure to corticosteroids: prospective cohort study and meta-analysis of epidemiological studies. Teratology 2000; 62: 385–92.

Peltoniemi OM, Kari MA, Lano A et al. Repeat Antenatal Betamethasone (RepeatBM) Follow-Up Study Group: Two-year follow-up of a randomised trial with repeated antenatal betamethasone. Arch Dis Child Fetal Neonatal Ed 2009; 94: F402–6.

Persson B, Swahn M-L, Hjertberg R et al. Insulin lispro therapy in pregnancies complicated by type 1 diabetes mellitus. Diab Res Clin Pract 2002; 58: 115–21.

Pesonen AK, Räikkönen K, Lano A et al. Antenatal betamethasone and fetal growth in prematurely born children: implications for temperament traits at the age of 2 years. Pediatrics 2009; 123: e31–7.

Pettitt DJ, Ospina P, Howard C et al. Efficacy, safety and lack of immunogenicity of insulin aspart compared with regular human insulin for women with gestational diabetes mellitus. Diabet Med 2007; 24: 1129–35.

Peyron R, Aubeny E, Targosz V et al. Early termination of pregnancy with mifepristone (RU 486) and the orally active prostaglandin misoprostol. N Engl J Med 1993; 328: 1509–13.

Pollex E, Moretti ME, Koren G, Feig DS. Safety of insulin glargine use in pregnancy: a systematic review and meta-analysis. Ann Pharmacother 2011; 45: 9–16.

Pons JC, Imber MC, Elefant E et al. Development after exposure to mifepristone in early pregnancy. Lancet 1991; 338: 763.

Pop VJ, Brouwers EP, Vader HL et al. Maternal hypothyroxinaemia during early pregnancy and subsequent child development: a 3-year follow-up study. Clin Endocrinol (Oxf) 2003; 59: 282–8.

Porto AM, Coutinho IC, Correia JB et al. Effectiveness of antenatal corticosteroids in reducing respiratory disorders in late preterm infants: randomised clinical trial. BMJ 2011; 342: d1696.

Pradat P, Robert-Gnansia E, di Tanna GL et al. First trimester exposure to corticosteroids and oral clefts. Birth Defects Res A 2003; 67: 968–70.

Price N, Bartlett C, Gillmer M. Use of insulin glargin during pregnancy: a case-control pilot study. BJOG 2007; 114: 453–547.

Raman-Wilms L, Tseng AL, Wighardt S et al. Fetal genital effects of first trimester sex hormone exposure: a meta-analysis. Obstet Gynecol 1995; 85: 141–9.

Ramprasad M, Bhattacharyya SS, Bhattacharyya A. Thyroid disorders in pregnancy. Indian J Endocrinol Metab 2012; 16: S167–70.

Ray JG. DDAVP use during pregnancy: an analysis of its safety for mother and child. Obstet Gynecol Survey 1998; 53: 450–5.

Rayburn W, Piehl E, Sanfield J, Compton A. Reversing severe hypoglycemia during pregnancy with glucagon therapy. Am J Perinatol 1987; 4: 259–61.

Reece EA. Diabetes – induced birth defects: what do we know? What can we do? Curr Diab Rep 2012; 12: 24–32.

Reefhuis J, Honein MA, Schieve LA et al. National Birth Defects Prevention Study: Use of clomiphene citrate and birth defects, National Birth Defects Prevention Study, 1997–2005. Hum Reprod 2011; 26: 451–7.

Reefhuis J, Shaw G, Romitti PA et al. Ovulation stimulation, assisted reproductive techniques, and craniosynostosis – Atlanta, California, and Iowa, 1993–1997 {Abstract}. Teratology 2002; 65: 300.

Reid SM, Middleton P, Cossich MC et al. Interventions for clinical and subclinical hypothyroidism in pregnancy. Cochrane Database Syst Rev 2010; 7: CD007752.

Ringholm L, Secher AL, Pedersen-Bjergaad U et al. The incidence of severe hypoglycemia in pregnant women with type 1 diabetes mellitus can be reduced with unchanged HbA1c levels and pregnancy outcomes in a routine care setting. Diabetes Res Clin Pr 2013; 123–30.

Rivkees SA, Szarfman A. Dissimilar hepatotoxicity profiles of propythiouracil and methimazole in children. J Clin Endocrinol Metab 2010; 95: 3260–7.

Rodriguez-Pinilla E, Martinez-Frias ML. Corticosteroids during pregnancy and oral defects: a case-control study. Teratology 1998; 58: 2–5.

Rodriguez-Pinilla E, Prieto-Merino D, Dequino G et al. Grupo del ECEMC: [Antenatal exposure to corticosteroids for fetal lung maturation and its repercussion on weight, length and head circumference in the newborn infant]. Med Clin (Barc) 2006; 127: 361–7.

Rosenfeld H, Ornoy A, Shechtman S et al. Pregnancy outcome, thyroid dysfunction and fetal goitre after in utero exposure to propylthiouracil: a controlled cohort study. Br J Clin Pharmacol 2009; 68: 609–17.

Rowan JA, Hague WM, Gao W et al. MiG Trial Investigators: Metformin versus insulin for the treatment of gestational diabetes. N Engl J Med 2008; 358: 2003–15.

Sánchez-Luceros A, Meschengieser SS, Turdó K et al. Evaluation of the clinical safety of desmopressin during pregnancy in women with a low plasmatic von Willebrand factor level and bleeding history. Thromb Res 2007; 120: 387–90.

Scherbaum WA, Lankisch MR, Pawlowski B et al. Insulin lispro in pregnancy – retrospective analysis of 33 cases and matched controls. Exp Clin Endocrinol Diabetes 2002; 110: 6–9.

Simmonds CS, Kovacs CS. Role of parathyroid hormone (PTH) and PTH related protein (PTHrP) in regulating mineral homeostasis during fetal development. Crit Rev Eukaryot Gene Expr 2010; 20: 235–73.

Siristatidis C, Salamalekis E, Iakovidou H et al. Three cases of diabetes insipidus complicating pregnancy. J Matern Fetal Neonatal Med 2004; 16: 61–3.

Sitruk-Ware R, Davey A, Sakiz E. Fetal malformations and failed medical termination of pregnancy. Lancet 1998; 352: 323.

Sobiło-Jarek L, Popowska-Drojecka J, Muszytowski M et al. Anemia treatment with darbepoetin alpha in pregnant female with chronic renal failure: report of two cases. Adv Med Sci 2006; 51: 309–11.

Sohrabvand F, Shariat M, Haghollahi F et al. Effect of metformin on miscarriage in pregnant patients with polycystic ovary syndrome. West Indian Med J 2009; 58: 433–6.

Sørensen HT, Pedersen L, Skriver MV et al. Use of clomiphenee during early pregnancy and risk of hypospadias: population based case-control study. BMJ 2005; 330: 126–7.

Spellacy WN, Buhi WC. Glucagon, insulin, and glucose levels in maternal and umbilical cord plasma with studies of placental transfer. Obstet Gynecol 1976; 47: 291–4.

Storgaard L, Bonde JP, Olsen J. Male reproductive disorders in humans and prenatal indicators of estrogen exposure: a review of published epidemiological studies. Reprod Toxicol 2006; 21: 4–15.

Tabacova S, Szarfman A, Lyndly JM et al. Adverse developmental events reported to FDA in association with maternal use of drugs for treatment of hyperthyroidism in pregnancy {Abstract}. Birth Defects Res A 2010; 88: 411 WP4.

Tews G, Arzt W: Eine ausgetragene Schwangerschaft nach Einnahme von Cyproteronazetat im 1. Trimenon. Gynäkol Rundsch 1988; 28: 193–7.

Thangaratinam S, Tan A, Knox E et al. Association between thyroid autoantibodies and miscarriage and preterm birth: meta-analysis of evidence. BMJ 2011; 342: d2616.

Titus-Ernstoff L, Troisi R, Hatch EE et al. Offspring of women exposed in utero to diethylstilbestrol (DES): a preliminary report of benign and malignant pathology in the third generation. Epidemiology 2008; 19: 251–7.

Titus-Ernstoff L, Troisi R, Hatch EE et al. Birth defects in the sons and daughters of women who were exposed in utero to diethylstilbestrol (DES). Int J Androl 2010; 33: 377–84.

Toulis KA, Anastasilakis AD, Tzellos TG et al. Selenium supplementation in the treatment of Hashimoto's thyroiditis: a systematic review and a meta-analysis. Thyroid 2010; 20: 1163–73.

Trussell J, Raymond EG, Cleland K. Emergency Contraception: A Last Chance to Prevent Unintended Pregnancy. 2013; Available at: http://ec.princeton.edu/questions/ec-review.pdf

Tulandi T, Martin J, Al-Fadhli R et al. Congenital malformations among 911 newborns conceived after infertility treatment with letrozole or clomiphene citrate. Fertil Steril 2006; 85: 1761–5.

Van Loon K, Besseghir K, Eshkol A. Neural tube defects after infertility treatment: a review. Fertil Steril 1992; 58: 875–84.

Vanky E, Stridsklev S, Heimstad R et al. Metformin versus placebo from first trimester to delivery in polycystic ovary syndrome: a randomized, controlled multicenter study. J Clin Endocrinol Metab 2010; 95: E448–55.

Ventz M, Puhlmann B, Knappe G et al. Schwangerschaften bei hyperprolaktinämischen Patientinnen. Zentralbl Gynäkol 1996; 118: 610–5.

Verloop J, van Leeuwen FE, Helmerhorst TJ et al. Cancer risk in DES daughters. Cancer Causes Control 2010; 21: 999–1007.

Webster J. A comparative review of the tolerability profiles of dopamine agonists in the treatment of hyperprolactinaemia and inhibition of pregnancy. Drug Saf 1996; 14: 228–38.

West MC, Anderson L, McClure N et al. Dietary oestrogens and male fertility potential. Hum Fertil (Camb) 2005; 8: 197–207.

Wogelius P, Horváth-Puhó E, Pedersen L et al. Maternal use of oral contraceptives and risk of hypospadias – a population-based case-control study. Eur J Epidemiol 2006; 21: 777–81.

Wooltorton E. Diane-35 (cyproterone acetate): safety concerns. CMAJ 18, 2003; 168: 455–6.

Pregnancy

2.15 Hormones

Wyatt JW, Frais JL, Hoyme HE et al. Congenital anomaly rate in offspring of mothers with diabetes treated with insulin lispro during pregnancy. Diabet Med 2005; 22: 803–7.

Yaris F, Yaris E, Kadioglu M et al. Normal pregnancy outcome following inadvertent exposure to rosiglitazone, gliclazide, and atorvastatin in a diabetic and hypertensive woman. Reprod Toxicol 2004; 18: 619–21.

Young BE, McNanley TJ, Cooper EM et al. Maternal vitamin D status and calcium intake enteract to affect fetal skeletal growth in utero in pregnant adolescents. Am J Clin Nutr 2012; 95:1103–12.

Zhang L, Chen J, Wang Y et al. Pregnancy outcome after levonorgestrel-only emergency contraception failure: a prospective cohort study. Hum Reprod 2009; 24: 1605–11.

Zhu QX, Gao ES, Chen AM et al. Mifepristone-induced abortion and placental complications in subsequent pregnancy. Hum Reprod 2009; 24: 315–9.

General and local anesthetics and muscle relaxants

2.16

Stefanie Hultzsch and Asher Ornoy

2.16.1	Halogenated inhalational anesthetic agents	452
2.16.2	Ether (diethyl ether)	454
2.16.3	Nitrous oxide	454
2.16.4	Xenon	454
2.16.5	Occupational exposure to anesthetic gases	454
2.16.6	Injection anesthetics	455
2.16.7	Local anesthetics	457
2.16.8	Muscle relaxants	460

Due to their lipid solubility, general anesthetic agents rapidly cross the blood–brain barrier and the placenta. In addition to their sleep-inducing effect in the brain, they also frequently have a depressant effect on the respiratory center. Thus, during the perinatal phase, there is a risk of hypoxia from neonatal respiratory depression. Fortunately there is no indication that an uncomplicated general anesthetic can lead to developmental disorders. Based on our current knowledge, the commonly used injection or inhalation anesthetics do not have teratogenic properties. However, impairments of respiration and circulation arising in the course of maternal anesthesia, stronger uterine contractions or events such as malignant hyperthermia can also harm the fetus.

Although there are only limited epidemiological data on individual anesthetics, the effects of surgery under anesthesia on pregnant women have been examined in some larger studies. When various anesthetics were combined, none of these older studies found significant indications of damaging effects (Ebi 1994, Duncan 1986, Brodsky 1980). In animal experiments, some anesthetic agents have shown neurotoxic effects on the developing brain (Ikonomidou 2001, Paule 2011, Jevtovic-Todorovic 2003, Olney 2000), possibly through interaction at the glutamate N-methyl-D-aspartate (NMDA) receptor. Substantial debate continues as to whether these animal results are applicable to humans, because in humans, the exposure are generally a single anesthetic and are usually of shorter duration in relation to brain development than in these animal experiments (Cheek 2009, El-Beheiry 2006). The results from studies conducted in young children, mostly retrospective to date, are not uniform. It is difficult to control for confounders like pre-existing diseases which might contribute to the incidence of repeat operations (Sprung 2009, Wilder 2009). Large prospective multicenter studies are currently being conducted to clarify these questions, e.g. the PANDA study (Pediatric Anesthesia and Neurodevelopment Assessment, www.kidspandastudy.org)

Drugs During Pregnancy and Lactation. **http://dx.doi.org/10.1016/B978-0-12-408078-2.00017-2**

or the GAS study (compare also http://www.smarttots.org/research/related-studies.html). Results are not expected before 2015.

Local anesthetics that are either injected or sprayed on tissue were long considered the agents of choice during pregnancy because it was assumed that the anesthetics remain at the site of administration and so would not pass to the fetus. However, even with this form of anesthesia, complications cannot be ruled out since local anesthetics also reach the fetus following adsorption into the mother's circulation, depending on the location and vascularization at the injection site (de Barros Duarte 2011).

Muscle relaxants used in connection with surgical procedures are quaternary ammonia salts which, under physiological conditions, are available in a highly ionized form and therefore pass through the placenta only relatively slowly. Nevertheless, they reach the fetus in detectable amounts. Overall, no differences were found in the Apgar scores or the postpartum neurological adaptation of the newborns after caesarean section regardless of whether the mother had had general anesthesia with desflurane or sevoflurane or epidural anesthesia (Karaman 2006).

2.16.1   Halogenated inhalational anesthetic agents

Desflurane, enflurane, halothane, isoflurane and *sevoflurane* are halogenated inhalation agents. In the perinatal phase, attention should be paid to their relaxant effect on the uterus, which can lead to a reduction in contraction activity with increased risk of bleeding and to their respiratory depressant effect, especially with high risk births. The uterine relaxing effect is used for example during *ex utero* intrapartum treatment (EXIT procedure) to resuscitate a fetus with a difficult airway on placental support or in fetal surgery in order to carry out operations on the baby in the opened uterus (Moldenhauer 2013, Liechty 2010, Tran 2010). Even with uncomplicated caesarean section, uterine atony can lead to increased loss of blood, in this context the relaxant effect of the inhalation agents is unwanted. The rapid dispersal of the newer inhalation anesthetics (sevoflurane, desflurane) leads to a more rapid normalization of the uterine tone after the operation is finished (Yoo 2006).

▶ Desflurane

Of all the anesthetic agents, desflurane has the lowest blood/gas and tissue/blood distribution coefficients, as well as the least solubility. It is the weakest effective halogenated anesthetic gas. Desflurane is, like isoflurane, only minimally metabolized, so the toxic potential is low. Because of rapid induction and wake-up times, desflurane is frequently used for anesthesia for caesarean section with no known disadvantages for the newborn or the mother. No teratogenic effects in humans are known. Similar to the other halogenated inhalation anesthetics, the uterine relaxing effect is dependent on the depth of anesthesia and its strength is similar to that of halothane (Yoo 2006). Because of rapid diffusion and dispersal, however, the uterine tone is more easily regulated.

▶ Enflurane

Enflurane is a fluorinated ether, which is only 2–5% metabolized. The use in Caesarean anesthesia is well-tolerated by newborns

(Tunstall 1989, Abboud 1985). No teratogenic effects are known among humans. Due to the less favorable properties of enflurane in comparison to isoflurane it is now only rarely used for anesthesia.

▶ Halothane

Halothane is one of the oldest and most widely used of the halogenated inhalation anesthetics. There are no known teratogenic effects in humans. In animal studies, however, skeletal and other anomalies, fetal growth retardation, behavioral anomalies and death of the offspring have been found. These anomalies have not been observed in humans with normal use. When halothane is given at delivery (i.e. for caesarean section) there may be more pronounced uterine atony with an increased risk of bleeding as well as respiratory depression in the newborn. Among the inhalation anesthetics, halothane has the strongest circulatory depressive effect. High doses can cause cardiac arrythmias and cardiac arrest in the mother, especially with the use of β-sympathomimetic tocolytics or catecholamines. Halothane has the highest rate of metabolization (15–20%, mainly in the liver) of the inhalation anesthetics now still in use. There have been reports of liver toxicity after repeat anesthesia. Therefore it is mostly replaced by the newer agents (desflurane, sevoflurane) today.

▶ Isoflurane

Isoflurane is a structural isomer of enflurane. With a metabolization rate of only 0.2%, it belongs, like desflurane, to the halogenated inhalation anesthetics that are only minimally metabolized. In the course of *in vitro* fertilization under isoflurane anesthesia, no reduced implantation rate was seen (Beilin 1999). Anesthesia with isoflurane for a caesarean delivery is well-tolerated by the fetus. A slight increase in neonatal bilirubin values has been discussed (De Amici 2001). No teratogenic effects among humans are known.

▶ Sevoflurane

Sevoflurane has only fluoride as a halogen. The wash-in rate is somewhat slower than that of desflurane, but faster than that of all the other halogenated inhalation anesthetics. The metabolization rate is between 3 and 5%. It is used in many obstetrical centers today as the standard inhalation anesthetic for caesarean section with no known negative effects on the newborn. No teratogenic risks are known in humans. The uterine relaxing effect of sevoflurane is similar to that of halothane or desflurane and, due to the rapid diffusion and dispersal, just as easily regulated as with the use of desflurane (Yoo 2006).

> **Recommendation.** Halogenated anesthetics are among the standard anesthetic agents used in obstetrics. Being aware of the characteristic side-effects, they can be used at any time during the entire pregnancy. When used during labor, uterine relaxation and the related risk of hemorrhage and depressive effects on the newborn need to be kept in mind.

Pregnancy

2.16 General and local anesthetics and muscle relaxants

2.16.2   Ether (diethyl ether)

Ether (ether as anesthetic agent) has only historical significance today. Because of serious side-effects such as, for instance, the explosiveness of an ether-air mix, post-operative nausea and vomiting and agitation, ether is no longer used as an anesthetic in most industrialized countries. Ether reaches the fetus unimpeded. There are no indications of teratogenic properties in humans.

> **Recommendation.** Ether drip anesthesia is not indicated during pregnancy or in obstetrics. Due to serious side effects it should only be used in a setting when no other anesthetic possibility is available.

2.16.3   Nitrous oxide

Nitrous oxide (laughing gas, N_2O) is a slow reacting gas with good analgesic and limited anesthetic properties. Therefore, it has to be combined with other anesthetics and/or muscle relaxants to achieve good anesthetic results.

Compared to halogenated inhalation anesthetics, nitrous oxide is a well-tolerated anesthetic that has neither negative effects on the circulatory system nor on the uterus. In rare cases, nitrous oxide can be associated with neonatal respiratory depression requiring resuscitation (Langanke 1987). Comprehensive studies on the use of nitrous oxide on over 1,000 pregnant women have not identified any teratogenic effects (Crawford 1986, Heinonen 1977).

In England, and increasingly also in other countries, nitrous oxide is often used for control of labor pain in vaginal births in a 50:50 mix with oxygen (*Entonox*). Its use is largely harmless for the baby since the remaining nitrous oxide is quickly exhaled by the newborn via the lungs (Reynolds 2010). In a recent systematic review 59 studies on nitrous oxide use during labor were identified in 58 publications of variable quality and did not uncover severe neonatal side effects (Likis 2014).

> **Recommendation.** Nitrous oxide is an ideal inhalation anesthetic for small surgical procedures during pregnancy. With obstetrical procedures, attention should be paid to a possible respiratory depressant effect in the newborn. It is the fastest-acting analgesic during labor.

2.16.4   Xenon

The inert gas *xenon* can, similarly to nitrous oxide, be used as an anesthetic. Since it is expensive and is only available to a limited extent, its use has not become established. In animal experiments it has not proven to be either teratogenic or fetotoxic (Burov 2002).

2.16.5   Occupational exposure to anesthetic gases

Pregnant women working in the operating room (OR) are exposed to anesthetic gases despite modern gas extraction systems and air conditioning, as measurements have confirmed. Also women working in dentists offices or labor wards may be exposed to *nitrous oxide*.

The commonly used anesthetic gases cross the placental barrier easily (Herman 2000, Cordier 1992). Different countries have set limits on the OR air concentrations of anesthetic gases applicable not only to pregnant women. For example, in the USA, the recommended exposure limit is 25 ppm of nitrous oxide. In Germany the limit has been set at 100 ppm, and there is also a maximum air concentration for *halothane* (5 ppm) and *enflurane* (20 ppm) (Deutsche Forschungsgemeinschaft DFG 2013). However, it is often difficult to impose these limits; therefore routine and repeat monitoring is advisable. An increased rate of spontaneous abortions among anesthesia and OR personnel exposed occupationally was reported, and attributed to the chronic exposure to anesthetic gases (Hemminki 1985, Vessey 1980). This could not be confirmed later in extensive epidemiological studies as stress, coffee consumption, smoking, tense body positions as well as a pre-existing tendency to spontaneous abortion were assumed as confounding factors (Rowland 1992). A newer study (Lawson 2012) did not find a relationship between occupational exposure to anesthetic gases and an elevated risk of spontaneous abortion. They attribute this to better scavenging systems nowadays resulting in lower exposure to waste anesthetic gases at the workplace.

In many studies, a lower birth weight and a shorter gestational period have been noted (Ericson 1979, Rosenberg 1978, Pharoah 1977, Cohen 1971). Long-term development in 40 children up to the ages of 5 to 13 years, whose mothers were exposed to OR anesthesia gases as anesthetists or nurses, was studied by Ratzon (2004) and compared to 40 children whose mothers worked in other departments of the hospital. No differences in development were found in the newborns or the 5- to 13-year-olds, but limitations in gross motor skills, attention deficits and hyperactivity were observed more frequently in the exposed group. The level of exposure was significantly and negatively correlated with limitations in fine motor ability and lower IQ scores. However, these groups of children are too small to permit authoritative conclusions.

To summarize, the state of the data on the risk of birth defects and spontaneous abortion through occupational exposure to anesthetic gases is reassuring, while the effects on other developmental disorders need further studies. Care should be taken to observe the limits of exposure.

> **Recommendation.** It is safe for pregnant women to work in operating rooms with modern scavenging systems if the air concentrations are measured and the maximum permitted workplace concentrations are not exceeded. Alternatively, pregnant women may work in areas of the hospital in which anesthetic gases are not used, i.e. in ORs in which only total intravenous anesthesia (TIVA) is carried out or in pre-anesthesia consultation clinics.

2.16.6   Injection anesthetics

Among the injection anesthetics are *etomidate, ketamine/ketamine S, methohexital propofol* and *thiopental*. After intravenous injection, the concentration of an injectable anesthetic immediately reaches its maximum value in the blood, which then quickly falls again due to rapid redistribution and excretion. As a result of large blood flow to the brain, there is rapid onset and short duration of action. Due to their high lipid solubility, injectable anesthetics quickly pass through the placenta, but before they reach the fetal brain they are increasingly diluted in the fetal blood and, to some extent, metabolized by the fetal liver. Therefore, a single induction dose of an injectable anesthetic does not anesthetize the fetus or the newborn. A depressive effect on the fetus or newborn should only be expected after repeated doses. Concerning the neurotoxicity of anesthetic agents, see www.smarttots.org.

After use in labor, the serum concentration in the newborn and the risk of side effects will be lower the more time has elapsed between injection of the anesthetic and the delivery of the child (Flowers 1959). As a general rule all injectable anesthetics can be used during pregnancy. They are discussed below.

▶ Etomidate

Etomidate is an imidazole derivative that is inactivated by non-specific esterases. The rapid onset and short duration of action (half-life in the serum is 3 minutes) is, similar to barbiturates, dependent on redistribution from the well-vascularized brain into the less vascularized regions, such as muscle and fat. Due to its lower cardio-depressive action it is indicated, for instance, with pre-existing maternal cardiac disease.

▶ Ketamine

Ketamine is a fast-acting injectable anesthetic that has a good analgesic effect and little effect on respiration. Due to central stimulation of the sympathetic nervous system, it leads to indirect cardiovascular effects (increased heart rate, cardiac output and blood pressure). Ketamine has a dose-related stimulating effect on the uterine tone and the frequency of uterine contractions and must not be used with uterine hyperactivity and threatening fetal hypoxia. Due to these side-effects, it can impair fetal functions and may necessitate more intense fetal monitoring during labor (Baraka 1990, Reich 1989). Used in caesarean deliveries, ketamine has, in individual cases, led to states of anxiety in the mother, occasionally requiring therapy. Therefore, its use is limited despite its good analgesic properties. There has also been increasing concern about the neurotoxicity of ketamine as an anesthetic. Exposure of 5- to 6-day-old rhesus monkeys to 24 hours of ketamine anesthesia resulted in long-term learning disabilities (Paule, 2011). It is unclear whether these results are transferable to humans, as the brain development period is considerably longer and the usual exposure to anesthesia is shorter by comparison. Further studies are in progress (compare www.smarttots.org).

▶ Propofol

Next to *thiopental, propofol* is the preferred injectable anesthetic agent during pregnancy today. As an induction substance it is an appropriate alternative to thiopental (Abboud 1995, Gin 1990). For intubation, propofol is characterized by a rapid loss of consciousness. The brief wake-up time and limited side-effects are a great advantage to the pregnant patient. After injection, propofol quickly crosses the placenta.

The fetal blood concentrations are about 70% of the maternal values (Jauniaux 1998, Dailland 1989). Propofol is rapidly eliminated from the circulation of the newborn (Dailland 1989, Moore 1989, Valtonen 1989). In a study using the early neonatal neurobehavioral scale (ENNS) for evaluation, newborns after caesarean section have been shown to have less favorable results for some neurological functions after anesthesia with propofol compared to thiopental (Celleno 1989). However, these effects were transitory. By contrast, Gin (1990) found that propofol was superior to thiopental as an induction agent for a caesarean section. Cardiovascular side-effects were no more frequently observed than with thiopental. Using propofol for anesthesia for oocyte retrieval in assisted reproduction technologies had no effect on the success of pregnancy compared to other anesthetic agents or techniques (Beilin 1999), (Christiaens 1998). The fetal neurotoxicity found by some authors in animal experiments (Al-jahdari 2006) is considered by other authors as not applicable to humans (El-Beheiry 2006). In children and adults, a propofol infusion syndrome (PRIS) with fatal outcome was described after several days of sedation with propofol (Wong 2010, Roberts 2009). It is unclear whether propofol can also have similar effects on the fetus after intrauterine exposure. In a nationwide survey of pediatric intensive care units in Germany, it was seen that PRIS only occurred in pediatric patients if the sedation was prolonged over several days and no upper dose limit was in place (Kruessell 2012).

► **Thiopental**

Thiopental is the anesthetic induction agent most frequently used in obstetric anesthesia next to propofol. It is a thiobarbiturate characterized by its rapid action. The brief duration of action is determined by redistribution similar to the other injection anesthetics. Since thiobarbiturates do not influence the uterine tone and contraction activity, the ability of the uterus to contract after delivery is maintained. In addition, no interaction with α- or β-sympathomimetics has been described. Thiobarbiturates can be detected in fetal blood as early as 1 minute after injection. The concentration is only slightly lower than in the maternal blood. No fetal impairment is expected with maternal doses up to 5 mg/kg bodyweight. With higher or repeated doses, neonatal respiratory depression is more likely to be expected (Langanke 1987).

> **Recommendation.** Propofol and thiopental are among the drugs of choice for general anesthesia both for obstetrical anesthesia and for anesthesia during pregnancy. Because of the unclear data on propofol infusion syndrome, propofol should not be used for long-term sedation in pregnant women if alternatives are available. For special indications, etomidate may also be used. Attention should be paid to possible depressant effects on the newborn after use of these three anesthetics. Because of its blood pressure increasing effect, ketamine is contraindicated in pregnant women with high blood pressure and preeclampsia. All injectable anesthetics should be used in the lowest effective dose.

2.16.7　Local anesthetics

The most commonly used local anesthetics are *chloroprocaine, lidocaine, bupivacaine* and its levorotatory enantiomer *levobupivacaine,*

Pregnancy

2.16 General and local anesthetics and muscle relaxants

ropivacaine, prilocaine, articaine, mepivacaine, prilocaine and also *benzocaine* and *cinchocaine*, which are only used topically. Local anesthetics are characterized by varying durations of action which in turn lead to different indications for use. Local anesthetics do not remain at the site of administration but are absorbed, depending on the site of administration and vascularity, and also reach the fetus via the maternal blood. Local anesthetics inhibit nerve conduction through blockade of sodium channels. This may lead to characteristic side effects in overdose or accidental intravascular injection. Systemic toxicity of local anesthetic agents correlates well with their anesthetic potency. Early signs are central nervous system agitation or even seizures, cardiovascular toxicity includes conduction delays and vascular dilatation. In pregnant patients receiving epidural anesthesia for labor, the incidence of systemic toxic reactions to local anesthetics is 1% compared to 0.2–0.3% in nonpregnant women. The addition of vasoconstrictive substances such as adrenaline/epinephrine or noradrenaline/norepinephrine can prolong the duration of action of the local anesthetic and reduce the blood level by limiting the rate of systemic absorption. On the other hand, the risk for local complications such as tissue necrosis or gangrene increases. *Metabisulfite*, which is added to adrenaline-containing local anesthetic solutions as an antioxidant, is neurotoxic and is suspected as cause of cauda equina syndrome.

However, local anesthetics are generally well-tolerated in all stages of pregnancy. They appear to have no lasting effect on the neurophysiology of the newborn. No teratogenic damage following use in the first trimester has been observed. Care should be taken with pudendal anesthesia, as several reports of toxic effects on the newborn exist (see prilocaine, lidocaine).

In the following the most commonly used local anesthetics will be briefly presented.

▶ Articaine

Articaine is frequently used, primarily in dental medicine – also in combination with adrenaline. There is no evidence of embryo- or fetotoxic effects.

▶ Bupivacaine

Bupivacaine is frequently used in obstetrics. It has a strong effect and marked central nervous and cardiotoxic side-effects which are intensified during pregnancy through progesterone. Bupivacaine can lead to a re-entry phenomenon triggering ventricular tachycardia and fibrillation. The rate of toxic effects was significantly reduced after 0.75% bupivacaine was barred from use in obstetric units. The main advantage of this local anesthetic is its long-lasting effect (3 to 10 hours). Due to high protein binding, passage into the placenta is limited compared to lidocaine, a placental transfer of 32% for the R- and S-enantiomer was reported (de Barros Duarte 2011).

▶ Lidocaine

Lidocaine is the most commonly used local anesthetic agent. Due to its low pH-value (7.7–7.8) it is rapidly effective and easily crosses the placenta. A placental transfer of 60% for lidocaine and its metabolites was reported (de Barros Duarte 2011). No negative influence on pregnancy is known. In a study with more than 1,200 pregnant women, no increase in the rate of congenital birth defects was found (Heinonen 1977). Lidocaine is also used in obstetrics for peridural anesthesia. It alleviates birth pains without significantly affecting the strength of the contractions or the cooperation of the woman giving birth. One case of systemic lidocaine toxicity in the newborn after maternal pudendal anesthesia was reported (Bozynski 1987). Alterations in the brain-stem evoked potential (Bozynski 1989) and disturbances in temperature regulation with hyperthermia were seen after several hours of epidural analgesia (Macaulay 1992). In some studies epidural anesthesia was associated with changes in the behavior of newborns, which were, however, rare and only transient (Decocq 1997, Fernando 1997).

► Prilocaine

Prilocaine is used for infiltration and induction anesthesia and also, in combination with lidocaine, for surface anesthesia. With comparatively limited systemic toxicity, one of its metabolites, o-toluidine, is a toxic methemoglobin generator. Particularly after pudendal anesthesia in obstetrics, there have been several case reports of methemoglobinemia in newborns (Uslu 2013, Heber 1995, Hrgovic 1990). Another study found no increased methemoglobin values in the mothers and only minimally elevated levels in the newborns. Of the 17 women who had been given pudendal anesthesia with a dose of prilocaine limited to 200 mg, none developed symptomatic methemoglobinemia (Kirschbaum 1991). A literature review on methemoglobinemia caused by local anesthetic agents, found a higher risk with the use of prilocaine and benzocaine than with other local anesthetics (Guay 2009).

► Ropivacaine

Ropivacaine is a local anesthetic of the amide type. Its pharmacokinetic and pharmacodynamic properties are comparable to bupivacaine but with lower cardiovascular toxicity and an anesthetic potential that is about 30% lower. The preferable sensory blockade is more pronounced than with bupivacaine. Nevertheless, no advantage of ropivacaine compared to bupivacaine has been shown with respect to motor blockades (which may make an instrumental delivery necessary) with the same anesthetic quality (Eddleston 1996). Toxic and central nervous side-effects occur with ropivacaine compared to bupivacaine only with a higher total amount of the local anesthetic administered (Santos 1995).

► Combination of local anesthetics with other active substances

The addition of opiates to epidurally administered local anesthetics offers the advantages of a more rapid onset, improved analgesia and a reduction in the dose of local anesthetics. Thereby, the rate of motor blockades and instrumental deliveries can be reduced. In epidural or spinal anesthesia lipophilic opiates such as *sufentanil* and fentanyl are preferred because they are quickly taken up at the place of administration and have only limited side effects. The risk of respiratory depression is reduced due to a shorter liquor retention period. Other opiate-related side-effects such

Pregnancy

2.16 General and local anesthetics and muscle relaxants

as nausea, vomiting and pruritus occur less frequently (Gogarten 1997). Lipophilic opiates, such as sufentanil, are more easily absorbed into the vascular system and can be found in significant concentrations in the plasma. By comparison to fentanyl, sufentanil leads to more effective pain control and accumulates less in the newborn despite proven placental passage (Loftus 1995). Sufentanil 30 μg injected into the epidural space did not lead to clinically relevant neonatal impairment (Chapter 2.1). A recent case control study of 206 newborns with respiratory distress and 206 controls found a positive association between exposure to maternal epidural analgesia and respiratory distress in the immediate neonatal period in neonates ≥34 weeks gestation (Kumar 2014). Whether this is an effect of the Fentanyl administered epidurally, of the epidural in itself or residual confounding is not clear. No medication doses are cited in the article. Whether the administration of fentanyl epidurally during labor or the epidural itself has a negative effect on the start of breastfeeding or the duration of breastfeeding is discussed controversially (Reynolds 2010) (compare also Chapter 4.1). As Szabo (2013) points out in his comprehensive review, the discussion is limited by study deficiencies such as lack of randomization or control for potential confounding variables.

Adding clonidine to epidurally administered local anesthetics leads to a reduction of the need for local anesthetics with better analgesia and fewer opiate-related side-effects such as, for instance, pruritus (Wallet 2010). In the group treated with clonidine, the blood pressure values were lower during treatment, but no therapeutic measures were required. Dewandre (2008) found a comparable reduction of the minimum local anesthetic concentration with the addition of 5 μg sufentanil as well as of 75 μg clonidine to 0.2% ropivacaine as a bolus. However, clonidine was not recommended for routine use because of increased occurrence of hypotonia (Dewandre 2010). In a randomized, double-blind study comparing a study-solution of low-concentration levobupivacaine and sufentanil with or without the addition of clonidine for patient controlled epidural, Bazin (2011) found better control of labor pain with the addition of clonidine. In the clonidine-group blood pressure was lower and the rate of instrumental delivery higher with no difference in fetal outcome.

> **Recommendation.** Local anesthetics may be used during pregnancy for infiltration and conduction anesthesia. This also applies for preparations with an adrenaline additive. The substances of choice are, for example, bupivacaine in obstetrics and articaine in dentistry. Prilocaine should be avoided because of the comparatively high risk of methemoglobinemia, especially when used for pudendal anesthesia right before delivery. Mepivacaine should only be used when other local anesthetics cannot be considered. When clonidine is added to the epidural infusion, the blood pressure must be monitored even more carefully.

2.16.8   Muscle relaxants

Muscle relaxants are used for general anesthesia when anesthetics alone do not produce sufficient relaxation of the skeletal muscles which is especially important in rapid sequence induction of anesthesia for caesarean section.

Suxamethonium (*succinylcholine*) is the only depolarizing muscle relaxant in general use today. It is metabolized quickly by plasma cholinesterase. Due to its rapid onset and short duration of action, it is frequently used for rapid sequence intubation when a high risk of aspiration is expected, as is the case in pregnant patients undergoing caesarean delivery. Heinonen (1977) found no anomalies in 26 infants whose mothers were treated with succinylcholine during pregnancy. Transient respiratory depression in newborns after succinylcholine use in the mother during delivery has occasionally been described. In about 3–4% of the population the serum cholinesterase activity is low due to genetic variations. In addition, the activity of this enzyme declines by up to 30% between gestational week 10 and the end of pregnancy. In these patients prolonged neuromuscular blockade requiring respiratory assistance may occur after administration of succinylcholine (Cherala 1989). Such complications should be avoided by using the lowest effective dose. Succinylcholine given in a dose of 1 mg/kg can increase the uterine tone or stimulate contractions. This unwanted side-effect should be considered with threatening fetal hypoxia.

Alcuronium, atracurium, cisatracurium, mivacurium, pancuronium, rocuronium and *vecuronium* are, like *d-tubocurarine* competitive inhibiting muscle relaxants, also called non-depolarizing muscle relaxants. In contrast to general or local anesthetic agents, muscle relaxants cross the blood–brain barrier and only enter the placenta in limited amounts due to their high degree of ionization and low lipid solubility. In the cord blood or fetal tissue they only achieve about 10% of the concentration measured in the mother. These concentrations are thought to be well below the effective dose for inducing neuromuscular relaxation in the fetus or newborn. However, newborn paralysis has been reported after administration of 245 mg d-tubocurarine to the mother over 10 hours to treat an epileptic state (Older 1968). A case report exists of a newborn with arthrogryposis after treatment of maternal tetanus with tubocurarine for 2.5 weeks at the end of the first trimester (Jago 1970).

Teratogenic properties have not so far been observed. Pancuronium, in particular, has proven itself in obstetrics. No neonatal side-effects were observed after a maternal dose of 0.03 mg/kg in 800 caesarean deliveries (Langanke 1987). Due to its long duration of action and the availability of shorter acting muscle relaxants, it is only rarely used today for caesarean deliveries. It can also be used for neuromuscular relaxation in the fetus during intrauterine transfusion (Moise 1987).

Atracurium is said to be superior to pancuronium in directly relaxing the fetus when he or she is being prepared for intrauterine transfusions for anemia (Mouw 1999). In another study, vecuronium was recommended, as it seems to have less side effects on fetal cardiac function than pancuronium (Watson 1996). It may also be used for neuromuscular relaxation of the fetus in *ex utero* intrapartum treatment or fetal surgery (Tran 2010).

Rocuronium can also be used for rapid sequence intubation in general anesthesia during pregnancy. Up to now, the longer duration of action compared to succinylcholin, was a disadvantage in cases of difficult intubation. Thanks to *sugammadex*, a cyclodextrin, the neuromuscular blockade caused by rocuronium can be rapidly reversed (Sharp 2009). In two case series no patient showed evidence for recurarization and none of the newborns showed signs of muscular weakness after neuromuscular blockade with rocuronium was reversed with sugammadex (Pühringer 2010, Williamson 2011).

Mivacurium is a short-acting, non-depolarizing muscle relaxant also metabolized by serum cholinesterase similar to succinylcholine. Because of the short duration of a caesarean delivery, it is appropriate as a muscle relaxant, although its onset of action is slower than either succinylcholine or rocuronium. In case of a plasma cholinesterase deficiency, there is the risk of prolonged neuromuscular blockade.

Preparations with botulinum-neurotoxin (BoNT) have completely different indications and are administered for blepharospasm and other focal spasticity as well as for primary hyperhidrosis. There is also increasing use for cosmetic reasons (treatment of "the aging face"). There are no systematic studies, but several case reports of treatment during pregnancy (Aranda 2012, Li Yim 2010, Wataganara 2009) have been reported with normal pregnancy outcome. However, all authors caution against routine use in pregnant patients. In a survey of foodborne botulism in Canada between 1985 and 2005 three of the reported 205 cases with laboratory confirmed botulism occurred in pregnancy. None of the patients was diagnosed with pregnancy complications although one case had toxemia for ≥10 days. There was also no evidence that botulinum toxin can cross the placenta (Leclair 2013). Anaphylactoid reactions to the injections cannot be ruled out.

> **Recommendation.** In the course of anesthesia the usual muscle relaxants may be used during pregnancy. The lowest possible doses should be chosen. Botulinum neurotoxin is not recommended for use in pregnancy for cosmetic reasons as this is not a vital indication. For other indications a risk-benefit evaluation should be made including risks of using alternative substances. Accidental exposure does not require consequences if the mother does not have any appreciable side-effects.

References

Abboud TK, Kim SH, Henriksen EH et al. Comparative maternal and neonatal effects of halothane and enflurane for cesarean section. Acta Anaesthesiol Scand 1985; 29: 663–8.

Abboud TK, Zhu J, Richardson M et al. Intravenous propofol vs thiamylal-isoflurane for caesarean section, comparative maternal and neonatal effects. Acta Anaesthesiol Scand 1995; 39: 205–9.

Al-jahdari WS, Saito S, Nakano T, Goto F. Propofol induces growth cone collapse and neurite retractions in chick explant culture. Can J Anaesth 2006; 53: 1078–85.

Aranda MA, Herranz A, del Val J et al. Botulinum toxin A during pregnancy, still a debate. Eur J Neurol 2012; 19: e81–2.

Baraka A, Louis F, Dalleh R. Maternal awareness and neonatal outcome after ketamine induction of anaesthesia for Caesarean section. Can J Anaesth 1990; 37: 641–4.

Bazin M, Bonnin M, Storme B et al. Addition of clonidine to a continuous patient-controlled epidural infusion of low-concentration levobupivacaine plus sufentanil in primiparous women during labour. Anaesthesia 2011; 66: 769–79.

Beilin Y, Bodian CA, Mukherjee T et al. The use of propofol, nitrous oxide, or isoflurane does not affect the reproductive success rate following gamete intrafallopian transfer (GIFT): a multicenter pilot trial/survey. Anesthesiology 1999; 90: 36–41.

Bozynski ME, Rubarth LB, Patel JA. Lidocaine toxicity after maternal pudendal anesthesia in a term infant with fetal distress. Am J Perinatol 1987; 4: 164–6.

Bozynski ME, Schumacher RE, Deschner LS, Kileny P. Effect of prenatal lignocaine on auditory brain stem evoked response. Arch Dis Child 1989; 64: 934–8.

Brodsky JB, Cohen EN, Brown BW et al. Surgery during pregnancy and fetal outcome. Am J Obstet Gynecol 1980; 138: 1165–7.

Burov NE, Arzamastsev EV, Kornienko LI, Kudimova LA. Investigation of the teratogenic and embryotoxic action of xenon. Anesteziol Reanimatol 2002; 4: 69–70.

Celleno D, Capogna G, Tomassetti M et al. Neurobehavioural effects of propofol on the neonate following elective caesarean section. Br J Anaesth 1989; 62: 649–54.

Cheek TG, Baird E. Anesthesia for nonobstetric surgery: maternal and fetal considerations. Clin Obstet Gynecol 2009; 52: 535–45.

Cherala SR, Eddie DN, Sechzer PH. Placental transfer of succinylcholine causing transient respiratory depression in the newborn. Anaesth Intensive Care 1989; 17: 202–4.

Christiaens F, Janssenswillen C, Van Steirteghem AC et al. Comparison of assisted reproductive technology performance after oocyte retrieval under general anaesthesia (propofol) versus paracervical local anaesthetic block: a case-controlled study. Hum Reprod 1998; 13: 2456–60.

Cohen EN, Bellville JW, Brown BW Jr. Anesthesia, pregnancy, and miscarriage: a study of operating room nurses and anesthetists. Anesthesiology 1971; 35: 343–7.

Cordier S, Ha MC, Ayme S, Goujard J. Maternal occupational exposure and congenital malformations. Scand J Work Environ Health 1992; 18: 11–7.

Crawford JS, Lewis M. Nitrous oxide in early human pregnancy. Anaesthesia 1986; 41: 900–5.

Dailland P, Cockshott ID, Lirzin JD et al. Intravenous propofol during cesarean section: placental transfer, concentrations in breast milk, and neonatal effects. A preliminary study. Anesthesiology 1989; 71: 827–34.

De Amici D, Delmonte P, Martinotti L et al. Can anesthesiologic strategies for caesarean section influence newborn jaundice? A retrospective and prospective study. Biol Neonate 2001; 79: 97–102.

de Barros Duarte L, Dantas Moises EC, Cavalli RC et al. Distribution of bupivacaine enantiomers and lidocaine and its metabolite in the placental intervillous space and in the different maternal and fetal compartments in term pregnant women. J Clin Pharmacol 2011; 51: 212–7.

Decocq G, Brazier M, Hary L et al. Serum bupivacaine concentrations and transplacental transfer following repeated epidural administrations in term parturients during labour. Fundam Clin Pharmacol 1997; 11: 365–70.

Deutsche Forschungsgemeinschaft DFG "MAK- und BAT-Werte-Liste" 2013: Maximale Arbeitsplatzkonzentrationen und Biologische Arbeitsstofftoleranzwerte. Berlin: Wiley VCH. http://onlinelibrary.wiley.com/book/10.1002/9783527675135 (accessed December 8, 2013).

Dewandre PY, Decurninge V, Bonhomme V et al. Side effects of the addition of clonidine 75 microg or sufentanil 5 microg to 0.2% ropivacaine for labour epidural analgesia. Int J Obstet Anesth 2010; 19: 149–54.

Dewandre PY, Kirsch M, Bonhomme V et al. Impact of the addition of sufentanil 5 microg or clonidine 75 microg on the minimum local analgesic concentration of ropivacaine for epidural analgesia in labour: a randomized comparison. Int J Obstet Anesth 2008; 17: 315–21.

Duncan PG, Pope WD, Cohen MM, Greer, N. Fetal risk of anesthesia and surgery during pregnancy. Anesthesiology 1986; 64: 790–4.

Ebi KL, Rice SA. Reproductive and developmental toxicity of anesthetics in humans. In: Anesthetic Toxicity, edited by Rice SA, New York: Raven, 1994; pp. 175–98.

Eddleston JM, Holland JJ, Griffin RP et al. A double-blind comparison of 0.25% ropivacaine and 0.25% bupivacaine for extradural analgesia in labour. Br J Anaesth 1996; 76: 66–71.

El-Beheiry H, Kavanagh B. Is propofol neurotoxic to the developing brain? Can J Anaesth 2006; 53: 1069–73.

Ericson A, Kallen B. Survey of infants born in 1973 or 1975 to Swedish women working in operating rooms during their pregnancies. Anesth Analg 1979; 58: 302–5.

Fernando R, Bonello E, Gill P et al. Neonatal welfare and placental transfer of fentanyl and bupivacaine during ambulatory combined spinal epidural analgesia for labour. Anaesthesia 1997; 52: 517–24.

Flowers CE Jr. The placental transmission of barbiturates and thiobarbiturates and their pharmacological action on the mother and the infant. Am J Obstet Gynecol 1959; 78: 730–42.

Gin T, Gregory MA, Oh TE. The haemodynamic effects of propofol and thiopentone for induction of caesarean section. Anaesth Intensive Care 1990; 18: 175–9.

Gogarten W, Marcus MA, Van AH. Obstetrical pain therapy. Anaesthesist 1997; 46: S159–64.

Guay J. Methemoglobinemia related to local anesthetics: a summary of 242 episodes. Anesth Analg 2009; 108: 837–45.

Heber G, Hasenburg A, Jaspers V, Spatling L. Methemoglobinemia in the newborn infant – caused by prilocaine? A case report. Zentralbl Gynakol 1995; 117: 105–7.

Heinonen OP, Slone D, Shapiro S. Birth defects and drugs in pregnancy. Littleton, Massachusetts: Publishing Sciences Group, Inc., 1977.

Hemminki K, Vineis P. Extrapolation of the evidence on teratogenicity of chemicals between humans and experimental animals: chemicals other than drugs. Teratog Carcinog Mutagen 1985; 5: 251–318.

Herman NL, Li AT, Van Decar TK et al. Transfer of methohexital across the perfused human placenta. J Clin Anesth 2000; 12: 25–30.

Hrgovic Z. Methemoglobinemia in a newborn infant following pudendal anesthesia in labor with prilocaine. A case report. Anasth Intensivther Notfallmed 1990; 25: 172–4.

Ikonomidou C, Bittigau P, Koch C et al. Neurotransmitters and apoptosis in the developing brain. Biochem Pharmacol 2001; 62: 401–5.

Jago RH. Arthrogryposis following treatment of maternal tetanus with muscle relaxants. Arch Dis Child 1970; 45: 277–9.

Jauniaux E, Gulbis B, Shannon C et al. Placental propofol transfer and fetal sedation during maternal general anaesthesia in early pregnancy. Lancet 1998; 352: 290–1.

Jevtovic-Todorovic V, Hartman RE, Izumi Y et al. Early exposure to common anesthetic agents causes widespread neurodegeneration in the developing rat brain and persistent learning deficits. J Neurosci 2003; 23: 876–82.

Karaman S, Akercan F, Aldemir O et al. The maternal and neonatal effects of the volatile anaesthetic agents desflurane and sevoflurane in caesarean section: a prospective, randomized clinical study. J Int Med Res 2006; 34: 183–92.

Kirschbaum M, Biscoping J, Bachmann B, Kunzel W. Fetal methemoglobinemia caused by prilocaine – is use of prilocaine for pudendal block still justified? Geburtshilfe Frauenheilkd 1991; 51: 228–30.

Kruessell MA, Udink ten Cate FE, Kraus AJ et al. Use of propofol in pediatric intensive care units: a national survey in Germany. Pediatr Crit Care Med 2012; 13: e150–4.

Kumar M, Chandra S, Ijaz Z, Senthilselvan A. Epidural analgesia in labour and neonatal respiratory distress: a case-control study. Arch Dis Child Fetal Neonatal Ed 2014; 99: F116–F119.

Langanke D, Jährig K. Narkotika, Muskelrelaxantien und Lokalanästhetika. In: Arzneimittelanwendung in Schwangerschaft und Stillperiode, Huller H, Jährig D, Göretzlehner G, Träger A (eds), 1987; pp. 105–17. Berlin: Volk und Gesundheit.

Lawson CC, Rocheleau CM, Whelan EA et al. Occupational exposures among nurses and risk of spontaneous abortion. Am J Obstet Gynecol 2012; 206: 327–8.

Leclair D, Fung J, Isaac-Renton JL et al. Foodborne botulism in Canada, 1985–2005. Emerg Infect Dis 2013; 19: 961–8.

Li Yim JF, Weir CR. Botulinum toxin and pregnancy-a cautionary tale. Strabismus 2010; 18: 65–6.

Liechty KW. Ex-utero intrapartum therapy. Semin Fetal Neonatal Med 2010; 15: 34–9.

Likis FE, Andrews JC, Collins MR, Lewis RM, Seroogy JJ, Starr SA, Walden RR, McPheeters ML. Nitrous oxide for the management of labor pain: a systematic review. Anesth Analg 2014; 118: 153–167.

Loftus JR, Hill H, Cohen SE. Placental transfer and neonatal effects of epidural sufentanil and fentanyl administered with bupivacaine during labor. Anesthesiology 1995; 83: 300–8.

Macaulay JH, Bond K, Steer PJ. Epidural analgesia in labor and fetal hyperthermia. Obstet Gynecol 1992; 80: 665–9.

Moise KJ Jr, Carpenter RJ Jr, Deter RL et al. The use of fetal neuromuscular blockade during intrauterine procedures. Am J Obstet Gynecol 1987; 157: 874–9.

Moldenhauer JS. Ex utero intrapartum therapy. Semin Pediatr Surg 2013; 22: 44–9.

Moore J, Bill KM, Flynn RJ et al. A comparison between propofol and thiopentone as induction agents in obstetric anaesthesia. Anaesthesia 1989; 44: 753–7.

Mouw RJ, Klumper F, Hermans J et al. Effect of atracurium or pancuronium on the anemic fetus during and directly after intravascular intrauterine transfusion. A double blind randomized study. Acta Obstet Gynecol Scand 1999; 78: 763–7.

Older PO, Harris JM. Placental transfer of tubocurarine. Case Report. Br J Anaesth 1968; 40: 459–63.

Olney JW, Farber NB, Wozniak DF et al. Environmental agents that have the potential to trigger massive apoptotic neurodegeneration in the developing brain. Environ Health Perspect 2000; 108: 383–8.

Paule MG, Li M, Allen RR et al. Ketamine anesthesia during the first week of life can cause long-lasting cognitive deficits in rhesus monkeys. Neurotoxicol Teratol 2011; 33: 220–30.

Pharoah PO, Alberman E, Doyle P, Chamberlain G. Outcome of pregnancy among women in anaesthetic practice. Lancet 1977; 1: 34–6.

Pühringer FK, Kristen P, Rex C. Sugammadex reversal of rocuronium-induced neuromuscular block in Caesarean section patients: a series of seven cases. Br J Anaesth 2010; 105: 657–60.

Ratzon NZ, Ornoy A, Pardo A et al. Developmental evaluation of children born to mothers occupationally exposed to waste anesthetic gases. Birth Defects Res, A Clin Mol Teratol 2004; 70: 476–82.

Reich DL, Silvay G. Ketamine: an update on the first twenty-five years of clinical experience. Can J Anaesth 1989; 36: 186–97.

Reynolds F. The effects of maternal labour analgesia on the fetus. Best Pract Res Clin Obstet Gynaecol 2010; 24: 289–302.

Roberts RJ, Barletta JF, Fong JJ et al. Incidence of propofol-related infusion syndrome in critically ill adults: a prospective, multicenter study. Crit Care 2009; 13: R169.

Rosenberg PH. Vanttinen H. Occupational hazards to reproduction and health in anaesthetists and paediatricians. Acta Anaesthesiol Scand 1978; 22: 202–7.

Rowland AS, Baird DD, Weinberg CR et al. Reduced fertility among women employed as dental assistants exposed to high levels of nitrous oxide. N Engl J Med 1992; 327: 993–7.

Santos AC, Arthur GR, Wlody D et al. Comparative systemic toxicity of ropivacaine and bupivacaine in nonpregnant and pregnant ewes. Anesthesiology 1995; 82: 734–40.

Sharp LM, Levy DM. Rapid sequence induction in obstetrics revisited. Curr Opin Anesthesiol 2009; 22: 357–61.

Sprung J, Flick RP, Wilder RT et al. Anesthesia for cesarean delivery and learning disabilities in a population-based birth cohort. Anesthesiology 2009; 111: 302–10.

Szabo AL. Review article: Intrapartum neuraxial analgesia and breastfeeding outcomes: limitations of current knowledge. Anesth Analg 2013; 116: 399–405.

Tran KM. Anesthesia for fetal surgery. Semin Fetal Neonatal Med 2010; 15: 40–5.

Tunstall ME, Sheikh A. Comparison of 1.5% enflurane with 1.25% isoflurane in oxygen for caesarean section: avoidance of awareness without nitrous oxide. Br J Anaesth 1989; 62: 138–43.

Uslu S, Comert S. Transient neonatal methemoglobinemia caused by maternal pudendal anesthesia in delivery with prilocaine: report of two cases. Minerva Pediatr 2013; 65: 213–7.

Valtonen M, Kanto J, Rosenberg P. Comparison of propofol and thiopentone for induction of anaesthesia for elective caesarean section. Anaesthesia 1989; 44: 758–62.

Vessey MP, Nunn JF. Occupational hazards of anesthesia. Br Med J 1980; 281: 696–8.

Wallet F, Clement HJ, Bouret C et al. Effects of a continuous low-dose clonidine epidural regimen on pain, satisfaction and adverse events during labour: a randomized, double-blind, placebo-controlled trial. Eur J Anaesthesiol 2010; 27: 441–4.

Wataganara T, Leelakusolvong S, Sunsaneevithayakul P, Vantanasiri C. Treatment of severe achalasia during pregnancy with esophagoscopic injection of botulinum toxin A: a case report. J Perinatol 2009; 29: 637–9.

Watson WJ, Atchison SR, Harlass FE. Comparison of pancuronium and vecuronium for fetal neuromuscular blockade during invasive procedures. J Matern Fetal Med 1996; 5: 151–4.

Wilder RT, Flick RP, Sprung J et al. Early exposure to anesthesia and learning disabilities in a population-based birth cohort. Anesthesiology 2009; 110: 796–804.

Williamson RM, Mallaiah S, Barclay P. Rocuronium and sugammadex for rapid sequence induction of obstetric general anaesthesia. Acta Anaesthesiol Scand 2011; 55: 694–9.

Wong JM. Propofol infusion syndrome. Am J Ther 2010; 17: 487–91.

Yoo KY, Lee JC, Yoon MH et al. The effects of volatile anesthetics on spontaneous contractility of isolated human pregnant uterine muscle: a comparison among sevoflurane, desflurane, isoflurane, and halothane. Anesth Analg 2006; 103: 443–7.

Dermatological medications and local therapeutics

2.17

Gudula Kirtschig and Christof Schaefer

2.17.1	Typical skin changes during pregnancy	468
2.17.2	Antiseptics and disinfectants	468
2.17.3	Glucocorticoids and non-steroid antiphlogistics	471
2.17.4	Astringents	471
2.17.5	Antipruritics and essential oils	472
2.17.6	Coal tar and slate oil preparations	472
2.17.7	Local immunomodulators as therapy for atopic eczema	473
2.17.8	Keratolytics	473
2.17.9	Retinoids for acne and psoriasis therapy	475
2.17.10	Ultraviolet light	479
2.17.11	Fumaric acid preparations	479
2.17.12	Biologicals	480
2.17.13	Wart therapeutics	480
2.17.14	Lithium	481
2.17.15	Lice medications	481
2.17.16	Anti-scabies	482
2.17.17	Vein therapeutics	483
2.17.18	Antihidrotica	483
2.17.19	Eflornithine, finasteride and minoxidil	484
2.17.20	Repellents	485
2.17.21	Cosmetics	485
2.17.22	Eye, nose and ear drops	486
2.17.23	Hemorrhoid medications	488
2.17.24	Vaginal therapeutics	488

In this chapter, the most important dermatological medications as well as other frequently used topical therapeutics will be discussed. More extensive information on individual medications can be found under the substance headings in other chapters. Anti-infectives are discussed in Chapter 2.6.

Drugs During Pregnancy and Lactation. **http://dx.doi.org/10.1016/B978-0-12-408078-2.00018-4**

2.17.1   Typical skin changes during pregnancy

The adaptation of the woman during pregnancy leads to typical morphological and functional changes in the skin. These are completely normal and do not require treatment. Among them are:

- *Pigmentation*: Particularly striking is the appearance of a spotty hyperpigmentation of the face (melasma) which usually disappears spontaneously after birth. This is intensified by exposure to UV light (i.e. to direct sunlight) and can be minimized by using a sun block. Pigmented areas like the nipples and the areola, the area around the navel (linea alba), the armpits, and the anogenital regions may get darker in pregnant women. Moles may also become darker in some women. In general, sensitivity to light is increased during pregnancy.
- *Striae*: During the second half of pregnancy, striae distensae appear frequently on the stomach, hips, thighs and also on the breasts. As body size increases, these become broader and more plentiful. They begin as reddish purple lines and with time, they become white atrophic (cigarette paper like wrinkled) scars. They are more frequently seen in young women and in women who are overweight and have large babies; there is probably a genetic relationship. There is no known effective medical prophylaxis. Daily massage of the skin with a simple moisturizer or olive oil may be tried and also the control of excess weight gain may partly help to prevent the development of stretch marks (Brennan 2012).
- *Fibroma*: Soft fibromata appear more frequently especially in the neck and axillary regions.
- *Blood vessel changes*: Circulation in the skin is increased. The skin feels warmer, and the vasomotor excitability of the vessels in the face increases. This leads to quick blushing and blanching and to increased dermographism. In addition, the veins in the breast and stomach skin are much more visible and varicosities in the legs and the vulva as well as hemorrhoids may appear.
- *Skin glands, hair and nails*: Especially in early pregnancy, the secretion of the sebaceous glands can increase significantly. Existing acne frequently improves. On the other hand, an acute pregnancy acne (*acne gravidarum*) can occur from the third month forward, which disappears during the postpartum period. The growth of the nails is generally enhanced during pregnancy, and more hair goes into the resting phase. This causes diminished shedding of the hair and is perceived as thickening of the hair. Three months after delivery the hair cycle normalizes producing temporarily more loss of hair in many women (*postpartum effluvium*). This is called *telogen effluvium*. This process is usually completed 6 to 12 months after delivery. Thereafter, the hair will usually be the same as before pregnancy. Treatment is not required.

Topically applied substances are better absorbed during pregnancy. This applies especially to skin that has been altered by inflammation and open wounds and may lead to the exposure of the fetus to the ingredients.

2.17.2   Antiseptics and disinfectants

Disinfectants should have a strong bactericidal or bacteriostatic action, on one hand, but good local tolerance by the skin, mucosa and wounds on the other hand. In addition, they should not lead to toxic effects if absorbed.

► **Alcohol**

No toxic effects have been observed, as yet, from topical use of alcohols during pregnancy. In practice only ethanol and isopropyl alcohol (isopropanol) are of importance.

> **Recommendation.** Alcohol derivatives are not dangerous and can be used as disinfectants during pregnancy.

► **Benzoyl peroxide**

Benzoyl peroxide is used, in particular, for external treatment of acne. About 5% is absorbed (Leachman 2006). To some extent, it is converted to benzoic acid in the skin. Simultaneous topical therapy with retinoids increases the absorption. Benzoyl peroxide is also used in the food and plastics industries. There are insufficient epidemiological data for a risk assessment. Despite the broad use, there are no indications of any teratogenic effects.

> **Recommendation.** Benzoyl peroxide may be used for acne treatment in pregnant women on a limited basis (i.e. the face).

► **Povidone iodine**

When using *povidone iodine* as a local disinfectant on intact skin, on wounds and on the mucosa, as well as in body cavities, iodine transfer to the fetus must be assumed. This can lead to functional disturbances of the fetal thyroid. A vaginal douche during labor can lead to a temporary TSH increase in the newborn – a sign of a transient hypothyroidism (Weber 1998), but also to effects on the maternal thyroid metabolism and maternal iodine excretion (Velasco 2009). A study of 42 mother–child pairs found significantly increased iodine excretion in the urine of both mother and child when povidone iodine was used as disinfectant before Caesarean section, but the TSH values of the children were not different compared with a control group disinfected with alcoholic solutions (Tahirović 2009). In a retrospective comparative study of children with birth defects and healthy children, there were no indications of teratogenic effects after vaginal use during pregnancy (Czeizel 2004). However, an undisturbed thyroid status is necessary for the differentiation of the central nervous system. Therefore, even slight imbalances should be avoided.

> **Recommendation.** Iodine-containing disinfectants may only be used during pregnancy on small areas for a few days. Body cavities should not be cleansed with iodine-containing solutions. However, in the light of current knowledge, its use is not connected with any irreversible damage, and it is not clear what specific skin preparation may be most efficient for preventing post-caesarean wound and surgical site infection (Hadiati 2012).

Pregnancy

2.17 Dermatological medications and local therapeutics

► Phenol derivatives

Phenol derivatives are used primarily in over-the-counter preparations for rinsing the mouth, disinfecting the skin, and treating perianal infections. Solutions of phenol derivatives, such as cresol and thymol as well as chlorinated phenol derivatives are viewed as relatively safe during pregnancy. They should not be used in a concentration stronger than 2% and should only be used on intact skin. With higher concentrations, incremental absorption must be assumed.

Chlorhexidine is appropriate for pregnant women to disinfect the skin and mucosa. In a study of 2,500 mother–child pairs, however, following disinfection of the vagina with chlorhexidine, no superiority in the maternal and child postpartum course was observed compared to a placebo (Saleem 2010). Daily use of chlorhexidine mouthwash for the treatment of periodontal disease was associated with a reduction of preterm birth (Boutin 2013).

By contrast, caution should be exercised during pregnancy with the neurotoxic phenol derivative, hexachlorophene, because, when larger areas are treated with concentrations of more than 3%, resorptive poisoning, with central nervous system symptoms, has been observed in treated patients. In some animal experiments, hexachlorophene has been shown to be teratogenic. In many publications over the last decades, workplace contact with hexachlorophene has been controversially discussed with respect to fetotoxic effects. An older study involving 3,000 pregnant women who were occupationally exposed did not find anything remarkable (Baltzar 1979). A further retrospective study postulated a connection between mental retardation and occupational exposure in the last trimester of pregnancy (Roeleveld 1993).

> **Recommendation.** Hexachlorophene should be avoided during pregnancy. However, accidental use requires no action. The other phenol derivatives such as, for instance, chlorhexidine, may be used by pregnant women for appropriate indications for disinfection of the skin and mucosa.

► Mercury compounds

Mercury can be substantially absorbed after external use and is a potential developmental toxin (Lauwerys 1987).

> **Recommendation.** Mercury-containing disinfectants are contraindicated during pregnancy. However, their (accidental) use does not require any action (Chapter 1.15).

► Other antiseptics

Quinoline sulfate has shown mutagenic properties experimentally. *Clioquinol* is one of the iodine-containing antiseptics. Additional antiseptics are dequalinium salts, hexetidine for throat or vaginal use, gentian violet or crystal violet, pyoktanin, ethacridine and hydrogen peroxide.

There is evidence of carcinogenic properties and contradictory data on teratogenicity for gentian violet in animal studies. Hydrogen peroxide is naturally developed from bacteria of the vaginal flora. None of these substances has been systematically studied during pregnancy, but there have also been no serious indications of teratogenicity in human with any of these substances.

> **Recommendation.** Quinoline should be avoided. Small areas and brief use of the other antiseptic substances mentioned are unobjectionable for appropriate indications during pregnancy, but their use should be critically considered.

2.17.3   Glucocorticoids and non-steroid antiphlogistics

With long-term use of glucocorticoids (Chapter 2.15) and the non-steroid antiphlogistics or application to larger and, above all, inflamed skin areas, absorption and transfer to the fetus must be assumed. Topically used glucocorticoids are divided into four groups according to their potency. Among the mildly potent are hydrocortisone acetate, prednisolone and dexamethasone. Among the moderately potent are *clobetasone, flumetasone, fluocinolone* and *prednicarbate*. Among the most potent are *amcinonide, fluocinonide, fluticasone, hydrocortisone17-butyrate* and *mometasone* and a very potent topical steroid is, for example, *clobetasol propionate*.

Among 363 children whose mothers were treated with topical glucocorticoids during pregnancy (170 of them in the first trimester), neither an increased risk of malformations nor a difference in the birth parameters was found compared to an untreated control group (Mygind 2002). Also in a review, considering the heterogeneous and, to some extent, insufficient data, there was no indication found of teratogenic effects or effects on prematurity. At most, an association with low birthweight was discussed in connection with very potent corticosteroids (Chi 2009).

There are no systematic studies on the use in pregnancy of *bufexamac, levomenol* and *benzydamine*, and there is also no indication of teratogenic action. The non-steroid antiphlogistic bufexamac was removed from the market in 2010 because of its (allergic) side-effects. Non-steroid antiphlogistic substances have also not, as yet, been shown to be teratogenic with systemic use but due to their prostaglandin antagonistic effect they could be fetotoxic in the last trimester (Chapter 2.1).

> **Recommendation.** There is no objection to occasional use of topical glucocorticoids or topical antiphlogistics in limited areas. Very potent steroids such as clobetasol propionate should be avoided during pregnancy. However, their use may be favored to systemic steroids if required because of disease severity.

2.17.4   Astringents

On mucosa and in wounds, astringents lead, through protein precipitation of the surface layers, to sealing and shriveling of tissue. They are used for local treatment of inflamed mucosa and wounds. Two groups are used therapeutically – tannin-containing preparations (Chapter 2.5) and dilute solutions of metal salts, e.g. *aluminum aceticum* and aluminum acetate-tartrate-solution DAB) or *zinc salts*.

> **Recommendation.** There is no contraindication for therapy with astringents during pregnancy as their absorption is unlikely.

2.17.5   Antipruritics and essential oils

▶ Antiallergics and local anesthetics

Antiallergics and local anesthetics which are used as antipruritics for topical therapy are, as a rule, harmless during pregnancy (Chapter 2.2).

▶ Polidocanol

Macrogol lauryl ether (polidocanol) is used externally against itching. In addition, it is used intravenously to obliterate varicose veins, for lesions of the oral mucosa, in vaginal spermicides and in cosmetics (Reich-Schupke 2012). Further, it is used in wound therapeutics, in combination with benzethonium and urea. No teratogenic effects have been published for this widely used substance to date neither in animal nor human studies. However, systematic studies are lacking.

> **Recommendation.** Polidocanol may also be used by pregnant women against itching.

▶ Camphor and menthol

A small amount of *camphor* applied to the skin has a cooling and local anesthetic effect; while rubbing it in vigorously enhances the blood flow of the skin. Because of these effects, camphor and other essential oils are included in a large number of hyperemia-causing dermatological products (Chapter 2.19).

Menthol is used topically for itching.

No teratogenic action has, as yet, been published in either animal or human studies.

> **Recommendation.** Camphor and other essential oils may be used topically during pregnancy.

2.17.6   Coal tar and slate oil preparations

Coal tar preparations, which are used primarily for the treatment of eczema, in particular atopic eczema and psoriasis, have not been suspected of having a teratogenic effect. A retrospective study of 23 exposed women revealed nothing remarkable (Franssen 1999). Experimentally, coal tar products have, to some extent, shown mutagenic or carcinogenic properties. However, coal tar has been used as a dermatological treatment for decades and has not, as yet, shown any indication of this kind in humans (Roelofzen 2010).

The *slate oil extracts*, ammonium *bitumen sulfonate* and *sodium bitumen sulfonate* are used topically for both (sub)acute and chronically inflamed dermatitis as well as other skin conditions. There are no systematic studies on prenatal toxicity, but also no indications of replicable teratogenic effects in humans.

> **Recommendation.** Ideally, coal tar preparations should not be used during pregnancy. However, (accidental) use does not require any action. Topically limited use of slate oil extracts is acceptable.

2.17.7 Local immunomodulators as therapy for atopic eczema

▶ **Tacrolimus and pimecrolimus**

Tacrolimus and *pimecrolimus* are licensed for topical treatment of atopic eczema. There are no systematic studies on topical use during pregnancy but there is considerable experience on the systemic use of *tacrolimus* as an immune suppressant after transplants, which do not indicate a teratogenic risk (Hebert 2013).

There is insufficient experience on the use of *pimecrolimus* during pregnancy to assess teratogenic risk.

> **Recommendation.** Tacrolimus may be used on small areas of the skin during pregnancy for strict indications. Due to limited experience, therapy with pimecrolimus should be avoided.

2.17.8 Keratolytics

▶ **Salicylate and carbamide preparations**

Keratolytics are used to soften the keratin layer and for loosening scales. *Salicylates* are used as keratolytics in concentrations of 2–10% or 30–50% (i.e. in solutions or vaseline for therapy of verrucae vulgares (warts). *Carbamide* preparations are used in 10% solutions. Systemic effects are not expected if appropriately used, even during pregnancy.

> **Recommendation.** Topical use of the keratolytics mentioned is no cause for concern in pregnant women if the time period and areas of treatment are used as recommended.

▶ **Dithranol**

Dithranol (=anthralin, cignoline) is used for the treatment of psoriasis. Systematic studies on prenatal toxicity in humans are lacking. According to one manufacturer (American Dermal Corporation, Somerset NJ), no anthralin was detectable in the urine of subjects who had used this drug topically. A second manufacturer (Dermik Labs, Blue Bell PA) cites an unpublished animal study, performed in piglets, to suggest that the dermal absorption of anthralin is small or negligible. However, this antimitotic substance should on theoretical grounds be avoided during pregnancy, although a quantitative absorption of the usual 1–3% preparation is unlikely.

> **Recommendation.** Repeated use on large areas should be avoided in inflamed skin, like psoriatic skin, as absorption is enhanced.

▶ **Selenium disulfide**

Selenium disulfide is used topically as a supportive therapy for psoriasis as well as pityriasis vesicolor. There are no systematic studies on topical use during pregnancy. There are no substantial indications of a teratogenic risk as yet (Chapter 2.15).

> **Recommendation.** Topical use of selenium disulfide on small areas of the skin and for a limited period is acceptable during pregnancy.

▶ **Azelaic acid**

The antibacterial, antiphlogistic and keratolytic azelaic acid is used in acne therapy. It is also used for treatment of skin pigmentation including melasma and post-inflammatory hyperpigmentation, particularly in individuals with darker skin types. It has been recommended as an alternative to hydroquinone. As a tyrosinase inhibitor, *azelaic acid* reduces synthesis of melanin. About 4–8% of the topically applied substance is absorbed systemically. In animal experiments azelaic acid, even in high doses, is not teratogenic (Akhavan 2003). However, systematic studies on its use in humans are lacking.

> **Recommendation.** During pregnancy, azelaic acid should only be used for strict indications on small skin surfaces, e.g. facial acne, preferably not in the first trimester.

▶ **Sulfur-containing preparations**

Sulfur is used as an additive (2–10%) to lotions, creams, powders and ointments. It has mild keratolytic and bacteriostatic properties. The bioavailability of topically applied sulfur is about 1% (Akhavan 2003). There are no data on its use during pregnancy.

> **Recommendation.** Sulfur may also be used during pregnancy on small areas for relevant indications. Systemic effects after local therapy are unlikely.

► Resorcin

Resorcin is an aromatic alcohol used in local acne therapy, seborrheic eczema and psoriasis. It is also contained in hair dye and cosmetics. As yet, there is no indication of teratogenic effects. However, systematic studies on its use during pregnancy are lacking. After (accidental) oral intake serious complications with cramps and unconsciousness were reported and, in one incident with a pregnant woman, intrauterine fetal death (Duran 2004).

> **Recommendation.** Topical treatment with resorcin on small areas of skin is acceptable during pregnancy for relevant indications.

2.17.9 Retinoids for acne and psoriasis therapy

Pharmacology

Isotretinoin (13-cis-retinoic acid) and *tretinoin* (all-trans-retinoic acid) are natural derivatives of vitamin A (retinol). They have been used with great success externally and systemically for the treatment of acne. Tretinoin is, in addition, approved as a systemic preparation for treating promyelocytic leukemia (Chapter 2.13). Oral alitretinoin is approved for use in patients with severe chronic hand eczema unresponsive to treatment with potent topical corticosteroids (Garnock-Jones 2009, Ruzicka 2008). Retinoic acid is identical to the body's own growth factor, which is present in all cells and is bound to retinoid receptors. Retinoic acid has a particularly important function during the embryonic phase, because it is responsible for the development of the brain, heart, thymus and the spinal cord via migration of neural crest cells.

Retinoids stimulate the proliferation of epidermal cells. In the skin, they loosen the keratin layer and, in this way, ease the scaling process. Isotretinoin also leads to atrophy of sebaceous glands. These properties explain their effectiveness in acne therapy. The half-life of isotretinoin and its metabolite, 4-oxo-isotretinoin, is on average 29 and 22 hours, respectively. In extreme cases, it can be up to 1 week (Nulman 1998).

Acitretin and *etretinate* (which has, meanwhile, been taken off the market) have proved themselves in the treatment of psoriasis. Both lead to prolonged high concentrations of retinoids in the body. Acitretin is metabolized to etretinate, which has a half-life of 80–175 days. The use of alcohol increases the conversion to etretinate (Larsen 2000).

Among the synthetic polyaromatic, receptor-selective retinoids are *adapalene*, which is used for severe acne vulgaris and *tazarotine* for the treatment of psoriasis.

For topical treatment of AIDS-associated Kaposi sarcoma, 0.1% *alitretinoin*-gel is available. By activating the retinoid receptors, it blocks the growth of tumor cells.

Toxicology

The marked teratogenic properties of retinoids were known experimentally even before they were introduced to the market. Today, retinoids are the strongest teratogenic-acting medications since thalidomide. Their use during pregnancy increases the risk of spontaneous abortion and leads to the characteristic retinoid syndrome: anomalies of the ears, including agenesis or stenosis of the auditory canal, facial and palatine defects, micrognathia, cardiovascular defects and developmental defects of the thymus and the central nervous system which can range from involvement of the eyes and the inner ear to hydrocephalus (Lammer 1985, 1988). Intelligence deficits have also been observed even in children without recognizable birth defects (Adams 2010). With the reported risk of 30% birth defects, they have a tenfold higher risk for major birth defects if used systemically during the first trimester. Follow-up examination of 5- to 10-year-old children with intrauterine exposure showed an increased rate of mental retardation and special weaknesses in visual-spatial processing and this, to some extent, also among children without major visible birth defects (Adams 2010).

Damaged children are reported from many countries in association with prenatal *isotretinoin* exposure – and this, although scientific societies, e.g. the Teratology Society (1991) in the USA, had forcefully drawn attention to the teratogenic risk and helped establish intensified birth control programs. Even the demand to prescribe retinoids only after a negative pregnancy test every month along with two complementary methods of birth control be used, only monthly prescriptions of one package and the demand of effective contraception 4 weeks after cessation of treatment still resulted in exposed pregnancies (Teichert 2010). Countless publications still report on individual cases or small case series of isotretinoin exposure. The majority of pregnancies conceived during isotretinoin treatment are interrupted out of fear of developmental defects. Only a minority of pregnancies are carried to term (Honein 2001). Moerike (2002) describe two fetuses after interruption of pregnancy, without any external malformations but with middle and inner ear anomalies. A Canadian study reported on 90 pregnancies among 8,600 women who were prescribed isotretinoin between 1984 and 2002, of which 76 were interrupted. Only one malformation was found among the nine children born alive (Bérard 2007).

An Australian study reporting on undesirable occurrences during isotretinoin therapy described two pregnancies among 1,743 patients in a 6-year period (Rademaker 2010). A study in France between 1999 and 2006 reported on two children of a group of 44 children or fetuses with typical anomalies after isotretinoin intake during the sensitive period. The authors calculated an anomaly rate of 4.5%. During the 7-year observation period, they reported a 30% increase in pregnancies during isotretinoin therapy (Autret-Leca 2010). A study from The Netherlands determined from pharmacy data that only 59% of the women of child-bearing age received contraceptives whilst on isotretinoin.

A German study reported on 115 women who were treated with isotretinoin during pregnancy or within 4 weeks before conception (Schaefer 2010). Among the pregnancies for which the outcome was known, 76% were interrupted. Among them there was no case with an embryopathic diagnosis according to ultrasound investigation. Of the 18 live-born children only one child showed an (unspecific) small ventricular septum defect. These recent figures give the impression that if the exposure took place up to nidation (implantation), the malformation risk is significantly lower than 30%. However, there are not enough documented reports in order to make a statement on the long-term development of exposed children who were unremarkable at birth. Astonishingly, in the German study, women with higher education, including university education, were overrepresented, when educational levels of women who had not used birth control were evaluated. Nine of the 49 women who had not practiced adequate contraception even worked in health care. Such findings demonstrate the difficulty of effectively implementing pregnancy prevention programs for high-risk medications. In a review evaluating 17 publications on the occurrence of pregnancies during isotretinoin therapy in Europe, Crijns (2011) reported a frequency of 0.2–1.0 pregnancies per 1,000 treated women of childbearing age; 65–87% of these pregnancies were interrupted, and only 6–26% of isotretinoin is prescribed in complete concordance with pregnancy prevention programs.

There are many case reports available on multiple birth defects after *acitretin* exposure (de Die-Smulders 1995, Barbero 2004). Geiger (1994) reported on a total of eight pregnancies and acitretin of which two ended in interruptions, four in spontaneous abortions and two were born alive. One of the aborted fetuses showed typical malformations. The two live-born babies were healthy, though one of the children had a hearing disturbance for high frequencies. Of 67 pregnancies with preconception acitretin treatment (on average 5 months before conception), nine ended in spontaneous abortion, 18 in interruptions and 40 were born alive. Four children showed non-specific birth defects.

A Korean study reported on 18 pregnant women who received a transfusion from a blood donor who was treated with acitretin. None of the nine live-born babies showed any birth defects or was neurologically remarkable (Han 2009).

Of 75 women with *etretinate* therapy during pregnancy, 29 live-births were reported of which six showed typical retinoid and three unspecific birth defects. Among the 41 interrupted pregnancies five fetuses showed retinoid-specific and two showed other birth defects. A further five pregnancies ended in spontaneous abortions. Among 88 live-born babies of 173 pregnancies exposed to etretinate before conception (on average 15 months), five children with typical and 13 with unspecific malformations were documented. In addition, three fetuses of interrupted pregnancies showed retinoid specific malformations (Geiger 1994).

Paternal exposure

In post marketing studies, 11 cases of *acitretin* treatment of the father at the time of conception are documented. Five pregnancies delivered healthy children, five ended in spontaneous abortions and one in an interruption of the pregnancy (Geiger 2002).

External use

Five case descriptions have raised the suspicion that birth defects cannot be ruled out after topical use of *tretinoin* (vitamin A derivate, retinoic acid) (Selcen 2000, Colley 1998, Navarre-Belhassen 1998, Lipson 1993, Camera 1992). However, two controlled studies with a total of 300 pregnant women gave no indication of teratogenic effects (Shapiro 1997, Jick 1993). The larger of these studies was based on prescription protocols and does not allow the conclusion that the medication was, in fact, used

Pregnancy

2.17 Dermatological medications and local therapeutics

by all women. The design and number of cases in this study therefore does not allow the assumption that tretinoin is harmless (Martinez-Frias 1999). A further prospective study with 106 topically-treated women during the first trimester neither indicated a higher spontaneous abortion rate nor an increased risk of malformations. There was also no indication of an increased incidence of suspected small retinoid anomalies compared to a control group. In this study, however, no data on the dose or frequency of topical tretinoin treatment is presented (Loureiro 2005).

Based on pharmacokinetic data, an appreciable teratogenic risk after external use is unlikely if the area treated is not too large (e.g. the face only): the usual daily dose of about 2 g of 0.05% tretinoin cream contains 1 mg of the active ingredient. The rate of absorption is about 2% on average and about 6% at maximum (van Hoogdalem 1998). No appreciable increase of the endogenous plasma retinoid concentrations (2–5 µg/L) were observed after treatment. However, it must be kept in mind that, in severely inflamed skin or with the use of additional (disinfectant) substances (i.e. with benzoyl peroxide; see Section 2.17.2), the absorption rate may be increased.

Topical use of *isotretinoin* should be evaluated exactly in the same way as that of tretinoin.

There is a case report on *adapalene* used until the thirteenth week of pregnancy, in which the pregnancy was terminated based upon an ultrasonographic diagnosis of anophthalmia and agenesis of the chiasma opticum. The authors judged these anomalies as not typical for retinoids (Autret 1997).

In a French prospective study, 94 pregnancies with topical retinoid therapy (tretinoin, isotretinoin or adapalene) were evaluated. There was neither an indication of an increased risk of spontaneous abortion nor was a teratogenic effect demonstrable (Carlier 1998). However, there was no differentiation according to substances nor were details on the time and duration of the therapy provided.

When *tazarotene* is used topically, 6% of the dose applied is absorbed through the skin. Its half-life is 17–18 hours. Its metabolites are hydrophilic so that there is no accumulation in the fat tissue. Healthy children were reported after treatment during pregnancy; however, details on the duration of therapy and the dose were not presented (Menter 2000).

There is no experience with topical treatment with *alitretinoin* gel during pregnancy.

Recommendation. Systemic therapy with the retinoids, acitretin, etretinate, isotretinoin, alitretinoin and tretinoin, is absolutely contraindicated during pregnancy. For women of childbearing age, treatment is only permitted with sufficient contraceptive protection and after a pregnancy has been ruled out in accordance with the current contraceptive program, and only if other retinoid-free therapeutic approaches have not been effective. After using acitretin and etretinate, reliable contraception must be continued for 2 years after cessation of therapy and after isotretinoin use for 1 month. If the period of contraception was insufficient, especially if there was treatment in early pregnancy, severe damage of the embryonic development is possible. Each individual case of a clear deviation from these time periods must be assessed individually. External/topical use of retinoids should also be strictly avoided during pregnancy. In the case of a systemic or topical exposure, a risk-grounded termination of the pregnancy (Chapter 1.15) is not necessarily indicated, but individual consultation should take place. In any case, a detailed fetal ultrasound investigation must be offered. For the use of tretinoin in hematology/oncology see Chapter 2.13.

2.17.10   Ultraviolet light

Ultraviolet light therapy (UV light) produces an immunomodulatory effect on the skin and is widely used for the treatment of psoriasis, eczema and other conditions. UV light is important for vitamin D synthesis. A variety of reports have suggested that low levels of vitamin D in early pregnancy may be associated with adverse developmental effects. Whether ultraviolet light exposure decreases folic acid levels remains to be studied (Juzeniene 2010).

▶ **UV-B**

UV-B light has got a wave length of 290–320 nm; its effects are confined to the skin and it does not penetrate the uterus. Narrow band UV-B light with a wave length of 311 nm is less erythemogenic (sunburning potential) than broadband UV-B and since erythema is a risk factor for skin cancer, treatment with narrow band UV-B light should theoretically be less carcinogenic for the same therapeutic results.

▶ **UV-A and photochemotherapy**

UV-A1 with a wave length of 340–400 nm penetrates the skin more deeply than UV-B. UV-A1 radiation induces collagenase (matrix metalloproteinase-1) expression, T-cell apoptosis, and depletes Langerhans and mast cells in the dermis. UV-A1 exposure stimulates endothelial cells to undergo neovascularization. UV-A1 exerts significant therapeutic effects in atopic dermatitis and morphea; there is also evidence for its use in other skin diseases, including cutaneous T-cell lymphoma and mastocytosis.

Photochemotherapy (PUVA therapy) combines psoralens with UV-A light to treat, e.g. severe psoriasis and atopic dermatitis. The psoralen makes the skin more sensitive to UV light. PUVA therapy is given either orally or by external application of *methoxsalen (8-methoxypsoralen* followed by UV-A irradiation. A form of external use is the so-called bath-PUVA, through which the skin is sensitized with a psoralen-containing bath water. The psoralen is chemically activated by the UV light, binds more strongly to the DNA and damages the cells.

The European Network of Teratology Information Services (ENTIS) analyzed 41 pregnancies in which systemic PUVA therapy with 8-methoxypsoralen was administered (Garbis 1995). This study (Gunnarskog 1993) found no hint for embryotoxic effects.

> **Recommendation.** Sole UV-B and UV-A light treatment is considered safe in pregnancy. Although no fetotoxic effects have been documented to date, oral photochemotherapy with 8-methoxypsoralen and UV-A irradiation should be avoided during pregnancy because of possible mutagenic effects. External use like bath PUVA seems to be acceptable; however, data are limited.

2.17.11   Fumaric acid preparations

Fumaric acid is used in small amounts in the preparation of food, i.e. as an antioxidant. In the treatment of psoriasis, doses of several hundred mg are common. Among the side-effects are leucopenia and lymphopenia. Tolerance for the fetus has not been systematically studied, but the current unpublished experience of the authors on psoriasis treatment with fumaric acid *dimethyl fumarate + ethyl hydrogen fumarate* have given no indication of embryotoxic or teratogenic effects.

> **Recommendation.** Treatment with Fumaric acid cannot be recommended during pregnancy. However, if treatment was applied accidentally, this does not justify either a risk-grounded termination of the pregnancy nor invasive diagnostics (Chapter 1.15).

2.17.12   Biologicals

Anti-TNFα and anti-IL12/23 antibodies are licensed for the treatment of psoriasis (Bae 2012, Rustin 2012). Anti-CD 20 antibodies are used in the treatment of lymphoma and e.g. autoimmune bullous diseases (Hertl 2008); for their use in pregnancy, see Chapter 2.12.

2.17.13   Wart therapeutics

Twenty-nine pregnant women, two of them in the first trimester, were treated externally with the immune modulator or virustatic *imiquimod* for condylomata acuminata (genital warts) or other warts. All of them delivered healthy children (Ciavattini 2012, Audisio 2008, Einarson 2006, Maw 2004). However, these experiences are insufficient for a differentiated risk assessment.

Podophyllotoxin, a plant-based mitosis inhibitor for local treatment of condylomata acuminata (genital warts) is insufficiently studied during pregnancy. Systemic toxicity, as was observed earlier with the topically used raw product *podophyllin* (Chapter 2.22) is unknown after topical use of podophyllotoxin. There have been, as yet, no indications of teratogenicity.

The usual treatment options of laser therapy, cryotherapy, electrocautery or trichloroacetic acid have not been studied systematically during pregnancy but are not of concern on theoretical considerations (Robert 1994). The same applies to local treatment with green tea extract.

Between the twelfth and twenty-fourth weeks of pregnancy, condylomata acuminata frequently develop progressively and then often improve spontaneously from the twenty-fifth week onwards. Thus for minor complaints an invasive therapy can be postponed to the twenty-fifth week or later (Dunne 2011, Workowski 2010). However, in the last eight weeks of pregnancy methods that destroy the warts and harm the skin should be avoided over large areas so there is no damage to the skin before delivery.

For the treatment of verrucae vulgares (common warts) and other warts the cytostatics *fluorouracil* (Chapter 2.13) and bleomycin (Chapter 2.13), as well as interferon (Chapter 2.12) are used. These substances should not, as a rule, be used during pregnancy. There are safer, less questionable and better studied alternatives like salicylic acid or cryotherapy; furthermore, the therapy may also be postponed until after delivery. For keratolytics such as salicylic acid see Section 2.17.8.

> **Recommendation.** For condylomata acuminata, cryotherapy, trichloroacetic acid or electrocautery are the treatments of choice during pregnancy. Common warts can be treated with salicylic acid or cryotherapy. Also, they may regress spontaneously after pregnancy. All other substances cannot be recommended due to insufficient data during pregnancy.

2.17.14   Lithium

Lithium is not only used for oral therapy of bipolar disorders (Chapter 2.11) but also for topical treatment of seborrhoeic dermatitis. Percutaneous absorption is limited and plasma concentrations are substantially lower than after oral treatment (Sparsa 2004).

> **Recommendation.** External treatment with lithium is not advisable due to insufficient data during pregnancy, but nevertheless does not require any action after exposure.

2.17.15   Lice medications

With lice infestation (pediculosis), topical treatment with various mechanisms of action are used. There are two main choices: (1) the use of chemicals (i.e. *pediculicides*) that kill lice; and (2) the use of physical methods that remove lice and their eggs by repeated combing.

The primary representative of the latter group is *dimeticon*. Dimeticon is a silicone that acts as a physical agent to kill the head lice (Meda Pharma 2012). There is, in fact, a lack of systematic studies on use during pregnancy but teratogenic effects would not be expected due to the nature of the substance and the lack of absorption.

Among the plant-based pediculocides are preparations with coconut oil and other essential oils such as *neem oil*. This group has not been shown to be suspect during pregnancy. However, their tolerance and effectiveness are poorly documented.

Rinsing with *vinegar water* is said to loosen the adhesion of lice and nits to hair.

The chemical pediculocides are neurotoxic-acting insecticides. Available for this purpose are malathion and the natural extract of chrysanthemums, *pyrethrum*, as well as its synthetic derivates, *permethrin* and *allethrin* (*bioallethrin*), which are characterized particularly by longer half-lives. Some of the preparations contain *piperonyl butoxide* as an effectiveness enhancer. Due to increasing resistance and the risk of side-effects, these substances have lost significance over the past few years. *Lindane*, which also has a neurotoxic action is no longer on the market in many countries.

Malathion (organophosphorus insecticide) 0.5% lotion is used for the treatment of scabies, head lice and scrab lice. The risk of systemic effects associated with 1–2 applications is considered to be very low. No significant increase in risk of congenital defects was reported in a case-cohort study performed to examine pregnancy outcomes in 7,450 women potentially exposed to malathion during the 1981–1982 aerial spraying of large areas of the San Francisco Bay area (Thomas 1990). Similar results were reported in an earlier study on a cohort of 22,465 infants born to women who lived in areas where aerial malathion spraying had occurred during their first trimester of pregnancy (Grether 1987). No differences in birth weight, length, or head circumference were reported in 149 infants whose mothers had detectable urinary concentrations of malathion metabolites, and 233 infants whose mothers did not have detectable amounts of these metabolites in their urine (Eskenazi 2004).Neurodevelopmental outcome was not affected in a study of Mexican-American children of farm workers that evaluated maternal and child metabolites in urine and serum (Eskenazi 2007). Children were evaluated at 6, 12, and 24 months using the Bayley Scales of Infant Development and the Child Behavior Checklist. A case report from Holland described an amyoplasia congenita-like condition that was associated with maternal exposure to malathion during the eleventh and twelfth week of pregnancy (Lindhout 1987). Because malathion is an agent that acts on the neuromuscular system, the possibility of a causal association was considered. There is debate regarding the precise nature of the defect that was reported (Hall 1988), and conclusions about causation cannot be reached based on this case.

Permethrin is absorbed up to 2% percutaneously (Fölster-Holst 2000). Due to its long-term effect, it is considered more effective than *pyrethrum* for lice infestation, although there are no comparative studies available on the two substances. The prospective study of 113 pregnant women who used permethrin shampoo (31 in the first trimester) gave no indication of an embryotoxic risk (Kennedy 2005). Mytton (2007) also found nothing remarkable among 196 pregnant women treated with permethrin. A study on the environment and air pollution through permethrin and piperonyl butoxide, found a 3.9 point lower mental development index on the Bayley test among 3-year-old children exposed to higher concentrations of piperonyl butoxide (>4.34 ng/m^3) than among those children with lower exposures (Horton 2011). A hospital-based case-control study from Brazil reports an increased incidence of the development of acute leukemia in children <2 years of age after pesticide exposure during pregnancy (permethrin was one of the substances) (Ferreira 2013). However, these results are not relevant for the external, short contact medical use of permethrin (Mytton 2007).

> **Recommendation.** A very safe and effective treatment for lice is achieved by combing with dimeticon or, alternatively, coconut oil or vinegar water. For easier combing, conditioner (possibly containing tea tree oil) may be used. Malathion (lice resistance is reported) or pyrethrum extract and synthetic pyrethroids (permethrin topical 5% cream/scalp treatment) are the treatment of second choice. Pump sprays should be avoided because of the danger of higher systemic intake through the air.

2.17.16   Anti-scabies

Benzyl benzoate, crotamiton, malathion and *permethrin* (Section 2.17.13) are available for external treatment of scabies. External treatments with *lindane* are not recommended and have been removed from the market in many countries. Two studies from India found significantly higher concentrations of lindane in maternal and cord blood from pregnancies with intrauterine growth restriction in comparison to control pregnancies (Sharma 2012, Pathak 2011). *Ivermectin* – available for example in France – is used orally for scabies (Chapter 2.6).

Apart from irritation of the skin and mucosa, there has not been any indication of appreciable toxicity either in animal experiments or use in humans after external use of benzyl benzoate (Fölster-Holst 2000). In a study in Thailand, 444 pregnant women who had used a 25% benzyl benzoate preparation topically during their pregnancy, showed no increased risk for birth defects. However, treatment was mostly applied in the second and third trimesters (Mytton 2007).

Crotamiton is only absorbed percutaneously to a very limited degree. An accumulation of the substance has, up to now, not been documented. By comparison to other anti-scabies medications it is thought to be less effective (Fölster-Holst 2000). No teratogenic effects have been observed in animal experiments. While studies concerning use during pregnancy are lacking, a substantial risk with topical use is unlikely.

Permethrin is more effective in the treatment of scabies compared to Benzyl benzoate 25%, Crotamiton 10% or Malathion 0.5% lotion. Because in medical treatments the skin is only exposed twice for a short period of time teratogenic effects are not expected.

Recommendation. The treatment of choice for scabies is permethrin because of its better effect. Pump sprays should be avoided because of the danger of higher systemic intake through the air.

Malthion, benzyl benzoate and crotamiton may be used as reserve treatments.

2.17.17   Vein therapeutics

Aescin preparations (*horse chestnut extract*) for vein complaints during pregnancy have not, as yet, appeared to be a problem. However, systematic studies are lacking.

Sclerotherapy for varicosities as with *polidocanol* (*macrogol lauryl ether*) may also – if urgently needed – be used during pregnancy (Reich-Schupke 2012). However, as spontaneous improvement of varicose veins after delivery is possible, any treatment, other than prophylaxis, should be postponed.

2.17.18   Antihidrotica

Aluminum-containing deodorants consist of aluminum *chlorhydrate*. Aluminum constricts the pores through denaturing of the proteins in the skin cells and thereby minimizes the production of sweat, which can lead to toxic skin irritation. There are no hints for adverse effects during pregnancy, but this substance has not been systematically studied.

Methinamine is used in excessive transpiration. There are no systematic studies on its use during pregnancy. Systemic use is controversial (Chapter 4.4); however, with local application, absorption of larger amounts of the active ingredient are not expected. Systematic studies on intracutaneous application of preparations with *clostridium botulinum toxin* for hyperhydrosis during pregnancy are lacking; 25 case reports of botulinum toxin injections, for example painful cervical dystonia, have not shown any adverse effects on the unborn child (Aranda 2012; Chapter 2.16).

The anticholinergic substance, *methanthelinium bromide*, is approved for, among other things, systemic treatment of hyperhydrosis (Chapter 2.5), but is insufficiently investigated during pregnancy.

> **Recommendation.** Deodorants can be used during pregnancy. Aluminum-containing substances should, for theoretical safety considerations, not be used long-term. Methinamine may also be used on small areas during pregnancy with good indications. Clostridium botulinum toxin should not be used for hyperhydrosis or cosmetic indications during pregnancy. However, inadvertent exposure does not require action, especially if the mother had no appreciable side-effects.

2.17.19   Eflornithine, finasteride and minoxidil

Minoxidil is used orally as an antihypertensive. It has a vasodilatory effect and is used topically for androgenetic alopecia and other kinds of hair loss. The substance is lipophilic and its absorption rate is 2–3%. Thereby, serum concentrations are reached that are far below a therapeutic, antihypertensive concentration for adults.

With *eflornithine*, which is available for the treatment of hirsutism, less than 1% is absorbed and systemically available, according to information from the manufacturer. There is no experience available for use during pregnancy.

Finasteride inhibits the enzyme, 5-α-reductase, which converts testosterone into the active dihydrotestosterone. It is approved for hair loss in men and benign prostate hypertrophy. It is also occasionally taken by women for both hair loss and hirsutism. Its effectiveness is controversial. In animal experiments, it disturbs the development of male rat fetuses. Among other things, hypospadia occurs more often, and the distance from the anus to the genitals is reduced as an expression of the anti-androgenic effect. In humans, its use at the end of the first trimester could lead to hypospadia. Up to now, however, there are no available studies in humans. There is merely a case report on a malformation of the extremities on the right hand and left foot of a child whose mother took finasteride because of hair loss (Sallout and Al Wadi 2009). However, this observation does not justify any causal connection.

In a prospective study, 17 pregnant women were treated with a minoxidil solution. One of the live-born children had a heart malformation (Shapiro 2003). In one woman who had applied minoxidil topically to her scalp at least twice a day, brain, heart and vascular malformations were diagnosed in her fetus. Pathology showed a significantly enlarged heart with distal stenosis of the aorta, a considerably longer colon sigmoideum, a ventricular broadening of the brain, and cerebral hemorrhages as well as an ischemic area in the placenta (Smorlesi 2003). In a further publication, a significant caudal regression syndrome in the fetus with aplasia of the lower spine, malformation of the lower extremities and of the urinary tract system, complete kidney agenesia and esophageal atresia were reported after topical 2% minoxidil treatment over many years (Rojansky 2002).

Multiple case reports also describe hypertrichosis in newborns of mothers after systemic minoxidil treatment.

> **Recommendation.** Finasteride and minoxidil is contraindicated during pregnancy. There is insufficient experience available for the topical use of minoxidil during pregnancy; however, long-term external use during pregnancy should be avoided. The same applies for eflornithine. An accidental intake of finasteride or minoxidil does not justify either a risk-grounded interruption of pregnancy nor invasive diagnostics (Chapter 1.15). However, a detailed ultrasound examination should be offered after intake during the first trimester.

2.17.20　Repellents

Mosquito-repelling substances (repellents), such as *diethyltoluamide* or *icaridin* are rubbed into or sprayed on the skin. Percutaneously about 8% to a maximum of 17% of DEET can be absorbed (Sudakin 2003). A mother in Africa who gave birth to a mentally retarded child had not only been using malarial prophylaxis (chloroquine) but had also been rubbing her arms and legs daily with a 25% DEET lotion (Schaefer 1992). Since DEET has neurotoxic properties and is absorbed through the skin, the authors cannot entirely eliminate a causal connection. However, there are no further reports of developmental toxic effects in humans.

A randomized prospective double-blind study found no differences in the development of the newborns of 449 women, who had used an average of 1.7 g of DEET daily in the second and third trimesters compared to the control group. In 8% of the treated women, DEET was detectable in the cord blood. However, no differences were found in the development of the children up to the first year of life. This was confirmed by a second study (Wickerham 2012, McGready 2001). There are merely three individual case observations with children who were born healthy (author's own data). *Icaridin* has a lower toxic potential than DEET. However, systematic studies in pregnancy are not available. A cohort study evaluated *chlorpyrifos, diazinon, carbofuran, chlorothalonil, dacthal, metolachlor, trifluralin* and *diethyl-m-toluamide* (DEET) in cord blood. A high ($\geq$ 75th percentile) metolachlor concentration in cord blood was found, this correlated with low birth weight (3605 g in upper quartile versus 3399 g; $p=0.05$). Furthermore, an increase in abdominal circumference with increasing cord dichloran concentrations ($p = 0.031$) was observed. These observations suggest that *in utero* exposure to certain pesticides may alter birth outcomes (Barr 2010).

> **Recommendation.** Pregnant women should be advised against the use of insect repellents of the DEET type over large areas of their bodies for a long period during the pregnancy. In areas with a high risk of malaria, which should only be visited during pregnancy when there are compelling grounds to do so, DEET should be used, because potential harms from DEET exposure for both mother and child are still lower than the potential harm due to a malarial infection. Pyrethroid-containing repellents should be avoided. Wherever possible, other repellents, including icaridin, should be preferred.

2.17.21　Cosmetics

Cosmetics, also hair cosmetics, including dyes and permanent waves, may be used in the usual quantities if they contribute to the well-being of the pregnant woman provided the hair products do not contain lead.

2.17.22   Eye, nose and ear drops

Eye, nose and ear drops may generally also be used during pregnancy. However, medication should be chosen carefully and questionable combination preparations as well as (pseudo) innovations should be avoided during pregnancy. Where there is some doubt, the recommendations on systemic therapy in the appropriate chapters can serve as orientation.

▶ **Ophthalmic medications**

With eye drops, in particular, quantitative absorption of the medication via the conjunctiva should be assumed. For this reason, the possibility cannot be ruled out that, for example, atropine-like substances and β-receptor blockers (Chapter 2.8), could increase or decrease the fetal heart frequency. Threatening situations are not expected with the usual doses of mydriatics for diagnosing long-sightedness or for glaucoma treatment.

Among the β-receptor blockers available as eye drops are *levobunolol* and *metipranolol*. While the carbonic anhydrase inhibitors, *brinzolamide*, *dorzolamide* and, for systemic use, *acetazolamide* have not been systematically studied, no negative effects on fetuses have been shown with the preparations that have been in use for a long time.

Maternal therapy with 750 mg/day acetazolamide during the last 3 days before delivery led to tachypnea and a combined respiratory-metabolic acidosis, hypoglycemia and hypokalemia in the child born in the thirty-fourth week of pregnancy. Serum concentrations in the child 5 hours after delivery were 2.9 μg/mL – almost a therapeutic concentration for adults (3–10 μg/mL). After normalization of the pH value, the clinical symptoms improved spontaneously. On the 11th day of life acetazolamide was no longer detectable. The further development of the child was uneventful (Ozawa 2001).

There were no birth defects or postnatal disorders observed in the newborns of 12 women treated for idiopathic increased intracranial pressure with an average of 500 mg acetazolamide daily. Nine of them were treated in the first trimester (Lee 2005).

With *latanoprost* 10 prospectively documented treatments were reported, nine of them in the first trimester. One pregnancy ended with a spontaneous abortion. The nine full-term babies had no birth defects (de Santis 2004b). Another publication described two cases of latanoprost treatment, both in the first trimester or, in one case, throughout the pregnancy. Both newborns were healthy. One of the patients was treated with *brimonidine* as well (see also below) and in both cases treatment was combined with *timolol* (Johnson 2001).

Also with bimatoprost, our own observations do not indicate embryotoxicity. There is no experience with *travoprost* during pregnancy.

According to a case report, a healthy baby was born after maternal treatment with *pilocarpin* during the entire pregnancy (Johnson 2001). While cholinergics such as pilocarpin, clonidine preparations or sympathomimetics such as brimonidine or *dipivefrin* have not been systematically studied, neither have yet been associated with congenital anomalies.

In a small study, six children of six pregnant patients with glaucoma were observed up to the age of 2 years; comparing them with a control group, no psycho-physical developmental anomalies were determined (Razeghinejad and Nowroozzadeh 2010).

Scopolamine, cyclopentolate and tropicamide are offered as mydriatics. And even though systematic studies are lacking, decades of experience and the available case studies do not indicate an appreciable risk of these anticholinergic substances for the embryo/fetus (Chapter 2.5).

Intravenous verteporfin is used for choroidal neovascularization. Three case reports with exposure in the first trimester did not reveal any anomalies in the children (Rodrigues 2009, Rosen 2009, de Santis 2004a). In animal experiments, congenital malformations of the eyes were found in rats after very high systemically administered doses.

Pegaptanib is injected intravitreally for moist macular degeneration. There is no experience on its use during pregnancy.

See Chapter 2.12 for the other biologics or monoclonal antibodies in ophthalmology.

> **Recommendation.** Generally speaking, there is no objection to glaucoma therapy during pregnancy. Since prostaglandins increase uterine tone and can cause reduced perfusion to the fetus, they should be seen as reserve medications. Should severe glaucoma require topical treatment with prostaglandin derivatives, the lowest possible dose should be selected. Theoretically, the other therapeutics used topically on the eye are also not regarded as problematic. This probably also applies to pegaptanib. In general, of course, proven medications should be given preference. Mydriatics may be used. After unavoidable treatment with verteporfin or treatment already administered during pregnancy, a detailed ultrasound investigation is advisable. Neither a risk-grounded interruption of pregnancy nor invasive diagnostics are justified.

▶ Nasal decongestants

There are no systematic studies on the embryotoxicity of nasal decongestant drops or sprays. The frequently used preparations containing *xylometazoline* or *oxymetazoline* have not, as yet, been shown to be a risk for the fetus. Although theoretically (with high doses) vasoconstriction could lead to reduced circulation to the fetus, this side-effect is no reason for concern with the usual doses. Many women (including pregnant women) take nasal decongestant preparations for many months instead of the recommended period of a few days. In order to avoid damage to the nasal mucosa, "withdrawal strategies" should be offered.

There is insufficient experience on *indanazoline, naphazoline, tetryzoline* and *tramazoline* during pregnancy.

▶ Other eye, nose and ear preparations

Glucocorticoids, cromoglicic acid, antihistamines, antibiotics and acyclovir as filming agents ("artificial tears") such as, for example, *povidone*, may be used by pregnant women for appropriate indications. *Chloramphenicol* should, on principle, be avoided.

Nasal or inhalative use of *budesonide* and other corticosteroids has not been associated with any appreciable teratogenicity (Källén and Olausson 2003).

Among 26 women who used *fluticasone* nasal spray in a randomized double blind study, no difference was found in the development of the newborns compared to the placebo group (Ellegard 2001).

There are no systematic studies available on the use of other cortico-steroid sprays, such as *flunisolide* or *fluorometholone, loteprednol* and *rimexolone*, containing eye drops during pregnancy. Perhaps they should be evaluated similarly to other topical gluocorticosteroids and regarded as acceptable for short-term use if no other therapeutic possibilities are available. See Chapter 2.15 for the glucocorticoids.

2.17.23   Hemorrhoid medications

Hemorrhoid medications (salves and suppositories) are topical thera-peutics which mostly contain local anesthetics, glucocorticoids, antibiot-ics and disinfectants, either as individual substances or in combination. These preparations are also used following surgical procedures in the rectal–anal area and frequently prescribed to pregnant women with hem-orrhoids. While such preparations have not been systematically studied, neither have they yet been associated with congenital anomalies.

> **Recommendation.** The usual medications for hemorrhoids may be used during pregnancy.

2.17.24   Vaginal therapeutics

Treatment of bacterial vaginosis may prevent premature births. In high risk pregnancies, systemic antibiotic treatment apparently has a protec-tive effect on the premature birth/miscarriage rate. An ascendant infec-tion cannot be adequately treated with local vaginal treatment. Systemic (oral) anti-infective therapy poses no toxic risk for the child's develop-ment if medications recommended for use during pregnancy are admin-istered (Chapter 2.6).

Povidone iodine as vaginal suppositories and iodine rinsing of the vagina should be avoided (Section 2.17.2.). Treatment with other vagi-nal therapeutics, which contain disinfectants, e.g. *dequalinium chloride, hexetidine, policresulenum* or with estrogens have not, as yet, been sus-pected of having a teratogenic potential. In an effort to find a rational therapy for vaginosis, one should, however, avoid old medications that are controversial with respect to their effectiveness. This also applies to nitrofurans such as *furazolidone* and *nifuratel* (Mendling and Mailland 2002) as well as the antimycotic, *chlorphenesin*, which should be viewed critically even though the risk of a teratogenic potential seems low.

References

Adams J. The neurobehavioral teratology of retinoids: a 50-year history. Birth Defects Res A Clin Mol Teratol 2010; 88: 895–905.
Akhavan A, Bershad S. Topical acne drugs. Am J Clin Dermatol 2003; 4: 473–92.
Aranda MA, Herranz A, del Val J et al. Botulinum toxin A during pregnancy, still a debate. Eur J Neurol 2012; 19: e81–2.
Audisio T, Roca FC, Piatti C. Topical imiquimod therapy for external anogenital warts in pregnant women. Int J Gynaecol Obstet 2008; 100: 275–6.

Autret E, Berjot M, Jonvile-Bera AP et al. Anophthalmia and agenesis of optic chiasma associated with adapalene gel in early pregnancy. Lancet 1997; 350: 339.

Autret-Leca E, Kreft-Jais C, Elefant E et al. Isotretinoin exposure during pregnancy: assessment of spontaneous reports in France. Drug Saf 2010; 33: 659–65.

Bae YS, Van Voorhees AS, Hsu S et al. National Psoriasis Foundation. Review of treatment options for psoriasis in pregnant or lactating women: from the Medical Board of the National Psoriasis Foundation. J Am Acad Dermatol 2012; 67: 459–77.

Baltzar B, Ericson A, Källén B et al. Delivery outcome in women employed in medical occupations in Sweden. J Occup Med 1979; 21: 543–8.

Barbero P, Lotersztein V, Bronberg R et al. Acitretin embryopathy: a case report. Birth Defects Res A Clin Mol Teratol 2004; 70: 831–3.

Barr DB, Ananth CV, Yan X et al. Pesticide concentrations in maternal and umbilical cord sera and their relation to birth outcomes in a population of pregnant women and newborns in New Jersey. Sci Total Environ 2010; 408: 790–5.

Bérard A, Azoulay L, Koren G et al. Isotretinoin, pregnancies, abortions and birth defects: a population-based perspective. Br J Clin Pharmacol 2007; 63: 196–205.

Boutin A, Demers S, Roberge S et al. Treatment of periodontal disease and prevention of preterm birth: Systematic review and meta-analysis. Am J Perinatol 2013; 30: 537–44.

Brennan M, Young G, Devane D. Topical preparations for preventing stretch marks in pregnancy. Cochrane Database Syst Rev 2012; 11: CD000066.

Camera G, Pregliasco P. Ear malformation in baby born to mother using tretinoin cream (letter). Lancet 1992; 339: 687.

Carlier P, Choulika S, Dally S. Topical retinoids exposure in pregnancy. Cooperative study from January 1992 to April 1997: 132 cases and 94 with known pregnancy outcome. Thérapie 1998; 53: 180.

Chi CC, Lee CW, Wojnarowska F et al. Safety of topical corticosteroids in pregnancy. Cochrane Database Syst Rev 2009; 3: CD007346.

Ciavattini A, Tsiroglou D, Vichi M et al. Topical Imiquimod 5% cream therapy for external anogenital warts in pregnant women: report of four cases and review of the literature. J Matern Fetal Neonatal Med 2012; 25: 873–6.

Colley S, Walepole I, Fabian VA et al. Topical tretinoin and fetal malformations. Med J Aust 1998; 168: 467.

Crijns HJ, Straus SM, Gispen-de Wied, C et al. Compliance with pregnancy prevention programmes of isotretinoin in Europe: a systematic review. Br J Dermatol 2011; 164: 238–44.

Czeizel AE, Kazy Z, Vargha P. Vaginal treatment with povidone-iodine suppositories during pregnancy. Int J Gynaecol Obstet 2004; 84: 83–5.

De Die-Smulders CE, Sturkenboom MC, Veraart J et al. Severe limb defects and craniofacial abnormalities in fetus conceived during acitretine therapy. Teratology 1995; 52: 215–9.

de Santis M, Carducci B, de Santis L et al. First case of post-conception verteporfin exposure: Pregnancy and neonatal outcome. Acta Ophthalmol Scand 2004a; 82: 623–4.

de Santis M, Lucchese A, Carducci B et al. Latanoprost exposure in pregnancy. Am J Ophthalmol 2004b; 138: 305–6.

Duran B, Gursoy S, Cetin M et al. The oral toxicity of resorcinol during pregnancy: a case report. J Toxicol Clin Toxicol 2004; 42: 663–6.

Dunne EF, Friedman A, Datta SD et al. Updates on human papillomavirus and genital warts and counseling messages from the 2010 Sexually Transmitted Diseases Treatment Guidelines. Clin Infect Dis 2011 Dec; 53: S143–52.

Einarson A, Costei A, Kalra S et al. The use of topical 5% imiquimod during pregnancy: A case series. Reprod Toxicol 2006; 21: 1–2.

Ellegard EK, Hellgren M, Karlsson NG. Fluticasone propionate aqueous nasal spray in pregnancy rhinitis. Clin Otolaryngol 2001; 26: 394–400.

Eskenazi B, Harley K, Bradman A et al. Association of in utero organophosphate pesticide exposure and fetal growth and length of gestation in an agricultural population. Environ Health Perspect 2004; 112: 1116–24.

Eskenazi B, Marks AR, Bradman A et al. Organophosphate pesticide exposure and neurodevelopment in young Mexican-American children. Environ Health Perspect 2007; 115: 792–8.

Ferreira JD, Couto AC, Pombo-de-Oliveira MS et al. In utero pesticide exposure and leukemia in Brazilian children <2 years of age. Environ Health Perspect 2013; 121: 269–75.

Fölster-Holst R, Rufli T, Christophers E. Die Skabiestherapie unter besonderer Berücksichtigung des frühen Kindesalters, der Schwangerschaft und Stillzeit. Hautarzt 2000; 51: 7–13.

Franssen ME, van der Wilt GJ, de Jong PC et al. A retrospective study of the teratogenicity of dermatological coal tar products [letter]. Acta Derm Venereol 1999; 79: 390–1.

Garbis H, Elefant E, Bertolotti E et al. Pregnancy outcome after periconceptional and first-trimester exposure to methoxsalen photochemotherapy. Arch Dermatol 1995; 131: 492–3.

Garnock-Jones KP, Perry CM. Alitretinoin: in severe chronic hand eczema. Drugs 2009; 69: 1625–34.

Geiger JM, Baudin M, Saurat JH. Teratogenic risk with etretinate and acitretine treatment. Dermatology 1994; 189: 109–16.

Geiger JM, Walker M. Is there a reproductive safety risk in male patients treated with acitretine (neotigason®/soriatane®)? Dermatology 2002; 205: 105–7.

Grether JK, Harris JA, Neutra R et al. Exposure to aerial malathion application and the occurrence of congenital anomalies and low birthweight. Am J Public Health 1987; 77: 1009–10.

Gunnarskog JG, Källén BAJ, Lindelof BG et al. Psoralen photochemotherapy (PUVA) and pregnancy. Arch Dermatol 1993; 129: 320–3.

Hadiati DR, Hakimi M, Nurdiati DS. Skin preparation for preventing infection following caesarean section. Cochrane Database Syst Rev 2012; 9: CD007462.

Han JY, Choi JS, Chun JM et al. Pregnancy outcome of women transfused during pregnancy with blood products inadvertently obtained from donors treated with acitretin. J Obstet Gynaecol 2009; 29: 694–7.

Hebert MF, Zheng S, Hays K et al. Interpreting tacrolimus concentrations during pregnancy and postpartum. Transplantation 2013; 95: 908–15.

Hertl M, Zillikens D, Borradori L et al. Recommendations for the use of rituximab (anti-CD20 antibody) in the treatment of autoimmune bullous skin diseases. J Dtsch Dermatol Ges 2008; 6: 366–73.

Hall JG. Comments on "Amyoplasia congenita-like condition and maternal malathion exposure: Is all amyoplasia amyoplasia?" (letter). Teratology 1988; 38: 493–5.

Honein MA, Paulozzi LJ, Erickson JD. Continued occurrence of accutane® exposed pregnancies. Teratology 2001; 64: 142–7.

Horton MK, Rundle A, Camann DE et al. Impact of prenatal exposure to piperonyl butoxide and permethrin on 36-month neurodevelopment. Pediatrics 2011; 127: e699–706.

Jick SS, Terris BZ, Jick H. First trimester topical tretinoin. Lancet 1993; 341: 1181–2.

Johnson SM, Martinez M, Freedman S. Management of glaucoma in pregnancy and lactation. Survey Ophthalmol 2001; 45: 449–54.

Juzeniene A, Stokke KT, Thune P et al. Pilot study of folate status in healthy volunteers and in patients with psoriasis before and after UV exposure. J Photochem Photobiol B 2010; 101: 111–6.

Källén BAJ, Otterblad Olaussen P. Maternal drug use in early pregnancy and infant cardiovascular defect. Reproduct Toxicol 2003; 17: 255–61.

Kennedy D, Hurst V, Konradsdottir E et al. Pregnancy outcome following exposure to permethrin and use of teratogen information. Am J Perinat 2005; 22: 87–90.

Lammer EJ, Chen DT, Hoar RM et al. Retinoic acid embryopathy. N Engl J Med 1985; 313: 837–41.

Lammer EJ, Hayes AM, Schunior A et al. Unusually high risk for adverse outcomes of pregnancy following fetal isotretinoin exposure. Am J Hum Genet 1988; 43: A58.

Larsen FG, Steinkjer B, Jakobsen P et al. Acitretin is converted to etretinate only during concomitant alcohol intake. Br J Dermatol 2000; 143: 1164–9.

Lauwerys R, Bonnier C, Eurard P et al. Prenatal and early postnatal intoxication by inorganic mercury resulting from maternal use of mercury containing soap. Human Toxicol 1987; 6: 253–6.

Leachman SA, Reed BR. The use of dermatologic drugs in pregnancy and lactation. Dermatol Clin 2006; 24: 167–97.

Lee AG, Pless M, Falardeau J et al. The use of acetazolamide in idiopathic intracranial hypertension during pregnancy. Am J Ophthalm 2005; 139: 855–9.

Lindhout D, Hageman G. Amyoplasia congenita-like condition and maternal malathion exposure. Teratology 1987; 36: 7–10.

Lipson AH, Collins F, Webster WS. Multiple congenital defects associated with maternal use of topical tretinoin. Lancet 1993; 341: 1352–3.

Loureiro KD, Kao KK, Jones KL et al. Minor malformations characteristic of the retinoic acid embryopathy and other birth outcomes in children of women exposed to topical tretinoin during early pregnancy. Am J Med Gen 2005; 136A: 117–21.

Martinez-Frias ML, Rodriguez-Pinilla E. First-trimester exposure to topical tretinoin: its safety is not warranted (letter). Teratology 1999; 60: 5.

Maw RD. Treatment of external genital warts with 5% imiquiod cream during pregnancy: a case report. BJOG 2004; 111: 1475.

McGready R, Hamilton KA, Simpson JA et al. Safety of the insect repellent N,N-diethyl-m-toluamide (DEET) in pregnancy. Am J Trop Med 2001; 65: 285–9.

Meda Pharma. 2012. http://www.youtube.com/watch?v=XQlscXS0iaE

Mendling W, Mailland F. Microbiological and pharmaco-toxicological profile of nifuratel and its favourable risk/benefit ratio for the treatment of vulvo-vaginal infections. A review. Arzneimittelforschung 2002; 52: 8–13.

Menter A. Pharmacokinetics and safety of tazaroten. J Am Acad Dermatol 2000; 43: 31–5.

Moerike S, Pantzar JT, de Sa D. Temporal bone pathology in fetuses exposed to isotretinoin. Pediatr Dev Pathol 2002; 5: 405–9.

Mygind H, Thulstrup AM, Pedersen L et al. Risk of intrauterine growth retardation, malformations and other bad outcomes in children after topical use of corticosteroid in pregnancy. Acta Obstet Gynaecol Scand 2002; 81: 234–9.

Mytton OT, McGready R, Lee SJ. Safety of benzyl benzoate lotion and permethrin in pregnancy: a retrospective matched cohort study. BJOG 2007; 114: 582–7.

Navarre-Belhassen C, Blancehet P, Hillaire-Buys D et al. Multiple congenital malformations associated with topical tretinoin. Ann Pharmacother 1998; 32: 505–6.

Nulman I, Berkovitch M, Klein J et al. Steady-state pharmacokinetics of isotretinoin and its 4-oxo metabolite: implications for fetal safety. J Clin Pharmacol 1998; 38: 926–30.

Ozawa H, Azuma E, Shindo K et al. Transient renal tubular acidosis in a neonate following transplacental acetazolamide. Eur J Pediatr 2001; 160: 321–2.

Pathak R, Mustafa MD, Ahmed T et al. Intra uterine growth retardation: association with organochlorine pesticide residue levels and oxidative stress markers. Reprod Toxicol 2011; 31: 534–9.

Rademaker M. Adverse effects of isotretinoin: A retrospective review of 1,743 patients started on isotretinoin. Australas J Dermatol 2010; 51: 248–53.

Razeghinejad MR, Nowroozzadeh MH. Anti-glaucoma medication exposure in pregnancy: an observational study and literature review. Clin Exp Optom 2010; 93: 458–65.

Reich-Schupke S, Leiste A, Moritz R et al. Sclerotherapy in an undetected pregnancy – a catastrophe? Vasa 2012; 41: 243–7.

Robert E, Scialli AR. Topical medications during pregnancy. Reprod Toxicol 1994; 8: 197–202.

Rodrigues M, Meira D, Batista S et al. Accidental pregnancy exposure to verteporfin: obstetrical and neonatal outcomes: a case report. Aust N Z J Obstet Gynaecol 2009; 49: 236–7.

Roeleveld N, Zielhuis GA, Gabreels F. Mental retardation and parental occupation: A study on the applicability of job exposure matrices. Br J Ind Med 1993; 50: 945–54.

Roelofzen JH, Aben KK, Oldenhof UT et al. No increased risk of cancer after coal tar treatment in patients with psoriasis or eczema. J Invest Dermatol 2010; 130: 953–61.

Rojansky N, Fasouliotis SJ, Ariel I et al. Extreme caudal agenesis. J Reproduct Med 2002; 47: 241–5.

Rosen E, Rubowitz A, Ferencz JR. Exposure to verteporfin and bevacizumab therapy for choroidal neovascularization secondary to punctate inner choroidopathy during pregnancy. Eye (Lond) 2009; 23: 1479.

Rustin MH. Long-term safety of biologics in the treatment of moderate-to-severe plaque psoriasis: review of current data. Br J Dermatol 2012; 167: 3–11.

Ruzicka T, Lynde CW, Jemec GB et al. Efficacy and safety of oral alitretinoin (9-cis retinoic acid) in patients with severe chronic hand eczema refractory to topical corticosteroids: results of a randomized, double-blind, placebo-controlled, multicentre trial. Br J Dermatol 2008; 158: 808–17.

Saleem S, Rouse DJ, McClure EM et al. Chlorhexidine vaginal and infant wipes to reduce perinatal mortality and morbidity: a randomized controlled trial. Obstet Gynecol 2010; 115: 1225–32.

Sallout BI, Al Wadi KA. Aphalangia possibly linked to unintended use of finasteride during early pregnancy. Ann Saudi Med 2009; 29: 155–6.

Schaefer C, Meister R, Weber-Schoendorfer C. Isotretinoin exposure and pregnancy outcome: an observational study of the Berlin Institute for Clinical Teratology and Drug Risk Assessment in Pregnancy. Arch Gynecol Obstet 2010; 281: 221–7.

Schaefer C, Peters PWJ. Intrauterine diethyltoluamide exposure and fetal outcome. Reprod Toxicol 1992; 6: 175–6.

Selcen D, Seidman S, Nigro MA. Otocerebral anomalies associated with topical tretinoin use. Brain Dev 2000; 22: 218–20.

Shapiro J. Safety of topical minoxidil solution: a one-year, prospective, observational study. J Cutan Med Surg 2003; 7: 322–9.

Shapiro L, Pastuszak A, Cutro G et al. Safety of first-trimester exposure to topical tretinoin: prospective cohort study. Lancet 1997; 350: 1143–4.

Sharma E, Mustafa M, Pathak R et al. A case control study of gene environmental interaction in fetal growth restriction with special reference to organochlorine pesticides. Eur J Obstet Gynecol Reprod Biol 2012; 161: 163–9.

Smorlesi C, Caldarella A, Caramelli L et al. Topically applied minoxidil may cause fetal malformation: a case report. Birth Defects Res A 2003; 67: 997–1001.

Sparsa A, Bonnetblanc JM. Lithium. Ann Dermatol Venereol 2004; 131: 255–61.

Sudakin DL, Trevathan WR. DEET: a review and update of safety and risk in the general population. J Toxicol Clin Toxicol 2003; 41: 831–9.

Tahirović H, Toromanović A, Grbić S et al. Maternal and neonatal urinary iodine excretion and neonatal TSH in relation to use of antiseptic during cesarean section in an iodine sufficient area. J Pediatric Endocrinol Metab 2009; 22: 1145–9.

Teichert M, Visser LE, Dufour M et al. Isotretinoin use and compliance with the Dutch Pregnancy Prevention Programme: a retrospective cohort study in females of reproductive age using pharmacy dispensing data. Drug Saf 2010; 33: 315–26.

Teratology Society: Recommendations for isotretinoin use in women of child-bearing potential. Teratology 1991; 44: 1–6.

Thomas D, Goldhaber M, Petitti D et al. Reproductive outcome in women exposed to malathion. Am J Epidemiol 1990; 132: 794–5.

van Hoogdalem EJ. Transdermal absorption of topical anti-acne agents in man; review of clinical pharmacokinetic data. J Europ Acad Dermatol Venereol 1998; 11: 13–9; 28–9.

Velasco I, Naranjo S, López-Pedrera C et al. Use of povidone-iodine during the first trimester of pregnancy: a correct practice? BJOG 2009; 116: 452–5.

Weber G, Vigone MC, Rapa A et al. Neonatal transient hypothyroidism: aetiological study. Italian collaborative study on transient hypothyroidism. Arch Dis Childhood Fet Neonat Ed 1998; 79: 70–2.

Wickerham EL, Lozoff B, Shao J et al. Reduced birth weight in relation to pesticide mixtures detected in cord blood of full-term infants. Environ Int 2012; 47: 80–5.

Workowski KA, Berman S. Centers for Disease Control and Prevention (CDC). Sexually transmitted diseases treatment guidelines, 2010. MMWR Recomm Rep 2010; 59: 1–110.

Vitamins, minerals and trace elements

2.18

Richard K. Miller and Paul Peters

2.18.1	Vitamin A (retinol)	494
2.18.2	Vitamin B_1 (thiamine)	496
2.18.3	Vitamin B_2 (riboflavin)	496
2.18.4	Vitamin B_3 (nicotinamide)	497
2.18.5	Vitamin B_6 (pyridoxine)	497
2.18.6	Vitamin B_{12} (cyanocobalamin)	497
2.18.7	Vitamin C (ascorbic acid)	498
2.18.8	Folic acid	498
2.18.9	Vitamin D group	501
2.18.10	Vitamin E (tocopherol)	502
2.18.11	Vitamin K	503
2.18.12	Multivitamin preparations	503
2.18.13	Iron	503
2.18.14	Calcium	504
2.18.15	Fluoride	505
2.18.16	Strontium	506
2.18.17	Biphosphonates and other osteoporosis drugs	506
2.18.18	Iodide	507
2.18.19	Trace elements	507

Vitamins and minerals are organic foods found only in plants and animals, and are essential to the normal functioning of the body. However, the actual definition of the term "essential" is not applied to all vitamins. Vitamin imbalances can be divided into three categories:

1. Hypovitaminosis – shortage of one or more vitamins.
2. Avitaminosis – depletion of one or more vitamins.
3. Hypervitaminosis – excess of selected vitamins by overdose, and hence intoxication.

Altered maternal metabolism, growth of the conceptus and additional storage of some vitamins in the yolk sac and placenta, in particular vitamins A, B_1, B_2, B_3, B_6, B_{12}, C, folic acid and minerals (calcium and iron), increase vitamin and mineral requirements during pregnancy.

Drugs During Pregnancy and Lactation. **http://dx.doi.org/10.1016/B978-0-12-408078-2.00019-6**

A varied and balanced composition of the daily diet is the preferred basis for supplying vitamins and minerals. Folic acid may be the only vitamin identified to date that must be supplemented before and during pregnancy to prevent birth defects. However, questions have arisen with regard to additional supplementation of Vitamins A and D where an absence in the diet or lack of exposure to sunshine before and during pregnancy may occur. Researchers have demonstrated in countries with low dietary intake of vitamin A that supplementation with retinyl esters is critical for continued pregnancy and normal development (Emmett 2014, Murguia-Peniche 2013). Alternate sources of vitamin A are being developed as food sources, e.g. "golden" rice (www.goldenrice.org; Tang 2012). There is always a concern that hypervitaminosis may produce toxicity for the newborn based upon animal studies; however, the dosages for producing such birth defects are usually extraordinarily high compared with the RDA.

In many countries, multivitamins/mineral tablets are used prior to, and during pregnancy, in order to provide coverage for any deficiencies in diet. It is commonly recommended that a daily prenatal vitamin tablet be taken and is recommended by the health care provider (HCP); as mentioned earlier the need for the multivitamin is often related to the need for prenatal folic acid supplementation (see Section 2.18.7). These recommendations may be especially important for the vegan and vegetarian who may not receive sufficient vitamins in their diets as well as appropriate amounts of iron.

A special note is added concerning gastric bypass surgery and pregnancy. Little information is specifically available for pregnant women; however, Saltzman (2013) reviewed the population and stated: "The most common clinically relevant micronutrient deficiencies after gastric bypass include thiamine, vitamin B_{12}, vitamin D, iron, and copper. Reports of deficiencies of many other nutrients, some with severe clinical manifestations, are relatively sporadic. Diet and multivitamin use are unlikely to consistently prevent deficiency, thus supplementation with additional specific nutrients is often needed. Though optimal supplement regimens are not yet defined, most micronutrient deficiencies after gastric bypass currently can be prevented or treated by appropriate supplementation." This chapter will not directly address pregnant women following gastric bypass surgery; however, the reader will hopefully incorporate the above advise in the care of these women who may be planning a pregnancy or already pregnant.

Also, the use of dietary supplements for preventing postnatal depression does not appear to be effective based upon a recent Cochrane Report assessment (Miller 2013). In contrast, in another National Birth Defects Prevention Study (Carmichael 2013), results implied an association of nutrient intake with preterm deliveries.

2.18.1   Vitamin A (retinol)

Pharmacology

Vitamin A is a fat-soluble vitamin that occurs in two forms in nature. It (*retinol/retinal*) is found in food derived from animals, such as fish oils and liver. The body readily converts these forms to retinoids. Vitamin A values are expressed in different ways.

The nutrient was originally measured in IU (international units). In 1974, the United States began using a measurement called Retinol Equivalents (REs), where 1 RE = 1 μg of retinol, or 6 μg of β-carotene, or 3.333 IU of vitamin A. The recommended daily allowance for pregnant women is 700 RE.

Vitamin A can also be found in vegetables in the form of β-carotene or provitamin A. This form is found in plants, and is the precursor of the actual vitamin (retinol/retinal). Vitamin A is the basic substance needed for rhodopsin (visual purple). In addition, epithelial cells need vitamin A for growth and functional maintenance. Vitamin A, like vitamin C, accumulates in the embryo. The endogenous concentration of vitamin A metabolites in the serum is reduced in pregnant women during the first trimester, and amounts to between 0.26 and 7.7 μg/L. Even after 3 weeks of supplementation with 30,000 IU vitamin A per day, the peak values of the metabolites – retinoic acids (*tretinoin* and *isotretinoin*) are, at most, slightly above the concentrations measured previously (Wiegand 1998), or no different than noted in pregnant women who were not taking supplements (Miller 1998). During the second half of pregnancy, the endogenous concentration increases to about 150% of the level in nonpregnant women (Malone 1975).

Toxicology

The teratogenic action on humans of vitamin A derivatives, such as the retinoids (isotretinoin and *acitretin*), which are used as therapy for severe forms of acne and psoriasis, is discussed in Chapter 2.17. Retinoids are absolutely contraindicated during pregnancy.

About three decades ago, the possibility was first discussed that vitamin A preparations in doses over 25,000 IU daily might have a teratogenic action on humans similar to that of retinoids, and could cause characteristic "retinoid effects" (Rosa 1986). At the end of the 1980s, manufacturers of multivitamin preparations in many countries changed the composition of their products, following the opinions of the Teratology Society and at the insistence of regulatory authorities, so that a daily dose did not contain more than 6,000 IU (Teratology Society 1987). The safety of such doses has been confirmed repeatedly in many studies, among them the Dudas (1992) study on pregnant women in Hungary. Amazingly, a later study from the European Network of Teratology Information Services (ENTIS) gave no indication of a teratogenic effect, even with higher vitamin A doses (10,000–300,000, mean 50,000 IU per day), taken in the first trimester. In particular, the observations in another study that doses over 15,000 IU daily cause neural crest anomalies (Rothman 1995) has been discredited based upon subjects not having the neural crest anomalies (Miller 1998). The ENTIS study of 423 pregnant women is the largest vitamin A study to date (Mastroiacovo 1999). There was no increase in the rate of birth defects either among the 311 live-born children, or within the high-dose group of 120 children whose mothers took 50,000 IU daily. Nevertheless, looking at these case numbers statistically, they only allow for a relative risk above 2.8 to be ruled out.

A retrospective study discussed a higher risk for transposition of the great vessels with maternal vitamin A intake >10,000 IU daily during the 12 months prior to conception (Botto 2003). However, the number of affected children was low, and these results were not confirmed by other studies. Another retrospective study found no association between oral clefts and the (normal) vitamin A levels of women taking supplementation or consuming liver (Mitchell 2003).

There is a general warning against eating liver because a meal portion (100 g) may contain up to 400,000 IU; however, there is no clear indication yet of teratogenic effects from liver consumption. According to a pharmacokinetic study by Buss (1994), the peak value of vitamin A or of the ultimate teratogen, all-trans-retinoic acid, in the serum after eating liver is only 1/20 of that measured after taking vitamin A tablets. However, the three- to five-fold observed increase in plasma concentrations and the dose-dependent increase in exposure to 13-cis and 13-cis-4-oxo retinoic acid support the current safety recommendation: that women should be cautious regarding their consumption of liver-containing meals during pregnancy (Hartmann 2005).

β-carotene, also called pro-vitamin A, is converted as needed by the organism to vitamin A (retinol). Even high doses of β-carotene do not increase the retinol concentration in the serum and do not pose any teratogenic risk (Miller 1998, Polifka 1996).

It must be re-emphasized that vitamin A deficiency is a serious condition as mentioned in the introduction above. Besides regions of the world deficient in vitamin A, another condition pregnancy following bariatric surgery may lead to vitamin A deficiency and should be monitored (Chagas 2013).

> **Recommendation.** A pregnant woman is recommended not to take more than 6,000 IU of vitamin A as retinyl esters, retinal or retinol per day. Basically, there is no reason to consume a vitamin A supplement, particularly when nutrition is reasonably well-balanced. Exceptions are, of course, illnesses where there is a proven deficiency – for example, as a result of limited intestinal absorption or living in an environment where food stuffs do not have adequate Vitamin A. If, however, a dosage of more than 25,000 IU per day has been given by accident, interruption of the pregnancy is not indicated. An individual risk assessment should be made using detailed fetal ultrasound. Potentially pregnant women should not eat liver. However, single liver meals do not require any action. β-carotene is safe to ingest during pregnancy.

2.18.2   Vitamin B$_1$ (thiamine)

Pharmacology and toxicology

Thiamine is important as a co-enzyme in carbohydrate metabolism. The need for *vitamin B$_1$* (1–1.2 mg daily) does increase slightly during pregnancy, and there is a higher concentration in the fetal blood than in that of the mother. Even though thiamine supplementation is not usually discussed for *hyperesis gravidarum* treatment (Maltepe 2013), thiamine deficiency can induce clinical symptoms within 1 week. Severe polyneuropathy (Wernicke's encephalopathy) can occur with chronic hyperemesis during pregnancy, and must be treated with thiamine supplementation (Kotha 2013, Sonkusare 2011) (see Chapter 2.4.6).

> **Recommendation.** Supplementation with vitamin B$_1$ during pregnancy is, as a rule, unnecessary; however, for chronic *hyperemesis gravidarum*, thiamine supplementation should be instituted to prevent polyneuropathies. There are no clinical data suggesting teratogenicity with overdoses of thiamine.

2.18.3   Vitamin B$_2$ (riboflavin)

Pharmacology and toxicology

Riboflavin is an important co-enzyme in energy metabolism. No developmental disorders could be demonstrated in newborns whose mothers had clinical or laboratory signs of riboflavin deficiency (Heller 1974). In the same study, vitamin B$_2$ concentrations in the cord blood were four times higher than in the maternal blood. It would appear that there may be an active transplacental transport of vitamin B$_2$, which prevents deficiency in the fetus. A suggestion has been made that riboflavin hypovitaminosis might be an additional risk factor for preeclampsia (Wacker 2000).

> **Recommendation.** Supplementation with vitamin B$_2$ during pregnancy is, as a rule, unnecessary when adequate dietary intake is available. Embryo- or fetotoxicity with an overdose of riboflavin has not been reported.

2.18.4   Vitamin B$_3$ (nicotinamide)

Pharmacology and toxicology

Nicotinamide is a constituent in many important enzymes. Deficiencies in pregnancy have not been reported.

> **Recommendation.** Supplementation with vitamin B$_3$ during pregnancy is, as a rule, unnecessary. No adverse reactions are known.

2.18.5   Vitamin B$_6$ (pyridoxine)

Pharmacology and toxicology

Pyridoxine is the co-enzyme for some amino acid decarboxylases and transaminases. In North America, vitamin B$_6$ is used in combination with *doxylamine* as therapy for excessive vomiting in pregnancy (hyperemesis) (see Chapter 2.4). The vitamin B$_6$ concentration in the mother's blood is reduced throughout the entire pregnancy. By contrast, the concentrations in the fetal blood are about three times higher (Cleary 1975). There is no indication as yet for teratogenicity (see Chapter 2.4.5).

> **Recommendation.** Supplementation with vitamin B$_6$ is only necessary in exceptional cases; for example, during tuberculostatic treatment with isoniazid (see Chapter 2.6). For treatment of nausea and vomiting in pregnancy, see Chapter 2.4.

2.18.6   Vitamin B$_{12}$ (cyanocobalamin)

Pharmacology and toxicology

Vitamin B$_{12}$ (cyanocobalamin) is a factor in animal proteins necessary for the maturation of the erythroblasts. Its absence leads to megaloblastic (pernicious) anemia, with neurological consequences. Although the concentration of vitamin B$_{12}$ in the maternal serum drops slightly during the pregnancy, there is no reduction in the vitamin B$_{12}$ stored in the mother's liver (about 3,000 µg). The newborn's need for about 50 µg of stored vitamin B$_{12}$ is comparatively modest.

Diets in Western Europe commonly include 5–15 µg vitamin B_{12} per day. The daily requirement for vitamin B_{12} is 2 µg for nonpregnant women; during pregnancy this rises to 3 µg per day. Low vitamin B_{12} levels have been discussed as a risk factor for early recurrent abortion (Reznikoff-Etiévant 2002). Another genetic problem is transcobalamin II deficiency, which reduces the transfer of vitamin B_{12} into the cell because of a lack of the carrier protein Transcobalamin II binding to Transcobalamin II receptors on cells especially the placenta. Interestingly, the placenta produces transcobalamin II and can provide sufficient transcobalamin II for the mother to overcome her transcobalamin II deficiency and thus low cellular levels of Vitamin B_{12}. Low vitamin B_{12} levels are measured directly in the blood; however, with vitamin B_{12} deficiency in cells, one must monitor methylmalonic acid levels.

> **Recommendation.** Because vitamin B_{12} deficiency is not caused by pregnancy, supplementation with this vitamin is not routinely necessary. At most, it might be indicated with an unbalanced vegetarian or vegan diet. Anemia in the pregnancy caused by a vitamin B_{12} deficiency should, of course, be treated.

2.18.7   Vitamin C (ascorbic acid)

Pharmacology and toxicology

Vitamin C is important in cellular metabolism for the maintenance of oxidation–reduction balance. The daily requirement is set at 100 mg.

Vitamin C deficiency leads to scurvy, with disturbances in the collagen metabolism, and to a tendency to bleed. Vitamin C concentration in the fetal blood is three times as high as in the maternal blood because vitamin C accumulates in the fetus after the placental transfer of dehydroascorbic acid (Malone 1975). It is not known whether giving vitamin C affects the fetal reduction–oxidation balance. Recently, the association of vitamin C deficiency with gestational diabetes has been discussed (Zhang 2004a, 2004b), as has vitamin C supplementation during second and third trimesters to prevent premature rupture of membranes (Casanueva 2005, Tejero 2003) and most recently with selected birth defects (limb, cleft palate and heart defects) and exposure to notrosatable drugs (Shinde, 2013). This association with drug/chemical induced birth defects is among the first for human exposures and certainly requires further study. A recent meta-analysis did not find that supplementation with Vitamins C and E could prevent or improve maternal preeclampsia (Conde-Agudelo 2011).

> **Recommendation.** Vitamin C supplementation is not necessary during pregnancy, if the diet is balanced.

2.18.8   Folic acid

Pharmacology and toxicology

Folic acid, a *pteridine* derivate, is a B vitamin that is essential for nucleoprotein synthesis in general, and especially for growing tissues – i.e. for blood synthesis, embryonic and fetal development. It also keeps homocysteine levels low. The organism metabolizes folic acid in its biologically effective form, *folinic acid*. With a balanced diet, the effects on the maternal blood production produced by a deficiency should not be of any concern. However, with the rare, marked, folic acid deficiency, macrocytic anemia can develop.

As with all vitamin and nutritional standards, committees of experts set folate requirement. This explains the differences among countries and at various times. For example, in 1970 the US Food and Nutrition Board (FNB 1970) set the recommended folate intake for pregnant women at 0.4 mg/day. This was reduced to 0.270 mg per day in 1989, mainly because of data showing that healthy folate-replete adults ingested this amount. The recommendation was increased to 0.450 mg/day in 1999 by the same authority, in order to maintain adequate folate status in pregnant women (Tamura 2006). In the UK, the recommended daily intake of folic acid for pregnant women is set at 0.6 mg/day in 2006.

In the UK in 1965, an association between a relative folic acid deficiency in the mother and a high rate for neural tube defects (NTDs), especially open spina bifida and anencephaly, was reported for the first time (Hubbard 1965). In 1980, the first studies seemed to indicate that these serious birth defects could be prevented by giving multivitamin preparations (Smithells 1980), or by supplementation with folic acid (Laurence 1981) in pregnancies with a recurrent risk (Teratology Society 1994, Rosenberg 1992, MRC 1991). Since there are no clinical studies that indicate prevention of NTDs in a recurrent risk situation with less than 4 mg folic acid per day, it is ethically and practically not common to use lower daily doses in such a situation.

Comprehensive studies in the USA (Mulinare 1988), Australia (Bower 1989), Cuba (Vergel 1990), England (MRC 1991), Hungary (Czeizel 1992), and China (Berry 1999) suggested a possible protective action of folic acid supplementation for NTDs in cases where there is no recurrent risk. A meta-analysis by Blom 2009 further demonstrated the effectiveness of preconceptual folate administration for reducing NTDs. It is emphasized that the original studies were only for open NTDs and not all NTDs as later studies have included. However, in the Hungarian study, there was probably a selection bias in the control group, since the risk of NTDs in that control group was higher than in the general Hungarian population (ICBDMS 1991). Apart from NTDs, there have been studies that found a protective effect with respect to other birth defects (Bailey 2005, Czeizel 2004), such as cardiac defects (Czeizel 2004, Botto 2003, Bailey 2005), anal atresia (Myers 2001), and miscarriage (Gindler 2001, Nelen 2000).

The role of methylation, genetics (methylenetetrahydrofolate dehydrogenase, methionine synthase reductase, methylenetetrahydrofolate reductase) and autoantibodies to folate receptors have been proposed as sites for perturbation in producing associated birth defects (Van der Linden, 2006; van Gelder 2010, Blom 2009, Molloy 2009) (Figure 2.18.1). However, the importance of vitamins B_{12} and B_6 should be included (Blom 2009). It has to be stressed that folding of the neural walls and closure of the neural tube (neural tube formation) takes place between about 22 and 28 days post-conception – i.e. before the pregnant woman is about 14 days "overdue," and before she is 42 days pregnant (counting from the first day of the last menstruation). Thus, folic acid supplementation must be taken prior to conception and during conception and during the first 2 months of pregnancy. The role of the placenta in the transfer of folic acid may be of less interest because during the critical window of neural tube

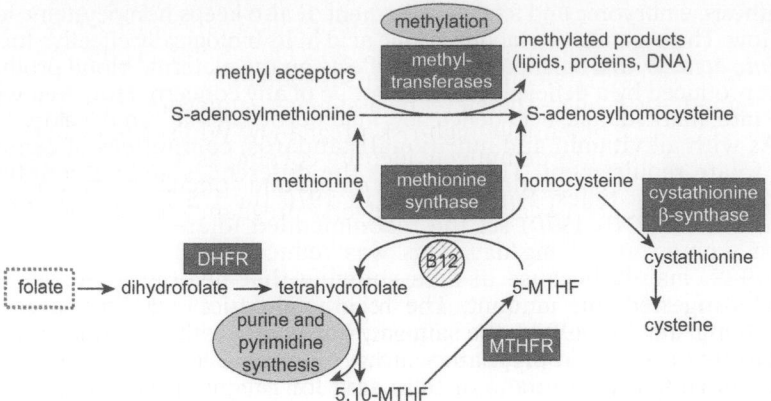

Figure 2.18.1 Folate – homocysteine – methionine metabolism. B$_{12}$, vitamin B$_{12}$; DHFR, reductase; MTHF, methyltetrahydrofolate; MTHFR, methyltetrahydrofolate reductase. Modified from van Gelder 2010.

morphogenesis, the functioning of the yolk sac may be primary (Garbis-Berkvens 1987). Shaw (1997) and others have discussed the relation of methionine and folic acid with respect to neural tube formation – for example, they observed that a higher dietary intake of methionine was associated with a reduction in NTD risk irrespective of maternal folate intake.

Based on current experience, a dose of folic acid of up to 5 mg daily is not dangerous for embryonic development. The possible masking of a rare vitamin B$_{12}$ deficiency anemia, repeatedly mentioned as a risk of taking folic acid, is possible, but in light of the recommended temporary supplementation this is not relevant.

In the USA, the Food and Drug Administration (FDA) has required folic acid fortification of foods (grain-based products) with 1.4 mg/kg since January 1988. This ruling is also true in Canada (0.15 mg per 100 g flour), in Chile (2.2 mg per kg flour) and Costa Rica. In the UK, enrichment has been assessed at 0.240 mg folic acid per 100 g flour, and a final decision to fortify bread with folic acid has yet to be made.

Food fortification was introduced in Hungary, but was not successful because of the higher price of the enriched bread and flour (Czeizel 2006). The issue of food fortification is still being discussed in other European countries, since only a small number of pregnant women actually take the supplementary tablets, and the average diet contains only 0.2 mg per day.

Occasionally there has been discussion regarding whether or not a balanced diet would provide sufficient folic acid anyway. Moreover, the decrease of NTD prevalence observed in line with the implementation of food fortification with folic acid might well also be correlated with the genetic and/or nutritional characteristics of the population involved. For example, Ireland, Wales, and North China were, in the past, high risk areas for NTDs, and it may be that changing nutritional habits in those countries explains a lowering of NTDs (Rosano 1999). However, reports from the CDC have demonstrated that the incidence of spina bifida and anecephaly have been reduced by 27% since fortification of flour has occurred in the US (CDC 2004a).

Finally, even with the many public health initiatives, the most recent evidence available (Khodr 2014) from the United States that in the most compliant group less than 60% of the women are taking folate prior to pregnancy. Further efforts are needed to tailor the message of preconceptional use of folate to prevent birth defects to every woman regardless of ethnicity/race, education, or age (CDC 2014b). However, fortification of grain, corn and other flour with folic acid can be an excellent adjunct to reduce the incidence of neural tube defects sensitive to folic acid.

We agree with the statement of Källén (2002) that folic acid should not be promoted as a teratologic panacea; however, as indicated above, a number of birth defects including neural tube, cardiac and cleft palate have all been associated with a reduction in incidences when the women had taken folate prior to pregnancy.

It should be noted that concomitant use of the high dosage of 1–5 mg folic acid supplementation compromises the efficacy of *sulfadoxine–pyrimethamine* for the treatment of uncomplicated malaria in pregnant women. Countries that use this medication for treatment or prevention of malaria in pregnancy need to evaluate their antenatal policy on the timing or dosage of folic acid supplementation (Ouma 2006) (see also Chapter 2.6).

In the US, prenatal vitamins now contain 0.8 mg/pill and are often recommended for the women not at identifiable risk for birth defects. For those women at recurrent risk, 1–5 mg per day is recommended. It should be noted that pre-pregnancy prenatal vitamins with 0.8 mg of folic acid/pill are often recommended instead of the usual women's multivitamin supplementation which contains 0.4 mg/pill.

Finally, even though evidence continues to accrue concerning the importance of adequate folic acid both preconceptually and during pregnancy for altering the incidences of NTD, we should not promote folic acid as a teratologic panacea; certainly a woman having a child with spina bifida should not feel guilty for not having taken enough folic acid pills before and during pregnancy.

> **Recommendation.** For the protective action of folic acid against open NTDs to be effective, supplementation with 0.4–0.8 mg folic acid per day should begin as early as possible when a pregnancy is planned, and be continued throughout the first 8 weeks of pregnancy, especially where flour fortification is unavailable. Pregnant women should also be encouraged to consume foods high in folate, such as green leafy vegetables, and fruit. If the mother has already given birth to a child with a NTD (i.e. has a recurrent risk), the supplementary dosage should be 1–5 mg per day. This is also suggested in connection with the intake of certain medications with a folic acid antagonist action. Folic acid deficiency/anemia should be treated in the usual way during pregnancy. However, fortification of grains with folic acid is an optimal method to provide folic acid for all pregnant women who are not at risk for neural tube defects.

2.18.9   Vitamin D group

Pharmacology and toxicology

Several fat-soluble vitamins with a central role in calcium metabolism are referred to collectively as *vitamin D*. Vitamin D promotes the resorption of calcium and phosphate from the intestines. New definitions for vitamin D levels have been proposed by the Institute of Medicine (IOM 2011): Sufficiency is 25(OH)D serum levels of ≥50 nmol/L (20 ng/mL); it should be noted that >75 nmol/L (>30 ng/mL) have not been consistently associated with enhanced benefit. Risk of Deficiency is <30 nmol/L (<12 ng/mL) and Potential Risk for Inadequacy is 30–50 nmol/L (12–20 ng/mL).

Vitamin D deficiency produces a disturbance in bone growth and development, which manifests itself as rickets in children and as osteo-malacia in adults. Vitamin D_2 (*ergocalciferol*) and vitamin D_3 (*colecal-ciferol*), are found in milk, cod-liver oil, and butter. Colecalciferol and ergocalciferol are transformed into the active form of vitamin D under the influence of UV rays. In the fetus, the active form of vitamin D is related to the maternal concentration – i.e. it is normally about 70–90% of this concentration, but increases significantly to over 100% when the maternal vitamin D concentration is deficient (Murguia-Peniche 2013, Uriu-Adams 2013, Pitkin 1975). The American College of Obstetricians and Gynecologists does not recommend screening of all pregnant women for vitamin D deficiency but rather suggests those women who appear at risk be screened and then given 1,000–2,000 IU/day (ACOG 2011).

A longitudinal study up to the age of 9 years, covering 198 mother–child pairs, indicated that vitamin D deficiency in late pregnancy may lead to significantly reduced ossification of the whole skeleton, and in particular of the lower spine. A lower than normal calcium concentra-tion in the cord blood may also predict poorer ossification (Javaid 2006). In a recently published case-cohort study from the Collaborative Perina-tal Project, maternal vitamin D deficiency may be a risk factor for severe preeclampsia but not for its mild subtypes (Bodnar 2014).

Other derivatives of vitamin D are *alfacalcidol* and *calcitriol. Dihydrot-achysterol* is a vitamin D analog for the treatment of hypoparathyroid-ism. There have been no studies on its use during pregnancy. However, dihydrotachysterol dosages are adjusted to maintain physiological condi-tions. Therefore, developmental toxicity is unlikely.

Paricalcitol is a synthetic vitamin D derivative used for the preven-tion and treatment of secondary hyperparathyroidism and osteoporosis. There is no experience with treatment during pregnancy.

> **Recommendation.** During pregnancy, very high doses of vitamin D are contrain-dicated because they can lead to hypercalcaemia in both the mother and the new-born. For healthy women, the need for vitamin D does not increase in pregnancy. When the diet is balanced, there is no need for supplementation. However, if there is a documented deficiency, supplementation, vitamin D may – or even must – be given until the maternal plasma concentrations are normal. This also applies to high doses for inherited dominant X-chromosomal vitamin D-resistant rickets needing treatment. In this case, it seems that a genetically healthy fetus is not damaged even with daily doses as high as 20,000 IU. Where there is phosphate diabetes, interruption of the vitamin D therapy should be discussed if the maternal symptoms allow this. Generally speaking, with these diseases the calcium and phosphate concentrations in the blood of both mother and newborn should be measured regularly.

2.18.10   Vitamin E (tocopherol)

Pharmacology and toxicology

Vitamin E is not essential for human beings, and deficiencies are unknown. The usual requirement for vitamin E is provided by a normal diet (10–20 IU). There have not been any observations of vitamin E defi-ciency during pregnancy.

Among 82 prospectively ascertained pregnancies exposed to high doses of vitamin E during the first trimester (400–1200 IU daily), the birth weight was significantly lower than among non-exposed controls. However, it was not clear whether the authors adjusted for gestational age at birth. There were no increased rates of prematurity, miscarriage, or birth defects (Boskovic 2004a, 2004b).

Additional studies have explored whether vitamin E with and without vitamin C can reduce the incidence and symptoms of preeclampsia. Much controversy has resulted about the intended benefits of such supplementation. A 2011 meta-analysis has not supported a therapeutic benefit in the treatment of preeclampsia (Conde-Agudelo 2011).

> **Recommendation.** Routine supplementation with vitamin E is not necessary.

2.18.11   Vitamin K

See Chapter 2.9.

2.18.12   Multivitamin preparations

Pharmacology and toxicology

Multivitamin preparations are frequently prescribed during pregnancy, or are taken by patients without a doctor's prescription. There is controversy over whether or not supplementation of additional vitamins might prevent birth defects (Källén 2009, Groenen 2004, Krapels 2004, Shaw 2000). However, there is no proven indication as yet for using multivitamins, either as supplements or as a preventive measure, with the exception of folic acid supplementation. Despite the lack of scientific justification, it has become common practice to prescribe certain vitamin (and mineral) combinations.

It should be noted that the formulation of prenatal vitamins has been changed to be supportive of the perceived need for additional folate to prevent NTDs. Especially in the US, the prenatal vitamins now have 0.8 mg of folate/pill. This is why many health care providers are recommending that prior to pregnancy, a prenatal vitamin be taken instead of a typical over the counter multivitamin preparation which contains 0.4 mg folate/pill.

> **Recommendation.** Prophylactic administration of multivitamin preparations to healthy pregnant women is controversial, because a balanced diet should be sufficient, and vitamins A and D may be toxic for the embryo in higher doses (when preparations are used inappropriately). However, most multivitamins include a combination of beta-carotene and a retinyl ester for vitamin A to reduce risk.

2.18.13   Iron

The total amount of *iron* in the human body is 4–5 g. Of this, about 70% is bound to hemoglobin (Hb). With the help of a protein, ferritin, iron is actively absorbed from the intestine. In the blood, iron is bound to the transport protein, transferrin, and reaches the unborn in this form through the placenta. During pregnancy, the need for iron increases due to the increase in the maternal blood volume as well as the increased need of the fetus and the placenta. The maternal plasma volume increases more than the number of erythrocytes (hemodilution), and this in turn leads to a relative decline in the hemoglobin value. The need of the embryo (and later the fetus) for iron increases during pregnancy, from 4 mg to 6.6 mg per day. Keeping in mind that the daily rate of excretion of iron is 1.5 mg, a pregnant woman needs about 5 mg of iron per day. The increased need for iron in pregnancy is not sufficiently covered by food. For this reason, stored iron is mobilized from the mother's degraded hemoglobin. Over the course of the pregnancy, the hemoglobin level drops by 20 g/L, primarily because of the increase in blood volume. With uncomplicated labor and normalization of the blood volume, the hemoglobin value returns to a normal level by the end of the postpartum period. It is recommended that total iron be measured (Ferritin) and not just hematocrit to obtain an accurate measure of iron adequacy.

Pharmacology

Iron (II) salts are well-absorbed after oral intake, and are suitable for supplementation prior to and during pregnancy. The addition of vitamins and trace elements to oral iron (II) preparations has no proven value. Combination preparations with folic acid cannot be recommended, because iron absorption with these preparations is reduced by up to 60%. About 15–20% of the patients who take iron (II) preparations complain of gastrointestinal problems, which may force a change to another preparation or even cessation of iron supplementation, especially in the presence of morning sickness. Parenteral administration of iron preparations (Singh 2000) such as iron (III)-gluconate complex is only indicated with marked anemia, for instance, and, in combination with other anti-anemics, eliminates, for the most part, the need for transfusions in pregnancy.

Toxicology

The suspicion that the birth defect rate could increase slightly with routine iron supplementation in pregnancy has not been confirmed by comprehensive prospective studies (Royal College of General Practitioners 1975). For iron overdose, see Chapter 2.22.

Recommendation. Iron supplementation prior to and during pregnancy is indicated if the hemoglobin level is ≥100 g/L. However, any indication of iron deficiency should be evaluated with total iron measurements (Ferritin). It should be given orally, using an iron (II) preparation. If for some reason parenteral iron supplementation is necessary, this should be given intravenously with an iron (III) preparation. For iron overdose, see Chapter 2.22.

2.18.14   Calcium

Pharmacology and toxicology

Nearly all *calcium* in the body, totaling about 1,100–1,200 g, is found in the bones, bound in complexes with phosphate and hydroxyapatite. The daily calcium requirement is 800–1,000 mg. Calcium metabolism and fetal bone development are dependent on the maternal vitamin D metabolism and pregnancy-related changes in the activity of different hormones (parathormone, calcitonin, cortisteroids, estrogens) (IOM 2011). Calcium is actively transported through the placenta to the fetus. In the last trimester, bone development is enhanced as a result of low parathormone concentrations and high calcitonin concentrations in the fetus. Over the course of the pregnancy, the fetus takes in about 30 g of calcium. This amount is normally mobilized during pregnancy from maternal storage, without additional administration of calcium salts. However, it is generally advised that a supplement of about 500 mg per day be taken to ensure the daily requirement is met. Calcium should not be given as a phosphate salt because of leg muscle cramps. Organic salts, such as calcium citrate, calcium aspartate, calcium globionate and calcium gluconate, are more appropriate for calcium supplementation. Also, if there is known lead poisoning/exposure anytime in the life of the mother, 1000 mg per day should be given to compete with the lead leached from mother's bones in the second and third trimesters (see Lead, Chapter 2.23).

> **Recommendation.** It makes sense to take 500 mg of calcium per day orally, or to drink a liter of milk; milk has the advantage that it supplies not only the calcium but also the daily vitamin D requirement.

2.18.15 Fluoride

Pharmacology and toxicology

Whether a *fluoride* supplement during pregnancy of about 1 mg/day in tablet form (equivalent to about 2 mg sodium fluoride), or ingested via fluoridated drinking water (about 1 mg/L), actually reduces the incidence of caries in the baby is still not validated. However, such fluoride prophylaxis does not appear to harm the fetus. Earlier suspicions regarding the possible toxic effect of regular fluoride on reproduction – for example, an increased rate of Down syndrome – is biologically implausible. Even higher fluoride doses as a result of environmentally contaminated drinking water (above 10 mg/L) do not apparently produce any increase in birth defects. Prenatally induced fluorosis of the teeth and bones in the second half of pregnancy is theoretically possible, and has been described in individual cases after extreme continuous exposure, but would not be expected after (as has occasionally happened) accidental intake of an osteoporosis preparation containing about 25 mg of fluoride.

> **Recommendation.** Fluoride supplementation of about 1 mg per day can be given during pregnancy without risk. Calcium (including milk products) and fluoride must not be taken together because of the formation of insoluble calcium fluoride, which cannot be absorbed. High-dose fluoride therapy for osteoporosis is contraindicated. However, accidental intake of higher doses does not justify either interruption of the pregnancy or additional diagnostic procedures.

2.18.16   Strontium

Pharmacology and toxicology

Strontium is prescribed in cases of postmenopausal osteoporosis. There are insufficient data concerning the use of strontium in pregnancy. Experimental data on bone marrow cells have given indications for clastogenic effects. Strontium also has an effect on capacitation, both in humans and animals (Sharma 1989), and on the activation of oocytes in rodents (Fraser 1987). It is currently been evaluated for use in intracytoplasmic sperm injections (Chen 2010).

> **Recommendation.** Indications for treatment with strontium are outside the scope of this book. Therefore, and because of the possible mutagenic activity, the use of strontium is not indicated in pregnancy. In cases of unintended strontium use, invasive diagnostics or interruption of pregnancy is not justified.

2.18.17   Biphosphonates and other osteoporosis drugs

Pharmacology and toxicology

Alendronatic acid, clodronic acid, etidronic acid, ibandronic acid, pamidronic acid, risedronic acid, tiludronic acid and *zoledronic acid* are among the osteolysis inhibitors. They are used for Morbus Paget, postmenopausal osteoporosis, and other osteolytic processes. There are no systematic studies on their use during pregnancy. Animal experiments suggest a possible placental transfer and effect on fetal skeletal development (Ornoy 1998).

In one study, there was no major congenital anomaly among 24 pregnancies with pre-pregnancy or early pregnancy exposure to alendronate (Ornoy 2006). Another case report describes a healthy newborn, with normal bone structure and uneventful development until the age of 1 year, who was exposed to 10 mg per day throughout pregnancy (Rutgers-Verhage 2003). Another report was on a woman receiving zoledronic acid during the second and third trimesters, after chemotherapy for breast cancer during the first trimester. The child was born at 35 weeks' gestation, and was followed until the age of 1 year, during which time development was normal (Andreadis 2004). A prospective study covering 15 pregnancies where the mothers underwent biphosphonate treatment (alendronatic acid, 7; etidronic acid, 5; pamidronic acid, 1; risedronic acid, 2), and where nine of the mothers were being treated during the first trimester, resulted in 14 live births and 1 spontaneous abortion. There was no indication of developmental toxicity (Levy 2004). There are insufficient data on the use of *calcitonin, cinacalet*, and *raloxifen* during pregnancy.

> **Recommendation.** Biphosphonates and the other osteoporosis drugs are not indicated during pregnancy. Accidental acute use of individual doses in the first trimester does not justify either interruption of the pregnancy or additional diagnostic procedures.

2.18.18   Iodide

See Chapter 2.15.2.

2.18.19   Trace elements

Pharmacology and toxicology

Trace elements such as *chromium, copper, selenium,* or *zinc* are not normally supplemented in pregnancy. However, zinc is used therapeutically in cases of Wilson's disease. In a prospective study of 26 pregnancies (in 19 women) with this condition, the mothers received 25–50 mg zinc three times daily. All the pregnancies resulted in live-born children; one child had a cardiac disorder and another had microcephaly (Brewer 2000). Additional studies from the same investigative team in the Philippines and Utah produced contradictory results, which suggests that poor maternal zinc status may become a risk factor only when the status in highly compromised (Munger 2009, Tamura 2005).

Chromium is, according to some investigators, associated with glucose intolerance which commonly develops during late pregnancy (Saner 1981). This theory has been criticized as poorly supported by available data (Knopp 1982).

Selenium (see also Chapter 2.17) is an essential trace element. Selenium poisoning can be caused by high concentrations in drinking water. In this respect, it has been associated with miscarriages (Robertson 1970). No definitive data are available – certainly not to evaluate the use of selenium as an antioxidant.

> **Recommendation.** Supplementation with trace elements such as chromium, copper, and zinc is not necessary during pregnancy, apart from those instances when there is a documented deficiency or particular treatment indication (e.g. Wilson's disease). "Detoxification treatment" with selenium should not be undertaken either. However, the accidental use of these trace elements does not require any action.

References

ACOG. Vitamin D: Screening and supplementation during pregnancy. Committee Opinion No. 495. Obstet Gynecol 2011; 118: 197–8.

Andreadis C, Charalampidou M, Diamantopoulos N et al. Combined chemotherapy and radiotherapy during conception and first two trimesters of gestation in a women with metastatic breast cancer. Gynecol Oncol 2004; 95: 252–5.

Bailey LB, Berry RJ. Folic acid supplementation and the occurrence of congenital heart defects, orofacial clefts, multiple births, and miscarriage. Am J Clin Nutr 2005; 81: 1213–7.

Berry RJ, Li Z, Erickson JD et al. Prevention of neural-tube defects with folic acid in China. China–US Collaborative Project for Neural Tube Defect Prevention. N Engl J Med 1999; 341: 1485–90.

Blom HJ. Folic acid, methylation and neural tube closure in humans. Birth Defects Res A 2009; 85: 295–302.

Bodnar LM, Simhan HN, Catov JM, Roberts JM, Platt RW, Diesel JC, Klebanoff MA. Vitamin D status and the risk of mild and severe preeclampsia, Epidemiology 2014; 25:207–214.

Boskovic R, Cargaun L, Dulus J et al. High doses of vitamin E and pregnancy outcome. Reprod Toxicol 2004a; 18: 722.

Boskovic R, Cargaun L, Oren D et al. Pregnancy outcome following high doses of vitamin E supplementation; a prospective controlled study. Birth Def Res A 2004b; 70: 358.

Botto LD, Mulinare J, Erickson JD. Do multivitamin or folic acid supplements reduce the risk for congenital heart defects? Evidence and gaps. Am J Med Genet 2003; 121A: 95–101.

Bower C, Stanley FJ. Dietary folate as a risk factor for neural-tube defects: evidence from a case-control study in Western Australia. Med J Aust 1989; 150: 613–9.

Brewer GJ, Johnson VD, Dick RD et al. Treatment of Wilson's disease with zinc. XVII: Treatment during pregnancy. Hepatology 2000; 31: 364–70.

Buss NE, Tembe EA, Prendergast BD et al. The teratogenic metabolites of vitamin A in women following supplements and liver. Hum Exp Toxicol 1994; 13: 33–43.

Carmichael SL, Yang W, Shaw GM, Maternal Dietary Nutrient Intake and Risk of Preterm Delivery. Am J Perinatol 2013; 30: 579–88.

Casanueva E, Ripoll C, Tolentino M et al. Vitmin C supplementation to prevent premature rupture of the chorioamniotic. Am J Clin Nutr 2005; 81: 859–63.

CDC (Center for Disease Control). Spina bifida and anencephaly before and after folic acid mandate – United States 1995–1996 and 1999–2000. MMWR 2004a; 53: 362–5.

CDC (Centers for Disease Control) http://m.cdc.gov/en/HealthSafetyTopics/LifeStages-Populations/Pregnancy/QAfolicAcid, 2014b.

Chagas CB, Saunders C, Pereira S et al. Vitamin A deficiency in pregnancy: perspectives after bariatric surgery. Obes Surg 2013; 23: 249–54.

Chen J, Qian Y, Tan Y, Mima H. Successful pregnancy following oocyte activation by strontium in normozoospermic patients of unexplained infertility with fertilization failures during previous intracytoplasmic sperm injection treatment. Reprod Fertil De 2010; 22: 852–5.

Cleary RE, Lumeng L, Li T. Maternal and fetal plasma levels of pyridoxal phosphate at term: adequacy of vitamin B6 supplementation during pregnancy. Am J Obstet Gynecol 1975; 121: 25–8.

Conde-Agudelo A, Romero R, Kusanovic JP, Hassan SS. Supplementation with vitamins C and E during pregnancy for the prevention of preeclampsia and other adverse maternal and perinatal outcomes: a systematic review and metanalysis. Am J Obstet Gynecol 2011; 204: 503, e1–12.

Czeizel AE. Folic acid: a public health challenge. Lancet 2006; 367: 2056.

Czeizel AE, Dobo M, Varga P. Hungarian cohort control trial of periconceptional multivitamin supplementation shows a reduction in certain congenital abnormalities. Birth Def Res A 2004; 70: 853–61.

Czeizel AE, Dudas I. Prevention of the first occurrence of neural-tube defects by periconceptional vitamin supplementation. N Engl J Med 1992; 327: 1832–5.

Dudas I, Czeizel AE. Use of 6,000 IU vitamin A during early pregnancy without teratogenic effect. Teratology 1992; 45: 335–6.

Emmett, SD, West KP Jr. Gestation vitamin A deficiency: a novel cause of sensorineural hearing loss in the developing world? Med Hypotheses 2014; 82: 6–10.

FNB, NRC. Maternal nutrition and the course of pregnancy. Washington, DC: NAS, 1970.

Fraser LR. Strontium supports capacitation and the acrosome reaction in mouse sperm and rapidly activates mouse eggs. Gamete Res 1987; 18: 363–74.

Garbis-Berkvens JM, Peters PWJ. Comparative morphology and physiology of embryonic and fetal membranes. In: H Nau, WJ Scott (eds), Pharmacokinetics in Teratogenesis, Vol. I. Boca Raton, FL: CRC Press, 1987, pp. 13–44.

Gindler J, Li Z, Berry RJ et al. Folic acid supplements during pregnancy and the risk of miscarriage. Lancet 2001; 358: 796–800.

Groenen PM, van Rooij IA, Peer PG et al. Low maternal dietary intake of iron, magnesium, and niacin are associated with spina bifida in the offspring. J Nutr 2004; 134: 1516–22.

Hartmann S, Brors O, Bock J et al. Exposure to retinoic acids in non-pregnant women following high vitamin A intake with a liver meal. Intl J Vit Nutr Res 2005; 75:187–94.

Heller SP, Salkeld RM, Korner WE. Riboflavin status in pregnancy. Am J Clin Nutr 1974; 27: 1225–39.

Hubbard ED, Smithells RW. Folic acid metabolism and human embryopathy. Lancet 1965; 1: 1254.

ICBDMS (International Clearinghouse for Birth Defects Monitoring Systems). Congenital Malformations Worldwide, A Report from the International Clearinghouse for Birth Defects Monitoring Systems. Amsterdam: Elsevier, 1991.

IOM (Institute of Medicine). Committee to Review Dietary Reference Intakes for Vitamin D and Calcium. Dietary Reference Intakes for Calcium and Vitamin D. Washington, DC National Academics Press, 2011.

Javaid MK, Crozier SR, Harvey NC et al. Maternal vitamin D status during pregnancy and childhood bone mass at age 9 years: a longitudinal study. Lancet 2006; 367: 36–43.

Källén BA. Drugs During Pregnancy, Nova Biomedical Books, 2009, New York.

Källén BAJ, Otterblad Olausson P. Use of folic acid and delivery outcome: a prospective registry study. Reprod Toxicol 2002; 16: 327–32.

Krapels IP, van Rooij IA, Ocke MC et al. Maternal nutritional status and the risk for orofacial cleft in humans. J Nutr 2004; 134: 3106–13.

Khodr AG, Lup PJ, Agopian AJ et al. Preconceptional folic acid-containing supplement use in the national birth defects prevention study Birth Defects Res. Part A Clin Mol Teratol. 2014; E-print ahead of press (DOI: 10.1002/bdra.23238).

Knopp RH. Altered chromium excretion in pregnancy: a physiological change? Am J Clin Nutr 1982; 35: 776–7.

Kotha VK, DeSouza A. Wernicke's encephalopathy following Hyperemesis Gravidarum. A report of three cases. Neuroradiol J 2013; 26: 35–40.

Laurence KM, James N, Miller MH et al. Double-blind randomised controlled trial of folate treatment before conception to prevent recurrence of neural-tube defects. Br Med J 1981; 282: 1509–11.

Levy S, Fayez I, Han JY et al. Fetal outcome after intrauterine exposure to biphosphonates. Birth Def Res A 2004; 70: 359–60.

Malone JM. Vitamin passage across the placenta. Clin Perinatol 1975; 2: 295–307.

Maltepe C, Koren G. The management of nausea and vomiting of pregnancy and hyperemesis gravidarum – A 2013 update. J Popul Ther Clin Pharm 2013; 20: 184–92.

Mastroiacovo P, Mazzone T, Addis A et al. High vitamin A intake in early pregnancy and major malformations: a multicenter prospective controlled study. Teratology 1999; 59: 7–11.

Miller BJ, Murray L, Beckmann MM et al. Dietary supplements for preventing postnatal depression. Cochrane Database Syst Rev 2013; 10: CD009104.

Miller RK, Hendrickx AG, Mills JL. Periconceptional Vitamin A use: how much is teratogenic? Reprod Toxicol 1998; 12: 75–88.

Mitchell LE, Murray JC, O'Brien S et al. Retinoic acid receptor alpha gene variants, multivitamin use, and liver intake as risk factors for oral clefts: a population-based case-control study in Denmark, 1991–94. Am J Epidemiol 2003; 158: 69–76.

Molloy AM, Brody LC, Miller, JL et al. The search for genetic polymorphism in the homocysteine/folate pathway that contribute to the etiology of human neural tube defects. Birth Defects Research A 2009; 85: 285–94.

MRC (Medical Research Council), Vitamin Study Research Group. Prevention of neural tube defects: results of the MRC vitamin study. Lancet 1991; 338: 131–7.

Mulinare J, Cordero JF, Erickson JD et al. Periconceptional use of multivitamins and the occurrence of neural tube defetcts. J Am Med Assoc 1988; 260: 3141–5.

Munger RG, Tamura T, Johnston, KE et al. Plasma Zinc Concentrations of Mothers and the Risk of Oral Clefts in their Children in Utah. Birth Defects Res A 2009; 85: 151–5.

Murguia-Peniche T. Vitamin D, Vitamin A, maternal-perinatal considerations: old concepts, new insights, new questions. J Ped 2013; 162: S26–30.

Myers MF, Li S, Correa-Villasenor A et al. Folic acid supplementation and risk for imperforate anus in China. Am J Epidemiol 2001; 154: 1051–6.

Nelen WLDM, Blom HJ, Steegers EAP et al. Homocysteine and folate levels as risk factors for recurrent early pregnancy loss. Obstet Gynecol 2000; 95: 519–24.

Ornoy A, Patlas N, Pinto T et al. The transplacental effects of alendronate on the fetal skeleton in rats. Teratology 1998; 57: 242.

Ornoy A, Wajnberg R, Diav-Citrin O. The outcome of pregnancy following pre-pregnancy or early pregnancy alendronate treatment. Reprod Toxicol 2006; 22: 578–9.

Ouma P, Parise ME, Hamel MJ et al. A randomized controlled trial of folate supplementation when treating malaria in pregnancy with sulfadoxine-pyrimethamine. PLoS Clin Trials 2006; 6: 20–1.

Pitkin RM. Vitamins and minerals in pregnancy. Clin Perinatol 1975; 2: 221–32.

Polifka JE, Donlan CR, Donlan MA et al. Clinical teratology counseling and consultation report: high-dose ®-carotene use during early pregnancy. Teratology 1996; 54: 103–7.

Reznikoff-Etiévant MC, Zittoun J, Vaylet C et al. Low vitamin B12 level as a risk factor for early recurrent abortion. Eur J Obstet Gynecol 2002; 104: 156–9.

Robertson DSF. Selenium a possible teratogen? Lancet 1970; 1: 518–19.

Rosa EW, Wilk AL, Kelsey EO. Vitamin A congeners. Teratology 1986; 33: 355–64.

Rosano A, Smithells D, Cacciani L et al. Time trends in neural tube defects prevalence in relation to preventive strategies: an international study. J Epidemiol Community Health 1999; 53: 630–35.

Rosenberg IH. Folic acid and neural-tube defects time for action? N Engl J Med 1992; 327: 1875–7.

Rothman KJ, Moore LL, Singer MR et al. A. Teratogenicity of high vitamin A intake N Engl J Med 1995; 333: 1369–73.

Royal College of General Practitioners. Morbidity and drugs in pregnancy. J R Coll Gen Pract 1975; 25: 631–5.

Rutgers-Verhage AR, de Vries TW. No effects of biphosphonates on the human fetus. Birth Def Res A 2003; 67: 203–4.

Saltzman E, Karl JP. Nutrient deficiencies after gastric bypass surgery. Ann Rev Nutr 2013; 33: 183–203.

Saner G. Urinary chromium excretion during pregnancy and its relationship with intravenous glucose loading. Am J Clin Nutr 1981; 34: 1676–9.

Sharma A, Talukder G. Effects of metals on chromosomes of higher organisms. Environ Mut 1989; 9: 191–226.

Shaw GM, Croen LA, Todoroff K et al. Periconceptional intake of vitamin supplements and risk of multiple congenital anomalies. Am J Med Genet 2000; 93: 188–93.

Shaw GM, Velie EM, Schaffer DM. Is dietary intake of methionine associated with a reduction in risk for neural tube defect-affected pregnancies? Teratology 1997; 56: 295–9.

Shinde MU, Voung AM, Brender JD et al. Prenatal exposure to nitrosatable drugs, vitamin C and risk of selected birth defects. Birth Defects Res A 2013; 97: 515–31.

Singh K, Fong YF. Letter to the editor: Intravenous iron polymaltose complex for treatment of iron deficiency anaemia in pregnancy resistant to oral iron therapy. Eur J Haematol 2000; 64: 272–4.

Smithells RW, Sheppard S, Schorah CJ et al. Possible prevention of neutral-tube defects by periconceptional vitamin supplementation. Lancet 1980; 1: 339–400.

Sonkusare S. The Clinical management of hyperemesis gravidarum. Arch Gyn Obstet 2011; 283: 1183–92.

Tamura T, Munger MG, Corcoran. Plasma Zinc Concentrations of mothers and the risk of nonsydromic oral clefts in the children: A cas-Control study in the Philippines. Birth Defects Res A 2005; 73: 612–6.

Tamura T, Picciano F. Folate and human reproduction. Am J Clin Nutr 2006; 83: 993–1016.

Tang G, Hu Y, Yin S et al. Beta-carotene in Golden Rice is as good as beta-carotene in oil at providing vitamin A to children. Amer J Clin Nutr 2012; 96: 658–64.

Tejero E, Perichart O, Pfeffer F et al. Collagen snthesis during pregnancy, vitamin C availability, and risk of premature rupture of fetal membranes. Intl J Gynaecol Obstet 2003; 81: 29–34.

Teratology Society. Position Paper: Recommendations for Vitamin A use during pregnancy. Teratology 1987; 35: 269–75.

Teratology Society. Summary of the 1993 Teratology Society. Public Affairs Committee Symposium: folic acid prevention of neural tube defects – public policy issues. Teratology 1994; 49: 239–41.

Uriu-Adams JY, Obican SG and Keen CL. Vitamin D and Maternal and Child Health: Overview and Implications for Dietary Requirements. Birth Defects Res C Embryo Today 2013; 99: 24–44.

Van der Linden IJM, Den Heijer M, Afman LA et al. The methionine synthase reductase 66a→G polymorphism is a maternal risk factor for spina bifida. J Mol Med 2006; 84: 1047–54.

van Gelder MMHJ, van Rooij IAQLM, Miller R et al. Teratogenic mechanisms of medical drugs. Hum Reprod Update 2010; 16: 378–94.

Vergel RG, Sanchez LR, Heredero BL et al. Primary prevention of neural tube defects with folic acid supplementation: Cuban experience. Prenatal Diagn 1990; 10: 149–52.

Wacker J, Fruhauf J, Schulz M et al. Riboflavin deficiency and pre-eclampsia. Obstet Gynecol 2000; 96: 38–44.

Wiegand UW, Hartmann S, Hummler H. Safety of vitamin A: recent results. Intl J Vit Nutr Res 1998; 68: 411–6.

Zhang C, Williams MA, Sorensen TK et al. Maternal plasma ascorbic acid (vitamin C) and risk of gestational diabetes mellitus. Epidemiol 2004a; 15: 597–604.

Zhang C, Williams MA, Frederick IO et al. Vitamin C and the risk of gestational diabetes mellitus: a case-control study. J Reprod Med 2004b; 49: 257–66.

Herbs during pregnancy

2.19

Henry M. Hess and Richard K. Miller

2.19.1	The safety of herbs during pregnancy	511
2.19.2	Counseling a pregnant woman about herbs	512
2.19.3	General concepts regarding the use of herbs during pregnancy	513
2.19.4	Herbs used as foods	514
2.19.5	Essential oils that are safe during pregnancy	514
2.19.6	Herbs frequently used during pregnancy	514
2.19.7	Herbs controversially used during pregnancy	515
2.19.8	Herbs contraindicated during pregnancy	520

Plants and plant extracts have been used for medicinal purposes since before recorded time. Many pharmaceutical agents have their origins in plant-based compounds. In a trend towards returning to the "natural," and believing that such agents are safer, patients worldwide are more and more frequently consulting natural therapists and taking herbs to enhance their nutrition, stay healthy, and treat their illnesses. Women taking herbs can and do get pregnant. They take herbal therapies to ensure that they are healthy prior to and during their pregnancy, and also to treat medical conditions during their pregnancy. A 2003 study of 578 pregnant women in the United States showed that 45% of respondents used herbal medicines (Glover 2003). Other studies reported similar high usage (Lapi 2012, Nordeng 2011, Cuzzolin 2011, Bercaw 2010, Low Dog 2009, Moussally 2009, Holst 2008, 2009, 2010, Fugh-Berman 2003).

2.19.1 The safety of herbs during pregnancy

The difficulties in evaluating the safety and risk of herbal therapies are known, and are faced by everyone who takes, or is considering taking, herbs. These concerns are enhanced in pregnant women, and risks are even more difficult to evaluate. The problems of determining the safety of herbs in this context are as follows:

- There are few published clinical trials or investigations of these substances establishing the efficacy and/or toxicity of the preparations at specific doses.
- There are no clinical studies of a sufficient number of women to evaluate meaningful safety effects of an herb or herbs on pregnancy outcomes (Low Dog 2009).

Drugs During Pregnancy and Lactation. http://dx.doi.org/10.1016/B978-0-12-408078-2.00020-2

- There are limited standards for the preparation and for the established amounts of specific ingredients in the products marketed, and there are few regulating bodies that certify the products sold or doses used (for example, the US Food and Drug Administration (FDA), the European Medicines Agency (EMEA) and the European Evaluation Food Safety Authority (EFSA)). The German Commission E does provide some oversight on selected herbal products (Blumenthal 1998, 2003).
- There are differing health claims made by the agencies in Europe, the United States, and other countries around the world.
- Some of the products available worldwide may contain (and in some instances have been shown to contain) contaminants such as lead and/or arsenic from the agricultural or manufacturing processes. These could have devastating effects on the pregnant woman.
- It is always important to know the potential side effects of anything we take, and this is even more significant during pregnancy. The fetus grows rapidly, and is vulnerable to substances that affect cellular growth and division. In addition, certain herbs and natural substances can affect the muscle tone and circulation of the uterus, and some can act as uterine stimulants, abortifacients or teratogens (Low Dog 2005, 2009).

2.19.2   Counseling a pregnant woman about herbs

For the above reasons, it is difficult even for an experienced healthcare provider to counsel a pregnant woman on the use of herbal preparations. As providers, evidence-based medicine is expected. However, few herbs and natural therapies even have good scientific evidence, never mind the evidence-based medicine that people expect today. Rather, herbal therapies use more traditional evidence as their proof of safety. This is evidence passed down by culture and tradition, and is often only oral. There is almost no solid scientific evidence regarding the benefits or the risks of herbs in pregnancy to the mother or fetus. It is difficult to reassure patients under these circumstances.

There is some good news, though. There is a considerable body of traditional evidence that can be used as a basis for a discussion with patients. This is traditional evidence – a different kind of evidence-based medicine. It can be very helpful to patients, when put in the proper perspective and used with appropriate understanding. This chapter presents the latest and best evidence that is available, to help counsel pregnant patients, and is organized to optimize the thinking and approach to understanding the most up-to-date knowledge regarding the safety of herbs during pregnancy.

Following a general discussion of herbs during pregnancy, descriptions of some of the frequently used herbs during pregnancy are presented here, along with the best evidence available regarding their safety and risk assessment during pregnancy. Next, there is a description of some common herbs where there is controversy over their use during pregnancy. Again, there is a description and discussion of the latest known evidence for these herbs. Finally, there is a list of herbs thought to be contraindicated during pregnancy. These are organized into groups according to how they might negatively affect a pregnant woman. This can be helpful in terms of counseling a patient.

This chapter focuses on herbal preparations for the pregnant woman. It does not include information on *ayurvedic* preparations (Sharma 2007), Chinese herbs (Wang 2012) and/or medicines, or *homeopathy*, where evidence-based safety data for the pregnant woman are even more limited.

Sections and tables are presented identifying herbs where there is some evidence supporting the safety of their use during pregnancy, but only at the doses and in the preparations mentioned. It should be emphasized that any product can have potential adverse effects, based upon the quantity or doses used. Since manufacturing standards have not yet been established, it is impossible to be certain of the dosage in many products manufactured around the world. While manufacturers in developed countries have tried to establish more defined preparations, this still remains an area of concern. In addition, the stability of products and possible contamination of the plant or product grown in other parts of the world may still be an issue because of the lack of regulatory standards. Therefore, it is a requirement for any consumers of these products, and the provider counseling them, to evaluate carefully the stated preparation of each product used, focusing upon the reported concentrations of the ingredients, the country of origin, the manufacturer and its reputation, and any reported incidents of contamination for that type of product. For pregnant or lactating women, or any woman of reproductive age, further caution is necessary because of the potential for enhanced effects of these substances on the mother, the embryo/fetus, and the breastfed baby. With regard to purity and the safety of specific products, there are two valuable and important resources. Consumer Labs (www.ConsumerLab.com) is an independent laboratory for the testing of herbal, vitamin, and mineral supplements. A subscription service at ConsumerLab.com is a valuable resource for any provider who counsels patients, including pregnant women, about the purity of specific brands of natural substances.

The United States Pharmacopeia (USP) is also a useful reference.

2.19.3   General concepts regarding the use of herbs during pregnancy

There are a few points that are important for consideration of the use of herbs in pregnancy:

1. Herbs should only be recommended by a competent and qualified provider caring for the pregnant woman, and one who is comfortable with, and knowledgeable about, the efficacy and risk assessment of herbs in pregnancy. It is well worth becoming familiar with Hess (2013), Mills (2000, 2006), Blumenthal (2003), Rotblatt (2002) and www.ConsumerLab.com.
2. Herbs are extracts of plants or plant roots, and they contain numerous compounds. Different forms of the herbal preparation will have different compounds in its preparation, as well as differing concentrations. How the herb is prepared is very important to the effect and safety of the pregnant woman and fetus. Herbal preparations come in the following forms:
   - teas or infusions (infusions are hot-water extracts of dried herbs)
   - capsules
   - dried extracts
   - tinctures (tinctures are alcohol extracts of dried herbs).

   The most commonly used herbs in pregnancy are teas or infusions (which are similar to teas). These usually have the lowest concentrations and contain the least amount of compounds. Capsules and dried extracts are less commonly used; examples include ginger and echinacea. Tinctures should be avoided in pregnancy because of their higher concentrations as well as the use of alcohol as a carrier.

Pregnancy

2.19 Herbs during pregnancy

3. The effects and safety of herbs will depend on the trimester. One of the most important concepts is that herbs – just like pharmaceuticals – should be used with caution in the first trimester. In general, there is no pharmaceutical or herb that is absolutely safe in the first trimester, based upon our current knowledge. It is important to be aware that the rapid cellular development in organogenesis can be altered by any compound, and that some herbs may increase uterine tone, increasing the risk of pregnancy loss.

The pregnant woman has an altered physiological state. Drugs and herbs may therefore behave differently in the pregnant woman's body compared to in a nonpregnant woman (see Low Dog 2005, Blumenthal 2003).

2.19.4   Herbs used as foods

The safest herbs in pregnancy are, in general, those considered to be food. Herbs commonly used as food or food additives are usually safe for use during pregnancy, and can be used daily (at the levels generally used as food ingredients) without affecting the pregnant woman or fetus (see Low Dog 2005, Fleming 2004, Blumenthal 2003, Weed 1986).

2.19.5   Essential oils that are safe during pregnancy

Some essential oils can be safely used as aromatherapy during pregnancy, based on traditional and historic use. There are no evidence-based studies that will assure their safety. They should always be used carefully, in a well-diluted form, and should not be ingested. They should be used in an aromatherapy diffuser. Such oils, and their uses, are listed in Table 2.19.1 (see Low Dog 2005, Fleming 2004, Blumenthal 2003, Weed 1986).

Table 2.19.1 Essential oils considered safe during pregnancy

Essential oil	Common usage
Chamomile	Respiratory tract disorders
Tangerine	Antispasmodic, decongestant, general relaxant
Grapefruit	Stimulant, antidepressant
Geranium	Dermatitis, hormone imbalances, PMS, menstrual problems, viral infections
Rose	Astringent, used for mild inflammation of the oral and pharyngeal mucosa
Jasmine	Stimulant, antidepressant, anxiety
Ylang-ylang	Antispasmodic, cardiac arrhythmias, anxiety, antidepressant, hair loss, intestinal problems
Lavender	Loss of appetite, nervousness, and insomnia

2.19.6   Herbs frequently used during pregnancy

Herbs are frequently used as teas or infusions. Although there are no clinical trials available, and there is no evidence-based proof in terms of Western medical standards, some herbal teas/infusions have been used for many years without adverse effects, and are considered to be safe. The evidence of their safety comes from their traditional use and from traditional evidence passed down through history by traditional users. Although there are no data to suggest how much is "safe," it is suggested that consumption of herbal teas be limited to two cups per day during pregnancy. This is similar to the safety data regarding coffee in pregnancy. Their safety is unknown when used at higher levels, so the use of herbs above these amounts is not recommended. If the quantities consumed are above these recommended levels, no special action is required except stopping usage at high doses (see Low Dog 2005, Blumenthal 2003, Weed 1986). Table 2.19.2 lists those herbs that are frequently used during pregnancy.

Table 2.19.2 Herbs frequently used during pregnancy

Herb	Usage	Form
1. Red raspberry	Relief of nausea, increase in milk leaf production, increase in uterine tone, and ease of labor pains; there is some controversy over its use in the first trimester, primarily because of concern of stimulating uterine tone and causing miscarriage (McFarland 1999, Parsons 1999, Brinker 1997).	Tea or infusion
2. Peppermint	Nausea, flatulence.	Tea or infusion is the most common; enteric-coated tablets (187 mg) three times a day (maximum), are also used; peppermint may cause gastroesophageal reflux
3. Chamomile	Gastrointestinal irritation, insomnia, and (German) joint irritation; a higher incidence of threatening miscarriage or preterm labor with regular use has been reported (Cuzzolin 2011).	Tea or infusion
4. Dandelion	A mild diuretic, and to nourish the liver; dandelion is known for high amounts of vitamins A and C, and elements of iron, calcium, and potassium, as well as trace elements.	Tea or infusion
5. Alfalfa	General pregnancy tonic; a source of high levels of vitamins A, D, E, and K, minerals, and digestive enzymes; thought to reduce the risk of postpartum hemorrhage in late pregnancy.	Tea or infusion
6. Oat and oat straw	Sources of calcium and magnesium; helps to relieve anxiety, restlessness, insomnia, and irritable skin.	Tea or infusion
7. Nettle leaf	All-around pregnancy tonic; sources of high amounts of vitamins A, C, K, and calcium, potassium; and iron. NB: Nettle root (different from nettle leaf) is used for inducing abortions and is not safe in pregnancy; nettle-leaf tea is a traditional tea in pregnancy and lactation.	Tea or infusion
Slippery elm bark	Nausea, heartburn, and vaginal irritations.	Tea or infusion

2.19.7   Herbs controversially used during pregnancy

These herbs, listed in Table 2.19.3, are commonly used during pregnancy and, with some controversy, are considered effective and safe by the preponderance of both evidence based and traditional evidence.

Table 2.19.3 Herbs controversially used during pregnancy

Herb	Usage	Form and dosage	Safety
1. Ginger	Nausea and vomiting, or morning sickness.	250 mg four times a day maximum; ginger is also frequently used as a tea or infusion.	Ginger is the only herb with reasonable evidence-based data regarding its benefit and safety during pregnancy. In several studies, it is estimated to be safe when used at doses of 250 mg four times a day or less (Low Dog 2005, Blumenthal 2003). Three published placebo-controlled trials have addressed the safety and efficacy of ginger for morning sickness. In 1990, Fischer-Rasmussen reported 30 pregnant women, randomly assigned, who were admitted to the hospital before 20 weeks' gestation, and received either 250 mg of powdered ginger capsules or placebo four times a day over a 4-day period. No adverse effects on the pregnancy and outcome were noted. Vutyavanich (2001) conducted a randomized double-blind placebo-controlled study of 70 women with nausea of pregnancy with or without vomiting before the seventeenth week. Again, either 250 mg powdered ginger capsules or placebo four times a day was used. Good efficacy was reported, and no adverse effects were noted on pregnancy outcomes. A study by Willetts (2003), in a double-blind placebo-controlled trial, randomly assigned 120 women before the twentieth week of gestation who had experienced morning sickness daily for at least a week. These patients received either 125 mg of ginger extract or placebo four times a day. Again, the efficacy was excellent, and outcomes were normal. Follow-up of the pregnancies revealed normal ranges of birth weight, gestational age, Apgar scores, and frequencies of congenital abnormalities when the study group infants were compared to the general population of infants born that year. Surprisingly, the German Commission E (Blumenthal 1998) and the American Herbal Products Association (McGaffin 1997) contraindicate the use of ginger during pregnancy. This is definitely not supported by the popular data, popular experience, or traditional-based evidence. Their advice appears to be based on two concerns. The first is that inhibition of thromboxane synthetase may affect testosterone binding in the fetus, although this usually happens at much higher doses than those practically used or used in the studies (Backon 1991). The second concern is *in vitro* evidence that gingerol and shogoal, isolated components of ginger, exhibit mutagenic activity in certain salmonella strains (Nagabhushan 1987). However, researchers have also found potential anti-mutagenic compounds in ginger (Fudler 1991). In that regard, however, a study of rats failed to find malformations in the offspring of animals administered 20 g/l or 50 g/L of ginger tea in their drinking water in early pregnancy. Researchers at the Hospital For Sick Children in Toronto, Canada, studied 187 pregnant women who used some form of ginger in the first trimester (Portnoi 2003). In this small study, there were no increased risks in babies with congenital malformations compared to a control group. With the vast number of women taking ginger during pregnancy, it is reasonable to assume that it is safe for women to use small amounts (up to 250 mg four times a day) of ginger during pregnancy. However, it is prudent to use ginger in moderation (Low Dog 2005, Blumenthal 2003, Muller 1997, Fudler 1991). See also chapter 2.4.3.

2.	Cranberry	Prevention and treatment of urinary tract infection (Wing 2008, Mills 2006, Low Dog 2005, Blumenthal 2003)	300–400 mg three times daily	There is a long history of the safe and effective use of cranberry during pregnancy but only a few studies confirming this.
3.	Evening primrose oil	Mastalgia, mood swings (Hibbeln 2002)	500 mg daily	There are no known restrictions on the use of evening primrose oil during pregnancy (Chen 1999, Brown 1996, Harrobin 1992, 1991). No teratogenic effects have been seen, based on animal studies. According to The World Health Organization, pregnant and lactating women should obtain 5% of their total daily caloric intake from evening primrose, from EFA (essential fatty acids).
4.	Aloe vera gel	Topical use (only), for burns (Low Dog 2005, Blumenthal 2003)	Gel	Although there is a long history of safe topical use during pregnancy, there are no studies showing its safety.
5.	Echinacea	Prevention and treatment of upper respiratory tract infections, vaginitis, and herpes simplex virus (Gallo 2000, Blumenthal 1998, McGaffin 1997, Mengs 1991).	900 mg of dried root (or equivalent) three times daily.	Although there is a long history of safe use during pregnancy, there are very few studies (Gallo 2000, Mengs 1991) showing its safety. Early animal studies have failed to demonstrate evidence of mutagenicity or carcinogenicity after 4 weeks of ingestion of the expressed use of Echinacea at doses that far exceed normal human consumption. A prospective study of 206 pregnant women found no increased risk for fetal malformations when Echinacea was ingested during pregnancy, even during the first trimester (Gallo 2000). The authors of these studies suggest that gestational use of Echinacea during organogenesis is not associated with a detectable increased risk of malformations, but these studies did not have the statistical power or sufficient scientific rigor to assure this. The British Herbal Compendium, The German Commission E Monograph (Blumenthal 1998), and The American Herbal Products Association (McGaffin 1997) have listed the use of Echinacea as not contraindicated during pregnancy.

(Continued)

2.19 Herbs during pregnancy

Table 2.19.3 (*Continued*)

Herb	Usage	Form and dosage	Safety
6. St John's wort	Mild to moderate depression (Low Dog 2005, Blumenthal 2003).	300 mg three times daily, of a standardized extract.	Although its safety in pregnancy has not been scientifically evaluated, the German Commission E (Blumenthal 1998, 2003) and the American Herbal Products Association (Blumenthal 2003, McGaffin 1997) state that St John's wort is not contraindicated. Its use in pregnant women is commonly reported. However, there have not been any adequate clinical trials using evidence-based principles that can absolutely reassure of safety of St John's wort for the pregnant or lactating woman. In one study in mice (Fudler 1991), maternal administration of 180 mg/kg of hypericum before and throughout gestation did not affect the long-term growth or physical maturation of exposed mouse offspring. In another study, no adverse effects were noted in the offspring of animals given 1.5 g/kg per day of hypericum. No chromosomal aberrations have been found on *in vitro* or animal testing. In one published case report, low levels of hyperforin were found in the breast milk of a woman who had been taking 300 mg three times a day of a standard extract of St John's wort while nursing (a standard dose). No adverse effects were noted in the mother or the infant (Rayburn 2001, Mills 2000, Okpanyi 1991). It should be noted that St John's wort induces CYP 3A4 and P-glycoprotein, which can result in decreased action of many drugs. Photosensitization has also been reported.
7. Valerian root	Anxiety, insomnia (Low Dog 2005, Blumenthal 2003).	Tea/capsule: 2–3 g of crude herb at bedtime	No contraindications have been found in the literature, including The German Commission E (Blumenthal 2003, McGaffin 1997) and the Botanical Safety Handbook (McGaffin 1997). Several articles and books support the use of valerian during pregnancy, and generally conclude that occasional use, for insomnia, is safe. Traditional clinical use supports its safety, and therapists use it for pregnant and lactating women. The World Health Organization (WHO) (Low Dog 2005), on the other hand, contraindicates the use of valerian during pregnancy and lactation as a general precaution, because its safety has not been established clinically – i.e. there are no clinical trials available using evidence-based medicine to prove its safety. In one study, *valepotriates*, the key constituent in valerian, was given orally for 30 days to pregnant rats, and there were no adverse findings in the pregnant rats or in their offspring. To date, there have been no studies of human pregnancies (Low Dog 1005, Blumenthal 1998, Tufik 1994).
8. Milk thistle (Silymarin)	Intrahepatic cholestasis of pregnancy, alcoholic and non-alcoholic liver cirrhosis, chronic and acute viral hepatitis, drug induced liver toxicity, fatty degeneration of the liver (Giannola 1998, Reys 1992, 1993).	400 mg of standardized silymarin extract in two to three divided doses per day. Second and third trimester only.	There are many references in the literature for the use of milk thistle in pregnancy for liver dysfunctions. There are also concerns and warnings about possible significant side effects. There are limited evidence-based studies to recommend milk thistle in pregnancy. However, the few evidence – based studies do support the safety and efficacy for use in these specific situations. In four studies, no evidence of adverse effects was reported in mothers and offspring (Reys 1992, 1993, Giannola 1998).

	Usage	Dosage	Comments
9. Senna	Constipation (Gattuso 1994).	10–60 mg at bedtime for a maximum of 10 days – in second and third trimester only.	Controversial because senna is a member of the anthraquinone laxative group thought contraindicated in pregnancy because of the potential to stimulate the uterus. The Compendium in Herbal Safely recommends to avoid in pregnancy; but there are no reports in the literature showing it is contradicted. A literature review (Gattuso 1994, Mills 2006, Hess 2013) and traditional use recommends senna as the stimulant laxative of choice in pregnancy.
10. Horse chestnut	Chronic venous insufficiency.	300 mg divide daily of venistatin (reg)retard (240 to 290 mg horse chestnut seed extract standardized to 50 mg escin) DO NOT use RAW horse chestnut preparations, which can be toxic and lethal when ingested.	Been shown to significantly reduce leg edema, varicose veins, chronic venous insufficiency. One very good randomized placebo controlled trial of 52 women showed improvements without serious side effects after 2 weeks of use (Reys 1992, 1993).
11. Horse chestnut gel	Hemorrhoids (Steiner 1991, Mills 2006)	Topical 2% (escin) gel 2–4 times per day	The few studies have shown horse chestnut gel safe and efficacious, particularly with severe hemorrhoids in pregnancy (Steiner 1991, Mills 2006).

2.19 Herbs during pregnancy

2.19.8 Herbs contraindicated during pregnancy

There are numerous herbs that are thought to be contraindicated during pregnancy, or that traditional herbalists consider potentially contraindicated during pregnancy. Studies are minimal, however (see Low Dog 2005, Blumenthal 2003, Blumenthal 1998, Weed 1986). These herbs can be classified into five subgroups for an understanding of their potential effect on a pregnant woman:

1. Herbs used traditionally to stimulate menstruation (Table 2.19.4). Herbs that may stimulate the smooth muscle of the uterus may be risky during pregnancy, as they may cause a pregnancy loss.
2. Alkaloid-containing herbs (Table 2.19.5). Alkaloids are a diverse group of chemical plant constituents that have a wide range of pharmacological impacts on the body. Some alkaloids have been shown to be hepatotoxic and potentially carcinogenic. In some instances these compounds can be very potent, and they have been isolated as medications or as the active ingredients in many pharmaceuticals and herbs.

Table 2.19.4 Herbs used traditionally to stimulate menstruation (not recommended during pregnancy)

Herb	Usage
Angelica	Diuretic and diaphoretic
Celandine	Loss of appetite; liver and gallbladder complaints
Goldenseal	Dyspepsia, gastritis, diarrhea, menorrhagia
Shepherd's purse	Arrhythmia, hypertension, hypotension, nosebleeds, PMS
Barberry	Constipation, loss of appetite, heartburn
Dong Quai	Hormone imbalance, PMS, menopause
Motherwort	Arrhythmia, hyperthyroid, flatulence, PMS
Southernwood	Anxiety, depression
Black Cohosh	Menstrual irregularity, PMS, menopause
Ephedra	Bronchospasms (bronchodilator), nasal congestion, weight loss
Mugwort	Gastrointestinal complaints, sedative
Tansy	Migraines, antihelminthic, neuralgia, rheumatism, loss of appetite
Blue Cohosh*	Gynecologic disorders, dysmenorrhea, dyspareunia, menorrhagia, labor induction, antispasmodic symptoms during labor
Feverfew	Migraines; nausea and vomiting associated with migraines
Rue	Menstrual disorders, contraception, abortifacient, anti-inflammatory
Yarrow	Loss of appetite, dyspepsia, liver and gallbladder complaints
Nettle root	Urinary tract infections, kidney and bladder stones, rheumatism
Baldo	Depression, stimulant
Andrographis	Anxiety, gastritis

*Blue Cohosh has been used by some medical providers to induce labor at the end of a pregnancy (Weed 1986, Dugoua 2008).

3. Essential oils (Table 2.19.6). Essential oils are frequently used by patients in many situations. Some essential oils are potentially very dangerous during pregnancy when ingested. All essential oils should be appropriately diluted when used, and none should be taken internally. In some instances, especially with external use, essential oils may be safe, but in general – especially during pregnancy – they are contraindicated.
4. Anthraquinone laxatives (Table 2.19.7). Anthraquinones are very potent compounds which can stimulate bowel peristalsis. They are frequently used as potential laxative agents. In pregnancy, overstimulation of the bowel or bladder has the potential to irritate/stimulate the uterus in some women, and may cause premature labor.
5. Herbs thought to have an effect on the hormonal system (Table 2.19.8). Herbs that may have an effect on the hormonal system, and that have potential estrogen-like properties, give scientists cause for concern regarding the possible effects on the fetus.

Table 2.19.5 Alkaloid-containing herbs (contraindicated during pregnancy)

Herb	Usage
Autumn crocus	Digestion stimulation
Broom	Hypertension, edema, menorrhagia, postpartum hemorrhage
Comfrey	Gastritis, gastrointestinal ulcers, external bruises, and blunt injuries
Mandrake (podophyllin)*	One of the oldest medicinal plants; stomach ulcers, colic, hay fever
Barberry	Constipation, loss of appetite, heartburn
Coffee**	Stimulation, increased performance, migraines, diarrhea, inflammation of the mouth/pharynx, weight loss
Goldenseal	Dyspepsia, gastritis, diarrhea, and menorrhagia
Tansy	Migraines, antihelminthic, neuralgia, rheumatism, loss of appetite
Blood root	Expectorant, antiplaque agent, mouthwash
Colt's foot	Treatment and prevention of diseases of the respiratory tract

*Animal studies have suggested risks of reproductive and developmental toxicity (Joneja 1974, Dwornik 1967, Thiersch 1963).
**More than two cups per day of freshly brewed coffee (Christian 2001, Mills 1993).

Table 2.19.6 Essential oils (contraindicated during pregnancy when taken orally)

Herb	Usage
Arbor vitae	Liver cleanse, loss of appetite, anxiety
Juniper	Acne, liver problems, urinary tract infections, fluid retention
Pennyroyal	Digestive disorders, colds, increased micturition
Nutmeg	Stomach complaints
Catnip	Colds, colic, migraines, nervous disorders, gynecologic disorders
Rosemary	Loss of appetite, blood pressure problems, liver and gallbladder complaints, rheumatism
Baldo	Depression, stimulant

Table 2.19.7 Anthraquinone laxatives (not recommended during pregnancy)

Herb	Usage
Alder buckthorn	Constipation, anal fissures, hemorrhoids, diuretic
Cascara	Constipation, anal fissures, hemorrhoids
Purging buckthorn	Constipation, anal fissures, hemorrhoids
Senna*	Constipation, anal fissures, hemorrhoids

*In general, Senna as an anthraquinone laxative would not be recommended. But, studies indicate it is effective and probably safe in the second and third trimester (see Section 2.19.3).

Table 2.19.8 Herbs with potential hormonal action (not recommended during pregnancy)

Herb	Usage
Ginseng	Adaptogen, general tonic, fatigue
Licorice	Gastric disorders, upper respiratory disorders, menorrhagia, menopause
Chasteberry (Vitex)*	Menstrual disorders
Saw palmetto	Benign prostatic hyperplasia, menopause
Passion flower	Nervousness and insomnia
Isoflavones	PMS, menstrual disorders, menopause
Red clover	Coughs, respiratory conditions, PMS, menopause
Flaxseed	Hyperlipidemia, atherosclerosis, breast cancer, constipation, IBS, diverticulitis, gastritis
Hops	Anxiety, insomnia

*Chasteberry is sometimes used by experienced practitioners to treat and/or prevent postpartum bleeding.

> **Recommendation.** It is important to remember, and to remind patients, that it is critical to know the safety issues regarding particular herbs during pregnancy, and also critical to know the doses, stability, and purity of the product. www. ConsumerLab.com is an extremely helpful resource in this regard.

▶ Useful websites

American Botanical Council (www.herbalgram.org).
CAM On Pubmed http://nccam.nih.gov/research/camonpubmed and www.pubmed.gov).
HerbMed (www.herbmed.org).
International Bibliographic Information On Dietary Supplements (IBIDS) Database (http://ods.od.nih.gov/health_information/ibids.aspx).
Natural Medicines Comprehensive Data Base (www.naturaldatabase.com).
Natural Standard (www.naturalstandard.com).
United States Pharmacopeia Dietary Supplement Verification Program (www.uspveri-fied.org).
www.ConsumerLab.com (for evaluating preparations).

References

Backon J, Fischer-Rasmussen W. Ginger in preventing nausea and vomiting of pregnancy; a caveat do to its thromboxane synthetase activity and effect on testosterone binding. Eur J Obstet Gynecol Reprod Biol 1991; 42: 163–4.

Bercaw J, Maheshwari B, Sangi-Hangpeykar H. The use during pregnancy of prescription, over-the-counter, and alternative medications among hispanic women. Birth 2010; 37: 211.

Blumenthal M. (ed.) The ABC Clinical Guide To Herbs. New York: Thieme Medical Publishing, 2003.

Blumenthal M, Gruenwald J, Hall C et al. (eds). The Complete German Commission E Monographs: Therapeutic Guide To Herbal Medicine. Boston, MA: Integrative Medicine Communications, 1998.

Brinker F. Herb Contraindications And Drug Interactions. Sandy, OR: Eclectic Institute, 1997.

Brown D. Herbal Prescriptions for Better Health. Rockland, CA: Prima Publishing, 1996, pp. 79–89.

Chen J. Evening Primrose Oil – Continuing Education Module. Bolder, CO: University of Southern California School of Pharmacy, 1999.

Christian MS, Brent RL. Teratogen update: evaluation of the reproductive and developmental risks of caffeine. Teratology 2001; 64: 51–78.

Cuzzolin L, Francini-Pesenti F, Veriato G et al. Use of herbal products among 392 Italian Pregnant women: focus on pregnancy outcome. Pharmacoepidemiol Drug Saf 2011; Nov 19: 1151–8.

Dugoua JJ, Seely D, Perri D et al. Safety and efficacy of cranberry [vaccinium macrocarpon] during pregnancy and lactation. Can J Pharmacol 2008; 15: e80–6.

Dwornik JJ, Moore KL. Congenital anomalies produced in the rat by podophyllin. Anat Rec 1967; 157: 237.

Fischer-Rasmussen W. Ginger treatment of hyperemesis gravidarum. Eur J Obstet Gynecol Reprod Biol 1990; 38: 19–24.

Fleming T. (ed.) PDR For Herbal Medicines, 3rd edn. Montvale, NJ: Medical Economics Company, 2004.

Fudler S, Tenne M. Ginger as an anti-nausea remedy in pregnancy; the issue of safety. Herbalgram 1991; 38: 47–50.

Fugh-Berman A, Kronenberg F. Complementary and alternative medicine(CAM) in reproductive-age women: A review of randomized controlled trials. Reproductive Toxicology 2003; 17: 137–52.

Gallo M, Sarkarm M, Au W. Pregnancy outcome following gestational exposure to Echinacea: a prospective controlled study. Arch Intern Med 2000; 160: 3141–3.

Gattuso JM, Kamm MA. Adverse effects of drugs used in the management of constipation and diarrhea. Drug Saf 1994; 10: 47–65.

Giannola C, Buogo F, Forestiere G. A two centered study on the effects of silymarin in pregnant women and adult patients with so-called minor hepalic insuffiency. Clin Ther 1998, 114: 129–35.

Glover DG, Amonkar M, Rybeck BF. Prescription, over-the-counter, and herbalmedicine use in a rural, obstetric population. Am J Obstet Gynecol 2003; 88: 1039–45.

Harrobin N. Nutritional and medical importance of gamma-linolenic acid. Progn Lipid Reis 1992; 31: 163–94.

Harrobin N, Alice K, Morris-Fisher. The effects of evening primrose oil, safflower oil and paraffin on plasma fatty acid levels in humans: choice of an appropriate placebo for clinical studies on primrose oil. Prostagland Leukot Essent Fatty Acids 1991; 42: 245–9.

Hess HM. Herbs and Alternative Remedies. In Clinical Pharmacology During Pregnancy (Mattison DR, Ed) San Diego: Academic Press, 2013, pp. 383–94.

Hibbeln JR. Seafood consumption, the DHA content of mother's milk and prevalence rates of postpartum depression: a cross-national, ecological analysis. J Affect Disord 2002; 69: 15–29.

Holst L, Nordeng H, Haavik S. Use of herbal drugs during early pregnancy in relation to maternal characteristics and pregnancy outcomes. Pharmacoloepidemiol Drug Saf 2008; 17: 151–9.

Holst L, Wright D, Haavik S et al. The use and the user of herbal remedies during pregnancy. J Altern Complement Med 2009; 15: 787–92.

Holst L, Wright D, Haavik S et al. Safety and efficacy of herbal remedies in obstetrics – review and clinical implications. Midwifery 2010; 27: 80–6.

Joneja MG, LeLiever WC. Effects of vinblastine and podophyllin on DBA on mouse fetuses. Toxicol Appl Pharmacol 1974; 27: 408–14.

Lapi F, Vaunacci A, Moschini M et al. Use, attitudes and knowledge of complementary and alternative drugs (CADs) among pregnant women: a preliminary survey in Tuscany. Evid Based Complement Alternat Med 2012; 7: 477–86.

Low Dog T. The use of botanicals during pregnancy and lactation. Altern Ther Health Med 2009: 15: 54–8.

Low Dog T, Micozzi MS. Women's Health in Complementary and Integrative Medicine: a Clinical Guide. Oxford: Elsevier, 2005.

McFarland BC, Gilson MH, O'Rear J et al. A national survey of herbal preparation use by nurse midwives for labor stimulation. Review of the literature and recommendations for practice. J Nurse Midwif 1999; 44: 205–16.

McGaffin M, Hobb C, Upton R et al. American Herbal Products Association's Botanical Safety Handbook. Boca Raton, FL: CRC Press, 1997.

Mengs U, Clare CB, Poiley JA. Toxicity of Echinacea purpurea. Acute, subacute and genotoxicity studies. Arzneim-Forsch Drug Res 1991; 41: 1976–81.

Mills S, Bone K. Principles and Practice of Phytotherapy. London: Churchill Livingstone, 2000; 548–9.

Mills E, Dugoua J, Perri D et al. Herbal Medicines in Pregnancy and Lactation. An Evidence-Based Approach. Boca Raton: Taylor and Francis, 2006.

Mills JL, Holmes LB, Aarons JH et al. Moderate caffeine use and the risk of spontaneous abortion and intrauterine growth retardation. J Am Med Assoc 1993; 269: 593–7.

Moussally K, Oraichiu D, Berard A. Herbal products use during pregnancy: Prevalance and predictors. Pharmacoepidemiol Drug Saf 2009; 18: 454–61.

Muller J, Clauson KA. Pharmaceutical considerations of common herbal medicine. Am J Managed Care 1997; 3: 1753–70.

Nagabhushan M. Mutagenicity of gingerol and shogoal and antimutagenicity of zingerone, in Parsons Salmonella/microsome assay. Cancer Lett 1987; 36: 221–3.

Nordeng H, Bayne K, Haynen GC, Paulsen BS. Use of herbal drugs during pregnancy among 600 Norwegian women in relation to concurrent use of conventional drugs and pregnancy outcome: Complement Ther Clin Pract 2011; 17: 147–51.

Okpanyi SN, Lidzba H, Scholl BC. Genotoxicity of standardized Hypericum extract. Arzneimettl-Forsch 1991; 40: 851–5.

Parsons M, Simpson M, Ponton TJ. Raspberry leaf and its effect on labour: safety and efficacy. Aust Coll Midwives 1999; 12: 20–25.

Portnoi G, Chng LA, Karimi-Tabesh L et al. Prospective comparative study of the safety and effectiveness of ginger for the treatment of nausea and vomiting in pregnancy. Am J Obstet Gynecol 2003; 189: 1374–7.

Rayburn WF, Gonzalez CL, Christense HB. Effect of prenatally administered hypericum (St John's wort) on growth and physical maturation of mouse offspring. Am J Obstet Gynecol 2001; 184: 191–5.

Reys H. The spectrum of liver and gastrointestinal diseases seen in cholestasis of pregnancy. Gastrointestinal Clin North Am 1992; 21: 905–21.

Reys H, Simm FR. Intrahepatic cholestasis of pregnancy.An estrogen-related disease. Semin Liver Dis 1993; 13: 289–301.

Rotblatt M, Zimint I. Evidence-Based Herbal Medicine. Philadelphia, PA: Lippincott Williams & Wilkins, 2002.

Sharma H, Chandola HM, Singh G et al. Utilization of Ayurveda in health care: An approach for prevention, health promotion, and treatment for disease. Part 2. Ayurveda in primary health care. J Altern Complement Med. 2007; 13: 1135–50.

Steiner, M. "Untersuchungen Zur odemvermindernden und odemportektiven wirking von ro kastanienoamenextrakt. Phlebol Prookto 1991; 19: 239–42.

Thiersch JB. Effect of podophyllin and podophyllotoxine on the rat litter in utero. Proc Soc Exper Biol 1963; 113: 124–7.

Tufik S, Fujita K, Seabra M de L. Effects of a prolonged administration ofvalepotriates in rats on the mothers and their offspring. J Ethnophamacol 1994; 41: 39–44.

Vutyavanich T, Kraisarint T. Ginger for nausea and vomiting in pregnancy: randomized, double-masked, placebo-controlled trial. Ruangsrira Obstet Gynecol 2001; 97: 577–82.

Wang CC, Li L, Tang LY et al. Safety evaluation of commonly used Chinese herbal medicines during pregnancy in mice. Hum Reprod 2012; 27: 2448–56.

Weed S. Wise Woman Herbal For The Childbearing Year. Woodstock, NY: Ash Tree Publishing, 1986.

Willetts KE, Ekangahi A, Eden JA. Effect of a ginger extract on pregnancy-induced nausea: a randomised controlled trial. Aust NZ J Obstet Gynaecol 2003; 43: 139–44.

Wing DA, Rumney PJ, Preslicka CW, Chung JH. Daily cranberry juice for prevention of asymptomatic bacteriuria in pregnancy: A randomized controlled pilot study. J Urol 2008; 180: 367–72.

Diagnostic agents

Stefanie Hultzsch

2.20

2.20.1	Diagnostic imaging	527
2.20.2	Contrast media	531
2.20.3	Radioactive isotopes	534
2.20.4	Stable isotopes	536
2.20.5	Dyes	537
2.20.6	Other diagnostic agents	538

Before exposing a woman who is, or may be, pregnant to diagnostics, a pertinent risk-benefit estimation should be made, as exposure towards ionizing radiation must be minimized. Magnetic resonance tomography (MRT) can be safely used but ultrasonography remains the imaging method of choice. Contrast agents should only be applied if the diagnosis cannot be made without their use. After 12 weeks of gestation, intrauterine exposure to iodinated contrast agents can result in disturbances of fetal thyroid function. Radioactive isotopes should be avoided if possible, especially radioactive iodine. After inadvertent exposure to radioactive isotopes, a calculation of the radiation dose should be made to estimate any risk to the embryo/fetus.

Diagnostic dyes should be used with caution. When used for marking twin pregnancies in amniocentesis, small bowel atresia as a fetotoxic effect has been described in the literature. For the diagnosis of a ruptured membrane, indigo carmine is the agent of choice, if the leak cannot be ruled out by any other method.

2.20.1   Diagnostic imaging

Before any examination of a pregnant woman with imaging procedures, the benefits and risks of the respective examination should be assessed.

▶ X-ray examinations

X-rays are ionizing radiation

The energy dose is expressed in Gray (Gy). (The old dose unit was rad: 1 Gray = 100 rad.) During pregnancy the uterus dose resp. the embryo/fetus dose is relevant. The actual effective equivalent dose in the target organ (embryo) is expressed in Sievert (Sv). (The old dose designation was rem: 1 Sv = 100 rem.) For a simpler calculation of the effective organ dose a dimensionless radiation-weighting factor is used, which describes the effect of radiation on the human body. It is determined experimentally and fixed at 1, i.e. 1 Sv = 1 Gy for X-ray or γ- and β-rays, respectively. Generally, in practice milli-Sievert (1 mSv = 0.001 Sv) is used.

The dose range of usual X-ray studies

The embryo/fetus dose with usual X-ray examinations (including the lower abdomen) typically lies significantly under 50 mSv. For an individual abdominal, pelvic or lumbar spinal picture without shielding the uterus, the gonad dose is frequently even lower than 2 mSv (ICRP 2000). With multiple radiograms with the uterus in the primary radiation beam, the total uterine dose must be calculated. For this purpose, it is important to know the tube voltage in kilovolts (kV), the thickness of the aluminum filter, the filter-skin distance, and the beam direction. Longer fluoroscopy times in imaging of the gastrointestinal tract or kidneys and urinary tract, could actually lead to a uterus load of 20 mSv. Table 2.20.1 provides dose values per minute for the worst case when the uterus lies in the primary radiation beam. The values vary depending the patient's constitution (diameter) and the direction of exposure.

Table 2.20.1 Maximum value of the equivalent dose level for the uterus in mSv/min during X-ray screening with image enhancing television chain (according to the DGMP-Report 2002, www.dgmp.de)

Projection	a.p.	a.p.	a.p.	p.a.	p.a.	p.a.	Lateral
Constitution	thin cm	normal, 22 cm	thick 6 cm	thin, 17 cm	normal, 22 cm	thick, 26 cm	normal, 36 cm
Equivalent-dose	16	24	40	8	12	20	32

a.p. = anterior-posterior.
p.a. = posterior-anterior.

With computerized tomographic (CT) studies, the location of the examination is of primal importance. When the uterus is in the primary X-ray beam a uterus dose between 20 and 40 mSv – very rarely over 50 mSv – is calculated with a CT examination in modern multi-layer-spiral CT consoles. The dose is dependent upon the number of scans, the collimation, the pitch, the tube voltage, and the tube current. For a simplified estimate of the uterus dose, the volume computed tomography index ($CTDI_{vol}$), i.e. the mean radiation dose in the volume of a rotation, can be used (Huda 2010, Jaffe 2009). This value is given on all modern CT consoles. Only when the $CTDI_{vol}$ lies significantly over 20 mGy, and the uterus is in the primary X-ray beam, should a specialized center be consulted for a detailed individual estimate of the uterus dose through patient- and equipment-specific data. The scattered radiation from examinations of other body regions, such as the upper abdomen, thorax, extremities or head, can be ignored because it is generally below 1 mSv. Nevertheless, attention should always be paid to using a lead apron to protect against scattered radiation because this further reduces the total dose (Kennedy 2007). Modern CT consoles have several mechanisms that reduce patient dose without sacrificing diagnostic power, e.g. dose modulation protocols. In contrast to the American Thoracic Society, which recommends lung scintigraphy for pregnant women with suspected pulmonary embolism (PE) and normal chest X-rays (Leung 2012), other experts recommend CT pulmonary angiography as first line diagnostic imaging modality before scintigraphy (Browne 2014, Duran-Mendicuti 2011). During CT of the chest, the fetus is outside the primary X-ray beam and receives only indirect, scattered irradiation. Iodinated contrast agents should only be used if clearly indicated because of the added risk of fetal hypothyroidism (compare Section 2.20.2) and the exposure to ionizing radiation should be kept as low as possible.

▶ Effects of radiation

With X-rays – as with other ionizing rays – two categories of biological radiation effects are distinguished: deterministic and stochastic effects. Deterministic effects only appear above a certain threshold dose and lead to a reduction or a complete loss of organ or tissue function due to cellular death (Minkov 2009). Teratogenic effects belong to these deterministic effects. Depending on the dose and the embryonic developmental stage, this may result in the death of the embryo, or malformation of various organ systems, specifically the eyes, general growth retardation, microcephaly and mental retardation. This has been documented both in animal experiments as well as empirically in humans (Brent 1999a). During the first 5 days after conception (i.e., during the "all-or-nothing phase") the lowest lethal dose is calculated at 100 mGy. During actual embryogenesis, this value is estimated at 250–500 mGy, then later at >1 Gy (Brent 1999a). Severe CNS malformations during the early embryogenesis period (18–36 days after conception) are only to be expected beginning at 200 mGy. Permanent growth retardation can be expected at 250–500 mGy. Microcephaly and mental retardation is observed, above all, after doses >200 mGy between gestational weeks 10 and 17.

With a radiation dose of <50 mGy most studies conclude that no substantially increased malformation risk in humans is expected (Brent 1999a; Sternberg 1973). One study observed a lower birth weight after dental X-rays during pregnancy. The authors speculated that impairment of maternal thyroid function by X-rays was responsible for these findings (Hujoel 2004). Other authors discuss the underlying dental illness as causal (Lockhart 2004).

Much more difficult than estimating the teratogenic X-ray risk is assessing the stochastic mutagenic and carcinogenic effects, because there is no threshold dose under which no effect would be expected. Damage of a single cell can lead to an illness which, with higher exposure may result in a greater incidence of, for example, leukemia following prenatal X-ray exposure (Brent 2009). Point mutations might also occur spontaneously. The radiation dose leading to a doubling of the point mutation rate is given as 1.2 Gy (Brent 1999a; Neel 1999). A doubling of the mutation rate of a certain gene does not necessarily mean a doubling of the associated frequency of the disease. On the other hand, the completely inadequate knowledge of the effects on later generations must lead to greater caution in the definition of safe exposure values for the population at large (Brent 1999a).

Empirical evidence on the risk for stochastic X-ray effects in the literature is still inconsistent. Among the parents of some 500 children with neuroblastomas, the use of X-ray examinations before pregnancy was no more frequent than that in a healthy control group (Patton 2004). In a case

Pregnancy

2.20 Diagnostic agents

control study no significant association between a history of radiography in pregnancy and a risk of childhood leukemia was found (Kumar 2014). A study of twin pregnancies reported a 2.4 factor increase in the risk of leukemia with a fetal dose of 0.01 Sv or more (Harvey 1985). Lengfelder (1990) already considers an increased leukemia risk when additional prenatal X-ray exposure of the embryo lies in the range of the natural background radiation of about 0.001 Sv/year. By contrast, other authors assume there is no risk for the embryo with exposure of 0.02–0.05 Sv (Boice 1999). In a case control study from the USA, an increased risk for rhabdomyosarcoma was found in the children of mothers who had had an X-ray examination during pregnancy (Grufferman 2009). However, due to methodological irregularities, these results should be interpreted with necessary caution.

Wakeford (2003) calculated the relative and absolute risk for children under the age of 15 years to become affected by a cancer after intrauterine X-ray exposure. They gave the absolute risk as 8% per Gray. Their detailed calculation was based on the largest world-wide data collection on the risk of cancer through intrauterine X-ray exposure, primarily pelvimetry, in the Oxford Survey of Childhood Cancers (Wakeford 2003). The authors derive comparable risk coefficients from the Japanese data on the atomic bomb victims and conclude that there is also an increased risk from a comparatively low fetal dose of 10 mSv, which, in the 1950s, was reached during a pelvic X-ray. Other authors consider such an assumption of risk to be too high and suggest that the risk of an exposure lower than 100 mSv is negligible compared to the background risk for cancer (Brent, 2013). They also point to the group of intrauterine-exposed Hiroshima victims comprising not even 1,000 survivors, and to the data of the experience of exposed children in Hiroshima. However, these studies, frequently cited as proof for a rather low risk of cancer after radioactive exposure, should be critically evaluated in the light of the methodological shortcomings and the political interests of the American researchers at that time.

▶ Ultrasound

For about 30 years, ultrasound has been used during all phases of pregnancy. Numerous animal experiments (overview in Jensh 1999) and epidemiological studies (overview in Ziskin 1999) have analyzed the effects on the fetus. Negative effects could be caused mainly by local hyperthermia. Although anomalies such as an increase in fetal activity, reduced birth weight, delayed speech development and increased left-handedness, have been mentioned by individual researchers (Newnham 1993, Visser 1993) as consequences of ultrasound examinations, these effects cannot be confirmed (Sheiner 2012). Follow-up studies on considerably more than 1,000 children between the ages of 1–8 years, whose mothers had received ultrasound examinations between the eighteenth and thirty-eighth week, showed no differences related to weight gain and other developmental parameters between children whose mothers were examined by ultrasound five times and those whose mothers had only one ultrasound examination (Newnham 2004). Pulsed doppler studies, flow measurements, and studies in the first trimester require a higher dose of energy and, theoretically, can damage embryonic tissue by warming. Thermal or non-thermal damage of the fetus cannot be ruled out, especially with the modern high output devices, and is theoretically conceivable (Abramowicz 2008, Stratmeyer 2008). The AIUM (2013) sees the available data as insufficient for proving a causal relationship between medically indicated ultrasound examinations and damaging effects on the fetus. Using ultrasound only when medically indicated, as well as adhering to the ALARA principle (as low as reasonably achievable), is recommended for obstetrical ultrasound.

► Magnetic resonance imaging (MRI)

With MRI, magnetic fields, which do not differ from other electrical appliances (including radio waves) are created. The magnetic field strength cited for patients is 1.5–3 Tesla (T) and for the examining staff 5 to 100 mT.

MRI has also been used in pregnancies for about 20 years. For example, through MRI, the placenta can be localized, fetal pathologies diagnosed, and the pelvic diameter can be measured (de Wilde 2005). The experience acquired primarily in the second and third trimesters has not found any negative effects on the fetus after exposure to the electromagnetic fields created and to the noise of the device (Kok 2004, Brent 1999b, overviewed in Robert 1999). This also applies to follow-up examinations, including hearing and visual tests in children at the ages of 3 and 8 to 9 years (Kok 2004, Baker 1994). Studies on MRI personnel have given no indication of a reproductive risk (Evans 1993). No statistically significant difference in the diagnostic sensitivity between MRI and CT for the evaluation of acute nontraumatic abdominal pain in pregnancy was found (Baron 2012). Given its lack of ionizing radiation, MRI should be preferred over CT (Khandelwal 2013).

Recommendation. When using diagnostic imaging procedures in pregnancy, ultrasound is the method of choice, especially for questions in the abdominal region. However, video films and pictures made with ultrasound for the family album are not medically indicated. X-ray procedures in the lower abdominal area should be used with caution in women of childbearing age, especially if a pregnancy cannot definitely be ruled out. Apart from life-threatening situations, X-ray examination of the lower abdomen should only be carried out in the first half of the menstrual cycle. For unavoidable X-ray examinations in the uterine region, only the most modern devices should be used, with optimal protection for the uterus. X-ray examinations outside of the genital region are neither an indication for a risk-justified termination of the pregnancy nor for any additional diagnostic procedures (Chapter 1.15). This also applies to the usual X-ray examinations, which may have (inadvertently) included the pregnant uterus. When considering the potential risks of CT and MRI, MRI is preferable at all stages of pregnancy. In cases of CT with uterine exposure during pregnancy a Teratology Information Service should be contacted to calculate and estimate the dosage and the potential risk.

2.20.2   Contrast media

► Bariumsulfate contrast medium

Barium sulfate is used for radiologic opacification of the stomach and intestinal tract. This insoluble compound is not absorbed by the digestive tract. Therefore, no damage to the fetus is expected from this contrast medium during pregnancy. A small prospective cohort study found no increased risk after diagnostic upper gastrointestinal tract fluoroscopic examination with barium swallow in pregnancy (Han 2011).

▶ Iodine-containing contrast media

Iodine-containing contrast agents include: *iobitridol, iodamide, iodixanol, iohexol, iomeprol, iopamidol, iopanoic acid, iopentol, iopodate, iopromide, iotalamic acid, iotrolan, iotroxic acid, ioversol, ioxaglic acid, ioxitalamic acid, lysine amidotrizoate, meglumine amidotrizoate* and *sodium amidotrizoate, metrizamide* and *metrizoate*.

Iodinated contrast media can be separated into two groups: ionic or non-ionic preparations. Ionic hyperosmolaric contrast media may no longer be used intravenously due to their high osmolality with related side effects and are thus used primarily in gastrointestinal diagnostic procedures. The newer, non-ionic preparations have a lower osmolality and are better tolerated. Renal and biliary preparations should also be differentiated. Biliary contrast media are lipophilic and have a high plasma protein binding. This facilitates their elimination by the liver, but also aids transplacental passage. However, nowadays, mostly ultrasound is used for examining the bile ducts. For kidney and urinary tract representation as well as angiography, intravenously administered hydrophilic non-ionic iodinated contrast media are used, which have a low plasma protein binding and are quickly excreted through the kidneys. Case studies have been published which describe transplacental passage following the intravenous administration of non-ionic contrast media to the mother during pregnancy. For example, ioversol, which was seen in high-contrast in the newborn's intestine in a postpartum X-ray (Hill 2007, Saigal 2007). In both case descriptions an anomaly of the placenta (hematoma or infarct) was found, which the authors see as a possible causal etiology. Another case describes radiocontrast material seen on abdomen X-ray of a newborn after iopamidol was applied to the mother twice in the last two weeks of pregnancy (Huang 2014). No details about any placental abnormalities are given. In all three cases the contrast medium was excreted without negative effects.

The amount of free iodine in the contrast medium is normally under 1‰ of the amount of the contrast medium, but can increase with storage. After administration, a further enzymatic release through deiodases is possible. Free iodine can reach the fetal thyroid and be stored there, possibly causing fetal hypothyroidism, when the fetal thyroid starts its endocrine function. In a study the neonatal outcome of 61 pregnant women, who received iodinated contrast agents at eight to thirty-seven weeks of gestation was compared to that of six women, who did not receive any contrast agent during pregnancy. Outcome was assessed by medical chart review only. One of the 64 exposed infants had abnormal thyroid function results (normal thyroid stimulating hormone but low T4), and all the unexposed infants had normal results in the standard neonatal screening program (Kochi 2012). Since the infant with abnormal values was also premature and septic, the authors conclude that no significant clinical effect on the fetus should be expected after the administration of iodinated contrast agents to pregnant women. However, the American College of Radiology (ACR 2013) as well as the European Society of Urogenital Radiology (ESUR 2013) recommend using iodinated contrast agents only if the diagnosis cannot be made any other way and the care of the patient is affected.

Recommendation. After the twelfth week of gestation at the latest, the use of iodine-containing contrast media should be limited to urgent diagnostic indications. The thyroid function of the newborn should be checked postpartum if such treatment was used later in the pregnancy.

▶ **Magnetic resonance contrast media**

Gadopentetic acid, gadobenic acid, gadodiamide, gadofosveset triso-dium, gadoteridol, gadoteric acid, gadoversetamide, and *gadoxetic acid* are ionic paramagnetic contrast media used for MRI. Within a few seconds after maternal injection these substances are detectable in the fetal bladder and are excreted into the amniotic fluid, which, in turn, is ingested orally by the fetus. In the contrast medium, the highly poisonous *gadolinium* is present in a chelate-bound, well-tolerated form. Theoretically, with a longer stay in the body, toxic gadolinium could be freed from the complex, and hence damage the fetus. The available case studies on the administration of gadolinium complex in human beings (De Santis 2007, Marcos 1997) gave no indication of embryonic or fetal toxicity; however, a recent report has found high levels of gadolium +3 (the toxic form) in the placentae of about six% of women in a control population. It is not known if the gadolinium +3 is the result of a previous MRI with contrast (Darrah 2014).

In 2006 a causal relationship between nephrogenic systemic fibrosis (NSF), a fibrosing disease mainly of the skin and subcutaneous tissues, and gadolinium-based contrast agents was discussed (Grobner 2006). The European Society of Urogenital Radiology (Thomsen 2013) therefore recommends that the smallest possible dose of one of the most stable gadolinium contrast agents should be used only when there is a very strong indication for an enhanced MRI. Other publications advise preferentially using the more stable macrocyclic preparations, which are thought to have a lower risk for NSF, in pregnant women (Fröhlich 2013). The American College of Radiology (ACR 2013) recommends that gadolinium-based contrast agents are administered only when there is significant benefit to the patient or fetus that outweighs the possible risk of exposure of the fetus to free gadolinium ions.

Ferristen is considered safe from a theoretical point of view. No human data is available for *Ferucarbotran* and *Ferumoxsil*. In animal experiments, they were not embryotoxic at normal therapeutic doses, although Ferucarbotran proved to be toxic in higher doses. Ferumoxsil should be used only with caution due to possible side effects of additives (Fröhlich 2013).

Manganiferous mangafodipir was shown to be teratogenic in animal experiments. Due to insufficient experience it should not be used in pregnancy. According to ESUR (2013), its use in pregnancy is contraindicated.

In order to avoid contrast agents in neuroimaging in patients with absolute or relative contraindications to their use, time-of-flight magnetic resonance angiography with 3D reconstruction (TOF MRA with 3DR) might also be an option where it is technically possible (Yanamadala 2013).

> **Recommendation.** Gadolinium-containing contrast media should be used at the lowest possible dose and only if the benefits outweigh the risks when the diagnosis cannot be made without their use and the treatment of the patient would be impaired. Ferristen may be used if the benefits outweigh the risks. Ferucarbotran, Ferumoxsil and Mangafodipir should be avoided because of insufficient experience.

▶ **Ultrasound/ultrasonographic-contrast media**

D-Galactose, from which no prenatal toxic risk is to be expected, is used for ultrasound diagnostic procedures. There are no data on *perflutren,*

Pregnancy

2.20 Diagnostic agents

which is used in echocardiography, or *perflubutane* in pregnancy. Experimental animal studies do not permit a conclusion on direct or indirect effects on prenatal development.

Recommendation. D-Galactose may be used for specific indications for diagnostic procedures. Due to insufficient experience, perflutren or perflubutane should be used with caution, if the diagnosis cannot be made without their use.

2.20.3   Radioactive isotopes

Most radiopharmaceuticals today are marked with *technetium-99m*. Also in thyroid scintigraphy technetium has largely replaced iodine. Radioactive iodine compounds are used almost exclusively for thyroid diagnostic procedures (radio-iodine test) in connection with a planned radioactive iodine therapy. For *positron-emissions-tomography* (PET) ^{18}FDG (2-Fluoro-2-Desoxy-D-Glucose) is administered intravenously

The activity of a radiopharmaceutical is given in Becquerels, which gives the median number of atoms, which decay in 1 second ($1\ Bq = 1\ s^{-1}$) In medical use, it is mostly MegaBecquerel ($1\ MBq = 106\ Bq$) that are spoken of. The radiation dose for the embryo during *scintigraphy* is dependent on the radiation characteristics of the radionuclide, the applied activity (dose in MBq) as well as the distributional patterns and elimination behavior of the radiopharmaceutical. It cannot be measured, but must be calculated with simplified assumptions considering the anatomy of the patient and the biokinetics of the radiopharmaceutical, including its half-life. Dose coefficients for the embryo or fetus in the different stages of pregnancy are used (0, 3, 6, 9 months). In Table 2.20.2, the highest presumed values are presented. Yet, unusual individual kinetics may cause higher values. As a rule, the dose coefficient and the dose decline from the beginning to the end of pregnancy.

Table 2.20.2 Energy dose for the embryo/fetus with selected diagnostic and therapeutic nuclear medicine procedures. For applied activities that deviate from this, the dose values should be modified accordingly (according to the DGMP-Report 2002 www.dgmp.de, ICRP 2000 Publication 84)

Organ or method	Radionuclide	Radiopharma-ceutical	Dose coefficient μGy/MBq	Applied activity MBq	Energy dose (embryo/fetus) mGy
Bone scan	^{99m}Tc	MDP, HDP	6.1	750	4.6
Thyroid scan	^{131}I	Iodide	72	2	0.1
Thyroid scan	^{99m}Tc	Pertechnetate	11	75	0.8
Kidney scan	^{99m}Tc	MAG3	18	200	3.6
Lung scan	^{99m}Tc	Microspheres	2.8	200	0.6
Therapy for hyperthyroidism	^{131}I	Iodide	72	750	54
Therapy for thyroid carcinoma	^{131}I	Iodide	72	4,000	288

Iodine metabolism is a distinctive feature. Accumulation of iodine, and also radioiodine, in the fetal thyroid begins around 90 days after conception. In the case of radioiodine application to the mother, this internal radiation exposure must be taken into account in addition to the external radiation when calculating the effective fetal dosage (Minkov 2009). Although there are studies on accumulation in fetal thyroids, dosimetry is still marked by great uncertainty. When giving radioiodine, the maximum dose for the fetal thyroid is reached by the end of the second trimester. When using iodine-131 (^{131}I) for therapy of hyperthyroidism, the thyroid dose is about the same for the fetus as for the mother. Table 2.20.3 summarizes the results of the relevant calculations. The results in Table 2.20.2 indicate that diagnostic uses cause a comparatively low fetal dose. However, radio iodine therapy with ^{131}I for hyperthyroidism and thyroid cancer will generate a fetal dose of 50–300 mGy, resulting in a substantial risk to the fetus. The DGMP-Report (2002) gives more detailed information, in tables, concerning the embryo or fetal dose with radioiodine therapy than the corresponding ICRP 2000 publication 84. It has to be remembered, however, that all these calculations are only model calculations. As Table 2.20.3 shows, ^{131}I can lead to an excessive fetal thyroid dose even with diagnostic use. A therapeutic dose of ^{131}I to the mother after the first trimester carries a high risk for fetal thyroid abnormalities. Nevertheless, there have also been unremarkable outcomes observed after accidental use in early pregnancy. The fetal thyroid stimulating hormone collected by umbilical cord puncture can provide information about the effect of the maternal ^{131}I-therapy, also in still (compensated) euthyroid fetuses and gives indications for a possibly necessary postnatal thyroxin supplementation (Welch 1997).

Today the radioiodine test is used almost exclusively before radioiodine therapy. The usual nuclear medicine diagnostic procedure mostly involves values of less than 10 mGy for the embryo or fetus (ICRP 2000, Adelstein 1999).

Therapeutic (ablative) use of ^{131}I in the years before a pregnancy for hyperthyroidism or thyroid cancer has, according to several studies with some 100 evaluated pregnancies, no adverse effects on the pre- and postnatal development of the child (Bal 2005, Chow 2004, Read 2004, Schlumberger 1996). Of the numerous children in these studies, there are reports on their development right up to adulthood, from which there is no indication of late effects such as development of cancer or genetic defects. However, Schlumberger (1996) did observe an increased rate of miscarriages when the treatment took place within a year before the

Table 2.20.3 Fetal thyroid dose with one-time intake of radiopharmaceutical at different stages of pregnancy (according to the DGMP-Report 2002, www.dgmp.de)

Method	Radiopharmaceutical	Applied activity MBq	Fetal thyroid dose mSv; 95 days	Fetal thyroid dose mSv; 130 days	Fetal thyroid dose mSv; 250 days
Thyroid scintigraphy	^{99m}Tc-pertechnetate	75	0.7	1.7	0.6
Thyroid scintigraphy	^{123}Iodine	10	29	70	27
Radioiodine-test	^{131}Iodide	2	810	1,950	760
Therapy for hyperthyroidism	^{131}Iodide	750	300,000	730,000	280,000

Pregnancy

2.20 Diagnostic agents

pregnancy. The authors discuss both exposure of the gonads as well as inadequate thyroid hormone adjustment as a cause after nuclear medicine therapy. Read (2004) found no birth defects in 36 pregnancies after paternal exposure to ablative treatment with [131]I.

After technetium-scintigraphy of the thyroid or the bones, no increase in the risk of malformations was found (Schaefer 2009). Gropper (2014) found sentinel lymph node biopsy after localization with either 99m-technetium or methylene blue to be a safe and an accurate method in pregnancy. In calculating the dosage after lymphangioscintigraphy for sentinel-lymph node localization (breast cancer or melanoma), a minimal fetal dose, below the annual background load, was found (Spanheimer 2009, Pandit-Taskar 2006).

The dose calculation is more difficult after PET-CT with [18]FDG; here, the radiation load from the CT is added to the estimated load from the radiopharmaceutical. The dose coefficient for [18]FDG is still under discussion. Stabin (2004) gives 22 µGy/MBq for early pregnancy and the first trimester, and 17 µGy/MBq for the second and third trimesters and refers to measurements on primates. Zanotti-Fregonara (2010) calculated the radiation dose for a human fetus in the 10th week of pregnancy and reported a dose coefficient of 40 µGy/MBq. In a report on six stand- alone PET studies (without CT) in five pregnant women using [18]FDG the dose to the fetus was estimated to range from 1.1 to 2.43 mGy for various trimesters in pregnancy (except for one patient in early pregnancy, where uptake of the whole uterus was measured and the fetal dose was estimated to be 9.04 mGy) (Takalkar 2011). All patients delivered healthy infants with no visible abnormalities at term. For a PET-CT with [18]FDG at 21 weeks of pregnancy a fetal dose of 3.6 mGy was calculated (Zanotti-Fregonara 2012). The author explains the lower dose in the second trimester compared to the first trimester with a high glucose turnover in the embryo due to rapid cell proliferation in early pregnancy.

It has to be remembered, however, that all these calculations are only model-calculations which might only be an order of magnitude estimation of the real value.

> **Recommendation.** Diagnostic and therapeutic administration of radioisotopes during pregnancy is contraindicated. Nevertheless, exposure for diagnostic purposes is neither a risk-justified indication for termination of pregnancy nor for invasive diagnostic procedures (Chapter 1.15). When administering a therapeutic dose of ^{131}I for hyperthyroidism or thyroid carcinoma the resulting diagnostic and therapeutic consequences must be discussed individually. A teratology information center should be consulted for advice.

2.20.4   Stable isotopes

Stable isotopes, which are not radioactive and differ from the original element in their atomic weight, have been developed for different elements. After the inclusion of stable isotopes into chemical compounds, for example medications, they can be detected with analytical methods such as, for instance, mass spectrometry. So far, no embryotoxic effects have been observed, either in animal experiments (Spielmann 1986) or in humans.

> **Recommendation.** From a reproductive toxicological perspective, there are no concerns about the use of diagnostic procedures with stable isotopes.

2.20.5   Dyes

Specially developed dyes are used for the determination of heart, liver and kidney function. They include *bromsulphthalein, Evans blue, indigo carmine, Congo red, methylene blue, phenol red* (also known as *phenolsulphthalein*), *toluidine blue* (also known as *tolonium chloride*), *tricarbocyanin* and *trypaflavin*.

Methylene blue and toluidine blue are used to treat methemoglobinemia but can also produce mild methemoglobinemia themselves. Methylene blue and toluidine blue as well as indigo carmine and Evans blue are also used in twin pregnancies to mark one twin during amniocentesis as well as for antepartum localization of leakage from the amniotic sac. Especially with the use of methylene blue and toluidine blue small bowel atresias have been described as fetotoxic effects (e.g. Dinger 2003, Glüer 1995). These are likely consequences of a disturbed perfusion in the small intestine, which is either due to hemolysis or can be explained by the vasoactive effect of the compounds. Especially after the use of methylene blue, but also after toluidine blue, in late pregnancy for the diagnosis of ruptured membranes, newborns may develop hemolysis with neonatal hyperbilirubinemia, skin discoloration and respiratory distress syndrome (Gauthier 2000, overviewed in Cragan 1999, Mehler 2013). Indigo carmine is an analog of serotonin and therefore an indirect vasoactive effect cannot be excluded. So far no effects comparable to those of methylene blue have been reported in over 150 documented pregnancies (Cragan 1993). The American College of Obstetricians and Gynecologists recommends the use of indigo carmine only if leakage of amniotic fluid cannot be excluded any other way (ACOG 2013).

Phenolred is intravenously injected for the PSP (phenolsuphthalein) kidney function test which is no longer regularly used. There is insufficient experience with it or any of the other compounds in pregnancy.

▶ Fluorescent dyes

Fluorescein is administered as a diagnostic agent in the eye, orally and intravenously (angiography). In a case series of over 100 pregnant women who had angiography with fluorescein, no indication of undesirable fetal effects was seen (Halperin 1990). Animal experiments have also shown no teratogenic effects. The substance was documented in the amniotic fluid of a pregnant woman after administration to her eye.

There is also no indication of undesirable effects for the unborn baby with retinal angiography for measuring the micro-circulation and the hepatic blood flow with *indocyanine green* and *sodium iodide*. Indocyanine green could not be demonstrated in the umbilical cord blood (Fineman 2001). The sodium iodide part of 5% of the dry mass can, with the usual dose, lead to an iodide dose of 700 µg/day which, with the usual brief or one-time usage should not lead to any fetal thyroid gland suppression.

Recommendation. In pregnant women, the use of diagnostic dyes should be avoided except for vital indications. The use of methylene blue for marking in amniocentesis is contraindicated. Inadvertent administration does not justify either elective termination of pregnancy or invasive diagnostic procedures (Chapter 1.15). Fluorescent dyes may be used during pregnancy.

Pregnancy

2.20 Diagnostic agents

2.20.6   Other diagnostic agents

Skin tests such as tuberculin tests, or allergy tests are considered to be harmless. The same applies to enzyme tests, e.g. with secretin.

> **Recommendation.** The diagnostic agents mentioned may be used in pregnancy.

References

Abramowicz JS, Barnett SB, Duck FA, et al. Fetal thermal effects of diagnostic ultrasound. J Ultrasound Med 2008; 27: 541–59.

ACOG (American College of Obstetricians and Gynecologists). Practice bulletin no. 139: Premature rupture of membranes. Obstet Gynecol 2013; 122: 918.

ACR (American College of Radiology) Manual on Contrast Media (2013). http://www.acr.org/~/media/ACR/Documents/PDF/QualitySafety/Resources/Contrast%20Manual/2013_Contrast_Media.pdf.

Adelstein SJ. Administered radionuclides in pregnancy. Teratology 1999; 59: 236–9.

AIUM (American Institute of Ultrasound in Medicine). AIUM practice guideline for the performance of obstetric ultrasound examinations. J Ultrasound Med 2013; 32: 1083–101.

Baker PN, Johnson IR, Harvey PR et al. A three-year follow-up of children imaged in utero with echo-planar magnetic resonance. Am J Obstet Gynecol 1994; 170: 32–3.

Bal C, Kumar A, Tripathi M et al. High-dose radioiodine treatment for differentiated thyroid carcinoma is not associated with change in female fertility or any genetic risk to the offspring. Int J Radiat Oncol Biol Phys 2005; 63: 449–55.

Baron KT, Arleo EK, Robinson C, Sanelli PC. Comparing the diagnostic performance of MRI versus CT in the evaluation of acute nontraumatic abdominal pain during pregnancy. Emerg Radiol 2012; 19: 519–25.

Boice JD, Miller RW. Childhood and adult cancer after intrauterine exposure to ionizing radiation. Teratology 1999; 59: 227–33.

Brent RL. Utilization of developmental basic science principles in the evaluation of reproductive risks from pre- and postconception environmental radiation exposures. Teratology 1999a; 59: 182–204.

Brent RL. Reproductive and teratologic effects of low-frequency electromagnetic fields: a review of in vivo and in vitro studies using animal models. Teratology 1999b; 59: 261–86.

Brent RL. Saving lives and changing family histories: appropriate counseling of pregnant women and men and women of reproductive age, concerning the risk of diagnostic radiation exposures during and before pregnancy. Am J Obstet Gynecol 2009; 200: 4–24.

Brent RL. Carcinogenic risks of prenatal ionizing radiation. Semin Fetal Neonatal Med 2013 Dec 27; pii: S1744–165X(13)00118-2.

Browne AM, Cronin CG, NiMhuircheartaigh J et al. Evaluation of imaging quality of pulmonary 64-MDCT angiography in pregnancy and puerperium. AJR Am J Roentgenol 2014; 202: 60–4.

Chow SM, Yau S, Lee SH et al. Pregnancy outcome after diagnosis of differentiated thyroid carcinoma: no deleterious effect after radioactive iodine treatment. Int J Radiat Oncol Biol Phys 2004; 59: 992–1000.

Cragan JD. Teratogen update: methylene blue. Teratology 1999; 60: 42–8.

Cragan JD, Martin ML, Khoury MJ et al. Dye use during amniocentesis and birth defects. Lancet 1993; 341: 1352.

Darrah T, Miller RK, Stodgell CJ et al. Exploring the biometal composition of human placentae from the U.S. National Childrens Study (NCS), Placenta 2014 (in press).

De Santis SM, Straface G, Cavaliere AF et al. Gadolinium periconceptional exposure: pregnancy and neonatal outcome. Acta Obstet Gynecol Scand 2007; 86: 99–101.

De Wilde JP, Rivers AW, Price DL. A review of the current use of magnetic resonance imaging in pregnancy and safety implications for the fetus. Prog Biophys Mol Biol 2005; 87: 335–53.

DGMP-Report (Deutsche Gesellschaft für Medizinische Physik und Deutsche Röntgengesellschaft) German Society for Medical Physics: Report Nr. 7: Pränatale Strahlenexposition aus medizinischer Indikation. Dosisermittlung, Folgerungen für Arzt und Schwangere, 2002. www.dgmp.de.

Dinger J, Autenrieth A, Kamin G et al. Jejunal atresia related to the use of toluidine blue in genetic amniocentesis in twins. J Perinatal Med 2003; 31: 266–8.

Duran-Mendicuti A, Sodickson A. Imaging evaluation of the pregnant patient with suspected pulmonary embolism. Int J Obstet Anesth 2011; 20: 51–9.

ESUR (European Society of Urogenital Radiology) Guidelines on Contrast Media, v. 8.1. http://www.esur.org/guidelines/en/index.php (accessed March 28, 2014).

Evans JA, Savitz DA, Kanal E, et al. Infertility and pregnancy outcome among magnetic resonance imaging workers. J Occup Med 1993; 35: 1191–5.

Fineman MS, Maguire JI, Fineman SW, et al. Safety of indocyanine green angiography during pregnancy: a survey of the retina, macula, and vitreous societies. Arch Ophthalmol 2001; 119: 353–5.

Fröhlich JM, Kubik-Huch RA. Radiographic, MR or ultrasound contrast media in pregnant or breast-feeding women: what are the key issues? Rofo 2013; 185: 13–25.

Gauthier TW. Methylene blue-induced hyperbilirubinemia in neonatal glucose-6-phosphate dehydrogenase (G6PD) deficiency. J Matern Fetal Med 2000; 9: 252–4.

Glüer S. Intestinal atresia following intraamniotic use of dyes. Eur J Pediatr Surg 1995; 5: 240–2.

Grobner T. Gadolinium – a specific trigger for the development of nephrogenic fibrosing dermopathy and nephrogenic systemic fibrosis? Nephrol Dial Transplant 2006; 21: 1104–8.

Gropper AB, Calvillo KZ, Dominici L et al. Sentinel Lymph Node Biopsy in Pregnant Women with Breast Cancer. Ann Surg Oncol 2014 [Epub ahead of print].

Grufferman S, Ruymann F, Ognjanovic S et al. Prenatal X-ray exposure and rhabdomyosarcoma in children: a report from the Children's Oncology Group. Cancer Epidemiol Biomarkers Prev 2009; 18: 1271–6.

Halperin LS, Olk RJ, Soubrane G, Coscas G. Safety of fluorescein angiography during pregnancy. Am J Ophthal 1990; 109: 563–6.

Han BH, Lee KS, Han JY et al. Pregnancy outcome after 1st-trimester inadvertent exposure to barium sulphate as a contrast media for upper gastrointestinal tract radiography. J Obstet Gynaecol 2011; 31: 586–88.

Harvey EB, Bolce JD, Honeyman M et al. Prenatal x-ray exposure and childhood cancer in twins. N Engl J Med 1985; 312: 541–5.

Hill BJ, Saigal G, Patel S et al. Transplacental passage of non-ionic contrast agents resulting in fetal bowel opacification: a mimic of pneumoperitoneum in the newborn. Pediatr Radiol 2007; 37: 396–8.

Huang TK, Reese J, Weitkamp JH, Stancombe BB et al. Congenital radiocontrast agent in the neonatal gut. J Pediatr 2014; 164: 1236.

Huda W, Randazzo W, Tipnis S et al. Embryo dose estimates in body CT. AJR Am J Roentgenol 2010; 194: 874–80.

Hujoel PP, Bollen A-M, Noonan CJ et al. Antepartum dental radiography and infant low birth weight. JAMA 2004; 291: 1987–93.

ICRP. Pregnancy and Medical Radiation. ICRP Publication 84. Ann ICRP 2000; 30.

Jaffe TA, Neville AM, Anderson-Evans C et al. Early first trimester fetal dose estimation method in a multivendor study of 16- and 64-MDCT scanners and low-dose imaging protocols. AJR Am J Roentgenol 2009; 193: 1019–24.

Jensh RP, Brent RL. Intrauterine effects of ultrasound: animal studies. Teratology 1999; 59: 240–51.

Kennedy EV, Iball GR, Brettle DS. Investigation into the effects of lead shielding for fetal dose reduction in CT pulmonary angiography. Br J Radiol 2007; 80: 631–8.

Khandelwal A, Fasih N, Kielar A. Imaging of acute abdomen in pregnancy. Radiol Clin North Am 2013; 51: 1005–22.

Kochi MH, Kaloudis EV, Ahmed W, Moore WH. Effect of in utero exposure of iodinated intravenous contrast on neonatal thyroid function. J Comput Assist Tomogr 2012; 36: 165–9.

Kok RD, de Vries MM, Heerschap A et al. Absence of harmful effects of magnetic resonance exposure at 1.5 T in utero during the third trimester of pregnancy: a follow-up study. Magn Reson Imaging 2004; 22: 851–4.

Kumar A, Vashist M, Rathee R. Maternal factors and risk of childhood leukemia. Asian Pac J Cancer Prev 2014; 15: 781–4.

Lengfelder E. Strahlenwirkung - Strahlenrisiko: Daten, Bewertung und Folgerungen aus ärztlicher Sicht (Radiation action - radiation risk: data, assessment, and consequences from aphysician's point of view). 2nd ed. Landsberg/Lech: ecomed, 1990.

Leung AN, Bull TM, Jaeschke R et al. American Thoracic Society documents: an official American Thoracic Society/Society of Thoracic Radiology Clinical Practice Guideline – Evaluation of Suspected Pulmonary Embolism in Pregnancy. Radiology 2012; 262: 635–46.

Lockhart PB, Brennan MT, Sasser H et al. Antepartum dental radiography and low birth weight [letter]. JAMA 2004; 292: 1020.

Pregnancy

2.20 Diagnostic agents

Marcos HB, Semelka RC, Worawattanakul S. Normal placenta: gadolinium-enhanced, dynamic MR imaging. Radiology 1997; 205: 493–6.

Mehler K, Oberthuer A, Weisshaar G et al. Hemolytic anemia and methemoglobinemia in a preterm baby as a complication of antenatal intraamnial injection of toluidine blue. Klin Padiatr 2013; 225: 263–5.

Minkov V, Nekolla EA, Nobke D et al. Nuclear-medical irradiation during pregnancy Risk assessment for the offspring. Nuklearmedizin 2009; 48: 10–6.

Neel JV. Changing perspectives on the genetic doubling dose of ionizing radiation for humans, mice, and drosophila. Teratology 1999; 59: 216–21.

Newnham JP, Doherty DA, Kendal GE et al. Effects of repeated prenatal ultrasound examinations on childhood outcome up to 8 years of age: follow-up of a randomised controlled trial. Lancet 2004; 364: 2038–44.

Newnham JP, Evans SF, Michael CA et al. Effects of frequent ultrasound during pregnancy: a randomized controlled trial. Lancet 1993; 342: 887–91.

Pandit-Taskar N, Dauer LT, Montgomery L et al. Organ and fetal absorbed dose estimates from 99mTc-sulfur colloid lymphoscintigraphy and sentinel node localization in breast cancer patients. J Nucl Med 2006; 47: 1202–8.

Patton T, Olshan AF, Neglia JP et al. Parental exposure to medical radiation and neuroblastoma in offspring. Paediatr Perinat Epidemiol 2004; 18: 178–85.

Read CH Jr, Tansey MJ, Menda Y. A 36-year retrospective analysis of the efficacy and safety of radioactive iodine in treating young Graves' patients. J Clin Endocrinol Metab 2004; 89: 4229–33.

Robert E. Intrauterine effects of electromagnetic fields (low frequency, mid frequency RF, and microwave): review of epidemiologic studies. Teratology 1999; 59: 292–8.

Saigal G, Abdenour GE. Another case of transplacental passage of the non-ionic contrast agent ioversol. Pediatr Radiol 2007; 37: 726–7.

Schaefer C, Meister R, Wentzeck R et al. Fetal outcome after technetium scintigraphy in early pregnancy. Reprod Toxicol 2009; 28: 161–6.

Schlumberger M, de Vathaire F, Ceccarelli C et al. Exposure to radioactive iodine-131 for scintigraphy or therapy does not preclude pregnancy in thyroid cancer patients. J Nucl Med 1996; 37: 606–12.

Sheiner E, Abramowicz JS. A symposium on obstetrical ultrasound: is all this safe for the fetus? Clin Obstet Gynecol 2012; 55; 188–98.

Spanheimer PM, Graham MM, Sugg SL et al. Measurement of uterine radiation exposure from lymphoscintigraphy indicates safety of sentinel lymph node biopsy during pregnancy. Ann Surg Oncol 2009; 16: 1143–7.

Spielmann H, Nau H. Embryotoxicity of stable isotopes and use of stable isotopes in studies of teratogenic mechanisms. J Clin Pharmacol 1986; 26: 474–80.

Stabin MG. Proposed addendum to previously published fetal dose estimate tables for 18F-FDG. J Nucl Med 2004; 45: 634–5.

Sternberg J. Radiation risk in pregnancy. Clin Obstet Gynecol 1973; 16: 235–78.

Stratmeyer ME, Greenleaf JF, Dalecki D et al. Fetal ultrasound: mechanical effects. J Ultrasound Med 2008; 27: 597–605.

Takalkar AM, Khandelwal A, Lokitz S et al. 18F-FDG PET in pregnancy and fetal radiation dose estimates. J Nucl Med 2011; 52: 1035–40.

Thomsen HS, Morcos SK, Almen T et al. Nephrogenic systemic fibrosis and gadolinium-based contrast media: updated ESUR Contrast Medium Safety Committee guidelines. Eur Radiol 2013; 23: 307–18.

Visser GHA, de Vries JIP, Mulder EJH et al. Effects of frequent ultrasound during pregnancy. Lancet 1993; 342: 1360.

Wakeford R, Little MP. Risk coefficients for childhood cancer after intrauterine irradiation: a review. Int J Radiat Biol 2003; 79: 293–309.

Welch CR, Hocking M, Franklyn JA et al. Fetal thyrotrophin: the best indicator of long term thyroid function after in utero exposure to iodine-131. Fetal Diagn Ther 1997; 13: 176–8.

Yanamadala V, Sheth SA, Walcott BP et al. Non-contrast 3D time-of-flight magnetic resonance angiography for visualization of intracranial aneurysms in patients with absolute contraindications to CT or MRI contrast. J Clin Neurosci 2013; 20: 1122–6.

Zanotti-Fregonara P, Jan S, Taieb D et al. Absorbed 18F-FDG dose to the fetus during early pregnancy. J Nucl Med 2010; 51: 803–5.

Zanotti-Fregonara P, Koroscil TM, Mantil J, et al. Radiation dose to the fetus from [(18)F]-FDG administration during the second trimester of pregnancy. Health Phys 2012; 102: 217–9.

Ziskin MC. Intrauterine effects of ultrasound: human epidemiology. Teratology 1999; 59: 252–60.

Recreational drugs

Sally Stephens and Laura M. Yates

2.21

Introduction	541
2.21.1	Alcohol	542
2.21.2	Caffeine and other xanthines	547
2.21.3	Tobacco and smoking	549
2.21.4	Drugs of abuse in general (excluding caffeine)	555
2.21.5	Sedating drugs	562

Introduction

Use of recreational drugs and other substances by women of childbearing potential, and during pregnancy varies widely across different populations. Whilst some women discontinue, or attempt to reduce use of alcohol, nicotine and other recreational drugs once pregnant, a significant number continue use throughout pregnancy. With half of all pregnancies being unplanned, exposure in the weeks prior to identification of pregnancy is therefore common.

Despite these exposures, robust scientific data on the fetal effects for many of these drugs are severely lacking as a consequence of the ethical barriers to conducting epidemiological studies concerning drug misuse in pregnancy and the prevalence in existing studies of multiple confounding factors such as researcher bias, lack of reliable information regarding dose and purity of the substance being studied, pattern of use and concomitant use of alcohol and/or other recreational drugs. Not only is inaccurate maternal recall a concern, so is underreporting or non-reporting of misuse. Furthermore, use of illicit drugs may be associated with maternal nutritional deficiencies, infectious diseases, failure to access antenatal care as well as psychosocial factors that independently influence fetal outcome. For these reasons, selection of a control group is difficult, and as a result many studies do not include one. Follow-up studies for longer term outcome are often limited by low recruitment rates and subsequent poor retention of study participants.

As a consequence of these issues, study findings may be inaccurate and interpretation of the data difficult, particularly in terms of ascribing causality to a particular exposure. For many substances, no clear evidence of increased fetal risk is documented. However, the data are often not sufficient to demonstrate a lack of adverse fetal, neonatal or longer term effects of recreational drug use during pregnancy and may not examine the additional risks to fetus and child that are associated with maternal addiction, withdrawal and overdose.

Interventions for both the mother and child are important in not only reducing usage but also in controlling withdrawal. The World Health Organization (WHO 2014) has published guidelines for providing support for mother and child by describing best practices. It is critical that the health care team work closely with the pregnant woman and her family to impact the usage of recreational drug use during pregnancy and breastfeeding.

2.21.1   Alcohol

The detrimental effects of maternal alcohol (ethanol) consumption on the developing fetus have long been recognized. The connection is documented both in the Bible and in William Hogarth's famous painting "Gin Lane" which depicts a typical scene from the gin-epidemic in England between 1720 and 1750. Despite this, alcohol exposure *in utero* remains the most common preventable cause of learning and disability in developed countries (Astley 2013), and is highly prevalent amongst certain populations in developing countries. The detrimental effects of alcohol on the fetus are life-long, and manifest in intellectual, physical, behavioral, social and emotional difficulties.

Research into the epidemiology, prevention, diagnosis and treatment of what are now commonly referred to as *fetal alcohol spectrum disorders* (FASD) has increased dramatically over recent years and the published literature on the topic is extensive. The following is a brief overview of current thinking and practice; however, this is an evolving field and readers are advised to access information and international expertise such as that provided by The National Organization for Fetal Alcohol Syndrome (www.NOFAS.org) and World Health Organization (WHO 2014).

Pharmacokinetics

Alcohol is rapidly absorbed through mucosa of the mouth, stomach and upper duodenum where absorption is greatest (70–80%). Peak serum concentrations are attained 30–60 minutes after ingestion but will be influenced by variation in interindividual metabolism and physical characteristics, and the circumstances under which the alcohol has been consumed (e.g. full versus empty stomach). The pharmacokinetics of alcohol are further influenced by pregnancy, and differ depending upon stage of gestation. Alcohol dissolves equally well in all body fluids, passes unhindered across the placenta and, due to the high permeability of the blood-cerebral-spinal-fluid-barrier, reaches the same concentration in the fetal brain and blood as in the maternal circulation. Fetal exposure may be prolonged as a result of delayed clearance of alcohol from the amniotic fluid. In some studies several hours after alcohol is no longer detectable in the maternal circulation, it is still detectable in the fetus (Zelner 2013a).

Mechanism of teratogenesis

The adverse fetal effects of maternal alcohol consumption during pregnancy are thought to result from the direct teratogenic effects of ethanol and its breakdown product, acetaldehyde. Proposed mechanisms of teratogenesis include increased oxidative stresses, altered glucose, lipid, protein and DNA metabolism, decreased neurogenesis and increased apoptosis, endocrinological actions and altered gene expression. It is likely that multiple mechanisms are involved (Ornoy 2010).

Fetal effects of alcohol – Fetal alcohol spectrum disorders (FASD)

Alcohol and its metabolites are teratogenic and impact both structural and functional fetal development. The effects of *in utero* exposure are reviewed in Jones (2011) and include:

- Dysmorphic features – short palpebral fissures, smooth philtrum, thin upper lip, short fifth finger and hypoplastic nail, "hockey-stick" palmar crease, "railroad track" pinnae
- Structural anomalies of the brain, heart, kidneys, limbs, skeleton
- Reduced intrauterine and postnatal growth
- Microcephaly
- Neurobehavioral impairment – learning difficulties, ADHD, visual and hearing impairment
- Infant death.

The degree to which the fetus is affected is dependent on the duration and intensity of the maternal alcohol consumption during pregnancy, and on the timing of exposure. Alcohol misuse in early pregnancy carries a risk of the facial dysmorphisms and birth defects described above in addition to neurobehavioural effects. However, heavy drinking beyond the first 12 weeks of pregnancy has been shown to induce neuronal damage in the rapidly growing brain and heavy alcohol exposure at any gestational time may result in significant neurobehavioral changes.

The term *Fetal Alcohol Syndrome* (FAS) was coined in the 1970s to describe the specific pattern of dysmorphic facial features and associated growth and central nervous system anomalies amongst children of women with chronic alcohol-dependency. However, it is now recognized that this triad of features represents the most severe form of alcohol teratogenesis and accounts for the minority of children affected by *in utero* exposure. Prospectively collected data suggest that 80% of children exposed to high levels of alcohol prenatally are affected with at least one or more features of FAS, with neurodevelopmental problems identified in 40% of cases who did not fulfill criteria for a diagnosis of classical FAS (Kuehn 2012). The term fetal alcohol spectrum disorder (FASD), which encompasses the full spectrum of alcohol teratogenicity, has therefore been introduced. This classification includes "classic" FAS, partial FAS (growth not affected), alcohol-related neurodevelopmental disorder (ARND), alcohol-related birth defects (ARBD), and fetal alcohol effects (FAE).

Several different guidelines have been developed in an attempt to improve the diagnosis of FASD, each with its own terminology and system of classification. This has introduced a further layer of complexity both in terms of diagnostic clinical application and in the interpretation and comparison of study findings. The use of classification systems that imply a causal relationship between maternal alcohol consumption and problems in a specific child have, however, been criticized given the complex circumstances under which exposure often occurs. Therefore, diagnostic codes such as neurobehavioral disorder/alcohol-exposed (ND/ AE) are increasingly being adopted in place of ARND (Astley 2013). The need for a single set of diagnostic guidelines to be developed was highlighted at the 2013 International FASD conference in Vancouver British Columbia (Astley 2013).

Pregnancy

2.21 Recreational drugs

The longer term consequences of FASDs are a concern. Whilst the facial features of classical FAS may become less obvious with time, microcephaly, growth retardation, attention deficit disorders, cognitive and motor deficits remain unchanged (i.e. Rasmussen 2011, Simmons 2011). In a 10-year long-term study, school performances grew worse despite considerable support (and encouragement) by their foster parents as well as social integration. During puberty, the problems of the affected children increased as a rule so that even at this age the diagnosis of FAS should be considered (Streissguth 1996). The consequences of intrauterine alcohol damage stretch right into adulthood with physical growth retardation (more frequent with male patients), impaired mental development and adjustment disorders presenting challenges particularly in the workplace (Larkby 2011, Autti-Ramo 2006, Barr 2006, Steinhausen 1998).

Only about 30% of FAS/FAE patients diagnosed in childhood were able to live independently as adults and only 20% had a job. For the prognosis in adulthood, the diagnosis of FAE was no different to that of FAS: the FAE patients had a less favorable prognosis because they were often only diagnosed very late (Spohr 2007). In an uncontrolled retrospective study, an approximately 10-fold increased prevalence of epilepsy in 425 FASD patients was determined compared to the normal population. However, this result should be considered to be provisional and the connection with prenatal alcohol exposure must still be confirmed in further studies (Bell 2010).

Quantifying fetal risk on the basis of exposure

Although the embryotoxic effects of alcohol are dose dependent, no "safe" level of alcohol consumption in pregnancy has been defined. Various studies have attempted to define fetal risk by pattern of drinking or quantity of alcohol consumed. The following categories have been proposed for this purpose: heavy alcohol consumption (more than 48–60 g/day), moderately high consumption (about 24–48 g/day) and binge-drinking, i.e., the occasional drinking of more than four to five drinks daily (Ornoy 2010). However, alcohol intake in studies is often reported by number of drinks or pattern of drinking, but definitions used to categorize exposure differ among countries, as does the quantity of alcohol in what is considered to be a "standard drink" (Zelner 2013b).

Whilst risk of classic FAS and the other FASDs with heavy consumption is well established, the reliability of the available data in terms of informing risk with low-moderate or binge drinking is questionable. In addition to the limitations described above, inter-individual variation in alcohol metabolism and susceptibility to teratogenic effects as a result of genetic polymorphisms in both mother and fetus are likely to significantly influence risk at the individual level (review Ramsay 2010). Consumption of equivalent quantities of alcohol by different women therefore may affect their fetuses differently. Underreporting or denial of alcohol use in pregnancy also is not uncommon, leading to the risk of an underestimation of effect. Lastly, and perhaps most importantly is the concern that many studies of neurological effect focus on IQ, or measure the effect against diagnostic parameters developed for diagnosing conditions such as autism; and therefore will not identify issues relating to social functioning and behavior, or those arising from autistic-traits that do not meet the criteria for a formal diagnosis of autism.

The studies summarized below are not exhaustive and findings should be considered in the context of the limitations described above.

Light to moderate alcohol consumption

Consumption of more than four alcoholic drinks a week has been associated with an increased rate of stillbirth and offspring mortality in the first year of life (Strandberg-Larsen 2009, Aliyu 2008). However, a meta-analysis found no association between increased rates of low birth weight (LBW), preterm birth or the infant being small for gestational age (SGA) with light to moderate consumption of alcohol in pregnancy (Patra 2011). Neither was an increased risk or dose-response relationship observed for infant LBW and SGA with maternal consumption up to 10 g of pure alcohol (approximately one drink) per day when compared to infants of women who did not drink alcohol in pregnancy. No effect on preterm birth rates was observed with maternal consumption of up to 18 g of alcohol per day (approximately 1.5 drinks per day).

A meta-analysis involving 24,000 pregnancies did not report an increased risk for birth defects among women who had consumed between two drinks/week and two drinks/day during the first trimester of pregnancy (Polygenis 1998). In the multi-center European Maternal Alcohol Consumption Study (EUROMAC 1992), in which alcohol consumption during pregnancy of 6,000 women was recorded, and newborns were examined by a pediatrician, average maternal alcohol consumption of 120 g a week (approximately 0.2 liters of wine a day), was associated with a significant reduction in the body length of newborns in comparison to the newborns of pregnant women who abstained from drinking alcohol.

No significant associations between light, light to moderate, or moderate prenatal alcohol exposure and various neuropsychological outcomes (including impaired attention, behavior, cognition, visual and motor development and language skills) were seen in a recent meta-analysis of 22 studies (Flak 2014). However, when analysis was limited to the only three studies that were considered to be of high quality, a statistically significant association was demonstrated between moderate prenatal alcohol exposure and detrimental effects on child behavior. In addition, a small but positive association between mild to moderate prenatal alcohol exposure and decreased cognition was seen, but disappeared when one large study was removed or when only data relating to moderate consumption was included.

One study has noted an increased risk of anxiety and depression in children and young people of non-alcoholic mothers who regularly consumed moderate amounts of alcohol (10 g occasion/day) during pregnancy (O'Leary 2010).

A meta-analysis of 21 case control studies which compared any alcohol intake during pregnancy with no reported alcohol consumption, found a statistically significantly association with childhood acute myeloid leukemia but not with acute lymphoblastic leukemia (Latino-Martel 2010). The dose of alcohol was not taken into account in this analysis and it therefore is not possible to draw conclusions regarding the risk to children who are only exposed to modest amount of alcohol in pregnancy. It should be noted that the absolute risk of childhood AML following prenatal exposure to alcohol remained very small.

"Binge drinking"

Risk to the unborn child of *in utero* exposure to alcohol is thought to depend both on the absolute amount consumed in each episode, as well as the pattern of maternal alcohol ingestion during pregnancy (Bailey 2004). Occasional heavy drinking, commonly referred to as "binge drinking" is likely to be associated with high maternal peak blood concentrations of alcohol which may coincide with key fetal developmental time-points. The exact definition of the amount of alcohol which constitutes a binge varies among studies but is generally regarded as the occasional ingestion of 4–5 units of alcohol in a 24-hour period as defined above.

Chiodo (2012) and Strandberg-Larsen (2008) did not find any association with spontaneous abortion and binge drinking although the latter study did find an association with an increased risk for stillbirth.

A systematic review of 14 studies considered the evidence for a number of birth outcomes. Although, overall, no significant effect of binge drinking on birth weight, gestational age, growth, or congenital anomaly rates (which included fetal alcohol syndrome) (Henderson 2007) was evident, the authors raised concerns regarding the variability in quality of the studies which made interpretation of the findings difficult. A recent study investigating alcohol consumption in early pregnancy (<15 weeks) also found no association with alcohol consumption, including binge drinking, in pregnancy and the infant being small for gestational age or of low birth weight, maternal preeclampsia, or spontaneous preterm birth (McCarthy 2013).

Feldman (2012) reported infants with microcephaly, a smooth philtrum and a thin vermillion border in association with increasing numbers of binge episodes in the second half of the first trimester of pregnancy.

Whilst certain structural anomalies have been reported more commonly in children with features of classical fetal alcohol syndrome, increased risk with binge drinking in the first trimester of pregnancy has not been conclusively demonstrated. Whilst DeRoo (2008) reported an increased risk for cleft lip and palate in the offspring of mothers who binged on alcohol during pregnancy, Romitti (2007) found only a slight increase in rate of oral clefts with maternal binge drinking which did not reach statistical significance. After controlling for confounders Richardson (2011) reported a significant increase in the incidence of omphalocele and gastroschisis, but not craniosynostosis, in infants of women who had consumed more than four alcoholic drinks per occasion in pregnancy. A recent study (Makelarski 2013) found no association between neural tube defects and any alcohol consumption patterns, including binging in pregnancy. There was also no significant increase in the prevalence of cryptorchidism (Strandberg-Larsen 2009) or isolated ventricular septal defects (VSD) and atrial septal defects (ASD) in the offspring of women who reported occasional binge drinking during the early pregnancy (Strandberg-Larsen 2011).

The Danish National Birth Cohort study reported an increased mortality rate amongst term infants, of women who had three or more binge-drinking episodes during pregnancy (Strandberg-Larsen 2009). In another study, a single episode of binge-drinking between the 11th and 16th weeks of pregnancy was associated with an increased risk of seizures and epilepsy in the child (Sun 2009).

A recent meta-analysis of 34 cohort studies, of which 15 included data from children aged 6 months to 4 years of women who binge drank during pregnancy showed a significant association between binge drinking in pregnancy and reduced cognitive ability in the child. However, this finding was of borderline significance when only studies of high quality were included in the analysis (Flak 2014). No effects on other neuropsychological outcomes, including behavior, visual and motor development were observed. However, others found increased inattention and hyperactivity behaviours in offspring, but no effect on IQ, with maternal binge drinking in the second and thrid trimester (Sayal et al 2009).

Therapeutic use of alcohol in pregnancy

Ethanol inhibits the release of the hormones, oxytocin and vasopressin, from the posterior pituitary gland and administration of high doses was one of the first methods of tocolysis in the management of preterm labor. Ethyl alcohol has been used in the past for tocolysis, for its presumed inhibition of oxytocin release by the posterior pituitary gland. To be effective, substantial maternal serum levels are needed! The harmful effects of alcohol on the development of the child are well known, and thus alcohol is an obsolete tocolytic (Chapter 2.14.4).

Intravenous administration of alcohol is used in the treatment of ethylene glycol poisoning where the alternative antidote, fomepizole, is not available. In this context, use may be justified as the risk to both mother and fetus of untreated toxicity is likely to exceed that posed by the ethanol (see Chapter 2.22).

Recommendation. Guidelines regarding consumption of alcohol in pregnancy are inconsistent. Whilst some guidelines advise abstinence periconceptually and throughout pregnancy, others recommend a maximum daily exposure. There is, however, no proven level of exposure which is "safe" and as alcohol is a known teratogen with lifelong effects on the fetus, avoidance of alcohol in pregnancy is strongly recommended.

During and before pregnancy: It is imperative that all pregnant women are asked about drug and alcohol use as early on in pregnancy as possible so that the appropriate interventions can be initiated to minimize fetal and maternal risk. In some areas, maternal screening programs are established to routinely detect alcohol and drug use. The use of alcohol-containing tonics and medications with an alcohol base (with concentrations >10%) although not comparable with abuse, should, nevertheless, be avoided in pregnancy.

Diagnosis of FASD: Where a diagnosis of fetal alcohol syndrome disorder is suspected clinically, assessment of the child by a clinical geneticist or pediatrician with expertise in this area is recommended to ensure that an underlying genetic syndrome has been excluded, especially where antenatal exposure to alcohol has not been confirmed (as is often the case when a child has been adopted). Where available, genetic investigation such as microarray CGH analysis should be considered for all dysmorphic or developmentally delayed children, especially if associated with multiple congenital anomalies.

2.21.2   Caffeine and other xanthines

The xanthines, *caffeine* and *theobromine* are the pharmacologically active components of a range of drinks such as coffee, tea, cocoa and soft drinks. The caffeine content of a cup of coffee is generally estimated to be approximately 100 mg, and a cup of tea approximately 50 mg but may be greater depending on how the drink is prepared. For instance, an espresso is likely to have a higher caffeine concentration than a cup of instant coffee. Cola drinks contain up to 25 mg of caffeine per 100 mL. Energy drinks are likely to have an even higher caffeine content, and often contain other stimulants. Caffeine is also a component of certain medications, such as analgesic preparations and over the counter cold and flu preparations. Xanthines also include medicines such as theophylline, used in the treatment of asthma (Chapter 2.3).

Pregnancy

2.21 Recreational drugs

Caffeine, as a lipophilic substance, is well absorbed from the gastrointestinal tract, crosses the placenta and can exert its stimulant effects on the fetus resulting in increased fetal activity and heart rate, and in some cases fetal arrhythmia.

Regular use of large amounts of caffeine have been associated with reduced fertility in both women and men (Jensen 1998). A meta-analysis of studies involving approximately 50,000 pregnant women in total suggested a slightly elevated rate of spontaneous abortion amongst women who drank more than 150 mg of caffeine per day during pregnancy (Fernandes 1998). Stefanidou (2011) reported a dose-response relationship between caffeine ingestion and recurrent miscarriage. After controlling for confounders, the odds ratio for recurrent miscarriage increased with increased daily caffeine intake in the periconceptional period and in early gestation. A prospective Danish study found a slight elevated rate of stillbirth amongst pregnant women who had consumed more than eight cups of coffee a day (Wisborg 2003). A follow-up study by the same authors demonstrated that women who drank more than eight cups of coffee per day were at increased risk of a fetal death (Bech 2005). However, further studies have been unable to confirm these risks and there are concerns regarding confounding by pregnancy symptoms (where women tend to reduce their caffeine intake in response to morning sickness) (review in Peck 2010).

A number of studies have demonstrated an increased rate of cryptorchidism, anal atresia and cleft lip/palate amongst infants whose mothers consumed caffeine during pregnancy; however, these studies were limited by retrospective exposure assessment, small sample size and failure to adjust for other potential confounders including maternal smoking and alcohol consumption (Peck 2010, Mongraw-Chaffin 2008, Bille 2007). A study by Schmidt (2010) identified an association between infant neural tube defect (NTD) risk and polymorphisms in a fetal and maternal gene involved in caffeine metabolism. The authors suggested that risk of NTDs may be increased in genetically susceptible individuals with caffeine consumption.

The data relating to the effects of caffeine on fetal growth *in utero* are mixed. Numerous studies have suggested a link between intrauterine growth restriction (IUGR) or low infant birth weight and caffeine consumption in pregnancy. A meta-analysis from 1998, which included approximately 50,000 pregnant women, suggested a slightly increased risk of having a baby with IUGR, if the mother had consumed more than 150 mg of caffeine per day (Fernandes 1998). More recent studies have also found a positive correlation between caffeine intake and low birth weight (Sengpiel 2013, Bakker 2010). Bakker (2010) found reduced infant birth weight with maternal daily caffeine intake of more than 540 mg, whilst Sengpiel (2013) reported that maternal caffeine intake of more than 200 mg to 300 mg/day increased the odds for having a small for gestational age infant. Other studies have suggested that effects of maternal caffeine consumption on birth weight are restricted to male offspring only (Vik 2003), or to infants of women who are rapid caffeine metabolizers (Grosso 2006). However, a review of the literature in 2000 demonstrated no evidence of an effect of even moderate to high caffeine consumption on *in utero* growth (Brent 2011) and another concluded that low infant birth weight cannot be clearly attributed to caffeine and cannot be separated from effects of other exposures such as maternal smoking and alcohol consumption (Peck 2010).

The hypothesis that the methylxanthine, *theobromine*, which is found particularly in cocoa, could reduce the rate of preeclampsia, has not been confirmed (Klebanoff 2009). A meta-analysis of 22 studies found no clear connection between coffee consumption during pregnancy and preterm delivery (Maslova 2010). In a study by Barr (1991) no effect on physical development parameters and IQ up to the age of 7.5 years in the children of 500 pregnant women who had consumed more than 150 mg of caffeine daily was found. One prospective study reported a weak association between the occurrence of hyperactivity at 18 months in children whose mothers had consumed caffeine-containing drinks during the pregnancy (Bekkhus 2010). Another study found no connection between caffeine use during pregnancy and attention deficit disorders (Linnet 2009).

Regular coffee consumption during pregnancy has recently been associated with childhood acute leukemia in the offspring in a single study, with the risk increasing linearly with daily intake (Bonaventure 2013).

In summary, the data regarding caffeine consumption during pregnancy are highly confounded and for some outcomes contradictory. An association between caffeine intake and increased miscarriage risk, and possibly fetal demise has been reported but remains unproven. Similarly, various structural anomalies have been reported following caffeine exposure *in utero* but a causal association or consistent embryopathy has not been demonstrated.

Maternal caffeine consumption of less than 150 mg caffeine a day in pregnancy does not appear to affect fetal growth, and although an adverse effect on birth weight has been reported at higher doses by some, these data are inconsistent with respect to identifying a threshold dose for this effect. Single studies have suggested a possible association with childhood acute leukemia and hyperactivity, but these findings remain to be confirmed.

Recommendation. There is insufficient robust scientific evidence on which to provide a specific recommendation regarding the amount of caffeine that can be consumed during pregnancy without causing harm to the fetus. Some practitioners advise no more than 300 mg of caffeine (around three cups of coffee) per day. The caffeine content of medications and other foods, such as chocolate should also be considered. Where caffeine ingestion is considered to be excessive or is associated with maternal symptoms, additional fetal monitoring may be indicated.

2.21.3   Tobacco and smoking

▶ **Tobacco and nicotine replacement therapy**

Pharmacology

Tobacco smoke consists of a mixture of numerous gases (primarily carbon monoxide) (see also Chapter 2.22.2) a particulate phase which contains nicotine and the so-called "tobacco tar" which comprises over 4,000 different substances (Rogers 2008), and taste and olfactory corrigents. Nicotine is the primary toxin in tobacco. In 2000, a new directive stipulated that cigarettes sold in the EU should each contain no more than 10 mg of tar and 1 mg of nicotine. Nicotine is absorbed through the mucosa of the oral cavity, the respiratory tract and the gastrointestinal tract.

Cigarette smoke is embryo- and fetotoxic. Nicotine crosses the placenta, and accumulates in fetal blood and amniotic fluid to reach concentrations in excess of those in the mother, resulting in an increased fetal heart rate. In addition to the heavy metal, *cadmium*, the organochlorine pesticide, *hexachlorbenzene* (HCB) and *polychlorinated biphenyls* (PCBs) have been documented in serum from newborns obtained before the first oral feed (Lackmann 2000). Concentrations of PCB and HCB were significantly increased among infants of active and passive smokers in comparison to those born to women from non-smoking households.

Birth defects

Whilst studies which analyzed overall birth defect rates amongst infants of women who smoked in pregnancy do not demonstrate that these are significantly increased, an association between smoking during the first trimester and an increased risk of cleft lip and palate specifically has been reported by a number of authors (i.e. Shi 2008, Zeiger 2005, Little 2004a, 2004b, Wyszynski 1997). Risk of orofacial clefts appears to correlate with maternal exposure, and there is evidence to support an increased risk amongst fetuses harboring certain variations in genes which encode molecules involved in the detoxification of cigarette smoke; for example, *GSST1* (Shi 2007). A meta-analysis of 24 international publications found that maternal smoking during pregnancy is associated with an increased risk for non-syndromic orofacial clefts. The association for cleft lip, with or without palate involvement, was stronger and more consistent than for isolated cleft palate (Little 2004a, 2004b). A previous meta-analysis of 11 studies reported a significantly increased risk of both cleft lip and palate, and cleft palate without cleft lip with maternal smoking in pregnancy (Wyszynski 1997).

Other studies have reported an elevated risk for craniosynostosis (Honein 2000, Källén 1999), gastroschisis (Draper 2008, Martinez-Frias 1997),urinary tract defects (Li 1996), heart defects (Patel 2012, Malik 2008), defects of the extremities (Caspers 2013, Källén 1997, Wasserman 1996), congenital diaphragmatic hernia (Caspers 2010) and talipes (Sommer 2011, Skelly 2002) with maternal smoking; however, the data are limited and an increased risk for birth defects other than orofacial clefts remains to be proven.

Pregnancy complications

- Women who had smoked at any time during their reproductive years were more likely to experience spontaneous abortion, stillbirth or tubal ectopic pregnancies (Hyland 2014). Smoking during pregnancy increases the risk of spontaneous abortion (Ness 1999). This finding remains when other risk factors, such as alcohol consumption, pregnancy history, social status and genetic predisposition, are taken into account. In a Swedish case-control study, the spontaneous abortion risk was increased 2-fold in active smokers and to about 1.7-fold in passive smokers after controlling for risk factors (George 2006).
- Other than infection of the pelvic organs, smoking is the main risk factor for an extrauterine pregnancy. Rogers (2009) reported a dose-dependent effect with a doubling of the risk associated with smoking 10 cigarettes a day.
- Placenta previa occurs more frequently among smokers and an increased risk for placental abruption has also been attributed to maternal smoking with risk increasing with the number of cigarettes smoked per day (Ananth 1999). Perinatal mortality as a result of placental abruption is two to three times higher among the children of

smokers than among those of non-smokers. Smoking in pregnancy is responsible for 10% of these two functional placental disturbances (Werler 1997).

■ Smoking in pregnancy is associated with a reduction in infant birth weight of, on average, 200 g but depends on the number of cigarettes smoked daily. This effect is thought to be caused by pathophysiological changes in the placenta which limit uterine blood flow thereby causing fetal growth restriction. The hypoxemic effect of carbon monoxide is also proposed to be a contributing factor. Maternal smoking is thought to account for low infant birth weight in 20% of all underweight babies. When gestational age is taken into account intrauterine growth restriction (IUGR) is 2.5 times higher amongst the offspring of smokers compared to those of non-smokers. Primiparae and older women appear to be at greatest risk of this effect. Importantly, cessation of smoking in the early weeks of pregnancy has been shown to remove the increased risk of reduced intrauterine growth (review in Rogers 2009, Werler 1997).

■ Preterm delivery (<37 weeks) is, on average, 30% more common amongst smokers even once the effects of the placental complications described above are taken into account. Once again, there is a dose-response relationship with the risk for preterm rupture of the membranes before the 33rd week of pregnancy which is doubled amongst women who smoke 20 cigarettes per day. Multiparous women are particularly at increased risk of delivery of an infant before the 33rd week of pregnancy (Werler 1997).

■ Perinatal mortality (fetal death after the 20th week or infant death up to 28 days after birth) is increased by about 30% amongst women who smoke in pregnancy. This increase is likely to be explained by higher rates of low infant birth weight, prematurity and placental impairment. Risk of perinatal mortality remains raised amongst offspring of smokers compared to those of non-smokers when birth weight is standardized according to gestational age at delivery. In contrast, no increased mortality was observed amongst the offspring of women who live at high altitudes and smoke in pregnancy, i.e. under conditions of limited oxygen availability (reviewed in Werler 1997).

■ Smoking, both during and after pregnancy is considered the primary risk factor for sudden infant death syndrome (SIDS) (Fleming 2007). A systematic review involving 39 studies showed the pooled odds ratio for maternal smoking was 2.77 (Anderson 1997). A large prospective study from Denmark, involving over 25,000 pregnancies, showed that the risk of both stillbirth and infant mortality (death within the first year of life), was approximately doubled amongst women who smoked during pregnancy compared to non-smokers. Cessation of smoking in the first trimester, reduced the risk for stillbirth and infant death to that of the control group (Wisborg 2001). A recent meta-analysis of 96 studies that investigated risk factors for still birth attributed 4–7% of stillbirths to maternal smoking (Flenady 2011).

■ A study of pregnant women with borderline iodine intake suggested that, smoking in pregnancy may be a major etiological factor for thyroid enlargement in the newborn (Chanoine 1991).

Illnesses in childhood

The relationship between childhood morbidity and mortality and maternal smoking in pregnancy is hard to determine because in almost every case both prenatal and postnatal exposure has occurred (reviewed in Bruin 2010).

- A meta-analysis of 17 studies involving 94,997 pregnancies collectively identified a significant association between maternal smoking and obesity in the exposed offspring aged between 3 and 33 years (Ino 2010). A further study suggests that postnatal exposure may also play a part in this finding (Florath 2014).
- Passive exposure to tobacco smoke is well documented as a risk factor for respiratory tract infection and otitis media in children. An association with prenatal exposure is less clear. Cotinine in meconium has been demonstrated to be predictive of increased risk of early childhood respiratory infection (Nuesslein 1999) in one study. However, whilst another study showed that pre- and postnatal exposure to tobacco smoke increased sensitization to food allergens during the first 3 years of life, this was not observed for inhaled allergens (Kulig 1999).
- Smoking in pregnancy has been associated with an increased risk of infantile colic (Shenassa 2004, Søndergaard 2001).
- A marginally, but statistically significant, increased risk of high blood pressure has been demonstrated amongst adolescents of women who smoked during pregnancy and was not thought to be attributable to familial confounding (Brion 2007).
- In two recent case control studies, offspring of mothers who smoked in pregnancy exhibited a two-fold greater risk for bipolar disorder (Talati 2013) and a significant increased risk of developing schizophrenia (Stathopoulou 2013).
- Metabolites of the tobacco-specific carcinogen, 4-(methylnitrosamino)-1-(3-pyridyl) 1-butanone (NNK), are detectable in newborns of smoking mothers. The average metabolite concentration in the first urine is about 10% of that found in urine of adult smokers and correlates positively with the number of cigarettes smoked and urinary nicotine and cotinine concentration (Lackmann 1999).

Various studies, which used differing methodologies, have investigated the potential for maternal smoking to increase the risk of cancer in the offspring. Whilst many found no evidence of an association, others have suggested an increased risk for childhood brain tumors, leukemia and lymphomas (review in Sasco 1999). A prospective Swedish study of 1.4 million births found a significant increase in the frequency of benign and malignant brain tumors, with the greatest effect observed for astrocytomas (Brooks 2004).

An increased frequency of lymphocytes containing mutations at the hypoxanthine phosphoribosyltransferase (hprt) locus was observed in the cord blood of babies whose mothers smoked in pregnancy compared to babies of mothers who did not. It should, however, be noted that the sample size for this study was extremely small (10 smokers and 10 non-smokers), and that the sensitivity of using hprt mutation frequency as a biomarker for genotoxic effect has been questioned (Ammenheuser 1994). Data relating to a possible mutagenic effect of maternal smoking on fetal lymphocytes are conflicting. Whilst increased micronuclei have been demonstrated in cord blood samples from neonates of smokers, another study showed no association between maternal smoking and increased rates of chromosome translocation in the mother or the newborn infant (Bennett 2010, Zalacain 2006, de la Chica 2005).

Cognitive development

Although not conclusive, several studies now suggest that smoking in pregnancy has an adverse effect on fetal neurodevelopment and contributes to cognitive and behavioral disturbances in childhood, and potentially into adulthood.

- Smoking 10 or more cigarettes a day during pregnancy doubled the risk that the exposed child was not yet "babbling" at 8 months of age (Obel 1998).
- A review of the published literature from 2000 to 2011 which included 20 reports from 18 studies found that measures of academic achievement and intellectual ability were poorer amongst children who had been prenatally exposed to tobacco. Testing was conducted at an early age and into young adulthood. Two papers found significant associations with intelligence in male offspring only (Clifford 2012).
- A study of 1,265 children in New Zealand (Fergusson 1998) found an association between smoking during pregnancy and behavioral problems, specifically "conduct disorder", in the exposed offspring at 16 and 18 years. The effect was more pronounced in males than females Cornelius 2011, 2001). The authors reported that prenatal tobacco exposure was associated with deficits at 10 years of age in verbal learning, design memory and hand–eye coordination as well as with disturbances in attention and behavior. Follow-up of the same cohort at 22 years of age (Cornelius 2012) found that exposed individuals had significantly higher scores on externalizing, internalizing, aggression, and somatic scales of a behavioral problem self-assessment. These individuals were also more likely to have a history of arrests and a higher rate of smoking and nicotine dependence themselves.
- In another study, children whose mothers smoked during pregnancy had an increased prevalence of childhood hyperkinetic syndrome (Linnet 2005) and a high hyperactivity–inattention score (Obel 2009) when compared with children of non-smokers after controlling for certain confounders. However, a further analysis using a sibling-based comparison showed a significantly weaker association with smoking suggesting an environmental or genetic basis for these outcomes (Obel 2011). A study of 14-year-olds, whose mothers had smoked during pregnancy, found a higher occurrence of psychological symptoms, aggressive behavior and social problems amongst these children in comparison to non-exposed children of the same age (Indredavik 2007).
- A long-term observational study of 808 children who were followed up to the age of 12 years found persisting sleep disturbances to be more frequent, amongst children of mothers who had smoked during pregnancy. The effect was dose-dependent and remained after adjusting for other factors but was interpreted by the authors as only an indication of a possible connection (Stone 2010).

Passive smoking

Maternal "passive smoking", the term used to describe indirect exposure to secondhand smoke (SHS) has also been shown to adversely affect fetal outcome. Women who had never smoked, but had experienced a high level of lifetime exposure to SHS, had a significantly increased risk for spontaneous abortion, stillbirth, and tubal ectopic pregnancy when compared to women who had never smoked or been exposed to SHS (Hyland 2014). A recent study which undertook a combined analysis

Pregnancy

2.21 Recreational drugs

of 17 studies showed that maternal exposure to SHS during pregnancy increased the risk of miscarriage by 11% (Pineles 2014).

Another meta-analysis found a 22% increased risk for low infant birthweight with maternal exposure to SHS (Leonardi-Bee 2008). A significantly higher risk of preterm delivery has also been reported amongst pregnant women who were exposed to SHS for at least 7 hours a day (Hanke 1999).

Chen (2013) reviewed the literature published between 1989 and 2012 which investigated the association between *in utero* SHS exposure and performance in neurocognitive and academic tests. They concluded that even after controlling for postnatal SHS exposure there were strong associations with reduced neurodevelopment, especially in children aged <5-years-old. Much weaker associations between SHS exposure *in utero* and IQ in older children (>5 years) were reported, although language and attention performance was reduced in SHS exposed children aged 6 to 7 years.

Medicinal therapy for nicotine dependency

The main benefit of nicotine replacement therapy (NRT) use in pregnancy is that mother and baby are exposed to nicotine alone, and not to the hundreds of other chemicals in tobacco smoke.

Whilst a Danish study found a slight, but statistically significant, increased risk of birth defects in users of substitution therapy in the first trimester who reported not smoking cigarettes during this period (Morales-Suárez-Varela 2006), another study found no increased risk of birth defects (Forinash 2010).

Two recent meta-analyses have investigated the efficacy and safety of NRT use to support smoking cessation in pregnancy. The Coleman (2011) meta-analysis included five trials in which NRT was used with or without behavioral support to promote smoking cessation. Although some pregnancy safety outcomes (including spontaneous abortion, prematurity, perinatal mortality, fetal death and admissions to neonatal intensive care units) were generally better among those infants born to women who had received NRT compared to women who did not, none of these observed differences reached statistical significance. The authors concluded that there is currently insufficient evidence to demonstrate efficacy or safety of NRT use in pregnancy.

A year later, Myung (2012) published a similar meta-analysis which included an additional two studies, one relating to use of *buproprion*, the other to NRT. They also found no significant difference in mean birth weight, low birth weight rate, mean gestational age, and preterm delivery rate between the pharmacotherapy and control groups.

Varenicline is a nicotine acetylcholine receptor partial agonist and is approved as a therapy for smoking cessation. There are limited data concerning use of varenicline in pregnancy but, in principle, similar effects to those caused by nicotine may be expected, given its mode of action, although risk of teratogenicity remains unpredictable (Maritz 2009). In animal experiments, whilst reduced fertility and an increased startle reflex in response to noise was shown in offspring of treated rats, no evidence of structural teratogenesis was observed in rats or in rabbits. Human data are limited to 24 gestational varenicline exposures (nine in monotherapy), 22 (91.6%) of which occurred in the first trimester. Pregnancy outcomes included four elective terminations, seven spontaneous abortions and one intrauterine death. The only adverse outcome reported amongst 13 live-born infants was a dilated renal pelvis in one of a twin pair (Richardson 2013b).

The antidepressant, *bupropion*, is also approved for use as a smoking cessation therapy in the nonpregnant population. For a review of use in pregnancy please see Chapter 2.11.5.

There is thus no evidence of efficacy or safety regarding use of any of the available smoking cessation therapies in pregnancy. A blanket recommendation that women who smoke use NRT or other pharmacotherapies such as varenicline or buproprion whilst pregnant to support smoking cessation can, therefore, not be made. Use of these interventions in heavy smokers may, however, be considered to offer clinical benefit and should be decided on an individual basis in discussion with the patient.

> **Recommendation.** Smoking at any stage of pregnancy is potentially harmful not only to the fetus, but also to the mother, her partner and other children at home. Women should be strongly advised to discontinue smoking before pregnancy and to abstain from smoking throughout the entire pregnancy and after birth. The decision as to whether or not to use a nicotine replacement therapy or other pharmacological smoking cessation therapy during pregnancy should be made individually, taking the available data into account. In some situations, use of nicotine replacement therapy may be preferable to continued exposure to tobacco smoke. However, where possible, smoking cessation during pregnancy should be achieved using non-pharmacological interventions such as cognitive behavioral therapy (CBT) and clinical support from healthcare providers if available.
>
> Smoking in pregnancy is not in itself an indication for interruption of the pregnancy. The need for additional monitoring of fetal growth and wellbeing may be indicated where maternal smoking is heavy but will need to be decided on a case-by-case basis

2.21.4   Drugs of abuse in general (excluding caffeine)

▶ Amphetamines

Amphetamines increase catecholamine concentrations in the brain via various mechanisms and are therefore referred to as CNS stimulants. In addition to potential adverse effects on the developing fetal brain, vaso-constrictive effects of amphetamines like cocaine or nicotine, can lead to reduced perfusion of the fetoplacental unit or of individual fetal organs. Fetal harm may also occur secondary to maternal malnutrition as a consequence of the appetite suppressant effects of these drugs.

Amphetamine-containing drugs are usually ingested, sniffed, smoked or injected. Whereas *Methylamphetamine* (*Methamphetamine*), also termed *crystal, ice, meth* or *yaba* is generally used in pure form, the term "speed" generally refers to preparations containing a variable mixture of amphetamines. Although there are no specific studies which investigate the maternofetal effects of different amphetamine derivatives (i.e. 2-CB, methylthioamphetamine, dimethoxymethylamphetamine, dimethyltryptamine among others), adverse effects with use in pregnancy must be considered to be at least equivalent in risk to those associated with methamphetamine use due to the similarity in their mechanisms of action. The same is true for the use of Khat-plant (*Catha edulis*, herbal ecstasy) leaves and derivatives which contain toxins that are structurally similar to amphetamines. Although regular use of Khat is common in parts of Africa and Arabia, the fetal risks associated with use in pregnancy are undocumented; however, hypertension has been induced in a case report (Kuczkowski 2005).

Pregnancy

2.21 Recreational drugs

Retrospective case control studies have suggested an increase in specific congenital malformations including congential heart defects (Nora 1967), billary atresia (Levin 1971) and gastroschisis (Elliott 2009, Draper 2008) with use of amphetamines or related substances in early pregnancy, and one case report describes cholestasis in a newborn after prenatal methamphetamine exposure (Dahshan 2009). More recent prospective studies have, however, not identified an overall increased risk of congenital malformation or any specific pattern of anomalies that would suggest a teratogenic embryopathy (Felix 2000, Little 1988).

However, a meta-analysis of 10 studies of pregnancy outcome following amphetamine exposure identified significantly increased risks of prematurity, low infant birth weight and infants being small for gestational age (Ladhani 2011).

Significantly increased rates of neonatal withdrawal symptoms including agitation, tachypnea, vomiting, tremor, excoriation and temperature instability were reported amongst neonates who were exposed to amphetamines *in utero* when compared to unexposed neonates (Chomchai 2004).

A study which followed up 65 children who were exposed to amphetamines *in utero* until the age of 14, identified a significantly increased number with learning difficulties, when compared to the national average for their age group. However, a large percentage of the mothers not only abused amphetamines during their pregnancies but also consumed opiates and alcohol, smoked more than 10 cigarettes a day and were in challenging psychosocial situations. Only 22% of the children still lived with their biological mothers at the age of 14 (Cernerud 1996). A further study of 49 methamphetamine exposed and 49 unexposed children between the ages of 3 and 4, found significantly lower neuropsychological scores in the exposed compared to the unexposed children (Chang 2009). In contrast, a study by Smith (2011) found no difference in cognitive abilities between infants of mothers who abused amphetamines during pregnancy compared to a control group; although a slight effect on fine motor performance was observed at 1 year of age, this was no longer present at 3 years of age. Changes in specific brain structures, including a reduction in hippocampus volume, have been documented in children who were exposed to methamphetamine prenatally; however, the imaging procedures used were limited, reducing the reliability of these data (Chang 2007).

▶ MDMA (Ecstasy)

Ecstasy is jargon for various illicit drugs including the hallucinogenic amphetamine, MDMA (*methylendioxymethylamphetamine*). Animal experiments have shown impaired fetal growth with maternal exposure to high doses. A case series based on prospectively reported MDMA exposure of 136 pregnant women described 12 children with congenital anomalies amongst a total of 78 live-born infants. Some of these were minor anomalies, i.e. foot deformities, no consistent pattern was observed. About half of the mothers had also consumed alcohol or other drugs (McElhatton 1999).

"Bath salts"

Many of the actions of these synthetic cathionines are thought to mimic amphetamines and may result in cardiovascular effects as noted for Khat chewing (see above). Unfortunately, the obstetrical literature is almost non-existent concerning exposures to synthetic cathionines and thus, little guidance can be provided except to recommend avoidance because of the number of deaths reported in nonpregnant users (NIDA 2014).

> **Recommendation.** Pregnant women should avoid amphetamines and related compounds in all trimesters of pregnancy due to the potential for adverse effects on neurodevelopment even after the first trimester. Exposure to amphetamines would not in itself be considered justification for termination of the pregnancy. The need for a detailed fetal anomaly or growth scan should be considered on a case-by case basis where this is not offered as part of routine care.

▶ Cocaine

Pharmacology

Cocaine (coke, snow) or *benzoecgonine methyl ester* is an alkaloid of the coca bush (*Erythroxylon coca*). It is chemically related to local anesthetics, but has only been proven to be of medical value in the topical treatment of conditions affecting the eyes, ears, nose and throat. Crack, the free base of cocaine, is a recreational drug that is smoked, sniffed, ingested or injected for its euphoric effects. Cocaine is a serotonin-noradrenaline-dopamine reuptake inhibitor associated with sympathomimetic and central stimulating effects such as vasoconstriction, tachycardia, tachypnea, and may, therefore, induce hypertension and cardiac dysrhythmias.

Taken orally, cocaine is absorbed very slowly due to its vasoconstrictor action and hydrolytic breakdown in the stomach. It is metabolized in the liver within 2 hours of ingestion to the ineffective primary metabolite, benzoecgonine and about 20% is excreted unchanged via the kidneys. Intranasal absorption occurs within 20 minutes and intravenous use of smoking crack causes an effect within a few minutes with risk of maternal toxicity at lower doses than with other routes of exposure. Cocaine crosses the placenta and is found in relatively high concentrations in the amniotic fluid. The amniotic fluid concentration decreases very slowly as clearance is limited. Fetal exposure may therefore be significant as a result of ingestion of the amniotic fluid and absorption of cocaine through the skin which is relatively permeable until the 22nd week of pregnancy (Woods 1998).

Toxicology

In the US during the 1980s and early 1990s a "crack baby epidemic" received much attention, in part due to a number of case reports and small case series documenting adverse pregnancy outcomes and a range of abnormalities in children who were exposed prenatally. However, despite these multiple reports no typical "cocaine-syndrome" or characteristic pattern of persisting morphological and/or neurobehavioral effects (sometimes termed "crack-baby") has been defined (Bandstra 2010).

Documented consequences of cocaine use which appear to be independent of effects of other drugs include an increased risk of placental abruption and spontaneous rupture of membranes (Addis 2001). Studies which investigated a risk of spontaneous abortion have shown inconsistent findings (Bingol 1987, Chasnoff 1985). A meta-analysis of 31 studies demonstrated a significant association between prenatal cocaine exposure and prematurity, low birth weight and small for gestational age infants (Gouin 2011).

Various congenital anomalies and neonatal complications including cardiac defects, cleft palate, gastroschisis, defects of the urogenital and skeletal systems, cerebral seizures, intestinal atresia and infarction, and neonatal necrotizing enterocolitis, have been reported in individual cases after *in utero* exposure to cocaine (Hoyme 1990, Schaefer 1990, Draper 2008, Forrester 2007, Eyler 1998a, Mercado 1989, Chasnoff 1988). However, a prospective study of 717 children who were exposed to cocaine antenatally found no significant increase in the birth defect rate, but did show an increased risk of growth retardation and temporary postpartum neurological symptoms such as trembling and excitability in the neonate (Bauer 2005).

The broad spectrum of morphological changes described above have been attributed by some to cocaine induced vasoconstriction resulting in reduced circulation in the placenta and the fetal organs. Altered expression of key developmental genes due to altered neurotransmitter concentrations has also been proposed as a mechanism of cocaine embryopathy (review in Lester 2009).

Postnatal development

Neonatal withdrawal. Cocaine-induced withdrawal symptoms in the newborn include sleep disturbances, tremor, weak suck, vomiting, shrill crying, sneezing, tachypnea, soft stools and fever. Some studies also report abnormalities on neurological examination of newborns as well as behavioral and developmental disturbances later on in life. EEG-changes and sudden infant deaths have also been reported (Eyler 1998b).

Postnatal growth

A reduction in growth (weight, height and head circumference) was found at ages 7 and 10 years, but not at 1 and 3 years in a prospective long-term study of children exposed to cocaine in the first trimester compared to unexposed children (Richardson 2007, 2013a).

Neurodevelopment

Findings of studies investigating longer term neurodevelopmental effects of cocaine exposure *in utero* are conflicting for anomalies of muscle tone, behavior and orientation in the infant at 6 months (Chiriboga 2007) and diminished adaptation to stressful situations at 7 months (Eiden 2009).

In a longitudinal study of 200 children up to the age of 7 years, Bandstra (2002, 2004) found that even marked cocaine exposure during pregnancy could not be clearly documented as an independent risk factor for abnormal mental and psychomotor or behavioral development amongst exposed children. Beeghly (2006) came to a similar conclusion in a study on speech development at the ages of 6 and 9.5 years. In a further study, discreet effects on neuro-cognitive development at the age of 12 following antenatal cocaine exposure, were not detected (Hurt 2009).

Conversely, an evaluation of 31 long-term studies of five different cohorts reported an association between prenatal cocaine exposure and attention and behavioral regulation deficits, but not with general developmental parameters such as growth or cognitive disturbance (Ackerman 2010).

A further review of 42 studies involving 14 cohorts reported a dose-response between prenatal cocaine exposure and attention, cognition, language and behavioral disorders, with a weaker association observed for poor school performance and achievement and lower IQ scores (Lester 2010). It was, however, noted that it was not always possible to differentiate the effects of cocaine exposure from those of the maternal and environmental factors, which are often associated with cocaine use. Richardson (1996) and Messinger (2004) identified that women who took cocaine during pregnancy were more likely to suffer from stress and eating disorders, were often single and had a tendency to consume *marijuana*, tobacco, alcohol and other substances.

In summary, it must, therefore, be assumed that cocaine consumption is a marker of a potentially high-risk pregnancy. Whilst the evidence is not robust enough to definitively identify cocaine as a teratogen *per se*, the likelihood of co-existing maternal illness and concurrent exposure to substances that are associated with adverse pregnancy outcomes is high.

> **Recommendation.** Pregnant women should avoid cocaine in all circumstances. However, exposure to cocaine in pregnancy would not in itself be regarded as an indication to interrupt the pregnancy. In the case of repeated use, a psychosocial assessment is advisable and the need for additional antenatal monitoring such as a detailed fetal ultrasound scan considered on a case-by-case basis.

▶ Cannabis

Street terminologies for drugs containing marijuana are extensive and generally describe products containing dried leaves or resin of *Cannabis sativa*, or the related *Cannabis indica* (Indian Hemp) plant.

Along with alcohol, nicotine and opiates, cannabinoids are the drugs of abuse most frequently consumed during pregnancy. When smoked, cannabis results in blood carbon monoxide concentrations and tar content five-fold and three-fold in excess of those reached from smoking cigarettes. Δ9-Tetrahydrocannabinol (THC), is the main toxin of the 100 chemicals in cannabis, and causes intoxication through interaction with the endocannabinoid system of the CNS.

Animal and clinical studies do not indicate that maternal use of cannabis or THC causes an overall increase in the risk of birth defects or a pattern of specific birth defects. There are inconsistent data regarding risk of low birth weight, prematurity and intrauterine growth restriction after maternal cannabis use (Hayatbakhsh 2012, Gray 2010, Shiono 1995, Fried 1987, Linn 1983). A meta-analysis of 10 observational studies did not provide any conclusive indication of a decrease in mean birth weight with moderate or occasional use of cannabis (English 1997). A review of the literature by Huizink (2014) concluded that low birth weight appeared to be associated with *in utero* exposure to cannabis from mid-pregnancy onwards, but that the data for other birth outcomes, including birth length, gestational age, and head circumference were inconsistent.

Newborns, exposed to cannabis *in utero*, have been reported to show withdrawal signs and neurological symptoms such as restlessness and excitability after birth (de Moraes Barros 2006). The published data on cognitive development in childhood, derived from three prospective longitudinal studies which followed-up children prenatally exposed to cannabis, are inconsistent. Each used different methods and measurements of child development and only two of the three studies have followed up children beyond infancy. A study using data from the Ottawa Prenatal

Prospective Study (OPPS) found significantly impaired speech and memory performance in 4-year-old children whose mothers had consumed cannabis regularly – i.e. several times a week – during the pregnancy (Fried 1990). However, effects on cognitive development in these children were described as subtle (Fried 1999). Similar impairment of memory and verbal functioning were also seen in infants at 3 years of age in The Maternal Health Practices and Child Development (MHPCD) cohort (Day 1994).

At 6 years of age, lower verbal reasoning was associated with heavy use of prenatal cannabis (more than one joint per day) in the first trimester amongst children in the MHPCD cohort (Goldschmidt 2008). At the same age, exposed children were also significantly more likely to display behaviors suggestive of attention deficit such as impulsivity and hyperactivity than their unexposed peers (Goldschmidt 2000, Leech 1999, Fried 1992). Assessment at the ages of 9 and 12 in two of the cannabis exposed cohorts highlighted increased problems in abstract and visual reasoning and impaired visuoperceptual functioning compared with unexposed matched controls (Richardson 2002, Fried 2000). Anxiety and depressive symptoms were also frequently reported in one cohort of children who were exposed to cannabis *in utero* (Gray 2005). These findings remained significant after adjusting for abuse of other substances including alcohol, nicotine and cocaine.

The most recent analysis of data from the MHPCD cohort showed an association between *in utero* exposure to cannabis and lower achievement at school at 14 years of age. After controlling for confounders, the overall score on a test designed to assess reading, mathematics and spelling was significantly lower in those prenatally exposed to cannabis compared to children who were not exposed. Further analysis of scores for each area assessed showed that exposed children scored worse for basic reading, with an association present with maternal use of one or more joints a day during the first trimester of pregnancy (Goldschmidt 2012).

Synthetic cannabanoids such as *dronabinol* and *Sativex®* are used in the treatment of anorexia and chemotherapy-induced vomiting, and multiple sclerosis related spasticity. A case report describes a 26-year-old patient with hyperkinetic disease and anorexia who was treated throughout the entire pregnancy with 25 mg of dronabinol daily. The therapy was successful in terms of weight gain, labor and delivery. The infant was born healthy and there were no complications (Farooq 2009). No information on the long-term health of the infant has been reported and use in pregnancy needs to be decided on an individual basis. There are no studies on the cannabinoid preparation Sativex® during pregnancy.

A case control study which included 538 children found that maternal use of any illicit or recreational drug around pregnancy was associated with an increased risk of neuroblastoma in the offspring, with a weak association after use of marijuana in the first trimester of pregnancy Bluhm 2006).

Recommendation. Cannabis and THC-containing preparations should not be used recreationally during pregnancy. Where such preparations have been used therapeutically, other treatments should be considered unless the benefit of cannaboid use is considered to outweigh the potential risk of lasting neurodevelopmental effects of the fetus. Where use in pregnancy has occurred no additional fetal monitoring would usually be indicated, but neonatal monitoring for symptoms of withdrawal is advised with exposure near term.

▶ **LSD**

Malformation of the eyes, brain and skeleton have been reported following *in utero* exposure to the hallucinogen, *LSD* (*lysergic acid diethylamide*) (review in Schardein 2000). A study of 140 women who used LSD in a total of 148 pregnancies reported that 53 pregnancies were electively terminated, 12 (43%) of first trimester exposures resulted in a spontaneous abortion, and 83 exposed pregnancies resulted in a live-born infant. A birth defect was reported in eight of the live-born infants and 14 of the terminated fetuses were described as having gross anomalies, although no pattern of birth defects was noted. These data were, however, heavily confounded by maternal exposure to other illicit drugs, as well as maternal infection and poor nutrition (Jacobson 1972).

Spontaneous abortion following LSD exposure with associated maternal toxicity has been described in a few case reports and in a small study (McGlothlin 1970, Idänpään-Heikkilä 1969, Cohen 1968).

Mescaline

Mescaline is a hallucinogen that is derived from Mexican cacti (peyote-cactus, *Lophophora williamsii*) and is structurally related to amphetamines (Section 2.21.5). Synthetic forms of mescaline are also available. There are no published reports of fetal outcome following use in human pregnancy. Suicidal ideation and systemic effects including rhabdomyolysis in severe cases have been reported with mescaline use in nonpregnant patients. Mescaline use in pregnancy should, therefore, be avoided.

▶ **Phencyclidine**

Phencyclidine piperidine (PCP, *Angel dust*) is taken orally or smoked in combination with marijuana, tobacco and *oregano*. Severe intoxication may be associated with anticholinergic side effects, and severe respiratory depression, cardiovascular and CNS effects requiring treatment. Phencyclidine is rapidly absorbed in the small intestine following oral ingestion. It crosses the placenta and can accumulate in fetal tissue. Animal experiments have shown degeneration of fetal cortical neurons (review in Schardein 2000). Microcephaly, facial asymmetry and a complex intra- and extra-cranial birth defect syndrome have been described in single case reports of human maternal phencyclidine abuse during pregnancy. Intrauterine growth restriction and disordered postnatal neurological adjustment have also been observed in addition to typical opiate withdrawal symptoms. A follow-up study of 57 phencyclidine exposed children showed that 65% experienced neonatal narcotic withdrawal syndrome. At 1 year of age there was no difference in a behavioral assessment compared to a control group (Wachsman 1989).

▶ **Psilocybin**

Psilocybin is a hallucinogen and is the active component of "magic mushrooms," *Psilocybe semilanceata* and *cyanescens*. The mushrooms are often dried and powdered, but are sometimes ingested fresh. Although no structural anomalies have been reported in connection with psilocybin exposure in human pregnancy or in animal experiments, use may be associated with severe toxicity and is therefore not advised in pregnancy.

Pregnancy

2.21 Recreational drugs

> **Recommendation.** Pregnant women should avoid hallucinogens under all circumstances. In view of the limited available data regarding the fetal effects of use in human pregnancy, a detailed antenatal ultrasound is recommended following first trimester exposure if not already offered as part of routine antenatal care.

2.21.5   Sedating drugs

▶ Opiates

Dependency on opiates such as *morphine* and *heroin* (*diacetylmorphine*) is not uncommon amongst pregnant women. Heroin is more lipophilic than morphine and therefore penetrates the CNS more rapidly. The high potential for dependency is due to the rapid onset of euphoric effects with intravenous use.

Heroin and other opiates do not appear to induce fetal structural malformation; however, an effect on the fetus is evidenced by reduced fetal breathing movements and heart frequency with maternal exposure.

Concurrent use of other drugs, alcohol, the mother's nutritional status, maternal infections (HIV, Hepatitis B and C) and trauma ("drug related crime") in addition to other lifestyle factors more prevalent amongst women who use recreational drugs will also influence pregnancy outcome. Acute opiate withdrawal during pregnancy can cause fetal death and premature labor and is therefore not recommended (Mawhinney 2006).

In newborns, severe withdrawal symptoms, such as respiratory distress, hyperirritability, tremor, diarrhea, vomiting, fever, disturbances in the sleep–wake rhythm and, to some extent, therapy-resistant seizures, may occur after birth and, if left untreated, may lead to death. In a study from the UK, up to 80% of infants exposed to recreational drugs, the majority of which were opiates in combination with other drugs, showed symptoms within the first 5 days of life (Goel 2011). The risk of life-threatening withdrawal symptoms in the neonate is particularly high if the mother's dependency is not known, and the appropriate monitoring and therapeutic prophylaxis with opiates (*opium tincture, morphine*) is not started in time (review in Bandstra 2010). There is no clear correlation between the severity of the withdrawal symptoms and the extent of the maternal opiate use (Thajam 2010).

Where withdrawal symptoms are adequately treated, permanent neurological deficits as a consequence of the "detox" are not expected. However, sudden infant deaths have been more commonly reported amongst babies exposed to opiates prenatally than amongst a control cohort of unexposed babies (Kandall 1991, Finnegan 1979, Rajegowda 1978). Adverse longer term effects of fetal opiate exposure on neurodevelopment and behavior have also been reported, although it remains unclear as to how much these findings reflect postnatal environmental factors and a causal association with prenatal opiate exposure is unproven (Ornoy 1996, 2001, Hayford 1988, Hutchings 1982, Wilson 1979).

Substitution therapy

Where use of heroin in pregnancy is identified, substitution therapies such as methadone or its active enantiomer, *levomethadone* are advisable and are associated with better fetal outcome. Both methadone and levomethadone are long acting opioids with half-lives of 13–60 hours and 48–72 hours in the nonpregnant patient respectively, but may be significantly reduced in pregnancy (Jarvis 1999). Methadone crosses the placenta although fetal concentrations are dependent on gestational age, and maternal dose and plasma concentration. Newborns of mothers who are treated with methadone have a higher birth weight and reduced mortality compared to those of untreated heroin-using mothers, although neonatal respiratory depression and withdrawal symptoms also occur with methadone. There is evidence that the withdrawal symptoms related to methadone use in pregnancy are more severe and last for longer than those associated with intrauterine heroin exposure (review in Farid 2008). Neonatal treatment with oral opiates appears to be the most effective and well-tolerated therapy for neonatal withdrawal syndrome (Arlettaz 2005, Jackson 2004, Siddappa 2003). Although a correlation between neonatal withdrawal symptom severity and maternal opiate dose at the end of the pregnancy would be expected, Berghella (2003) did not identify any significant difference in the severity and/ or duration of neonatal withdrawal symptoms amongst neonates of pregnant women substituted with 40, 60 or 80 mg of methadone.

Buprenorphine is also used in the treatment of opioid dependence and is administered sublingually, transdermally or intravenously. The half-life varies depending on route of administration (1.2–7.2 hours intravenously, 20–36 hours transdermally or sublingually); however, the duration of action is significantly longer due to high μ-opioid receptor affinity and slow dissociation. In comparison to the other opiates, the placental transfer is lower (Nanovskaya 2002, Rohrmeister 2001) and a prospective, randomized, double-blind study of 113 newborns reported milder withdrawal symptoms in comparison to methadone (Jones 2010). The 58 infants in the buprenorphine group needed significantly lower doses of morphine in the treatment of neonatal withdrawal symptoms, were treated for a shorter period, and could be discharged from hospital more quickly. A prospective study of 117 pregnant women who used methadone, buprenorphine or heroin also found that the most severe withdrawal symptoms occurred in neonates of women in the methadone group. By contrast, women in the heroin group had the highest risk for low birthweight (Binder 2008). These results are consistent with those of older studies involving a total of more than 300 pregnant women (Kakko 2008; review by Johnson 2003). Conversely, Lejeune (2006) did not find any significant difference in the incidence or severity of neonatal withdrawal symptoms in a prospective study involving a total of 259 pregnant women. A retrospective evaluation of 23 neonates of women receiving buprenorphine therapy for opioid dependence during the pregnancy saw no significant relationship between maternal buprenorphine dose and infant birth-weight, severity of neonatal withdrawal symptoms or the interval between onset of withdrawal symptoms (O'Connor 2011).

Oral *naltrexone* formulations or naltrexone implants have also been used in the treatment of heroin-dependent pregnant women (Hulse 2001, 2004). However, the results of these studies are insufficient to assess their effectiveness and safety during pregnancy. Hartwig (2008) report a single case where *diamorphine* substitution was successfully used preconceptually and during pregnancy to manage a pregnant woman with multiple dependencies and morbidities. Regardless of the therapy chosen, pregnant women with dependencies or who are receiving substitution therapy should be closely monitored and supported by a multidisciplinary team.

Long-term studies

In contrast to the clearly documented developmental and behavioral effects of fetal alcohol spectrum disorder, no clear pattern of cognitive and/or neurological problems has been identified amongst children whose mothers abused drugs during pregnancy once factors relating to the child's social environment in the first years of life are taken into account. No difference in intellectual development was noticed between a cohort of heroin exposed children who were adopted and a non-exposed cohort, whereas the children who were raised by a parent who was a heroin user were more likely to be developmentally delayed (Ornoy 2001). However, follow-up of this cohort at age 6–11 years demonstrated that attention deficit and hyperactivity disorders (ADHD) occurred more frequently in all heroin-exposed children than in unexposed children in the control group although children who remained in a drug-taking environment (67%) were significantly more likely to have ADHD (37%) than those who were adopted out (Ornoy 2001). A case-control study of 133 children aged 3 years who were exposed to opiates prenatally, Hunt (2008) reported reduced growth, and deficits in mental, speech and social development. Long-term behavioral effects of fetal methadone exposure such as increased aggression and delayed cognitive and social development at the age of 7 have also been reported. By contrast, other studies did not determine any long-term effects of opiate exposure *in utero* (review in Farid 2008).

> **Recommendation.** Acute opiate withdrawal should not be conducted during pregnancy. In cases of heroin dependency, substitution with methadone or buprenorphine is recommended. Some feel that use of buprenorphine is preferable. Substitution requires careful dose titration and should only be undertaken by experienced physicians. Concurrent use of recreational or addictive drugs may be detectable on urine screening. A comprehensive assessment of the social environment is recommended and intensive support may be required both during pregnancy to optimize maternal health, as well as postnatally in situations where adoption or foster care of the infant is deemed appropriate. Newborn infants require careful monitoring and observation, in some instances for several weeks, so that withdrawal symptoms, some of which may be fatal, can be treated with opiates and other supportive therapies.

▶ Gamma-hydroxybutyric acid (GHB)

Gamma-hydroxybutyrate (γ or GHB) is also a sedative drug that is approved for use in the treatment of narcolepsy with cataplexy. It is structurally related to the neurotransmitter – GABA. In the 1960s, it was also used in obstetrical anesthesia for Caesarean births (Laget-Corsin 1972). It is more frequently taken as a drug of abuse as *liquid ecstasy*, and as a body building agent. Transplacental transfer of GHB has been described; however, there are no systematic studies on use in pregnancy therapeutically or recreationally. A single case study described the birth of a healthy newborn to a GHB-abusing mother who, herself, developed respiratory depression during the birth (Kuczkowski 2004).

> **Recommendation.** GHB should not be used recreationally in pregnancy. Where exposure has occurred in the first trimester a detailed fetal anomaly scan is recommended if not already offered as routine antenatal care at around 12 and 20 weeks.

References

Ackerman JP, Riggins T, Black MM. A review of the effects of prenatal cocaine exposure among school-aged children. Pediatrics 2010; 125: 554–65.

Addis A, Moretti ME, Ahmed SF et al. Fetal effects of cocaine: an updated meta-analysis. Reprod Toxicol 2001; 15: 341–69.

Aliyu MH, Wilson RE, Zoorob R et al. Alcohol consumption during pregnancy and the risk of early stillbirth among singletons. Alcohol 2008; 42: 369–74.

Ammenheuser MM, Berenson AB, Stiglich NJ et al. Elevated frequencies of hprt mutant lymphocytes in cigarette-smoking mothers and their newborns. Mutat Res 1994; 304: 285–94.

Ananth CV, Smulian JC, Vintzileos AM. Incidence of placental abruption in relation to cigarette smoking and hypertensive disorders during pregnancy: a meta-analysis of observational studies. Obstet Gynecol 1999; 93: 622–8.

Anderson HR, Cook DG. Passive smoking and sudden infant death syndrome: review of the epidemiological evidence. Thorax 1997; 52(11): 1003–9.

Arlettaz R, Kashiwagi M, Das Kundu S et al. Methadone maintenance in a Swiss perinatal center: II. Neonatal outcome and social resources. Acta Obstet Gynecol Scand 2005; 84: 145–50.

Astley SJ. Validation of the fetal alcohol spectrum disorder (FASD) 4-Digit Diagnostic Code. J Popul Ther Clin Pharmacol 2013; 20: e416–67.

Autti-Ramo I, Fagerlund A, Ervalahti N et al. Fetal alcohol spectrum disorders in Finland: Clinical delineation of 77 older children and adolescents. Am J Med Genet A 2006; 140: 137–43.

Bailey BN, Delaney-Black V, Covington JH et al. Prenatal exposure to binge drinking and cognitive and behavioral outcomes at age 7 years. Am J Obstet Gynecol 2004; 191: 1037–43.

Bakker R, Steegers EA, Obradov A et al. Maternal caffeine intake from coffee and tea, fetal growth, and the risks of adverse birth outcomes: the Generation R Study. Am J Clin Nutr 2010; 91: 1691–8.

Bandstra ES, Morrow CE, Mansoor E et al. Prenatal drug exposure: infant and toddler outcomes. J Addict Dis 2010; 29: 245–58.

Bandstra ES, Morrow CE, Vogel AL et al. Longitudinal influence of prenatal cocaine exposure on child language functioning. Teratology 2002; 24: 297–308.

Bandstra ES, Vogel AL, Morrow CE et al. Severity of prenatal cocaine exposure and child language functioning through age seven years: a longitudinal latent growth curve analysis. Subst Use Misuse 2004; 39: 25–59.

Barr HM, Bookstein FL, O'Malley KD et al. Binge drinking during pregnancy as a predictor of psychiatric disorders on the Structured Clinical Interview for DSM-IV in young adult offspring. Am J Psychiatry 2006; 163: 1061–5.

Barr HM, Streissguth AP. Caffeine use during pregnancy and child outcome: a 7-year prospective study. Neurotoxicol Teratol 1991; 13: 441–8.

Bauer CR, Langer JC, Shankaran S et al. Acute neonatal effects of cocaine exposure during pregnancy. Arch Pediatr Adolesc Med 2005; 159: 824–34.

Bech B, Nohr E, Vaeth M et al. Coffee and fetal death: a cohort study with prospective data. American Journal of Epidemiology, 2005; 162: 983–90.

Beeghly M, Martin B, Rose-Jacobs R et al. Prenatal cocaine exposure and children's language functioning at 6 and 9.5 years: moderating effects of child age, birthweight, and gender. J Pediatr Psychol 2006; 31: 98–115.

Bekkhus M, Skjothaug T, Nordhagen R et al. Intrauterine exposure to caffeine and inattention/overactivity in children. Acta Paediatr 2010; 99: 925–8.

Bell SH, Stade B, Reynolds JN et al. The remarkably high prevalence of epilepsy and seizure history in fetal alcohol spectrum disorders. Alcohol Clin Exp Res 2010; 34: 1084–9.

Bennett LM, Wang Y, Ramsey MJ et al. Cigarette smoking during pregnancy: chromosome translocations and phenotypic susceptibility in mothers and newborns. Mutat Res 2010; 696: 81–8.

Berghella V, Lim PJ, Hill MK et al. Maternal methadone dose and neonatal withdrawal. Am J Obstet Gynecol 2003; 189: 312–7.

Bille C, Olsen J, Vach W et al. Oral clefts and life style factors – a case-cohort study based on prospective Danish data. Eur J Epidemiol 2007; 22: 173–81.

Binder T, Vavrinkova B. Prospective randomised comparative study of the effect of buprenorphine, methadone and heroin on the course of pregnancy, birthweight of newborns, early postpartum adaptation and course of the neonatal abstinence syndrome (NAS) in women followed up in the outpatient department. Neuro Endocrinol Lett 2008; 29, 80–6.

Bingol N, Fuchs M, Diaz V, Stone RK, Gromisch DS. Teratogenicity of cocaine in humans. J Pediatr 1987; 110: 93–6.

Bluhm EC, Daniels J, Pollock BH et al. Maternal use of recreational drugs and neuroblastoma in offspring: a report from the Children's Oncology Group (United States). Cancer Causes Control 2006; 17: 663–9.

Bonaventure A, Rudant J, Goujon-Bellec S et al. Childhood acute leukemia, maternal beverage intake during pregnancy, and metabolic polymorphisms. Cancer Causes Control 2013; 24: 783–93.

Brent RL, Christian MS, Diener RM. Evaluation of the reproductive and developmental risks of caffeine. Birth Def Res B 2011; 92: 152–87.

Brion MJ, Leary SD, Smith GD et al. Similar associations of parental prenatal smoking suggest child blood pressure is not influenced by intrauterine effects. Hypertension 2007; 49: 1422–8.

Brooks DR, Mucci LA, Hatch EE et al. Maternal smoking during pregnancy and risk of brain tumors in offspring. Cancer Causes Control 2004; 15: 997–1005.

Bruin JE, Gerstein HC, Holloway AC. Long-term consequences of fetal and neonatal nicotine exposure: a critical review. Toxicol Sci 2010; 116: 364–74.

Caspers KM, Oltean C, Romitti PA et al. Maternal periconceptional exposure to cigarette smoking and alcohol consumption and congenital diaphragmatic hernia. Birth Defects Res A Clin Mol Teratol 2010; 88: 1040–9.

Caspers KM, Romitti PA, Lin S et al. National Birth Defects Prevention Study. Maternal periconceptional exposure to cigarette smoking and congenital limb deficiencies. Paediatr Perinat Epidemiol 2013; 27: 509–20.

Cernerud L, Eriksson M, Jonsson B et al. Amphetamine addiction during pregnancy: 14 year follow-up of growth and school performance. Acta Paediatr 1996; 85: 204–8.

Chang L, Alicata D, Ernst T et al. Structural and metabolic brain changes in the striatum associated with methamphetamine abuse. Addiction 2007; 102: 16–32.

Chang L, Cloak C, Jiang CS et al. Altered neurometabolites and motor integration in children exposed to methamphetamine in utero. Neuroimage 2009; 48: 391–7.

Chanoine JP, Toppet V, Bordoux P et al. Smoking during pregnancy: a significant cause of neonatal thyroid enlargement. Br J Obstet Gynaecol 1991; 98: 65–8.

Chasnoff IJ, Burns WJ, Schnoll SH, Burns KA. Cocaine use in pregnancy. N Engl J Med 1985; 313: 666–9.

Chasnoff IJ, Chisum GM, Kaplan WE. Maternal cocaine use and genitourinary tract malformations. Teratology 1988; 37: 201–4.

Chen R, Clifford A, Lang L, Anstey KJ. Is exposure to secondhand smoke associated with cognitive parameters of children and adolescents? A systematic literature review. Ann Epidemiol 2013; 23: 652–61.

Chiodo, L.M., Bailey, B., Sokol, R.J., Janisse, J., Delaney-Black, V., Hannigan, J.H. Recognized spontaneous abortion in mid-pregnancy and patterns of pregnancy alcohol use. Alcohol 2012; 46:261–267.

Chiriboga CA, Kuhn L, Wasserman GA. Prenatal cocaine exposures and dose-related cocaine effects on infant tone and behavior. Neurotoxicol Teratol 2007; 29: 323–30.

Chomchai C, Na Manorom N, Watanarungsan P et al. Methamphetamine abuse during pregnancy and its health impact on neonates born at Siriraj Hospital, Bangkok, Thailand. Southeast Asian J Trop Med Public Health 2004; 35: 228–31.

Clifford A, Lang L, Chen R. Effects of maternal cigarette smoking during pregnancy on cognitive parameters of children and young adults: a literature review. Neurotoxicol Teratol 2012; 34: 560–70.

Cohen MM, Hirschhorn K, Verbo S et al. The effect of LSD-25 on the chromosomes of children exposed in utero. Pediatr Res. 1968; 2: 486–92.

Coleman T, Chamberlain C, Cooper S et al. Efficacy and safety of nicotine replacement therapy for smoking cessation in pregnancy: systematic review and meta-analysis. Addiction 2011; 106: 52–61.

Cornelius MD, De Genna NM, Leech SL et al. Effects of prenatal cigarette smoke exposure on neurobehavioral outcomes in 10-year-old children of adolescent mothers. Neurotoxicol Teratol 2011; 33: 137–44.

Cornelius MD, Goldschmidt L, Day NL. Prenatal cigarette smoking: Long-term effects on young adult behavior problems and smoking behavior. Neurotoxicol Teratol 2012; 34: 554–9.

Cornelius MD, Ryan CM, Day NL et al. Prenatal tobacco effects on neuropsychological outcomes among preadolescents. J Dev Behav Pediatr 2001; 22: 217–25.

Dahshan A. Prenatal exposure to methamphetamine presenting as neonatal cholestasis. J Clin Gastroenterol 2009; 43: 88–90.

Day NL, Richardson GA, Goldschmidt L et al. Effect of prenatal marijuana exposure on the cognitive development of offspring at age three. Neurotoxicol Teratol 1994; 16: 169–75.

de la Chica RA, Ribas I, Giraldo J et al. Chromosomal instability in amniocytes from fetuses of mothers who smoke. JAMA 2005; 293: 1212–2.

de Moraes Barros MC, Guinsburg R, de Araujo PC et al. Exposure to marijuana during pregnancy alters neurobehavior in the early neonatal period. J Pediatr 2006; 149: 781–7.

DeRoo LA, Wilcox AJ, Drevon CA et al. First-trimester maternal alcohol consumption and the risk of infant oral clefts in Norway: a population-based case-control study. Am J Epidemiol 2008; 168: 638–46.

Draper ES, Rankin J, Tonks AM et al. Recreational drug use: a major risk factor for gastroschisis? Am J Epidemiol 2008; 167: 485–91.

Eiden RD, McAuliffe S, Kachadourian L et al. Effects of prenatal cocaine exposure on infant reactivity and regulation. Neurotoxicol Teratol 2009; 31: 60–8.

Elliott L, Loomis D, Lottritz L et al. Case-control study of a gastroschisis cluster in Nevada. Arch Pediatr Adolesc Med 2009; 163: 1000–6.

English DR, Hulse GK, Milne E et al. Maternal cannabis use and birth weight: a meta-analysis. Addiction 1997; 92: 1553–60.

EUROMAC. A European Concerned Action: Maternal alcohol consumption and its relation to the outcome of pregnancy and child development at 18 months. Int J Epidemiol 1992; 21: 1–87.

Eyler FD, Behnke M, Conlon M et al. Birth outcome from a prospective, matched study of prenatal crack/cocaine use: I. Interactive and dose effects on health and growth. Pediatrics 1998a; 101: 229–37.

Eyler FD, Behnke M, Conlon M et al. Birth outcome from a prospective, matched study of prenatal crack/cocaine use: II. Interactive and dose effects on neurobehavioral assessment. Pediatrics 1998b; 101: 237–41.

Farid WO, Dunlop SA, Tait RJ et al. The effects of maternally administered methadone, buprenorphine and naltrexone on offspring: review of human and animal data. Curr Neuropharmacol 2008; 6: 125–50.

Farooq MU, Ducommun E, Goudreau J. Treatment of a hyperkinetic movement disorder during pregnancy with dronabinol. Parkinsonism Relat Disord 2009; 15: 249–51.

Feldman HS, Jones KL, Lindsay S. Prenatal alcohol exposure patterns and alcohol-related birth defects and growth deficiencies: a prospective study. Alcohol Clin Exp Res 2012; 36: 670–6.

Felix RJ, Chambers CD, Dick LM et al. Prospective pregnancy outcome in women exposed to amphetamines. Teratology 2000; 61: 441.

Fergusson DM, Horwood LJ, Lynskey MT. Maternal smoking before and after pregnancy: effect on behavioral outcomes in middle childhood. Pediatrics 1998; 97: 815–22.

Fernandes O, Sabharwal M, Smiley T et al. Moderate to heavy caffeine consumption during pregnancy and relationship to spontaneous abortion and abnormal fetal growth: a meta-analysis. Reprod Toxicol 1998; 12: 435–44.

Finnegan LP. In utero opiate dependence and sudden infant death syndrome. Clin Perinatol 1979; 6: 163–180.

Flak AL, Su S, Bertrand J et al. The association of mild, moderate, and binge prenatal alcohol exposure and child neuropsychological outcomes: a meta-analysis. Alcohol Clin Exper Res 2014; 38: 214–26.

Fleming P, Blair PS. Sudden Infant Death Syndrome and parental smoking. Early Hum Dev 2007; 83: 721–5.

Flenady V, Koopmans L, Middleton P et al. Major risk factors for stillbirth in high-income countries: a systematic review and meta-analysis. Lancet 2011; 377: 1331–40.

Florath, Kohler M, Weck MN et al. Association of pre- and post-natal parental smoking with offspring body mass index: an 8-year follow-up of a birth cohort. Pediatr Obes 2014; 9: 121–34.

Forinash AB, Pitlick JM, Clark K et al. Nicotine replacement therapy effect on pregnancy outcomes. Ann Pharmacother 2010; 44: 1817–21.

Forrester MB, Merz RD. Risk of selected birth defects with prenatal illicit drug use, Hawaii, 1986–2002. J Toxicol Environ Health A 2007; 70: 7–18.

Fried PA, O'Connell CM. A comparison of the effects of prenatal exposure to tobacco, alcohol, cannabis and caffeine on birth size and subsequent growth. Neurotoxicol Teratol 1987; 9: 79–85.

Fried PA, Watkinson B, Gray R. A follow-up study of attentional behavior in 6-year-old children exposed prenatally to marihuana, cigarettes, and alcohol. Neurotoxicol Teratol 1992; 14: 299–311.

Fried PA, Watkinson B, Gray R. Growth from birth to early adolescence in offspring prenatally exposed to cigarettes and marijuana. Neurotox Teratol 1999; 21: 513–25.

Fried PA, Watkinson B. 36- and 48-month neurobehavioral follow-up of children prenatally exposed to marijuana, cigarettes and alcohol. Develop Behavioral Pediatrics 1990; 11: 49–58.

Fried PA, Watkinson B. Visuoperceptual functioning differs in 9- to 12-year olds prenatally exposed to cigarettes and marihuana. Neurotoxicol Teratol 2000; 22: 11–20.

George L, Granath F, Johansson AL et al. Environmental tobacco smoke and risk of spontaneous abortion. Epidemiology 2006; 17: 500–5.

Goel N, Beasley D, Rajkumar V et al. Perinatal outcome of illicit substance use in pregnancy-comparative and contemporary socio-clinical profile in the UK. Eur J Pediatr 2011; 170: 199–205.

Goldschmidt L, Day NL, Richardson GA. Effects of prenatal marijuana exposure on child behavior problems at age 10. Neurotoxicol Teratol 2000; 22: 325–36.

Goldschmidt L, Richardson GA, Willford J et al. Prenatal marijuana exposure and intelligence test performance at age 6. J Am Acad Child Adolesc Psychiatry 2008; 47: 254–63.

Goldschmidt L, Richardson GA, Willford JA et al. School achievement in 14-year-old youths prenatally exposed to marijuana. Neurotoxicol Teratol 2012; 34: 161–7.

Gouin K, Murphy K, Shah PS. Effects of cocaine use during pregnancy on low birthweight and preterm birth: systematic review and metaanalyses. Am J Obstet Gynecol 2011; 204: 340–12.

Gray KA, Day NL, Leech S, Richardson GA. Prenatal marijuana exposure: effect on child depressive symptoms at ten years of age. Neurotoxicol Teratol 2005; 27: 439–48.

Gray TR, Eiden RD, Leonard KE et al. Identifying prenatal cannabis exposure and effects of concurrent tobacco exposure on neonatal growth. Clin Chem 2010; 56: 1442–50.

Grosso LM, Triche EW, Belanger K et al. Caffeine metabolites in umbilical cord blood, cytochrome P-450 1A2 activity, and intrauterine growth restriction. Am J Epidemiol 2006; 163:1035–1041.

Hanke W, Kalinka J, Florek E et al. Passive smoking and pregnancy outcome in central Poland. Hum Experiment Toxicol 1999; 18: 265–71.

Hartwig C, Haasen C, Reimer J et al. Pregnancy and birth under maintenance treatment with diamorphine (heroin): a case report. Eur Addict Res 2008; 14: 113–4.

Hayford SM, Epps RP, Dahl-Regis M. Behavior and development patterns in children born to heroin-addicted and methadone-addicted mothers. J Natl Med Assoc 1988; 80: 1197–200.

Hayatbakhsh MR, Flenady VJ, Gibbons KS, Kingsbury AM, Hurrion E, Mamun AA, Najman JM. Birth outcomes associated with cannabis use before and during pregnancy. Pediatr Res 2012; 71(2): 215–9.

Henderson J, Kesmodel U, Gray R. Systematic review of the fetal effects of prenatal binge-drinking. J Epidemiol Community Health 2007; 61: 1069–1073.

Honein MA, Rasmussen SA. Further evidence for an association between maternal smoking and craniosynostosis. Teratology 2000; 62: 145–6.

Hoyme HE, Jones KL, Dixon SD et al. Prenatal cocaine exposure and fetal vascular disruption. Pediatrics 1990; 85: 743–51.

Huizink AC. Prenatal cannabis exposure and infant outcomes: Overview of studies. Prog Neuropsychopharmacol Biol Psychiatry 2014 Jul 3; 52: 45–52.

Hulse GK, O'Neil G, Arnold-Reed DE. Methadone maintenance vs. implantable naltrexone treatment in the pregnant heroin user. Int J Gynaecol Obstet 2004; 85: 170–1.

Hulse GK, O'Neill G, Pereira C et al. Obstetric and neonatal outcomes associated with maternal naltrexone exposure. Aust N Z J Obstet Gynaecol 2001; 41: 424–8.

Hunt RW, Tzioumi D, Collins E et al. Adverse neurodevelopmental outcome of infants exposed to opiate in-utero. Early Hum Dev 2008; 84: 29–35.

Hurt H, Betancourt LM, Malmud EK et al. Children with and without gestational cocaine exposure: a neurocognitive systems analysis. Neurotoxicol Teratol 2009; 31: 334–41.

Hutchings DE. Methadone and heroin during pregnancy: a review of behavioral effects in human and animal offspring. Neurobehav Toxicol Teratol 1982; 4: 429–34.

Hyland A, Piazza KM, Hovey KM et al. Associations of lifetime active and passive smoking with spontaneous abortion, stillbirth and tubal ectopic pregnancy: a cross-sectional analysis of historical data from the Women's Health Initiative. Tob Control 2014 (Epub ahead of print).

Idänpään-Heikkilä JE. LSD-effect on chromosomes and fetus. Duodecim 1969; 85: 274–82.

Indredavik MS, Brubakk AM, Romundstad P et al. Prenatal smoking exposure and psychiatric symptoms in adolescence. Acta Paediatr 2007; 96: 377–82.

Ino T. Maternal smoking during pregnancy and offspring obesity: meta-analysis. Pediatr Int 2010; 52: 94–9.

Jackson L, Ting A, McKay et al. A randomised controlled trial of morphine versus phenobarbitone for neonatal abstinence syndrome. Arch Dis Child Fetal Neonatal Ed 2004; 89: F300–4.

Jacobson CB, Berlin C M. Possible reproductive detriment in LSD users. JAMA 1972; 222: 1367–73.

Jarvis MA, Wu-Pong S, Kniseley JS, Schnoll SH. Alterations in methadone metabolism during late pregnancy. J Addict Dis 1999; 18: 51–61.

Jensen TK, Henriksen TB, Hjollund NHI, et al. Caffeine intake and fecundability: A follow-up study among 430 Danish couples planning their first pregnancy. Reprod Toxicol 1998, 12: 289–95.

Johnson RE, Jones HE, Fischer G. Use of buprenorphine in pregnancy: patient management and effects on the neonate. Drug Alcohol Depend 2003; 70: 87–101.

Jones HE, Kaltenbach K, Heil SH et al. Neonatal abstinence syndrome after methadone or buprenorphine exposure. N Engl J Med 2010; 363: 2320–31.

Jones KL. The effects of alcohol on fetal development. Birth Def Res C 2011; 93: 3–11.

Kakko J, Heilig M, Sarman I. Buprenorphine and methadone treatment of opiate dependence during pregnancy: comparison of fetal growth and neonatal outcomes in two consecutive case series. Drug Alcohol Depend 2008; 96: 69–78.

Källén K. Maternal smoking and craniosynostosis. Teratology 1999; 60: 146–50.

Källén K. Maternal smoking during pregnancy and limb reduction malformations in Sweden. Am J Public Health 1997; 87: 29–32.

Kandall SR, Gaines J. Maternal substance use and subsequent sudden infant death syndrome (SIDS) in offspring. Neurotoxicol Teratol 1991; 13: 235–40.

Klebanoff MA, Zhang J, Zhang C, Levine RJ. Maternal serum theobromine and the development of preeclampsia. Epidemiology 2009; 20: 727–32.

Kuczkowski KM. Herbal Ecstasy: cardiovascular complications of khat chewing in pregnancy. Acta Anaesthesiol Belg 2005; 56: 19–21.

Kuczkowski KM. Liquid ecstasy during pregnancy. Anaesthesia 2004; 59: 926.

Kuehn D1, Aros S, Cassorla F et al. A prospective cohort study of the prevalence of growth, facial, and central nervous system abnormalities in children with heavy prenatal alcohol exposure. Alcohol Clin Exp Res 2012; 36: 1811–9.

Kulig M, Luck W, Wahn U. Multicenter Allergy Study Group, Germany: The association between pre- and postnatal tobacco smoke exposure and allergic sensitization during early childhood. Hum Experiment Toxicol 1999; 18: 241–44.

Lackmann GM, Angerer J, Töllner U. Parental smoking and neonatal serum levels of polychlorinated biphenyls and hexachlorobenzene. Pediatr Res 2000; 47: 598–601.

Lackmann GM, Salzberger U, Chen M et al. Tabakspezifische transplazentare Kanzerogene, Nikotin und Cotinin im Urin von Neugeborenen rauchender Mütter. Monatsschr Kinderheilkd 1999; 147: 333–8.

Ladhani NN, Shah PS, Murphy KE; Knowledge Synthesis Group on Determinants of Preterm/LBW Births. Prenatal amphetamine exposure and birth outcomes: a systematic review and metaanalysis. Am J Obstet Gynecol 2011; 205: 219, e1–7.

Laget-Corsin L, Baroche J. L'anesthésie au gamma-hydroxybutyrate de sodium dans l'opération cesarienne. Anesth Anal Rean 1972; 29: 43–9.

Larkby CA, Goldschmidt L, Hanusa BH et al. Prenatal alcohol exposure is associated with conduct disorder in adolescence: findings from a birth cohort. J Am Acad Child Adolesc Psychiatry 2011; 50: 262–71.

Latino-Martel P, Chan DS, Druesne-Pecollo N et al. Maternal alcholo consumption during pregnancy and risk of childhood leukemia: systematic review and meta-analysis. Cancer Epidemiol Biomarkers Prev 2010; 19: 1238–60.

Leech SL1, Richardson GA, Goldschmidt L, Day NL. Prenatal substance exposure: effects on attention and impulsivity of 6-year-olds. Neurotoxicol Teratol 1999; 21: 109–18.

Lejeune C, Simmat-Durand L, Gourarier L et al. Prospective multicenter observational study of 260 infants born to 259 opiate-dependent mothers on methadone or high-dose buprenophine substitution. Drug Alcohol Depend 2006; 82: 250–7.

Leonardi-Bee J, Smyth A, Britton J et al. Environmental tobacco smoke and fetal health: systematic review and meta-analysis. Arch Dis Child Fetal Neonatal Ed 2008; 93: F351–61.

Pregnancy

2.21 Recreational drugs

Lester BM, Lagasse LL. Children of addicted women. J Addict Dis 2010; 29: 259–76.

Lester BM, Padbury JF. Third pathophysiology of prenatal cocaine exposure. Dev Neurosci 2009; 31: 23–35.

Levin JN. Amphetamine ingestion with biliary atresia. J Pediatr 1971; 79: 130–1.

Li D-K, Mueller BA, Hickok DE et al. Maternal smoking during pregnancy and the risk of congenital urinary tract anomalies. Am J Public Health 1996; 86: 249–53.

Linnet KM, Wisborg K, Obel C et al. Smoking during pregnancy and the risk for hyperkinetic disorder in offspring. Pediatrics 2005; 116: 462–7.

Linnet KM, Wisborg K, Secher NJ et al. Coffee consumption during pregnancy and the risk of hyperkinetic disorder and ADHD: a prospective cohort study. Acta Paediatr 2009; 98: 173–9.

Little BB, Snell LM, Gilstrap LC 3rd. Methamphetamine abuse during pregnancy: outcome and fetal effects. Obstet Gynecol 1988; 72: 541–4.

Little J, Cardy A, Arslan MT et al. United Kingdom-based case-control study. Smoking and orofacial clefts: a United Kingdom-based case-control study. Cleft Palate Craniofac J 2004a; 41: 381–6.

Little J, Cardy A, Munger RG. Tobacco smoking and oral clefts: a meta-analysis. Bull World Health Organ 2004b; 82: 213–8.

Makelarski JA, Romitti PA, Sun L et al. Periconceptional maternal alcohol consumption and neural tube defects. Birth Defects Res Part A: Clin Mol Teratol 2013; 97: 152–60.

Malik S, Cleves MA, Honein MA et al. Maternal smoking and congenital heart defects. Pediatrics 2008; 121: e810–6.

Maritz GS. Are nicotine replacement therapy, varenicline or bupropion options for pregnant mothers to quit smoking? Effects on the respiratory system of the offspring. Ther Adv Respir Dis 2009; 3: 193–210.

Martinez-Frias ML, Rodriguez-Pinilla E, Prieto L. Prenatal exposure to salicylates and gastroschisis: a case-control study. Teratology 1997; 56: 241–3.

Maslova E, Bhattacharya S, Lin SW et al. Caffeine consumption during pregnancy and risk of preterm birth: a meta-analysis. Am J Clin Nutr 2010; 92: 1120–32.

Mawhinney S, Ashe RG, Lowry J. Substance abuse in pregnancy: opioid substitution in a northern Ireland maternity unit. Ulster Med J 2006; 75: 187–91.

McCarthy FP, O'Keeffe LM, Khashan AS et al. Association between maternal alcohol consumption in early pregnancy and pregnancy outcomes. Obstet Gynecol 2013; 122: 830–7.

McElhatton PR, Bateman DN, Evans C et al. Congenital anomalies after prenatal ecstasy exposure. Lancet 1999; 354: 1441–2.

McGlothlin WH, Sparkes RS, Arnold DO. Effect of LSD on human pregnancy. JAMA 1970; 212: 1483–7.

Mercado A, Johnson G, Calver D et al. Cocaine, pregnancy and postpartum intracerebral hemorrhage. Obstet Gynecol 1989; 73: 467–72.

Messinger DS, Bauer CR, Das A et al. The maternal lifestyle study: cognitive, motor and behavioral outcomes of cocaine-exposed and opiate-exposed infants through three years of age. Pediatrics 2004; 113: 1677–85.

Mongraw-Chaffin ML, Cohn BA, Cohen RD et al. Maternal smoking, alcohol consumption, and caffeine consumption during pregnancy in relation to a son's risk of persistent cryptorchidism: a prospective study in the Child Health and Development Studies cohort, 1959–1967. Am J Epidemiol 2008; 167: 257–61.

Morales-Suárez-Varela MM, Bille C, Christensen K et al. Smoking habits, nicotine use, and congenital malformations. Obstet Gynecol 2006; 107: 51–7.

Myung SK, Ju W, Jung HS et al. Korean Meta-Analysis (KORMA) Study Group. Efficacy and safety of pharmacotherapy for smoking cessation among pregnant smokers: a meta-analysis. BJOG 2012; 119: 1029–39.

Nanovskaya T, Deshmukh S, Brooks M et al. Transplacental transfer and metabolism of buprenorphine. J Pharmacol Exp Ther 2002; 300: 26–33.

Ness RB, Grisso JA, Hirschinger N et al. Cocaine and tobacco use and the risk of spontaneous abortion. N Engl J Med 1999; 340: 333–9.

NIDA (National Institute for Drug Abuse) 2014. http://www.drugabuse.gov/publications/drugfacts/synthetic-cathinones-bath-salts

Nora JJ, McNamara DG, Fraser FC. Dexamphetamine sulphate and human malformations. Lancet 1967; 1: 570–1.

Nuesslein TG, Beckers D, Rieger CHL. Cotinine in meconium indicates risk for early respiratory tract infections. Hum Experiment Toxicol 1999; 18: 283–90.

O'Connor A, Alto W, Musgrave K et al. Observational study of buprenorphine treatment of opioid-dependent pregnant women in a family medicine residency: reports on maternal and infant outcomes. J Am Board Fam Med 2011; 24: 194–201.

O'Leary CM, Nassar N, Zubrick SR et al. Evidence of a complex association between dose, pattern and timing of prenatal alcohol exposure and child behaviour problems. Addiction 2010; 105: 74–86.

Obel C, Henriksen TB, Heedegard M et al. Smoking during pregnancy and babbling abilities of the 8-month-old infant. Paediatr Perinat Epidemiol 1998; 12: 37–48.

Obel C, Linnet KM, Henriksen TB et al. Smoking during pregnancy and hyperactivity-inattention in the offspring – comparing results from three Nordic cohorts. Int J Epidemiol 2009; 38: 698–705.

Obel C, Olsen J, Henriksen TB et al. Is maternal smoking during pregnancy a risk factor for hyperkinetic disorder? – Findings from a sibling design. Int J Epidemiol 2011; 40: 338–45.

Ornoy A, Ergaz Z. Alcohol abuse in pregnant women: effects on the fetus and newborn, mode of action and maternal treatment. Int J Environ Res Public Health 2010; 7: 364–79.

Ornoy A, Michailevskaya V, Lukashov I et al. The developmental outcome of children born to heroin-dependent mothers, raised at home or adopted. Child Abuse Negl 1996; 20: 385–96.

Ornoy A, Segal J, Bar-Hamburger R, Greenbaum C. Developmental outcome of school-age children born to mothers with heroin dependency: importance of environmental factors. Dev Med Child Neurol 2001; 43: 668–75.

Patel SS, Burns TL, Botto LD et al. National Birth Defects Prevention Study. Analysis of selected maternal exposures and non-syndromic atrioventricular septal defects in the National Birth Defects Prevention Study, 1997–2005. Am J Med Genet A 2012; 158A: 2447–55.

Patra J, Bakker R, Irving H et al. Dose-response relationship between alcohol consumption before and during pregnancy and the risks of low birthweight, preterm birth and small for gestational age (SGA)-a systemic review and meta-analyses BJOG 2011; 118: 1141–21.

Peck JD, Leviton A, Cowan LD. A review of the epidemiologic evidence concerning the reproductive health effects of caffeine consumption: a 2000–2009 update. Food Chem Toxicol 2010; 48: 2549–76.

Pineles BL, Park E, Samet JM. Systematic review and meta-analysis of miscarriage and maternal exposure to tobacco smoke during pregnancy. Am J Epidemiol 2014; 179: 807–23.

Polygenis D, Wharton S, Malmberg C et al. Moderate alcohol consumption during pregnancy and the incidence of fetal malformations: a meta-analysis. Neurotox Teratol 1998; 20: 61–7.

Rajegowda BK, Kandall SR, Falciglia H. Sudden unexpected death in infants of narcotic-dependent mothers. Early Hum Dev 1978; 2: 219–225.

Ramsay M. Genetic and epigenetic insights into fetal alcohol spectrum disorders. Genome Med 2010; 28; 2: 27.

Rasmussen C, Soleimani M, Pei J. Executive functioning and working memory deficits on the CANTAB among children with prenatal alcohol exposure. J Popul Ther Clin Pharmacol 2011; 18: e44–e53.

Richardson GA, Conroy ML, Day N. Prenatal cocaine exposure: effects on the development of school-age children. Neurotoxicol Teratol 1996; 18: 627–34.

Richardson GA, Goldschmidt L, Larkby C, Day NL. Effects of prenatal cocaine exposure on child behavior and growth at 10 years of age. Neurotoxicol Teratol 2013a; 40: 1–8.

Richardson JL, Jones D, Dunstan HJ et al. Gestational exposure to varenicline. Reproductive Toxicology 2013b; 37: 85.

Richardson GA, Goldschmidt L, Larkby C. Effects of prenatal cocaine exposure on growth: a longitudinal analysis. Pediatrics 2007; 120: e1017–e1027.

Richardson GA, Ryan C, Willford J et al. Prenatal alcohol and marijuana exposure: effects on neuropsychological outcomes at 10 years. Neurotoxicol Teratol 2002; 24: 309–20.

Richardson S, Browne ML, Rasmussen SA et al. Associations between periconceptional alcohol consumption and craniosynostosis, omphalocele, and gastroschisis. Birth Defects Res Part A: Clin Mol Teratol 2011; 91: 623–30.

Rogers JM. Tobacco and pregnancy. Reprod Toxicol 2009; 28: 152–60.

Pregnancy

2.21 Recreational drugs

Rogers JM. Tobacco and pregnancy: overview of exposures and effects. Birth Defects Res C Embryo Today 2008; 84: 1–15.

Rohrmeister K, Bernert G, Langer M et al. Opiatabhängigkeit in der Schwangerschaft – Konsequenzen für das Neugeborene. Ergebnisse eines interdisziplinären Betreuungsmodells. Z Geburtshilfe Neonatol 2001; 205: 224–30.

Romitti PA, Sun L, Honein MA, et al. Maternal periconceptional alcohol consumption and risk of orofacial clefts. Am J Epidemiol. 2007; 166: 775–85.

Sasco AJ, Vainio H. From in utero and childhood exposure to parental smoking to childhood cancer: a possible link and the need for action. Hum Experiment Toxicol 1999; 18: 192–201.

Sayal K, Heron J, Golding J et al. Binge pattern of alcohol consumption during pregnancy and childhood mental health outcomes: longitudinal population-based study. Pediatrics 2009; 123: e289–96.

Schaefer C, Spielmann H. Kokain in der Schwangerschaft: ein zweites Contergan? Geburtsh Frauenheilk 1990; 50: 899–900.

Schardein JL. Chemically Induced Birth Defects, 3rd edn. New York: Marcel Dekker, 2000.

Schmidt RJ, Romitti PA, Burns TL et al. Caffeine, selected metabolic gene variants, and risk for neural tube defects. Birth Defects Res A Clin Mol Teratol 2010; 88: 560–9.

Sengpiel V, Elind E, Bacelis J et al. Maternal caffeine intake during pregnancy is associated with birth weight but not with gestational length: results from a large prospective observational cohort study. BMC Med 2013; 11–42.

Shenassa ED, Brown MJ. Maternal smoking and infantile gastrointestinal dysregulation: the case of colic. Pediatrics 2004; 114: 497–505.

Shi M, Christensen K, Weinberg CR et al. Orofacial cleft risk is increased with maternal smoking and specific detoxification-gene variants. Am J Hum Genet 2007; 80: 76–90.

Shi M, Wehby GL, Murray JC. Review on genetic variants and maternal smoking in the etiology of oral clefts and other birth defects. Birth Defects Res C Embryo Today 2008; 84: 16–29.

Shiono PH, Klebanoff MA, Nugent RP et al. The impact of cocaine and marijuana use on low birth weight and preterm birth: a multicenter study. Am J Obstet Gynecol 1995; 172: 19–27.

Siddappa R, Fletcher J, Heard A et al. Methadone dosage for prevention of opioid withdrawal in children. Paediatr Anaesth 2003; 13: 805–10.

Simmons RW, Madra NJ, Levy SS et al. Co-regulation of movement speed and accuracy by children with heavy prenatal alcohol exposure. Percept Mot Skills 2011; 112: 172–82.

Skelly AC, Holt VL, Mosca VS et al. Talipes equinovarus and maternal smoking: a population-based case-control study in Washington State. Teratology 2002; 66: 91–100.

Smith LM, Lagasse LL, Derauf C et al. Motor and cognitive outcomes through three years of age in children exposed to prenatal methamphetamine. Neurotoxicol Teratol 2011; 33: 176–84.

Sommer A, Blanton SH, Weymouth K et al. Smoking, xenobiotic pathway and clubfoot. BDR A 2011; 91: 20–8.

Søndergaard C, Henriksen TB, Obel C, Wisborg K. Smoking during pregnancy and infantile colic. Pediatrics 2001; 108: 342–6.

Spohr HL, Willms J, Steinhausen HC. Fetal alcohol spectrum disorders in young adulthood. J Pediatr 2007; 150: 175–9.

Stathopoulou A, Beratis IN, Beratis S. Prenatal tobacco smoke exposure, risk of schizophrenia, and severity of positive/negative symptoms. Schizophr Res 2013; 148: 105–10.

Stefanidou EM, Caramellino L, Patriarca A, Menato G. Maternal caffeine consumption and sine causa recurrent miscarriage. Eur J Obstet Gynecol Reprod Biol 2011; 158: 220–4.

Steinhausen HC, Spohr HL. Long-term outcome of children with fetal alcohol syndrome: Psychopathology, behavior and intelligence. Alcohol Clin Exp Res 1998; 22: 334–8.

Stone KC, Lagasse LL, Lester BM et al. Sleep problems in children with prenatal substance exposure: the Maternal Lifestyle study. Arch Pediatr Adolesc Med 2010; 164: 452–6.

Strandberg-Larsen K, Grønboek M, Andersen AM et al. Alcohol drinking pattern during pregnancy and risk of infant mortality. Epidemiology 2009; 20: 884–91.

Strandberg-Larsen K, Nielsen NR, Grønboek M et al. Binge drinking in pregnancy and risk of fetal death. Obstet Gynecol 2008; 111: 602–9.

Strandberg-Larsen K, Skov-Ettrup LS, Grønbaek M et al. Maternal alcohol drinking pattern during pregnancy and the risk of an offspring with an isolated congenital heart defect and in particular a ventricular septal defect or an atrial septal defect. Birth Defects Res A Clin Mol Teratol 2011; 91: 616–22.

Streissguth AP, Bookstein FL, Barr HM. A dose-response study of the enduring effects of prenatal alcohol exposure: Birth to 14 years. In: Spohr HL, Steinhausen HC (eds.) Alcohol, pregnancy and the developing child. New York: Cambridge University Press, 1996, pp. 141–68.

Sun Y, Strandberg-Larsen K, Vestergaard M et al. Binge drinking during pregnancy and risk of seizures in childhood: a study based on the Danish National Birth Cohort. Am J Epidemiol 2009; 169: 313–22.

Talati A, Bao Y, Kaufman J et al. Maternal smoking during pregnancy and bipolar disorder in offspring. Am J Psychiatry 2013; 170: 1178–85.

Thajam D, Atkinson DE, Sibley CP et al. Is neonatal abstinence syndrome related to the amount of opiate used? J Obstet Gynecol Neonatal Nurs 2010; 39: 503–9.

Vik T, Bakketeig LS, Trygg KU et al. High caffeine consumption in the third trimester of pregnancy: gender-specific effects on fetal growth. Paediatr Perinat Epidemiol 2003; 17: 324.

Wachsman L, Schuetz S, Chan LS et al. What happens to babies exposed to phencyclidine (PCP) in utero? Am J Drug Alcohol Abuse 1989; 15: 31–9.

Wasserman CR, Shaw GM, O'Malley CD et al. Parental cigarette smoking and risk for congenital anomalies of the heart, neural tube, or limb. Teratology 1996; 53: 261–7.

Werler MM. Teratogen update: smoking and reproductive outcomes. Teratology 1997; 55: 382–8.

WHO (World Health Organization). Guidelines for the Identification And Management Of Substance Use and Substance Use Disorders in Pregnancy, WHO, Geneva Switzerland, 2014.

Wilson GS, McCreary R, Kean J, Baxter JC. The development of preschool children of heroin-addicted mothers: a controlled study. Pediatrics 1979; 63: 135–41.

Wisborg K, Kesmodel U, Hammer Beck B et al. Maternal consumption of coffee during pregnancy and stillbirth and infant death in first year of life: prospective study. BMJ 2003; 326: 420–2.

Wisborg K, Kesmodel U, Henriksen TB et al. Exposure to tobacco smoke in utero and the risk of stillbirth and death in the first year of life. Am J Epidemiol 2001; 154: 322–7.

Woods JR. Maternal and transplacental effects of cocaine. Ann New York Acad Sci 1998; 46: 1–11.

Wyszynski DF, Duffy DL, Beaty TH. Maternal cigarette smoking and oral clefts: a meta-analysis. Cleft Palate Craniofac J 1997; 34: 206–10.

Zalacain M, Sierrasesumaga L, Larrannaga C et al. Effects of benzopyrene-7,8-diol-9,10-epoxide (BPDE) in vitro and of maternal smoking in vivo on micronuclei frequencies in fetal cord blood. Pediatr Res 2006; 60: 180–4.

Zeiger JS, Beaty TH, Liang KY. Oral clefts, maternal smoking, and TGFA: a meta-analysis of gene-environment interaction. Cleft Palate Craniofac J 2005; 42: 58–63.

Zelner I, Koren G. Pharmacokinetics of ethanol in the maternal-fetal unit. J Popul Ther Clin Pharmacol 2013a; 20: e259–65.

Zelner I, Koren G. Alcohol consumption among women. J Popul Ther Clin Pharmacol 2013b; 20: e201–6.

Poisonings and toxins

Laura M. Yates and Sally Stephens

2.22

2.22.1	The general risk of poisoning in pregnancy	575
2.22.2	Treatment of poisoning in pregnancy	576
2.22.3	Medicines	582
2.22.4	Animal toxins	590
2.22.5	Mushrooms	592
2.22.6	Other plant toxins	592
2.22.7	Bacterial endotoxins	592

2.22.1   The general risk of poisoning in pregnancy

Poisoning in pregnancy may be accidental or intentional, and may reflect acute (e.g. deliberate overdose, therapeutic error) or chronic (e.g. environmental or occupational) exposure to one or more substances. Whilst risk to both mother and fetus will be determined primarily by the nature of the exposure(s) involved, the greatest risk in managing such patients is likely to arise from delayed, or incomplete treatment of the pregnant woman due to theoretical concerns regarding possible teratogenicity of an antidote or intervention. Whilst it is true that human pregnancy safety data for many of the commonly used antidotes are scarce, that which is available suggests that inadequately treated maternal and/or fetal toxicity correlates with poor fetomaternal outcome.

Robust epidemiological data on fetal and maternal outcome following maternal poisoning are lacking, partly due to the significant number of cases lost to follow-up in this setting. As a result of preferential reporting of cases involving highly toxic substances or which resulted in poor maternal or fetal outcome, any estimates of general risk associated with poisoning in pregnancy are likely to be highly biased towards adverse outcome. Furthermore, much of the published data relates to poisoning in the context of deliberate self-harm or attempted suicide, and data relating to a specific exposure are therefore often highly confounded as co-ingestion of multiple substances, and high rates of elective termination of pregnancy are common in this context (McClure 2011a).

Risk to the fetus will depend on factors such as the gestational age at which the poisoning occurred, the presence of maternal toxicity, the time interval between poisoning and maternal treatment, evidence of a change in the fetal biophysical profile or wellbeing, and the half-life of the exposure(s) as well as risks due to direct fetal effects of the drug or chemical concerned. Increased risk of miscarriage following overdose periconceptually or in early pregnancy, and of preterm birth, low birth

Drugs During Pregnancy and Lactation. http://dx.doi.org/10.1016/B978-0-12-408078-2.00023-8

weight, congenital malformation, fetal death or impaired neurodevelopment following poisoning in pregnancy have been reported by some, whereas others have shown no overall increased risk of adverse outcome (McClure 2011b, Timmerman 2008, Czeizel 1988). These data are however highly limited and confounded. A recent study assessed risk of learning difficulties amongst offspring of mothers who ingested high doses of prescription drugs in an attempted suicide in pregnancy. Although the authors suggest that preparations containing three component medicines may increase the risk of mental retardation in the absence of structural defects, and that this increased risk is not observed for the component medicines when taken alone, these findings are based on one particular preparation and provide little insight into risks for other exposures (Petik 2012).

Chronic poisoning may involve exposure over a long period of time, and therefore carries the potential to disrupt structural, functional or neurological aspects of fetal development over more than one trimester of pregnancy. The dose involved in an episode of acute poisoning, although restricted to a narrow window of fetal development, may be more likely to exceed the threshold for a particular adverse effect. In addition to the limitations described above, published and unpublished data on fetal outcome following poisoning in pregnancy are often further compromised due to reports for individual substances being retrospective and few in number; with critical details regarding dose or toxicity scores and presence of maternal toxicity and treatment lacking.

In summary, assessment of risk must be on a case-by-case basis. A thorough assessment of both maternal and fetal condition and possible risk should be made at presentation, and then again following treatment of maternal symptoms. Review by a psychiatrist should be considered in all cases of deliberate poisoning, particularly where the mother is known to have a prior history of mental illness.

2.22.2   Treatment of poisoning in pregnancy

There are no published evidence-based guidelines on the treatment of pregnant women who have been poisoned. Recommendations are generally based on the collective experiences gleaned over many years from specialist poisons and teratology centers worldwide, and from analysis of case reports or small case series on specific exposures, although these data are limited. Application of these data to the development of current guidelines is, however, not always appropriate, as in older cases the treatment regimes described are often no longer recommended or in use.

In most situations, treatment of the poisoned pregnant patient should be as for the nonpregnant patient and, where clinically indicated, antidotes or other interventions should not be withheld because of concerns regarding teratogenic effects. However, fetal well-being should be considered during any interventions and procedures. Direct or delayed effects of the toxic agent(s) on the fetus may also occur, and in such situations maternal treatment may need to be initiated or continued in the absence of maternal symptoms (see Carbon Monoxide below). Although the fetal effects of most antidotes are poorly documented, any theoretical risks to the fetus are likely to be less than those associated with failing to treat the mother adequately.

Despite differing opinions regarding the use of one antidote over another, or of a specific intervention, it is universally agreed that timely and adequate treatment of the mother to prevent or minimize maternal toxicity is essential. Maternal condition is a major predictor of fetal outcome and the priority is therefore to stabilize the mother. Maternal resuscitation should be in left tilt, ideally using a wedge or rolled blanket to avoid the obstruction of blood flow in the aorta and inferior vena cava by the gravid uterus. In some situations, early administration of an antidote is key to preventing maternal and fetal demise. Guidelines regarding antidote use, and hence availability may differ across units, and it is therefore advisable to obtain advice from a national or regional specialist poisons service as soon as possible. Early obstetric assessment, and where available, specialist teratological input, is also recommended as emergency delivery or close monitoring of the fetus may be necessary in situations where risk of intrauterine death is increased (see Ibuprofen below).

Once the maternal condition has been assessed and treated as appropriate, the possibility of delayed direct or indirect effects of the exposure on the fetus must be considered. These may occur even in the absence of maternal toxicity and prolonged or additional maternal treatment may be required despite complete recovery of the mother. The possibility of altered pharmacokinetic and pharmacodynamic effects of substances, on both mother and fetus, due to the physiological changes associated with pregnancy or differences in fetal metabolism of the substance should also be considered.

Until details of episodes of poisoning in pregnancy are accurately documented and systemically recorded through routine reporting to networks – such as the European Network of Teratology Information Services (www.ENTIS.org) or the Organization of Teratology Information Services (www.MotherToBaby.org) to enable longer term follow up of maternal and fetal outcome, evidence based guidance regarding treatment in pregnancy cannot be developed.

▶ **Arsenic**

Reports of *arsenic* poisoning in pregnancy all involve exposure after the first trimester with variable outcomes. The first describes maternal ingestion of 340 mg of *sodium arsenate* at 20 weeks, resulting in a healthy live-born at 36 weeks gestation after maternal treatment with 150 mg *dimercaprol* (4 hourly) 2 hours post ingestion. At birth, 24 hour urinary arsenic levels were <50 µg/L in the infant and <100 µg/L in the mother (Daya 1989). The second reports ingestion at 28 weeks of an unknown amount of arsenic with subsequent intrauterine fetal demise, and high arsenic concentrations documented in the fetus (Bolliger 1992). The last case involved a third-trimester ingestion of arsenic-based rat poison. The baby was born live 4 days post-ingestion but then died from hyaline membrane disease. An autopsy showed a high concentration of arsenic accumulation in the liver, brain and kidneys (Lugo 1969).

Chronic environmental exposure to arsenic may also occur, with populations in West Bengal, Bangladesh, China, Taiwan, Argentina and Chile exposed to drinking water from ground water wells with naturally occurring arsenic levels up to 3,000 mcg/L. A study of Mexican–American women who were exposed to arsenic >10 mcg/L in drinking water, and who lived within 2 miles of a facility with air emissions of heavy metals at the time of conception, showed no increased risk of NTD-affected pregnancies compared to women living near the Mexican border in Texas (Brender 2006). Data from other populations suggest an association between chronic exposure to arsenic in drinking water and an increased incidence of maternal anemia, spontaneous abortion, preterm birth and low birth weight (Bloom 2010, Rahman 2009, Vahter 2009, Hopenhayn 2006, Mukherjee 2005, Nordstrom 1979). See also Chapter 2.13.19.

> **Recommendation.** The treatment of suspected arsenic poisoning requires specialist expertise. The risk of toxicity will vary depending on the chemical form involved, and whether the exposure is acute or chronic. Early advice should be sought from a dedicated poisons unit where available. Poisoned pregnant women should be treated according to protocols for the treatment of nonpregnant patients.

▶ Carbon monoxide

Carbon monoxide (CO) crosses the placenta with maximum fetal blood concentrations likely to reach, and in some cases exceed, those of the mother. However, empirical observations, data from animal studies and theoretical models, show that there is a delay of up to 24 hours between maternal exposure and CO accumulating in the fetus. Maternal COHb (carboxyhemoglobin)-concentration may therefore not reflect fetal COHb-concentration at that time. Similarly, the elimination half-life in the fetus may be up to four to five times longer than in the mother.

Maternal COHb-concentrations and symptoms are proposed to predict risk of adverse fetal outcome, and risk of neurological damage in the fetus is thought to be increased if the mother was somnolent or lost consciousness. Fetal death occurred in 10 out of 15 cases where maternal toxicity was reported to be moderate to severe, and associated with loss of consciousness or coma (Mathieu-Nolf 2006).

However, whilst severe maternal toxicity increases the risk of adverse fetal outcome, low maternal COHb-concentrations do not necessarily correlate with a good fetal outcome, and a threshold for fetal toxicity has not been established. In a case series by Caravati (1988), *in utero* death occurred in two women who were exposed to CO at 38 weeks gestation. Whilst COHb was high, 32% in one woman, it was only 5% in the other. It should, however, be noted that maternal loss of consciousness was reported in both cases.

Reports of acute first trimester CO poisoning are scarce. Pregnancy loss and congenital malformation have been described following early pregnancy exposure associated with moderate to severe maternal poisoning (loss of consciousness or coma) (Koren 1991, Norman 1990, Woody 1990). However, there are no large epidemiological studies on which to accurately assess these risks. Acute CO poisoning in the later stages of pregnancy has been associated with fetal or neonatal death, prematurity and low birth weight (Yildiz 2010, Koren 1991, Farrow 1990, Norman 1990, Caravati 1988, Cramer 1982).

Chronic exposure to CO in pregnancy (via ambient air pollution or cigarette smoking), has been associated with an increased risk of congenital heart defects (Dadvand 2011, Ritz 2002), sudden infant death syndrome (Omalu 2007, Watkins 1986), and prematurity (Stieb 2012).

Third trimester *in utero* exposure to CO via environmental sources (e.g. wood smoke) has been associated with poorer performance in various neuropsychological tests, including long- and short-term memory recall, and fine motor performance amongst school age children (Dix-Cooper 2012).

The use of hyperbaric oxygen therapy (HBO) is controversial in the nonpregnant patient, with use during pregnancy raising further concerns regarding toxic effects such as retinopathy, and premature closure of the ductus arterious in the fetus as a result of high oxygen concentrations. However, the limited published data do not indicate that treatment of pregnant women with HBO poses an increased risk to the fetus, and HBO is advised by some units in cases where maternal COHb-concentration is >20%, or associated with an altered level of consciousness.

Recommendation. There are no published guidelines for the treatment of CO monoxides poisoning in pregnancy.

- Maternal treatment as for the nonpregnant patient is advised and should ideally involve discussion with a specialist poisoning or teratology unit.
- High-dose oxygen should be administered immediately to reduce the carboxy-haemoglobin half-life. Some centers also advocate the use of HBO in the pregnant woman with severe CO intoxication (reduced consciousness resulting from CO and COHb-concentrations >20%, or abnormal fetal heart rate); however, this recommendation is not universally supported.
- Because of the lag in CO accumulation in the fetus, oxygen treatment should be continued even after the maternal condition and COHb-concentration have returned to normal, and should still be commenced following a delay in presentation or spontaneous improvement of maternal symptoms.
- The need for enhanced fetal or neonatal monitoring should be considered.

► Methanol

Maternal and fetal effects of *methanol* poisoning are not immediately evident, owing to the relatively slow metabolism of methanol to toxic metabolites like formaldehyde. Maternal acidosis may therefore be delayed for several hours following ingestion, particularly if alcohol has been consumed simultaneously.

Early treatment of maternal methanol poisoning is therefore key to preventing both maternal and fetal toxicity, and should be as for the nonpregnant patient. Where use of an antidote is clinically indicated, treatment with *ethanol* or *fomepizole* to reduce metabolism of methanol to its toxic metabolites should be initiated as soon as possible. Although adverse fetal effects are well described with both regular and "binge" consumption of alcohol during pregnancy, intravenous ethanol should not be withheld if fomepizole is not available and use of an antidote is clinically indicated in the treatment of methanol poisoning at any stage of pregnancy.

The published literature includes only three cases of methanol poisoning in pregnancy. Belson (2004) described a pregnant woman with HIV infection and asthma who presented at around 30 weeks of gestation with respiratory distress following methanol exposure due to assumed ingestion. She was acidotic (pH 7.17) with an anion gap of 26, and the fetus was reported to be bradycardic. An emergency caesarean section was performed. The male infant weighed 950 g and required aggressive resuscitation, but died 4 days later following a grade 4 intraventricular bleed. Maternal metabolic acidosis persisted despite treatment with fluids, bicarbonate, and dopamine. Laboratory tests included undetectable ethanol and salicylates and showed an osmolar gap of 41. Intravenous ethanol was only commenced at this stage (3 days post ingestion), when a methanol concentration of 54 mg/dL was detected. The regional poisons service recommended maternal hemodialysis and fomepizole. It is unclear from the report whether this treatment was implemented and maternal death occurred on day 10.

A further report describes mild acidosis in a woman who ingested 250–500 mL methanol during the 38th week of pregnancy. She was treated with ethanol, hemodialysis and alkalinization, and delivered a normal healthy infant 6 days after the exposure (Hantson 1997). The child was followed up for more than 10 years, during which time clinical course was uneventful and no visual disturbances were reported. The remaining report describes fomepizole treatment at 11 and again at 16 weeks gestation for chronic maternal abuse of methanol (Velez 2003). An ultrasound at week 16 did not show any gross congenital abnormalities; however, the case was lost to follow-up and the outcome of the pregnancy is unknown.

> **Recommendation.** Treatment of methanol poisoning in pregnancy should be the same as for the nonpregnant patient, where clinically indicated treatment with fomepizole or ethanol should not be withheld on account of pregnancy. Fomepizole is generally preferred, given the known teratogenic potential of ethanol, but where fomepizole is unavailable or considered to be inappropriate, the risks of untreated methanol poisoning are likely to be far greater than those of ethanol exposure and treatment should not be withheld.

▶ Organophosphorus pesticides

The published data detail approximately 30 pregnancies in which accidental or deliberate exposure to organophosphates (OPs) occurred (Adhikari 2011, Jajoo 2010, Solomon 2007, Kamha 2005, Sebe 2005, Shah 1995, Romero 1989, Karalliedde 1988, Midtling 1985). Maternal antidote treatment with either *atropine* ($n = 23$) or atropine and *pralidoxime* ($n = 4$) was reported in 27 of these cases.

A case series of 21 women who ingested OPs in pregnancy and were treated with atropine, reported two maternal and fetal deaths, one spontaneous abortion, and 15 healthy live-born infants. Three women were lost to follow-up. In five cases, ventilatory support was needed. In two cases, where exposure occurred at 10 and 20 weeks gestation, the mothers died. Although no congenital malformations were reported, only three exposures occurred in the first trimester (Adhikari 2011). Dilated unresponsive pupils were reported in an infant following maternal ingestion of 15 to 20 mL of *diazinon* at 40 weeks of pregnancy, and treatment with 83 mg of atropine for 28 hours (Shah 1995). A further case report describes maternal ingestion of *chlorpyrifos* in a suicide attempt at 29 weeks of pregnancy. Atropine was administered over a period of 3 hours and the maternal symptoms resolved. However, premature labor ensued 2 days after the exposure, and the infant died 2 days later due to prematurity and hyaline membrane disease (Solomon 2007).

There are two published case reports of three normal healthy term infants following use of atropine and pralidoxime in the treatment of maternal ingestion of *fenthion* at 16 weeks gestation (Karalliedde 1988), *methamidophos* at 36 weeks (Karalliedde 1988), and maternal inhalation of undiluted diazinon fumes at 26 weeks (Kamha 2005). Fetal death has been reported in one case in which the mother was admitted to hospital 12 hours after the ingestion of chlorpyrifos at 19 weeks gestation, as she was unable to feel any fetal activity 2 hours post ingestion. Fetal blood chloropyrifos was 264 ppb (Sebe 2005).

> **Recommendation.** Treatment should be the same as for the nonpregnant patient, and may involve administration of an antidote such as atropine or pralidoxime. Where maternal OP poisoning occurs near to delivery, the risk of adverse neonatal effects should be considered. Monitoring or treatment of the neonate may be indicated.

▶ Paraquat

Paraquat has been withdrawn from the EU market. The literature regarding acute exposure to paraquat during pregnancy is limited. Eight published reports document paraquat exposure in the third trimester, associated with maternal toxicity which required hospitalization for treatment. Six cases resulted in maternal and fetal death (Chomchai 2007, Talbot 1988, Fennelly 1968), and survival of both the mother and the fetus was reported in only two (Chomchai 2007, Jenq 2005).

One case series documents four instances of first or second trimester exposure to paraquat. Maternal and fetal mortality occurred in two cases, maternal survival but fetal death in one, and maternal survival with an elective termination for social reasons in the last (Talbot 1988).

A case report described delivery of a normal term infant following a reported suicide attempt involving a few sips of Weedol, containing paraquat, at 20 weeks gestation (Musson 1982). The placenta showed signs of infarction in the absence of a maternal history of toxaemia or stroke. The child was reported to be healthy at 3 years of age. Maternal toxicity requiring hospital treatment occurred in all the above cases of acute exposure.

Paraquat was found in cord blood at about four times the maternal blood concentration (Talbot 1988), and ulceration of lips and oral mucosa, pulmonary toxicity and hepatic necrosis has been observed at fetal autopsy (Chomchai 2007) following severe maternal poisoning. In another case, paraquat concentrations in a conceptus were five times those present in the amniotic fluid, and greater than that in maternal blood. Even though maternal ingestion was considerable and accompanied by toxicity, the fetus was viable at three weeks after ingestion, at which stage the pregnancy was electively terminated (Tsatsakis 1996).

> **Recommendation.** There are no published guidelines concerning the management of paraquat poisoning during pregnancy. Maternal toxicity as a result of exposure in pregnancy is likely to be a major determinant of the risk posed to the developing fetus. Treatment should be in accordance with that recommended for the nonpregnant patient.

Pregnancy

2.22 Poisonings and toxins

▶ Thallium

Experience of *thallium* poisoning in the first 13 weeks of pregnancy is limited to a few published case reports. Most describe associated maternal toxicity. In three cases, healthy infants were delivered at term. Two pregnancies resulted in preterm delivery with respiratory insufficiency, cryptorchidism, imperforate anus, jaundice, alopecia and psychomotor impairment at 3 years of age reported in one infant (Hoffman 2000, Rangel Guerra 1980). No maternal symptoms were reported after thallium poisoning around the time of conception in a woman who was treated with gastric lavage, catharsis and *Prussian blue*, but subsequently miscarried at 9 weeks (Ghezzi 1979).

Around 13 cases of thallium poisoning in the second or third trimester of pregnancy have been published. All report associated maternal symptoms, and although the outcome for each was a live born infant. Features consistent with thallium toxicity were reported in some (alopecia in five, dermal effects in two and failure to thrive in three), with some infants having more than one of these features. In one case, maternal ingestion of thallium occurred at term and the neonate subsequently died (Hoffman 2000).

Use of the antidote Prussian blue has only been reported in two separate cases of thallium poisoning in pregnancy. The first resulted in the premature delivery of an infant at 6 months gestation after maternal thallium poisoning, and treatment with Prussian blue at an unknown stage of pregnancy (Pai 1987). The second case involved chronic intoxication from thallium-containing rodenticide in the workplace at 13 weeks gestation. The patient was treated with Prussian blue and nutritional support, but fetal loss was reported three weeks later and maternal symptoms of nausea, vomiting, and lumbar and epigastric pain persisted for 6 weeks after the exposure (Benavides 1997).

Recommendation. Although experience for use of Prussian blue in pregnancy is limited, it should not be withheld if clinically indicated. Prussian blue is not absorbed from the gastrointestinal tract, and the risk of fetal effects is therefore likely to be low, whereas the risks to both the mother and fetus of untreated thallium poisoning are significant. Enhanced antenatal monitoring of fetal viability and growth may be advisable following exposure at any stage of pregnancy, and newborn infants should be carefully assessed for systemic features of thallium toxicity, some of which may only manifest around 3 weeks post exposure.

2.22.3   Medicines

▶ Actylsalicylic acid

Outcome data prospectively collected by the UK Teratology Information Service for 90 pregnancies exposed to between 4.2 and 32 g of *aspirin* at different gestations included 19 live-born infants exposed in the first trimester (Stephens 2009). Malformations were reported in two, and comprised gastroschisis following a maternal overdose of 7.2 g of aspirin at 5 weeks gestation, and hypospadias following maternal overdose with 9.6 g of aspirin at 8 weeks gestation. The overall cohort malformation rate was however, not increased above that of the background population.

A few retrospective reports have also been published (Sezgin 2002, Velez 2001, Palatnick 1998, Rejent 1985, Bove 1979); two describe maternal overdose in the first trimester. One infant was diagnosed with cyclopia-astomia-agnathia-holoprosencephaly (thought to be genetic in aetiology), following maternal exposure to 500 g of aspirin twice daily for 1 week during the first trimester (Sezgin 2002), and one infant of a mother who took an aspirin overdose of 19 g at approximately 8 weeks gestation, had renal insufficiency at birth that progressed to renal failure (Bove 1979).

Three case-reports document aspirin overdose in late pregnancy. Fetal death occurred in two; the first at 33 weeks following ingestion of 32.5 g of aspirin (Rejent 1985), and the second at 37 weeks with 50 tablets of unknown strength aspirin per day, for 1 month (Palatnick 1998). Severe maternal toxicity and treatment with alkaline diuresis, IV fluids and haemodiaylysis was reported in both cases. The last case involved maternal overdose in late pregnancy (38 weeks) of 16.25 g, resulting in maternal tarchypnoea and fetal distress with bradycardia (HR 60). The infant was delivered by emergency caesarean and later discharged without complications (Velez 2001). See also Chapter 2.1.2.

Recommendation.

- Maternal treatment for aspirin overdose should be the same as for a non-pregnant patient.
- Maternal toxicity is likely to be a major determinant of risk to the fetus. There is some evidence to suggest that therapeutic use of aspirin in pregnancy increases the risk of gastroschisis in exposed offspring, and a fetal anomaly scan around 12 weeks gestation is advised following aspirin overdose in the first trimester – if this is not already offered routinely.
- If exomphalus, or any other malformations are identified, causality cannot be assumed and a co-incidental genetic syndrome should be considered.
- Therapeutic doses of NSAIDs after week 30 are associated with a risk of premature closure of the Ductus Arteriosus (DA), and exposure to *ibuprofen* or any other NSAID in overdose therefore warrants immediate assessment of fetal wellbeing, even in the absence of maternal toxicity or symptoms. Antenatal identification of premature closure of the DA may require expedited early fetal delivery or enhanced monitoring. Premature closure of the DA has also been associated with an increased risk of Persistent Pulmonary Hypertension of the Newborn (PPHN). Paediatricians should be made aware of the exposure at delivery. Maternal treatment of ibuprofen overdose in pregnancy at any stage should be in accordance with guidelines for nonpregnant patients.

▶ **Amitriptyline**

Supratherapeutic doses of tricyclic antidepressants like *amitriptyline* and *dothiepin* can cause severe maternal toxicity, including cardiac arrhythmia and seizures, which may be a risk to the fetus. There is also the risk of fetal cardiotoxicity.

The UK Teratology Information Service has followed up 24 enquiries to the service regarding overdoses in pregnancy where amitriptyline was taken alone in overdose, or in combination with other

Pregnancy

2.22 Poisonings and toxins

medications. Twenty of these cases were published in abstract form (McElhatton 2003). Dosage was not reported in all cases, but those included were reported to have involved ingestion of at least 200 mg on a single occasion, with recorded doses ranging from 350 to 1700 mg. Fetal outcomes included three spontaneous abortions, four elective terminations, and 17 live-born infants without major malformations, six of whom were exposed to amitriptyline in overdose during the first trimester. Details regarding maternal toxicity were not available.

There are seven reports of pregnancy outcome following amitriptyline overdose in the published literature (Timmerman 2008, Wertelecki 1980, Czeizel 1997). Five of the seven infants were reported to have congenital abnormalities, although the maternal overdose occurred in the first trimester in only one. In two infants, the anomalies were attributed to concomitant alcohol exposure *in utero*. Two of the remaining three infants were described as having very similar features, and were reported on different occasions by the same authors. It is likely that these reports relate to the same infant. The only case of first trimester exposure described an infant with multiple congenital anomalies (microcephaly, cleft palate, micrognathia, ambiguous genitalia, dermal ridges, and "cotton-like" hair), whose mother had ingested 725 mg amitriptyline and 58 mg perphenazine in a suicide attempt at 8 days gestation (Wertelecki 1980). No details of maternal toxicity were provided. See also Chapter 2.11.4.

> **Recommendation.** Amitryptyline is very toxic in overdose. Treatment in pregnancy should follow guidelines for treatment of nonpregnant patients, and should not be delayed or withheld on account of the pregnancy. Overdose close to delivery may result in neonatal toxicity and a careful assessment for features of toxicity in the newborn infant should be made (e.g. ECG, blood gas).

▶ Carbamazepine

There are two case reports in the published literature of suicide attempts involving *carbamazepine* overdose in pregnancy (Saygan-Karamursel 2005, Little 1993). The first documents a neural tube defect in the fetus after ingestion of approximately 4.8 g of carbamazepine during the third to fourth week post-conception in a non-epileptic woman. Maternal drug levels remained elevated above the therapeutic range for 2 days. Maternal serum α-fetoprotein was elevated, and a high-resolution fetal sonography demonstrated a large myeloschisis that was verified at autopsy. No family history of neural tube defects or any other malformations was reported by the patient. Use of periconceptual folic acid was not documented (Little 1993).

The second case involved ingestion of 40×200 mg carbamazapine tablets at week 33 of gestation, with suicidal intent. The mother was comatose and was treated with activated carbon and plasmapheresis. Delivery of a normal healthy baby occurred 48 hours later; the Apgar scores and umbilical artery pH were normal (Saygan-Karamursel 2005). See also Chapter 2.10.13.

> **Recommendation.** Toxicity may be associated with cardiac effects and ECG changes. Treatment should be as for the nonpregnant patient. Carbamazepine interferes with folic acid metabolism, and therapeutic use has been associated with an increased risk of neural tube defects. A fetal anomaly scan around 12 weeks gestation is advised following carbamazepine overdose in the first trimester, if not already offered routinely.

► **Clozapine**

There are only two cases of *clozapine* overdose in the published literature. The first reports an early neonatal death following an intentional maternal overdose of between 10 and 20 g of clozapine at 39 weeks of pregnancy. The patient had been exposed to clozapine in therapeutic doses during the first trimester and was also taking *valproate, promethazine, risperidone* and *fluoxetine*. As part of the maternal treatment, gastric lavage was performed. During assisted delivery the following day, she was administered *oxytocin* and *furosemide*. The male child died after 20 minutes of resuscitation immediately following delivery (Klys 2007).

The second case report documents a 16-year-old who took approximately 10 g of clozapine (not hers) at 32 weeks of pregnancy. She presented with a decreased level of consciousness and 28 hours later had developed hypotension and had an abnormal cardiotocogram tracing. Due to the maternal condition, an emergency caesarean section was performed resulting in a live-born infant. During the first day of life the infant developed abdominal distension which was investigated, but postulated to be due to delayed peristalsis as a consequence of the anti-cholinergic side effects of clozapine. The infant's symptoms resolved within a week, but over the next 42 days the mother developed complications of adult respiratory distress, hypotension and renal failure, and died in intensive care (Novikova 2009).

> **Recommendation.** Treatment is the same as for the nonpregnant patient. Effects of clozapine toxicity may be prolonged, and the neonate should be monitored for toxic effects when exposure has occurred in the weeks preceding delivery (there are no data which provide an indication of a "safe" interval).

► **Colchicine**

A woman took 8 mg/kg *colchicine* in week 34 of pregnancy. A healthy infant was delivered 10 hours later by caesarean section and was found to have very little colchicine in its serum (<5 ng/mL). Although given intensive care, the mother died (Blache 1982). See also Chapter 2.1.9.

> **Recommendation.** Treatment is as for the nonpregnant patient.

► **Diazepam**

A study compared 112 live-born infants of women who ingested more than 25 mg of *diazepam* as a suicide attempt (sometimes in combination with other medications) during pregnancy with 112 unexposed siblings

(Gidai 2008). There was no significant difference in congenital malformation rates between the two groups (OR 2.0, 95% CI 0.8–5.0), irrespective of when exposure occurred during pregnancy.

Malformations were reported in five of the 37 infants of mothers who took a diazepam overdose between the 4th and 12th week of gestation, and included undescended testis ($n = 2$), congenital dysplasia of the hip ($n = 1$), talipes equinovarus ($n = 1$), and congenital inguinal hernia ($n = 1$).

A case series described eight infants with craniofacial anomalies following maternal abuse of prescription medications, which included a minimum of 30 mg of diazepam and 75 mg *oxazepam* per day throughout pregnancy. All eight exposed offspring were described as having features similar to those of Fetal Alcohol Syndrome, although maternal consumption of alcohol was denied. Five of the infants, two of whom were microcephalic, demonstrated symptoms of neonatal withdrawal and subsequent intellectual impairment (Laegreid 1989). A further case report describes an infant with craniofacial asymmetry and cleft lip and palate following maternal ingestion of 580 mg of diazepam at 6 weeks gestation. The mother apparently slept for 30 hours and remained in a state of semi consciousness for a further 2 days post exposure (Rivas 1984). See also Chapter 2.10.4.

> **Recommendation.** Treatment of diazepam overdose in pregnancy is as for the nonpregnant patient. Where delivery occurs within a few days of the exposure, diazepam may still be present in the neonate at birth and careful assessment for withdrawal symptoms, drowsiness and respiratory depression ("floppy infant syndrome") is advised.

▶ Digitalis

One report deals with intoxication with *digitalis* (8.9 mg *digitoxin*) during the seventh month of pregnancy. After spontaneous delivery at week 30, the child died on its third day of life. Hemorrhagic infarctions in both kidneys and degenerative changes in the CNS were found, and were interpreted as hypoxic changes due to continuous intrauterine bradycardia (Sherman 1960). See also Chapter 4.6.9.

> **Recommendation.** Treatment of digitalis toxicity in pregnancy should be in accordance with guidelines for nonpregnant patients. If treatment with an antidote, such as digoxin antibodies is indicated, this should not be withheld because of pregnancy.

▶ Haloperidol

A single published case report describes an intentional overdose of 300 mg *haloperidol* at 34 weeks gestation. Some features of maternal toxicity occurred but resolved within 48 hours. Biophysical fetal effects including non-reactivity, profound depression and akinesia were also described. These resolved within 5 days of the overdose and a healthy infant was delivered following induction of labor at 39 weeks gestation (Hansen 1997). See also Chapter 2.11.6.

> **Recommendation.** Treatment is as for the nonpregnant patient.

▶ **Iron**

Publications on *iron* overdose in pregnancy consist of multiple case reports and a small cases series. The majority of these reports involve maternal iron overdose during the second and third trimesters of pregnancy (Tran 1998, Khoury 1995, McElhatton 1991, 1993, Turk 1993, Lacoste 1992, Schauben 1990, Tenenbein 1989, Van Ameyde 1989, Olenmark 1987, Blanc 1984, Rayburn 1983, Manoguerra 1976, Strom 1976) with only five published cases relating to overdose during the first trimester (McElhatton 1991, 1993, Tenenbein 1989).

Collectively, the published case reports document around 82 exposed pregnancies, resulting in the live births of 65 apparently healthy infants (including three preterm) with no congenital malformations, two spontaneous abortions, two maternal and fetal deaths (possible duplicate reporting of the same case), and five elective terminations. The case series of 66 maternal iron overdoses describes seven congenital malformations (six minor, one major – anencephaly). However, all exposures occurred in the second or third trimester of pregnancy (after the period of organogenesis), and a causal association with the exposure/overdose is therefore unlikely (McElhatton 1993).

Fetal death in association with maternal death following iron overdose in the second trimester has been reported in two separate case reports (Manoguerra 1976, Strom 1976). As alluded to above, the similarity in the details of each report suggest that both publications may relate to the same case, despite discrepancies between the reports regarding the dose and the maternal serum iron concentration.

Desferrioxamine was administered in 47 of the above cases (59%) (Tran 1998, Khoury 1995, McElhatton 1991, 1993, Turk 1993, Lacoste 1992, Schauben 1990, Tenenbein 1989, Van Ameyde 1989, Olenmark 1987, Blanc 1984, Rayburn 1983), suggesting severe maternal toxicity, although poison scores or maternal symptoms were often poorly documented. Data from case reports of pregnancy outcomes following desferrioxamine use provide no signal that it is harmful to the fetus. However, the data are extremely limited and in most cases of iron overdose, desferrioxamine use occurred during the second and third trimester (Tran 1998, Khoury 1995, Turk 1993, Lacoste 1992, McElhatton 1991, Schauben 1990, Van Ameyde 1989, Tenenbein 1989, Olenmark 1987, Blanc 1984, Rayburn 1983). See also Chapter 2.18.13.

> **Recommendation.** There are no published guidelines on the management of iron overdose during pregnancy. The patient should be managed as for the nonpregnant patient and use of antidotes such as desferrioxamine should not be withheld if clinically indicated.

▶ **Metoprolol**

A prospective, epidemiologic study of 559 self-poisoned pregnant women (Czeizel 1997) included two infants with congenital anomalies whose mothers had overdosed on *metoprolol*. One infant was exposed to *diaze-pam* (150 mg), *promethazine* (250 mg), *metoprolol* (1 g), and *meprobamate* (2 g) at 4 weeks gestation and was born (gestational age not reported) with undescended testes. The second infant was exposed to metoprolol (2 g) and *bromhexine* (160 mg) at 20 weeks gestation in addition to large amounts of alcohol throughout pregnancy. The baby was microcephalic and had seizures at birth. See also Chapter 2.8.

▶ Misoprostol

There are three published reports of misoprostol exposure involving doses above those that would normally be used to induce uterine contractions for termination of pregnancy.

The first details an attempted suicide with 6 mg *misoprostol* and 8 mg *trifluoperazine* at 31 weeks gestation resulting in maternal hyperthermia, tachycardia, tachypnoea, acidosis and a tetanic uterus. On examination, uterine ultrasound revealed no fetal movement or heart motion, and a stillborn baby with diffuse ecchymosis was delivered 1 hour later (Bond 1994).

The second case involved self-administration of 8 mg misoprostol (1 mg orally and 7 mg vaginally) to induce abortion at 5 weeks gestation. The patient developed agitation, tremors, hallucinations, tachycardia, fever, rhabdomyolysis, acute renal failure, raised liver enzymes and metabolic acidosis. Ultrasonography carried out 51 hours post-exposure (48 hours after admission) revealed a complete abortion (Barros 2011). The third report details an attempt to induce abortion by self-administration of 10.8 mg of misoprostol over a 6-week period (maximum daily dose was 800 mcg) from 5 weeks gestation. At 12 weeks the patient complained of mild to moderate pelvic pain. Ultrasonography at 16 weeks gestation revealed no fetal anomalies and the patient delivered an apparently healthy child at 38 weeks gestation (Rouzi 2010). See also Chapter 2.14.

▶ NSAID

Preliminary reports of data collected by the UK Teratology Service (Schaefer 2007), on *ibuprofen* overdose in 100 pregnant women documented the occurrence of cardiac malformations in three of the 73 live-born offspring. However, review of an expanded UKTIS dataset of over 150 exposures in 2010 (unpublished) does not suggest an increased risk of malformation following first trimester overdose. However, two infants with suspected premature closure of the ductus arteriosus (12.5%; 95% CI 2.2–39.5) were documented in a series of 16 confirmed cases of third trimester ibuprofen overdose (defined as ingestion of more than the maximum daily therapeutic amount of 2.4 g). The first infant was delivered at 34 weeks following maternal ingestion of at least 6 g ibuprofen during week 30 of pregnancy. The second infant was delivered by emergency caesarean section 36 hours after maternal ingestion of 7.2 g ibuprofen at week 37 of pregnancy. Ibuprofen doses ingested by the cohort ranged from 3.2 g to 28 g, and all 16 exposures resulted in live-born infants. Twelve of the infants in whom premature ductal closure was not reported were co-exposed to other medications (Jones 2010). See also Chapter 2.1.

Recommendation. Therapeutic doses of NSAIDs after week 30 are associated with a risk of premature closure of the Ductus Arteriosus (DA) and oligohydramnios. Exposure to ibuprofen or any other NSAID in overdose after 30 weeks gestation therefore warrants immediate assessment of fetal wellbeing, even in the absence of maternal toxicity or symptoms. Antenatal identification of premature closure of the DA may require expedited early fetal delivery or enhanced monitoring. Premature closure of the DA has also been associated with an increased risk of PPHN in the neonate. Pediatricians should be made aware of this at delivery. Maternal treatment of ibuprofen overdose in pregnancy at any stage should be in accordance with guidelines for nonpregnant patients.

▶ **Paracetamol**

Paracetamol is metabolized to an active metabolite which, in high concentration, is hepatotoxic. It is not known if the risk of maternal hepatotoxicity is increased in pregnancy. If untreated, paracetamol overdose may be fatal to both mother and fetus as a consequence of maternal toxicity. The fetal liver begins to metabolize paracetamol from around 18 weeks of pregnancy, and paracetamol overdose beyond this gestation therefore also carries a risk of direct fetal hepatotoxicity.

Prompt treatment with *acetylcysteine* (NAC) is very effective in the prevention of hepatotoxicity in nonpregnant patients. Data from a study of 60 pregnant women (Riggs 1989) and from individual case reports (Crowell 2008, Sancewicz-Pach 1999, Horowitz 1997, Wang 1997, Rosevear 1989, Ludmir 1986, Haibach 1984, Roberts 1984, Lederman 1983, Byer 1982, Stokes 1984), suggest that NAC is also effective in pregnancy, and that delayed treatment with NAC is associated with adverse pregnancy outcome. The available data, although limited, do not indicate that use of acetylcysteine as an antidote in human pregnancy is associated with fetal toxicity.

No significantly increased rate of congenital anomaly, or pattern of anomalies suggestive of a teratogenic embryopathy was observed amongst 604 cases of first trimester paracetamol overdose prospectively collected by the UK Teratology Information Service (reported in abstract form; Lawler 2004), and the study of 60 exposures referred to above (Riggs 1989). See also Chapter 4.1.1.

Recommendation. If clinically indicated, treatment with NAC should not be delayed or withheld on account of pregnancy. The UK National Poisons and Teratology Information Services (NPIS and UKTIS) recommend that the ingested paracetamol dose in mg/kg should be calculated using the woman's pre-pregnancy weight, but where indicated, the dose of NAC is calculated using actual maternal weight at the time of poisoning, up to a ceiling of 110 kg.

Whereas NPIS (UK) advises use of standard paracetamol normograms to assess whether treatment with NAC is indicated, others suggest use of an antidote at lower thresholds in pregnancy.

▶ **Podophyllotoxin**

Podophyllotoxin, externally applied in high doses, led to psychiatric symptoms in a few pregnant women. Furthermore, there was one maternal death, one fetal death (Stoudmire 1981, Slater 1978, Montaldi 1974, Chamberlain 1972, Ward 1954), and one malformation of extremities, heart and ear after exposure between weeks 5 and 9 of pregnancy (Karol 1980). See also Chapter 2.13.4.

▶ **Selective serotonin reuptake inhibitors (SSRIs)**

Only a single case report of SSRI overdose in pregnancy has been published (Tixier 2008). The 36-year-old patient experienced signs of acute serotonergic intoxication at 31 weeks gestation after ingestion of 280 mg of *escitalopram*. She was treated with activated charcoal at 5 hours post-ingestion, and due to regular uterine contractions indicating a risk of premature delivery, was also given intravenous *nicardipine* and an intramuscular corticosteroid. The contractions diminished and tocolytic treatment was withdrawn after 24 hours. She gave birth spontaneously at 37 weeks plus 4 days to a live-born infant who was well but extremely agitated. No other adverse events, including respiratory complications, were present. The infant remained irritable and nervous for several days and was discharged 17 days post-delivery. See also Chapter 2.11.3.

> **Recommendation.** Treatment of SSRI overdose in pregnancy is as for the nonpregnant patient. Therapeutic use of SSRIs in the latter half of pregnancy has been associated with an increased risk of neonatal withdrawal syndrome and Persistent Pulmonary Hypertension in the Newborn (PPHN). Neonatal observation following delivery may be advisable where maternal SSRI overdose has occurred within the preceding few weeks, although the risk period for these neonatal effects following overdose in pregnancy is unknown.

2.22.4   Animal toxins

▶ **Snake bites**

A literature review in 2010 identified 213 published cases worldwide of snake bite in pregnancy (Langley 2010). In 84 cases, the stage of pregnancy at which the bite occurred was not reported, and in 88 cases the identity of the snake was not known. Maternal death occurred in nine cases and fetal or neonatal death in 41 cases, the majority being intrauterine deaths. It is likely, however, that the retrospective nature of the publications included in this review has resulted in an over-estimation of fetomaternal mortality rate following snake bite in pregnancy, as a consequence of preferential and duplicate reporting of cases associated with an adverse outcome.

The authors found that in most reports details of the maternal and fetal deaths were scarce. Placental abruption was documented in eight cases and accounted for six fetal deaths. Two of the 96 pregnant women who were reported to have received antivenom died, and fetal or neonatal death occurred in 29 of these cases. Seven maternal deaths and 12 fetal/neonatal deaths occurred in the 106 cases where antivenom was not administered. Although the fetal death rate was higher in cases where the mother received antivenom (30.2 vs. 11.3%), this may reflect more significant envenomation, and the mother (and fetus) may have been more likely to die if antivenom was withheld.

Congenital malformation was reported in three cases, all of which involved the mother being bitten at or after 12 weeks of gestation. In addition to polydactyly in one and multiple unspecified anomalies in another, hydrocephalus or dilation of the cerebral ventricles was reported in all three infants. Death of one infant occurred at 4 days of age after apparent maternal anaphylaxis to antivenom therapy occurred during treatment of a snake bite at 28 weeks of gestation. The mother was also treated with epinephrine, isoproterenol, methylprednisolone and diphenhydramine.

Maternal and fetal outcome following a snake bite in pregnancy is likely to be determined by the species of snake involved, and whether or not envenoming occurs as a consequence of the bite.

Spider bites

The US National Poisons Control Centers reported on 97 black widow spider bites in pregnant women. Stage of pregnancy at the time of being bitten was known for 94 women, with 15% occurring in the first trimester. Symptoms were reported to be similar in pregnant women and nonpregnant women, and no pregnancy losses were reported (Wolfe 2011). The majority of women (72.2 %) received no treatment, 13.4% received *benzodiazepines*, 10.3% received *antihistamines*, 4.1% received *antivenom*, 5.2% received antibiotics and 2.1% received *calcium*.

There are four isolated case reports of black widow spider bites in the second and third trimester of pregnancy. Anxiolytics, morphine, calcium gluconate and antivenom were administered in all cases (Sherman 2000, Handel 1994, Scalzone 1994, Russell 1979). Two women who were bitten at 30 and 38 weeks gestation, respectively, were reported to have delivered healthy term infants (Sherman 2000, Scalzone 1994). Details regarding the pregnancy outcomes of the remaining two women who were bitten earlier in pregnancy, at 16 and 22 weeks, were not provided (Handel 1994, Russell 1979).

Stings from bees, wasps and ants

Only three retrospective case reports, each of which document outcomes from women who were stung by a bee, wasp or ant, are published in the literature (reviewed in Brown 2013). All three cases were associated with anaphylaxis and two resulted in premature deliveries, suspected by one author as being be due to a "post anaphylactic reaction." One preterm infant was healthy, but the second child was hypotonic and cyanotic at birth and died at 64 days of life. Autopsy identified cystic cavitation of the cerebral white matter consistent with hypoxic injury. The third case described anaphylaxis in a pregnant woman following an ant bite at 40 weeks gestation. She was treated but developed vaginal bleeding 16 hours later and ultrasound scan confirmed placental separation and fetal death.

Recommendation. Seek specialist advice regarding the likelihood of toxicity. Maternal treatment of toxicity due to a snake bite in pregnancy should be the same for the nonpregnant patient. Treatment with antitoxins following venomous snake or spider bites should not be withheld because of pregnancy.

Pregnancy

2.22 Poisonings and toxins

2.22.5   Mushrooms

There are only a few retrospectively reported cases, and one small study documenting mushroom poisoning in pregnancy in the published literature. Pregnancy outcomes of 22 pregnant women treated for *Amanita phalloides* ingestion compared with those of 40 non-exposed women, did not suggest any association between an increased risk of major congenital malformation or minor anomalies and mushroom toxicity (Tímár 1997). Ingestion occurred in five women during the first trimester, eight in the second and nine in the third trimester of pregnancy. Over half of the poisonings were documented as mild, with only two reported as severe. Compared to the control group, a significantly low birth weight (but no difference in gestational age) was observed in the exposed live-borns.

Single case reports document the birth of a normal infant following first trimester mushroom ingestion associated with moderate maternal intoxication (Boyer 2001), the birth of three normal infants following mushroom ingestion during the second trimester of pregnancy (Wacker 2009, Schleufe 2003, Nagy 1994), delivery of a premature infant at 36 weeks after ingestion of *Amanita phalloides* at 20 weeks associated with threatened miscarriage (Wu 2004), and delivery of a healthy baby following maternal plasmapheresis for *Amanita phalloides* poisoning in the eighth month of pregnancy (Belliardo 1983).

> **Recommendation.** Pregnant women who have ingested poisonous mushrooms, especially *Amanita phalloides* (death cap), should be treated as for nonpregnant women.

2.22.6   Other plant toxins

Although a large number of plant toxins have shown teratogenic effects in certain animal species (for example, *aflatoxins* and *cytochalasin* B and D), there is no evidence that these toxins cause malformations in humans (see survey in Schardein 2000). However, one report found a correlation between lower birth weight and aflatoxin in the maternal blood (de Vries 1989).

Potato blight is caused by a fungus, *Phytophthora infestans*. Renwick (1972) published a hypothesis that neural tube defects (NTD; i.e. anencephaly and spina bifida) were associated with maternal exposure to some component from potatoes, possibly *cytoclalasins*. A higher incidence of these defects among lower socioeconomic groups was suggested. Although the hypothesized potato-NTD association stimulated many research projects, it remains unproven (Allen 1977, Lemire 1977, Poswillo 1973, Roberts 1973).

2.22.7   Bacterial endotoxins

There are no reports regarding embryotoxic effects in humans of either bacterial toxins in *food poisoning* (e.g. staphylococcal, *E. coli*, and salmonella), or about other toxins (such as in diphtheria; see survey in

Schardein 2000). There are, however, reports about four mothers with *botulism* in the second or third trimester (Polo 1996, Robin 1996, St Clair 1975). None of the children were damaged by this illness, which is life-threatening to the mother. In one case (Polo 1996), it is explicitly mentioned that the only movements in the mother (who was totally paralyzed) were those of the fetus suggesting that the botulinum toxin does not cross the placenta.

References

Adhikari K, Ghosh A, Alauddin MD et al. Organophosphate poisoning in pregnancy. J Obstet Gynaecol 2011; 31: 290–292.

Allen JR, Marlar RJ, Chesney CF et al. Teratogenicity studies on late blighted potatoes in non-human primates (*Macaca mulatta* and *Saguinus labiatus*). Teratology 1977; 15: 17–24.

Barros JG, Reis I, Graca LM. Acute misoprostol toxicity during the first trimester of pregnancy. Int J Gynecol Obstet 2011; 113: 157–158.

Belliardo F, Massano G, Accomo S. Amatoxins do not cross the placental barrier. Lancet 1983; 1: 1381.

Belson M, Morgan BW. Methanol toxicity in a newborn. J Toxicol 2004; 42: 673–677.

Benavides I, Mercurio M, Hoffman R. Thallium overdose in pregnancy {Abstract}. J Toxicol Clin Toxicol 1997; 35: 522.

Blache JL, Jean Ph, Vigouroux C. Fatal colchicine poisoning. Two particular cases {Abstract}. Intensive Care Med 1982; 8: 249.

Blanc P, Hryhorczuk D, Danel I. Deferoxamine treatment of acute iron intoxication in pregnancy. Obstet Gynecol 1984; 64: 12S–14S.

Bloom MS, Fitzgerald EF, Kim K et al. Spontaneous pregnancy loss in humans and exposure to arsenic in drinking water. Int J Hyg Environ Health 2010; 213: 401–413.

Bolliger CT, van Zijl P, Louw JA. Multiple organ failure with the adult respiratory distress syndrome in homicidal arsenic poisoning. Respiration 1992; 59: 57–61.

Bond GR, Van Zee A. Overdosage of misoprostol in pregnancy. Am J Obstet Gynecol 1994; 171: 561–562.

Bove KE, Bhathena D, Wyatt RJ et al. Diffuse metanephric adenoma after *in utero* aspirin intoxication. A unique case of progressive renal failure. Arch Pathol Lab Med 1979; 103: 187–190.

Boyer JC, Hernandez F, Estorc J et al. Management of maternal Amanita phalloïdes poisoning during the first trimester of pregnancy: a case report and review of the literature. Clin Chem 2001; 47: 971–974.

Brender JD, Suarez L, Felkner M et al. Maternal exposure to arsenic, cadmium, lead, and mercury and neural tube defects in offspring. Environ Res 2006; 101: 132–139.

Brown SA, Seifert SA, Rayburn WF. Management of envenomations during pregnancy. Clin Toxicol (Phila) 2013; 51: 3–15.

Byer AJ, Traylor TR, Semmer JR. Acetaminophen overdose in the third trimester of pregnancy. Jama 1982; 247: 3114–3115.

Caravati EM, Adams CJ, Joyce SM et al. Fetal toxicity associated with maternal carbon monoxide poisoning. Ann Emerg Med 1988; 17: 714–717.

Chamberlain MJ, Reynolds AL, Yeoman WB. Toxic effect of podophylline application in pregnancy. Br Med J 1972; 3: 391–392.

Chomchai C, Tiawilai A. Fetal poisoning after maternal paraquat ingestion during third trimester of pregnancy: case report and literature review. J Med Toxicol 2007; 3: 182–186.

Cramer CR. Fetal death due to accidental maternal carbon monoxide poisoning. J Toxicol Clin Toxicol 1982; 19: 297–301.

Crowell C, Lyew RV, Givens M et al. Caring for the mother, concentrating on the fetus: intravenous N-acetylcysteine in pregnancy. Am J Emerg Med 2008; 26: 735.

Czeizel A, Szentesi I, Szekeres I et al. A study of adverse effects on the progeny after intoxication during pregnancy. Arch Toxicol 1988; 62: 1–7.

Czeizel AE, Tomcsik M, Timar L. Teratologic evaluation of 178 infants born to mothers who attempted suicide by drugs during pregnancy. Obstet Gynecol 1997; 90: 195–201.

Dadvand P, Rankin J, Rushton S et al. Ambient air pollution and congenital heart disease: a register-based study. Environ Res 2011; 111: 435–441.

Daya MR, Irwin R, Parshley MC et al. Arsenic ingestion in pregnancy. Vet Hum Toxicol 1989; 31: 347.

De Vries HR, Maxwell SM, Hendrickse RG. Foetal and neonatal exposure to aflatoxins. Acta Paediatr Scand 1989; 78: 373–378.

Dix-Cooper L, Eskenazi B, Romero C et al. Neurodevelopmental performance among school age children in rural Guatemala is associated with prenatal and postnatal exposure to carbon monoxide, a marker for exposure to woodsmoke 2012; 33: 246–254.

Farrow JR, Davis GJ, Roy TM et al. Fetal death due to nonlethal maternal carbon monoxide poisoning. J Forensic Sci 1990; 35: 1448–1452.

Fennelly JJ, Gallagher JT, Carroll RT. Paraquat poisoning in a pregnant woman. Br Med J 1968; 3: 722–723.

Ghezzi R, Bozza Marrubini M. Prussian blue in the treatment of thallium intoxication. Vet Hum Toxicol 1979; 21: 64–66.

Gidai J, Acs N, Banhidy F et al. No association found between use of very large doses of diazepam by 112 pregnant women for a suicide attempt and congenital abnormalities in their offspring. Toxicol Ind Health 2008; 24: 29–39.

Haibach H, Akhter JE, Muscato MS et al. Acetaminophen overdose with fetal demise. Am J Clin Pathol 1984; 82: 240–242.

Handel CC, Izquierdo LA, Curet LB. Black widow spider (Latrodectus mactans) bite during pregnancy. West J Med 1994; 160: 261–262.

Hansen LM, Megerian G, Donnenfeld AE. Haloperidol overdose during pregnancy. Obstet Gynecol 1997; 90: 659–661.

Hantson P, Lambermont J-Y, Mahieu P. Methanol poisoning during late pregnancy. J Toxicol Clin Toxicol 1997; 35: 187–191.

Hoffman RS. Thallium poisoning during pregnancy: a case report and comprehensive literature review. J Toxicol Clin Toxicol 2000; 38: 767–775.

Hopenhayn C, Bush HM, Bingcang A et al. Association between arsenic exposure from drinking water and anemia during pregnancy. J Occup Environ Med 2006; 48: 635–643.

Horowitz RS, Dart RC, Jarvie DR et al. Placental transfer of N-acetylcysteine following human maternal acetaminophen toxicity. J Toxicol Clin Toxicol 1997; 35: 447–451.

Jajoo M, Saxena S, Pandey M. Transplacentally acquired organophosphorus poisoning in a newborn: case report. Ann Trop Paediatr 2010; 30: 137–139.

Jenq CC, Wu CD, Lin JL. Mother and fetus both survive from severe paraquat intoxication. Clin Toxicol (Phila) 2005; 43: 291–295.

Jones D, Stephens S, Richardson JL et al. The fetal effects of ibuprofen overdose in the third trimester of pregnancy and the risk of premature closure of the ductus arteriosus. Clin Toxicol 2010; 48: 240–318.

Kamha AA, Al Omary IY, Zalabany HA et al. Organophosphate poisoning in pregnancy: a case report. Basic Clin Pharmacol Toxicol 2005; 96: 397–398.

Karalliedde L, Senanayake N, Ariaratnam A. Acute organophosphorus insecticide poisoning during pregnancy. Hum Toxicol 1988; 7: 363–364.

Karol MC, Connor CS, Murphy KJ. Podophyllum: suspected teratogenicity from topical application. Clin Toxicol 1980; 16: 283–286.

Khoury S, Odeh M, Oettinger M. Deferoxamine treatment for acute iron intoxication in pregnancy. Acta Obstet Gynecol Scand 1995; 74: 756–757.

Klys M, Rojek S, Rzepecka-Wozniak E. Neonatal death following clozapine self-poisoning in late pregnancy: an unusual case report. Forensic Sci Int 2007; 171: e5–10.

Koren G, Sharav T, Pastuszak A et al. A multicenter, prospective study of fetal outcome following accidental carbon monoxide poisoning in pregnancy. Reprod Toxicol 1991; 5: 397–403.

Lacoste H, Goyert GL, Goldman LS et al. Acute iron intoxication in pregnancy: case report and review of the literature. Obstet Gynecol 1992; 80: 500–501.

Laegreid L, Olegard R, Walstrom J et al. Teratogenic effects of benzodiazepine use during pregnancy. J Pediatr 1989; 114: 126–131.

Langley RL. Snakebite during pregnancy: a literature review. Wilderness Environ Med 2010; 21: 54–60.

Lawler JM, McElhatton P. Fetal outcome following maternal paracetamol overdose {Abstract}. European Association of Poisons Centres and Clinical Toxicologists XXIV International Congress. Clin Toxicol 2004; 42: 471.

Lederman S, Fysh WJ, Tredger M et al. Neonatal paracetamol poisoning: treatment by exchange transfusion. Arch Dis Child 1983; 58: 631–633.

Lemire RJ, Beckwith JB, Warkany J. Anencephaly, Incidences, Etiology and Epidemiology. New York: Raven Press, 1977, pp. 12–47.

Little BB, Santos-Ramos R, Newell JF et al. Megadose carbamazepine during the period of neural tube closure. Obstet Gynecol 1993; 82: 705–708.

Ludmir J, Main DM, Landon MB et al. Maternal acetaminophen overdose at 15 weeks of gestation. Obstet Gynecol 1986; 67: 750–751.

Lugo G, Cassady G, Palmisano P. Acute maternal arsenic intoxication with neonatal death. Am J Dis Child 1969; 117: 328–330.

Manoguerra AS. Iron poisoning: report of a fatal case in an adult. Am J Hosp Pharm 1976; 33: 1088–1090.

Mathieu-Nolf M, Mathieu D, Durak C et al. Acute carbon monoxide poisoning during pregnancy. Maternal and fetal outcome {Abstract}. Reprod Toxicol 2006; 22: 279.

McClure CK, Katz KD, Patrick TE et al. The epidemiology of acute poisonings in women of reproductive age and during pregnancy, California, 2000–2004. Matern Child Health J 2011a; 15: 964–973.

McClure CK, Patrick TE, Katz KD et al. Birth outcomes following self-inflicted poisoning during pregnancy, California, 2000 to 2004. J Obstet Gynecol Neonatal Nurs 2011b; 40: 292–301.

McElhatton PR, Easton T. The fetal effects of antidepressant overdose in pregnancy. J Toxicol-Clin Toxic 2003; 41: 445.

McElhatton PR, Roberts JC, Sullivan FM. The consequences of iron overdose and its treatment with desferrioxamine in pregnancy. Hum Exp Toxicol 1991; 10: 251–259.

McElhatton PR, Sullivan FM, Volans GN. Outcome of pregnancy following deliberate iron overdose by the mother {Abstract}. Hum Exp Toxicol 1993; 9: 579.

Midtling JE, Barnett PG, Coye MJ et al. Clinical management of field worker organophosphate poisoning. West J Med 1985; 142: 514–518.

Montaldi D, Giambrone JP, Courney NG. Podophyllin poisoning associated with the treatment of condyloma accuminatum. A case report. Am J Obset Gynecol 1974; 119: 1130–1131.

Mukherjee SC, Saha KC, Pati S et al. Murshidabad – one of the nine groundwater arsenic-affected districts of West Bengal, India. Part II: dermatological, neurological, and obstetric findings. Clin Toxicol (Phila) 2005; 43: 835–848.

Musson FA, Porter CA. Effect of ingestion of paraquat on a 20-week gestation fetus. Postgrad Med J 1982; 58: 731–732.

Nagy I, Pogátsa-Murray G, Zalányi S Jr et al. Amanita poisoning during the second trimester of pregnancy. A case report and a review of the literature. Clin Investig 1994; 72: 794–798.

Nordstrom S, Beckman L, Nordenson I. Occupational and environmental risks in and around a smelter in northern Sweden. V. Spontaneous abortion among female employees and decreased birth weight in their offspring. Hereditas 1979; 90: 291–296.

Norman CA, Halton DM. Is carbon monoxide a workplace teratogen? A review and evaluation of the literature. Ann Occup Hyg 1990; 34: 335–347.

Novikova N, Chitnis M, Linder V et al. Atypical antipsychotic (clozapine) self-poisoning in late pregnancy presenting with absent fetal heart rate variability without acidosis and delayed peristalsis in the newborn baby: a case report. Aust NZ J Obstet Gynaecol 2009; 49: 2–4.

Olenmark M, Biber B, Dottori O et al. Fatal iron intoxication in late pregnancy. J Toxicol-Clin Toxic 1987; 25: 347–359.

Omalu BI, Lindner JL, Janssen JK et al. The role of environmental factors in the causation of sudden death in infants: two cases of sudden unexpected death in two unrelated infants who were cared for by the same babysitter. J Forensic Sci 2007; 52: 1355–1358.

Pai V. Acute thallium poisoning. Prussian blue therapy in 9 cases. W Indian Med J 1987; 36: 256–258.

Palatnick W, Tenenbein M. Aspirin poisoning during pregnancy: increased fetal sensitivity. Am J Perinatol 1998; 15: 39–41.

Petik D, Czeizel B, Banhidy F et al. A study of the risk of mental retardation among children of pregnant women who have attempted suicide by means of a drug overdose. J Inj Violence Res 2012; 4: 10–19.

Polo JM, Martin J, Berciano J. Botulism and pregnancy. Lancet 1996; 348: 195.

Poswillo DE, Sopher D, Mitchell SJ et al. Further investigations into the teratogenic potential of imperfect potatoes. Nature 1973; 244: 367–368.

Rahman A, Vahter M, Smith AH et al. Arsenic exposure during pregnancy and size at birth: a prospective cohort study in Bangladesh. Am J Epidemiol 2009; 169: 304–312.

Rangel Guerra R, Martinez HR, Villarreal HJ. Thallium poisoning. Clinical experience with 14 cases. Rev Invest Clin 1980; 32: 381–389.

Rayburn WF, Donn SM, Wulf ME. Iron overdose during pregnancy: successful therapy with deferoxamine. Am J Obstet Gynecol 1983; 147: 717–718.

Rejent TA, Baik S. Fatal in utero salicylism. J Forensic Sci 1985; 30: 942–944.

Renwick JH. Spina bifida, anencephaly, and potato blight. Lancet 1972; 2: 976–986.

Riggs BS, Bronstein AC, Kulig K et al. Acute acetaminophen overdose during pregnancy. Obstet Gynecol 1989; 74: 247–253.

Ritz B, Yu F, Fruin S et al. Ambient air pollution and risk of birth defects in Southern California. Am J Epidemiol 2002; 155: 17–25.

Rivas F, Hernandez A, Cantu JM. Acentric craniofacial cleft in a newborn female prenatally exposed to a high dose of diazepam. Teratology 1984; 30: 179–180.

Roberts CJ, Revington CJ, Lloyd S. Potato cultivation and storage in South Wales and its relation to neural tube malformation prevalence. Br J Prevent Soc Med 1973; 27: 214–216.

Roberts I, Robinson MJ, Mughal MZ et al. Paracetamol metabolites in the neonate following maternal overdose. Br J Clin Pharmacol 1984; 18: 201–206.

Robin L, Herman D, Redett R. Botulism in a pregnant woman. N Engl J Med 1996; 335: 823–824.

Romero P, Barnett PG, Midtling JE. Congenital anomalies associated with maternal exposure to oxydemeton-methyl. Environ Res 1989; 50: 256–261.

Rosevear SK, Hope PL. Favourable neonatal outcome following maternal paracetamol overdose and severe fetal distress. Case report. Br J Obstet Gynaecol 1989; 96: 491–493.

Rouzi AA. Abortion failure after illegal use of misoprostol: A case report. Europ J Contracept Reprod Health Care 2010; 15: 376–378.

Russell FE, Marcus P, Streng JA. Black widow spider envenomation during pregnancy. Report of a case. Toxicon 1979; 17: 188–189.

Sancewicz-Pach K, Chmiest W, Lichota E. Suicidal paracetamol poisoning of a pregnant woman just before a delivery. Przegl Lek 1999; 56: 459–462.

Saygan-Karamursel B, Guven S, Onderoglu L et al. Mega-dose carbamazepine complicating third trimester of pregnancy. J Perinat Med 2005; 33: 72–75.

Scalzone JM, Wells SL. Latrodectus mactans (black widow spider) envenomation: an unusual cause for abdominal pain in pregnancy. Obstet Gynecol 1994; 83: 830–831.

Schaefer C. Poisonings and toxins. In: Drugs During Pregnancy and Lactation, Schaefer C. Ed., 2nd edn, London: Elsevier, 2007, pp. 552.

Schardein JL. Chemically Induced Birth Defects, 3rd edn. New York: Marcel-Dekker, 2000.

Schauben JL, Augenstein WL, Cox J et al. Iron poisoning: report of three cases and a review of therapeutic intervention. J Emerg Med 1990; 8: 309–319.

Schleufe P, Seidel C. Amanita poisoning during pregnancy. Anasthesiol Intensivmed Notfallmed Schmerzther 2003; 38: 716–718.

Sebe A, Satar S, Alpay R et al. Organophosphate poisoning associated with fetal death: a case study. Mt Sinai J Med 2005; 72: 354–356.

Sezgin I, Sungu S, Bekar E et al. Cyclopia-astomia-agnathia-holoprosencephaly association: a case report. Clin Dysmorphol 2002; 11: 225–226.

Shah AM, Chattopadhyay A, Khambadkone SM et al. Neonatal mydriasis due to effects of atropine used for maternal Tik-20 poisoning. J Postgrad Med 1995; 41: 21–22.

Sherman JL Jr, Locke RV. Transplacental neonatal digitalis intoxication. Am J Cardiol 1960; 6: 834–837.

Sherman RP, Groll JM, Gonzalez DI et al. Black widow spider (Latrodectus mactans) envenomation in a term pregnancy. Curr Surg 2000; 57: 346–348.

Slater GE, Rumack BH, Peterson RG. Podophllin poisoning: systemic toxicity following cutaneous application. Obset Gynecol 1978; 52: 94–96.

Solomon GM, Moodley J. Acute chlorpyrifos poisoning in pregnancy: a case report. Clin Toxicol (Phila) 2007; 45: 416–419.

St Clair EH, di Liberti JH, O'Brien ML. Observations of an infant born to a mother with botulism. J Pediatr 1975; 87: 658.

Stephens S, Jones D, Wilson G et al. The fetal effects of aspirin overdose during pregnancy. J Toxicol Clin Toxicol 2009; 47: 453–454.

Stieb DM, Chen L, Eshoul M et al. Ambient air pollution, birth weight and preterm birth: A systematic review and meta-analysis. Environ Res 2012; 117: 100–111.

Stokes IM. Paracetamol overdose in the second trimester of pregnancy. Case report. Br J Obstet Gynaecol 1984; 91: 286–288.

Stoudmire A, Baker N, Thompson TL. Delirium induced by topical application of podophyllin: a case report. Am J Psychiatry 1981; 138: 1505–1506.

Strom RL, Schiller P, Seeds AE et al. Fatal iron poisoning in a pregnant female. Minn Med 1976; 59: 483–489.

Talbot AR, Fu CC, Hsieh MF. Paraquat intoxication during pregnancy: a report of 9 cases. Vet Hum Toxicol 1988; 30: 12–17.

Tenenbein M. Iron overdose during pregnancy [Abstract]. Vet Hum Toxicol 1989; 31: 346.

Tímár L, Czeizel AE. Birth weight and congenital anomalies following poisonous mushroom intoxication during pregnancy. Reprod Toxicol 1997; 11: 861–866.

Timmermann G, Acs N, Banhidy F et al. A study of the potential teratogenic effects of large doses of drugs rarely used for a suicide attempt during pregnancy. Toxicol Ind Health 2008; 24: 121–131.

Tixier H, Feyeux C, Girod S et al. Acute voluntary intoxication with selective serotonin reuptake inhibitors during the third trimester of pregnancy: therapeutic management of mother and fetus. Am J Obstet Gynecol 2008; 199: e9–12.

Tran T, Wax JR, Steinfeld JD et al. Acute intentional iron overdose in pregnancy. Obstet Gynecol 1998; 92: 678–680.

Tsatsakis AM, Perakis K, Koumantakis E. Experience with acute paraquat poisoning in Crete. Vet Hum Toxicol 1996; 38: 113–117.

Turk J, Aks S, Ampuero F et al. Successful therapy of iron intoxication in pregnancy with intravenous deferoxamine and whole bowel irrigation. Vet Hum Toxicol 1993; 35: 441–444.

Vahter M. Effects of arsenic on maternal and fetal health. Annu Rev Nutr 2009; 29: 381–399.

Van Ameyde KJ, Tenenbein M. Whole bowel irrigation during pregnancy. Am J Obstet Gynecol 1989; 160: 646–647.

Velez LI, Keyes DC, Roth B et al. Aspirin overdose in mother and fetus. J Toxicol Clin Toxicol 2001; 39: 483–484.

Velez LI, Kulstad E, Shepherd G et al. Inhalational methanol toxicity in pregnancy treated twice with fomepizole. Vet Hum Toxicol 2003; 45: 28–30.

Wacker A, Riethmüller J, Zilker T et al. Fetal risk through maternal Amanita phalloides poisoning at the end of pregnancy. Am J Perinatol 2009; 26: 211–213.

Wang PH, Yang MJ, Lee WL et al. Acetaminophen poisoning in late pregnancy. A case report. J Reprod Med 1997; 42: 367–371.

Ward JW, Clifford WS, Monaco AR. Fatal systemic poisoning following podophylline treatment of condyloma accuminatum. South Med J 1954; 47: 1204–1206.

Watkins CG, Strope GL. Chronic carbon monoxide poisoning as a major contributing factor in the sudden infant death syndrome. Am J Dis Child 1986; 140: 619.

Wertelecki W, Purvis-Smith SG, Blackburn WR. Amitriptyline/perphenazine maternal overdose and birth defects. Teratology 1980; 21: 74A.

Wolfe MD, Myers O, Caravati EM et al. Black widow spider envenomation in pregnancy. J Matern Fetal Neonatal Med 2011; 24: 122–126.

Woody RC, Brewster MA. Telencephalic dysgenesis associated with presumptive maternal carbon monoxide intoxication in the first trimester of pregnancy. J Toxicol Clin Toxicol 1990; 28: 467–475.

Wu BF, Wang MM. Molecular adsorbent recirculating system in dealing with maternal Amanita poisoning during the second pregnancy trimester: a case report. Hepatobiliary Pancreat Dis Int 2004; 3: 152–154.

Yildiz H, Aldemir E, Altuncu E et al. A rare cause of perinatal asphyxia: maternal carbon monoxide poisoning. Arch Gynecol Obstet 2010; 281: 251–254.

Occupational, industrial and environmental agents

2.23

Susan M. Barlow, Frank M. Sullivan and
Richard K. Miller

2.23.1	Solvent exposure in general	601
2.23.2	Formaldehyde and formalin	607
2.23.3	Photographic/printing chemicals	607
2.23.4	Pesticides	608
2.23.5	Phenoxyacetic acid derivatives and polychlorinated dibenzo-dioxins	612
2.23.6	Polychlorinated biphenyls	614
2.23.7	Chlorinated drinking water by-products	614
2.23.8	Metals	616
2.23.9	Hazardous waste landfill sites and waste incinerators	622
2.23.10	Radiation associated with the nuclear industry	623
2.23.11	Cell/mobile phones	625
2.23.12	Other sources of electromagnetic radiation	625
2.23.13	Electric shocks and lightning strikes	627

It is ambitious to describe the risk assessment of occupational, industrial and environmental agents, since they are the sum total of all agents which are potentially capable of producing an effect, whether physical, chemical or biological. They are found everywhere and influence the development of an individual. Both synthetic and naturally occurring substances may have significant pharmacological and toxicological properties, but few have been tested. Among the millions of synthetic chemicals registered with national or regional authorities, fewer than 100,000 are currently in commercial or industrial use, and most of these have not been tested for developmental toxicity. Similarly, very few toxins from microorganisms, fungi, plants, and animals have been systematically characterized for effects on development. The agents highlighted in this chapter may be of importance if there is occupational or environmental exposure to women who are pregnant or to men and women in their reproductive years.

In principle, it is difficult to distinguish between industrial and environmental chemicals. Environmental pollutants are usually industrial chemicals released as pollutants into the environment (air, water, or soil) during production, use, waste disposal, recycling, and combustion processes. Others are released from naturally high sources – for example, *arsenic* in regions with substantial granite deposits or copper smelting, or *dioxins* from burning of wood. The concentration of a

Drugs During Pregnancy and Lactation. **http://dx.doi.org/10.1016/B978-0-12-408078-2.00024-X**

particular industrial chemical may normally be higher in the workplace than in the general environment. However, when an accident occurs, the environmental pollution may exceed the typical workplace exposure. A number of reviews have been published on the reproductive toxicity of industrial and environmental chemicals (see overviews in Stillerman 2008, Miller 2004, Schardein 2000, Gilstrap 1998, Paul 1993, Sullivan 1993, Barlow 1982), but these cover only a small fraction of the total number of chemicals to which women may be exposed in the workplace.

Individual risk characterization is much more difficult with occupational or environmental exposure to chemical or physical agents than with a particular drug treatment, because:

- a pregnant woman is rarely exposed to a single agent;
- quantifying workplace or environmental/household exposure levels is difficult, expensive, time-consuming, and often would have to be done prospectively to be useful;
- there is a lack of data regarding kinetic properties (absorption, distribution, metabolism, excretion) of most chemicals in the mother and the embryo/fetus.

There is legislation in most developed countries preventing gender discrimination in employment and protecting the rights of women to work during pregnancy. Alongside this, there is the need for adequate information on the possible risks of exposure to chemicals in the workplace. Most jurisdictions require the production of Materials Safety Data Sheets (MSDSs). These should include any information that exists on the reproductive and developmental toxicity of the chemical. However, in practice, MSDSs rarely provide a useful reference source other than identification of the constituents of the product; the same lack of information on potential for reproductive effects holds true for physical and biological agents.

Since it is difficult to specify the upper safe limits of workplace exposure for pregnant women because of the lack of data, general occupational exposure limits (OELs) for the agent in question are often used as a guide. An OEL is the amount of a workplace health hazard that most workers can be exposed to without harming their health. They are advisory, not regulatory limits. Most OEL values are for time-weighted average (TWA) exposures over an 8-hour working day. For some agents, higher short-term exposure limits (STELs) are also recommended. These are 15 minute TWAs that should not be exceeded at any point during the working day. In the USA, 8-hour OELs are recommended by the American Conference of Governmental Hygienists (termed threshold limit values – TLVs) and by the National Institute for Occupational Safety and Health. The Occupational & Safety Health Administration refers to these recommendations in setting enforceable permissible exposure limits (PELs) to protect workers against the health effects of exposure to hazardous substances. PELs are regulatory limits on the amount or concentration of a substance in the air. They may also contain a skin designation (see http://www.osha.gov/dsg/topics/pel/index.html). In the EU, Directives recommend indicative occupational exposure limit values (IOELVs), which can be implemented nationally into values that are usually, but not always, identical to IOELV recommendations; national values may or may not be legally binding. For an overview of global OELs for over 6000 specific chemicals, see Brandys (2008); for EU IOELVs, see, for example, the British workplace exposure limits (Health and Safety Executive, 2011). OELs are regularly updated in many countries, but they are not, in the main, based upon reproductive health data or concerns.

In accordance with the maternal protection laws in many countries, pregnant women should not be exposed to toxic, infectious, ionizing or carcinogenic substances. However, in practice many workplaces require women to handle potentially toxic compounds and do not take into account the possibility that workers might already be pregnant. In addition, non-specific symptoms have to be considered when discussing the tolerability of workplace or household contaminants. If pregnant women complain of repeated symptoms in the workplace – such as headaches, emesis, vertigo – this should be taken seriously. Such recurrent disorders can endanger the normal course of pregnancy. Women may also have exaggerated responses to exposure simply because they are pregnant. This is often reported in relation to nausea and vomiting in pregnancy. For evaluating approaches to exposure during pregnancy, see Miller (2004).

With respect to awareness of an increased risk of birth defects from environmental pollution, birth defect monitoring systems would be of help. However, birth defect monitoring and surveillance systems seldom methodically measure environmental exposure. Only in the case of a cluster of defects with suggestions for pollution-related causation might such studies be performed. Absence of a change in the prevalence of birth defects in a population is not sufficient to exclude a (new) environmental developmental toxicant *per se*, since these monitoring systems are considered too insensitive. Similarly, general population studies (e.g. on rural populations exposure to a variety of pesticides) are seldom sufficiently sensitive to identify any specific chemicals that may be involved. In the case of linkage of occupational exposures to reproductive hazards, the epidemiologist has to demonstrate that reproductive outcome is worse than expected when the mother or father has a specific occupational exposure, and that this is not due to confounders such as disease, maternal age, cigarette smoking, etc. (Källén 1988).

2.23.1   Solvent exposure in general

Toxicology

Many solvents are lipid soluble and well absorbed. Common organic solvents include *alcohols* (see Chapter 2.21), *glycol ethers*, *ethylether*, *hexane, tetrachloroethane, toluene*, and *xylene*. Products such as degreasers, paint thinners, varnish removers, lacquers, silk-screening inks, and paints, also contain solvents. Exposure to one single solvent is rare; more frequently exposure is to mixed solvents by the inhalational and/or dermal routes. Hence, much of the epidemiology has been conducted on mixed or unspecified solvent exposure both at work and at home.

Exposure to solvents has been associated with significant reductions in fertility in women working in agriculture (Sallmén 2006), shoe manufacturing, dry cleaning, the metal industry (Sallmén 1995, 2008), and the pharmaceutical industry (Attarchi 2012).

Spontaneous abortions have also been reported to be significantly increased in solvent-exposed women working in various occupations and industries (see Taskinen 1990, for review). These include pharmaceutical manufacture (Attarchi 2012, Taskinen 1986), graphics and shoe manufacturing, (Lindbohm 1990), laboratories (Taskinen 1994), and semiconductor manufacture (reviewed by Lin 2008). In some of these occupations, exposure is to several solvents, and in some specifically to glycol ethers, toluene, xylene, or aliphatic hydrocarbon solvents.

Pregnancy

2.23 Occupational, industrial and environmental agents

The influence of maternal occupational exposure to solvents on fetal growth has been studied in specific industries and in population-based studies. The evidence from the former is inconsistent but evidence from the latter shows an increase in the risk of small-for-gestational-age babies (see review by Ahmed 2007).

Early studies on the Finnish population reported an association between maternal occupational exposure to solvents in the first trimester and CNS defects in the offspring (Holmberg 1979, 1982), but later studies on the same population did not show an association (Kurppa 1983). In a meta-analysis of pregnancy outcome following maternal occupational exposure to organic solvents in the first trimester, it was concluded to be associated with a tendency towards an increased risk of spontaneous abortion (from five studies with 2899 subjects) and with a significantly increased risk of major malformations (from five studies with 7036 subjects) (McMartin 1998). An increased risk of major malformations and previous miscarriage was found in a Canadian study of women exposed occupationally to solvents in the first trimester through employment as factory workers, laboratory technicians, artists, graphic designers, and printing industry workers; importantly, maternal symptoms during exposure were predictive of an increased risk of malformations (Khattak 1999). An increased risk of major malformations was also reported in a cohort of Danish laboratory technicians with exposure to organic solvents (Zhu 2006). French studies on maternal occupational exposure to single organic solvents or to mixtures of solvents during the first trimester have reported a significantly increased risk of cleft lip with/without cleft palate (Chevrier 2006), and of major malformations, including oral clefts, urinary malformations and male genital malformations (Garlantézec 2009). In both studies, the risk was related to the level of exposure and in the latter study the risk was associated with detection of metabolites of glycol ether and chlorinated solvents in maternal urine collected during early pregnancy (Cordier 2012). Previous studies have not found an association between exposure to glycol ethers and malformations (see Maldonado 2003 for review, Lin 2008). Significant increases in the risk of neural tube defects and congenital heart defects (but not orofacial clefts) in association with maternal occupational exposure to solvents, particularly chlorinated solvents, has been reported in the US National Birth Defects Prevention Study (Desrosiers 2012, Gilboa 2012).

Some solvents are known to be neurotoxic and there have been a few studies on the neurodevelopment of children born to women with occupational exposure to solvents during pregnancy (Hjortebjerg 2012). Outcomes studied included general developmental neurobehavioral assessments, motor function, vision, language, attention, hyperactivity, and intelligence. Five of the six studies showed some deleterious effects (see Julvez 2009 for review), as has a more recent study (Pelé 2013).

Non-occupational exposure to organic solvents in the form of paint fumes in the home environment have been studied in the large Danish National Birth Cohort, comprising 19,000 mothers, of which 45% reported exposure to paint fumes during pregnancy when interviewed around the 30th week. No relationship was found between exposure to paint fumes and birth weight or preterm birth (Sørensen 2010); in the 7% reporting exposure in the first trimester, the risk of some types of malformations showed increased odds ratios, but the confidence intervals did not indicate statistical significance.

Exposure of men to solvents may also affect reproductive success. Weak associations between solvent exposure in various occupations and reductions in male fertility have been reported but no specific solvents could be identified (Sallmén 1998, 2006). Spontaneous abortions and congenital malformations in offspring among wives of men exposed to organic solvents have been studied in Finland. A significantly increased risk of spontaneous abortions but not malformations was found in Finland in wives of men exposed to organic solvents for 80 days before conception, but no significant effect was found in association with direct maternal exposure to organic solvents in the first trimester (Taskinen 1989). Male painters in the Netherlands exposed to organic solvents for 3 months before a conception had a significantly increased risk for malformations in their offspring compared to carpenters with little or no solvent exposure (Hooiveld 2006). An Egyptian study reported a significant increase in the risk of congenital malformations in the offspring of men occupationally exposed to solvents during the periconceptional period (El-Helaly 2011). A meta-analysis to assess the risks of spontaneous abortions and major malformations after paternal exposure to organic solvents concluded that paternal exposure was associated with an increased risk for neural tube defects, but not for spontaneous abortions (Logman 2005).

In summary, occupational exposure to solvents, especially if associated with maternal toxicity, has been reported to cause reduced fertility and an increased risk of spontaneous abortion, fetal growth retardation, malformations and neurobehavioral effects in offspring. The effect of exposure of males on pregnancy outcomes in their partners is less clear. Reports on specific solvents are given below.

Recommendation. In general, exposure to solvents should be avoided during pregnancy. At a minimum, exposure should be well below the permissible exposure or general occupational exposure limits (PELs and OELs). Acute exposure is not an indication for termination of pregnancy; neither are additional prenatal diagnostic tests required as long as the mother demonstrates no symptoms. If continuous and significant exposure has occurred, a detailed fetal ultrasound may be offered and fetal growth should be monitored.

► **Carbon disulfide**

Toxicology

Carbon disulfide is neurotoxic. It is used in the manufacture of rayon textiles, cellophane, rubber and agricultural fumigants.

Placental transfer in human pregnancy has been demonstrated (Cai 1981). Carbon disulfide-exposed women have been reported to have alterations in their menstrual cycles suggestive of hormonal abnormalities (Zhou, 1988). The results of Finnish studies suggested that female rayon workers exposed to carbon disulfide or wives of male rayon workers have an increased incidence of spontaneous abortion; however, no causal relationship with carbon disulfide exposures could be established (Hemminki 1982b, 1980). A higher incidence of congenital anomalies (e.g. heart defects, inguinal hernia, and CNS abnormalities) of 2.4% compared to 1.4% in controls has been briefly reported in a Chinese study of female workers exposed to carbon disulfide (Bao 1991). A review of OELs for carbon disulfide, which vary between 1 and 100 ppm concluded that female reproduction may not be adequately protected at exposures around 10 ppm or above (Gelbke 2009). The data are inadequate to assess its reproductive toxicity in humans. There is no clear evidence to indicate that maternal exposure is associated with an increased risk of fetal toxicity.

> **Recommendation.** In view of the possibility of fetal toxicity, exposure to carbon disulfide should be avoided in pregnancy. When there has been significant exposure, this is not an indication for the termination of pregnancy. However, if the mother has had symptoms of toxicity and/or continuous exposure, she may be offered additional prenatal diagnostic measures – e.g. a detailed fetal ultrasound – and should also be removed from exposure, as well as having the workplace monitored for carbon disulfide concentrations.

▶ Chloroform (trichloromethane)

Toxicology

Chloroform is a widely used industrial and laboratory solvent. Interference with implantation and fetal growth retardation has been reported after exposure to chloroform in human pregnancy. Chloroform is also one of the prominent by-products from chlorination of drinking water (see Section 2.23.7).

There are a small number of epidemiological studies on pregnancy outcomes following chloroform exposure, but they are difficult to interpret (Williams 1998, Reif 1996). Exposure in these studies was usually to chloroform and a varying number of other chemicals. In a study of 492 children of laboratory workers exposed to organic solvents during the first trimester of pregnancy, 148 were exposed to chloroform. The frequency of congenital anomalies was no greater than expected compared with the general population (Axelsson 1984). However, with multi-chemical exposure, establishing a cause-effect relationship is difficult. For spontaneous abortion, no increase in risk was found in 206 women exposed to chloroform in the pharmaceutical industry (Taskinen 1994), but an increased risk was found in women exposed to chloroform in biomedical research laboratories (Wennborg 2000).

> **Recommendation.** Exposure to chloroform should be avoided in pregnancy wherever possible. Certainly, atmospheric levels should be kept to a minimum well below the recommended OELs. Exposure *per se* is not an indication for termination of pregnancy. In cases where there is chronic exposure and/or severe maternal toxicity, a detailed fetal ultrasound should be offered and fetal growth monitored. The patient should be removed from exposure, and the workplace monitored for chloroform concentrations.

▶ Dichloromethane (methylene chloride)

Toxicology

The main uses of *dichloromethane*, a halogenated organic solvent, are as a solvent in paint removers, degreasing fluids, aerosol propellants and hair lacquers. It is also used in shoe manufacturing. As a consequence of its widespread use, many workers may be exposed for prolonged periods (Sullivan 1993). Dichloromethane is metabolized readily to carbon monoxide, which may have toxic effects on the developing fetal brain (see Chapter 2.20).

There are three published studies on the effects of occupational exposure to dichloromethane in human pregnancy (Taskinen 1986, Axelsson 1984, Kurppa 1983). Data from these studies indicate that there was no overall increase in the incidence of congenital malformations or any syndrome of defects. However, there was no significant increase in the incidence of spontaneous abortion.

A single study on environmental exposure to dichloromethane, due to emissions from a manufacturing facility in the USA, found no significant effect on birth weight among 91,302 births when comparing high exposure to low exposure areas (Bell 1991).

> **Recommendation.** Exposure to dichloromethane should be avoided in pregnancy wherever possible. When there has been significant exposure this is not an indication for termination of pregnancy. However, if the mother has had symptoms of toxicity and/or continuous exposure, she may be offered additional prenatal diagnostic measures, such as a detailed fetal ultrasound. The patient should be removed from exposure, and the workplace monitored for dichloromethane concentrations.

► Tetrachloroethylene (perchloroethylene, PERC)

Toxicology

Tetrachloroethylene is widely used in the dry-cleaning industry, and exposure of women is common, especially in small businesses where industrial hygienic practices may be inadequate. There are experimental and epidemiological data suggesting a carcinogenic potential of PERC (IARC 1995). A number of studies have shown an increased risk for spontaneous abortion of about two-fold in women exposed to tetrachloroethylene in the laundry and dry-cleaning industry, and the risk is increased in more heavily exposed women (Doyle 1997, Windham 1991, Olsen 1990, Kyyrönen 1989, Bosco 1987, Hemminki 1980).

No increase in the incidence of low birth weight children or congenital malformations was reported in a Canadian study (McDonald 1987). None of the other studies were adequate to draw any conclusions about these outcomes.

Maternal exposure to volatile organic compounds, such as PERC, was found to influence the immune status of the newborn (Lehman 2002). In summary, the data indicate an increased risk of spontaneous abortion associated with occupational exposure, but data are inadequate regarding other outcomes of pregnancy.

> **Recommendation.** Exposure to tetrachloroethylene should be avoided during pregnancy wherever possible. Nevertheless, when there has been significant exposure this is not an indication for termination of pregnancy. However, if the mother has had symptoms of toxicity and/or continuous exposure, she may be offered additional prenatal diagnostic measures, such as a detailed fetal ultrasound including control of fetal growth. The patient should be removed from exposure, and the workplace monitored for tetracholorethylene concentrations.

► Toluene

Toxicology

Toluene (*toluol, methylbenzene*) is a widely used solvent in the paint, metal-cleaning products and adhesive applications (shoes) industries. Besides the industrial applications, toluene has been used as a

Pregnancy

2.23 Occupational, industrial and environmental agents

recreational drug as an alternative to ethanol (see Chapter 2.21). Toluene is a difficult product to regulate in the workplace and elsewhere because an individual can detect the sweet odor at approximately 3 ppm and the TLV is 25 ppm. Thus, only solvent monitoring of the workplace can establish exposure levels.

Symptoms in the pregnant woman can be the first evidence of substantive exposure – dizziness, headaches and hallucinations can be one sign associated with the workplace or with use of the product. It is often difficult to separate the symptoms of pregnancy nausea and vomiting from toxic effects of the solvent. In either case, it will be necessary, if the symptoms persist, to remove the woman from the specific work area. As with ethanol, dose is a principal concern.

The majority of information on toluene exposure in pregnancy comes from recreational use (solvent abuse). High exposures are associated with intrauterine growth retardation and with congenital anomalies (Wilkins-Haug 1997). In more than 30 cases of exposure to toluene via chronic recreational use to the point of "getting high," both maternal effects (e.g. acute intoxication, chronic ataxia, and atrophy of the cerebellum upon MRI examination) and fetal effects similar to the fetal alcohol syndrome have been regularly noted (Bowen 2006). In 56 patients with reported solvent abuse, 12 patients (21.4%) delivered preterm infants, nine infants (16.1%) had major anomalies, seven (12.5%) had fetal solvent syndrome facial features, and six (10.7%) had hearing loss (Scheeres 2002).

Occupational exposure has been associated with reduced fertility (Plenge-Bönig 1999) and spontaneous abortion (Ng 1992). A Canadian occupational exposure study on maternal solvent exposure and the occurrence of birth defects noted that most of the excess in defects was associated with toluene exposure (McDonald 1987).

A review on the reproductive effect of toluene highlights that maternal solvent abuse, with intermittent high-level exposures, is more detrimental to fetal development than occupational exposures in which there is relatively constant low-level exposures (Hannigan 2010).

Recommendation. The difficulty with occupational and environmental exposure to toluene compared with its abuse is similar to the use of alcohol (ethanol). Chronic abusive high levels resulting in persistent and acute symptoms, for both ethanol and toluene, result in impaired children. Chronic exposure in the workplace to levels resulting in substantive maternal symptoms is thought to place the offspring and mother at risk. Thus, it is recommended that if the pregnant woman is having symptoms (whether exaggerated responses to noxious odors during pregnancy or intoxication because of the excessive levels of solvent), she should not return to the workplace in her usual capacity until environmental monitoring data demonstrate that levels of toluene and any other solvents are well below the regulated levels (PEL, OEL), remembering that odor detection is very low at 3 ppm, while regulatory levels are 25 ppm. Even if the levels of toluene are below the acceptable 8-hour threshold, the patient still may have to be moved to a non-solvent area because of enhanced sensitivity to odors and persistent and regular vomiting and nausea. It is recommended that the status of both mother and conceptus be more closely monitored throughout the pregnancy. Nevertheless, when there has been significant exposure this is not an indication for termination of pregnancy. However, if the mother has had symptoms of toxicity and/or continuous exposure, she may be offered additional prenatal diagnostic measures, such as a detailed fetal ultrasound including control of fetal growth.

2.23.2   Formaldehyde and formalin

Toxicology

Formaldehyde is a hydrocarbon that is widely used as a disinfectant and tissue preservative. *Formalin* is a solution of formaldehyde in water, often with 10–15% methanol to prevent polymerization.

One study reported that occupational exposure to formaldehyde was significantly associated with delayed conception (Taskinen 1999). Information on spontaneous abortion is inconsistent. In female hospital workers, some have reported no effect (Hemminki 1985, 1982a), while others have found a significant effect (Saurel-Cubizolles 1994). However, in addition to formaldehyde, such workers are also likely to have been exposed to other hazardous agents, such as anesthetics and ionizing radiation. Weak associations between spontaneous abortions and formaldehyde exposure have been reported in cosmetologists (John 1994), laboratory workers (Taskinen 1994), and wood workers (Taskinen 1999).

No significant association was observed between maternal occupational exposure to formaldehyde during the first 3 months of pregnancy and congenital anomalies (Hemminki 1985, 1982a).

A systematic review of epidemiological studies on occupational exposure to formaldehyde and reproduction found 16 studies relating to exposure of women. While recall bias and confounding could not be ruled out, the meta-analysis showed a significantly increased risk of spontaneous abortion from nine studies, and of all adverse pregnancy outcomes combined (spontaneous abortion, low birth weight, congenital malformation) from 12 studies (Duong 2011).

Non-occupational exposure to formaldehyde through ambient air has also been studied. Higher ambient air exposures to formaldehyde tended to increase the risk of low birth weight and of unspecified congenital heart defects (Dulskiene 2005, Maroziene 2002).

> **Recommendation.** Exposure to chronic or high concentrations of formaldehyde and formalin should be avoided in pregnancy wherever possible. Atmospheric levels should be kept to a minimum, well below the recommended OELs. Exposure *per se* is not an indication for termination of pregnancy; as a rule, additional prenatal diagnostic tests are not required.

2.23.3   Photographic/printing chemicals

Toxicology

Many substances used in photography and printing are highly irritant and corrosive (see overview in Schardein 2000, Gilstrap 1998, Paul 1993). The most commonly used chemicals are: *acetic acid, ammonium sulfate, ammonium thiocyanate, ammonium thiosulfate, bromine/potassium bromide, citric acid, diethylenetriaminepenta acetic acid (DTPA), ethylenediamine tetra acetic acid (EDTA; ferric ammonium salt of EDTA), glycol ethers, hydrocarbon solvents, hydroxylamine, 3-phenylenediamine, 4-phenylenediamine, potassium carbonate, sodium benzoate, sodium sulfite,* and *sulfur dioxide.*

There are no data available on the potential toxic effects in human pregnancy for the majority of chemicals used in the photographic/printing industry.

Pregnancy

2.23 Occupational, industrial and environmental agents

Exposure to ammonia gas is also common, due to accidental spills in photographic processing. Because ammonia is an irritant, it is difficult for workers to remain in the workplace. Therefore, most exposure to ammonia is acute. Ammonia is rapidly metabolized in humans with normal liver function. There is no information on occupational ammonia exposure and human pregnancy outcomes. High doses of *bromine salts* are toxic. There is one case report concerning an infant who was found to have high serum bromide levels at birth. The mother had handled photographic chemicals during her pregnancy. At birth the child was hypotonic, but once the bromism had resolved the early childhood development was normal (Mangurten 1982). Work in printing and related trades has been associated with reduced fertility in men (Ford 2002), and with no effect in men, but reduced fertility in women in association with exposure to toluene (Plenge-Bönig 1999; see also Section 2.23.1).

> **Recommendation.** Based on the very limited data available, exposure to high concentrations of photographic and printing chemicals should be avoided in pregnancy, wherever possible. If spills do occur, it is recommended that pregnant women avoid the area and allow others with appropriate protective gear to clean up the spillage. It is important that the atmospheric levels are well below the recommended OELs. Exposure *per se* is not an indication for termination of pregnancy.

2.23.4   Pesticides

▶ Pesticides in general

There is a lot of literature on male and female occupational and non-occupational exposure to pesticides in relation to fertility and pregnancy outcomes (for reviews, see Shirangi 2011, Roeleveld 2008, Hanke 2004, Arbuckle 1998, 2001, García 1998). These reviews concluded that while there is some evidence that exposure to pesticides contributes to male and female infertility, the evidence on spontaneous abortion, preterm birth, birth weight, stillbirth, and congenital malformations are inconsistent, and firm conclusions cannot be drawn, either for occupational exposure (gardening, farming, agriculture, horticulture, greenhouse work, etc.) or for those living in areas where pesticides are applied. A review of eight studies on maternal occupational exposure to pesticides and neurodevelopment in offspring concluded that there was a negative impact; exposures were usually to mixtures of pesticides from the organophosphate, carbamate, or organochlorine groups and specific pesticides were not identified (Julvez 2009). Studies that ascertain all pesticide exposures may be insensitive with regard to identifying individual pesticides that may carry a risk. They also do not assess exposures to other agents (e.g. solvents), and do not differentiate between workers that do or do not use personal protective equipment.

A number of studies have focused on the genital tract abnormalities, cryptorchidism and hypospadias, in male offspring of pesticide workers because of the role of an endocrine mechanism in the etiology of these conditions, and the endocrine modulating properties of some pesticides, such as organochlorines. A meta-analysis of 16 epidemiological studies on maternal and/or paternal occupational exposure to pesticides and cryptorchidism in sons indicated that while there were weak associations (often not statistically significant) with relevant occupations or maternal serum, milk or fat levels of certain pesticides, there were other studies showing no association (Virtanen 2012). Two ecological studies in geographical areas with varying levels of pesticide use also showed associations with higher levels of pesticide use and cryptorchidism (Virtanen 2012). A meta-analysis of nine studies on hypospadias showed marginally significant, increased risks from maternal or paternal exposure to pesticides (Rocheleau 2009). More recent studies not included in the above-mentioned meta-analyses have reported significantly increased risk of male genital malformations in sons of women occupationally exposed to pesticides (Gaspari 2011), and of cryptorchidism (Gabel 2011), and no increased risk for hypospadias (Rocheleau 2011).

Carbamates

Toxicology

Carbamates are rapidly metabolized by mammals and inactivate acetylcholinesterase by carbamylating the enzyme. *Bendiocarb* (*Ficam*) is a derivative of *carbamic acid*. *Benomyl* (*carbendazim*) is a benzimidazole carbamate that is widely used as a fungicide in agriculture and home gardening, and as an antihelminthic in veterinary medicine (IPCS 1993). Benomyl acts as a mitotic poison by altering tubulin binding and microtubule formation. This has been proposed as a possible mechanism of action for the developmental abnormalities seen in animal studies with high concentrations.

In 1993, small clusters of births of children with eye defects (anophthalmia or microphthalmia), allegedly related to garden and agricultural use of benomyl, were reported in the UK. Investigations were set up (Dolk 1993, Gilbert 1993); no evidence for geographic clustering was found in England among 444 cases of anophthalmia or microphthalmia found in the National Registry of Birth Defects data, although a higher prevalence of anophthalmia or microphthalmia was found in rural compared with urban areas (Dolk 1998a). Evaluation of data from several other national registries showed no secular changes in the frequency of anophthalmia or microphthalmia that would support an association with benomyl exposure (Bianchi 1994, Castilla 1994, Kristensen 1994, Spagnolo 1994, Gilbert 1993). Furthermore, the epidemiological evidence suggested that the background incidence of anophthalmia or microphthalmia originally used for comparison in the English clusters had limitations because of substantial underascertainment (Busby 1998, Källén 1996). A relatively small Italian study of 63 children with anophthalmia or microphthalmia showed no association with parental (either maternal, paternal or both) occupation in agriculture (Spagnolo 1994).

Recommendation. Exposure to carbamate pesticides should be avoided in pregnancy wherever possible. When here has been significant exposure, this is not always an indication for termination of pregnancy. Even though a large risk from the carbamate pesticides is unlikely, a small risk cannot be excluded. If the mother has had symptoms of toxicity and/or continuous exposure, she may be offered additional prenatal diagnostic measures such as a detailed fetal ultrasound.

Pregnancy

2.23 Occupational, industrial and environmental agents

▶ Organochlorines

Toxicology

Organochlorine pesticides, such as *dichlorodiphenyltrichlorethane* (DDT), *hexachlorobenzene* (HCB), *dieldrin*, and α- *and* β-*hexachlorocyclohexane* (α- and β-HCH), were removed from the market several years ago because of their long persistence in nature with resulting accumulation in the human food chain, including high levels in body fat and mother's milk (see Chapter 4.18). *Lindane* (γ-BHC) has also been banned for agricultural use in recent years, but medical uses for the topical treatment of lice and scabies continue (see Chapter 2.17). Despite bans on use, organochlorine pesticides and their breakdown products have persisted in the environment, including the food chain, resulting in widespread human exposure, albeit a declining exposure.

Data from an Australian cross-sectional study (Khanjani 2006) of organochlorines in breast milk indicated that there was no association between low birth weight/small-for-gestational-age babies, and DDT or its main breakdown product, DDE (*dichlorodiphenyldichloroethylene*). Studies in India have reported significant associations between blood lindane levels and recurrent miscarriage or intrauterine growth restriction (Pathak 2010, 2011). Others have reported no association between maternal serum levels of organochlorine pesticides (DDT, DDE, HCB) and birth size or birth weight (Sagiv 2007, Fenster 2006).

For details of another group of persistent organochlorine compounds, the *polychlorinated biphenyls* (PCB), see Section 2.23.6 and Chapter 4.18.

Recommendation. Exposure to organochlorine pesticides should be avoided in pregnancy wherever possible. When there has been exposure, this is not an indication for termination of pregnancy. Even though a large risk from organochlorine pesticides is unlikely, a small risk cannot be excluded. If the mother has had symptoms of toxicity and/or continuous exposure, she may be offered additional prenatal diagnostic measures such as a detailed fetal ultrasound. For therapeutic lindane administration, see Chapter 2.17.

▶ Organophosphates

Toxicology

Organophosphorus pesticides (OPs), such as *chlorpyrifos, carbophenothion, endothion, malathion*, and *triamiphos*, exert their toxic effects by long-lasting inhibition of cholinesterases at many sites in the body. A number of OPs have been removed from the market in recent years due to their toxicity at low doses.

There are limited data available on the effects of OPs during human pregnancy. Some early, limited reports linked exposure to OPs with birth defects in humans. However, none of these implicated specific OPs (overview in Schardein 2000, Gordon 1981).

No studies on the possible reproductive toxicity of occupational exposure to malathion were found, but there are two very large cohort studies involving agricultural use. There were no significant increases in the incidence of congenital anomalies in infants born to women who lived in areas where aerial malathion spraying had occurred (Thomas 1992, Grether 1987).

Chlorpyrifos is an insecticide that has been permitted for residential use indoors in the past, and is still used in agriculture, and has some public health uses. In a rigorous, comprehensive review of the strength of the evidence on prenatal exposure to chlorpyrifos and birth weight, birth length and head circumference, eight epidemiological reports on four different cohorts were identified (Mink 2012). No consistent effects were found across the four cohorts and the authors concluded that these studies did not support a causal association between prenatal chlorpyrifos exposure and impaired fetal growth.

OPs in general, and chlorpyrifos in particular, have also been highlighted as possible causes of adverse effects on neurodevelopment. Increasing levels of maternal urinary OP metabolites during pregnancy were associated with negative effects on cognitive development, particularly perceptual reasoning, in city children (Engel 2011) and with IQ deficits in children of farmworkers (Bouchard 2011). Maternal environmental exposure to chlorpyrifos, measured in umbilical cord blood at birth, was associated with delays in psychomotor and mental development, IQ deficits, and changes in brain morphology (e.g. cortical thinning) in a cohort of inner city children assessed between 3 and 11 years of age (Rauh 2006, 2011, 2012). The influence of chlorpyrifos was independent of the contribution of neighbourhood characteristics to adverse neurobehavioral development (Lovasi 2011). However, a review of four epidemiological studies on neurobehavioral outcomes from three cohorts (including that of Rauh 2006) concluded that they did not support a causal association between prenatal chlorpyrifos exposure and adverse neurobehavioral outcomes in infants or young children up to 36 months of age (Li 2012). See also Chapter 2.22.

> **Recommendation.** Exposure to organophosphorus pesticides should be avoided in pregnancy wherever possible. When there has been significant exposure, this is not an indication for the termination of pregnancy. However, if the mother has had symptoms of toxicity and/or continuous exposure, or reduced blood cholinesterase activity, she may be offered additional prenatal diagnostic measures, e.g. a detailed fetal ultrasound. Severe poisoning, especially if associated with features of cholinesterase inhibition, requires urgent medical attention.

▶ Pyrethrin (pyrethrum, pyrethroids)

Toxicology

Pyrethrins (*cypermethrin, deltamethrin, permethrin, tetramethrin*) are a group of synthetic analogs of the natural substance *pyrethrum*, which comes from dried chrysanthemum flowers. The pyrethrins are widely used as both domestic and agricultural insecticidal sprays and dusting powders. They have also been used in topical preparations for the treatment of pediculosis (see Chapter 2.17, and overview in Schardein 2000). Low toxicity for human subjects has been reported following pyrethroid exposure.

The National Teratology Information Service in the UK obtained follow-up data (unpublished) on the outcomes of pregnancy in 48 women exposed to this group of pesticides during pregnancy (35 permethrin, 5 deltamethrin, 4 cypermethrin and 4 tetramethrin). There were 41 normal babies, two spontaneous abortions (no post-mortem data available), and five children with anomalies (mild talipes, unilateral inguinal hernia, an abnormal right little toe, bilateral talipes,

Pregnancy

2.23 Occupational, industrial and environmental agents

a heart murmur). No cause-effect relationship with the pyrethroid exposure could be established in any of these infants. A teratogen information program in Australia (Kennedy 2005) published about the safety of permethrin exposure. The data on 113 pregnancies where the mothers had used 1% creme permethrin in the treatment of lice some time during pregnancy indicated that the use of such products was relatively safe. In summary, there are few data on the effects of the pyrethroids in human pregnancy and none that allow any firm conclusions to be drawn.

> **Recommendation.** Exposure to pyrethrins should be minimized in pregnancy. When there has been significant exposure, this is not an indication for termination of pregnancy, and additional prenatal diagnostic tests are not required. Occupational or environmental exposure to pyrethrins at or below accepted safety limits is unlikely to produce a teratogenic risk, but the data are insufficient to state that there is no risk for therapeutic pyrethrum/pyrethroid administration (see Chapter 2.17).

2.23.5   Phenoxyacetic acid derivatives and polychlorinated dibenzo-dioxins

Toxicology

Agent Orange, the active constituents of which are *2,4-dichlorophe-noxyacetic acid* (2,4-D) and *2,4,5-trichlorophenoxyacetic acid* (2,4,5-T), was widely used as a defoliant in the USA, and in Southeast Asia during the Vietnam War. There has been particular concern about one of its trace impurities, *2,3,7,8-tetrachlorodibenzo-p-dioxin* (TCDD, often referred to as *dioxin*, see below), and the epidemiology of Agent Orange is considered to be a reflection of dioxin exposure. Although the dioxin content in 2,4,5-T as a herbicide was considerably reduced, its use was phased out in the 1980s. 2,4-D is still in use and may contain dioxin impurities. Dioxins are widespread, persistent, environmental pollutants that can also be generated by natural processes, such as wood burning and volcanic eruption, but also by incomplete combustion of waste, and by industrial processes.

There is conflicting evidence for an association between Agent Orange and birth defects (see overview in Schardein 2000). There are three reports that suggest that there is an association with congenital malformations. The US Environmental Protection Agency (EPA) reported an increase in the incidence of spontaneous abortions in an area sprayed with herbicides including Agent Orange, compared with that found in two control areas (EPA 1979). However, there are serious methodological limitations in this study which make interpretation of the data very difficult (Tognoni 1982). The other two studies describe the incidence of neural tube defects (Field 1979) and congenital anomalies (Hanify 1981) in agricultural areas using 2,4,5-T herbicides.

There are several reports of investigations where no association between 2,4,5-T exposure and an increased incidence of either spontaneous abortions or any specific type of congenital anomalies was observed (Smith 1982, Townsend 1982, Thomas 1980, Nelson 1979).

Concerns have been raised regarding the possibility that paternal exposure to Agent Orange/TCDD may have increased incidences of congenital anomalies among the offspring of Vietnam veterans. Although there have been several reports of children with malformations allegedly due to paternal exposure to Agent Orange during the Vietnam War, the results of three comprehensive case-control studies indicate that no causal relationship could be established, and no pattern of congenital anomalies was observed (Wolfe 1995, Donovan 1984, Erickson 1984). Compared to the numerous studies on paternal exposure of US Vietnam veterans, there is little published material on the health of the exposed population of Vietnam (and their offspring). Moreover, a biologic plausibility regarding paternal teratogenicity, for example by indicating a mutagenic effect of Agent Orange/TCDD on spermatogonia and further developing sperm, has not been demonstrated.

Chlorinated dibenzodioxins are contaminants formed during the manufacture and combustion of organochlorine compounds. In July 1976, at Seveso in Italy, there was an accident at a pesticide manufacturing plant resulting in the release of TCDD into the environment. Numerous investigations followed this incident, involving the exposure of approximately 37,000 people, some of whom developed chloracne. The majority of studies found no association between exposure to TCDD/Agent Orange and an increased incidence of congenital anomalies (see overview in Schardein 2000, Smith 1982, Townsend 1982, Thomas 1980, Nelson 1979). Only one investigation indicated that the TCDD release was associated with an increase in adverse pregnancy outcome (Commoner 1977). Detailed analysis of this report indicates serious flaws in data collection, with no assessment of the relationship between exposure and stage of fetal development (Friedman 1984). More recent studies on the Seveso population have shown significantly increased neonatal blood TSH levels in children born to mothers living in the most contaminated zones 25 years after the accident (Baccarelli 2008), and increases in infertility and in time-to-pregnancy related to individual serum TCDD levels in women (Eskenazi 2010). In men, impaired semen quality in breast-fed sons of mothers exposed to TCDD during pregnancy and lactation (Mocarelli 2011), reduced sperm quality in men exposed as infants, but increased sperm quality in men exposed during puberty at the time of the accident, with reduced estradiol and increased FSH in both groups, have been reported (Mocarelli 2008).

As a result of widespread environmental pollution, including from natural sources, dioxins are present as low-level contaminants in foods, particularly fatty foods and most human exposure comes from the diet. There is no definitive information about the effects of background exposures, but from the human data on Agent Orange and other industrial/accidental exposures, background exposures are not expected to have adverse effects on pregnancy. Higher levels of contamination of foods have occurred from incidents in which contaminated feed has been given to food-producing animals.

Recommendation. Normal background exposure to dioxins via the diet is not expected to have adverse effects on pregnancy. Exposure to highly contaminated food or other sources of TCDD should be avoided in pregnancy. If exposure to high amounts has occurred this is not an indication for termination of pregnancy. It has to be decided case-by-case whether additional diagnostic measures should be undertaken.

Pregnancy

2.23 Occupational, industrial and environmental agents

2.23.6   Polychlorinated biphenyls

Toxicology

Polychlorinated biphenyls (PCBs) are man-made chemicals that have been banned for industrial use for some years, but they remain widespread, persistent, environmental pollutants due to their many former industrial uses, including in electrical transformers, capacitors and motors. Some have dioxin-like toxicological properties. Non-dioxin-like PCBs are less toxic. Like dioxins, PCBs accumulate in the food chain and the major route for exposure to PCBs for most of the population is via the diet. The literature on PCBs and pregnancy outcomes is extensive. PCBs are ubiquitous and found in humans. A recent study of the human placenta from multiple regions in the US demonstrated that PCBs levels were decreasing with an estimated half-life of 5 years (Nanes 2014).

An industrial accident in Japan in 1968 resulted in contamination of rice oil with high levels of PCBs and polychlorinated dibenzofurans, producing a disease known as "Yusho." It caused adverse effects on pregnancies, including stillbirth, low birth weight, and staining of the skin, gingiva, and nails for the first few months of life (reviewed by Barlow 1982).

Effects reported in human studies from prenatal or prenatal and early postnatal exposure to PCBs (see reviews by EPA 2013, EFSA 2005) include reduced birth weight and shorter duration of gestation in women occupationally exposed; neurobehavioral, developmental and immune function deficits in children of mothers consuming PCB-contaminated fish; and changes in neonatal thyroid hormone levels (reduced thyroxine, raised TSH). In a review of nine cohort studies on PCB exposure from the diet (mainly via maternal fish consumption), it was concluded that prenatal exposure is associated with a specific profile of cognitive deficits related to executive function (learning and retrieval strategies, adaptation to new situations; Boucher 2009). A systematic review and meta-analysis of 20 epidemiological studies has concluded that there is no significant association between current environmental exposure to PCBs, as measured by total PCBs in maternal blood lipids, and low birth weight (El Majidi 2012). A review of 21 studies on perinatal exposure to endocrine active substances concluded that there is an association between exposure to PCBs and attention deficit hyperactivity disorder (de Cock 2012).

> **Recommendation.** Normal background exposure to PCBs via the diet is unlikely to have adverse effects on pregnancy outcomes, with the exception of cognitive development in populations consuming high amounts of fish. Exposure to food highly contaminated with PCBs should be avoided during pregnancy. Many national authorities issue advisories for fish consumption in pregnant women, based mainly on mercury contamination (see FDA 2004); such advisories are also likely to protect against possible effects of PCBs.

2.23.7   Chlorinated drinking water by-products

Toxicology

In recent years, reports have raised concerns about possible pregnancy risks from *chlorinated drinking water by-products*. Drinking water is chlorinated to kill disease-causing microorganisms. However, when chlorine combines with other substances in water, it forms *trihalomethanes* (THM), the main ones of which are chloroform and *bromodichloromethane*, and *haloacetic acids* (HAA). The concentrations of these chemicals in water supplies vary. There are conflicting data concerning the possible adverse effects of THM and HAA in drinking water; a few studies suggest that the risk of miscarriage and poor fetal growth may be increased when levels of these chemicals are high, while other studies have not found an increased risk. In a prospective study of 5,144 pregnant women, there was an association between spontaneous abortion and maternal consumption of five or more glasses per day of water that contained 75 µg/L of THM (Waller 1998). The increased risk was related to the content of bromodichloromethane. There was no such association with the chloroform content of the water.

Some, but not all reports have shown an increased risk of low birth weight in term infants whose mothers drank water in the third trimester with high THM concentrations. Significant associations have been reported at total THM concentrations >60 µg/L (Gallagher 1998), >80 µg/L (Savitz 1995), or >100 µg/L (Bove 1995), or with chloroform concentrations >10 µg/L (Kramer 1992). In a very large US population study comprising 196,000 births, reductions in birth weight of between 9 and 19 g were found in association with exposure to concentrations of bromodichloromethane >5 µg/L, chloroform >20 µg/L, and total THM >40 µg/L (Wright 2004). In a similarly large study on over 900,000 births from three different regions of the UK, there was considerable heterogeneity between regions and while the risk for low and very low birth weight was elevated in areas with total THM >60 µg/L, the increases were not statistically significant (Toledano 2005). An Australian study on over 314,000 births showed that third trimester exposure to total THM, chloroform, and bromodichloromethane were all associated with a higher risk of small-for-gestational-age babies (Summerhayes 2012). In a prospective cohort study on 4,161 pregnant women in Kaunas, Lithuania, internal exposure to four specific THMs and nine HAAs was measured in blood; only the internal dose of chloroform (the most predominant THM) was associated with a significant reduction in birth weight (Grazuleviciene 2011). In a study in Arizona, USA, that included over 48,000 births, an association was found between reduced birth weight and exposure to the HAAs *dibromoacetic acid* and *dichloroacetic acid* in late gestation, but no association with other HAAs or THMs (Hinckley 2005).

Some have reported weak associations between elevated THM exposure through drinking water and increases in the length of gestation, the risk or preterm delivery (Wright 2004) and stillbirth (Toledano 2005, Dodds 1999). A systematic review yielding 37 epidemiological studies on total THM exposure and birth outcomes, of which 15 were suitable for meta-analysis, concluded that there was some evidence for an association with small-for-gestational-age babies, but little or no evidence for associations with low birth weight, term low birth weight, or preterm delivery (Grellier 2010).

In a case-control study of 1,039 infants with congenital anomalies, no association with maternal consumption of chlorinated drinking water during pregnancy was found (Aschengrau 1993). In contrast, data from an ecological study found an association between congenital abnormalities and maternal residence in an area in which the water supply contained >80 µg/L of trihalomethanes (Bove 1995). A significant increase in neural tube defects, but not in other birth defects, was reported in women exposed to bromodichloromethane at concentrations above 20 µg/L, but there were no significant associations with chloroform exposure (Dodds 2001). However, the data sets in all the above studies were small.

> **Recommendation.** The data on chlorinated drinking water by-products and pregnancy outcomes do not allow firm conclusions to be reached, but low exposure does not seem to carry risks. In areas where drinking water is known to contain higher levels of chlorinated drinking water by-products, pregnant women who are concerned may choose to drink bottled water.

2.23.8   Metals

▶ **Arsenic (see also Chapter 2.22)**

Toxicology

Arsenic (As) is an element. Some commonly encountered inorganic arsenic salts include the trivalent *sodium arsenite* and the pentavalent *sodium arsenate*. Arsenic is a by-product of smelting, and a contaminant in hazardous waste sites. It also occurs naturally in certain types of rock – e.g. granite – resulting in substantially elevated levels of arsenic in aquifers used for drinking water; it is a particular problem for unfiltered well water. *Arsine* (AsH_3) is an arsenical that is used as a gas in manufacturing semiconductors. *Monomethylarsonic acid* is present in some herbicides but its use is now very restricted due to environmental concerns.

Both inorganic arsenic salts and organic arsenicals cross the human placenta and have been shown to accumulate in the placenta and the fetus. Trivalent arsenite demonstrates enhanced cytotoxicity compared with the pentavalent arsenate.

Occupational and environmental exposure to arsenic has been associated with adverse effects on pregnancy. Nordstrom (1978) studied spontaneous abortions, birth weight of offspring, and congenital defects in Swedish workers in and around a smelter. Significant increases in malformation rates in the fetuses and newborns of the female workers, as compared to other women living in the region, were found. Birth weights were reduced, and spontaneous abortions increased.

Some epidemiological studies and reviews on inorganic arsenic in drinking water have reported increased risks of spontaneous abortion, stillbirth, low birth weight, infant death, impaired neurodevelopment, reduced thymic function, and increased lower respiratory tract infections in infancy, but the data are inconsistent (Bellinger 2013, Ahmed 2012, Rahman 2011, Myers 2010, Hamdani 2010, Bloom 2010, Vahter 2009, Smith 2009, Cherry 2008, Yang 2003, Hopenhayn 2003). Adverse effects have been associated with arsenic concentrations in drinking water above 50 μg/L, such as that found in Bangladesh. Increased levels of arsenic in soil have been associated with an increase in malformation rates (Wu 2011) and neurodevelopmental problems in offspring (Liu 2010, McDermott 2012). Raised maternal blood arsenic levels at birth were associated with reductions in birth weight, height and chest circumference of the newborn (Guan 2012).

> **Recommendation.** There is growing evidence that arsenic can increase the incidence of pregnancy loss and reduced fetal growth, and possibly other adverse outcomes for the offspring. If arsenic is a known or potential contaminant of soil or water (especially private wells), both the water/soil and blood/urine levels should be monitored. Eliminating exposure is the recommended intervention (e.g. using filtered water or bottled water in cases of water contamination), and following the pregnancy closely to monitor fetal growth and development.

▶ Cadmium

Toxicology

Cadmium is widely distributed in industrialized countries. Besides occupational exposure, some of the most common sources of exposure are from tobacco smoke, old and poorly coated cookware, and from ingestion of foods such as shellfish, kidney and rice. For example, using an old silver-plated pitcher for an acidic drink like lemonade can lead to acute gastritis (Miller 2004), while 2–4 µg of cadmium per day can be absorbed from inhalation by a one-pack-a-day smoker.

Cadmium accumulates in the kidney. Cadmium levels are significantly increased in placentas of women who smoke during pregnancy (Eisenmann 1996). In the past, most toxicologists have considered cadmium to be initially a renal toxicant. However, evidence in both animal and human *in vitro* and *in utero* studies have demonstrated that the placenta is more sensitive to the toxic effects of cadmium than is the kidney (Miller 2004, Wier 1990); for example, by interfering with zinc transfer to the fetus (Kippler 2010), and with placental steroid production (Stasenko 2010). Cadmium is considered to be an endocrine disrupter (Iavacoli 2009).

Cadmium may reduce the likelihood of getting pregnant. Fecundability was reduced in women with increased blood cadmium levels (Buck Louis 2012), and in women undergoing *in vitro* fertilization who had increased urinary cadmium levels (Bloom 2012).

Occupational exposure is usually found in welders, and workers in foundries and cadmium battery factories. Two case reports identified cadmium intoxication in women who taught welding. They lost multiple pregnancies, could not carry a child beyond the second trimester and showed evidence of placental damage (Eisenmann 1996).

Studies from Bangladesh, Taiwan, Japan and China have shown reductions in birth weight and head circumference in children born to mothers with raised blood or urinary cadmium levels, which can persist to 3 years of age, and reductions in IQ at 4.5 years (Kippler 2012, Lin 2011, Shirai 2010, Tian 2009, Nishijo 2004).

> **Recommendation.** Current limited human studies indicate the potential for adverse effects on fertility, maintenance of pregnancy and fetal growth, but not malformations. If a pregnant woman is demonstrating signs of renal toxicity – increased β-microglobulins and cadmium in their urine – then very close monitoring of the pregnancy, with determination of the source of cadmium to eliminate any further exposure, is required to reduce risk of pregnancy loss.

▶ Lead

Toxicology

Lead toxicity has been recognized for over 1,000 years. Poisoning by organic lead (*tetraethyl lead*) is associated primarily with CNS toxicity which is distinguishable from that produced by inorganic lead. The overall toxicity of the organic form would seem to be due to the molecular species as a whole, rather than the metallic constituent alone.

Women who live in older homes may be exposed to higher levels of lead due to deteriorating lead-based paint. If paint needs to be removed (preferably by experts) from a home, pregnant women and children

Pregnancy

2.23 Occupational, industrial and environmental agents

should remain out of the way. Lead crystal glassware and some ceramic dishes may contain lead, and pregnant women and children should avoid frequent use of these items. Other unexpected sources of lead in the home may include such items as the wicks of scented candles and the plastic (polyvinylchloride) grips on some hand tools. Jobs that are related to lead, and thus contamination with lead, include painters, smelters, and workers in auto repair shops, battery manufacturing plants, and certain types of construction (Sallmén 1992).

Of particular concern regarding lead exposure are specialty food products produced in the home – for example, ethnic foods cooked in lead pots. These foods have a sweet taste provided by the lead (NYCDH 2004). Further, women are obtaining elevated levels of lead from ayurvedic medicines produced in non-health-inspected sites and some cosmetics. Careful monitoring of all cookware and knowing the origins of prepared foods and medicines can assist in reducing lead exposure. In New York (USA), there are mandatory requirements for all pregnant women to be screened for lead at their first prenatal visit (Miller 2004). Organic lead is much more rapidly absorbed than inorganic lead salts, by all routes, and is highly lipid-soluble, rapidly passing the blood–placenta barrier from 12 weeks onwards, and the fetal blood–brain barrier (Rabinowitz 1988). There have been many unsubstantiated reports that women who worked in occupations with high lead exposure (white lead industries, potteries) had high miscarriage and stillbirth rates and gave birth to stunted, abnormal babies, but there are no epidemiological studies or case reports specifically on organic lead. It was also a commonly held belief that lead was an abortifacient.

As lead is a cumulative poison and is ubiquitously distributed in the environment, it is potentially a reproductive hazard for men and women (ACOG 2012, Schardein 2000, Miller 1993, Manton 1992, Bornschein 1985, Barlow 1982, Scanlon 1975). There is no conclusive evidence to suggest that maternal exposure to lead is associated with an increased risk of major structural malformations. There have, however, been unconfirmed indications that there may be an increased risk of minor anomalies in women with high blood lead levels, which in some instances seemed to be a dose-related effect (Schardein 2000, Miller 1993, Rabinowitz 1988, Bornschein 1985, Needleman 1984, Barlow 1982, Scanlon 1975).

Other forms of fetal lead toxicity have been reported. Some studies have shown a significant association between chronic exposure to high concentrations of lead and premature delivery, decreased gestational maturity, low birth weight, and reduced postnatal growth (Kaul 2002). Exposure to high concentrations of lead in the third trimester has been associated with an increased risk of macrocephaly.

There are a number of case reports indicating neurological deficits and poor IQ scores in the offspring of lead-exposed mothers, even with a moderate increase of maternal blood lead level (<30 µg/dL) (see overviews in Schardein 2000, Miller 1993, Bellinger 1991, 1992, Davis 1990, Barlow 1982). However, other workers have reported no adverse effects of maternal lead on language development in children studied from birth to 3-years-old (Dietrich 1991, Ernhart 1989). Two other studies have found no association between prenatal lead exposure and intelligence at 4 years of age (Dietrich 1993, Davis 1990). Iron deficiency anemia often occurs in populations with high lead exposure, and has also been associated with lower scores on mental and psychomotor indices (McCann 2007). One study has reported an association between prenatal lead exposure (maternal blood lead >15 µg/dL) and the development of schizophrenia later in life (Opler 2008). A recent meta-analysis involving

33 studies and over 10,000 children demonstrated a significant association between lead exposure and attention deficit hyperactivity disorder (ADHD) symptoms (Goodlad 2013).

The results of two large prospective studies in the smelter town Port Pirie (Australia) and in Boston showed no significant association between prenatal lead exposure and child intelligence during the preschool period (Bellinger 1991, McMichael 1988). A third prospective study of lead exposure and early postnatal development was performed in two groups of pregnant women, one group from a smelter town and the other group from a non-lead-exposed town in Yugoslavia (Wasserman 1994). The children were followed until they were 4 years old. The authors concluded that continuing lead exposure is associated with cumulative losses in cognitive function, particularly those involving perceptual-motor integration, during the preschool years. Collectively, the findings of these three prospective studies indicate that the most sensitive period for exposure to lead occurs from the age of 18 months onwards.

Previously, maternal blood lead concentrations within the normal range (i.e. <10 µg/dL) were not thought to be associated with an increased risk of fetal toxicity. However, US Centers for Disease Control have refined their consideration of exposures with a statement for lead exposure in children, and there is now a reference level of 5 µg/dL (CDC 2014). Questions continue to be raised for values >5 µg/dL. In adults, blood lead concentrations regarded as toxic and requiring chelation therapy are in the range of >60 µg/dL; however, symptoms in the mother should be the deciding factor for chelation. In pregnant women, blood lead concentrations >30 µg/dL would be cause for concern. At concentrations which cause severe maternal toxicity (>100 µg/dL), an increased risk of fetal loss may occur. In such circumstances, the uterine muscles relax and the fetus is expelled from the uterus. It is not known whether this is due entirely to the high concentrations of lead *per se*, or whether it is secondary to the maternal toxicity (ACOG 2012, see overview in Schardein 2000, Rabinowitz 1988, Barlow 1982, Scanlon 1975). In children with brain dysfunction following *in utero* exposure to lead, the blood concentrations of lead are usually >35 µg/dL. Lead concentrations of >40 µg/dL in children are regarded as toxic, and require chelation therapy; however, for women during pregnancy, one must monitor mother's symptoms and be cautious concerning chelation in mothers for fear of exacerbating levels in the fetus due to additional lead being released from the maternal skeleton.

If mothers are found to have elevated blood lead levels, the source should be eliminated. The mothers should be followed monthly to determine if there is a falling blood lead level consistent with the half-life of approximately 30 days. If levels are highly elevated, calcium supplementation 1–2 gm per day should be considered, especially in the third trimester to reduce previously accumulated lead from leaching from the bone into the fetus.

Recommendation. Low exposure levels have been shown to influence mental development. A water supply running through lead pipes with the usual water pH value is not a major concern; however, standing water in lead-sealed containers can lead to significant exposure. Accidental exposure is not an indication for termination of pregnancy. However, all (occupational, environmental, home, medicines, foods) exposure to lead should be avoided, wherever possible. If there is any known exposure to lead, women who are planning a pregnancy or currently pregnant should, as a minimum, have their blood lead level checked. A factor that influences judgment regarding

Pregnancy

2.23 Occupational, industrial and environmental agents

lead exposure is whether the lead exposure is acute or chronic. If any time in her life, a mother was lead intoxicated, her blood levels of lead should also be monitored during the third trimester. If significant (continuous) exposure has occurred before or during pregnancy, maternal blood lead concentrations should be determined. Measuring bone lead with K-X-ray fluorescence (K-XRF) can provide a history of chronic exposure (Miller 2006). Tibia and patellar bone lead provides the index for chronic versus acute exposure to lead. This assessment can be helpful in predicting whether large amounts of lead will be mobilized from the bone as the pregnancy continues and a supplementation of calcium should be considered.

▶ Mercury

Toxicology

Mercury enters the environment from natural and man-made sources (such as coal-burning, and other industrial pollution). There are two main types of mercury: inorganic (metallic mercury, used in thermometers, sphygmomanometers and dental amalgam), and organic mercury (e.g. *methylmercury, ethylmercury, phenylmercuric acetate*), which can be formed from inorganic mercury by bacterial conversion. Ethylmercury is used as an antifungal agent in seed dressings. Methylmercury (MeHg) is accumulated in the fatty tissues of fish. While trace amounts of MeHg are present in many types of fish, it is most concentrated in large fish which eat other fish, such as bonito (tuna), swordfish, and shark; these fish may contain more than 1 mg/kg of mercury (EFSA 2012). There is an extensive amount of literature on the reproductive toxicology of mercury both in humans and animals (Clarkson 2006). While there are many studies showing that mercury is available to the fetus, there are conflicting data regarding whether or not the placenta concentrates mercury (Yoshida 2002, Barlow 1982). Acute inhalation of mercury vapor by pregnant women has resulted in comparable levels of mercury in maternal and neonatal blood samples (Lien 1983). According to a recent review of a large number of studies published since 2000 on European populations, average concentrations of total mercury in blood ranged from 0.2–4.85 µg/L in adults (including pregnant women); from 0.12–0.94 µg/L in children; and from 0.86–13.9 µg/L in cord blood (EFSA 2012). Blood concentrations appear to be related to fish consumption and the number of dental amalgam fillings. These ranges exclude data from the Faroe Islands where, in the past, MeHg concentrations in adults and children have been high due to consumption of whale meat.

The effects on pre- and postnatal development of exposure to high amounts of MeHg from maternal consumption of contaminated fish have been well documented as Minamata disease, the main feature of which is CNS damage. Exposure to organic mercury from eating contaminated fish in Japan, flour made from treated grain in Iraq, or contaminated pork have all resulted in poisoning. Spontaneous abortion and stillbirth rates both increased as a result of the Japanese poisoning incidents (Itai 2004).

Concerning exposure to lower levels of MeHg from fish consumption, there is inconsistency in the evidence regarding fetal growth and neurodevelopmental effects in children after maternal normal-to-moderate fish intake (EFSA 2012, Karagas 2012, Trasande 2006, Oken 2005, Myers 2003, Grandjean 1997). A number of studies and reviews indicate the complexity of evaluations of the effects of low-level exposure to methylmercury from fish consumption on neurodevelopment (EFSA 2012, Karagas 2012, Oken 2008). They have emphasized the importance of timing of exposure, precision of exposure assessment, age of the child at assessment, specific neurobehavioral outcome, sex differences, differing approaches to dose–response modeling, and particularly confounding, such as by beneficial constituents in fish (e.g. n-3 long-chain polyunsaturated fatty acids), in determining the observed results (Stokes-Rines 2011). The current consensus is that pregnant women should receive advice on the benefits and risks of fish consumption and on which species of fish are high in MeHg (see, for example, NHS 2011, FDA 2004, 2009).

Regarding *thiomersal* (*thimerosal*) (see also Chapter 2.7), which is metabolized to ethylmercury, studies on children have found no evidence that early exposure to mercury in thiomersal has any deleterious effect on neurologic or psychological outcome up to 10 years of age (Thompson 2007, Heron 2004).

There is conflicting evidence whether or not metallic mercury causes reduced fertility, spontaneous abortions, low birth weight, or birth defects. The majority of studies report no association between occupational exposure to mercury and adverse effects on pregnancy (Hujoel 2005, Ratcliffe 1996, Rowland 1994, Matte 1993, Ericson 1989, Brodsky 1985, de Rosis 1985), but a few report some effects (Ratcliffe 1996, Rowland 1994).

Recommendation. Occupational exposure to mercury should be avoided during pregnancy. However, acute, inadvertent exposure to inorganic/metallic mercury is not necessarily grounds for termination of pregnancy, and, as a rule, no additional prenatal diagnostic tests are required.

The clinical data and experimental results of studies concerning the potential teratogenic risks associated with the inhalation of mercury vapor from dental amalgam do not warrant restriction of amalgams in pregnant women. If indicated, dental amalgam fillings may be restored during pregnancy. However, if it is available and applicable, substitute material may be preferred. Dental amalgam fillings are by no means grounds for "detoxification" with chelating agents.

Prenatal exposure to organic mercury from maternal consumption of seafood may influence mental development. Consumption of seafood known for having higher levels of mercury contamination (shark, swordfish, tilefish, whaleblubber, and, to a lesser degree, tuna) should be avoided. If chronic, significant mercury exposure has occurred before or during pregnancy, maternal blood levels should be monitored. Several national authorities have issued advice on fish consumption for pregnant women. An example is the advice issued in 2004 by the US FDA (Food and Drug Administration) and EPA (Environmental Protection Agency). They made three recommendations for women who might become pregnant, women who are pregnant, and nursing mothers (see also Chapter 4.18) so they can gain the benefits of eating fish while reducing exposure to the harmful effects of mercury:

1. Do not consume fish that contain high levels of mercury, e.g. shark, swordfish, king mackerel or tilefish.
2. Consume up to 12 ounces (2 average meals) a week of a variety of fish and shellfish that are lower in mercury, e.g. shrimp, canned light tuna, salmon, pollock and catfish. Albacore ("white") tuna has more mercury than canned light tuna. Consume no more than 6 ounces (one average meal) of albacore tuna per week.

3. Check local advisories about the safety of fish caught by family and friends in your local lakes, rivers, and coastal areas. If no advice is available, eat up to 6 ounces (one average meal) per week of fish you catch from local waters, but don't consume any other fish during that week.

2.23.9   Hazardous waste landfill sites and waste incinerators

Toxicology

Waste disposal sites may be a potential hazard to health. There has been a series of publications to assess reproductive disorders and birth defects in communities near hazardous chemical sites (Boyle 1997, Goldman 1997, Holmes 1997, Kimmel 1997, Savitz 1997, Scialli 1997, Wyrobek 1997). These studies investigated structural anomalies, genetic changes, mutagenesis, stillbirth and infant death, functional deficits, and growth retardation. Menstrual dysfunction, infertility, pregnancy loss, pregnancy complications, and effects on lactation were also investigated (Scialli 1997). Problems involved in epidemiological studies of congenital anomalies incorporating measurements of both environmental and genetic factors have also been reviewed (Shaw 1997, Kipen 1996). Such studies are difficult to perform and interpret because of the numerous confounding factors.

A multicenter (21) case-control study (EUROHAZCON) on the risks of congenital anomalies associated with residential living within a 7 km radius of hazardous landfill sites in Europe indicated that residents living within 3 km of a landfill site were at a significantly increased risk of having a child with congenital anomalies and the risk deceased considerably with distance from the sites (Dolk 1998b).

Adverse birth outcomes were studied in populations living within 2 km of 9,565 landfill sites in Great Britain (Elliott 2001). Over 8.2 million live births, nearly 125,000 congenital anomalies (including terminations of pregnancy) and more than 40,000 stillbirths were involved. It concluded that there was a small excess of congenital anomalies and low and very low birth weight in populations living near landfill sites, without causal mechanisms available to explain the findings. Alternative explanations included (*inter alia*) data artefacts and residual confounding. Hence, for primary prevention interventions there are no indications. In two further studies by the same group, birth outcomes in populations living within 2 km of 61 special waste landfill sites in Scotland showed no statistically significant excess risks for all congenital anomalies, specific anomalies, stillbirths or low birth weight (Morris 2003), nor for the risk of giving birth to a child with Down syndrome in association with living within 2 km of 6,289 landfill sites in England and Wales (Jarup 2007).

The debate on possible risks from living near landfill sites was enriched by Vrijheid (2002), who suggested an increase in risk of chromosomal anomalies similar to that found for non-chromosomal anomalies from 245 cases of chromosomal anomalies whose mothers lived within 0–3 km of 23 hazardous landfill sites in Europe. Pregnancy outcomes in women living near municipal waste incinerators have also been studied with a focus on exposure to dioxins (see also Section 2.23.5), although emissions from incinerators may include other hazardous substances. Vinceti (2008, 2009) reported no increase in miscarriages or birth defects in women residing close to a municipal solid waste incinerator in relation to exposure to dioxins. Cordier (2010) reported a significant increase in the risk of urinary tract defects in association with increased exposure to dioxins in births to women living near 21 waste incinerators.

> **Recommendation.** None of the studies on hazardous waste landfill sites or emissions from municipal waste incinerators have shown conclusive or causally related links to adverse outcomes of pregnancy. Therefore, no advice can be given other than the obvious: no dwellings should be built on or close to a (hazardous) landfill site.

2.23.10   Radiation associated with the nuclear industry

Adverse effects

Information on *ionizing radiation* associated with the nuclear industry comes from nuclear accidents and occupational exposure. Although background ionizing radiation is a known mutagen, few studies have examined transgenerational effects in humans. No information is available concerning pregnancy and increased exposure to environmental ionizing radiation associated with travel flights or exposure to indoor radon (e.g. in houses built on rock/soil emitting radon gas).

Nuclear accidents

Chernobyl, Ukraine, was the site in 1986 of one of the worst accidents ever to have occurred at a nuclear plant. Considerable quantities of radioactivity were released into the atmosphere, much of which was dispersed over the former Soviet Union and Western and Northern Europe. The radioactivity from the accident was washed from the skies and entered the food chain, notably in areas of high rainfall. Subsequent to the accident, people in the area around Chernobyl were evacuated; they have not been allowed to return.

Twenty-five years after the accident, a clear increase in the risk of thyroid cancer has been confirmed for those who were children or adolescents at the time of the accident (Cardis 2011), and this is now regarded as the main adverse health consequence for those living in the region of the accident. A possible increase in the risk of thyroid cancer has been reported for fetuses exposed via the mother at the time, or 2 months after the accident (Hatch 2009). There is no indication that the incidence of other types of cancer increased following prenatal exposure.

There are few studies on the possible effects of the accident on congenital malformation rates. One study indicates high malformation rates in an area of the Ukraine that was subject to chronic low-dose radiation following the accident (Wertelecki 2010). There is limited evidence for an increase in Trisomy 21 (Down syndrome) in 1987/88 in several north European countries that experienced increases in radiation fallout following the Chernobyl accident (Sperling 2012).

In March 2011, following an earthquake and a tsunami, three nuclear reactors at Fukushima, Japan, experienced meltdown. This is the most serious nuclear disaster since Chernobyl. As yet, no adverse health effects as a result of radiation exposure have been reported for the population now evacuated from the area, or living around the evacuation area, but the possibility of thyroid cancer in children is a concern and the population is being closely monitored (UNSCEAR 2013).

Pregnancy

2.23 Occupational, industrial and environmental agents

UK nuclear facilities

A study on the male workforce at the Sellafield nuclear reprocessing plant in Cumbria in the UK, which was considered to be the most highly exposed workforce in Western Europe and North America, investigated whether there was any association between risk of stillbirth and paternal exposure to ionizing radiation (Parker 1999). Data from birth registration documents for all singleton live births (248,097) and stillbirths (3,715) in Cumbria between 1950 and 1989 were analyzed. Within this cohort, the 9,078 live births and 130 stillbirths to partners of male radiation workers employed at Sellafield were identified. A significant positive association was found between the risk of a baby being stillborn and the father's total exposure to external ionizing radiation before conception. There was a higher risk for stillbirths with congenital anomalies (nine stillbirths with neural tube defects). In contrast, another study of similarly exposed workforces from across the UK nuclear industry (UK Atomic Energy Authority, Atomic Weapons Establishment, British Nuclear Fuels) showed no increase in fetal death and congenital malformations in babies born to nuclear industry employees (Doyle 2000). This study analyzed a total of 23,676 singleton pregnancies reported by male workers and 3,585 pregnancies by women workers. Among the pregnancies in female workers, the risk of early miscarriage before 13 weeks' gestation was higher if the mother had been monitored before conception, but this finding was not dose-related, and was based on a small number of cases, of which 13 of 29 were exposed. The risk of any major malformation or of specific groups of malformations was not associated with maternal monitoring, the dose received during pregnancy, or the dose received before conception. There was no evidence of a link between exposure to low-level ionizing radiation before conception and an increased risk of adverse reproductive outcome in men working in the nuclear industry. The findings relating maternal preconceptual monitoring to increased risk of fetal death remain equivocal, and require ongoing investigation (Doyle 2000). In a second study, the hypothesis linking exposure to low-level ionizing radiation among men with primary infertility was not supported (Doyle 2001).

In a critique of the first study, it was pointed out that 12% of the pregnancies reported by male radiation workers and 15% reported by female workers ended in fetal death. However, the female workers were on average 10 years younger than the male workers at the time of the survey. Moreover, pregnancies reported by female workers were more recent than those reported by the men. Both of these factors contribute to a much lower expected fetal death rate in female workers than in male workers, especially for late events such as stillbirths (Parker 2001).

Recommendation. There is no clear evidence of adverse effects on fertility or pregnancy outcomes from working in the nuclear industry. The main health effects following nuclear accidents have been on the thyroid, with children and adolescents particularly susceptible to thyroid cancer, illustrating the importance of immediate potassium iodide prophylaxis following such accidents. If a new nuclear accident happens exposing a population to low-level radiation, data from UNSCEAR, the United Nations study group evaluating the measures and decisions taken after the Chernobyl and Fukushima accidents, may help to make the right decisions – including, for example, restricting food intake and distribution from an exposed area.

2.23.11   Cell/mobile phones

Adverse effects

Cell/mobile phones are low-power radio devices that transmit and receive radio-frequency (RF) radiation in the microwave range of 900–1,800 MHz through an antenna in the phone (Maier 2000). Analog systems have been replaced by digital models.

Concerns have been expressed that microwaves might induce or promote cancer, along with symptoms such as sleep disturbance, memory problems, headaches, nausea, and dizziness. Changes in the permeability of the blood–brain barrier, blood pressure, and electroencephalographic activity have also been reported. There is uncertainty about the validity of many of these findings and the underlying mechanism of action. A series of studies on the effects of pre- and postnatal exposure to cell phones has been published using the Danish National Birth Cohort which recruited pregnant women between 1996–2002 (Divan 2008, 2011, 2012). Assessments were based on questionnaires filled in by the mothers. When children were examined at the ages of 6 and 18 months for developmental milestone delays, less than 5% of the children had cognitive/language or motor delays and no significant association or dose-response relationship with prenatal cell phone use was observed. In a subset of 13,000 children examined at the age of 7 years, behavioral difficulties such as emotional and hyperactivity problems at school entry age were associated with pre-natal cell phone exposure. In a different subset of over 28,000 children examined 2 years later, also at 7 years of age, and with more control for possible confounders, the association between behavioral problems and cell phone use was confirmed. The highest odds ratio of 1.5 (95% CI 1.4–1.7) for behavioral problems was for children who had both pre- and postnatal exposure to cell phones, compared with children who had neither exposure. The authors comment that the association may be due to uncontrolled confounding.

On the other hand, a birth cohort study in the Netherlands examined the association between behavioral problems in children aged 5 years, as reported by teachers and mothers, and the use of cell phones and cordless phones by the mothers during pregnancy (Guxens 2013). A total of 2,618 children were studied, and there was no significant or dose-related association between behavioral problems and cell or cordless phone use by the mothers.

> **Recommendation.** As there is some evidence from the data available to indicate that the children of women who use cell/mobile phones during pregnancy may have an increased risk of behavioral problems, women should be advised to limit where possible their use of mobile phones during pregnancy.

2.23.12   Other sources of electromagnetic radiation

Adverse effects

Proximity to electric current involves exposure to weak electromagnetic fields (EMF). Very low-frequency magnetic fields are generated by a large number of electrical appliances in the home and office (Breysse 1994). EMF from magnetic resonance imaging is discussed elsewhere (see Chapter 2.20).

Pregnancy

2.23 Occupational, industrial and environmental agents

One of the highest exposure sources, both in homes and factories, is the sewing machine (Sobel 1994). There is a report of a weak association between childhood diagnosis of acute lymphoblastic leukemia and maternal work at home during pregnancy (Infante-Rivard 1995). Most of the pregnant women were thought to have used electric sewing machines, and thus exposed the fetus to electromagnetic fields. Childhood exposure to sewing machines or other factors in the home was also mentioned.

In a survey of 372 married couples in which the man worked at one of two Swedish power companies between 1953 and 1979, an increase in the incidence of congenital anomalies was found, but no pattern of anomalies (Nordstrom 1983). The mechanism by which these anomalies might have been transmitted via paternal exposure is not clear. However, in this study the finding could not be explained by confounding or reporting biases (Coleman 1988).

A seasonally related increase in spontaneous pregnancy loss was reported in users of electric blankets and heated waterbeds (Wertheimer 1986). The authors concluded that either thermal or electromagnetic field effects might be involved. Similar results were reported by the same authors following exposure to ceiling heating coils (Wertheimer 1989). A small increase in risk of pregnancy loss associated with electric blanket use at the time of conception and in early pregnancy has also been reported (Belanger 1998). However, Lee (2000) found no association between electric blanket use and spontaneous abortions. A brief report on pregnant women with a history of subfertility implied that there was an association between electric blanket use and congenital urinary tract anomalies (Li 1995). However, an increased risk of congenital anomalies or fetal loss associated with electric bed heating was not confirmed by the results of an epidemiological study in New York State (Jansson 1993, Dlugosz 1992), nor with neural tube defects or orofacial clefts (Shaw 1999). Similarly, a comprehensive prospective study of 2,967 pregnant women that included some use of personal monitors to measure exposure to electromagnetic fields did not find a biologically significant increase in risk in relation to birth weight and fetal growth retardation associated with the use of electrically heated beds (Bracken 1995). Overall, the majority of evidence indicates that electromagnetic fields are unlikely to cause adverse effects on pregnancy in women under normal exposure conditions (Brent 1999).

Concern has been expressed about possible effects on fetal development of living in an area close to high-voltage power lines. However, the results of studies in France and Norway did not identify an excess of congenital anomalies among children whose parents lived within 500 m of a high-voltage power line (Blaasaas 2004, Robert 1993, 1996, 1999). It was emphasized that the field strength drops rapidly with distance from the line, and that few people live directly below a power line. Therefore, most of the index children were exposed to electromagnetic field levels *in utero* that were not much different from those to which the non-exposed children were subjected. In a subsequent study, no significant association with residence within 100 or 50 m of a high-voltage power line was found in a subsequent study (Robert 1996). Similarly, in an Iranian study, living near high-voltage electricity towers and cables was found to have no effects on pregnancy duration, birth weight, length, head circumference, gender or congenital malformations (Mahram 2013). No association was found with congenital malformations in an Italian study (Malagoli 2012). A possible increase in the risk of stillbirth has been reported for those living within 25 m of power transmission lines in Quebec, Canada, but there was no relation with longer distances from power lines, and no association with preterm birth, low birth weight, or small-for-gestational age babies (Auger 2011, 2012).

> **Recommendation.** As the majority of evidence indicates that electromagnetic fields are unlikely to cause adverse effects on pregnancy in women under normal exposure conditions, such exposures do not require any additional prenatal diagnostic intervention.

2.23.13   Electric shocks and lightning strikes

Adverse effects

Electric shocks during pregnancy have been reviewed by Goldman (2003). There are published data on 15 pregnant women who received electric shocks when their fetuses were between 12 and 40 weeks' gestation (Mehl 1992, Leiberman 1986, Peppier 1974). Only one mother, who had been shot with a Taser (electro-weapon), lost consciousness and sustained injuries and burns (Mehl 1992). Fetal death occurred in 11 (73%) of the pregnancies, possibly due to changes in fetal heart conduction leading to cardiac arrest. The adverse outcomes may also be due to lesions to the uteroplacental bed. Two of the surviving fetuses had oligohydramnios, a clinical sign that is also consistent with impaired cardiac function (Leiberman 1986). In cases of accidental electric shock, the most common sign of adverse fetal effects was immediate cessation of fetal movements. It is possible that there is a reporting bias with these cases, in that only those with the most serious adverse outcomes are more likely to be reported. Nevertheless, these reports do indicate that even an apparently harmless maternal electric shock may cause fetal death.

In 1997, the results were published of a small case-control study of 31 women who received electrical shocks during pregnancy, matched with control subjects (Einarson 1997). Of these women, 26 had been exposed to 110V, two to 220V, two to high voltage (from electrified fences), and one to 12 V (from a telephone wire). In the exposed group there were 28 normal infants, one infant with ventricular septal defect, and two miscarriages. In the unexposed control, there were 30 normal infants and one miscarriage. The authors reported that in this study the pathway of electric current was only likely to have passed through the uterus in three of the 31 women, in contrast with previously published case reports. Adverse effects on the fetus are considered more likely to occur when the current is reported to have passed from hand to foot, or electrical burn marks suggest such a route.

Eleven case reports of lightning strikes of pregnant women were found (Flannery 1982, Chan 1979, Guha-Ray 1979, Weinstein 1979, Rees 1965). There was a wide range of maternal symptoms reported, from no loss of consciousness to brief loss of consciousness in those in whom the electrical injury caused maternal cardiovascular collapse and uterine rupture at 6 months' gestation. Five (45%) of the exposed fetuses died.

> **Recommendation.** Any work that could expose a pregnant woman to the risk of electrical shock must be avoided during pregnancy. If an electrical shock has occurred, the fetal status should be evaluated immediately.

Pregnancy

2.23 Occupational, industrial and environmental agents

References

ACOG. Lead screening during pregnancy and lactation. Committee Opinion no. 533, American College of Obstetricians and Gynecologists. Obstet Gynecol 2012; 120: 416–20.

Ahmed S, Ahsan KB, Kippler M et al. In utero arsenic exposure is associated with impaired thymic function in newborns possibly via oxidative stress. Toxicol Sci 2012; 129: 305–14.

Ahmed P, Jaakkola JJK. Exposure to organic solvents and adverse pregnancy outcomes. Human Reprod 2007; 22: 2751–7.

Arbuckle TE, Lin Z, Mery LS. An exploratory analysis of the effect of pesticide exposure on the risk of spontaneous abortion in an Ontario farm population. Environ Health Perspect 2001; 109: 851–7.

Arbuckle TE, Sever LE. Pesticide exposures and fetal death: a review of the epidemiologic literature. Crit Rev Toxicol 1998; 28: 229–70.

Aschengrau A, Zierler S, Cohen A. Quality of community drinking water and the occurrence of late adverse pregnancy outcomes. Arch Environ Health 1993; 48: 105–13.

Attarchi MS, Ashouri M, Labbafinejad Y et al. Assessment of time to pregnancy and spontaneous abortion status following occupational exposure to organic solvents mixture. Int Arch Occup Environ Health 2012; 85: 295–303.

Auger N, Joseph D, Goneau M et al. The relationship between residential proximity to extremely low frequency power transmission lines and adverse birth outcomes. J Epidemiol Community Health 2011; 65: 83–5.

Auger N, Park AL, Yacouba S et al. Stillbirth and residential proximity to extremely low frequency power transmission lines: a retrospective cohort study. Occup Environ Med 2012; 69: 147–9.

Axelsson G, Lutz C, Rylander R. Exposure to solvents and outcome of pregnancy in university laboratory employees. Br J Ind Med 1984; 41: 305–12.

Baccarelli A, Giacomini SM, Corbetta C et al. Neonatal thyroid function in Seveso 25 years after maternal exposure to dioxin. PLoS Med 2008; 5: e161.

Bao YS, Cai S, Zhao SF et al. Birth defects in the offspring of female workers occupationally exposed to carbon disulfide in China. Teratology 1991; 43: 451–2.

Barlow SM, Sullivan FM. Reproductive Hazards of Industrial Chemicals. Academic Press, London, 1982.

Belanger K, Leaderer B, Hellenbrand K et al. Spontaneous abortion and exposure to electric blankets and heated water beds. Epidemiology 1998; 9: 36–42.

Bell BP, Franks P, Hildreth N et al. Methylene chloride exposure and birthweight in Monroe County, New York. Environ Res 1991; 55: 31–9.

Bellinger DC. Prenatal exposures to environmental chemicals and children's neurodevelopment: an update. Saf Health Work 2013; 4: 1–11.

Bellinger D, Needleman HL. Neurodevelopmental effects of low level lead exposure in children. In: Needleman HL. (ed.), Human Lead Exposure. CRC Press, Ann Arbor, MI, 1992, pp. 191–208.

Bellinger D, Sloman J, Leviton A et al. Low level lead exposure and children's cognitive function in the preschool years. Pediatrics 1991; 87: 219–27.

Bianchi F, Calabro A, Calzolari E et al. Clusters of anophthalmia. No link with benomyl in Italy or in Norway. Br Med J 1994; 308: 205.

Blaasaas KG, Tynes T, Lie RT. Risk of selected birth defects by maternal residence close to power lines during pregnancy. Occup Envon Med 2004; 61: 174–6.

Bloom MS, Fitzgerald EF, Kim K et al. Spontaneous pregnancy loss in humans and exposure to arsenic in drinking water. Int J Hyg Environ Health 2010; 213: 401–13.

Bloom MS, Fujimoto VY, Steuerwald AJ et al. Background exposure to toxic metals in women adversely influences pregnancy during in vitro fertilization (IVF). Reprod Toxicol 2012; 34: 471–81.

Bornschein RL, Rabinowitz MB (eds). The Second International Conference on Prospective Studies of Lead, Cincinnati, Ohio, April 1984. Environ Res 1985; 38: 1–210.

Bosco MG, Figa-Talamanca I, Salerno S. Health and reproductive status of female workers in dry cleaning shops. Intl Arch Occup Environ Health 1987; 59: 295–301.

Bouchard MF, Chevrier J, Harley KG et al. Prenatal exposure to organophosphate pesticides and IQ in 7-year-old children. Environ Health Perspect 2011; 119: 1189–95.

Boucher O, Muckle G, Bastien CH. Prenatal exposure to polychlorinated biphenyls: a neuropsychologic analysis. Environ Health Perspect 2009; 117: 7–16.

Bove FJ, Fulcomer MC, Klotz JB et al. Public drinking water contamination and birth outcomes. Am J Epidemiol 1995; 141: 850–62.

Bowen SE, Hannigan JH. Developmental toxicity of prenatal exposure to toluene. AAPS J 2006; 8: E419–24.

Boyle CA. Surveillance of developmental disabilities with an emphasis on special studies. Reprod Toxicol 1997; 11: 271–4.

Bracken MB, Belanger K, Hellenbrand K et al. Exposure to electromagnetic fields during pregnancy with emphasis on electrically heated beds: association with birthweight and intrauterine growth retardation. Epidemiology 1995; 6: 263–70.

Brandys RC, Brandys GM. Global occupational exposure limits for over 6,000 specific chemicals. Hinsdal: OEHCS Inc., 2008.

Brent RL. Reproductive and teratologic effects of low-frequency electromagnetic fields: a review of in vivo and in vitro studies using animal models. Teratology 1999; 59: 261–86.

Breysse P, Lees PS, McDiarmid MA et al. ELF magnetic field exposures in an office environment. Am J Ind Med 1994; 25: 177–85.

Brodsky JB, Cohen EN, Whitcher C et al. Occupational exposure to mercury in dentistry and pregnancy outcome. J Am Dent Assoc 1985; 111: 779–80.

Buck Louis GM, Sundaram R, Schisterman EF et al. Heavy metals and couple fecundity, the LIFE Study. Chemosphere 2012; 87: 1201–7.

Busby A, Dolg H, Collin R et al. Compiling a national register of babies born with anophthalmia/microphthalmia in England 1988–94. Arch Dis Child Fetal Neonatal Ed 1998; 79: F168–173.

Cai SX, Bao YS. Placental transfer secretion into mothers' milk of carbon disulfide and the effects on maternal function of female viscose rayon workers. Indust Health 1981; 19: 15–30.

Cardis E, Hatch M. The Chernobyl accident – an epidemiological perspective. Clin Oncol (R Coll Radiol) 2011; 23: 251–60.

Castilla EE. Clusters of anophthalmia. No further clues from global investigation. Br Med J 1994; 308: 206.

CDC. Fact Sheet on Lead Exposure in Children. http://www.cdc.gov/nceh/lead/ACCLPP/Lead_Levels_in_Children_Fact_Sheet.pdf, 2014.

Chan Y-F, Sivasamboo R. Lightning accidents in pregnancy. J Obstet Gynecol Br Commonw 1979; 79: 761–2.

Cherry N, Shaikh K, McDonals C et al. Stillbirth in rural Bangladesh: arsenic exposure and other etiological factors: a report from Gonoshasthaya Kendra. Bull World Health Organ 2008; 86: 172–7.

Chevrier C, Dananché B, Bahuau M et al. Occupational exposure to organic solvent mixtures during pregnancy and the risk of non-syndromic oral clefts. Occup Environ Med 2006; 63: 617–23.

Clarkson TW, Magos L. The toxicology of mercury and its chemical compounds. Crit Rev Toxicol 2006; 36: 609–62.

Coleman M, Beral V. A review of epidemiological studies of the health effects of living near or working with electricity generation and transmission equipment. Intl J Epidemiol 1988; 17: 1–13.

Commoner B. Seveso: The tragedy lingers on. Clin Toxicol 1977; 11: 479–82.

Cordier S, Garlantézec R, Labat L et al. Exposure during pregnancy to glycol ethers and chlorinated solvents and the risk of congenital malformations. Epidemiology 2012; 23: 806–12.

Cordier S, Lehébel A, Amar E et al. Maternal residence near municipal waste incinerators and the risk of urinary tract birth defects. Occup Environ Med 2010; 67: 493–9.

Davis JM, Otto DA, Weil DE et al. The comparative developmental neurotoxicity of lead in humans and animals. Neurotoxicol Teratol 1990; 12: 215–29.

De Cock M, Maas YG, van de Bor M. Does perinatal exposure to endocrine disruptors induce autism spectrum and attention deficit hyperactivity disorders? Review. Acta Paediatr 2012; 101: 811–8.

De Rosis F, Anastasio SP, Selvaggi L et al. Female reproductive health in two lamp factories: effects of exposure to inorganic mercury vapour and stress factors. Br J Ind Med 1985; 42: 488–94.

Desrosiers TA, Lawson CC, Meyer RE et al. Maternal occupational exposure to organic solvents during early pregnancy and risks of neural tube defects and orofacial clefts. Occup Environ Med 2012; 69: 493–9.

Dietrich KN, Berger OG, Succop PA et al. The developmental consequences of low to moderate prenatal and postnatal lead exposure: intellectual attainment in the Cincinnati lead study cohort following school entry. Neurotoxicol Teratol 1993; 15: 37–44.

Dietrich KN, Succop PA, Berger OG et al. Lead exposure and the cognitive development of urban preschool children: The Cincinnati lead study cohort at 4 years. Neurotoxicol Teratol 1991; 13: 203–11.

Divan HA, Kheifets L, Obel C et al. Prenatal and postnatal exposure to cell phone use and behavioral problems in children. Epidemiology 2008; 19: 523–9.

Divan HA, Kheifets L, Obel C et al. Cell phone use and behavioural problems in young children. J Epidemiol Community Health 2012; 66: 524–9.

Divan HA, Kheifets L, Olsen J. Prenatal cell phone use and developmental milestone delays among infants. Scand J Work Environ Health 2011; 37: 341–8.

Dlugosz L, Vena J, Byers T et al. Congenital defects and electric bed heating in New York State: a register-based case-control study. Am J Epidemiol 1992; 135: 1000–11.

Dodds L, King WD. Relation between trihalomethane compounds and birth defects. Occup Environ Med 2001; 58: 443–6.

Dodds L, King W, Woolcott C et al. Trihalomethanes in public water supplies and adverse birth outcomes. Epidemiology 1999; 10: 233–7.

Dolk H, Busby A, Armstrong BG et al. Geographical variation in anophthalmia and microphthalmia in England, 1988–94. Commentary: clustering of anophthalmia and microphthalmia is not supported by the data. Br Med J 1998a; 317: 905–10.

Dolk H, Elliott P. Evidence for "clusters of anophthalmia" is thin. Br Med J 1993; 307: 203.

Dolk H, Vrijheid M, Armstrong B et al. Risk of congenital anomalies near hazardous-waste landfill sites in Europe: the EUROHAZCON study. Lancet 1998b; 352: 423–7.

Donovan JW, MacLennan R, Adena M. Vietnam service and the risk of congenital anomalies a case-control study. Med J Aust 1984; 140: 394–7.

Doyle P, Roman DP, Beral V et al. Spontaneous abortion in dry cleaning workers potentially exposed to perchloroethylene. Occup Environ Med 1997; 54: 848–53.

Doyle P, Maconochie N, Roman E et al. Fetal death and congenital malformation in babies born to nuclear industry employees: report from the nuclear industry family study. Lancet 2000; 356: 1293–9.

Doyle P, Roman E, Maconochie N et al. Primary infertility in nuclear industry employees: report from the nuclear industry family study. Occup Environ Med 2001; 58: 535–9.

Dulskiene V, Grazuleviciene R. Environmental risk factors and outdoor formaldehyde and risk of congenital heart malformations. Medicina (Kaunas) 2005; 41: 787–95.

Duong A, Steinmaus C, McHale CM et al. Reproductive and developmental toxicity of formaldehyde: a systematic review. Mutat Res 2011; 728: 118–38.

EFSA. Opinion of the scientific panel on contaminants in the food chain on a request from the commission related to the presence of non-dioxin-like polychlorinated biphenyls (PCB) in feed and food. EFSA J 2005; 284: 1–137.

EFSA. Scientific Opinion on the risk for public health related to the presence of mercury and methylmercury in food. EFSA J 2012; 10: 2985.

Einarson A, Bailey B, Inocencion G et al. Accidental electric shock in pregnancy: a prospective cohort study. Am J Obstet Gynecol 1997; 176: 678–81.

Eisenmann CJ, Miller RK. Placental transport, metabolism and toxicity of metals. In: Toxicology of Metals, Chang LW, Ed., pp. 1003–26. CRC Press, Boca Raton, 1996.

El-Helaly M, Abdel-Elah K, Haussein A et al. Paternal occupational exposures and the risk of congenital malformations – a case-control study. Int J Occup Med Environ Health 2011; 24: 218–27.

El Majidi N, Bouchard M, Gosselin NH et al. Relationship between prenatal exposure to polychlorinated biphenyls and birth weight: a systematic analysis of published epidemiological studies through a standardization of biomonitoring data. Regul Toxicol Pharmacol 2012; 64: 161–74.

Elliott P, Briggs D, Morris S et al. Risk of adverse birth outcomes in populations living near landfill sites. Br Med J 2001; 323: 363–8.

Engel SM, Wetmur J, Chen J et al. Prenatal exposure to organophosphates, paraoxonase 1, and cognitive development in childhood. Environ Health Perspect 2011; 119: 1182–8.

EPA. Health effects of PCBs. Available at: http://www.epa.gov/osw/hazard/tsd/pcbs/pubs/effects.htm, 2013.

EPA. Epidemiology Studies Division, US EPA. Six years' spontaneous abortion rates in Oregon areas in relation to forest 2,4,5-T spray practices. Fed Register 1979; 44: 874.

Erickson JD. Vietnam veterans' risk for fathering babies with birth defects. J Am Med Assoc 1984; 252: 903–12.

Ericson A, Källén B. Pregnancy outcome in women working as dentists, dental assistants or dental technicians. Intl Arch Occup Environ Health 1989; 61: 329–33.

Ernhart C. Low lead level exposure and early preschool periods: intelligence prior to school entry. Neurotoxicol Teratol 1989; 11: 161–70.

Eskenazi B, Warner M, Marks AR et al. Serum dioxin concentrations and time to pregnancy. Epidemiology 2010; 21: 224–31.

FDA. What You Need to Know About Mercury in Fish and Shellfish. Advice forWomen Who Might Become Pregnant, Women Who are Pregnant, Nursing Mothers,Young Children from the U.S. Food and Drug Administration and U.S. Environmental Protection Agency FDA, 2004. Available at: http://www.fda.gov/Food/ResourcesForYou/Consumers/ucm110591.htm (accessed 29 March 2014).

FDA. Draft Report of Quantitative Risk and Benefit Assessment of Consumption of Commercial Fish, Focusing on Fetal Neurodevelopmental Effects (Measured by Verbal Development in Children) and on Coronary Heart Disease and Stroke in the General Population. January 15, 2009. Available at: http://www.fda.gov/Food/FoodborneIllness-Contaminants/Metals/ucm088794.htm (accessed 29 March 2014).

Fenster L, Eskenazi B, Anderson B et al. Association of in utero organochlorine pesticide exposure and fetal growth and fetal length of gestation in agricultural population. Environ Health Perspect 2006; 114: 597–602.

Field B, Kerr C. Herbicide use and incidence of neural tube defects. Lancet 1979; 1: 1341–2.

Flannery DB, Wiles H. Follow-up of a survivor of intrauterine lightning exposure. Am J Obstet Gynecol 1982; 142: 238–9.

Ford WC, Northstone K, Farrow A et al. Male employment in some printing trades is associated with prolonged time to conception. Int J Androl 2002; 25: 295–300.

Friedman JM. Does Agent Orange cause birth defects? Teratology 1984; 29: 193–221.

Gabel P, Jensen MS, Andersen HR et al. The risk of cryptorchidism among sons of women working in horticulture in Denmark: a cohort study. Environ Health 2011; 10: 100.

Gallagher MD, Nuckols JR, Stallones L et al. Exposure to trihalomethanes and adverse pregnancy outcomes. Epidemiology 1998; 9: 484–9.

García AM. Occupational exposure to pesticides and congenital malformations: a review of mechanisms, methods, and results. Am J Ind Med 1998; 33: 232–40.

Garlantézec R, Monfort C, Rouget F et al. Maternal occupational exposure to solvents and congenital malformations: a prospective study in the general population. Occup Environ Med 2009; 66: 456–63.

Gaspari L, Paris F, Jandel C et al. Prenatal environmental risk factors for genital malformations in a population of 1442 French male newborns: a nested case-control study. Hum Reprod 2011; 26: 3155–62.

Gelbke HP, Göen T, Mäurer M et al. A review of health effects of carbon disulphide in viscose industry and a proposal for an occupational exposure limit. Crit Rev Toxicol 2009; 39: 1–126.

Gilbert R. "Clusters" of anophthalmia in Britain. Difficult to implicate benomyl on current evidence. Br Med J 1993; 307: 340–1.

Gilboa SM, Desrosiers TA, Lawson C et al. Association between maternal occupational exposure to organic solvents and congential heart defects, National Birth Defects Prevention Study, 1997–2002. Occup Environ Med 2012; 69: 628–35.

Gilstrap LC, Little BB. Drugs and Pregnancy, 2nd edn. Chapman & Hall, London, 1998.

Goldman LR. New approaches for assessing the etiology and risks of developmental abnormalities from chemical exposure. Reprod Toxicol 1997; 11: 443–51.

Goldman RD, Einarson A, Koren G. Electric shock during pregnancy. Can Fam Physician 2003; 49: 297–8.

Goodlad JK, Marcus DK, Fulton JJ. Lead and Attention-Deficit/Hyperactivity Disorder (ADHD) symptoms: A meta-analysis. Clin Psychol Rev 2013; 33: 417–25.

Gordon JE, Shy CM. Agricultural chemical use and congenital cleft lip and/or palate. Arch Environ Health 1981; 36: 213–20.

Grandjean P, Weihe P, White RF et al. Cognitive deficit in 7-year-old children with prenatal exposure to methylmercury. Neurotoxicol Teratol 1997; 19: 417–28.

Grazuleviciene R, Nieuwenhuijsen MJ, Vencloviene J et al. Individual exposures to drinking water trihalomethanes, low birth weight and small for gestational age risk: a prospective Kaunas cohort study. Environ Health 2011; 10: 32.

Grellier J, Bennett J, Patelarou E et al. Exposure to disinfectant by-products, fetal growth, and prematurity: a systematic review and meta-analysis. Epidemiology 2010; 21: 300–13.

Grether JK, Harris JA, Neutra R et al. Exposure to aerial malathion application and the occurrence of congenital anomalies and low birthweight. Am J Public Health 1987; 77: 1009–10.

Guan H, Piao F, Zhang X et al. Prenatal exposure to arsenic and its effects on fetal development in the general population of Dalian. Biol Trace Elem Res 2012; 149: 10–5.

Guha-Ray DK. Fetal death at term due to lightning. Am J Obstet Gynecol 1979; 134: 103–5.

Guxens M, van Eijsden M, Vermeulen R et al. Maternal cell phone and cordless phone use during pregnancy and behaviour problems in 5-year-old children. J Epidemiol Community Health 2013; 67: 432–8.

Hamdani JD, Grantham-McGregor SM, Tofail F et al. Pre- and postnatal arsenic exposure and child development at 18 months of age: a cohort study in rural Bangladesh. Int J Epidemiol 2010; 39: 1206–16.

Hanify JA, Metcalf P, Nobbs CL et al. Aerial spraying of 2,4,5-T and human birth malformations: an epidemiological investigation. Science 1981; 212: 349–51.

Hanke W, Jurewicz J. The risk of adverse reproductive and developmental disorders due to occupational pesticide exposure: an overview of current epidemiological evidence. Int J Occup Med Environ Health 2004; 17: 223–43.

Hannigan JH, Bowen SE. Reproductive toxicology and teratology of abused toluene. Syst Biol Reprod Med 2010; 56: 184–200.

Hatch M, Brenner A, Bogdanova T et al. A screening study of thyroid cancer and other thyroid diseases among individuals exposed in utero to iodine-131 from Chernobyl fallout. J Clin Endocrinol Metab 2009; 94: 899–906.

Health and Safety Executive. EH40/2005 Workplace Exposure Limits. 2nd edition, 2011. Available at: http://www.hse.gov.uk/pubns/priced/eh40.pdf (accessed 29 March 2014).

Hemminki K, Franssila E, Vainio H. Spontaneous abortions among female chemical workers in Finland. Intl Arch Occup Environ Health 1980; 46: 93–8.

Hemminki K, Kyyronen P, Lindbohm M-L. Spontaneous abortions and malformations in the offspring of nurses exposed to anaesthetic gases, cytostatic drugs, and other potential hazards in hospitals, based on registered information of outcome. J Epidemiol Commun Health 1985; 39: 141–7.

Hemminki K, Mutanen P, Saloniemi I et al. Spontaneous abortions in hospital staff engaged in sterilizing instruments with chemical agents. Br Med J 1982a; 285: 1461–3.

Hemminki K, Niemi ML. Community study of spontaneous abortions: relation to occupation and air pollution by sulfur dioxide, hydrogen sulfide, and carbon disulfide. Intl Arch Occup Environ Health 1982b; 51: 55–63.

Heron J, Golding J, ALSPAC Study Team. Thimerosal exposure in infants and developmental disorders: a prospective cohort study in the United Kingdom does not support a causal association. Pediatrics 2004; 114: 577–83.

Hinckley AF, Bachand AM, Reif JS. Late pregnancy exposures to disinfection by-products and growth-related birth outcomes. Environ Health Perspect 2005; 113: 1808–13.

Holmberg PC. Central-nervous-system defects in children born to mothers exposed to organic solvents during pregnancy. Lancet 1979; 2: 177–9.

Holmberg PC, Hernberg S, Kurppa K et al. Oral clefts and organic solvent exposure during pregnancy. Intl Arch Occup Environ Health 1982; 50: 371–6.

Holmes LB. Impact of the detention and prevention of developmental abnormalities in human studies. Reprod Toxicol 1997; 11: 267–9.

Hooiveld M, Haveman W, Roskes K et al. Adverse reproductive outcomes among male painters with occupational exposure to organic solvents. Occup Environ Med 2006; 63: 538–44.

Hopenhayn C, Ferreccio C, Browning SR et al. Arsenic exposure form drinking water and birth weight. Epidemiology 2003; 14: 592–602.

Hjortebjerg D, Nybo Andersen A-M, Garne E et al. Non-occupational exposure to paint fumes during pregnancy and risk of congenital anomalies: a cohort study. Environ Health 2012; 11: 54.

Hujoel PP, Lydon-Rochelle M, Bollen AM et al. Mercury exposure from dental filling placement during pregnancy and low birth weight risk. Am J Epidemiol 2005; 161: 734–40.

IARC. Tetrachloroethylene. In: Dry Cleaning, Some Chlorinated Solvents and Other Industrial Chemicals. IARC Monographs on the Evaluation of Carcinogenic Risks to Humans, Vol 63. International Agency for Research on Cancer, Lyon, France, 1995.

Iavicoli I, Fontana L, Bergamaschi A. The effects of metals as endocrine disruptors. J Toxicol Environ Health B Crit Rev 2009; 12: 206–23.

Infante-Rivard C. Electromagnetic field exposure during pregnancy and childhood leukaemia. Lancet 1995; 346: 177.

IPCS (International Programme on Chemical Safety). Benomyl. Environmental Health Criteria 1993; 148: 13–8.

Itai Y, Fujino T, Ueno K et al. An epidemiological study of the incidence of abnormal pregnancy in areas heavily contaminated with methylmercury. Environ Sci 2004; 1: 83–97.

Jansson E. Re: "Congenital defects and electric bed heating in New York State: a register-based case-control study" (Letter; comment). Am J Epidemiol 1993; 137: 585–7.

Jarup L, Morris S, Richardson S et al. Down syndrome in births near landfill sites. Prenat Diagn 2007; 27: 1191–6.

John EM, Savitz DA, Shy CM. Spontaneous abortions among cosmetologists. Epidemiology 1994; 5: 147–55.

Julvez J, Grandjean P. Neurodevelopmental toxicity risks due to occupational exposure to industrial chemicals during pregnancy. Indust Health 2009; 47: 459–68.

Källén B. Epidemiology of Human Reproduction. CRC Press, Boca Raton, 1988.

Källén B, Robert E, Harris J. The descriptive epidemiology of anophthalmia and microphthalmia. Intl J Epidemiol 1996; 25: 1009–16.

Karagas MR, Choi AL, Oken E et al. Evidence on the human health effects of low-level methylmercury exposure. Environ Health Perspect 2012; 120: 799–806.

Kaul PP, Srivastava R, Srivastava SP. Relationships of maternal blood lead and disorders of pregnancy to neonatal birthweight. Vet Hum Toxicol 2002; 44: 321–3.

Kennedy D, Hurst V, Konradsdottir E et al. Pregnancy outcome following exposure to permethrin and use of teratogen information. Am J Perinatol 2005; 22: 87–90.

Khanjani N, Sim MR. Maternal contamination with dichlorophenyltrichloroethane and reproductive outcomes in an Australian population. Environ Res 2006; 101: 37–9.

Khattak S, K-Moghtader G, McMartin K et al. Pregnancy outcome following gestational exposure to organic solvents: a prospective controlled study. J Am Med Assoc 1999; 281: 1106–9.

Kimmel CA. Introduction to the symposium. Reprod Toxicol 1997; 11: 261–3.

Kipen HM. Assessment of reproductive health effects of hazardous waste. Toxicol Ind Health 1996; 12: 211–24.

Kippler M, Hoque AM, Raqib R et al. Accumulation of cadmium in human placenta interacts with the transport of micronutrients to the fetus. Toxicol Lett 2010; 192: 162–8.

Kippler M, Tofail F, Gardner R et al. Maternal cadmium exposure during pregnancy and size at birth: a prospective cohort study. Environ Health Perspect 2012; 120: 284–9.

Kramer MD, Lynch CF, Isacson P et al. The association of waterborne chloroform with intrauterine growth retardation. Epidemiology 1992; 3: 407–13.

Kristensen P, Irgens LM. Clusters of anophthalmia. No link with benomyl in Italy… or in Norway. Br Med J 1994; 308: 205–6.

Kurppa K, Holmberg PC, Hernberg S et al. Screening for occupational exposures and congenital malformations. Scand J Work Environ Health 1983; 9: 89–93.

Kyyrönen P, Taskinen H, Lindbohm ML et al. Spontaneous abortions and congenital malformations among women exposed to tetrachloroethylene in dry cleaning. J Epidemiol Commun Health 1989; 43: 346–51.

Lee GM, Neutra RR, Hristova L et al. The use of electric bed heaters and the risk of clinically recognized spontaneous abortion. Epidemiology 2000; 11: 406–15.

Lehman I, Thoelke A, Rehwagen M et al. The influence of maternal exposure to volatile organic compounds on the cytokine secretion profile of neonatal T cells. Environ Toxicol 2002; 17: 203–10.

Leiberman JR, Mazor M, Molcho J et al. Electrical accidents during pregnancy. Obstet Gynecol 1986; 67: 861–3.

Li D-K, Checkoway H, Mueller BA. Electric blanket use in relation to the risk of congenital urinary tract anomalies among women with a history of subfertility. Teratology 1995; 51: 90.

Li AA, Lowe KA, McIntosh LJ et al. Evaluation of epidemiology and animal data for risk assessment: chlorpyrifos developmental neurobehavioral outcomes. J Toxicol Environ Health B Crit Rev 2012; 15: 109–84.

Lien DC, Todoruk DN, Rajani HR et al. Accidental inhalation of mercury vapor: respiratory and toxicologic consequences. Can Med Assoc J 1983; 129: 591–5.

Lin CM, Doyle P, Wang D et al. Does prenatal cadmium exposure affect fetal and child growth? Occup Environ Med 2011; 68: 641–6.

Pregnancy

2.23 Occupational, industrial and environmental agents

Lin CC, Wang JD, Hsieh GY et al. Health risk in the offspring of female semiconductor workers. Occup Med (Lond) 2008; 58: 388–92.

Lindbohm ML, Taskinen H, Sallmén M et al. Spontaneous abortions among women exposed to organic solvents. Am J Ind Med 1990; 17: 449–63.

Liu Y, McDermott S, Lawson A et al. The relationship between mental retardation and developmental delays in children and the levels of arsenic, mercury and lead in soil samples taken near their mother's residence during pregnancy. Int J Hyg Environ Health 2010; 213: 116–23.

Logman JF, de Vries LE, Hemels ME et al. Paternal organic solvent exposure and adverse pregnancy outcomes: a meta-analysis. Am J Ind Med 2005; 47: 37–44.

Lovasi GS, Quinn JW, Rauh VA et al. Chlorpyrifos exposure and urban residential environment characteristics as determinants of early childhood neurodevelopment. Am J Public Health 2011; 101: 63–70.

Mahram M, Ghazavi M. The effect of extremely low frequency electromagnetic fields on pregnancy and fetal growth, and development. Arch Iran Med 2013; 16: 221–4.

Maier K Sr. Mobile phones: are they safe? Lancet 2000; 355: 1793.

Malagoli C, Crespi CM, Rodolfi R et al. Maternal exposure to magnetic fields from high-voltage power lines and the risk of birth defects. Bioelectromagnetics 2012; 33: 405–9.

Maldonado G, Delzell E, Tyl RW et al. Occupational exposure to glycol ethers and human congenital malformations. Int Arch Occup Environ Health 2003; 76: 405–23.

Mangurten HM, Kaye CI. Neonatal bromism secondary to maternal exposure in photographic laboratory. J Pediatr 1982; 100: 596–8.

Manton WI. Postpartum changes to maternal blood lead concentrations (Letter). Br J Ind Med 1992; 49: 671–2.

Maroziene L, Grazuleviciene R. Maternal exposure to low-level air pollution and pregnancy outcomes: a population-based study. Environ Health 2002; 1: 6.

Matte TD, Mulinare J, Erickson JD. Case-control study of congenital defects and parental employment in health care. Am J Ind Med 1993; 24: 11–23.

McCann JC, Ames BN. An overview of evidence for a causal relation between iron deficiency during development and deficits in cognitive or behavioral function. Am J Clin Nutr 2007; 85: 931–45.

McDermott S, Bao W, Aelion CM et al. When are fetuses and young children most susceptible to soil metal concentrations of arsenic, lead and mercury? Spat Spatiotemporal Epidemiol 2012; 3: 265–72.

McDonald AD, McDonald JC, Armstrong B et al. Occupation and pregnancy outcome. Br J Ind Med 1987; 44: 521–6.

McMartin KI, Chu M, Kopecky E et al. Pregnancy outcome following maternal organic solvent exposure: a meta-analysis of epidemiologic studies. Am J Ind Med 1998; 34: 288–92.

McMichael AJ, Baghurst PA, Wigg NR et al. Port Pirie cohort study: environmental exposure to lead and children's abilities at the age of four years. N Engl J Med 1988; 319: 468–75.

Mehl LE. Electrical injury from tasering and miscarriage. Acta Obstet Gynecol Scand 1992; 71: 118–23.

Miller RK. Environmental and occupational exposures involving reproduction. In: Primary Care for Women, 2nd edn., Leppert P, Ed. Lippincott, New York, 2004.

Miller RK, Bellinger D. Metals: occupational and environmental. In: Reproductive Hazards: A Guide for Clinicians, Paul M, Ed., Williams & Wilkins, Baltimore, MD, 1993.

Miller RK, Hu H, Peterson J et al. Lead Exposures During Pregnancy: Importance of Blood Leads and K-XRF Assessments. OTIS Annual Meeting, p. 2, 2006.

Mink PJ, Kimmel CA, Li AA. Potential effects of chlorpyrifos on fetal growth outcomes: implications for risk assessment. J Toxicol Environ Health B Crit Rev 2012; 15: 281–316.

Mocarelli P, Gerthoux PM, Needham LL et al. Perinatal exposure to low doses of dioxin can permanently impair human semen quality. Environ Health Perspect 2011; 119: 713–8.

Mocarelli P, Gerthoux PM, Patterson DG Jr et al. Dioxin exposure, from infancy through puberty, produces endocrine disruption and affects human semen quality. Environ Health Perspect 2008; 116: 70–7.

Morris S, Thompson AO, Jarup L et al. No excess risk of adverse birth outcomes in populations living near special waste landfill sites in Scotland. Scott Med J 2003; 48: 105–7.

Myers GJ, Davidson PW, Cox C et al. Prenatal methylmercury exposure from ocean fish consumption in the Seychelles child development study. Lancet 2003; 361: 1686–92.

Myers SL, Lobdell DT, Liu Z et al. Maternal drinking water arsenic exposure and perinatal outcomes in inner Mongolia, China. J Epidemiol Community Health 2010; 64: 325–9.

Nanes JA, Xia Y, Dassanayake RM et al. Selected persistent organic pollutants in human placental tissue from the United States. Chemosphere 2014; 106: 20–7.

Needleman H, Rabinowitz M, Leviton A et al. The relationship between prenatal exposure to lead and congenital anomalies. J Am Med Assoc 1984; 251: 2956–9.

Nelson CJ, Holson JF, Green HG et al. Retrospective study of the relationship between agricultural use of 2,4,5-T and cleft palate occurrence in Arkansas. Teratology 1979; 19: 377–83.

Ng TP, Foo SC, Yoong T. Risk of spontaneous abortion in workers exposed to toluene. Br J Ind Med 1992; 49: 804–08.

NHS. Should pregnant and breastfeeding women avoid some types of fish? 2011. Available at: http://www.nhs.uk/chq/Pages/should-pregnant-and-breastfeeding-women-avoid-some-types-of-fish.aspx?CategoryID=54&SubCategoryID=216 (accessed 29 March 2014).

Nishijo M, Tawara K, Honda R et al. Relationship between newborn size and mother's blood cadmium levels, Toyama, Japan. Arch Environ Health 2004; 59: 22–5.

Nordstrom S, Beckman L, Nordenson I. Occupational and environmental risks in and around a smelter in northern Sweden. VI. Congenital malformations. Hereditas 1978; 90: 297–307.

Nordstrom S, Birke E, Gustavsson L. Reproductive hazards among workers at high voltage substations. Bioelectromagnetics 1983; 4: 91–101.

NYCDH (New York City Department of Health) Report. Guidelines for the Identification and Management of Pregnant Women with Elevated Lead Levels in New York City, October 4, 2004.

Oken E, Bellinger DC. Fish consumption, methylmercury and child neurodevelopment. Curr Opin Pediatr 2008; 20: 178–83.

Oken E, Wright RO, Kleinman KP et al. Maternal fish consumption, hair mercury, and infant cognition in a US Cohort. Environ Health Perspect 2005; 113: 1376–80.

Olsen J, Hemminki K, Ahlborg G et al. Low birthweight, congenital malformations, and spontaneous abortions among dry-cleaning workers in Scandinavia. Scand J Work Environ Health 1990; 16: 163–8.

Opler MG, Buka SL, Groeger J et al. Prenatal exposure to lead, delta-aminolevulinic acid, and schizophrenia: further evidence. Environ Health Perspect 2008; 116: 1586–90.

Parker L. Fetal death and radiation exposure. Lancet 2001; 357: 556–7.

Parker L, Pearce MS, Dickinson HO et al. Stillbirths among offspring of male radiation workers at Sellafield nuclear reprocessing plant. Lancet 1999; 354: 1407–14.

Pathak R, Mustafa MD, Ahmed RS et al. Association between recurrent miscarriages and organochlorine pesticide levels. Clin Biochem 2010; 43: 131–5.

Pathak R, Mustafa MD, Ahmed T et al. Intrauterine growth retardation: association with organochlorine pesticide residue levels and oxidative stress markers. Reprod Toxicol 2011; 31: 534–9.

Paul M. Occupational and Environmental Reproductive Hazards. Baltimore, MD: Williams & Wilkins, 1993.

Pelé F, Muckle G, Costet N et al. Occupational solvent exposure during pregnancy and child behaviour at age 2. Occup Environ Med 2013; 70: 114–9.

Peppier RD, Labranche FJ, Comeaux JJ. Intrauterine death of a fetus in a mother shocked by an electric current: a case report. J LA State Med Soc 1974; 124: 37–8.

Plenge-Bönig A, Karmaus W. Exposure to toluene in the printing industry is associated with subfecundity in women but not in men. Occup Environ Med 1999; 56: 443–8.

Rabinowitz M. Lead and pregnancy. Birth 1988; 15: 236–41.

Rahman A, Vahetr M, Ekström EC et al. Arsenic exposure in pregnancy increases the risk of lower respiratory tract infection and diarrhea during infancy in Bangladesh. Environ Health Perspect 2011; 119: 719–24.

Ratcliffe HE, Swanson GM, Fischer LJ. Human exposure to mercury – a critical assessment of the evidence of adverse health effects. J Toxicol Environ Health 1996; 49: 221–70.

Rauh V, Arunajadai S, Horton M et al. Seven-year neurodevelopmental scores and prenatal exposure to chlorpyrifos, a common agricultural pesticide. Environ Health Perspect 2011; 119: 1196–1201.

Rauh VA, Garfinkel R, Perera FP et al. Impact of prenatal chlorpyrifos exposure on neurodevelopment in the first 3 years of life among inner-city children. Environ Health Perspect 2006; 118: 1845–59.

Rauh V, Perera F, Horton M et al. Brain anomalies in children exposed prenatally to a common organophosphate pesticide. Proc Natl Acad Sci USA 2012; 109: 7871–6.

Rees WD. Pregnant woman struck by lightning. Br Med J 1965; 1: 103–4.

Reif JS, Hatch MC, Bracken M et al. Reproductive and developmental effects of disinfection byproducts in drinking water. Environ Health Perspect 1996; 104: 1056–61.

Robert E. Birth defects and high voltage power lines: an exploratory study based on registry data. Reprod Toxicol 1993; 7: 283–7.

Robert E. Intrauterine effects of electromagnetic field–(low frequency, mid frequency RF, and microwave): review of epidemiologic studies. Teratology 1999; 59: 292–8.

Robert E, Harris JA, Robert O et al. Case-control study on maternal residential proximity to high voltage power lines and congenital anomalies in France. Paediatr Perinat Epidemiol 1996; 10: 32–8.

Rocheleau CM, Romitti PA, Dennis LK. Pesticides and hypospadias: a meta-analysis. J Pediatr Urol 2009; 5: 7–24.

Rocheleau CM, Romitti PA, Sanderson WT et al. Maternal occupational pesticide exposure and risk of hypospadias in the National Birth Defects Prevention Study. Birth Defects Res A Clin Mol Teratol 2011; 91: 927–36.

Roeleveld N, Bretveld R. The impact of pesticides on male fertility. Curr Opin Obstet Gynecol 2008; 20: 229–33.

Rowland AS, Baird DD, Weinberg CR et al. The effect of occupational exposure to mercury vapour on the fertility of female dental assistants. Occup Environ Med 1994; 51: 28–34.

Sagiv SK, Tolbert PE, Altshul LM et al. Organochlorine exposures during pregnancy and infant size at birth. Epidemiology 2007; 18: 120–9.

Sallmén M, Baird DD, Hoppin JA et al. Fertility and exposure to solvents among families in the Agricultural Health Study. Occup Environ Med 2006; 63: 469–75.

Sallmén M, Lindbohm ML, Anttila A et al. Paternal occupational lead exposure and congenital malformations. J Epidemiol Commun Health 1992; 46: 519–22.

Sallmén M, Lindbohm ML, Anttila A et al. Time to pregnancy among the wives of men exposed to organic solvents. Occup Environ Med 1998; 55: 24–30.

Sallmén M, Lindbohm ML, Kyyrönen P et al. Reduced fertility among women exposed to organic solvents. Am J Ind Med 1995; 27: 699–713.

Sallmén M, Neto M, Mayan ON. Reduced fertility among shoe manufacturing workers. Occup Environ Med 2008; 65: 518–24.

Saurel-Cubizolles MJ, Hays M, Estryn-Behar M. Work in operating rooms and pregnancy outcome among nurses. Intl Arch Occup Environ Health 1994; 66: 235–41.

Savitz DA, Andrews KW, Pastore LM. Drinking water and pregnancy outcome in central North Carolina: source, amount and trihalomethane levels. Environ Health Perspect 1995; 103: 592–6.

Savitz DA, Bornschein RL, Amler RW et al. Assessment of reproductive disorders and birth defects in communities near hazardous chemical waste sites. I. Birth defects and developmental disorders. Reprod Toxicol 1997; 11: 223–30.

Scanlon JW. Dangers to the human fetus from certain heavy metals in the environment. Rev Environ Health 1975; 2: 39–64.

Schardein J. Chemically Induced Birth Defects, 3rd edn. Marcel Dekker, New York, 2000.

Scheeres JJ, Chudley AE. Solvent abuse in pregnancy: a perinatal perspective. J Obstet Gynaecol Can 2002; 24: 22–6.

Scialli AR, Swan SH, Amler RW et al. Assessment of reproductive disorders and birth defects in communities near hazardous chemical waste sites. II. Female reproductive disorders. Reprod Toxicol 1997; 11: 231–42.

Shaw GM, Lammer EJ. Incorporating molecular genetic variation and environmental exposures into epidemiological studies of congenital anomalies. Reprod Toxicol 1997; 11: 275–80.

Shaw GM, Nelson V, Todoroff K et al. Maternal periconceptional use of electric bed-heating devices and risk for neural tube defects and orofacial clefts. Teratology 1999; 60: 124–9.

Shirai S, Suzuki Y, Yoshinaga J et al. Maternal exposure to low-level heavy metals during pregnancy and birth size. J Environ Sci Health A Tox Hazard Subst Environ Eng 2010; 45: 1468–74.

Shirangi A, Nieuwenhuijsen M, Vienneau D et al. Living near agricultural pesticide applications and the risk of adverse reproductive outcomes: a review of the literature. Paediatr Perinat Epidemiol 2011; 25: 172–91.

Smith AH, Fisher DO, Pearce N et al. Congenital defects and miscarriages among New Zealand 2,4,5-T sprayers. Arch Environ Health 1982; 37: 197–200.

Smith AH, Steinmaus CM. Health effects of arsenic and chromium in drinking water: recent human findings. Annu Rev Publ Health 2009; 30: 107–22.

Sobel E, Davanipour Z, Sulkava R. Occupational exposure to electromagnetic fields as a risk factor for Alzheimer's disease. Proceeding of the Annual Review of Research on Biological Effects of Electric and Magnetic Fields from the Generation, Delivery and Use of Electricity. US Dept of Energy, 6–10 November 1994, Albuquerque, NM.

Spagnolo A, Bianchi F, Calabro A et al. Anophthalmia and benomyl in Italy: a multicenter study based on 940,615 newborns. Reprod Toxicol 1994; 8: 397–403.

Sperling K, Neitzel H, Scherb H. Evidence for an increase in trisomy 21 (Down syndrome) in Europe after the Chernobyl reactor accident. Genet Epidemiol 2012; 36: 48–55.

Stasenko S, Bradford EM, Piasek M et al. Metals in human placenta: focus on the effects of cadmium on steroid hormones and leptin. J Appl Toxicol 2010; 30: 242–53.

Stillerman KP, Mattison DR, Giudice LC et al. Environmental exposures and adverse pregnancy outcomes: a review of the science. Reprod Sci 2008; 15: 631–50.

Stokes-Rines A, Thurston SW, Myers GJ et al. A longitudinal analysis of prenatal exposure to methylmercury and fatty acids in the Seychelles. Neurotoxicol Teratol 2011; 33: 325–8.

Sørensen M, Andersen AM, Raaschou-Nielsen O. Non-occupational exposure to paint fumes during pregnancy and fetal growth in a general population. Environ Res 2010; 110: 383–7.

Sullivan FM, Watkins WJ, van der Venne M-Th. The Toxicology of Chemicals – Series Two. Reproductive Toxicology, Vol 1, pp. 81–91. Commission of European Communities. EUR. 14991 EN 1993.

Summerhayes RJ, Morgan GG, Edwards HP et al. Exposure to trihalomethanes in drinking water and small-for-gestational-age births. Epidemiology 2012; 23: 15–22.

Taskinen H. Effects of parental occupational exposures on spontaneous abortion and congenital malformation. Scand J Work Environ Health 1990; 16: 297–314.

Taskinen H, Anttila A, Lindbohm ML et al. Spontaneous abortions and congenital malformations among the wives of men occupationally exposed to organic solvents. Scand J Work Environ Health 1989; 15: 345–52.

Taskinen H, Lindbohm ML, Hemminki K. Spontaneous abortions among women working in the pharmaceutical industry. Br J Med 1986; 43: 199–205.

Taskinen H, Kyyrönen P, Hemminki K et al. Laboratory work and pregnancy outcome. J Occup Med 1994; 36: 311–9.

Taskinen H, Kyyrönen P, Sallmén M et al. Reduced fertility among female wood workers exposed to formaldehyde. Am J Ind Med 1999; 36: 206–12.

Thomas HE. 2,4,5-T use and congenital malformation rates in Hungary. Lancet 1980; 2: 214–5.

Thomas DC, Petitti DB, Goldhaber M et al. Reproductive outcomes in relation to malathion spraying in the San Francisco Bay Area, 1981–1982. Epidemiology 1992; 3: 32–9.

Thompson WW, Price C, Goodson B et al. Early thimerosal exposure and neuropsychological outcomes at 7 to 10 years. N Engl J Med 2007; 357: 1281–92.

Tian LL, Zhao YC, Wang XC et al. Effects of gestational cadmium exposure on pregnancy outcome and development in the offspring at age 4.5 years. Biol Trace Elem Res 2009; 132: 51–9.

Tognoni G, Bonaccorsi A. Epidemiological problems with TCDD (a critical view). Drug Metab Rev 1982; 13: 447–69.

Toledano MB, Nieuwenhuijsen MJ, Best N et al. Relation of trihalomethane concentrations in public water supplies to stillbirth and birth weight in three water regions in England. Environ Health Perspect 2005; 113: 225–32.

Townsend JC, Bodneri K, van Peenen PFD et al. Survey of reproductive events of wives of employees exposed to chlorinated dioxins. Am J Epidemiol 1982; 115: 695–713.

Trasande L, Schechter CB, Haynes KA et al. Mental retardation and prenatal methylmercury toxicity. Am J Ind Med 2006; 49: 153–8.

UNSCEAR. The Fukushima-Daiichi nuclear power plant accident. UNSCEAR's assessment of levels and effects of radiation exposure due to the nuclear accident after the 2011 great east-Japan earthquake and tsunami, 2013. Available at: http://www.unscear.org/unscear/en/fukushima.html.

Vahter M. Effects of arsenic on maternal and fetal health. Annu Rev Nutr 2009; 29: 381–99.

Vinceti M, Malagoli C, Fabbi S et al. Risk of congenital anomalies around a municipal solid waste incinerator: a GIS-based case-control study. Int J Health Geogr 2009; 8: 8.

Vinceti M, Malagoli C, Teggi S et al. Adverse pregnancy outcomes in a population exposed to the emissions of a municipal waste incinerator. Sci Total Environ 2008; 407: 116–21.

Virtanen HE, Adamsson A. Cryptorchidism and endocrine disrupting chemicals. Mol Cell Endocr 2012; 355: 208–20.

Pregnancy

2.23 Occupational, industrial and environmental agents

Vrijheid M, Dolk H, Armstrong B et al. Chromosomal anomalies and residence near hazardous waste landfill sites. Lancet 2002; 359: 320–2.

Waller K, Swan SH, de Lorenze G et al. Trihalomethanes in drinking water and spontaneous abortion. Epidemiology 1998; 9: 134–40.

Wasserman GA, Graziano JH, Factor-Litvak P et al. Consequences of lead exposure and iron supplementation on childhood development at age 4 years. Neurotoxicol Teratol 1994; 16: 233–40.

Weinstein L. Lightning: a rare cause of intrauterine death with maternal survival. South Med J 1979; 72: 632–3.

Wennborg H, Bodin L, Vainio H et al. Pregnancy outcome of personnel in Swedish biomedical research laboratories. J Occup Environ Med 2000; 42: 438–46.

Wertelecki W. Malformations in a Chornobyl-impacted region. Pediatrics 2010; 125: e836–843.

Wertheimer N, Leeper E. Possible effects of electric blankets and heated waterbeds on fetal development. Bioelectromagnetics 1986; 7: 13–22.

Wertheimer N, Leeper E. Fetal loss associated with two seasonal sources of electromagnetic field exposure. Am J Epidemiol 1989; 129: 220–4.

Wier PJ, Miller RK, Maulik D et al. Cadmium toxicity in the perfused human placenta. Toxicol Appl Pharm 1990; 105: 156–71.

Wilkins-Haug L. Teratogen update: toluene. Teratology 1997; 55: 145–51.

Williams MA, Weiss NS. Drinking water and adverse reproductive outcomes. Epidemiology 1998; 9: 113–4.

Windham GC, Shusterman D, Swan SH et al. Exposure to organic solvents and adverse pregnancy outcome. Am J Ind Med 1991; 20: 241–59.

Wolfe WH, Michalek JE, Miner JC et al. Paternal serum dioxin and reproductive outcomes among veterans of Operation Ranch Hand. Epidemiology 1995; 6: 17–22.

Wright JM, Schwartz J, Dockery DW. The effect of disinfection by-products and mutagenic activity on birth weight and gestational duration. Environ Health Perspect 2004; 112: 920–5.

Wu J, Chen G, Liao Y et al. Arsenic levels in the soil and risk of birth defects: a population-based case-control study using GIS technology. J Environ Health 2011; 74: 20–5.

Wyrobek AJ, Schrader SM, Perreault SD et al. Assessment of reproductive disorders and birth defects in communities near hazardous chemical waste sites. III. Guidelines for field studies of male reproductive disorders. Reprod Toxicol 1997; 11: 243–59.

Yang CC, Chang CC, Tsai SS et al. Arsenic in drinking water and adverse pregnancy outcome in an arseniasis-endemic area in northeastern Taiwan. Environ Res 2003; 91: 29–34.

Yoshida M. Placental to fetal transfer of mercury and fetotoxicity. Tohoku J Exp Med 2002; 196: 79–88.

Zhou SY, Liang YX, Chen ZQ et al. Effects of occupational exposure to low-level carbon disulfide on menstruation and pregnancy. Indust Health 1988; 26: 203–14.

Zhu JL, Knudsen LE, Andersen A-MN et al. Laboratory work and pregnancy outcomes: a study within the National Birth Cohort in Denmark. Occup Environ Med 2006; 63: 53–8.

General commentary on drug therapy and drug risk during lactation

3

Ruth A. Lawrence and Christof Schaefer

3.1	The advantages of breastfeeding versus the risks of maternal medication	639
3.2	The passage of medications into the mother's milk	641
3.3	Infant characteristics	642
3.4	Milk plasma ratio	643
3.5	Amount of medication in the milk and relative dose	644
3.6	Toxicity of medications in the mother's milk	645
3.7	Medications that affect lactation	647
3.8	Breastfeeding support	648

3.1 The advantages of breastfeeding versus the risks of maternal medication

No discussion of the risks of maternal medications can be undertaken without an understanding of the benefits of being breastfed for the child. Advantages to breastfeeding have been recognized in general terms for decades. However, new information and evidence-based studies following breastfed infants for months and even years have identified many additional advantages and protections provided by human milk and the process of breastfeeding.

The nutrient advantages can be simply stated by "species specificity" (see Table 3.1). The nutrient needs of the human infant are specifically met by the nutrient content of human milk. The most dramatic evidence of this is demonstrated by the comparative advantages to brain growth, visual acuity, auditory acuity, and scores on developmental tests related to infants who are exclusively breastfed, compared to infants who receive traditional formulas. These data are substantiated by multiple studies in both premature and full-term infants. Along with the ideal nutrients, such as omega-3 fatty acids, whey protein, and high levels of lactose, the energy for the brain, are the presence of enzymes and ligands that facilitate the digestion and absorption of nutrients, including the micronutrients.

The other well-documented advantages of human milk are the infection-protection qualities that protect the breastfed infant from respiratory infections, otitis media, gastrointestinal infections, and even urinary tract and meningeal infections and necrotizing enterocolitis (NEC) (Hanson 2004). The study of the immunologic properties of human milk has shown that infants who are exclusively breastfed for at least 4 months

Table 3.1 Composition of human breast milk and of cow's milk

	Cow's milk	Colostrum	Mature milk
Total protein (g/L)	33	23	11
Casein (g/L)	25	12	3.7
Lactalbumin (g/L)	2.4	–	3.6
Lactoglobulin (g/L)	1.7	35	–
Secretory IgA (g/L)	0.03	6	1
Lactose (g/L)	47	57	71
Fat (g/L)	38	30	45
Polyunsaturated fatty acids (%)	20	70	80
Calories (kcal/L)	701	671	747

Mean values; adopted from Behrman (2000).

have a reduced risk of childhood onset diabetes, Crohn's disease, celiac disease, and childhood-onset cancers – especially leukemia. Hundreds of articles testing the allergy protection of human milk have shown a clear advantage in being breastfed for potentially allergic children (Eidelman 2012).

There are many advantages to breastfeeding for the mother herself. The process facilitates a rapid recovery postpartum, with a reduced loss of blood and prompt involution of the uterus to its pre-pregnant state. Further breastfeeding prevents postpartum depression (Ip 2009), and reduces the long-term risk of obesity and osteoporosis for the nursing mother. Studies of specific diseases show that there is a reduced risk of breast cancer and ovarian cancer for women who breastfeed (Lawrence 2010). Finally, the special relationship between mother and infant that develops while the infant suckles at the breast has always been a prime reason to breastfeed.

Determining the risk–benefit ratio of maternal medication for a given infant, requires taking all of the tremendous advantages under consideration and understanding the specific risk of the medication to a given child. For example, if the child is in a developing country where the risk of dying of an infectious disease in the first year of life is 50% for those infants who receive formula, then the risk of a maternal medication is relatively insignificant by comparison.

The World Health Organization (WHO) and the Innocenti Declaration state clearly the importance of infants being breastfed. The Innocenti Declaration was reaffirmed in 2006 at its fifteenth-year anniversary, once again urging exclusive breastfeeding for the first 6 months of life followed by continued breastfeeding with the addition of solid foods through to 12 months of age, and for as long thereafter as mother and child wish.

The incidence of breastfeeding decreased significantly throughout the 1970s and 1980s and is now slowly increasing worldwide because of a vigorous effort on the part of many supportive organizations to reverse the trend of bottle feeding. The most extensive program is the Baby Friendly Hospital Initiative (BFHI), which was begun by the United Nations International Children's Emergency Fund (UNICEF). The BFHI has spread throughout most of the developing world, but has been slowly accepted in Western cultures. BFHI requires that all hospitals have a breastfeeding policy and that all staff be thoroughly trained in the introduction and management of breastfeeding. In addition to adequate training of the staff, all infants should be put to breast within the first hour of life. It is also required that dummies or pacifiers not be provided to breastfeeding infants, and that BFHI hospitals pay for any formula utilized, accept no free samples, and distribute no free samples to their patients.

While encouraging mothers and babies to breastfeed in the hospital, support needs to be provided at home as well by the mother's physician, the pediatrician, the nurse midwife, and office staff, as well as licensed, board-certified lactation consultants. With respect to medications, however, proper information is essential. Many mothers are told to wean because of the medication that they must take. This is actually very rarely necessary. The information available to the practitioner, however, may often be incorrect. Package inserts and the physician's desk reference, for instance, almost always suggests that the drug is not recommended during lactation, not because there is negative information but because the manufacturer has not provided any studies or information that would permit them to say it is safe. This may also lead to poor compliance – that is, the mothers do not follow medical advice. In a prospective study carried out at a counseling center among 203 breastfeeding mothers who were prescribed an antibiotic compatible with breastfeeding, 15% of the women did not take the medication prescribed and 7% stopped breastfeeding (Ito 1993b). It therefore becomes the responsibility of the practitioner, using relevant medical literature, to adequately inform the breastfeeding mother, and to determine whether the drug will enter the milk in a relevant quantity or present any problems for the child. The AAP Committee on Drugs (Sachs 2013) has published a new statement proclaiming that "The benefits of breastfeeding outweigh the risk of exposure to most therapeutic agents via human milk."

3.2   The passage of medications into the mother's milk

It is important to be aware of the characteristics of the drug itself, the ability of a given mother to absorb, metabolize, and excrete the medication, and the infant's ability to absorb, detoxify, and excrete the agent. The infant's age influences the latter ability, and no decision can be made about a given drug without knowing the age of the infant.

The significant characteristics of the drug include the route of administration, the absorption rate, the half-life or peak serum time, the dissociation constant, and the volume of distribution. The passage of a drug is influenced by the size of the molecule, its ionization, and the pH of the substrate (plasma 7.4, milk 6.8), the solubility in water and in lipids, and the protein binding. The distribution of a compound may follow one of several pathways (Figure 3.1).

The solubility of a drug is important because the alveolar and epithelial layer of the breast is a lipid barrier that is most permeable in the first few days of lactation, when colostrum is being produced. The solubility of a compound in water and in lipid is a determining factor for its transfer throughout lactation (see Table 3.2).

Drugs pass into milk by five identified pathways: (1) simple diffusion, (2) carrier mediated diffusion, (3) active transport, (4) pinocytosis, and (5) reverse pinocytosis. If it is assumed that the body is a single compartment and the blood is distributed in the compartment uniformly, then an important characteristic of the drug is the volume of distribution (Vd)

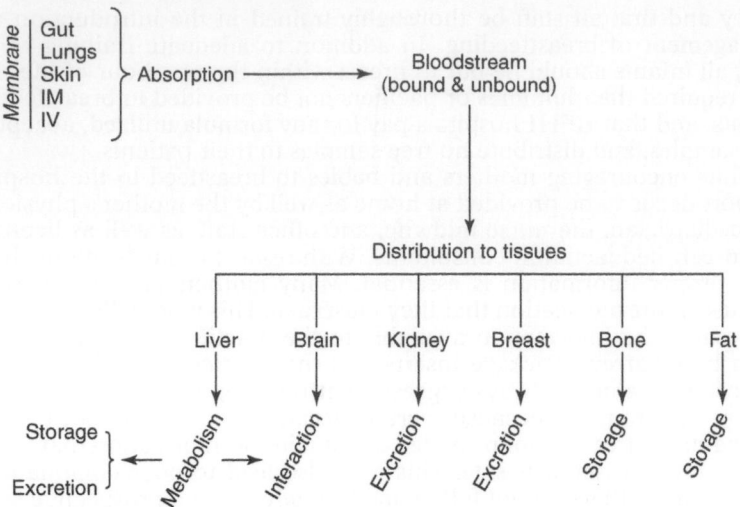

Figure 3.1 Distribution pathways for drugs absorbed during lactation (see Figure 12-1, Page 366, Lawrence 2010).

Table 3.2 Predicted distribution ratios of drug concentrations in milk and plasma

General drug type	Milk/plasma (M/P) ratio
Highly lipid-soluble drugs	~1
Highly protein-bound drugs in maternal serum	<1
Small (mol wt <200) water-soluble drugs	~1
Weak acids	=1
Weak bases	=1
Actively transported drugs	>1

Modified from Lawrence (2010).

which can be calculated as the quotient of the total amount of drug in the body/concentration of drug in the plasma. Thus, drugs with a large volume of distribution do not get into the milk in any amount as compared to drugs with a low volume of distribution which pass into the milk from the plasma in greater amounts.

$$Vd = \frac{\text{Total amount of drug in body}}{\text{concentration of drug in plasma}}$$

3.3   Infant characteristics

In addition to the parameters of the drug and the dose in mother's serum, and the amount in the milk, the characteristics of the infant are essential.

The most important is the age and maturity of the infant, because the infant's ability to absorb, metabolize, and excrete the drug are dependent on this. Therefore, medications in the milk are of greater concern in the first weeks of life than with a month or a year of age. For example, when a mother is taking a medication that is poorly excreted by a neonate, such as aminophylline, it may be well excreted by a 1-year-old and is not accumulated.

Absorption from the infant's gastrointestinal tract is dependent on the bioavailability of the drug, the effect of gastric pH and gastric enzymes, and the presence of food, which may impair absorption. Obviously, drugs in breast milk are present with food. If a medication can be given directly to an infant (for example, *acetaminophen*), it can be given to the nursing mother. Infants tolerate acetaminophen very well, detoxifying it in the sulfhydryl pathway rather than the glucuronidase pathway.

Infants' liver and kidneys are immature at birth. Thus, a drug that depends on liver metabolism, such as *sulfadiazine*, will compete with the bilirubin metabolism. A drug such as aspirin competes for albumin-binding sites in the infant, displacing bilirubin in the first month of life. However, clinical relevance may be questionable, due to the small amounts of a drug transferred via breast milk. In the case of aspirin, it is salicylic acid that passes into the milk and not acetyl-salicylic acid; thus, it does not interfere with platelets in the infant.

Renal excretion is also immature early in life and a drug that depends on renal excretion, such as *caffeine*, *theophylline*, and some antibiotics, will accumulate in the infant in the first weeks and months of life but will gradually be better tolerated as the infant excretes it more effectively. These same drugs when given to an infant directly are given less frequently (daily instead of twice daily) in the first week of life.

3.4   Milk plasma ratio

The milk/plasma (M/P) ratio for drugs has been measured and reported for a number of medications. The milk plasma ratio is the concentration of the drug in the milk at the same moment that the concentration in maternal plasma is measured. It assumes that the relationship between the two remains constant, but in most cases it does not. Therefore, the M/P ratio is often calculated from the average concentrations in the blood and milk over a longer period of several hours. These average concentrations are the area under the respective concentration curves (area under curve, or AUC), which are constructed from individual concentrations reported over the course of the time interval. The latter method is preferred in the newer studies because the M/P values they establish are more representative. Nevertheless, to some extent there are considerable variations in the M/P ratios calculated, not only between different studies and subjects, but also with the same mother: the colostrum has different concentrations than the milk some weeks later, and the first milk of a breastfeed is different from a sample taken later in the same feed. Thus, the M/P ratios cited in the following chapters should be viewed only as approximate values. They represent the mean values of present experience, and are useful only for a rough comparison with other medications.

The M/P ratio is not suitable for comparison of drug risks. A milk/plasma ratio of 1 assumes that the levels are the same in both plasma and milk. If, however, the level is very low in the plasma, it will also be low in the milk, even though the milk plasma ratio is 1. Low M/P ratios

Lactation

3 General commentary on drug therapy and drug risk during lactation

(0.1) indicate that there is no accumulation in the mother's milk. However, significant concentrations in the milk can be reached even with low M/P ratios when there is a high maternal plasma value. On the other hand, relevant or even toxic amounts of medication cannot necessarily be assumed from a high M/P ratio with those drugs where the concentration in the maternal serum is very limited because of a high distribution volume typical for the particular medication. In such a case, even an M/P ratio of 8, which indicates a relative accumulation in the milk compared to the maternal plasma, means only a limited concentration of the medication in the milk, and consequently only a limited relative dosage (see below).

3.5   Amount of medication in the milk and relative dose

The simple calculation to determine the amount of the drug which the infant would consume via the milk in a day's time can be calculated by multiplying the concentration in the mother's milk (C_M) by the volume of milk consumed (V_M).

The amount of milk produced daily is between 500 and 900 mL. This amount is achieved about 4 days after birth. In order to better compare the different medications, the average daily amount per kg bodyweight that the infant takes in, rather than the individual total amount of milk consumed, is used as a basis for calculation. It is presumed that an infant receives about 150 mL/kg per day (=0.15 L/kg per day).

If, for example, the concentration of a medication in the milk is 50 μg/L, the exclusively breastfed baby receives:

$$50 \ \mu g/L \times 0.15 \ L/kg \ daily = 7.5 \ \mu g/kg \ daily$$

Sometimes there is also information about how much medication a child takes in with each meal. This method of calculating can make sense in the case of a single dosage of a drug with a short half-life. Based on the assumption of five breastfeeds a day, a child would drink 150/5 = 30 mL/kg per breastfeed (=0.03 L/kg per breastfeed). The amount of ingested drug is calculated analogous to the formula above (see also Bennett 1996):

$$\frac{50 \ \mu g/L \times 0.15 \ L/kg \ daily}{5} = 1.5 \ \mu g/kg \ per \ breastfeed$$

In the first month or so of life, infants breastfeed at least six to eight times a day.

The relative dose is the proportion of the maternal dosage per kg bodyweight that the breastfed baby takes in from the milk per kg of his bodyweight – i.e. the percentage of the maternal weight-related dosage:

$$Relative \ dosage \ (\%) = \frac{dosage \ via \ mother's \ milk/kg}{maternal \ dosage/kg} \times 100$$

Using the above example, and assuming that the maternal daily dosage of medication is 150 mg (=150,000 μg), the mother weighs 60 kg, and the baby takes in 7.5 μg/kg daily as calculated above, then the relative dosage is:

$$\text{Relative dosage} = \frac{7.5\ \mu g/kg\ \text{daily}}{150,000\ \mu g\ \text{daily}/60} \times 100 = 0.3\%$$

Compared to the M/P ratio, the "Relative dose" is more appropriate for estimating the exposure risk for the child via breast milk because it considers the distribution volume of the drug (see Table 3.3).

3.6   Toxicity of medications in the mother's milk

Via breast, most medications reach the child in limited amounts of under 3% of a therapeutic dosage per kg bodyweight. Thus, a toxic effect is unlikely. However, some aspects have to be considered: firstly, metabolites of the medication may also have pharmacological effects; and secondly, medications with longer half-lives can accumulate, especially in younger or premature newborns (Hale 2003). In such cases, a relative dosage of 3% may cause serum concentrations in the child that by far exceed 3% of the therapeutic serum concentration in the mother.

When the baby's feeding behavior changes while the mother is taking medication, this does not necessarily mean that there has been a toxic effect. Just like maternal diet, a medication can alter the sensory qualities of the milk and lead to "feeding problems."

Most medications reach concentrations in the mother's milk far below a therapeutic level for an infant. Only very rarely are toxic amounts measured. However, when medication is taken over a long period, even drugs with a low relative dosage may accumulate as a result of the prolonged half-life in infancy, and lead to symptoms. For this reason, the repeated administration of a medication must be more critically viewed than a single dosage.

Of a group of 838 mothers who had drug therapy while breastfeeding, about 11% reported symptoms in their infants that were possibly caused by the medication. In no case did this involve serious symptoms needing

Table 3.3 Comparison of the M/P ratio and relative drug dose

Drug	M/P ratio	Relative dose (%)
Atenolol	3	8–19
Chlortalidone	0.06	15.5
Captopril	0.03	0.014
Sotalol	4	42
Iodine	15–65	49
Pentoxyverin	10	1.4
Propylthiouracil	0.1	1.5
Carbimazole	1	27
Valproic acid	0.05	7
Lithium	1	80

Lactation

3 General commentary on drug therapy and drug risk during lactation

therapeutic intervention. The following associations were observed by the mothers (Ito 1993a):

- Antibiotics decreased stool consistency.
- Analgesics, narcotics, sedatives, antidepressants, antiepileptics: sedation.
- Antihistamines: irritability.

Toxic effects need to be considered more with very young infants than with those above 2 months of age, or even with an older baby who is only breastfed once or twice a day. Newborns and especially premature infants are more at risk because neither the clearance nor the functional competency of barriers, such as the blood–brain barrier, is completely developed (Hale 2003). Particularly in the case of long-term therapy, attention must be paid to symptoms in the infant.

In a review of all published reports on toxic symptoms in breastfed infants, Anderson (2003) evaluated 100 eligible case descriptions. Causality between maternal exposure and symptoms in the infant was categorized as "possible" in 53 cases, and "probable" in 47. In three of 100 cases the infants died; their mothers were all exposed to psychotropic substances and to additional risk factors like drugs of abuse. Of the 100 children, 63 were younger than 1 month, 78 were a maximum of 2 months old, and only four were older than 6 months.

In some cases, an interruption of breastfeeding following the administration of medication may make sense. This may be easier to adhere to if the mother chooses, for instance, to take the medication in the evening after the breastfeed. By avoiding the peak plasma times, the maternal drug levels that reach the milk can be minimized. To "clean" the milk by pumping makes no sense since the maternal reservoir is too large. In the case of *paracetamol* (acetaminophen), it was even demonstrated that there was a higher concentration of medication if the breast had been frequently pumped (Notarianni 1987).

The risk of an increased icterus in the newborn as a result of medication in the milk is often overestimated. For example, a bilirubin measurement does not reflect the amount of free bilirubin; the minimal amounts of medication and today's established control and phototherapy make the possibility of any damage less likely. In an otherwise healthy newborn, the risk for bilirubin encephalopathy as a result of medication in the mother's milk is low, even in the presence of the rare metabolic disorder glucose-6-phosphate-dehydrogenase deficiency, in which patients are disposed to hemolysis.

There is very little experience regarding the question of long-term effects caused by medications that the baby receives through the milk. However, it is theoretically possible, for example, for specific sensitization through antibiotics and an increase of allergies as a result of various sorts of chemicals. Psychotropic medications and drugs could have a negative effect on later behavior and intellectual development, and potentially carcinogenic substances could promote the development of a tumor at a later stage. At present, however, there is no serious suspicion of such damage resulting exclusively from the mother's milk, and independently from intrauterine exposure or direct postnatal exposure. However, studies of long-term effects are rare.

The following exposures are known to be problematic in breastfeeding and require individual decisions:

- Antineoplastic drugs.
- Radionuclides.

- Combination therapy with several psychotropic drugs or antiepileptics.
- Iodine-containing contrast media, iodine-containing expectorants, and broad-based iodine-containing disinfectants.
- Opioids if more than single doses up to 2 days.

When administration cannot be avoided in an individual case, it must be decided whether to abandon breastfeeding temporarily or permanently. For details, see the appropriate chapters.

The provision of pain relief in the post-partum woman has been challenging. *Codeine* has been a popular and presumably safe option. There are, however, women who are rapid metabolizers and others who are poor metabolizers of codeine into *morphine* (Etwel 2014). Pharmacogenetics have helped identify the metabolic issues. Codeine is a prodrug which is transformed into morphine by the highly polymorphic cytochrome P450 enzyme. Individuals who are ultra-rapid metabolizers have 50% higher plasma concentrations of morphine and its glucuronides than the average person. Poor metabolizers usually have no benefit from codeine. The safe use of codeine during breastfeeding is dependent on knowing how the mother handles the drug. Life threatening CNS depression can occur in breastfeeding infants. A case reported by Koren (2006) demonstrated a lethal effect when one mother continued taking codeine after discharge from hospital. Neonates metabolize morphine very slowly for the first 2 to 6 months of age.

It is recommended that maternal codeine use be limited to four days. Careful observation for signs and symptoms of CNS depression in the breastfeeding infant is mandatory (Kelly 2013). Similar metabolic issues exist with ultra-rapid metabolizers of merperidine (Etwel 2014).

3.7 Medications that affect lactation

Medications with an antidopamine effect, such as *phenothiazine, haloperidol*, and other neuroleptics, such as *sulpiride* and *risperidone*, as well as the antihypertensive α-*methyldopa*, and medications used to stimulate intestinal peristalsis, *domperidone* and *metoclopramide*, can, as a result of increasing the secretion of prolactin, stimulate milk production. The sympatholytic action of *reserpine* can have the same effect. Growth hormone and thyrotrophin-releasing hormone can also enhance milk production. Domperidone and metoclopramide are used for this purpose – for example, 10 mg metoclopramid three times a day (for a maximum of 7–10 days) and then tapering off the dosage for 2–5 days is recommended. Domperidone (not available in the USA) is less capable of crossing the blood–brain barrier, and therefore the risk of extrapyramidal symptoms is remote. Due to a molecular mass of 426, protein binding of 90%, and poor oral bioavailability, the relative dose for a fully breastfed child is only 0.4% (see Chapter 4.3). A dose of 50 mg of sulpiride two to three times a day, or 10 mg of *chlorpromazine* three times a day, have also been tried (Hallbauer 1997). Extrapyramidal symptoms and tiredness in the mother make use of the latter two medications questionable. In addition, it has been repeatedly reported that individual psychological and technical support of the mother is as successful as prolactin-activating medication in resolving breastfeeding problems, or even with relactation (see, for example, Seema 1997).

Oxytocin stimulates the milk ejection reflex (also called the letdown reflex). For this reason, and because it also encourages uterine involution, it is the drug of choice for the often painful engorgement. *Amphetamines, diuretics, estrogen* and *dopamine agonists* from the group of *ergotamine derivatives* – such as, for instance, *bromocriptine, cabergolin, lisuride, methylergometrine (methylergonovine), pergolide,* and the drug *quinagolide,* all of which have an antiprolactin action – can reduce the production of milk. The various *prostaglandins* have been observed both to enhance and impede milk production. *Alcohol* and *opiates* cause a decline in the milk ejection due to reduction in the release of oxytocin.

Bromocriptine has been used especially for weaning. However, the possible risks for the mother led to its cautious use and FDA restriction in the United States. Because of the possible cardiovascular side effects, the American Food and Drug Administration (FDA) has rescinded the (earlier) permission to prescribe bromocriptine for weaning. Physical measures such as well-fitted supportive clothing, cooling, and emptying the breasts until the mother feels relieved are preferable to ergotamine derivatives. In the case of mastitis, recommendations are bed rest, frequent emptying of the breast (after first using heat), and cooling it afterwards, as well as antibiotic therapy in some cases. Binding the breasts is no longer recommended because of the danger of engorgement. However, mothers are instructed to wear firm-fitting brassieres.

High-dosage *estrogen* is no longer used for weaning because of the risk of thromboembolism. The low estrogen content in the oral contraceptives which are available today limit milk production, if at all, only then when lactation is already poorly established. Pure *gestagen* contraceptives have no influence on the amount of milk produced. Progesterone compounds can inhibit milk production if used in the first 2 weeks postpartum.

3.8   Breastfeeding support

Inquiries from breastfeeding mothers about regional lactation consultants and self-help groups for questions and problems connected with breastfeeding can be addressed to the organizations listed below.

The following organizations are the International Centers from which local addresses can be obtained. Prescription of drugs and medications requires a license to practice (MDs and Nurse Practitioners).

Medical organizations

1. Academy of Breastfeeding Medicine (ABM) (physician only), www.bfmed.org/
2. International Society for Research in Human Milk and Lactation (ISRHML) (doctoral level researchers). General Enquiries, Secretary/Treasurer, Dr. Michelle (Shelley) McGuire, smcguire@wsu.edu

Lactation organizations

1. International Board of Lactation Consultant Examiners (IBLCE), http://iblce.org/
2. International Lactation Consultant Organization (ILCA), www.ilca.org
3. La Leche League International (LLLI), www.lalecheleague.org/

References

Anderson PO, Pochop SL, Manoguerra AS. Adverse drug reaction in breastfed infants: less than imagined. Clin Pediatrics 2003; 42: 325–40.

Behrman RE, Kliegman RM, Jenson HB (eds). Nelson Textbook of Pediatrics, 16th edn. Philadelphia, PA: Saunders, 2000.

Bennett PN (ed.). Drugs and Human Lactation, 2nd ed. Amsterdam: Elsevier, 1996.

Etwel F, Hutson JR, Madadi P, et al. Fetal and perinatal exposure to drugs and chemicals: novel biomarkets of risk. Annu Rev Pharmacol Toxicol 2014; 54: 295–315.

Eidelman AI, Schanler RJ. Section on Breastfeeding Committee. Breastfeeding and the use of human milk. Pediatrics 2012; 129: e287–841.

Hale TW. Medications in breastfeeding mothers of preterm infants. Pediatric Annals 2003; 32: 337–47.

Hallbauer U. Sulpiride (Eglonyl) – use to stimulate lactation. SA Med J 1997; 87: 774–5.

Hanson L. Immunobiology of human milk. Amarillo, TX: Pharmasoft Publishing, 2004.

Ip S, Chung M, Raman G et al. A summary of the Agency for Healthcare Research and Quality's evidence report on breastfeeding in developed countries. Breastfeed Med 2009; 4: S17–30.

Ito S, Blajchman A, Stephenson M et al. Prospective follow-up of adverse reactions in breastfed infants exposed to maternal medication. Am J Obstet Gynecol 1993a; 168: 1393–9.

Ito S, Koren G, Einarson TR. Maternal noncompliance with antibiotics during breastfeeding. Ann Pharmacother 1993b; 27: 40.

Kelly LE, Chaudhry SA, Rieder MJ et al. A Clinical tool for reducing central nervous system depression among neonates exposed to codeine through breastmilk. PLoS One 2013; 8: e70073.

Koren G, Cairns J, Chitayat D et al. Pharmacogenetics of morphine poisoning in a breastfed neonate of a codeine-prescribed mother. Lancet 2006; 368: 704.

Lawrence RA, Lawrence RM. Breastfeeding: A Guide for the Medical Profession. St Louis, MI: Mosby, 7th Ed, 2010.

Notarianni LJ, Oldham HG, Bennett PN. Passage of paracetamol into breast milk and its subsequent metabolism by the neonate. Br J Clin Pharmacol 1987; 24: 63–7.

Sachs C. Committee on Drugs. The transfer of drugs and therapeutics into human breast milk: An update on selected topics. Pediatrics 2013; 132: e796–809.

Seema, MD, Patwari AK, Satyanarayana L. Relactation: an effective intervention to promote exclusive breastfeeding. J Trop Pediatrics 1997; 43: 213–16.

Specific drug therapies during lactation

4

4.1 Analgesics, antiphlogistics and anesthetics (Maria Ellfolk and Stefanie Hultzsch)   653

4.2 Antiallergics, antiasthmatics and antitussives (Paul Merlob and Corinna Weber-Schöndorfer)   671

4.3 Gastrointestinal drugs (Paul Merlob and Corinna Weber-Schöndorfer)   677

4.4 Anti-infectives (Stephanie Padberg)   687

4.5 Vaccines and immunoglobulins (Ruth A. Lawrence and Mary Panse)   705

4.6 Cardiovascular drugs and diuretics (Paul Merlob and Corinna Weber-Schöndorfer)   711

4.7 Anticoagulants, thrombocyte aggregation inhibitors and fibrinolytics (Paul Merlob and Juliane Habermann)   725

4.8 Antiepileptics (Paul Merlob and Christof Schaefer)   731

4.9 Psychotropic drugs (Paul Merlob and Christof Schaefer)   743

4.10 Immunomodulating and antineoplastic agents (Paul Merlob and Corinna Weber-Schöndorfer)   775

4.11 Hormones and hormone antagonists (Gerard H.A. Visser and Corinna Weber-Schöndorfer)   783

4.12 Dermatological medication and local therapeutics (Christof Schaefer and Gudula Kirtschig)   797

4.13 Alternative remedies, vitamins, and minerals (Ruth A. Lawrence and Eleanor Hüttel)   803

4.14 Contrast media, radionuclides and diagnostics (Stefanie Hultzsch)   813

4.15 Infections during breastfeeding (Bernke te Winkel and Christof Schaefer)   821

4.16 Recreational drugs (Mark Anderson and Marc Oppermann)   835

4.17 Plant toxins (Ruth A. Lawrence and Christof Schaefer)   845

4.18 Industrial chemicals and environmental contaminants (Ruth A. Lawrence and Christof Schaefer)   847

Please note that in the following chapters drugs are discussed under their generic names. For trade names, refer to the Physician's Desk Reference or comparable pharmacopoeias of your country.

Only a limited number of drugs have been studied with respect to their quantitative passage into mother's milk. Over the years, analytic methods have been considerably refined. Results of older studies (such as for propylthiouracil) needed to be revised. In the following sections, medications, arranged according to indications, are evaluated with the proviso that the currently available results are by no means definitive. Wherever possible, the amount of medication that the infant receives with the milk is given as a percentage of the maternal therapeutic daily dosage (per kilogram bodyweight; see Chapter 3). The terms "percentage of weight-related maternal dosage" and "relative dosage" used in the text are synonymous. Sometimes the percentage of the drug that the baby takes in per feeding is given. This way of calculating can make sense in the case of a single dose with active ingredients that have a short half-life. When there is a recommended dosage for therapeutic use in infancy or childhood, the relative dosage will, in some cases, be compared to this instead of to the maternal dosage.

Presuming an average daily breastmilk intake of 150 mL/kg of the child's bodyweight, the infant's weight-related exposure to the medication is identical to the amount of medication in 150 mL of milk (again, see Chapter 3). When protein binding and the half-life of a particular drug are mentioned, these values refer to the relationships in adults (i.e. in the mother) unless otherwise indicated. For some medications, the reference "Bennett 1996" is given for the sake of an overview. This is a standard publication of the European WHO Working Group. We refer less often to the classification of the American Academy of Pediatrics, Committee on Drugs (2001), cited more frequently in other places, because there is, for the most part, no additional information in this source.

References

American Academy of Pediatrics, Committee on Drugs. The transfer of drugs and other chemicals into human milk. Pediatrics 2001; 108: 776–89.
Bennett PN (ed.). Drugs and Human Lactation, 2nd edn. Amsterdam: Elsevier, 1996.

Analgesics, antiphlogistics and anesthetics

4.1

Maria Ellfolk and Stefanie Hultzsch

4.1.1	Paracetamol	653
4.1.2	Acetylsalisylic acid	654
4.1.3	Pyrazolone and phenylbutazone derivatives	655
4.1.4	Non-steroidal anti-inflammatory drugs (NSAID)	655
4.1.5	Selective COX-2 inhibitors	657
4.1.6	Other antirheumatics	658
4.1.7	Migraine medications	659
4.1.8	Opioids and opioid derivatives	660
4.1.9	Local anesthetics	664
4.1.10	Other medications used in connection with anesthesia	665
4.1.11	Myotonolytics and other analgesics	666
4.1.12	Gout therapy	666

Paracetamol and ibuprofen are the drugs of choice for treating pain and their use requires no limitation of breastfeeding. Continuous treatment with acetylsalicylic acid is not recommended and selective COX-2 inhibitors should be avoided because of limited experience on their use during breastfeeding. Sumatriptan or eletriptan can be used to treat migraine. Muscle relaxants should not be taken during breastfeeding.

Opiates can be used for a few days, if paracetamol or ibuprofens are not effective. However, close observation of the baby is essential as many cases of opiate-induced toxic effects in breastfed infants have been reported. Particular care should be taken if the baby is born preterm or is less than a month old as opiate metabolism and excretion is undeveloped in neonates and drug accumulation and toxicity is possible.

Neither general nor local anesthesia requires interruption of breastfeeding.

4.1.1   Paracetamol

The half-life of *paracetamol* is 2.6 hours, both in the mother's plasma and milk, and the milk/plasma ratio is close to unity (Bitzén 1981, Berlin 1980). After a single dose of 650 mg paracetamol to 12 nursing mothers, maximum milk concentrations were 10–15 mg/L recorded 1–2 hours

Drugs During Pregnancy and Lactation. **http://dx.doi.org/10.1016/B978-0-12-408078-2.00026-3**

post-dose. The maximum exposure for a fully breastfed infant would be 0.45 mg/kg, which corresponds to 4% of the weight-related therapeutic dose for infants (Berlin 1980). Another study including three nursing mothers reported that after a single dose of 500 mg paracetamol, the maximum measured concentration in breast milk was 4.39 mg/L, and the authors estimated infant exposure to be less than 0.1% of maternal dose (Bitzén 1981). One report of adverse effects in the breast-fed infant has been reported to date: a case of reproducible maculopapular rash following a maternal dose of 1 g of paracetamol, suggesting causal association (Matheson 1985). The concentration in breast milk was low and the dose ingested by the infant would only amount to 1 mg per feed. Further, one study including 43 infants whose mothers were treated with paracetamol were followed and no side effects were observed in any of the infants (Ito 1993). Even though drug metabolism is not fully developed in newborns, and an accumulation of paracetamol in the breastfed infant could theoretically be possible, it has not been reported. Paracetamol is used to treat pain and fever in neonates and it can even be given to premature infants (van Lingen 1999).

> **Recommendation.** *Ibuprofen* and paracetamol are the analgesics/antiphlogistics of choice during breastfeeding.

4.1.2   Acetylsalisylic acid

Only small amounts of *acetylsalicylic acid* (ASA) are excreted in milk, with a milk/plasma ratio of <0.1 (Bailey 1982). Peak values in breast milk are reached in 2–6 hours post dose but may delay even more (Bailey 1982, Jamali 1981). In a study of five breastfeeding mothers the highest salicylate concentration in breast milk after a 500 mg dose was 7.8 mg/L, after a 1,000 mg dose was 21 mg/L, and after a 1,500 mg dose was 48 mg/L (Jamali 1981).

One case report describes a 16-day old infant with serum concentrations of 240 mg/L salicylate suffering from tachypnea, metabolic acidosis and tachycardia. The mother used 3.9 g ASA daily. Because of the unexpectedly high drug concentration, the authors also considered the possibility that the child herself was given ASA (Clark 1981). Another case report describes a woman using 2.4 g ASA daily for rheumatic disease during pregnancy and postpartum. The child was born slightly preterm at 36 gestational weeks. At the age of 2 months, while only partially breast-fed, the infant serum salicylate concentration was nearly 30% of maternal drug concentration (0.47 mmol/L versus 1.63 mmol/L, respectively). The child did not have any symptoms. The authors concluded that the neonatal immature hepatic metabolism and renal excretion capacity might have predisposed to the high serum drug concentration (Unsworth 1987). In a study based maternal interviews, 15 mothers used ASA during breastfeeding and none of the infants were reported to have any symptoms; however, no data on dose or length of treatment was recorded (Ito 1993). In users, aspirin in analgesic doses (>500 mg/day) is associated with risk of platelet dysfunction and possibly also with Reye's syndrome in children. Repeated analgesic doses should therefore be avoided during breastfeeding. Adverse effects would not be expected in the breastfed infant if the mother uses low-dose therapy (100–300 mg/day) or takes occasional analgesic doses.

> **Recommendation.** Ibuprofen and paracetamol are the analgesics/antiphlogistics of choice during breastfeeding. Occasional use of ASA is acceptable but repeated use with analgesic doses should be avoided. Low-dose ASA (50–300 mg/day) is considered safe.

4.1.3   Pyrazolone and phenylbutazone derivatives

Little documented experience exists on the use of drugs from this group during breastfeeding.

Dipyrone or *metamizol* is excreted in milk, the M/P-ratio being close to unity, including the four main metabolites (Zylber-Katz 1986). Breast milk and plasma levels of dipyrone were investigated in eight lactating women after a single oral dose of 1.0 g. Concentration-time curves were presented for two mothers, indicating that the peak levels for the different metabolites occurred at 2–18 hours post-dose, and none of the metabolites were detected in milk samples after 48 hours (Zylber-Katz 1986). One case report describes cyanotic attacks in an infant of a mother who had taken three doses of 500 mg dipyrone. A milk sample, and blood samples from both mother and infant were taken 24 hours after the last dose. The concentration of dipyrone in milk was 4.3 µg/mL, and the serum concentration was similar in the mother and the infant (3.3 µg/mL and 3.2 µg/mL, respectively) (Rizzoni 1984). Dipyrone is no longer widely used due to the potential serious hematological adverse effects, as safer alternatives are available.

Phenylbutazone has a half-life of 30–170 hours. No detailed information on the passage to human milk is available. No adverse effects have been reported and the American Academic of Pediatrics (AAP) Committee on Drugs considers its occasional use compatible with breastfeeding (AAP 2001). However, due to the long half-life and the potentially serious adverse effects which include hematological disturbances and renal and liver toxicity, use during breast feeding is not justifiable. One report describes a case of hemolytic anemia in the breastfed infant when the mother was taking propyphenazone after delivery. *Propyphenazone* was detected in infant plasma during the acute phase of hemolysis, and could still be detected in the milk 8 days after stopping treatment (Frei 1985). Similarly to phenylbutazone, propyphenazone has been largely replaced by newer non-steroidal anti-inflammatory drugs (NSAIDs) with a more favorable safety profile.

No information on *famprofazone* and breast-feeding is available. Famprofazone is metabolized to metamphetamine and amphetamine. Use is contraindicated during breast feeding, as safer alternatives are available.

> **Recommendation.** Ibuprofen and paracetamol are the analgesics/antiphlogistics of choice during breastfeeding. Pyrazolone and phenylbutazone derivatives should be avoided. Accidental intake of the other above-mentioned drugs does not require any limitations of breastfeeding but the medication should be changed.

4.1.4   Non-steroidal anti-inflammatory drugs (NSAID)

Non-steroidal anti-inflammatory drugs (NSAIDs) are acidic, have limited lipofilicity and are highly plasma protein bound (up to 99%), resulting

Lactation

4.1 Analgesics, antiphlogistics and anesthetics

in low M/P-ratios. The AAP has evaluated that *ibuprofen, naproxen, diclofenac, indomethacin, ketorolac, piroxicam, mefenamic acid* and *flufenamic acid* are all compatible with breastfeeding (AAP 2001).

Ibuprofen has a half-life of 2 hours. Transfer to milk is minimal and no adverse events related to exposure via breast milk have been reported. Following daily administration of 800–1600 mg ibuprofen to 13 lactating women, no ibuprofen could be detected in the milk. The detection limit in the studies were 0.5 µg/mL and 1 µg/mL and, respectively (Townsend 1984, Weibert 1983). In a further report, 400 mg ibuprofen was given every 6–8 hours to a lactating woman for dental surgery, confirming minimal exposure to the infant (Walter 1997). Ibuprofen is also widely used in pediatrics.

The half-life for naproxen is 10–18 hours and much longer than for several other NSAIDs. In a study of a breastfeeding mother receiving long-term naproxen therapy (250–375 mg × 2), the maximum relative infant dose was calculated as 3.6% (Jamali 1983). Another study based on maternal interviews included 20 mothers who used naproxen while breastfeeding (Ito 1993). Two of the mothers reported symptoms (slight sleepiness) in their children. However, no data on dose or length of treatment were reported, and no conclusions about causal association can be made on the basis of these results (Ito 1993).

Diclofenac has a short half-life (1–2 hours). No original data on transfer to milk have been published. However, due to the pharmacokinetic profile, exposure via breast milk is expected to be minimal and no adverse effects have been reported.

Indomethacin has a half-life of 4 hours. One study, including 16 mothers who received 75–300 mg indomethacin daily for several days during the postpartum period reported low drug transfer to milk (M/P ratio 0.37). Plasma concentration was measured in seven of the infants and was above the detection limit in only one infant, the highest weight-related dose calculated as 1% for any of the infants (Lebedevs 1991). While exposure is probably minimal, the potential adverse effects on renal function, and the prolonged half-life of indomethacin in neonates and preterm infants make indomethacin less suitable for repeated use during breast feeding.

Keterolac has a half-life of 3–9 hours and is excreted into breast milk in small amounts. After 10 mg dose four times daily, the maximum milk concentration was 7.9 ng/mL, corresponding to a relative infant dose of 0.2%. In four out of ten mothers no ketorolac could be detected in milk (Wischnik 1989).

Piroxicam has a relatively long half-life of 30–60 hours. Small amounts are excreted in milk. Milk and plasma samples were analyzed in four women who received 20 mg piroxicam once a day for arthritis (Østensen 1988). At steady state the relative infant dose was calculated to average 3.5% and at most 6.3% of the weight-related maternal dose (Østensen 1988). A urine sample from one of the infants did not show any traces of piroxicam or its metabolites. Piroxicam is poorly absorbed from intact skin.

Flufenamic acid and mefenamic acid both have a short half-life, 2–3 hours. Minimal amounts of both drugs were detected in milk and infant serum in two studies both including ten mother/infant pairs, but using insensitive assay methods (Buchanan 1968, 1969).

There are no data for etofenamate and breast feeding. Systemic absorption through intact skin is 20%.

Flurbiprofen has a half-life of 3 hours. In a study of 12 women given 100–200 mg flurbiprofen daily, only three milk samples from two women contained detectable drug concentrations, the highest level measured 0.08 mg/mL. This corresponds to maximal infant exposure of 0.012 mg/kg/day or 0.5% of the maternal dose per kg. No toxic effects have been reported (Smith 1989, Cox 1987).

Ketoprofen has a short half-life, 1.5–2.5 hours. Low levels of ketoprofen in mother's milk were reported in a study where a combination of ketoprofen and nalbuphine was given to 18 mothers. The calculated relative infant dose of ketoprofen was 0.31% (Jacqz-Aigrain 2007). Tenoxicam has a long half-life of 42–100 hours and no apparent advantages over other NSAIDs. No published information on administration during breast feeding is available.

A single dose of tiaprofen 300 mg was given to three mothers in one study published only as an abstract. Transfer to milk was minimal and the relative infant dose was estimated as 1.7% (Jones 1986). No further conclusions can be made on the safety of tiaprofen use on the basis of this report.

There is no documented experience on the use of *acemethacin, dexketoprofen, lornoxicam, meloxicam, nabumetone* or *proglumetacin* during breastfeeding.

> **Recommendation.** Among the NSAIDs during breastfeeding, ibuprofen is the drug of first choice. For systemic therapy, diclofenac, indometacin and ketoprofen are also acceptable for short-term therapy. Repeated administration of piroxicam and naproxen should be avoided because of their relatively long half-lives but single doses are acceptable. Single doses of the other NSAID mentioned do not require any limitation of breastfeeding. Local application does not represent any hindrance to breastfeeding.

4.1.5   Selective COX-2 inhibitors

Celecoxib is a lipophilic substance and could therefore easily pass into mother's milk. However, it is 97% bound to plasma protein and it has a high volume of distribution, both of which limit passage into milk.

A case report describes a breastfeeding mother taking 100 mg celecoxib twice a day for 2 days. Milk sampling was started 5 hours after the last dose. The highest milk concentration was from the first sample (133 ng/mL), which would result in 20 µg/kg/day infant exposure (Knoppert 2003). Milk concentrations were further studied in two mothers after a single dose of 200 mg celecoxib, and in three mothers who had been using 200 mg celecoxib daily for several weeks. Two children were breastfed during the study and neither of them had any symptoms. The average dose transferred to the infant was minimal and corresponded to 0.3% of the weight-adjusted maternal daily dose (Hale 2004). In yet another study six women were given a single dose of 200 mg celecoxib. Similarly to other studies, the average relative infant dose was low, 0.23% (Gardiner 2006).

One study has been published on the transfer of rofecoxib into milk. Six women at weaning were given single doses of 25 mg rofecoxib. Milk-plasma ratio was 0.25, and the median relative infant dose was 2.1% (Gardiner 2005).

The analgesic effect of valdecoxib following a caesarean section was investigated in a study including 24 women. There was no difference in

Lactation

4.1 Analgesics, antiphlogistics and anesthetics

breastfeeding success when compared to the control group, however, no data were provided for the number of women actually breastfeeding their infants. No milk concentrations were measured but no adverse effects in the breastfed infants were reported (Carvalho 2006).

Parecoxib is a prodrug rapidly converted to the active moiety *valdecoxib*. The excretion of parecoxib and valdecoxib into milk was studied in 40 mothers receiving a single intravenous dose of 40 mg parecoxib (Paech 2012). Median milk concentrations were 0.75 µg/L for parecoxib and 31 µg/L for valdecoxib. The median combined relative infant dose for parecoxib and valdecoxib was 0.63% (Paech 2012).

There is no information on the use of the other selective COX-2 inhibitors during breastfeeding.

> **Recommendation.** Selective COX-2 inhibitors should be avoided due to the potential adverse effects on infant renal function and the limited experience with these substances during breastfeeding. However, short-term use of celecoxib can be considered if the infant is born full-term. Single doses of other COX-2 inhibitors do not require any limitation of breastfeeding.

4.1.6   Other antirheumatics

Gold compounds exist in an injectable form (*aurothiomalate*) and in an oral form (*auranofin*). Aurothiomalate has a half-life of 120–160 hours in serum but is stored in deep compartments in the body and can be detected in urine after 1 year after cessation of therapy. A mother receiving monthly intramuscular injections of 10 mg sodium aurothiomalate had gold concentrations varying between 15–30 µg/L in milk samples taken 5–21 days after gold administration. The infant's monthly gold intake would amount to 130 µg/kg, which is equivalent to or even higher than the maternal weight-related gold dose (Bennett 1990). Comparable milk levels have been reported by other groups: 50 mg weekly intramuscular aurothiomalate injections resulting in 22–40 µg/L milk gold concentrations (Bell 1976), and 20 mg weekly intramuscular aurothiomalate injections resulting in gold milk concentrations of 10–185 µg/L (Østensen 1986). Contrary to these findings, in one case report no gold could be detected in either the serum or the urine of a breastfed infant whose mother had received gold therapy for 20 weeks (Rooney 1987). Despite these conflicting data, it is apparent that systemic absorption occurs to some extent, exposing the infant to gold for long periods. There are no published data on auranofin and breast feeding.

Data for *hydroxychloroquine* suggest that the drug can be used relatively safely during breast feeding. One mother took 310 mg hydroxychloroquine daily for 6 weeks for SLE. The highest measured milk concentration was 1.46 mg/L and the mean concentration was calculated as 1.1 mg/L. The relative infant dose calculated for the 9-month-old infant was estimated as 2% (Nation 1984). Similar concentrations have been found in other reports: long term therapy with daily doses of 200–400 mg hydroxychloroquine in four women produced milk concentrations of 0.34–1.4 mg/L, with a relative infant dose calculated as 3% (Costedoat-Chalumeau 2002, 2004). Significantly lower hydroxychloroquine milk concentrations were reported in a woman who started on 200 mg of hydroxychloroquine twice a day. The highest milk concentration measured was 10.6 ng/mL (i.e. 10.6 µg/L). The total amount of hydroxy-chloroquine excreted into the milk over 48 hours was 3.2 µg, corresponding to 0.0003% of the maternal dose (Østensen 1985). Because of the potential retinotoxicity of hydroxychloroquine, long-term follow-up has been performed to children exposed in utero and during breast-feeding. Normal results in electroretinography were reported in six infants (age range 3–30 months) exposed prenatally to hydroxychloroquine, all but one exposed also via mother's milk (Cimaz 2004). Further, normal visual function and neurodevelopment during the first year of life was reported in 24 infants exposed to hydroxychloroquine during pregnancy, 13 of whom were also exposed by mother's milk (Motta 2005).

Leflunomide is considered a prodrug with the active metabolite M1 reported to have a half-life of 2 to 4 weeks. It is highly plasma protein bound, which makes significant milk transfer unlikely. There is no experience on its use during breastfeeding, however, due to the potent immunosuppressive activity, even small amounts reaching the infant could be hazardous.

D-Penicillamine is used today chiefly as a chelating agent and antidote in metal poisonings, and to treat Wilson's disease. One case report describes a mother suffering from cystinurea treated with 1.5 g pencillamine a day. She breastfed her infant for 3 months and the child developed normally (Gregory 1983). Another case report describes a mother suffering from Wilson's disease who was treated with penicillamine during two pregnancies and while breastfeeding. She breastfed her children for 3 months while taking 750 mg penicillamine a day. No adverse reactions were observed in the infants (Messner 1998).

> **Recommendation.** Among the basic antirheumatics, sulfasalazine, glucocorticoids and hydroxychloroquine are preferable during breastfeeding. Gold therapy should be avoided. *Azathioprine* and *cyclosporine* may also be prescribed . With certain restrictions, the biological agents adalimumab, etanercept and infliximab are apparently acceptable. Leflunomide is contraindicated. Ibuprofen is the antirheumatic of first choice.

4.1.7   Migraine medications

Sumatriptan exposure via mother's milk appears to be minimal. Five women were given a single subcutaneous dose of 6 mg sumatriptan. The mean relative infant dose was 3.5% of the maternal dose, but considering the low oral bioavailability of sumatriptan (14%) the exposure via milk is probably even lower (Wojnar-Horton 1996). *Eletriptan*, with a half-life of 4 hours, is also considered compatible with breast feeding. One study has been reported to include eight women given 80 mg eletriptan with no adverse effects observed in the infants. Drug concentration in breast milk was reported to be minimal at 24 hours (Hutchinson 2013).

There are no studies on *almotriptan, frovatriptan, naratriptan, rizatriptan* and *zolmitriptan* during breast feeding.

There are no data on the passage of the ergotamines into mother's milk. *Ergotamine* and *ergotamine tartrate* are more fat soluble than dihydroergotamine and their secretion into mother's milk is more likely. Ergotamine derivatives have antiprolactin action and their use may decrease milk production. No difference was observed in milk production between mothers receiving ergot therapy for 6 days and the control group receiving no treatment (Jolivet 1978).

Lactation

4.1 Analgesics, antiphlogistics and anesthetics

Recommendation. If ibuprofen, diclofenac, naproxen, ketoprofen or parac-etamol (in combination with *caffeine* or *codeine*) are not sufficiently effective for a migraine attack, ASA is also acceptable. When conventional treatment fails, single doses of sumatriptan or eletriptan are considered relatively safe during breast-feeding. The accompanying nausea can be treated with metoclopramide. Use of ergot alkaloids is not recommended but single doses do not require any limita-tion of breastfeeding. Medications compatible with breastfeeding for preventive migraine treatment include tricyclic antidepressants (amitriptyline, nortriptyline), beta-blockers (metoprolol, propranolol, bisoprolol); and when other treatment options fail, *valproic acid* is also acceptable.

4.1.8   Opioids and opioid derivatives

▶ **Morphine and hydromorphone**

Morphine has low oral bioavailability (26%) which limits infant expo-sure (Bar-Oz 2003). Excretion of morphine into milk was studied in five women undergoing surgery earliest a month after delivery. The highest milk concentration of morphine (500 μg/L) was found in a mother 30 minutes after she was given 15 mg morphine (10 mg i.v. and 5 mg i.m.). The amount per feed would add up to 10–20 μg morphine, assuming that the oral bioavailability of morphine in infants is the same as in adults (Feilberg 1989). One case report describes significant exposure to the nursing infant when the mother was taking 5 mg morphine four times a day (Robieux 1990). The mother had been using morphine regu-larly for arthritic back pain, and the dose was gradually lowered during breast-feeding, being 40 mg/day the day before the study. The infant serum morphine concentration was in the analgesic range (4 μg/L). The highest concentration in milk, 100 μg/L, was measured before feeding and 4 hours after dosing. Calculating from the highest milk levels, some discrepancy exists with the unexpectedly high serum concentration in the infant. The authors concluded that exposure via mother' milk may be substantial (Robieux 1990). Limited amounts of morphine and its active metabolite morphine-6-glucuronide were found in the colostrum of seven women after postpartum patient-controlled analgesia with mor-phine following a caesarean section (Baka 2002). To conclude, infant exposure is limited by the poor oral bioavailability of morphine, however, substantial absorption may occur in the neonate. Further, repeated expo-sure may result in accumulation due to slower elimination in neonates resulting from immature drug metabolism and urinary excretion capacity (Bouwmeester 2004). Genetic differences in the capacity to convert mor-phine to the active metabolite morphine-6-glucuronide may also influence risk (Koren 2007). Due to the serious potential adverse effects, including central nervous system and respiratory depression, great caution is justified.

Eight breastfeeding women were given a single intranasal dose of hydro-morphone 2 mg. The relative infant dose was 0.67%. Based on these results a fully breastfed infant would receive a total of 2.2 μg/kg/day of hydromor-phone, which is less than 10% of the therapeutic dose for infants. The infants were not nursed during the study (Edwards 2003).

Recommendation. Opiate analgesics should only be used for short periods (1–2 days) during breastfeeding. Because of the potential for central nervous system and respiratory depression, particular caution is justified in premature infants and in infants with pre-existing conditions increasing vulnerability. Long-term use is contraindicated.

▶ Codeine, oxycodone and hydrocodone

Codeine is a prodrug. It is converted by the enzyme *CYP2D6* to *morphine*, which is responsible for the analgesic effect. The enzyme CYP2D6 displays a large degree of polymorphism. Ultrarapid metabolizers have several functional copies of the gene and they convert codeine to morphine extensively and quickly. Both codeine itself and its metabolite morphine are glucuronidated and then excreted from the body. Around 10% of the morphine is converted by the enzyme UGT2B7 to morphine-6-glucuronide which is pharmacologically active (Coller 2009). The glucuronidation capacity of the liver is limited at birth and increases gradually by 2–6 months of age. The elimination half-life of morphine and codeine is thus extended in newborns and accumulation may occur (Madadi 2009).

Codeine has a half-life of 3 hours in adults, low protein binding (7–25%) and oral bioavailability of 100%. A single dose of 60 mg codeine given to two nursing mothers indicated that codeine passes easily into mother's milk with a M/P-ratio of 1.3–2.5. Peak milk concentration was reached in 1 hour (Findlay 1981).

Maternal codeine use is usually well tolerated by breastfed infants. In a study of seven mothers and their eleven breastfed neonates the codeine concentration in milk varied between 34–314 µg/L in samples taken 20–240 min after drug dosing. The mothers had taken 1–12 doses of 60 mg codeine every 4–6 hours before giving the milk samples. Codeine concentration in infant plasma varied between 0.8–4.5 µg/L in samples taken 1–4 hours after breastfeeding. Morphine concentration in milk varied between 1.9–20.5 µg/L and in infant plasma between 0.5–2.2 µg/L (Meny 1993).

However, there are also many case reports on adverse effects in breastfed infants following maternal codeine use. Most of them describe apnea (Lam 2012a, Naumburg 1988, Davis 1985) and lethargy (Lam 2012a). Bradycardia has also been reported (Davis 1985, Smith 1982). In the case reported by Smith, the observed bradycardia was probably not connected to maternal codeine use. A 1-week-old infant had bradycardia 6 days after the mother had taken a single oral dose of 30 mg codeine. The infant's bradycardia dissolved in 24 hours (Smith 1982).

There is also a report of death in an infant following maternal codeine use during breastfeeding. The mother was prescribed a paracetamol-codeine combination after birth. Due to side-effects she reduced the prescribed dose on the second day of treatment to 30 mg twice daily. When the child was 7-days-old he showed signs of lethargy and began to breast-feed poorly. On day 12 his skin color was grey and milk intake had fallen. On day 13 the infant was found dead. Post-mortem serum concentration of morphine was 70 ng/mL. The mother had stored milk on day 10 for later use, with a morphine concentration of 87 ng/mL, and much higher than previously reported. A genotype analysis on CYP2D6 was carried out and the mother turned out to be an ultra-rapid metabolizer (Koren 2006). The causal relationship between maternal codeine use and the death of her infant in this case has been questioned by some authors (Bateman 2008, Ferner 2008). Postmortem serum samples are difficult to interpret as drug from the tissues redistribute into serum after death. There have also been reports of infants exposed to similar concentrations of morphine in milk without displaying any symptoms (Bateman 2008, Ferner 2008).

In a retrospective study interviewing 72 mothers who used codeine during breastfeeding, 17 infants were reported to have signs of central nervous system depression. Two of the mothers of symptomatic infants were ultra-rapid metabolizers of codeine (duplication of CYP2D6), one of them the case previously described (Koren 2006). Twelve mothers of symptomatic infants had also symptoms themselves (Madadi 2009). The Motherisk guidelines state that the occurrence of central nervous system depression is consistent between the mother and the baby. Therefore, if the mother suffers from symptoms of CNS depression the infant should also be examined (Kelly 2013).

Oxycodone 10 mg as needed (up to every 2 hours) was given to 50 mothers after a caesarean section and the milk and infant plasma levels were measured. The M/P-ratio was 3.2 and the highest milk concentration 168 µg/L. Serum samples from 41 neonates were also analyzed and oxycodone was detected in only one of the samples (Seaton 2007).

In a retrospective study a total of 533 mother-child pairs were contacted after use of oxycodone, codeine or paracetamol during breastfeeding. Of 139 mothers who used oxycodone, 28 reported that the child had symptoms of lethargy and sleepiness. The mothers of symptomatic infants took larger doses of oxycodone than those whose infants did not show any signs of CNS depression. All mothers took doses within the recommended range (not exceeding 40 mg/day) (Lam 2012b). There is also a case report describing lethargy and poor feeding in a 4-day-old infant whose mother had taken 15 mg oxycodone during the previous day. When the infant was given naloxone, the symptoms disappeared and the infant did well during the next 24 hours in follow-up at the hospital (Timm 2013).

Hydrocodone secretion into milk was studied in two breastfeeding women taking varying doses (5–35 mg/day) of hydrocodone. The absolute infant doses were 3.07 µg/kg/day and 8.57 µg/kg/day, corresponding to a relative infant dose of 3.1 and 3.7% (Anderson 2007). Hydrocodone excretion in milk was further studied in 30 postpartum women, indicating that the average relative infant dose was 1.6% (range 0.2–9.0%) (Sauberan 2011).

Recommendation. For an urgent indication, codeine can be taken temporarily (not longer than 2–3 days) in an analgesic combination preparation or as an antitussive. Longer-term therapy with the drugs discussed here (Codeine, oxycodone and hydrocodone) should not be undertaken during breastfeeding and should be critically viewed, especially in the first postpartum weeks. In any case, attention must be paid to any adverse symptoms in the breastfed baby, but also in the mother. Analgesics of first choice are paracetamol or ibuprofen.

► **Fentanyl, alfentanil, remifentanil, sufentanil**

The half-life of i.v. *fentanyl* is 3–12 hours, and for transdermal preparations 20–27 hours. Half-life in neonates is prolonged due to immature drug metabolism and renal excretion. Concentration of fentanyl in milk and mother's serum was determined in a study of 13 women who received fentanyl in analgesic dose (2 µg/kg i.v.) during caesarean section or postpartum tubal ligation (Steer 1992). Ten hours after administration virtually no fentanyl could be detected in milk. The maximum amount the infant could receive over a 24-hour period was determined as 16 ng/kg (Steer 1992). In another study, five women were given 100 µg i.v. fentanyl for surgery and milk was collected over the following 24 hours. The average amount of fentanyl excreted into the milk was 24 ng, corresponding to 0.024% of the maternal dose of 100 μg, and a relative infant dose 0.6% (Nitsun 2006). Further, the concentration of fentanyl in colostrum was measured in 100 women undergoing caesarean section and given fentanyl either epidurally or intravenously. The amounts found in milk were low (mean concentration 0.4 ng/mL 45 min after dosing) (Goma 2008). A further report describes a woman using transdermal fentanyl 100 μg/h throughout pregnancy and lactation. One month postpartum fentanyl concentration in milk was 6.4 ng/mL and neither fentanyl nor its metabolite could be detected in the infant's serum. The infant had been breastfed for 2 weeks by the time of the study (Cohen 2009).

Several studies suggesting negative effects of fentanyl neuraxial analgesia on the start and duration of breastfeeding have been reported, however, without a definitive conclusion yet (Szabo 2013).

The half-life of *alfentanil* (1 hour) is shorter than that of fentanyl and sufentanil. Alfentanil is also highly protein-bound (>90%) and therefore likely to have limited passage into milk. Nine women were given intravenous alfentanil 50 μg and then 10 μg as needed during anesthesia in the postpartum period. At 4 hours after the last dose, the average level of alfentanil in colostrum was 0.88 μg/L and the highest measured level was 1.5 μg/L. According to these results, published only as abstract, an exclusively breastfed infant would receive alfentanil 0.2 μg/kg daily (Giesecke 1985).

No reliable data on estimation of infant exposure to *sufentanil* are available. The half-life is short (2–3 hours). Sufentanil is highly protein bound (>90%), therefore passage into milk is probably very limited.

There are no data on the passage of *remifentanil* into mother's milk. However, it has a short half-life (between 3 to 6 minutes) reducing the potential risks for a breastfed infant.

> **Recommendation.** Fentanyl and sufentanil are the opiate analgesics of choice during breastfeeding. Brief therapy seems unproblematic and an interruption of breastfeeding following anesthesia in general is not required. Long-term therapy, i.e. with a fentanyl patch, is not recommended but may in individual cases and with close observation of the infant be allowed.

▶ Other opiate derivatives and centrally acting analgesics

Pethidine is excreted into breast milk in small amounts. After i.v. pethidine was given to maintain anesthesia during surgery, the relative infant dose was low varying between 1% and 3.5%. Pethidine was undetectable in milk by 24 hours (Borgatta 1997). In another study 20 mothers received pethidine through patient-controlled epidural analgesia. The relative infant dose was calculated as 0.7% based on samples taken 2 hours after pethidine administration stopped. Infant behavior was assessed by midwives and no untoward effects were observed (Al-Tamimi 2011). Pethidine has a half-life of 7–40 hours in neonates, and the half-life of the active metabolite norpethidine is 48 hours, making accumulation with continuous exposure possible. Therefore particular care should be taken if breastfeeding a newborn, especially if the child is born prematurely (Bar-Oz 2003). The AAP considers pethidine to be usually compatible with breastfeeding (AAP 2001).

Tramadol 100 mg every 6 hours was given to 75 breastfeeding mothers 2–4 days after a caesarean section. A relative infant dose of 2.24% was reported (Ilett 2008).

Lactation

4.1 Analgesics, antiphlogistics and anesthetics

There is no information on the transfer of *piritramide* into milk. However, it is frequently used for analgesia in newborns.

Nalbuphine 0.2 mg was given intravenously every 4 hours to 14 mothers after caesarean section and milk samples were collected during the second day of treatment. The highest measured milk concentration was 98 ng/mL and the average relative infant dose was 0.59% (Jacqz-Aigrain 2007).

There are no data on the milk transfer of *flupirtin, meptazinol, tilidine, tapentadol* and *ziconotide*.

One case report describes transfer of naltrexone into milk. At the time of the study the mother had used naltrexone for 3 months and her infant was 1.5 months old. The baby had been breastfed from birth and had not suffered any ill effects and was developing normally. Milk sampling started 4 hours after the mother had taken her oral daily dose of 50 mg of naltrexone. The relative infant dose was 0.86% and no naltrexone could be detected in the infant plasma. The authors point out that the results should be interpreted with some caution as naltrexone could be quantitated in only two of the milk samples (Chan 2004).

There are no data on the transfer of naloxone into milk.

Recommendation. When analgesic therapy with paracetamol and /or NSAID is not sufficient, short-term administration of tramadol is possible. Single doses of pethidine or piritramide do not require any limitation of breastfeeding, but repeated use is not recommended. The opiate analgesics with no information on drug transfer into milk should not be used while breastfeeding. However, single doses do not require either weaning or an interruption of breastfeeding.

4.1.9   Local anesthetics

Lidocaine passes into milk in small amounts. Seven breastfeeding mothers received lidocaine for local analgesia prior to a dental procedure. Lidocaine concentration was highest in the first sample taken 3 hours after injection (average 120.5 μg/L). The average infant dose of lidocaine would be 73 μg/day, assuming a milk intake of 90 mL every 3 hours (Giuliani 2001).

In one study, 27 women undergoing caesarean section received epidural anesthesia with 0.5% *bupivacaine* and 2% lidocaine. On average the women received a total of 82 mg bupivacaine and 183 mg lidocaine. The average milk concentrations in the 2 hour sample were 0.86 mg/L lidocaine, 0.09 mg/L bupivacaine and 0.14 mg/L PPX (the main metabolite of bupivacaine), while the average milk/serum ratios were 0.85, 0.36 and 1.32, respectively. All infants were breastfed and no untoward effects were observed during 24 hours after delivery. Oral bioavailability of both lidocaine and bupivacaine is low and the amount excreted into milk is not expected to cause any adverse effects in the breastfed infant (Ortega 1999). A mother who was 10 months postpartum was given 25 mg/hour of bupivacaine interpleurally for a cholecystectomy, starting immediately before the operation and continuing for 5 days. Breastfeeding was restarted 22 hours after the start of the infusion and 30 hours later a blood sample from the infant was taken. No bupivacaine could be detected in the infant (Baker 1989).

Women undergoing caesarean delivery ($n = 25$) were given a combination of *ropivacaine* and *fentanyl* for patient-controlled epidural analgesia during

24 hours. The basal rate was 9 mg ropivacaine per hour; the on-demand dose was 6 mg/20 min. The ropivacaine concentration in breast milk was 246 μg/L in the 18-hour sample and 301 μg/L in the 24 hour sample. The M/P-ratio was 0.25 and 0.23, respectively. All the neonates were breastfed by their mothers and no adverse effects were noted (Matsota 2009).

There are no data on the use of *articaine, benzocaine, chlorethane, cinchocaine, levobupivacaine, mepivacaine, oxybuprocaine, prilocaine, procaine* and *tetracaine* during breastfeeding. Adrenalin use in combination with local anesthetics reduces systemic absorption.

> **Recommendation.** Local anesthesia can be used for dental procedures and other minor surgery during breastfeeding, also in combinations with adrenalin/epinephrine. Prilocaine and benzocaine should primarily be avoided but when used, interruption of breastfeeding is not required.

4.1.10   Other medications used in connection with anesthesia

After administration of 120–150 mg of *methohexital* to nine women for anesthesia induction, the peak concentration in mother's milk was 407 ng/mL 1 hour after anesthesia induction. By 10 hours methohexital was no longer detectable in half of the samples and could not be detected in any of the samples at 24 hours. The relative infant dose was determined for each mother–child pair and varied between 1–2% (Borgatta 1997).

Propofol appears in limited amounts in the colostrum when administered before a caesarean section. The highest milk concentration was measured from a sample taken 5 hours postoperatively (0.74 μg/mL). The amount reaching the fetus through placenta is much higher (Dailland 1989). Propofol was given as an induction to anesthesia (2.5 mg/kg) and maintenance for up to 30 minutes. Propofol concentration was 0.12–0.97 μg/mL after 4–8 hours, and the infant would receive 1.5% of the maternal weight-related dose per feed at most (review by Spigset 1994). Further, five post-partum women received propofol for general anesthesia. Less than 0.1% of the maternal dose was recovered in milk over the next 24 hours. The average propofol intake via milk was 0.052 mg/kg which is less than 1% of the average maternal weight-related dose of 2.5 mg/kg (Nitsun 2006). In another study, propofol concentration in milk was measured in two out of four women receiving propofol for anesthesia induction. The highest milk concentration (2.78 mg/L) was measured 90 minutes after extubation. All four mothers breastfed their infants (less than 6 months of age) and none of them showed any signs of drowsiness or dizziness (Stuttmann 2010).

Excretion of *thiopental* into mature milk and the colostrum was studied in eight women undergoing either minor surgery or caesarean section. The maximal concentration was 0.9 mg/L in mature milk 2 hours, and in colostrum 0.34 mg/L 4 hours after anesthesia induction. This would lead to infant daily doses of 0.135 mg/kg which is less than 3% of the maternal weight-related dose (Andersen 1987).

No information on transfer of inhalational anaesthetics (*desflurane, enflurane, halothane, isoflurane* and *sevoflurane*) is available but exposure is expected to be very low and generally not problematic for the breastfed infant (Chu 2013, Lee 1993).

Muscle relaxants of the curare type (*suxamethone, pancurone, vecurone, rocuroniumbromide*) are quaternary ammonium compounds and

Lactation

4.1 Analgesics, antiphlogistics and anesthetics

because being ionized at physiological pH, are not expected to pass in significant amounts into milk. They are also poorly absorbed from the gastrointestinal tract (review by Spigset 1994).

> **Recommendation.** As soon as the mother is able to put her child to breast again after general anesthesia, she may breastfeed. Neither the pharmacokinetic qualities connected to drugs used today for anesthesia nor clinical experience justifies interruption of breastfeeding. This also applies to anesthesia for a caesarean section.

4.1.11   Myotonolytics and other analgesics

In one case report, a single dose of 20 mg of *baclofen* was given to a breastfeeding mother 14 days postpartum. The highest milk concentration (0.13 mg/L) was measured 4 hours after baclofen administration. Milk was collected for 26 hours and the total amount of baclofen excreted into milk during this time was 22 μg (Eriksson 1981).

A woman was suspected of having developed malignant hyperthermia in connection with the general anesthesia for urgent caesarean section. She was given 160 mg dantrolene when the umbilical cord was clamped and the dantrolene therapy was continued for 3 days, when she had completely recovered. The highest dantrolene concentration in milk was 1.2 μg/mL and it was measured from a sample taken 36 hours after the first dose and when the mother had received in total 720 mg *dantrolene* (Fricker 1998). The authors concluded that with the half-life of 9 hours for dantrolene, a waiting period of 2 days after discontinuing treatment should be applied before continuing breastfeeding.

According to one case report, botulinum toxin is not transferred into milk. The toxin was identified from the serum of a woman suffering from botulism but not detected in milk. The 8-month-old child was breastfed during the mother's hospital stay and did not display any signs of botulism during this time. Botulism toxin could not be detected in the child's serum (Middaugh 1978).

There is no experience on the use of *methocarbamol, orphenadrine, pridinol tetrazepam, tizanidine* and *tolperisone* during breastfeeding. However, due to lipid solubility, transfer to milk is expected.

> **Recommendation.** Apart from emergency treatment with dantrolene for malignant hyperthermia, the indications for using a myotonolytic should be considered very critically. Physiotherapeutic measures and antiphlogistics or antirheumatics are preferable. In individual cases, the relaxant effect of low doses of the better-studied diazepam should be used in the short term. Use of botulinum toxin for cosmetic purposes is contraindicated.

4.1.12   Gout therapy

One case report has been published on the use of allopurinol during breastfeeding. Concentrations of *allopurinol* and its active metabolite *oxypurinol* were measured from the mother's milk and serum and the nursing infant's serum after 4 weeks treatment. The infant received 8 mg/

kg of oxypurinol via milk which is close to the therapeutic dose for children (10–20 mg/kg/day). No allopurinol could be found in the infant's plasma, but oxypurinol concentration was 6.6 µg/mL (Kamilli 1991). No untoward effects were reported.

There is no experience on the use of *benzbromaron* during breastfeeding. However, due to the potential serious adverse effects related to use and including fulminant liver failure, use during breastfeeding is contraindicated.

One case report describes a woman who received *probenecid* 500 mg four times daily together with cephalexin for the treatment of mastitis. On day 16 of treatment the average concentration of probenecid in milk was 964 µg/mL. The absolute infant dose was 145 µg/kg/day and the relative infant dose 0.7% (Ilett 2006). Passage of *colchicine* to milk was investigated in four breastfeeding women suffering from Familial Mediterranean Fever (FMF) and treated with 1–1.5 mg colchicine daily for several years. The highest concentration in milk was 8.6 ng/mL, and the calculated absolute infant dose 1.29 µg/kg/day. The infants were followed up for at least 10 months and no effects were observed. The authors also report of an additional six infants whose mothers used colchicine during breastfeeding. No adverse effects were observed in any of the infants over a follow up period of 2 years (Ben-Chetrit 1996). There are additional two case reports where the mothers were using colchicine 1–1.2 mg daily. The highest milk concentrations measured were 2.5 ng/mL (Milunsky 1991) and 31 ng/mL (Guilloneau 1995). No ill effects were observed in the one infant followed up until 6 months' of age (Milunsky 1991).

> **Recommendation.** Probenecid is the drug of choice for interval treatment of gout during breastfeeding, and ibuprofen is the drug of choice for acute gout attacks. Intra-articular or systemic corticoids are also safe. *Allopurinol, phenylbutazone* and *colchicine* should be avoided. Decisions about breastfeeding in women using long-term colchicine for Familial Mediterranean Fever should be decided individually. With good observation of the infant for potential hematological and gastrointestinal side-effects, therapy with colchicine seems acceptable.

References

AAP. The transfer of drugs and other chemicals into human milk. Pediatrics 2001; 108:776–89.

Al-Tamimi Y, Ilett KF, Paech MJ et al. Estimation of the infant dose and exposure to pethidine and norpethidine via breast milk following patient-controlled epidural pethidine for analgesia post caesarean delivery. Int J Obstet Anesth 2011; 20: 128–34.

Andersen LW, Qvist T, Hertz J et al. Concentrations of thiopentone in mature breast milk and colostrum following an induction dose. Acta Anaesthesiol Scand 1987; 31: 30–2.

Anderson PO, Sauberan JB, Lane JR et al. Hydrocodone excretion into breast milk: the first two reported cases. Breastfeed Med 2007; 2: 10–14.

Bailey DN, Weibert RT, Naylor AJ. A study of salicylate and caffeine excretion in the breast milk of two nursing mothers. J Anal Toxicol 1982; 6: 64–8.

Baka N-E, Bayoumeu F, Boutroy M-J et al. Colostrum morphine concentrations during postcesarean intravenous patient-controlled analgesia. Anesth Analg (Hagerstown, MD, US) 2002; 94: 184–87.

Baker PA, Schroeder D. Interpleural bupivacaine for postoperative pain during lactation. Anesth Analg (Hagerstown, MD, US) 1989; 69: 400–2.

Bar-Oz B, Bulkowstein M, Benyamini L et al. Use of antibiotic and analgesic drugs during lactation. Drug Saf 2003; 26: 925–35.

Bateman DN, Eddleston M, Sandilands E. Codeine and breastfeeding. Lancet 2008; 372: 625.

Bell RAF, Dale IM. Gold secretio in maternal milk. Arthritis Rheum 1976; 19: 1374.

Ben-Chetrit E, Scherrmann J.-M, Levy M. Colchicine in breast milk of patients with familial Mediterranean fever. Arthritis Rheum 1996; 39: 1213–7.

Bennett PN, Humphries SJ, Osborne JP et al. Use of sodium aurothiomalate during lactation. Br J Clin Pharmacol 1990; 29: 777–9.

Berlin CM Jr, Yaffe SJ, Ragni M. Disposition of acetaminophen in milk, saliva and plasma of lactating women. Pediatr Pharmacol (New York) 1980; 1: 135–41.

Bitzén P-O, Gustafsson B, Jostell KG et al. Excretion of paracetamol in human breast milk. Eur J Clin Pharmacol 1981; 20: 123–5.

Borgatta L, Jenny RW, Gruss L et al. Clinical significance of methohexital, Meperidine and diazepam in breast milk. J Clin Pharmacol 1997; 37: 186–92.

Bouwmeester NJ, Anderson BJ, Tibboel D. Developmental pharmacokinetics of morphine and its metabolites in neonates, infants and young children. Br J Anaesth 2004; 92: 208–17.

Buchanan RA, Eaton CJ, Koeff ST et al. The breast milk excretion of mefenamic acid. Curr Ther Res 1968; 10: 592–96.

Buchanan RA, Eaton CJ, Koeff ST et al. The breast milk excretion of flufenamic acid. Curr Res Ther 1969; 11: 533–8.

Carvalho B, Chu L, Fuller A et al. Valdecoxib for postoperative pain management after cesarean delivery: a randomized, double-blind, placebo-controlled study. Anesth Analg (Hagerstown, MD, US) 2006; 103: 664–70.

Chan CF, Page-Sharp M, Kristensen JH et al. Transfer of naltrexone and its metabolite 6:β-Naltrexol into human milk. J Hum Lact 2004; 20: 322–6.

Chu TC, McCallum J, Yii MF. Breastfeeding after anaesthesia: a review of the pharmacological impact on children. Anaesth Intens Care 2013; 41: 35–40.

Cimaz R, Brucato A, Meregalli E et al. Electroretinograms of children born to mothers treated with hyrdoxychloroquine during pregnancy and breast-feeding: comment on the article by Costedoat-Chalumeau. Arthritis Rheum 2004; 50: 3056–7.

Clark JH, Wilson WG. A 16-day-old breast-fed infant with metabolic acidosis caused by salicylate. Clin Pediatr (Philadelphia) 1981; 20: 53–4.

Cohen RS. Fentanyl transdermal analgesia during pregnancy and lactation. Journal of Human Lactation 2009; 25: 359–61.

Coller JK, Christrup LL, Somogyi AA. Role of active metabolites in the use of opioids. Eur J Clin Pharmacol 2009; 65: 121–39.

Costedoat-Chalumeau N, Amoura Z, Aymard G et al. Evidence of transplacental passage of hydroxychloroquine in humans. Arthritis Rheum 2002; 46: 1123–4.

Costedoat-Chalumeau N, Amoura Z, Sebbough D et al. Electroretinograms of children born to mothers treated with hydroxychloroquine during pregnancy and breast-feeding: author reply. Arthritis Rheum 2004; 50: 3057–8.

Cox RS, Forbes KK. Excretion of flurbiprofen into breast milk. Pharmacotherapy 1987; 7: 211–15.

Dailland P, Cockshott ID, Lirzin JD et al. Intravenous propofol during Cesarean section: placental transfer, concentrations in breast milk and neonatal effects. A preliminary study. Anesthesiology 1989; 71: 827–34.

Davis JM, Bhutani VK. Neonatal apnea and maternal codeine use. Pediatr Res 1985; 19: 170A.

Edwards JE, Rudy AC, Wermeling DP et al. Hydromorphone transfer into breast milk after intranasal administration. Pharmacotherapy 2003; 23: 153–8.

Eriksson G, Swahn C-G. Concentrations of baclofen in serum and breast milk from a lactating woman. Scand J Clin Lab Invest 1981; 41: 185–7.

Feilberg VL, Rosenborg D, Broen Christensen C et al. Excretion of morphine in human breast milk. Acta Anaesthesiol Scand 1989; 33: 426–8.

Ferner RE. Did the drug cause the death? Codeine and breastfeeding. Lancet 2008; 372: 606–8.

Findlay JWA, DeAngelis RL, Kearney MF et al. Analgesic drugs in breast milk and plasma. Clin Pharmacol Ther 1981; 29: 625–33.

Frei H, Bühlmann, U, Rudin O. Toxic hemolytic anemia in the newborn infant following ingestion of a phenazone derivative (Cibalgin) via breast milk. Z Geburtsh Perinatol 1985; 189: 11–12.

Fricker RM, Hoerauf, KH, Drewe J et al. Secretion of dantrolene into breast milk after acute therapy of a suspected malignant hyperthermia crisis during cesarean section. Anesthesiology 1998; 89: 1023–5.

Gardiner SJ, Begg EJ, Zhang M. Transfer of rofecoxib into human milk. Eur J Clin Pharmacol 2005; 61: 405–8.

Gardiner SJ, Doogue P, Zhang M et al. Quantification of infant exposure to celecoxib through breast milk. Br J Clin Pharmacol 2006; 61: 101–4.

Giesecke AH, Rice LJ, Lipton JM. Alfentanil in colostrum. Anesthesiology1985; 63: A284.

Giuliani M, Grossi GB, Pileri M et al. Could local anesthesia while breast-feeding be harmful to infants? J Pediatr Gastroenterol Nutr 2001; 32: 142–4.

Goma HM, Said RN, El-Ela AM. Study of the newborn feeding behaviors and fentanyl concentration in colostrum after an analgesic dose of epidural and intravenous fentanyl in cesarean section. Saudi Med J 2008; 29: 678–82.

Gregory MC, Mansell MA. Pregnancy and cysteinuria. Lancet 1983; 322: 1158–60.

Guillonneau M, Jacqz Aigrain E, Galliot M et al. Colchicine is excreted at high concentrations in human breast milk. Eur J Obstet Gynecol Reprod Biol 1995; 61: 177–8.

Hale TW, McDonald R, Boger J. Transfer of celecoxib into human milk. J Hum Lact 2004; 20: 397–403.

Hutchinson S, Marmura MJ, Calhoun A et al. Use of common migraine treatments in breast-feeding women: a summary of recommendations. Headache 2013; 53: 614–27.

Ilett KF, Hackett LP, Ingle B et al. Transfer of probenecid and cephalexin into breast milk. Ann Pharmacother 2006; 40: 986–9.

Ilett KF, Paech MJ, Page-Sharp M et al. Use of sparse sampling study design to assess transfer of tramadol and its O-desmethyl metabolite into transitional breast milk. Br J Clin Pharmacol 2008; 65: 661–6.

Ito S, Blajchman A, Stephenson M et al. Prospective follow-up of adverse reactions in breast-fed infants exposed to maternal medication. Am J Obstet Gynecol 1993; 168: 1393–9.

Jacqz-Aigrain E, Serreau R, Boissinot C et al. Excretion of ketoprofen and nalbuphine in human milk during treatment of maternal pain after delivery. Ther Drug Monit 2007; 29: 815–18.

Jamali F, Keshavarz E. Salicylate excretion in breast milk. Int J Pharm 1981; 8: 285–90.

Jamali F, Stevens RD. Naproxen excretion in milk and its uptake by the infant. Drug Intell Clin Pharm 1983; 17: 910–11.

Jolivet A, Robyn C, Huraux-Rendu C et al. Effects of ergot alkaloid derivatives on milk secretion in the immediate post-partum period. J Gynecol Obstet Biol Reprod 1978; 7: 129–34.

Jones RW, Freeman M. Tiaprofenic acid in human plasma and breast milk. Acta Pharmacol Toxicol Suppl 1986; 59, 183.

Kamilli I, Gresser U, Schaefer C et al. Allopurinol in breast milk. Adv Exp Med Biol 1991; 309A, 143–5.

Kelly LE, Chaudry SA, Rieder MJ et al. A clinical tool for reducing central nervous system depression among neonates exposed to codeine through breast milk. PLoS One 2013; 8: e70073.

Knoppert DC, Stempak D, Baruchel S et al. Celecoxib in human milk: a case report. Pharmacotherapy 2003; 23: 97–100.

Koren G. Morphine in breast milk: Response. Can Fam Physician 2007; 53: 1005–6.

Koren G, Cairns J, Chitayat D et al. Pharmacogenetics of morphine poisoning in a breastfed neonate of a codeine-prescribed mother. Lancet 2006; 368: 704.

Lam J, Matlow JN, Ross CJD et al. Postpartum maternal codeine therapy and the risk of adverse neonatal outcomes: the devil is in the details. Ther Drug Monit 2012a; 34: 378–80.

Lam J, Kelly L, Ciszkowski, C et al. Central nervous system depression of neonates breastfed by mothers receiving oxycodone for postpartum analgesia. J Pediatr 2012b; 160: 33–7.

Lebedevs TH, Wojnar-Horton RE, Yapp P et al. Excretion of indomethacin in breast milk. Br J Clin Pharmacol 1991; 32: 751–4.

Lee JJ, Rubin AP. Breast feeding and anaesthesia. Anaesthesia 1993; 48: 616–25.

Madadi P, Ross CJD, Hayden MR et al. Pharmacogenetics of neonatal opioid toxicity following maternal use of codeine during breast feeding: a case-control study. Clin Pharmacol Ther 2009; 85: 31–5.

Matheson I, Lunde PKM, Notarianni L. Infant rash caused by paracetamol in breast milk? Pediatrics 1985; 76: 651–2.

Matsota PK, Markantonis SL, Fousteri M-ZF et al. Excretion of ropivacaine in breast milk during patient-contrrolled epidural analgesia after cesarean delivery. Reg Anesth Pain Med 2009; 34: 126–9.

Messner U, Günter HH, Niesert S. Wilson disease and pregnancy. Review of the literature and case report. Z Geburtsh Neonatol 1998; 202: 77–9.

Meny RG, Naumburg EG, Alger LS et al. Codeine and the breastfed neonate. J Hum Lact 1993; 9: 237–40.

Middaugh J. Botulism and breast milk. N Engl J Med 1978; 298: 343.

Milunsky JM, Milunsky A. Breastfeeding during colchicine therapy for familial Mediterranean fever. J Pediatr 1991; 119: 164.

4.1 Analgesics, antiphlogistics and anesthetics   Lactation

Motta M, Tinciani A, Faden D et al. Follow-up of infants exposed to hydroxychloroquine given to mothers during pregnancy and lactation. J Perinatol 2005; 25: 86–9.

Nation RL, Hackett LP, Dusci LJ. Excretion of hydroxychloroquine in human milk. Br J Clin Pharmacol 1984; 17: 368–9.

Naumburg EG, Meny RG. Breast milk opioids and neonatal apnea. Am J Dis Child 1988; 142: 11–12.

Nitsun M, Szokol JW, Saleh J. Pharmacokinetics of midazolam, propofol and fentanyl transfer to human breast milk. Clin Pharmacol Ther 2006; 79: 549–57.

Ortega D, Viviand X, Lorec AM et al. Excretion of lidocaine and bupivacaine in breast milk following epidural anesthesia for cesarean delivery. Acta Anaesthesiol Scand 1999; 43: 394–7.

Østensen M, Brown ND, Chiang PK et al. Hydroxychloroquine in human breast milk. Eur J Clin Pharmacol 1985; 28: 357.

Østensen M, Matheson I, Laufen H. Piroxicam in breast milk after long-term treatment. Eur J Clin Pharmacol 1988; 35: 567–9.

Østensen M, Skavdal K, Myklebust G et al. Excretion of gold into human breast milk. Eur J Clin Pharmacol 1986; 31: 251–2.

Paech MJ, Salman S, Ilett KF et al. Transfer of parecoxib and its primary active metabolite valdecoxib via transitional breastmilk following intravenous parecoxib use after Cesarean delivery: a comparison of naïve pooled data analysis and nonlinear mixed-effects modeling. Anesth Analg (Hagerstown, MD, US) 2012; 114: 837–44.

Rizzoni G, Furlanut M. Cyanotic crises in a breast-fed infant from mother taking dipyrone. Hum Toxicol 1984; 3: 505–7.

Robieux I, Koren G, Vandenbergh H. Morphine excretion in breast milk and resultant exposure of a nursing infant. J Toxicol Clin Toxicol 1990; 28: 365–70.

Rooney TW, Lorber A, Veng-Pedersen P et al. Gold pharmacokinetics in breast milk and serum of a lactating woman. J Rheumatol 1987; 14: 1120–2.

Sauberan JB, Anderson PO, Lane JR et al. Breast milk hydrocodone and hydromorphone levels in mothers using hydrocodone for postpartum pain. Obstet Gynecol (Hagestown, MD, US) 2011; 117: 611–17.

Seaton S, Reeves M, McLean S. Oxycodone as a component of multimodal analgesia for lactating mothers after Cesarean section: relationships between maternal plasma, breast milk and neonatal plasma levels. Aust N Z J Obstet Gynaecol 2007; 47: 181–5.

Smith IJ, Hinson JL, Johnson VA et al. Flurbiprofen in post-partum women: plasma and breast milk disposition. J Clin Pharmacol 1989; 29: 174–84.

Smith JW. Codeine-induced bradycardia in a breast-fed infant. 1982; Clin Res 30: 259A.

Spigset O. Anaesthetic agents and excretion in breast milk. Acta Anaesthesiol Scand 1994; 38: 94–103.

Steer PL, Biddle C J, Marley WS et al. Concentration of fentanyl in colostrum after an analgesic dose. Can J Anaesth 1992; 39: 231–5.

Stuttmann R, Schäfer C, Hilbert P et al. The breast feeding mother and xenon anaesthesia: four case reports. Breastfeeding and xenon anaesthesia. BMC Anesthesiol 2010; 10: 1.

Szabo AL. Intrapartum neuraxial analgesia and breastfeeding outcomes: limitations of current knowledge. Anesth Analg 2013; 116: 399–405.

Timm NL. Maternal use of oxycodone resulting in opioid intoxication in her breastfed neonate. J Pediatr 2013; 162: 421–2.

Townsend RJ, Benedetti TJ, Erickson SH et al. Excretion of ibuprofen into breast milk. Am J Obstet Gynecol 1984; 149: 184–6.

Unsworth J, d'Assis-Fonseca A, Beswick DT et al. Serum salicylate levels in a breast fed infant. Ann Rheum Dis 1987; 46: 638–9.

van Lingen RA, Deinum JT, Quak JME et al. Pharmacokinetics and metabolism of rectally administered paracetamol in preterm neonates. Arch Dis Child Fetal Neonatal Ed 1999; 80: F59–F63.

Walter K, Dilger C. Ibuprofen in human milk. Br J Clin Pharmacol 1997; 44: 211–12.

Weibert RT, Townsend RJ, Kaiser DG et al. Lack of ibuprofen secretion into human milk. Clin Pharm 1983; 1: 457–8.

Wischnik A, Manth SM, Lloyd J et al. The excretion of ketorolac tromethanine into breast milk after multiple oral dosing. Eur J Clin Pharmacol 1989; 36: 521–4.

Wojnar-Horton RE, Hackett LP, Yapp P et al. Distribution and excretion of sumatriptan in human milk. Br J Clin Pharmacol 1996; 41: 217–21.

Zylber-Katz E, Linder N, Levy M. Excretion of dipyrone metabolites in human breast milk. Eur J Clin Pharmacol 1986; 30: 359–61.

Antiallergics, antiasthmatics and antitussives

4.2

Paul Merlob and Corinna Weber-Schöndorfer

4.2.1	Antihistamines (H₁-blocker)	671
4.2.2	Selective effective β₂-sympathomimetics	672
4.2.3	Inhalable corticosteroids (ICS)	673
4.2.4	Leukotrien-receptor antagonists	673
4.2.5	Theophylline	674
4.2.6	Mast cell inhibitors	674
4.2.7	Anticholinergics for asthma treatment	674
4.2.8	Omalizumab	675
4.2.9	Mucolytics, expectorants and cold remedies	675
4.2.10	Antitussives	675

Second-generation antihistamines which have practically no sedative effect are compatible during breastfeeding. First-generation antihistamines with sedating action should be reserved during breastfeeding for special conditions. Should adverse effects such as restlessness or mild sedation occur, the consequences are to be considered individually. Medications for local use can be used. Desensitization with allergen extracts is not known to negatively influence breastfeeding. For asthma control during breastfeeding the effective β_2-sympathomimetics such as terbutaline are well tolerated. Long-acting β_2-sympathomimetic formoterol or salmeterol can be used also. Should inhalation treatment and an adequate intake of fluid not be sufficiently effective, well-tried expectorants and mucolytics can be used during breastfeeding. With dry, severe coughing single doses of dextromethorphan or codeine are useful during breastfeeding. Individual counseling remains necessary.

4.2.1   Antihistamines (H₁-blocker)

Antihistamines are used to treat allergic illnesses, as antiemetics (Chapter 4.3) and as sleeping aids.

The newer antihistamines, which have practically no sedative effect, have also proven beneficial during breastfeeding. Following a single dose of 40 mg *loratadine* (four times the current therapeutic dose) transfer to the infant was calculated at approximately 1% of the effective ingredient (including metabolites) compared to the maternal weight-related

Drugs During Pregnancy and Lactation. **http://dx.doi.org/10.1016/B978-0-12-408078-2.00027-5**

dose (Hilbert 1988). Only two infants (3.9%) among 51 exposed to loratadine during breastfeeding showed sedation (Merlob 2002). There are no data on the passage into mother's milk of *cetirizine*, which has a half-life of 9 hours. Previous comprehensive experience, however, does not indicate any noteworthy intolerance while breastfeeding. Terfenadine with an M/P ratio of 0.2 has a half-life of 20 hours. A study of four breast-feeding women indicated less than 0.5% of the weight-related dose for the infant. Only the active metabolites, but not the maternal substance, were detectable in the milk (Lucas 1995). There is very limited experience with the following non-sedating H₁-blockers and no data on their passage into mother's milk: *desloratadine, ebastine, fexofenadine* and *levocetirizine*. There are no observations at all on *rupatadine* and *bilastine*.

The older antihistamines with sedating action have become less important and should be reserved during breastfeeding for special conditions. Mild restlessness that does not need treatment and irritability were described in around 10%, and sedation or weak suckling in 1.6% of the children exposed to various antihistamines (Moretti 1995, Ito 1993). None of the manufacturers have data on the relative dose. Twelve hours after the start of maternal treatment with *clemastine*, a stiff neck, hyper-excitability and sleepiness were observed in a 10-week-old infant; 5–10 µg/L of the drug was detected in the milk. No clemastine was found in the infant's serum (Kok 1982). In addition, the mother had long-term treatment with *phenytoin* and *carbamazepine*. Until a few years ago, *dimetindene* was a common antihistamine. It has a short half-life of 5 to 7 hours, was approved for children from age 1, and is comparatively non-sedating, but it has an atropine-like effect that should not be overlooked. Much less well studied are *cyproheptadine, dexchlorpheniramine, hydroxyzine, mizolastine* and *triprolidine*. *Azelastine* is available for systemic and local use. The latter is considered to be non-problematic but it could alter the milk taste leading to rejection by the infant.

Used exclusively for local therapy are *bamipine, chlorphenoxamine* and *levocabastine* as well as the newer substances *epinastine* and *olopatadine*. There are no data on passage into the mother's milk for any of these substances. Their use during breastfeeding is considered unproblematic.

> **Recommendation.** The antiallergics of choice during breastfeeding are loratadine and cetirizine. Should a sedating effect be expressly desired, breastfeeding could also be continued with dimentindene without limitation. Should symptoms such as restlessness or mild sedation occur, the (possible) consequences must be considered in individual cases – first and foremost changing to another preparation. Due to the longer market testing, levocabastine and azelastine are preferable for local use. Desensitization with allergen extracts may also be conducted during breastfeeding.

4.2.2   Selective effective β₂-sympathomimetics

The inhalable broncholytics *fenoterol, salbutamol, albuterol* and *terbutaline*, as well as *reproterol*, which is only available in a combination preparation, are well-tolerated during breastfeeding.

Only for terbutaline is there data available regarding passage into the mother's milk – 3.5 µg/L of milk was measured with oral medication of 2.5 or 5 mg, three times a day. The M/P ratio was between 1 and 2. The infant's intake was a maximum of 0.7µg/kg per day, which was about 0.7% of the maternal dosage per kg bodyweight. No toxic effects were observed (Boréus 1982, Lönnerholm 1982). With inhalation use, passage is less than with oral treatment. Excessive overdosing, however, can lead to restlessness and tachycardia in the infant.

The sympathomimetics *formoterol* and *salmeterol* are effective for longer but are less well studied. According to the experience to date, they are scarcely problematic for the breastfed infant. There are no observations available on *indacaterol*.

The oral or parenteral use of β_2-sympathomimetics such as, for instance, *bambuterol*, *clenbuterol* and *tulobuterol* should be reserved for exceptional conditions during breastfeeding.

> **Recommendation.** Terbutaline, salbutamol and fenoterol are the drugs of choice for asthma control during breastfeeding. If a long-acting β_2-sympathomimetic such as bambuterol, clenbuterol and tulobuterol (together with an inhalable corticosteroid) is indicated, formoterol or salmeterol can be used. Oral treatment with β_2-sympathicomimetics is not part of standard asthma treatment (see Chapter 2.3).

4.2.3   Inhalable corticosteroids (ICS)

ICS such as *budesonide* and the fluoridated ICS *beclomethasone*, *fluticasone*, *mometasone* and *ciclesonide* do not require any limitation of breastfeeding. The best studied is budesonide. The passage into the mother's milk and the serum concentrations were determined with eight mother–child pairs. The maternal oral dose was 200 or 400 µg 2 × daily, of which the infant received about 0.3%. No budesonide could be detected in the infant's serum (detection limit 9 mg/L); 1/600 of the maternal plasma levels were considered possible mathematically (Fält 2007).

> **Recommendation.** With maternal inhalable corticosteroid therapy, breastfeeding may continue without limitation. Budesonide is the best-studied drug (Chapter 4.11).

4.2.4   Leukotrien-receptor antagonists

The leukotrien-receptor antagonist *montelukast* is approved for children from 6 months. There are no published experiences during breastfeeding but, according to the manufacturer, among rats, the drug passes into the milk.

> **Recommendation.** When montelukast is necessary for asthma control in accordance with the guidelines, it can be used if the breastfed infant is closely monitored.

Lactation

4.2 Antiallergics, antiasthmatics and antitussives

4.2.5   Theophylline

Theophylline preparations are well tolerated during breastfeeding in moderate doses, and in the time-released form so commonly used today. After administration of higher doses, however, extreme restlessness in the infant can occur, particularly with injections or rectal preparations. Larger amounts of caffeine-containing drinks should also be avoided during therapy.

After administration of 300 mg of theophylline, maximum concentrations of 6 mg/L of milk were measured and an M/P ratio of 0.7 was calculated. At most, 0.9 mg/kg daily passes to the infant. With long-term therapy using 800 mg daily, 10% of the weight-related child dosage could pass to the infant (survey in Bennett 1996). Due to the extended plasma half-life of 15–40 hours in the infant, an accumulation in young babies is possible. Viewed realistically, plasma concentrations are not likely to exceed 4 mg/L. Even for the newborn this does not mean any risk since theophylline used for apnea prophylaxis in premature infants is well tolerated. Here, plasma concentrations of 6–13 mg/L are the goal.

> **Recommendation.** When necessary, theophylline can be used during breastfeeding in accordance with the guidelines for asthma control. The dose should be chosen to be as low as therapeutically possible. Further large amounts of caffeine containing beverages should be avoided during therapy.

4.2.6   Mast cell inhibitors

With *cromoglycic acid* less than 1% of the swallowed dose is absorbed. The plasma half-life is about 80 minutes. Transfer into the mother's milk can be practically ruled out.

> **Recommendation.** Cromoglycic acid can be used during breastfeeding when it is effective.

4.2.7   Anticholinergics for asthma treatment

The anticholinergic effect of *ipratropium bromide* and *tiotropium bromide* causes bronchodilatation through pulmonary vagolysis. There are no data available on the passage into the mother's milk. However, because only low maternal serum concentrations are achieved, the portion in the mother's milk is negligible.

> **Recommendation.** Ipratropium bromide may be used for asthma control in accordance with the guidelines.

4.2.8   Omalizumab

The monoclonal antibody binds to the IgE receptor and is reserved for severe asthma that cannot be treated any other way. According to the manufacturer, it passes into the milk of primates. Because oral bioavailability is limited, appreciable absorption from the mother's milk seems unlikely. So far, no experiences during breastfeeding are available.

> **Recommendation.** If possible, omalizumab should not be used during breastfeeding.

4.2.9   Mucolytics, expectorants and cold remedies

Acetylcysteine, ambroxol and *bromhexine* are established mucolytics and are also well tolerated during breastfeeding. Acetylcysteine is also used in high doses for infants as an antidote to paracetamol overdosing and is well tolerated by them.

Carbocisteine, guaifenesin and preparations with essential oils such as *cineol, myrtle, lime* or *eucalyptus* are probably well tolerated during breastfeeding, but there are no systematic studies available on this. Essential oils can change the taste of the milk and lead to feeding problems. Phytopharmaceuticals such as ivy leaves dried extract (*hedera helix*), *thyme, lamb's tongue* (*plantago lanceolata*) and *marshmallow* (*althea officinalis*) are not well-studied for use during breastfeeding. They are probably well tolerated.

Iodine from *potassium iodate*, formerly used as an expectorant, accumulates to a great extent in the milk and can, in this way, block the infant's thyroid (Chapter 4.11.6).

The antihistamine *chlorphenamine* is a component of a cold remedy which does not conform to any rational treatment. The sympathomimetics *pseudoephedrine* and *ephedrine* are also components of combination preparations that should be avoided.

> **Recommendation.** Should inhalation treatment and an adequate intake of fluid not be sufficiently effective, well-tried expectorants and mucolytics can be used during breastfeeding. Acetylcysteine, ambroxol and bromhexine are the drugs of choice. Potassium iodate is contraindicated during breastfeeding.

4.2.10   Antitussives

Codeine, dextromethorphan and *pentoxyverine* are centrally acting antitussives. For codeine see Chapter 4.1.

There are no data on the passage into mother's milk of dextromethorphan. The substance is a d-isomer of the codeine analog *levorphanol* with no analgesic properties. Sedative action and the potential for dependency are said to be lower than with codeine. Following short-term use, no undesirable side effects in the breastfed infant have been observed.

In connection with pentoxyverine, a child with apnea episodes lasting up to 15 seconds was described (Stier 1988). The mother had taken 90 mg daily. The levels measured in the infant's serum were higher than those in the maternal serum. The M/P ratio was given as 10; the half-life for the child was 5 days. Mathematically, 660 mL of mother's milk (the daily quantity) had only 93µg pentoxyverine. Apnea, sometimes with cyanosis, had already been observed earlier in young infants when pentoxyverine had been administered therapeutically (Mühlendahl 1996, Stier 1988).

The administration of 150 mg *noscapine* led to a concentration of a maximum of 83 µg/L milk (Olsson 1986). This represents 12.5 µg/kg daily for the infant, which is 0.5% of the maternal weight-related dosage. Following experimental results, mutagenic properties were attributed to noscapine.

There is no experience with *benproperine* and *levodropropizine* during breastfeeding.

Recommendation. With dry severe coughing, single doses of dextromethorphan or codeine are approved during breastfeeding. Pentoxyverin is contraindicated. Noscapine is approved during breastfeeding but on the basis of the mutagenic properties it appears not to be the ideal antitussive.

References

Bennett PN (ed). *Drugs and Human Lactation*. 2nd edn. Amsterdam, New York, Oxford: Elsevier, 1996.

Boréus LO, de Château P, Lindberg C et al. Terbutaline in breast milk. Br J Clin Pharmacol 1982; 13: 731–2.

Fält A, Bengtsson T, Kennedy BM et al. Exposure of infants to budesonide through breast milk of asthmatic mothers. J Allergy Clin Immunol 2007; 120: 798–802.

Hilbert J, Radwanski E, Affrime MB et al. Excretion of loratadine in human breast milk. J Clin Pharmacol 1988; 28: 234–9.

Ito S, Blajchman A, Stephenson M et al. Prospective follow-up of adverse reactions in breast-fed infants exposed to maternal medication. Am J Obstet Gynecol 1993; 168: 1393–9.

Kok THHG, Taitz LS, Bennett MJ et al. Drowsiness due to clemastine transmitted in breast milk. Lancet 1982; 1: 914–5.

Lönnerholm G, Lindström B. Terbutaline excretion into breast milk. Br J Clin Pharmacol 1982; 13: 729–30.

Lucas BD, Purdy CY, Scarim S et al. Terfenadine pharmacokinetics in breast milk in lactating women. Clin Pharmacol Ther 1995; 57: 398–402.

Merlob P, Stahl B. Prospective follow-up of adverse reactions in breast-fed infants exposed to maternal loratadine treatment (1999–2001). BELTIS Newsletter 2002; 10: 43–51.

Moretti ME, Liau-Chu M, Taddio A et al. Adverse events in breast-fed infants exposed to antihistamines in maternal milk. Reprod Toxicol 1995; 9: 588.

Mühlendahl KE, Oberdisse U, Bunjes R et al. Vergiftungen im Kindesalter. 2. Aufl. Stuttgart: Enke 1996.

Olsson B, Bolme P, Dahlström B et al. Excretion of noscapine in human breast milk. Eur J Clin Pharmacol 1986; 30: 213–5.

Stier BJ, Sieverding L, Moeller H. Pentoxyverin-Intoxikation über die Muttermilch bei einem voll gestillten Neugeborenen. Dtsch Med Wochenschr 1988; 113: 898–900.

4.3.1	Gastritis and ulcer medications	677
4.3.2	Peristaltic stimulators	679
4.3.3	Cholinergics	680
4.3.4	Anticholinergic spasmolytics	681
4.3.5	Laxatives	681
4.3.6	Agents used for chronic inflammatory bowel diseases	682
4.3.7	Antidiarrheals for acute diarrhea	683
4.3.8	Digestives and carminatives	683
4.3.9	Lipid reducers	683
4.3.10	Chenodeoxycholic acid and ursodeoxycholic acid	684
4.3.11	Appetite suppressants	684
4.3.12	Antiemetics	684

Medications used to treat gastrointestinal symptoms are often prescribed during breastfeeding. However, there is little information describing the transfer into human milk for many of these drugs. Some of the gastrointestinal agents can be administrated during breastfeeding: antacids, sulcrafate, *Helicobacter pylori* therapy, domperidone, metoclopramide and carminatives. Other groups of gastrointestinal medications are drugs of choice: famotidine as H2-receptor blocker, omeprazole and pantoprazole as proton-pump inhibitors, bulking agents and osmotic laxative as laxatives, and meclizine as an antiemetic. Lipid reducers, appetite suppressants and chenodeoxycholic acid are contraindicated during breastfeeding. As a general rule, the progress of infants exposed to maternal gastrointestinal drugs during breastfeeding should be monitored appropriately.

4.3.1   Gastritis and ulcer medications

▶ **Antacids**

Classic antacids such as *sodium hydrogen carbonate, aluminum phosphate, calcium carbonate* and *carbaldrate*, whose effect is similar to *aluminum hydroxide*, are only absorbed by the mother to a very limited degree. This also applies to the combination preparations of aluminum and magnesium such as *hydrotalcite, magaldrate* and *almasilate*. There

Drugs During Pregnancy and Lactation. **http://dx.doi.org/10.1016/B978-0-12-408078-2.00028-7**

are no available data on trials involving aluminum or other antacids during breastfeeding. Also, long-term use has not been evaluated.

Combinations of, for instance, calcium carbonate and magnesium salts, of an aluminum-containing substance such as algeldrate and magnesium salts, of alginic acid combinations, or combinations with licorice root, appear to be safe when therapeutic doses are used.

> **Recommendation.** Antacids can be used during breastfeeding. Fixed combinations of aluminum and magnesium salts as well as combination preparations are preferable, whereby attention should be paid to keeping to a therapeutic dose.

▶ H₂-Receptor-blocker

Cimetidine, famotidine and *ranitidine* block H$_2$-histamine-receptors in the stomach lining/gastric mucosa; this leads to reduced secretion of hydrochloric acid.

Cimetidine and ranitidine reach relatively high concentrations in mother's milk. According to a study of 12 women who received single doses of 100, 600 or 1200 mg, cimetidine was actively transported into the milk with an M/P ratio of about 5. An infant received, on average, 6–7% of the maternal weight-related dose, though at maximum it was as much as 20% (Oo 1995).

With nizatidine therapy, a maximum of 5% of the maternal weight-related dose can be secreted into the milk (Obermeyer 1990). This was reported in five mothers who received 150 mg every 12 hours for five doses.

Also with maternal therapy of ranitidine, 150–300 mg/day, a relative dose of up to 20% can reach the infant. The M/P ratio varies between 1 and over 20 (survey in Bennett 1996, Kearns 1985).

With famotidine the relative dose in the milk was lower than 2%, according to a study of eight mothers receiving a single dose of 40 mg (Courtney 1988).

> **Recommendation.** Famotidine is the H$_2$ blocker of choice during breastfeeding.

▶ Proton-pump inhibitors (PPIs)

PPIs, such as *omeprazole, esomeprazole*, an isomer of omeprazole, *lansoprazole, pantoprazole* and *rabeprazole* block acid secretion in the stomach.

In a case report on omeprazole, a maximum weight-adjusted dose for a fully breastfed infant was measured at less than 7% (Marshall 1998). According to a case report, pantoprazole only transfers into the mother's milk in small amounts (2.8% of the maternal plasma levels). After 40 mg maternal dose the relative infant dose was under 1% (Plante 2004). In both these cases, the infants were clinically unremarkable.

> **Recommendation.** Pantoprazole and omeprazole are the PPI of choice during breastfeeding.

▶ **Further ulcer medications**

Sucralfate is only minimally absorbed enterally. There are no data available on the passage into the mother's milk. This also applies to the so-called M1-receptor blocker, *pirenzepine*, the prostaglandin derivative, *misoprostol* and for *bismuth nitrate*.

> **Recommendation.** Sucralfate can be administered during breastfeeding. The other medications should be avoided.

▶ *Helicobacter pylori* **therapy**

> **Recommendation.** *Helicobacter* therapy consisting of a PPI, *clarithromycin* and *metronidazole* or *amoxicillin* can be carried out during breastfeeding (Chapter 4.4).

4.3.2   Peristaltic stimulators

The antiemetic *metoclopramide* eases the emptying of the stomach and increases milk production via its central antidopaminergic action. It may be used occasionally for 1 to 4 weeks in a dose of 3×10–15 mg/day to promote milk production (Zuppa 2010).

Numerous studies using metoclopramide to increase milk production were published. Many of them assessed a small sample size and used an inadequate clinical design. The young infant whose mother took 10–15 mg/3 × daily for many weeks received a maximum of 4.7% of a weight-related child's dose. In only one case among more than 20 mother–child pairs could the substance be measured in the infant's plasma (Kauppila 1983). No symptoms or disturbances of pituitary regulation were observed in breastfed children (Kauppila 1985). In a randomized double-blind study, Hansen (2005) investigated more than 60 mothers of preterm newborns who received either metoclopramide or a placebo, with respect to the amount of milk and duration of lactation. There were no significant differences between the two groups. In a more recent randomized double-blind study metoclopramide (10 mg/3 × daily) and placebo were taken for 8 days beginning within 36 hours of delivery (Fife 2011), with no significant difference between the two groups with regard to milk secretion. These two well-planned studies used metoclopramide early after delivery (within 96 hours and 36 hours), corresponding times of high plasma levels of prolactin. This means that metoclopramide should not be expected to work as a galactagogue when plasma prolactin levels are high. By contrast, in other cases, metoclopramide was used successfully (survey in Zuppa 2010). A woman with agenesis of the uterus, whose fertilized egg cells were successfully carried by a surrogate mother, expressed a wish during the pregnancy to breastfeed the baby after birth. She received 10 mg metoclopramide 3 × a day from week 28 until delivery. The effect was confirmed by concentrations of the serum prolactin and estradiol. In addition, the nipples were stimulated with a breast pump. The woman successfully breastfed the baby until the age of 3 months. However, due to insufficient milk, supplementation (with formula) was necessary (Biervliet 2001).

The peripheral dopamine antagonist *domperidone* is present only in a minimal concentration in the milk. No more than 0.4% of the maternal weight-related dose was calculated to be present in the milk (Hofmeyr 1985). The moderately high molecular mass of 426 and a protein binding of >90% are grounds for the low relative dose determined for the child. By comparison to metoclopramide, domperidone is less able to cross the blood–brain barrier. Therefore the risk for central nervous system side effects is low and such symptoms have not, as yet, been observed in breast-fed infants. The argument presented in the US as an objection against domperidone treatment – that it could lead to cardiac arrest – refers to experiences with patients treated with high doses administered by i.v., which are not comparable with the usual oral therapy of the mother and the breastfed infant. To increase milk production, 10 mg/3 × daily for 1–2 weeks (off-label) are recommended (Zuppa 2010). A double blind study of seven women exposed to domperidone, and nine women using a placebo while breastfeeding premature infants showed that with dom-peridone, the amount of milk could be increased by 49.5 mL per day (da Silva 2001). In a further study, the milk production and the milk com-position of mothers of premature infants who received either domperi-done ($n = 21$) or a placebo ($n = 24$) were compared (Campbell-Yeo 2010). The volume of milk with domperidone could be increased satisfactorily with only a minimal change in the composition of the milk. However, a significant difference was a somewhat higher proportion of calcium and carbohydrates in the domperidone milk samples. Two meta-analyses of randomized controlled trials on domperidone as a galactagogue con-cluded that it does indeed increase milk production in comparison with a placebo (Osadchy 2012, Donovan 2012).

Two small studies compared two dosages of domperidone (10 mg/3 × daily versus 20 mg/3 × daily). Both dosages increased milk production, but there was no statistically significant difference in milk volume between the two groups (Wan 2008, Knoppert 2013). Dosages greater than 30 mg daily should be used carefully because of the risk of arrhythmias.

> **Recommendation.** Domperidone and metoclopramide may be used during breastfeeding (preferably after complete initiation of lactation and/or measuring of plasma prolactin levels). Galactagogue medication should never replace evalu-ation and counseling on modifiable factors that affect milk production.

4.3.3   Cholinergics

In a case of myasthenia treatment with *neostigmine*, one child was observed with postprandial stomach cramps; others were unremarkable (Fraser 1963).

When using *pyridostigmine*, with a half-life of about 4 hours, the infant receives a maximum of 0.09% of the weight-related maternal dose per day. In the serum of two clinically unremarkable infants, no active ingre-dient was found (detection level 2 µg/L). The concentrations in the serum of the mothers were 25 and 80 µg/L. With an intravenous administration of 5 × 60 mg, up to 25 µg/L was found in the milk (Hardell 1982).

Occasionally discussed is whether patients with myasthenia gravis may breastfeed, or whether the increased level of maternal autoimmune fac-tors could cause symptoms in the infant. Today, the majority of authors do not discourage breastfeeding. Neonatal myasthenia is pregnancy-related.

It occurs in 10–20% of the newborns of ill mothers and is independent of the level of severity of the maternal illness. The symptoms are variable, consisting of mild hypotonia, weak crying, weak sucking and rarely, a ptosis and breathing insufficiency. They appear 12 to 48 hours after birth. Mostly they decline after 4 weeks but there are also instances of duration of up to 4 months (Klehmet 2010).

There are no data on transfer via mother's milk among the other cholinergics, *bethanechol*, *carbachol*, *distigmine* and the antidote *physostigmine*. Gastrointestinal discomfort (colics, nausea, diarrhea) were observed in several newborns of mothers taking bethanechol (Shore 1970).

> **Recommendation.** Neostigmine and pyridostigmine may also be used during breastfeeding for appropriate indications. It is preferable not to use other cholinergics.

4.3.4   Anticholinergic spasmolytics

Infants and small children react very sensitively to atropine-like preparations. As yet, there are no publications in which negative effects on the baby have been described as a result of giving atropine-like drugs to a breastfeeding mother. *Butylscopolamine* appears to be well tolerated by the breastfed infant, either as a single parenteral dose or with repeated oral or rectal administration.

Experience during breastfeeding with other anticholinergics such as *darifenacin, fesoterodine, glycopyrronium bromide, hymecromon, mebeverine, methanthelinium, tolterodine, trospium chloride* and *flavoxate* is insufficient. This also applies to *propiverine* with a half-life of 20 hours and for *solifenacin*, which is the only medication from this group with a long half-life of 55 hours.

Scopolamine is used as a mydriaticum as are cyclopentolate and tropicamide.

> **Recommendation.** Butylscopolamine may be administered for appropriate indications. The widely used oxybutynin also seems to be acceptable (preferably at the end of breastfeeding with a waiting period of 3–4 hours). Solifenacin should be avoided due to the danger of accumulation in the breastfed infant's serum. Should one of the other drugs mentioned be necessary after a critical look at the indications, an individual decision about further breastfeeding, with good observation of the infant can be made. *Mydriatica* can also be used diagnostically during breastfeeding.

4.3.5   Laxatives

All bulking agents (Chapter. 2.5), such as Indian psyllium seed husks, osmotic laxatives such as *macrogol* or *lactulose* as well as saline laxatives, are practically not absorbed and can be used during breastfeeding. According to the manufacturer's information, neither bisacodyl nor sodium sulfate with their metabolites pass into the mother's milk. Two groups of eight healthy lactating mothers who had stopped breastfeeding

Lactation

4.3 Gastrointestinal drugs

received multiple doses of *bisacodyl* or *sodium picosulfate* (Friedrich 2011). Their common active metabolite bis-(*p*-hydroxyphenyl)-pyridyl-2-methane (BHPM) was measured in the maternal plasma, urine and in breast milk. BHPM remained below the limits of detection in breast milk following single and multiple doses.

Multiple studies of senna preparations, which belong to the anthraquinone family and which used to be considered contraindicated, have shown that the risk of causing diarrhea in breastfed infants is apparently quite low (survey by Bennett 1996). However, the anthraquinones are insufficiently toxicologically investigated.

The inhibition of absorption of fat-soluble vitamins argues against giving castor oil. Moreover, use of high doses could produce diarrhea, tremor and insomnia in exposed infants (manufacturer's data 2009).

> **Recommendation.** Bulking agents and osmotic laxatives are the laxatives of choice during breastfeeding. Bisacodyl and sodium sulfate are also acceptable. The brief use of other laxatives can be supported.

4.3.6   Agents used for chronic inflammatory bowel diseases

A number of medications are available to treat chronic inflammatory bowel diseases (Chapter 2.5). In this section, 5-aminosalicylic acid preparations (5-ASA-preparations) and probiotics will be discussed. For other medications, the reader will be referred, for example, to Chapter 2.15 (corticosteroids) or Chapter 2.12 (immune modulators).

The sulfonamide, *salazosulfapyridine* (*sulfasalazine*) has an M/P ratio of 0.4. With a maternal dose of 3 g daily, up to 10% of the weight-related dose can reach the infant. In one case, bloody diarrhea occurred in a breastfed baby whose plasma concentration was 5.3 mg/L (therapeutic range 20–50 mg/L). With a maternal dose of 2 g/day, a significant lower relative dose was calculated for the infant (survey in Bennett 1996).

Mesalazine consists of 5-aminosalicylic acid, the anti-inflammatory part of sulfasalazine. With a daily intake of 3 g, an oral infant dose of 0.015 mg/kg bodyweight could be calculated. This represents less than 0.1% of the maternal weight-related dose (Klotz 1993, Jenss 1990). However, taking into consideration the metabolite, acetyl-5-aminosalicylic acid (about 12 mg/L of milk) it would be 7.5%. A further publication reports less than 15 mg of Ac-5-ASA per liter of milk (Christensen 1994). Silverman (2005) also found very low 5-ASA values in the milk of four breastfeeding mothers. However, the concentration of the inactive metabolite N-Ac-5-ASA was 1,000 fold higher. No symptoms were observed in any of these infants. Another case described an infant who developed diarrhea following repeated rectal administration of mesalazine to his mother. This ceased with the end of therapy (Nelis 1989). Among eight breastfed babies, one was observed with diarrhea (Ito 1993).

Olsalazine, which consists of two mesalazine molecules, has an intestinal absorption rate of about 2% and can only be detected in the mother's milk in the form of its acetylated metabolites (Miller 1993).

Probiotics with *E. coli*, *lactobacillus* or *enterococcus faecalis* strains are not absorbed orally and are unproblematic for the breastfed baby.

Lactation

> **Recommendation.** During therapy with the medications mentioned here, unlimited breastfeeding is permitted. However, follow-up for diarrhea is necessary especially for long period of treatment.

4.3.7 Antidiarrheals for acute diarrhea

Loperamide decreases intestinal motility by interacting with opiate receptors. In a study on loperamide, less than 0.1% of the maternal weight-related dose was reported for the infant after the mother had received two doses (Nikodem 1992). As yet, no toxic effects have been described.

Activated (medical) charcoal and apple pectin are not absorbed and the active ingredient, *tannin albuminate*, is not significantly absorbed. Oral *ethacridine* also remains largely in the gastrointestinal tract, with 0.1% eliminated with the urine. The new ingredient, *racecadotril*, is quickly absorbed after oral intake. There are no data available on passage into the mother's milk and its safety.

> **Recommendation.** Apple pectin and activated (medical) charcoal may be taken during breastfeeding. Oral tannin or ethacridine also do not harm the breastfed baby. Loperamide may be prescribed temporarily during breastfeeding if dietary measures are insufficient. Racecadotril should not be used as its safety has not yet been established.

4.3.8 Digestives and carminatives

Dimethicone or *simethicone* are practically not absorbed. Toxic effects are unlikely, as with caraway and anise preparations. This also applies to ingredients such as pancreatin with lipases, amylases and proteases, i.e. trypsin and chymotrypsin, and tilactase. With regard to these anti-flatulent drugs, no data are available for their use during breastfeeding. However, Simethicone has been safely used in many instances of colic in infants.

> **Recommendation.** All the substances mentioned here may also be taken during breastfeeding.

4.3.9 Lipid reducers

No toxic effects on the infant have been reported as yet in connection with maternal intake of lipid reducers. Among these are *bezafibrate, etofibrate, fenofibrate* and *gemfibrozil, atorvastatin, fluvastatin, lovastatin, pravastatin, rosuvastatin, simvastatin* and *ezetimibe*. There are data on the passage into the mother's milk only for pravastatin, which appears in negligible amounts in the milk. It was calculated as less than 0.4% of a weight-related dose (Pan 1988).

Cholestyramine is a resin used to bind bile acids into a non-absorbable complex. Thus, it is practically not absorbed from the maternal gastrointestinal tract and should, therefore, be considered not risky for the

4.3 Gastrointestinal drugs

breastfed infant. *Colesevelam* is a new bile acid chelating agent, which is not absorbed (manufacturer data).

> **Recommendation.** Lipid reducers should not be used during breastfeeding because their safety is not established and there would seem – as a rule – to be no disadvantage for the mother when therapy is stopped. Nevertheless, taking the medication does not require any limitation of breastfeeding. Continuation of treatment should, however, be critically reviewed. With urgent indications, colestyramine, colesevelam or also pravastatin, would be worth considering.

4.3.10   Chenodeoxycholic acid and ursodeoxycholic acid

There is no documented experience on tolerance for *chenodeoxycholic acid* during breastfeeding. With *ursodeoxycholic acid*, only limited amounts appear in the blood circulation and are overwhelmingly bound to albumin there. Among 10 breastfeeding mothers who took between 300 and 1,500 mg of ursodeoxycholic acid daily for primary biliary cirrhosis or intra-hepatic cholestasis, around 100 µg/L on average, and a maximum of 196 µg/L of the substance – insofar as it was detectable – was found in the milk. The breastfed babies developed age-appropriately (Vitek 2010, Goh 2001, Brites 1998).

> **Recommendation.** Ursodeoxycholic acid may be used for primary biliary cirrhosis during breastfeeding. The pregnancy cholestasis usually improves postpartum without further therapy. Treatment with chenodeoxycholic acid should be postponed if possible.

4.3.11   Appetite suppressants

Pharmacological effects of sympathomimetic appetite suppressants such as *amfepramone (diethylpropiorin)*, *norpseudoephedrine* or *cathinone* and *phenylpropanolamine* on the breastfed infant have barely been studied. There is also no information on the use of *orlistat* during breastfeeding. Even if this active ingredient is scarcely absorbed and thus only a limited concentration in the milk would be expected, it should not be used because significant weight loss in the mother releases contaminants from her fatty tissue, which could additionally burden the mother's milk.

> **Recommendation.** Appetite suppressants are contraindicated during breastfeeding. Accidental intake does not require any limitation of breastfeeding.

4.3.12   Antiemetics

Antihistaminics, prokinetics, such as *metoclopramide* (Section 4.3.2) and serotonin antagonists are used as antiemetics. During therapy with time-tested antihistamines such as *dimenhydrinate* the salt of *diphenhydramine*, occasional, mild, restlessness, which does not need treatment, sedation or weak sucking are described in the breastfed infant (Moretti 1995, Ito 1993).

For many antiemetics, there is no specific knowledge about the breast-feeding period available. This involves, above all, *dolasetron*, *granisetron*, *ondansetron* and *palonosetron*.

The short half-life of 2 to 3 hours and the long effectiveness of up to 24 hours argue for good tolerance of *meclizine* during breastfeeding. However, in many countries it is not available. *Diclectin* (*pyridoxine* and *doxylamine*) was used for the treatment of nausea and vomiting of pregnancy (Ashkenazi-Hoffnug 2013), but there are no data on breast-feeding.

> **Recommendation.** The antiemetic of choice during breastfeeding is meclizine. Metoclopramide and domperidone are safe. Dimenhydrinate may also be prescribed for short periods. Should single doses of a serotonin antagonist such as ondansetron be indicated, breastfeeding can be continued as long as the infant is observed for symptoms.

References

Ashkenazi-Hoffnug L, Merlob P et al. Evaluation of the efficacy and safety of bi-daily combination therapy with pyridoxine and doxylamine for nausea and vomiting of pregnancy. Isr Med Assoc J 2013; 15: 23–6.

Bennett PN (ed). Drugs and Human Lactation. 2nd ed. Amsterdam, New York, Oxford: Elsevier, 1996.

Biervliet FP, Maguiness SD, Hay DM et al. Induction of lactation in the intended mother of a surrogate pregnancy. Hum Reprod 2001; 16: 581–3.

Brites D, Rodrigues CMP. Elevated levels of bile acids in colostrum of patients with cholestasis of pregnancy are decreased following ursodeoxycholic acid therapy. J Hepatol 1998; 29: 743–51.

Campbell-Yeo ML, Allen AC, Joseph KS et al. Effect of domperidone on the composition of preterm human breast milk. Pediatrics 2010; 125: e107–14.

Christensen LA, Rasmussen SN, Hansen SH. Disposition of 5-aminosalicylic acid and N-acetyl-5-aminosalicylic acid preparations. Acta Obstet Gynecol Scand 1994; 74: 399–402.

Courtney TP, Shaw RW, Cedar E et al. Excretion of famotidine in breast milk. Proc Br Paed Soc 1988; 9: 639.

Da Silva OP, Knoppert DC, Angelini MM et al. Effect of domperidone on milk production in mothers of premature newborns: a randomized, double-blind, placebo-controlled trial. CMAJ 2001; 164: 17–20.

Donovan TJ, Buchanan K. Medications for increasing milk supply in mothers expressing breastmilk for their preterm hospitalised infants. Cochrane Database Syst Rev 2012; 3:CD005544. PMID: 22419310.

Fife S, Gill P, Hopkins M et al. Metoclopramide to augment lactation, does it work? A randomized trial. J Matern Fetal Neonatal Med 2011; 24: 1317–20.

Fraser D, Turner JWA. Myasthenia gravis and pregnancy. Proc R Soc Med 1963; 56: 379–81.

Friedrich C, Richter E, Trommeshauser D et al. Absence of excretion of the active moiety of bisacodyl and sodium picosulfate into human breast milk: an open-label, parallel group, multiple – dose study in healthy lactating women. Drug Metab Pharmacokinet 2011; 26: 458–64.

Goh SK, Gull SE, Alexander GJ. Pregnancy in primary biliary cirrhosis complicated by portal hypertension: report of a case and review of the literature. BJOG 2001; 108: 760–2.

Hansen WF, McAndrew S, Harrsi K et al. Metoclopramide effect on breastfeeding the preterm infant: a randomized trial. Obstet Gynecol 2005; 105: 383–9.

Hardell LI, Lindstrom B, Lonnerholm G et al. Pyridostigmine in human breast milk. Br J Clin Pharmacol 1982; 14: 565–67.

Hofmeyr GJ, van Iddekinge B, Blott JA. Domperidone: secretion in breast milk and effect on puerperal prolactin levels. Br J Obstet Gynecol 1985; 92: 141–4.

Ito S, Blajchman A, Stephenson M et al. Prospective follow-up of adverse reactions in breast-fed infants exposed to maternal infection. Am J Obstet Gynecol 1993; 168: 1393–9.

Jenss H, Weber P, Hartman F. 5-Aminosalicylic acid and its metabolite in breast milk during lactation. Am J Gastroenterol 1990; 85: 331.

Kauppila A, Anunti P, Kivinen S et al. Metoclopramide and breastfeeding: efficacy and anterior pituitary responses of the mother and the child. Eur J Obstet Gynecol Reprod Biol 1985; 19: 19–22.

Kauppila A, Arvela P, Koivisto M et al. Metoclopramide and breastfeeding: transfer into milk and the newborn. Eur J Clin Pharmacol 1983; 25: 819–23.

Kearns GL, McConnel Jr RF, Trang JM et al. Appearance of ranitidine in breast milk following multiple dosing. Clin Pharmacol 1985; 4: 322–4.

Klehmet J, Dudenhausen J, Meisel A. Verlauf und Behandlung der Myasthenia gravis in der Schwangerschaft. Nervenarzt 2010; 81: 956–62.

Klotz U, Harings-Kaim A. Negligible excretion of 5-aminosalicylic acid in breast milk. Lancet 1993; 342: 618–9.

Knoppert DC, Page A, Warren J et al. The effect of two different domperidone dosages on maternal milk production. J Hum Lact 2013; 29: 38–44.

Marshall JK, Thomson ABR, Armstrong D. Omeprazole for refractory gastroesophageal reflux disease during pregnancy and lactation. Can J Gastroenterol 1998; 12: 225–7.

Miller LG, Hopkinson JM, Motil KJ et al. Disposition of olsalazine and metabolites in breast milk. J Clin Pharmacol 1993; 33: 703–6.

Moretti ME, Liau-Chu M, Taddio A et al. Adverse events in breast-fed infants exposed to antihistamines in maternal milk. Reprod Toxicol 1995; 9: 588.

Nelis GF. Diarrhea due to 5-aminosalicylic acid in breast milk. Lancet 1989; 1: 383.

Nikodem VC, Hofmeyr GJ. Secretion of the antidiarrheal agent loperamide oxide in breast milk. Eur J Clin Pharmacol 1992; 42: 695–6.

Obermeyer BD, Bergstrom RF, Callaghan JT et al. Secretion of nizatidine into human breast milk after single and multiple doses. Clin Pharmacol Ther 1990; 47: 724–30.

Oo CY, Kuhn RJ, Desai N et al. Active transport of cimetidine into human breast milk. Clin Pharmacol Ther 1995; 58: 548–55.

Osadchy A, Moretti, Koren G. Effect of domperidone on insufficient lactation in puerperal women: a systematic review and meta-analysis of randomized controlled trials. Obstet Gynecol Int 2012; 642893.

Pan H, Fleiss P, Moore L et al. Excretion of pravastatin, an HMG CoA reductase inhibitor in breast milk of lactating women. J Clin Pharmacol 1988; 28: 942.

Plante L, Ferron GM, Unruh M et al. Excretion of pantoprazole in human breast. J Reprod Med 2004; 49: 825–7.

Shore MF. Drugs can be dangerous during pregnancy and lactation. Can Pharmacol J 1970; 103: 103–58.

Silverman DA, Ford J, Shaw I et al. Is mesalazine really safe for use in breast-feeding mothers? Gut 2005; 54: 170–1.

Vitek L, Zelenkova M, Bruha R. Safe use of ursodeoxycholic acid in a breast-feeding patient with primary biliary cirrhosis. Dig Liver Dis 2010; 42: 911–2.

Wan EW, Davey K, Page-Sharp M et al. Dose-effect study of domperidone as a galactagogue in preterm mothers with insufficient milk supply, and its transfer into milk. Br J Clin Pharmacol 2008; 66: 283–9.

Zuppa AA, Sindico P, Orchi C et al. Safety and efficacy of galactogogues: substances that induce, maintain and increase breast milk production. J Pharm Pharm Sci 2010; 13: 162–74.

Anti-infectives

Stephanie Padberg

4.4

4.4.1	Penicillins, cephalosporins and other β-lactam antibiotics	688
4.4.2	Erythromycin and other macrolides	688
4.4.3	Tetracyclines	689
4.4.4	Sulfonamides and trimethoprim	689
4.4.5	Quinolones	690
4.4.6	Nitrofurans and drugs for urinary tract infections	690
4.4.7	Nitroimidazole antibiotics	691
4.4.8	Aminoglycosides	692
4.4.9	Glycopeptide and polypeptide antibiotics	692
4.4.10	Other antibiotics	692
4.4.11	Tuberculostatics	693
4.4.12	Local antibiotics	694
4.4.13	Antimalarial medication	695
4.4.14	Systemic antifungal agents	696
4.4.15	Topical antifungal agents	696
4.4.16	Anthelmintics	697
4.4.17	Antiviral agents	697

With many antibiotics, a breastfed child receives less than 1% of the weight-related therapeutic dose when the mother is being treated. Thus only minimal concentrations – and in no case, bacteria-inhibiting concentrations – are achieved in the infant's plasma.

The following risks with antibiotic treatment during breastfeeding have been discussed repeatedly:

- Effects on the child's intestinal flora (a "thinner" stool consistency, but seldom diarrhea).
- Effects on bacteriological cultures, which may be necessary if the infant becomes ill.
- Development of bacterial resistance.
- Sensitization.

None of these side-effects has been proven to be clinically relevant or even requiring treatment. The most likely possibility is a temporary effect on the consistency of the infant's stool (Ito 1993).

Drugs During Pregnancy and Lactation. http://dx.doi.org/10.1016/B978-0-12-408078-2.00029-9

4.4.1   Penicillins, cephalosporins and other β-lactam antibiotics

The M/P ratio of all the commonly used penicillin derivatives is under 1. As a rule, the exclusively breastfed infant receives considerably less than 1% of a therapeutic dose (survey in Bennett 1996). Similarly, this also applies for the cephalosporins, which are, to some extent, inactivated in the infant's intestine (survey in Bennett 1996).

Benyamini (2005) asked 67 breastfeeding mothers, who were taking *amoxicillin* in combination with *clavulanic acid*, about side-effects in their breastfed children. Symptoms were reported more frequently (22%) than with amoxicillin therapy alone. The symptoms were dose-dependent, but did not need any intervention. In another group, which took *cefuroxim* while breastfeeding, mild side-effects were reported in just under 3% of the cases, which was no more frequently reported than in a control group with *cefalexin*.

With *sulbactam*, the relative daily dose transmitted was a maximum of 1% (Foulds 1985). With *aztreonam*, a 0.2% relative dose was reported for the baby at the next breastfeeding after the mother had taken a single dose (Ito 1990).

In a Japanese study on *imipenem* plus *cilastatin*, an average of 0.8% of a weight-related intravenously administered dose was measured in the daily amount of milk. Cilastatin was not detectable in the breastfed children (Ito 1988).

After administration of 1,000 mg *meropenem* every 8 hours, the maximum concentration in milk was 0.64 μg/mL; the infant weight-adjusted percentage of maternal dose was 0.18% (Sauberan 2012).

There are insufficient data on the breastfeeding period for the β-lactamase inhibitor, *tazobactam*, and the newer carbapenems (*doripenem* and *ertapenem*). Up to now, there have been no reports of toxic effects in the breastfed baby. The last-mentioned substances are scarcely absorbed. This argues against a biological availability to the breastfed baby.

Recommendation. Penicillin derivatives and cephalosporins are the antibiotics of choice during breastfeeding. When possible, therapies, e.g. cephalosporins, such as cefalexin and cefuroxim, that have been in use for a long time, are preferred. Should the use of other β-lactam antibiotics or β-lactamase inhibitors be necessary, breastfeeding may be continued.

4.4.2   Erythromycin and other macrolides

With *erythromycin* (M/P ratio about 0.5), the infant whose mother takes 2 g/day, receives a maximum of 0.48 mg/kg/day – just 2% of a weight-related therapeutic infant dose (Matsuda 1984). Pyloric stenosis, possibly caused by erythromycin via the mother's milk, has been reported (Sørensen 2003, Stang 1986), but a causal relationship has not been confirmed. Goldstein (2009) asked 55 breastfeeding mothers, who were treated with macrolides, about side-effects in their breastfed babies. Some 12% observed mild symptoms such as thinner stools or a skin rash, which, by comparison to *amoxicillin*, did not occur more frequently. In particular, no pyloric stenosis was observed.

In a case report on *azithromycin* (500 mg/day), a peak value of 2.8 mg/L of milk was cited. This represents 5% of the weight-related maternal dose (Kelsey 1994).

With 500 mg/day of *clarithromycin*, used to treat a puerperal infection, a maximum of 1.5 mg of the active substance per liter of milk was measured (Sedlmayr 1993). That is 2.7% of the maternal dosage per kg of bodyweight.

With *roxythromycin*, less than 0.05% is thought to pass into the milk (Lassman 1988).

There are no data on the breastfeeding period for *dirithromycin*, *josamycin*, *midecamycin*, *spiramycin*, *troleandomycin*, and the *ketolide telithromycin*. There are no reports of specific intolerance during breast-feeding to any of the macrolides described here.

> **Recommendation.** In addition to penicillin derivatives and cephalosporin antibiotics, macrolides are the antibiotics of choice during breastfeeding.

4.4.3   Tetracyclines

The older tetracyclines reach concentrations in the mother's milk that are significantly below the maternal plasma values. In addition, the calcium ions in the mother's milk reduce the absorption of the drug. There are no reports of breastfed infants having symptoms when mother is taking tetracyclines. In particular, there is no discoloration of the teeth as a result of exposure via mother's milk.

With *doxycycline* therapy initially with 200 mg followed by 100 mg after 24 hours, a maximum of 1.4 mg/L was detected in the milk (Morganti 1968).

One case report describes a brownish-black coloring of the milk after long-term intake of minocycline. Macrophages with iron-containing pigments were found in the milk. The authors believe that this is an iron chelate of minocycline or of a metabolite (Hunt 1996).

There is insufficient data on the breastfeeding period for the *glycylcycline, tigecycline*. The limited oral bioavailability of tigecycline, however, argues against an appreciable intake by the breastfed infant.

> **Recommendation.** Should the antibiotics of choice not be appropriate, breast-feeding may also continue with tetracycline. Local therapy with tetracyclines is not problematic.

4.4.4   Sulfonamides and trimethoprim

Sulfonamides pass into the mother's milk in various amounts. The percentage specifications, based on the weight-related maternal dosage, vary between 1 and over 50% (in the case of the old sulfonamide sulfanilamide).

Trimethoprim and *sulfamethoxazole*, used in combination in *co-trimoxazole*, are excreted in breast milk in small amounts. With the usual dose of trimethoprim 320 mg and sulfamethoxazole 800 mg daily, an exclusively breastfed infant would be expected to receive 0.3 mg/kg/day of trimethoprim and 0.68 mg/kg/day of sulfamethoxazole, which is much lower than the recommended dosage for children (Miller, 1974).

Since sulfonamides compete with bilirubin for albumin binding sites, there might be a risk of an increase in the newborn's bilirubin.

Lactation

4.4 Anti-infectives

> **Recommendation.** If the primary recommended antibiotics do not work suffi-
> ciently or cannot be tolerated, breastfeeding can continue with cotrimoxazole or
> trimethoprim monotherapy. For more severe indications, another sulfonamide can
> also be prescribed. With premature infants or newborns with hyperbilirubinemia
> or glucose-6-phosphate-dehydrogenase deficiency, the indication should be par-
> ticularly critically reviewed. Local therapy with sulfonamides does not require any
> limitation of breastfeeding.

4.4.5   Quinolones

Insofar as they have been studied at all, *nalidixic acid* and the newer
fluoroquinolones go into the mother's milk.

With *ciprofloxacin*, it has been calculated that between 2 and 7%
of the weight-related maternal dose reaches the infant (Cover 1990,
Giamarellou 1989). No ciprofloxacin could be detected in the serum of a
breastfed baby (maternal serum concentration 0.21 mg/L, detection limit
0.03 mg/L; Gardner 1992).

With *levofloxacin*, a mother received 500 mg/day over 3 weeks, first
administered parenterally and then orally, maximum concentrations in the
milk of 8.2 mg/L (5 hours after administration) and, at most, a relative dose
of 15% were calculated for an exclusively breastfed baby (Cahill 2005).

There are no data on the transfer of *enoxacin, lomefloxacin, moxifloxacin,
nadifloxacin, norfloxacin, ofloxacin* and *sparfloxacin* into mother's milk.

In animal research, quinolones irreversibly damage the cartilage in
the joints of juvenile animals. This has not as yet been observed with
exposure to quinolones via the mother's milk.

> **Recommendation.** Quinolones are not among the antibiotics of choice during
> breastfeeding. As a rule, a standard antibiotic with a lower potential for risk can
> be used. When a complicated infection really requires a quinolone, breastfeeding
> may continue. Ideally then, the most-tested ciprofloxacin should be chosen. With
> local therapy, breastfeeding may also be continued.

4.4.6   Nitrofurans and drugs for urinary tract infections

With *nitrofurantoin*, after a single dose of 100 mg to four women, an
average of 1.3 mg/L and a maximum (about 5 hours after administration)
of 3.2 mg/L was measured in the milk. An M/P ratio of 6 was calculated
(Gerk 2001). Based on these values, the relative dose for an exclusively
breastfed baby can reach 10%. Older investigations only reported 2.5%
(Pons 1990). Nitrofurantoin inhibits the glutathione reductase and should,
therefore, be used cautiously for breastfeeding mothers of newborns with
hyperbilirubinemia or glucose-6-phosphate-dehydrogenase deficiency.

One study estimated the exposure of *nifurtimox* through milk using
computer simulation (Garcia-Bournissen 2010). This population pharmacokinetic analysis calculated that a breastfed infant would receive less
than 10% of the maternal weight adjusted dose. In a study with 33 infants
whose mothers took nifurtimox, no serious adverse events were reported
in any of the breastfed infants (Schmid 2012).

The locally used nitrofurans, *furazolidone* and *nitrofural*, as well as *nifuratel* are insufficiently investigated for the breastfeeding period, and are not

among rational drug therapies. The same applies for nifuroxazide, which is used for diarrhea. For the same reasons, the urinary tract medications, methenamine and nitroxoline should be avoided during breastfeeding.

The limited experience with *fosfomycin* during breastfeeding permits the assumption that only a limited amount of the active ingredient passes into the mother's milk.

Recommendation. If nitrofurantoin is strongly indicated breastfeeding may continue during treatment. Local therapy with nitrofurans does not require any limitation of breastfeeding. Should it be unavoidable, breastfeeding might be continued with nifurtimox. Nifuroxazide and the urinary tract medications methenamine and nitroxoline should be avoided during breastfeeding. However, when use of the drug is short-term, whether it is justifiable to continue breastfeeding must be decided individually. Fosfomycin should only be prescribed during breastfeeding when the primary, recommended antibiotics are insufficiently effective or not tolerated. One-time oral administration does not require any limitation of breastfeeding.

4.4.7   Nitroimidazole antibiotics

Metronidazole passes into the mother's milk and is also detectable in the infant. Two to 4 hours after a single oral dose of 2 g for trichomoniasis, a maximum of 46 mg/L was measured in the milk. If the active metabolites in the milk are included, an average of 12% with a maximum of 20% of a weight-related therapeutic child's dose of 15 mg/kg/day is calculated for an exclusively breastfed infant. Metronidazole and its metabolite, *hydroxymetronidazole*, were detected in the plasma of breastfed babies with 2 mg/L. Comparable results were found with a 9-day course of 1,200 mg/day (Passmore 1988, Heisterberg 1983, Erickson 1981). The half-life of metronidazole is significantly extended in newborns. With adults it is up to 10 hours, and even up to 74 hours for premature infants.

Specific toxicity via the mother's milk has not been described among the 60 mother–child pairs published to date. Metronidazole is used therapeutically even with premature infants (e.g. for necrotizing enterocolitis) and is, in general, well-tolerated.

There has not, as yet, been any indication that the mutagenic and carcinogenic effects of metronidazole experimentally observed in animals occur in human beings.

With *tinidazole*, transfer via mother's milk can reach a maximum of 10% of the weight-related maternal dose administered intravenously (Mannisto 1983). *Nimorazole* and *ornidazole* have not been studied during breastfeeding.

Recommendation. When necessary, metronidazole may be used during breastfeeding. A single oral dose of 2 g is preferable to vaginal administration spread over several days. This is considered to be more effective therapeutically and limits the exposure for the infant. With intravenous treatment spread over several days, the administration should be, whenever possible, in the evening after the last breastfeed in order to limit the exposure during the nightly breastfeeding break. Weaning or interruption of breastfeeding no longer seems justifiable based on the available experience. Metronidazole should be used in preference to the other nitroimidazoles.

Lactation

4.4 Anti-infectives

4.4.8   Aminoglycosides

With an intramuscular *gentamicin* dose of 80 mg three times a day, a maximum of 0.78 mg/L of milk was measured (Celiloglu 1994). This is about 3% of the weight-related maternal dose. However, in five of the 10 newborns included in this study, gentamicin concentrations in the serum were measured, which were equivalent to 10% of the maternal values. This leads to the conclusion that newborns, to a degree that cannot be ignored, either absorb aminoglycosides enterally or accumulate them due to reduced excretion. *Amikacin, kanamycin* and *tobramycin* only appear in limited amounts (up to about 1%) in mother's milk (Festini 2006, Matsuda 1984).

The other aminoglycoside antibiotics, *framycetin, neomycin, netilmicin, paromomycin, ribostamycin, spectinomycin* and *streptomycin* are insufficiently researched. Possibly, they may be evaluated in an analogous way. Apart from the newborn period, aminoglycosides are scarcely absorbed.

> **Recommendation.** For urgent indications, breastfeeding may be permitted even with the parenteral administration of aminoglycosides. The indication should be critically reviewed, especially in the newborn period, since both quantitative absorption and accumulation by the infant must be reckoned with and, at least in the case of streptomycin, an ototoxic effect cannot be ruled out in this way. With local or oral aminoglycoside therapy breastfeeding may continue with no limitations.

4.4.9   Glycopeptide and polypeptide antibiotics

With 1 g of the glycopeptide antibiotic, *vancomycin*, administered intravenously, 12.7 mg/L were measured in the milk (Reyes 1989). Mathematically, such a concentration represents 5.8% of the maternal dose for an exclusively breastfed infant. There are no data on *teicoplanin* during breastfeeding.

In a breastfeeding woman who received 50 mg *daptomycin* daily, a maximum concentration of 0.045 mg/L was measured in the milk (Buitrago 2009). This extremely limited transfer and the limited enteral absorption, do not lead to an expectation of any risk for a breastfed infant.

There are no data on the primarily locally used polypeptide antibiotics *bacitracin, colistin, polymyxin B* and *tyrothricin* during breastfeeding.

All glycopeptides and polypeptides are absorbed either minimally or not at all. This leads to the assumption that an infant would not take in any relevant amount via the mother's milk.

> **Recommendation.** Should it be unavoidable, breastfeeding is permitted with glycopeptide and polypeptide antibiotics. With local therapy, breastfeeding may continue without limitations.

4.4.10   Other antibiotics

▶ **Chloramphenicol**

Chloramphenicol is suspected of causing dose-dependent bone marrow damage which, however, is not observed with exposure through the mother's milk. Refusal of food and vomiting in a breastfed infant were described in connection with maternal treatment (Havelka 1972).

> **Recommendation.** Due to its toxicity, chloramphenicol is contraindicated during breastfeeding. Local use should also be avoided if possible.

▶ Clindamycin and lincomycin

With *clindamycin* a maximum of 3.1 mg/L milk was measured. For the infant, this represents less than 2% of the weight-related dose taken by the mother, or just under 3% of a therapeutic infant dose (Steen 1982, Smith 1975). In a case report, hemorrhagic enteritis was described in an infant whose mother had taken clindamycin and *gentamicin*. The symptoms improved spontaneously after breastfeeding was interrupted (Mann 1980).

With *lincomycin*, a maximum of 1% of the maternal weight-related dose was measured in the milk (Medina 1963).

> **Recommendation.** Should it be unavoidable, breastfeeding is permitted with clindamycin and lincomycin. Clindamycin should not be prescribed routinely after dental procedures.

▶ Linezolid

A study showed a limited passage of *linezolid* into the mother's milk (Sagirli 2009). After taking 600 mg, the maximum concentration in the milk was 12.4 mg/L. The authors concluded that an exclusively breastfed infant would get a maximum of 2 mg/kg/day. That is about 7% of the recommended infant dose of 30 mg/kg/day.

> **Recommendation.** Linezolid should only be prescribed during breastfeeding where the primary, recommended antibiotics are insufficiently effective or not tolerated. In such a case, it must be decided individually whether to continue breastfeeding.

4.4.11   Tuberculostatics

The data on *ethambutol* during breastfeeding are limited (Snider 1984). With one woman, 1.4 mg/L were measured in the mother's milk 3 hours after taking 15 mg/kg ethambutol orally. From this, 1.5% of the maternal weight-related dose is calculated for the exclusively breastfed infant.

Isoniazid has an M/P ratio of about 1. A maximum of 16.6 mg/L was measured in the mother's milk (Singh 2008, Berlin 1979), which would hardly lead to any toxic effects on the baby. It has been discussed whether not only the mother, but also an exclusively breastfed infant who is not receiving therapy, should receive *pyridoxine* prophylactically (Blumberg 2003).

After oral administration of 1 g pyrazinamide, with an M/P ratio of 0.04, a maximum of 1.5 mg/L was measured in the milk. An exclusively breastfed baby would receive a maximum of 1.4% of the maternal weight-related dose (Holdiness 1984).

Lactation

4.4 Anti-infectives

Rifampicin is secreted into breast milk in low levels. After a single oral dose, milk levels were measured between 3.4 to 4.9 mg/L (Snider 1984).

Only a very limited amount of the aminoglycoside, *streptomycin*, would be expected in the milk and, apart from the newborn period, is not absorbed enterally to any significant degree (Section 4.4.8).

4-aminosalicylic acid seems to pass into the mother's milk only to a limited degree (Holdiness 1984).

With *dapsone* therapy, 10–20% of the weight-related dose could pass into the milk (Edstein 1986, Sanders 1982). One case describes a breast-fed infant with hemolytic anemia, whose mother was being treated with dapsone. Dapsone and the primary metabolite, *monoacetyldapsone*, were documented in his serum (Sanders 1982).

There is insufficient experience during the breastfeeding period for the reserve drugs *capreomycin, cycloserine, ethionamide, prothionamide rifabutin, rifapentine, terizidone* and *thioacetazone*.

The WHO (2010b) recommends that women who are ill with TBC receive therapy while they are breastfeeding according to the guideline. This is not only optimal for the mother who is ill, but also deters the baby from being infected. All tuberculostatics are, according to WHO, appropriate during breastfeeding. This recommendation rests on a risk-benefit-assessment which is oriented to the high risk countries.

Recommendation. During tuberculosis therapy with the first-line agents, isoniazid (+pyridoxine), rifampicin, ethambutol and pyrazinamide, breastfeeding is permitted. Should the breastfeeding mother need reserve medications due to resistance or intolerance, a limitation of breastfeeding must be decided on the individual case.

4.4.12   Local antibiotics

Up to now, there have been no indications of risks for the breastfed infant with topical use of anti-infectives. With longer treatment and greater areas, there may be relevant absorption. In such cases, one should orient oneself to the recommendations on systemic therapy.

There are no documented experiences on the breastfeeding period for *mupirocin*. As less than 1% of it is absorbed, a risk for the breastfed infant seems unlikely. There are also no data on the breastfeeding period for *fusidic acid, fusafungine* and *retapamulin*.

For local use of aminoglycosides, see the appropriate Section 4.4.8, chloramphenicol see Section 4.4.10, gyrase-inhibitors see Section 4.4.5, macrolides see Section 4.4.2, nitrofurans see Section 4.4.6, nitroimidazoles see Section 4.4.7, polypeptide antibiotics see Section 4.4.9, sulfonamides see Section 4.4.4, and tetracyclines see Section 4.4.3.

Recommendation. Fundamentally, every external antibiotic therapy should be critically reviewed. Should it be indicated, normally breastfeeding is permitted. Long-term treatment of larger areas should be avoided. For theoretical reasons, preparations that contain chloramphenicol should be avoided if possible. Should the breast need external treatment, it should be cleaned off before breastfeeding.

4.4.13 Antimalarial medication

Prophylaxis and treatment of malaria during breastfeeding are oriented primarily to the level of resistance in the affected area, and on the type of malaria diagnosed. Usually, treatment of malaria is short-term and most of the active ingredients are also approved for the newborn; therefore treatment with malarial drugs seldom requires an interruption of breastfeeding. With prophylaxis, the exposure continues for considerably longer than with acute therapy, so that general recommendations are difficult.

Chloroquine does pass into the mother's milk. In various studies, an average of 4 mg/L and a maximum of 7.5 mg/L have been documented in the milk. Depending on the study design, relative doses from 0.5–3% have been reported (Law 2008, Ette 1987, Ogunbona 1987, Edstein 1986). However, the main metabolite, *desmethylchloroquine*, also needs to be considered. With the very long half-life, continuing high plasma and milk levels can be expected despite a weekly intake of malaria prophylaxis. Chloroquine can be detected in the infant's urine (Witte 1990). Symptoms have not been reported as yet. In cases of using chloroquine for rheumatic illnesses see Chapter 4.1.

Mefloquine has a neurotoxic potential. There is one study on its use during breastfeeding, in which an M/P ratio of 0.15 and a transfer of a maximum of 4% of the weight-related dose were reported following a single dose of 250 mg of mefloquine (Edstein 1988).

Proguanil is a well-tested drug, apparently well-tolerated during breastfeeding and approved for children. There are no data on transfer into mother's milk.

For *pyrimethamine*, an M/P ratio of 0.4–0.6 and a relative dose of about 45% were reported in three women after oral administration of 12.5 mg/day (Edstein 1986).

Quinine which is currently experiencing a renaissance in malaria therapy because of increasing resistance, is well-tolerated during breastfeeding. Following oral administration, a maximum of 3.6 mg/L has been documented in the milk. After intravenous administration, it was a maximum of 8 mg/L. The authors estimate an M/P ratio of 0.2–0.5 (Phillips 1986).

For *artemisinin*, as well as its derivatives *artemether, artemotil, artesunate* and *dihydroartemisinin*, there are insufficient data on the breastfeeding period. There is also no documented experience for the breastfeeding period with the other malarial drugs such as *amodiaquine, atovaquone, halofantrine, lumefantrine, piperaquine* and *primaquine*. With primaquine, it should be reviewed whether the therapy can be postponed, particularly with newborns with glucose-6-phosphate-dehydrogenase deficiency (WHO 2010a). For *dapsone*, see Section 4.4.11, doxycycline see Section 4.4.3, clindamycin see Section 4.4.2, and sulfonamides see Section 4.4.4.

Recommendation. The usually short malaria therapy presents no medically based indication for interrupting breastfeeding. In the case of a malaria prophylaxis spread over several weeks, limitation of breastfeeding must be individually decided. At least chloroquine, mefloquine, proguanil and quinine are among the drugs for which there is the most experience, and which do not have substantial indications of potential for damage via the mother's milk.

4.4.14   Systemic antifungal agents

With *fluconazole*, a maximum of 2.9 mg/L of milk was measured following a single oral dose of 150 mg. Based on this, an exclusively breastfed infant would receive more than 18% of the maternal weight-related dose. A half-life of 30 hours was calculated for fluconazole (Force 1995). The mostly good tolerance of fluconazole after intravenous use in newborns is often used as an argument for continuing breastfeeding.

A Candida infection of the breast is a relatively frequent reason for systemic fluconazole therapy. The diagnosis is not easy and should be made with caution. It is estimated that 20% of lactating women complaining of breast pain have a Candida infection. Unfortunately, local treatment is usually insufficient, so that oral treatment with fluconazole for 2 to 3 weeks, or for 2 weeks after symptoms have resolved, is recommended. At the same time, the infant also needs antifungal treatment (e.g. with miconazole) because the amount transmitted through the milk is insufficient therapeutically.

In a case report on systemic administration of ketoconazole, an average of 0.4% and a maximum of 1.4% of the weight-related maternal dose was calculated for the infant (Moretti 1995). Because it is so poorly tolerated, ketoconazole is mostly replaced by systemically better tolerated drugs such as fluconazole.

There are no documented experiences during breastfeeding for the other systemically used azole derivatives such as *itraconazole, posaconazole* and *voriconazole*.

There are no publications about the use of *amphotericin B* during lactation. The high protein binding, the high molecular weight, and the poor oral absorption of this agent do not lead to an expectation of any appreciable transfer to the breastfed baby. Amphotericin B is also approved for infants.

There are insufficient data to evaluate *flucytosine, griseofulvin* and *terbinafine* during breastfeeding. The same applies for the *echinocandins anidulafungin, caspofungin* and *micafungin*.

> **Recommendation.** Should systemic antifungal therapy be unavoidable, fluconazole, the best studied during breastfeeding, should be selected when the pathogen spectrum permits. Interrupting breastfeeding is not justified. Breastfeeding is also permitted with amphotericin B. Other systemic antifungal agents should be avoided during breastfeeding if possible. When urgently therapy is indicated using one of these substances, a decision about breastfeeding should be made individually.

4.4.15   Topical antifungal agents

Clotrimazole and *miconazole* are not absorbed in relevant amounts. Extensive experience with their therapeutic use in infancy argues against any toxic potential. For ketoconazole see Section 4.4.14. The other azole derivatives *bifonazole, butoconazole, croconazole, econazole, fenticonazole, isoconazole, ketoconazole, omoconazole, oxiconazole, sertaconazole, sulconazole, terconazole*, and *tioconazole* are related to *clotrimazole* structurally and in their action, but they have been studied less.

Nystatin is not absorbed and is not available to the infant enterally. Although there are no relevant published data about its use during lactation, it is unlikely to be transferred in relevant amounts into the milk. With regard to the use of *amphotericin B* and *terbinafine* see Section 4.4.14.

There has been no experience with *amorolfin, butenafine, ciclopirox, haloprogin, clopirox, naftifin, natamycin, terbinafine, tolciclate* and *tolnaftate*. Most of these locally administered antifungals are only absorbed in limited amounts, so that a risk for the breastfed infant is unlikely.

> **Recommendation.** Local antifungals of choice during breastfeeding are clotrimazole, miconazole and nystatin. Amphotericin B is also acceptable. Should one of the other medications be indicated, breastfeeding may continue without limitation if they are only used temporarily, or if only small areas are being treated.

4.4.16   Anthelmintics

Most anthelmintic agents are poorly resorbed from the gastrointestinal tract and are only used briefly. Therefore a risk for the breastfed infant would not be expected.

In a study of 33 breastfeeding women following administration of 400 mg *albendazole*, only the anthelmintic-acting metabolite, *albendazole sulfoxide*, with an average concentration of 0.35 mg/L was detected in the milk (Abdel-Tawab 2009). From this the authors calculate a relative dose of <1.5%.

A single case report describes a reduction in the amount of milk after a 3-day therapy with *mebendazole* (Rao 1983). This observation was based on one case report and a causal relationship is not proven. Considering the poor enteral resorption it is unlikely that mebendazole reaches the breastfed infant in relevant concentrations.

For the other benzimidazole derivatives such as *flubendazole* and *triclabendazole*, no relevant reports about their use during lactation have been found.

By contrast *ivermectin* is well absorbed enterally. Following a single dose of 150 μg/kg to the mother, an average of 10 μg/L and a maximum of 23 μg/L was measured in the milk (Ogbuokiri 1994). Just considering the highest value, that is only 2% of the weight-related maternal dose for an exclusively breastfed infant.

With *praziquantel*, a maximum of 1.68 mg/L and, on average, 0.46 mg/L in the milk was found (Pütter 1979). These concentrations appear be too low to harm a breastfed infant.

There are no relevant data about the use of *niclosamide, pyrantel, pyrvinium* during lactation. As they are poorly absorbed enterally, it is unlikely that they would reach relevant concentrations in breast milk.

Due to insufficient data, no statements can be made on tolerance during breastfeeding of the other anthelmintic agents.

> **Recommendation.** *Pyrvinium* or *mebendazole* should be used to treat infections with pinworms (enterobiasis), and *niclosamide* for tapeworms (cestodes). The other anthelminthic agents should be reserved for specific compelling indications. If exposure is only short-term, breastfeeding may continue.

4.4.17   Antiviral agents

▶ **Herpes medications**

Acyclovir passes into the mother's milk. Multiple studies have shown higher concentrations in the milk than in the plasma (Bork 1995, Taddio 1994, Meyer 1988). Bork (2000) demonstrated that the accumulation of acyclovir in the mother's milk is due to passive diffusion and that no active transport mechanism is required, as was originally thought. If the results of the studies are summarized, after intravenous administration of 900 mg, the acyclovir concentrations in the milk reach a maximum of 7.3 mg/L. With oral intake of 800 mg, a maximum of 5.8 mg/L was measured in the milk. With this concentration, the relative dose via the mother's milk is a maximum of 7%. Since oral acyclovir is only about 20% absorbed, the baby would receive about 1% of the recommended infant dose via the mother's milk. Toxic symptoms have not been observed and seem unlikely, as acyclovir is used in neonates with mostly good tolerance.

Valacyclovir, is an easily available oral prodrug of acyclovir. In five mothers who received 500 mg twice daily, valacyclovir could not be detected either in the maternal serum or in the milk, because it is rapidly converted to acyclovir. The highest values of acyclovir in the milk were measured about 4 hours after administration. The M/P ratio was calculated at 3.4. Even considering the highest measured value in the milk, the relative dose for an exclusively breastfed baby amounts to only 5.7%. If the therapeutically used dose in neonatology is taken as a comparative basis, and the limited oral availability of acyclovir is considered, a maximum of 1% of a pediatric dose would be calculated for the infant via the mother's milk. In the urine of the infants studied, an average of 0.74 mg/L was found under steady-state conditions (Sheffield 2002).

There are no data on the breastfeeding period for *brivudine, cidofovir, famciclovir, fomivirsen, foscarnet, ganciclovir, idoxuridine, penciclovir, trifluridine, tromantadine,* and *valganciclovir.*

After the use of topical herpes medications, an adverse effect to the breastfed infant seems unlikely because of poor absorption. No side-effects for the infant via mother's milk would be expected with local therapy using *docosanol, zinc sulfate* or patches containing *hydrocolloid* particles.

> **Recommendation.** With external and systemic administration of acyclovir or valacyclovir, breastfeeding is permitted. The other herpes medications, if really indicated, require an individual decision about continuing breastfeeding. Topical application to small areas is compatible with breastfeeding if the exposure is short-term.

▶ Antiviral drugs for hepatitis

There are no documented experiences on the breastfeeding period for the *virustatics adefovir, boceprevir, entecavir, ribavirin, simeprevir, sofosbuvir, telaprevir,* and *telbivudine* used for chronic infectious hepatitis. For *lamivudine* and *tenofovir,* see under Antiretroviral agents in this section. For α-interferons see Chapter 4.10.

> **Recommendation.** The virustatics discussed here require an individual decision about continuing breastfeeding. For example, with an urgently required therapy for chronic hepatitis B, breastfeeding with lamivudine or tenofovir, after simultaneous hepatitis B immunization of the baby (Chapter 4.5), seems acceptable.

▶ Antiviral drugs for influenza

The neuraminidase inhibitor, *oseltamivir*, only passes into the mother's milk in limited amounts. A case report on a breastfeeding woman who took 75 mg of oseltamivir twice daily for 5 days determined a relative dose of 0.5% (Wentges-van Holthe 2008). Another publication analyzed the milk of seven postpartum women. Oseltamivir and its metabolite *oseltamivir carboxylate* were present in breast milk, but in concentrations significantly lower than considered therapeutic in infants (Greer 2011).

There is, in fact, no exact information on the inhalative use of *zanamivir*; however, the limited systemic intake and minimal oral bioavailability allow the assumption that there is no relevant transfer to the breastfed infant. One publication estimated the maximum amount of zanamivir that a 5 kg infant would ingest would be about 0.075 mg/day, which is much lower than the recommended prophylactic dosage for children of 10 mg/day inhalation (Tanaka 2009).

The dopamine agonist, *amantadine*, inhibits the production of prolactin and can, therefore, reduce the milk production. There are no data on *peramivir* during breastfeeding.

> **Recommendation.** With oseltamivir and zanamivir, breastfeeding is permitted. Should another anti-influenza agent be urgently indicated, it must be individually considered whether continuing breastfeeding is acceptable.

▶ Antiretroviral agents

In industrialized countries, breastfeeding is generally discouraged in the presence of a maternal HIV infection to avoid postnatal transmission. For this reason, there is scarcely any experience during breastfeeding for these medications.

Several publications report a transfer of *lamivudine* to human milk in biologically significant quantities. A relative infant dose of maximal 7% has been calculated. However, the serum levels in a completely breastfed infant are probably too low to produce adverse effects.

A study of 20 mother–child pairs with maternal antiretroviral therapy with lamivudine, *nevirapine*, and *zidovudine* calculated M/P ratios of 3.3, 0.7 and 3.2, respectively. For *lamivudine*, on average, 28 ng/mL was measured in the infant's serum, which is about 5% of a therapeutic concentration. The median infant serum concentration of nevirapine was high at 971 ng/mL, and similar to peak concentrations after a single 2-mg/kg dose of nevirapine. Thus the authors discussed both a preventive effect via the mother's milk, and potential toxicity or development of therapeutic resistance. The zidovudine transfer to the baby could not be evaluated, because the infants were also being treated with zidovudine for prophylaxis again infection (Shapiro 2005). Mirochnick (2009) also found an appreciable transfer of lamivudine and nevirapine to the breastfed infant among 67 mother–child pairs. In this study, lamivudine and nevirapine were detected in sub-therapeutic plasma concentrations. By contrast, zidovudine was not detectable in the children's plasma.

In another study involving 66 women with antiretroviral therapy (29 received zidovudine, lamivudine and nevirapine, 28 *stavudine*, lamivudine and nevirapine, and 9 zidovudine, lamivudine and *lopinavir/ritonavir*), only nevirapine reached significant levels in the breastfed infants and no adverse events due to medications were observed (Palombi 2012).

In mothers who were taking, among other medications *abacavir* and lopinavir, medium abacavir levels in breast milk were 0.057 µg/mL. Very low lopinavir levels were detected in breast milk (<0.25 µg/mL). Eight of nine infants had non-detectable abacavir plasma levels (<16 µg/L), and three of five infants had non-detectable lopinavir plasma levels (<1 mg/L; Shapiro 2013).

In a study of 13 mothers who were taking, among other medications, 600 mg *efavirenz* daily, the concentrations of the medication in the mother's milk and in the breastfed baby were determined. On average, the children had plasma concentrations of 0.86 mg/L (0.4–1.5 mg/L). This represented 13% of the maternal values. After 6 months of breastfeeding, the children had developed normally (Schneider 2008).

In a study of five mothers who took 200 mg *emtricitabine* and 300 mg *tenofovir* during the birth, and for 7 days postpartum, the concentrations of the medications in the mother's milk and in the breastfed children were determined. A maximum of 743 µg/L of emtricitabine was detected in the mother's milk. This represents a daily dose of 102 µg/kg for an exclusively breastfed infant and about 2% of a therapeutic infant dose. Tenofovir was detected with a maximum concentration of 16.25 µg/L in the mother's milk. An exclusively breastfed infant would, according to this, take in 2.44 µg/kg/day. This represents 0.03% of a therapeutic infant dose. By contrast to emtricitabine, the authors found extremely low plasma concentrations in the breastfed babies (Benaboud 2011).

Nelfinavir has been determined in low concentrations in breast milk. One publication calculated the M/P ratio for nelfinavir as 0.12, and for the active metabolite 0.03. The concentrations of nelfinavir and its metabolite were less than the limit of quantification for 20 of 28 infants (Weidle 2011).

Due to insufficient data, no statements can be made on tolerance during breastfeeding of the antiretroviral substances *atazanavir, darunavir, delavirdine, didanosine, elvitegravir, enfurvitide, etravirine, fosamprenavir, indinavir, maraviroc, raltegravir, rilpivirine, saquinavir,* and *tipranavir.*

> **Recommendation.** In addition to the potential toxicity of the drugs, it should be considered that in industrialized countries, HIV-infected women are generally advised against breastfeeding to prevent postnatal transmission of HIV via the mother's milk. Only in regions in which poor water hygiene when reconstituting infant formula, would pose a greater risk for the infant than the risk of infection via the mother's milk, is breastfeeding specifically recommended (Chapter 4.15). If chronic hepatitis B requires lamivudin or tenofovir therapy, breastfeeding seems acceptable after simultaneous hepatitis B immunization of the baby (Chapter 4.15).

References

Abdel-Tawab AM, Bradley M, Ghazaly EA et al. Albendazole and its metabolites in the breast milk of lactating women following a single oral dose of albendazole. Br J Clin Pharmacol 2009; 68: 737–42.

Benaboud S, Pruvost A, Coffie PA et al. Concentrations of tenofovir and emtricitabine in breast milk of HIV-1-infected women in Abidjan, Cote d'Ivoire, in the ANRS 12109 TEmAA Study, Step 2. Antimicrob Agents Chemother 2011; 55: 1315–7.

Bennett PN (ed). Drugs and Human Lactation. 2nd ed. Amsterdam, New York, Oxford: Elsevier, 1996.

Benyamini L, Merlob P, Stahl B et al. The safety of amoxicillin/clavulanic acid and cefuroxime during lactation. Ther Drug Monit 2005; 27: 499–502.

Berlin CM Jr, Lee C. Isoniazid and acetylisoniazid disposition in human milk, saliva and plasma. {Abstract 1044} Fed Proc 1979; 38: 426.

Blumberg HM, Burman WJ, Chaisson RE et al. American Thoracic Society/Centers for Disease Control and Prevention/Infectious Diseases Society of America: treatment of tuberculosis. Am J Respir Crit Care Med 2003; 167: 603–62.

Bork K, Benes P. Concentration and kinetic studies of intravenous acyclovir in serum and breast milk of a patient with eczema herpeticum. J Am Acad Dermatol 1995; 32: 1053–5.

Bork K, Kaiser T, Benes P. Transfer of aciclovir from plasma to human breast milk. Arzneimittelforschung 2000; 50: 656–8.

Buitrago MI, Crompton JA, Bertolami S et al. Extremely low excretion of daptomycin into breast milk of a nursing mother with methicillin-resistant Staphylococcus aureus pelvic inflammatory disease. Pharmacotherapy 2009; 29: 347–51.

Cahill JB Jr, Bailey EM, Chien S et al. Levofloxacin secretion in breast milk: a case report. Pharmacotherapy 2005; 25: 116–8.

Celiloglu M, Celiker S, Guven H et al. Gentamicin excretion and uptake from breast milk by nursing infants. Obstet Gynecol 1994; 84: 263–5.

Cover DL, Mueller BA. Ciprofloxacin penetration into human breast milk: a case report. DICP 1990; 24: 703–4.

Edstein MD, Veenendaal JR, Hyslop R. Excretion of mefloquine in human breast milk. Chemotherapy 1988; 34: 165–9.

Edstein MD, Veenendaal JR, Newman K et al. Excretion of chloroquine, dapsone and pyrimethamine in human milk. Br J Clin Pharmacol 1986; 22: 733–5.

Erickson SH, Oppenheim GL, Smith GH. Metronidazole in breast milk. Obstet Gynecol 1981; 57: 48–50.

Ette EI, Essien EE, Ogonor JI et al. Chloroquine in human milk. J Clin Pharmacol 1987; 27: 499–502.

Festini F, Ciuti R, Taccetti G et al. Breast-feeding in a woman with cystic fibrosis undergoing antibiotic intravenous treatment. J Matern Fetal Neonatal Med 2006; 19: 375–6.

Force RW. Fluconazole concentrations in breast milk. Pediatr Infect Dis J 1995; 14: 235–6.

Foulds G, Miller RD, Knirsch AK et al. Sulbactam kinetics and excretion into breast milk in postpartum women. Clin Pharmacol Ther 1985; 38: 692–6.

Garcia-Bournissen F, Altcheh J, Panchaud A et al. Is use of nifurtimox for the treatment of Chagas disease compatible with breast feeding? A population pharmacokinetics analysis. Arch Dis Child 2010; 95: 224–8.

Gardner DK, Gabbe SG, Harter C. Simultaneous concentrations of ciprofloxacin in breast milk and in serum in mother and breast-fed infant. Clin Pharm 1992; 11: 352–4.

Gerk PM, Kuhn RJ, Desai NS et al. Active transport of nitrofurantoin into human milk. Pharmacotherapy 2001; 21: 669–75.

Giamarellou H, Kolokythas E, Petrikkos G et al. Pharmacokinetics of three newer quinolones in pregnant and lactating women. Am J Med 1989; 87: 49S–51S.

Goldstein LH, Berlin M, Tsur L et al. The safety of macrolides during lactation. Breastfeed Med 2009; 4: 197–200.

Greer LG, Leff RD, Rogers VL et al. Pharmacokinetics of oseltamivir in breast milk and maternal plasma. Am J Obstet Gynecol 2011; 204: 524.

Havelka J, Frankova A. Adverse effects of chloramphenicol in newborn infants. Cesk Pediatr 1972; 27: 31–3.

Heisterberg L, Branebjerg PE. Blood and milk concentrations of metronidazole in mothers and infants. J Perinat Med 1983; 11: 114–20.

Holdiness MR. Antituberculosis drugs and breast-feeding. Arch Intern Med 1984; 144: 1888.

Hunt MJ, Salisbury EL, Grace J et al. Black breast milk due to minocycline therapy. Br J Dermatol 1996; 134: 943–4.

Ito S, Blajchman A, Stephenson M et al. Prospective follow-up of adverse reactions in breast-fed infants exposed to maternal medication. Am J Obstet Gynecol 1993; 168: 1393–9.

Ito K, Hirose R, Tamaya T et al. Pharmacokinetic and clinical studies on aztreonam in the perinatal period. Jpn J Antibiot 1990; 43: 719–6.

Ito K, Izumi K, Takagi H et al. Fundamental and clinical evaluation of imipenem/cilastatin sodium in the perinatal period. Jpn J Antibiot 1988; 41: 1778–5.

Kelsey JJ, Moser LR, Jennings JC et al. Presence of azithromycin breast milk concentrations: a case report. Am J Obstet Gynecol 1994; 170: 1375–6.

Lactation

4.4 Anti-infectives

Lassman HB, Puri SK, Ho I et al. Pharmacokinetics of roxithromycin (RU 965). J Clin Pharmacol 1988; 28: 141–52.

Law I, Ilett KF, Hackett LP et al. Transfer of chloroquine and desethylchloroquine across the placenta and into milk in Melanesian mothers. Br J Clin Pharmacol 2008; 65: 674–9.

Mann CF. Clindamycin and breast-feeding. Pediatrics 1980; 66: 1030–1.

Mannisto PT, Karhunen M, Koskela O et al. Concentrations of tinidazole in breast milk. Acta Pharmacol Toxicol (Copenh) 1983; 53: 254–6.

Matsuda S. Transfer of antibiotics into maternal milk. Biol Res Pregnancy Perinatol 1984; 5: 57–60.

Medina A, Fiske N, Hjelt-Harvey I et al. Absorption, diffusion, and excretion of a new antibiotic, lincomycin. Antimicrob Agents Chemother (Bethesda) 1963; 161: 189–96.

Meyer LJ, Miranda P, Sheth N et al. Acyclovir in human breast milk. Am J Obstet Gynecol 1988; 158: 586–8.

Miller RD, Salter AJ. The passage of trimethoprim/sulfamethoxazole into breast milk and its significance. In: Daikos CK (ed). Progress in Chemotherapy. Antibacterial chemotherapy. 1974; 1: 687–91.

Mirochnick M, Thomas T, Capparelli E et al. Antiretroviral concentrations in breast-feeding infants of mothers receiving highly active antiretroviral therapy. Antimicrob Agents Chemother 2009; 53: 1170–6.

Moretti ME, Ito S, Koren G. Disposition of maternal ketoconazole in breast milk. Am J Obstet Gynecol 1995; 173: 1625–6.

Morganti G, Ceccarelli G, Ciaffi G. Comparative concentrations of a tetracycline antibiotic in serum and maternal milk. Antibiotica (bilingual edition) 1968; 6: 216–23.

Ogbuokiri JE, Ozumba BC, Okonkwo PO. Ivermectin levels in human breast milk. Eur J Clin Pharmacol 1994; 46: 89–90.

Ogunbona FA, Onyeji CO, Bolaji OO et al. Excretion of chloroquine and desethylchloroquine in human milk. Br J Clin Pharmacol 1987; 23: 473–6.

Palombi L, Pirillo MF, Andreotti M et al. Antiretroviral prophylaxis for breastfeeding transmission in Malawi: drug concentrations, virological efficacy and safety. Antivir Ther 2012; 17: 1511–9.

Passmore CM, McElnay JC, Rainey EA et al. Metronidazole excretion in human milk and its effect on the suckling neonate. Br J Clin Pharmacol 1988; 26: 45–51.

Phillips RE, Looareesuwan S, White NJ et al. Quinine pharmacokinetics and toxicity in pregnant and lactating women with falciparum malaria. Br J Clin Pharmacol 1986; 21: 677–83.

Pons G, Rey E, Richard MO et al. Nitrofurantoin excretion in human milk. Dev Pharmacol Ther 1990; 14: 148–52.

Pütter J, Held F. Quantitative studies on the occurrence of praziquantel in milk and plasma of lactating women. Eur J Drug Metab Pharmacokinet 1979; 4: 193–8.

Rao TS. Does mebendazole inhibit lactation? NZ Med J 1983; 96: 589–90.

Reyes MP, Ostrea EM Jr, Cabinian AE et al. Vancomycin during pregnancy: does it cause hearing loss or nephrotoxicity in the infant? Am J Obstet Gynecol 1989; 161: 977–81.

Sagirli O, Onal A, Toker S et al. Determination of linezolid in human breast milk by high-performance liquid chromatography with ultraviolet detection. J AOAC Int 2009; 92: 1658–62.

Sanders SW, Zone JJ, Foltz RL et al. Hemolytic anemia induced by dapsone transmitted through breast milk. Ann Intern Med 1982; 96: 465–6.

Sauberan JB, Bradley JS, Blumer J et al. Transmission of meropenem in breast milk. Pediatr Infect Dis J 2012; 31: 832–4.

Schmid C, Kuemmerle A, Blum J et al. In-hospital safety in field conditions of nifurtimox eflornithine combination therapy (NECT) for TB gambiense sleeping sickness. PLoS Negl Trop Dis 2012; 6: e1920.

Schneider S, Peltier A, Gras A et al. Efavirenz in human breast milk, mothers', and newborns' plasma. J Acquir Immune Defic Syndr 2008; 48: 450–4.

Sedlmayr T, Peters F, Raasch W et al. Clarithromycin, a new macrolide antibiotic. Effectiveness in puerperal infections and pharmacokinetics in breast milk. Geburtshilfe Frauenheilkd 1993; 53: 488–91.

Shapiro RL, Holland DT, Capparelli E et al. Antiretroviral concentrations in breast-feeding infants of women in Botswana receiving antiretroviral treatment. J Infect Dis 2005; 192: 720–7.

Shapiro RL, Rossi S, Ogwu A et al. Therapeutic levels of lopinavir in late pregnancy and abacavir passage into breast milk in the Mma Bana Study, Botswana. Antivir Ther 2013; 18: 585–90.

Sheffield JS, Fish DN, Hollier LM et al. Acyclovir concentrations in human breast milk after valaciclovir administration. Am J Obstet Gynecol 2002; 186: 100–2.

Singh N, Golani A, Patel Z et al. Transfer of isoniazid from circulation to breast milk in lactating women on chronic therapy for tuberculosis. Br J Clin Pharmacol 2008; 65: 418–22.

Smith JA, Morgan JR, Rachlis AR et al. Clindamycin in human breast milk. Can Med Assoc J 1975; 112: 806.

Snider DE Jr, Powell KE. Should women taking antituberculosis drugs breast-feed? Arch Intern Med 1984; 144: 589–90.

Sørensen HT, Skriver MV, Pedersen L et al. Risk of infantile hypertrophic pyloric stenosis after maternal postnatal use of macrolides. Scand J Infect Dis 2003; 35: 104–6.

Stang H. Pyloric stenosis associated with erythromycin ingested through breastmilk. Minn Med 1986; 69: 669–70, 682.

Steen B, Rane A. Clindamycin passage into human milk. Br J Clin Pharmacol 1982; 13: 661–4.

Taddio A, Klein J, Koren G. Acyclovir excretion in human breast milk. Ann Pharmacother 1994; 28: 585–7.

Tanaka T, Nakajima K, Murashima A et al. Safety of neuraminidase inhibitors against novel influenza A (H1N1) in pregnant and breastfeeding women. CMAJ 2009; 181: 55–8.

Weidle PJ, Zeh C, Martin A et al. Nelfinavir and its active metabolite, hydroxy-t-butylamidenelfinavir (M8), are transferred in small quantities to breast milk and do not reach biologically significant concentrations in breast-feeding infants whose mothers are taking nelfinavir. Antimicrob Agents Chemother 2011; 55: 5168–71.

Wentges-van Hothe N, van Eijkeren M, van der Laan JW. Oseltamivir and breastfeeding. Int J Infect Dis 2008; 12: 451.

WHO. Guidelines for the treatment of malaria, 2010. http://whqlibdoc.who.int/publications/2010/9789241547925_eng.pdf (accessed on 14-3-2014).

WHO. Guidelines for treatment of tuberculosis, 2010. http://whqlibdoc.who.int/publications/2010/9789241547833_eng.pdf (accessed on 12-3-2014).

Witte AM, Klever HJ, Brabin BJ et al. Field evaluation of the use of an ELISA to detect chloroquine and its metabolites in blood, urine and breast-milk. Trans R Soc Trop Med Hyg 1990; 84: 521–5.

Vaccines and immunoglobulins

4.5

Ruth A. Lawrence and Mary Panse

4.5.1	Maternal immunization	705
4.5.2	Efficacy of immunization in breastfed infants	706
4.5.3	Hepatitis A vaccine	706
4.5.4	Hepatitis B vaccine	706
4.5.5	Human papillomavirus vaccine	707
4.5.6	Influenza vaccine	707
4.5.7	Polio vaccine	707
4.5.8	Rabies vaccine	708
4.5.9	Rubella vaccine	708
4.5.10	Smallpox vaccine	708
4.5.11	Typhoid vaccine	708
4.5.12	Immunoglobulins	709
4.5.13	CDC recommendations	709

4.5.1   Maternal immunization

A woman who has not received all the recommended immunizations before or during pregnancy may be immunized in the postpartum period even though she is breastfeeding. The presence of live viruses in the milk does not present a problem because the viruses have been attenuated. According to the statement of the American Academy of Pediatrics Committee on Infectious Diseases (Pickering 2012), breast-feeding women may be immunized with both killed and live vaccines. All vaccines and *immunoglobulins* used for mothers are considered safe for the infant during breastfeeding. Lactating women can be immunized, using standard recommended doses for adults, against measles, mumps, rubella, tetanus, diphtheria, pertussis, influenza, streptococcus pneumoniae, neisseria meningitis, hepatitis A, hepatitis B, and varicella. Often it is the need to travel to endemic countries that raises the issue.

A lactating woman can be given inactivated poliovirus vaccine, for instance, if necessary. The administration of live vaccine (oral vaccine) should be delayed in the mother (or parents) of a young infant until the infant has been vaccinated with killed virus regardless of the feeding mode.

Drugs During Pregnancy and Lactation. **http://dx.doi.org/10.1016/B978-0-12-408078-2.00030-5**

With some vaccines, i.e. against meningococcal or pneumococcal disease (Shahid 1995, 2002) and cholera, there is discussion on whether the relevant amounts of the maternal antibodies built up as a result of immunization appear in the milk.

4.5.2   Efficacy of immunization in breastfed infants

Many myths have circulated regarding the efficacy of immunization of the infant during breastfeeding. Actually, the immunogenicity of some vaccines is increased by breastfeeding, but long-range enhancement of efficacy has not been studied. In any case the response to vaccines while breastfeeding is not diminished, and the usual vaccination schedules should be followed. The American Academy of Pediatrics recommends that all infants should be vaccinated on the regular schedule regardless of the mode of feeding.

4.5.3   Hepatitis A vaccine

Experience

Hepatitis A vaccine is available in two preparations, which are prepared from cell culture-adapted hepatitis A virus which has in turn been cultured in human fibroblasts and inactivated. It has not been studied in breastfeeding or in children under 2 years of age.

> **Recommendation.** Hepatitis A vaccine is unlikely to present a problem during lactation and is not contraindicated.

4.5.4   Hepatitis B vaccine

Experience

Hepatitis B vaccine is a highly effective and safe vaccine which is produced by recombinant DNA technology. The vaccine is an inactivated non-infectious hepatitis B surface antigen vaccine, and contains between 10 and 40 μg of HB_sAg protein per mL with apparently similar rates of seroconversion. Pediatric vaccines contain no thimerosal. The vaccine is given to newborns at birth. Hepatitis B vaccine is also combined with other vaccines, and can be given concurrently with other vaccines but via a separate syringe and at another site. A total of three injections of Hepatitis B vaccine are required in the first 6 months of life.

> **Recommendation.** Hepatitis B vaccines are considered safe during lactation.

4.5.5   Human papillomavirus vaccine

Experience

Licensed in 2009, bivalent human papillomavirus vaccine (HPV2) Cervarix was made available for females 16 through 25 years. Quadrivalent
HPV vaccine (HPV4) Gardasil had been licensed in 2006 for a similar
group (CDC 2010). Both vaccines are composed of virus-like particles
but are not live vaccines. The dose is 0.5 mL administered intramuscularly, preferably in the deltoid on a 3-dose schedule. The second dose is
1 to 2 months after the first and the third dose administered 6 months
after the first dose. Vaccine administration during lactation is safe. The
target population is 11 years through 26 years (CDC 2010).

4.5.6   Influenza vaccine

Experience

Influenza vaccines come in two forms. One is the traditional killed virus
vaccine that is given by injection; the second is a live attenuated vaccine
available in a mist package to be administered via the nasal passages.
Both contain three virus strains, and typically one or two strains are
given each year to anticipate the strains circulating in that particular year.
Both are produced using embryonated hen eggs, and therefore cannot be
given to individuals sensitive to eggs. The inactivated vaccine (TIV) is
approved for individuals aged 6 months and older. The live attenuated
vaccine (LAIV) is cold adapted, developed by passing tissue cultures
through lower and lower temperatures. Thus, viral replication can only
occur in the upper respiratory tract, where it is cool. It is licensed for
individuals aged 5 years and older.

Both TIV and LAIV are considered safe during lactation. The live
attenuated vaccine is heat sensitive and does not survive in the plasma
or the milk. Whether the breastfed infant can be protected by maternal
immunization by either TIV or LAIV has not been studied.

4.5.7   Polio vaccine

Experience

Oral polio vaccine (Sabin) is a live attenuated vaccine combining three
strains of the virus. The transfer of these vaccine viruses to an unvac-
cinated contact person, i.e. via a smear infection, can lead to a normal
vaccination reaction and immunity against infection with the wild virus.
However, it is also possible that the person will become ill with contact
vaccine poliomyelitis. This complication – occurring once in 15.5 million immunizations – is very rare. In two cases, it has been reported in
infants (Mertens 1983, Heyne 1977). When immunization is urgent for
the mother, the killed virus vaccine can be given to her intramuscularly.
In the immunized mother, polio antibodies are present in the milk at a
level comparable to the mother's plasma levels. High concentrations of
anti-polio virus antibody in the milk could theoretically interfere with
the response of the breastfeeding infant to immunization, but no such
outcome has ever been reported.

Lactation

4.5 Vaccines and immunoglobulins

> **Recommendation.** Live oral vaccine should not be given to the mother until the infant has been immunized at 6 weeks or older.

4.5.8   Rabies vaccine

There are no breastfeeding data on the rabies vaccine. Since it is an inactivated rabies virus, it would not be a threat to the infant if it were to appear in the milk.

4.5.9   Rubella vaccine

Experience

Rubella vaccine is a live virus of the RA 27/3 strain grown in human diploid cell cultures and attenuated. It can be given in a combination vaccine (MMR). The early postpartum period, when risk of pregnancy is lowest, is the best time to be immunized. The risk to the breastfeeding infant is minimal with the recent techniques for vaccine preparation. The original preparations in the 1970s were associated with several cases of rubella. While the virus may appear in the milk, as reported in several studies (Losonsky 1982, Isacson 1971), symptoms in these infants were rare (Landes 1981). The Rubella virus has been found in the milk in 69% of the women immunized with live attenuated Rubella (HPV-77 DES or RA 27/3 strains; Losonsky 1982).

> **Recommendation.** Lactating mothers of normal full-term infants can receive rubella immunization during lactation.

4.5.10   Smallpox vaccine

A woman should not be vaccinated with smallpox vaccine while caring for an infant less than 1 year of age; unless she can be separated from the child until the site heals (at least 10 days). It is not known whether the virus passes into the milk.

> **Recommendation.** The killed-virus injectable form of the vaccine is recommended during lactation.

4.5.11   Typhoid vaccine

Protection is indicated when traveling to an endemic area. Typhoid vaccines are available both with killed and live attenuated viruses. The live attenuated vaccine is given orally. Although it has little potential for producing disease, there are no data about passage into milk. It is not recommended during lactation. The injectable form is a killed dried bacterium in a phenol inactivation preparation, and is preferable for a woman while lactating.

4.5.12   Immunoglobulins

Experience

Immunoglobulins are in general very large molecules and do not pass into milk. In addition, infants are given immunoglobulin directly. Immunoglobulins contain passive protective antibodies and are not contraindicated for newborns, and would not be contraindicated for a breastfeeding mother.

Immunoglobulin is used with specific immunoglobulins in high titer, such as immunoglobulin hepatitis B (Hepatitis B Immune Globulin; HBIG), which is used when there is known exposure to hepatitis B. If the mother is hepatitis-positive, the recommended regime is to give the newborn immunoglobulin within 12 hours of birth, plus the first dose of hepatitis B vaccine. If a mother is exposed to hepatitis B while breastfeeding, HBIG would not put the child at any risk via the breast milk. If the child required HBIG at the same time, it would be necessary to medicate the child directly.

Varicella Zoster Immune Globulin (VZIG) is obtained from the plasma of adult volunteer blood donors. VZIG is given during pregnancy and is also given directly to infants, so should pose no risk to the breastfed infant. As above, if there is the risk of varicella, the infant should receive a dose directly.

> **Recommendation.** Immunoglobulins are given directly to infants and are not contraindicated during lactation.

4.5.13   CDC recommendations

CDC recommendations for vaccines during breastfeeding are summarized:

"Neither inactivated nor live-virus vaccines administered to a lactating woman affect the safety of breastfeeding for women or their infants. Although live viruses in vaccines can replicate in vaccine recipients (i.e. the mother), the majority of live viruses in vaccines have been demonstrated not to be excreted in human milk. Varicella vaccine virus has not been found in human milk. Although rubella vaccine virus might be excreted in human milk, the virus usually does not infect the infant. If infection does occur, it is well tolerated because the virus is attenuated. Inactivated, recombinant, subunit, polysaccharide, and conjugate vaccines, as well as toxoids, pose no risk for mothers who are breastfeeding or for their infants."

(ACIP 2011)

"Breastfeeding is a contraindication for smallpox vaccination of the mother because of the theoretical risk for contact transmission from mother to infant. Yellow fever vaccine should be avoided in breastfeeding women.

However, when a nursing mother cannot avoid or postpone travel to areas endemic for yellow fever in which risk for acquisition is high, these women should be vaccinated."

(ACIP 2011)

References

ACIP (Advisory Committee on Immunization Practices). Guidance for Vaccine Recommendations in Pregnant and Breastfeeding Women MMWR; 60(No. 2): 26, www.cdc.gov/vaccines/pubs/preg-guide.htm, 2011.

CDC (Center for Disease Control). FDA Licensure of bivalent human papilloma virus vaccine (HPV2, Cervarix) for use in females and updated HPV vaccination recommendations from the Advisory Committee on Immunization Practices (ACIP) MMWR 2010; 59(No. 20): 624–6.

Heyne K. Paralytic poliomyelitis following vaccination contact in the 1st trimester of an infant {in German}. Med Welt 1977; 28: 1439–41.

Isacson P, Kehrer AF, Wilson H et al. Comparative study of life, attenuated rubella virus vaccines during the immediate puerperium. Obstet Gynecol 1971; 31: 332–7.

Landes RD, Bass JW, Millunchick EW et al. Neonatal rubella following postpartum maternal immunization. J Pediatr 1981; 98: 668–9.

Losonsky GA, Fishaut JM, Strussenberg J et al. Effect of immunization against rubella on lactation products. I. Development and characterization of specific immunologic reactivity in breast milk. J Infect Dis 1982; 145: 654–60.

Mertens T, Schürmann W, Gruppenbacher J et al. Problems of life virus vaccine associated poliomyelitis. Med Microbiol Immunol 1983; 172: 13–21.

Pickering L, Baker C, Kimberlin D et al. Red book : 2012 Report of the Committee on Infectious Diseases. Elk Grove Village, IL: American Academy of Pediatrics, 2012.

Shahid NS, Steinhoff MC, Hogue SS et al. Serum, breast milk, and infant antibody after maternal immunisation with pneumococcal vaccine. Lancet 1995; 346: 1252–7.

Shahid NS, Steinhoff MC, Roy E et al. Placental and breast transfer of antibodies after maternal immunization with polysaccharide meningococcal vaccine: a randomized, controlled evaluation. Vaccine 2002; 20: 2404–9.

Cardiovascular drugs and diuretics

4.6

Paul Merlob and Corinna Weber-Schöndorfer

4.6.1	β-Receptor blockers	711
4.6.2	Hydralazine	713
4.6.3	α-Methyldopa	713
4.6.4	Calcium antagonists	714
4.6.5	ACE inhibitors	715
4.6.6	Angiotensin-II receptor-antagonists (sartan)	715
4.6.7	Other antihypertensives	716
4.6.8	Antihypotensives	717
4.6.9	Digitalis	717
4.6.10	Antiarrhythmics	717
4.6.11	Vasodilators and circulatory drugs	719
4.6.12	Diuretics	720

There are cardiovascular drugs and diuretics that can be used during pregnancy and lactation. The decision to continue these medications during lactation depends on many factors. Some of these factors include the well-being of the mother, the blood/milk barrier, the pharmacological activity of the drug, and the consequences for the infant.

The recommended drugs of choice are those which are best studied and do not show unwanted adverse effects for either the mother or the child. Drugs should be avoided if there is insufficient experience, like the sartans. If not, the safest cardiovascular or diuretic drugs should be used and the therapeutic choice should be changed to the preferred agents. This can be possible without interrupting breastfeeding.

4.6.1   β-Receptor blockers

Circulatory symptoms and hypoglycemia have been cited in connection with the intake of β-receptor blockers via mother's milk. However, by contrast to prenatal exposure, such effects are less likely during breastfeeding, due essentially to the relatively low concentrations of these drugs in infant blood.

Bradycardia, hypotension and tachypnea have been seen in connection with *acebutolol*, which has a half-life of 3–4 hours and 26% plasma protein binding (PPB). Therefore, mathematically, the baby has received about 5–10% of the maternal dose per kg of bodyweight (Boutroy 1986).

Drugs During Pregnancy and Lactation. **http://dx.doi.org/10.1016/B978-0-12-408078-2.00031-7**

In particular, the active metabolite, *diacetolol* (half-life 8 to 13 hours), accumulates in the mother's milk with an unusually high milk/plasma (M/P) ratio of up to 24.7.

Atenolol has a half-life of 6 to 7 hours, a minimal PPB, and is hydrophilic. A recent study (Eyal 2010) examines the influence of atenolol on breastfed babies at 2 to 4 weeks of age ($n = 32$), 3 to 4 months ($n = 22$) and 6 to 8 months ($n = 17$). The maternal dose was between 25 and 200 mg/day. The M/P ratio was, on average, greater than 4.9, whereby the average relative infant dose was less than 15%. Infant doses of 34.8% (after 2 to 4 weeks) or 17.8% after 3 to 4 months were noted. Atenolol was not detected in the serum of any of the babies at 3 to 4 months. Further, whether maternal atenolol had a depressive effect on the heart rate in crying infants has been examined and no effect has been noted in this single study. However, Schimmel (1989) describes a breastfed infant who had toxic concentrations of atenolol acquired from her mother (dose 50 mg twice daily). This full-term infant at the age of 5 days had been transferred to the neonatal intensive care unit because of cyanosis and two episodes of bradycardia (80 beats/min). Forty-eight hours after discontinuing breastfeeding, the atenolol concentration in the baby's serum was 2010 ng/mL and 24 hours later it was 140 ng/mL. The possible accumulation of atenolol in human milk and infant serum should be considered before prescribing, because safer β-blockers can be used during breastfeeding.

Betaxolol has a half-life of 14 to 22 hours and a PPB of 50%. The relative dose transmitted by the milk reaches a maximum of 4.3% shortly after birth (Morselli 1990).

Labetalol, which is widely used in the USA, works as an α- and β-receptor blocker, has a half-life of 6 to 8 hours, and a PPB of 50%. With long-term treatment with 300 to 1,200 mg/day, a mother's maximum milk concentration of 0.7 mg/L and an M/P ratio between 0.2 and 1.5 are reported. Thus, an infant would receive, at most, 0.1 mg/kg daily. This represents 0.3% of the maternal dose per kg bodyweight (survey by Bennett 1996).

There is substantial experience available for *metoprolol* (half-life 3 to 4 hours, PPB 12%). With long-term therapy with 100 and 200 mg, a maximum of 0.7 mg/L is detected in the milk. The M/P ratio is 3. The daily dose for the infant is, nevertheless, 0.1 mg/kg at most. This represents 3.2% of the maternal weight-related dose. About 10% of the northern European population is thought to metabolize metoprolol slowly. This could be the reason why a plasma concentration of 45 μg/L is measured in one (symptom-free) infant. Among other breastfed infants, it is 0.5–3 μg/L (survey in Bennett 1996). The therapeutic concentration for adults is given as 93–881 μg/L.

With oxprenolol, up to 1.5% of the maternal weight-related dose is transmitted to the baby (Fidler 1983). Also, the low transfer of oxprenolol via the mother's milk (half-life 1 to 2 hours, PPB 80%) is confirmed in another study (Sioufi 1984).

Shortly after birth, 3.1 μg/L of S-enantiomers of *pindolol* and 1.9 μg/L of its R-enantiomers are found in the milk of three breastfeeding mothers who took 20 mg pindolol (half-life 3–4 hours, PPB 40–60%) daily. This represents 0.36% of a maternal weight-related dose (Goncalves 2007). The transfer of mepindolol can be 5% of the maternal weight-related dose (survey in Bennett 1996).

Among β-blockers propranolol is the most frequent studied and used drug.

Propranolol has a PPB of 90% and a half-life of 3 to 6 hours. The maximum transfer of 0.4% into the mother's milk is quite low (survey in Bennett 1996).

With oral use of *timolol*, the portion of the maternal weight-related dose that is transmitted is 3.3% (Fidler 1983). Timolol is used primarily in eye drops for glaucoma treatment (Chapter 4.12.8). This leads to limited concentrations in the milk. Madadi (2008) calculated a relative dose of 0.024% if the mother puts drops in both eyes twice daily.

There are insufficient data on bisoprolol (half-life 10–12 hours PPB 30%), carvedilol (half-life 6–10 hours PPB >98%), celiprolol half-life 5–6 hours, PPB 25%), nebivolol (half-life of 10–24 hours with slow metabolization, PPB of 98%), penbutolol (half-life of 20 hours PPB 80–98%), and talinolol to make a judgment. This also applies to esmolol (half-life 9 minutes, PPB 55%), which is indicated for i.v. injection with supraventricular tachycardias.

Sotalol has a high risk for accumulation in infants (see also Section 4.6.10).

> **Recommendation.** During therapy with β-receptor blockers, breastfeeding is allowed. Metoprolol, oxprenolol, pindolol, propranolol and labetalol are preferred. Therapy with other β-blockers should be changed to one of the preferred agents if possible.

4.6.2   Hydralazine

With 150 mg/day of hydralazine in the breast-feeding mother, a maximum of 130 µg/L is measured in the milk – which is 20 µg/kg per day or 1% of the therapeutic dose for an infant (Liedholm 1982). Following parenteral administration of 10–40 mg, an average of 47 µg/L, including the hydralazine metabolites, was measured in mother's milk. The M/P ratio was 0.5. With this therapy, up to 108 µg/L of hydralazine was found in the plasma of breastfed infants (Lamont 1986). By comparison, the plasma concentration in an infant being treated with 2 mg/kg was given as 1,700 µg/L. No toxic symptoms have been observed while breastfeeding. Dihydralazine can be evaluated as if hydralazine.

> **Recommendation.** Breastfeeding is permitted with hydralazine.

4.6.3   α-Methyldopa

With daily treatment with 250–2,000 mg of *α-methyldopa*, up to 1.14 mg/L is measured in the milk. The M/P ratio is 0.2– 0.5. For the infant, a daily dose of 0.17 mg/kg can be calculated, which represents 3.2% of the maternal dose per kg (survey in Bennett 1996). Only in one of three infants could the medication be detected in plasma (90 µg/L). For the mother, it is 4,250 µg/L. No toxic symptoms are observed in the infant. α-methyldopa can promote milk production as a result of increased prolactin secretion (Bennett 1996).

> **Recommendation.** Breastfeeding is permitted with α-methyldopa.

4.6.4   Calcium antagonists

There is no information on the transfer of *amlodipine* into the mother's milk. Two case reports describe age-appropriate development with a maternal dose of 5 and 10 mg/day (Szucs 2010, Ahn 2007).

In 11 mothers, only limited amounts of *nicardipine* are detected in mother's milk under steady-state conditions (Jarreau 2000). For a few days postpartum, seven mothers have received nicardipine in an hourly dose of 1–6.5 mg for treating preeclampsia. Less than 0.3 µg/day nicardipine in the mother's milk, or between 0.015 and 0.004% of a therapeutic infant dose, is calculated for these mother–child pairs (Bartels 2006).

With *nifedipine* and its active pyridine metabolites, a maximum of 2–10 µg/kg/day is transmitted to the infant when the mother has taken 30–90 mg/day. That is less than 5% of a weight-related child's dose (Ehrenkranz 1989). Average values of 2% and less are probably even more realistic (Manninen 1991, Penny 1989). Nifedipine is also used successfully to treat Raynaud phenomenon of the breast nipple. Anderson (2004) reports on 12 breastfeeding women complaining of pain in the nipple, which was finally diagnosed as Raynaud phenomenon. Those mothers, who chose nifedipine therapy, had rapid relief from the symptoms. Interestingly, eight of the 12 women and their children had previously been treated with antimycotics because of a suspected *Candida albicans* infection. A further case report describes good tolerance of nifedipine for vasospasms of the nipple (Page 2006). In a retrospective review of 22 cases of breastfeeding mothers diagnosed with Raynaud phenomenon of the nipple, previous treatment for Candida mastitis with oral or topical antifungals was ineffective in 20 cases (91%). Of the 12 patients who tolerated a trial with nifedipine, 10 (83%) report a decrease or resolved nipple pain during lactation. Thus, nifedipine and not the antifungal, appears to be an effective treatment of Raynaud phenomenon of the nipple (Barrett 2013).

With 6 × 60 mg of *nimodipine*, maximum concentrations of 3.5 µg/L in the mother's milk have been described (Tonks 1995). Mathematically, this would be only 0.01% of the weight-related maternal dose. A further case confirms this limited transfer of nimodipine (Carcas 1996).

With *nitrendipine*, a maximum relative dose of 0.6%, including its metabolites, can reach the infant (White 1989).

During therapy with the calcium antagonists mentioned, no intolerance in the breastfed infant has been described. By contrast *felodipine*, *gallopamil, isradipine, lercanidipine, manidipine, nilvadipine* and *nisoldipine* have been insufficiently studied.

For *verapamil* and *diltiazem*, see Section 4.6.10. Both have been considered as appropriate during breastfeeding by the American Academy of Pediatrics (2001).

The relative infant dose was 0.2% for verapamil and 0.9% for diltiazem and thus, the relative amount of these drugs transferred to the breastfed infant is quite small. In some cases no verapamil is detected in infant's plasma.

Recommendation. Breastfeeding is permitted during therapy with calcium antagonists. Depending on the indication, diltiazem, nicardipine, nifedipine, nitrendipine and verapamil are the calcium antagonists of choice while breastfeeding. Individual doses of other calcium antagonists do not require any limitation of breastfeeding, but the therapy should be changed.

4.6.5   ACE inhibitors

In nine mother–baby pairs with a daily dosage of 20 mg of benazepril, a maximum of 0.003 µg, including the active metabolite, *benazeprilate*, is measured per liter of milk. For an exclusively breastfed baby, this represents 0.00014% of the maternal weight-related dose (Kaiser 1989).

With 300 mg captopril daily, 4.7 µg/L milk is reported. The M/P ratio is 0.03. The infant receives up to 0.7 µg/kg/day. This represents about 0.014% of the maternal weight-related dose (Devlin 1981).

Enalapril can be similarly evaluated. The relative dose for the infant is about 0.1% (Rush 1991, Redman 1990, Huttunen 1989). By contrast to the maternal serum, there is no lowering of the angiotensin-converting enzyme found in milk samples (Huttunen 1989). No undesirable effects on the infant have been described.

Quinapril concentrations are reported for six mother-child pairs. The drug could not be detected in any of the milk samples. Based on the detection limit, the maximum estimated relative infant dose is 1.6% (Begg 2001).

There are insufficient data to evaluate *cilazapril, fosinopril, lisinopril, moexipril, perindopril, ramipril, spirapril, trandolapril* and *zofenopril*.

Following the use of ACE inhibitors in late pregnancy, kidney function disturbances as extreme as anuria requiring dialysis have been noted in the newborn (Chapter 2.8), but not during breastfeeding. For this reason, the American Academy of Pediatrics (2001) considers the use of those ACE inhibitors that have been tested extensively to be acceptable during breastfeeding.

> **Recommendation.** Benazepril, captopril, enalapril as well as quinapril may be prescribed during breastfeeding if β-blockers, calcium antagonists or methyldopa are not effective or indicated. As a safety measure, at least with premature infants and young infants under two months, attention should be paid to edema and the course of weight gain as indicators for disturbed kidney function. The accidental prescribing of another ACE inhibitor does not require any limitation of breastfeeding but changing the therapy is advisable.

4.6.6   Angiotensin-II receptor-antagonists (sartan)

There is insufficient experience with the use of *candesartan, eprosartan, irbesartan, losartan, olmesartan, telmisartan* and *valsartan* during breastfeeding.

Since very serious kidney function disturbances in the newborn can occur after using sartans in late pregnancy (Chapter 2.8.6) and there are no data on transfer into the mother's milk, this group of drugs should be avoided during breastfeeding. This applies particularly for premature and young infants.

> **Recommendation.** Sartans should be avoided during breastfeeding. The accidental administration of a single dose does not require weaning. However, the therapy should be changed.

Lactation

4.6 Cardiovascular drugs and diuretics

4.6.7   Other antihypertensives

▶ **Peripherally acting antiadrenergic agents**

With *prazosin*, the relative dose is a maximum of 3% in one mother–child pair studied (manufacturer's report).

There is no published experience with *bunazosin*, *doxazosin* and *terazosin*.

A single case report (Jensen 2013) provides the first quantitative data on the transfer of doxazosin into human milk. A 37-year-old woman receives two oral doses of 4 mg doxazosin 24 hours apart for urinary stones. Venous blood and milk are collected at different intervals after these two doses. The average and maximum milk concentrations are 2.9 and 4.2 μg/L. These values correspond to estimated relative infant doses of 0.06 and 0.09%, respectively. These very low results provide some reassurance for breastfeeding women who may benefit from doxazosin treatment.

Urapidil is well absorbed orally, has a PPB of 80%, and an elimination half-life of 5 hours after oral administration and 3 hours after i.v. injection. Two newborns, breastfed while their mothers were taking urapidil medication, did not develop any side effects (author's unpublished observations).

▶ **Centrally acting antiadrenergic agents**

In long-term clonidine therapy with 240–290 μg daily, clonidine is reported to levels of 2.8 μg/L in milk. For the infant, this means a maximum of 8% of the maternal, weight-related dose. With 0.3–0.6 μg/L in the infant's plasma, a near-therapeutic concentration is reached (Hartikainen-Sorri 1987). In another study involving on-going therapy with 75 μg/day, a maximum of 7% was measured for the exclusively breastfed infant in whose plasma no active ingredient could be detected (<0.096 ng/mL). There was 0.6 μg/L reported in milk and 0.3 μg/L in maternal plasma (Bunjes 1993). No undesirable effects, such as a drop in blood pressure, were observed in the infants.

Following daily administration of 200 μg *moxonidine* to five mothers during the first few postpartum days, a maximum of 2.7 μg/L was reported in milk. Mathematically, that is 12% of the maternal weight-related dose for an exclusively breastfed baby. The M/P ratio has been estimated to be 1–2 (cited in Schaefer 1998).

There are no data on the passage of reserpine into the mother's milk. The half-life of several days would suggest accumulation of reserpine in the infant.

▶ **Other antihypertensives**

Five percent of the weight-related dose of *minoxidil* passes into the milk. The exposed infant demonstrates no symptoms (Valdivieso 1985).

Aliskiren is a renin inhibitor, which should be avoided during breastfeeding.

Diazoxide is only approved for therapy for hypoglycemia. No information exists on the passage into the mother's milk of this drug or for sodium-nitroprusside, which is used in intensive medicine. *Phenoxybenzamine* is indicated for treatment of pheochromocytoma. However, there is no experience on its use during breastfeeding.

Recommendation. The antihypertensives mentioned in this section should not be prescribed during breastfeeding. If treatment has begun, this does not require weaning; however, a change in therapy should be arranged.

4.6.8 Antihypotensives

Ergotamine derivatives such as *dihydroergotamine* can, as prolactin inhibitors, reduce milk production. There is insufficient experience on *etilefrine, amezinium metilsulfate* and *midodrine*.

Recommendation. Hypotension should be treated primarily without medication. Individual dosing of dihydroergotamine during breastfeeding is acceptable. The accidental intake of other drugs does not require an interruption of breast-feeding.

4.6.9 Digitalis

With ongoing therapy of 250–750 µg *digoxin* daily (half-life about 36 hours), concentrations between 0.4 and 1.9 µg/L have been reported in mother's milk. With an M/P ratio of about 0.8, the dose transferred to the infant is, at most, 0.3 µg/kg/day. This is considerably lower than the usual maintenance dose in children of 10 µg/kg/day. No digoxin was measurable in the infant's plasma when the mother had taken 250 µg/day and with 750 µg/day, 0.2 µg/L (therapeutic level 0.5–2 µg/L) was detected (survey in Bennett 1996).

There are no studies on *digitoxin* and derivatives.

Recommendation. The use of digoxin is no cause for concern during breast-feeding.

4.6.10 Antiarrhythmics

Antiarrhythmics will be discussed below according to their classification (Chapter 2.8.15).

▶ Class IA

With daily administration of 1,800 mg *quinidine* (hydrochloride), a maximum of 9 mg/L is detected in milk. For exclusively breastfed infants, this is 1.3 mg/kg daily or about 4% of the maternal weight-related dose. The M/P ratio is 0.9 (Hill 1979). Despite possible accumulation due to the infant's delayed metabolization, the American Academy of Pediatrics (2001) stated that there is no cause for concern about using quinidine during breastfeeding. There are no case reports on symptoms in breastfed children.

Lactation

4.6 Cardiovascular drugs and diuretics

With *disopyramide*, up to 15% of the maternal weight-related dose can apparently be taken in by the infant. Between 0.1 and 0.5 mg/L are reported in the plasma of some children. The therapeutic level for adults is above 3 mg/L. No symptoms are described in breastfed children (survey in Bennett 1996). After a single dose of 100 mg, the relative dose is 3% of the maternal weight-related dose. There is no experience available for *ajmaline* and *prajmalium bitartrate* during breastfeeding.

▶ **Class IB**

Following i.v. administration of about 1,000 mg *lidocaine* and the resulting therapeutic plasma concentration of 5 μg/mL in the mother, a transfer of 1.8% of the weight-related dose has been observed (Zeisler 1986). A similar proportion is calculated following administration as a local anesthetic (Lebedevs 1993).

With long-term therapy using 600 mg *mexiletine* daily, a milk concentration to 0.96 mg/L has been reported for one mother. This represents 0.14 mg/kg/day or 1.4% of the maternal weight-related dose for the infant, whose plasma mexiletine was not detectable (Lewis 1981). For another infant, already prenatally exposed to mexiletine, growth disturbances and, 5 months after weaning, a questionable seizure has been reported. The development that followed has been reported as unremarkable (Lownes 1987). A connection with the exposure via the mother's milk was unlikely.

▶ **Class IC**

Flecainide is reported in milk from several mothers in long-term treatment with 2 × 100 mg daily at concentrations of 0.27–1.53 μg/mL (McQuinn 1990, Wagner 1990). Based on the highest value, an infant could get approximately 7% of the maternal weight-related dose. The American Academy of Pediatrics (2001) does not object to the use of this drug during breastfeeding as it is also used therapeutically in newborns. Propafenone has a PPB of 83%. After a single dose of 150 mg of propafenone, an M/P ratio of <1 and a weight-related dose of 0.1% were calculated (Wakaumi 2005).

▶ **Class II**

For β-receptor-blockers, see Section 4.6.1.

▶ **Class III**

Amiodarone has a very long half-life of 2–4 weeks. It consists of just about 40% iodide (see Chapter 4.11.6). In the mother's milk of one woman who had taken amiodarone at the end of her pregnancy for a number of reasons including fetal indications, only after 25 days was the active ingredient no longer detectable. Her breastfed infant had no side effects and the thyroid function was also normal (Hall 2003). With long-term therapy using 400 mg/day, a maximum of 16.4 mg/L of milk plus 6.5 mg/L of the metabolite, *desethylamiodarone* (DA), was reported (survey in Bennett, 1996). Based on this, the total amount of active substance, including the metabolite, which an infant could receive, would be a maximum of 3.5 mg/kg/day or 51.5% of the maternal weight-related dose. Up to 0.4 mg/L (therapeutic level 1.0–2.7 mg/L) was detected in the infant's plasma. In later studies, lower concentrations of amiodarone plus DA (up to 5 mg/L) were reported in mother's milk and infant's plasma (up to 0.15 mg/L) (Moretti 1995, Plomp 1992).

With *sotalol*, which has an M/P ratio of 3–5, an infant can receive 20–40% of the maternal weight-related dose, that is, up to 3 mg/kg daily (Hackett 1990, Wagner 1990). Because of a moderately long half-life, a high oral bioavailability, very low protein binding (0%) and 80 to 90% renal excretion, sotalol has a high risk for accumulation in infants. There is no experience on *dronedarone* available.

▶ **Class IV**

With on-going treatment using 240–360 mg verapamil daily, up to 0.3 mg/L is reported in milk. The M/P ratio lies between 0.2 and 0.9. The daily amount taken in by the infant is given as a maximum of 0.05 mg/kg. This represents about 1% of the maternal dose per kg of bodyweight. In the plasma of one of the breastfed infants, 2.1 µg/L is detected. No undesirable side effects have been described (survey in Bennett 1996).

For *diltiazem*, the results from only one patient are similar to those of *verapamil* including the drug measurement (Okada 1985). There is no experience on *gallopamil*.

Adenosine cannot be classified in any of the classic antiarrhythmic groups. Because of its extremely short half-life and the very brief time for which it is used, it should not be considered a cause for concern during breastfeeding. The anticholinergic, *ipratropium bromide* is available orally and by i.v. injection as a treatment for bradycardia. In the latter form, the elimination half-life is 1.6 hours. There are just not enough data available on its transfer into the mother's milk as for vernakalant.

Recommendation. In Class IA antiarrhythmics, quinidine can be used while breastfeeding. Long-term use requires careful monitoring especially of liver enzymes.

Lidocaine is the drug of choice in the Class 1B and mexiletine as a possible alternative.

Flecainide is the Class 1C drug of choice.

Within the Class II-antiarrhythmics (β-receptor blockers) propranolol and metoprolol are preferable (Section 4.6.1).

Should a representative of Class III be absolutely necessary, sotalol is preferable to the iodide-containing amiodaron but the follow-up of the infant is necessary for signs of β-blockade.

Verapamil and diltiazem, as representatives of Class IV, are well tolerated during breastfeeding. The same can be assumed for adenosine.

If treatment with an antiarrhythmic, which is not recommended, has begun, weaning is not necessarily required. We suggest only changing the treatment and continuing breastfeeding.

4.6.11   Vasodilators and circulatory drugs

The nitrates, *isosorbide mononitrates, isosorbide dinitrate* and *nitroglycerin* or *glyceryl trinitrate* and *pentaerythritol tetranitrate* are insufficiently investigated during breastfeeding. Short half-lives and the temporary use argue against a toxic risk for the breastfed baby.

Other cardiac/coronary therapeutics such as *molsidomine, ranolazine, ivabradine* and *trapidil* are insufficiently studied with respect to their tolerance during breastfeeding.

Naftidrofuryl and its primary metabolite LS74 appear only in trace levels in milk. Within 72 hours, only about 300 µg of the total 3,500 mg administered, had been excreted into milk. Thereby, an infant would receive 0.1% of the maternal weight-related dose per kg and day (report of the manufacturer Lipha). There are no known toxic effects on the infant.

Following a one-time oral administration of 400 mg of pentoxifylline, a maximum concentration of 1 mg/L milk, including the active metabolites, has been reported (Witter 1985). Based on this result, the infant would receive 0.5% of the weight-related adult dose per feed. No toxic effects have been described to date.

There is only little information on *ginkgo biloba* and, therefore, it should be avoided during pregnancy and lactation if possible (Dugoua 2006).

There is also no clinical experience available on a medication approved for improving the peripheral arterial circulation, *alprostadil alfadex*, a prostaglandin, that inhibits the thrombocyte aggregation and acts as a vasodilator or for *pentosan polysulfate*, a heparinoid with anticoagulatory and fibrinolytic properties. The substance passes into the milk of rats in negligible amounts.

There are also no data for the drugs *betahistine, cinnarizine* and *flunarizine* used for dizziness. Flunarizine has a very long half-life of 18 days and therefore should not be prescribed during breastfeeding, as an accumulation in the child's body cannot be eliminated.

Recommendation. Short-term use of nitrates is justifiable for relevant indications. Using the other drugs mentioned here does not require an interruption of breastfeeding, but the therapy should be changed.

4.6.12   Diuretics

With diuretic therapy, milk production can decrease, especially if there is already some lactational deficiency. Displacement of bilirubin from PPB in newborns has been discussed for *furosemide* and the thiazides. A risk for kernicterus is not considered a realistic possibility.

Chlortalidone has a half-life of 44 hours or more. Long-term treatment with 50 mg/day leads to comparatively high concentrations in the milk with values to 0.86 mg/L. The very high maternal plasma concentrations lead to an M/P ratio of only about 0.06. The maximum dose an infant would receive is given as 0.13 mg/kg/day. This represents 15.5% of the maternal weight-related dose. No symptoms of intolerance have been observed in breastfed infants (Mulley 1982).

Furosemide has an M/P ratio of 0.5–0.8 (Wilson 1980). There are no indications of any particular intolerance in breastfed infants.

With long-term treatment using 50 mg of *hydrochlorothiazide* daily, 0.12 mg/L at most is found in the milk. The dose received by the infant would be 0.02 mg/kg daily – that is, 2.2% of the maternal weight-related dose (Miller 1982).

Spironolactone is a potassium-saving diuretic. As soon as it is absorbed, it is changed into the active metabolite, *canrenone*, which is up to 98% bound to plasma protein. In animal studies, canrenone is carcinogenic at very high doses. No such carcinogenicity has been reported in human beings. The M/P ratio lies between 0.5 and 0.7. With ongoing treatment of 100 mg daily, a maximum milk concentration of 0.1 mg/L has been found. For the infant, this would mean a daily intake of 0.016 mg/kg, meaning only 1.2% of the maternal weight-related dose (Phelps 1977).

There arc insufficient data to make a judgment on *amiloride, bendroflumethiazide, bumetanide, clopamide, eplerenone, indapamide, mefruside, piretanide, torasemide, triamterene* and *xipamide*.

Recommendation. Diuretics should not be used primarily for treating hypertension during breastfeeding. However, when a diuretic is urgently needed, moderately dosed treatment with hydrochlorothiazide can be considered. Should furosemide be indicated, this can also be prescribed. Spironolactone should be reserved for special indications such as primary hyperaldosteronism, ascites, nephritic syndrome and the like. Chlortalidone is contraindicated because of its high relative dose. The other drugs mentioned should be avoided due to insufficient experience. Single doses, however, do not require limitation of breastfeeding, but the therapy should be changed.

References

Ahn HK, Nava-Ocampo AA, Han JY et al. Exposure to amlodipine in the first trimester of pregnancy and during breastfeeding. Hypertens Pregnancy 2007; 26: 179 87.

American Academy of Pediatrics, Committee on Drugs. The transfer of drugs and other chemicals into human breast milk. Pediatrics 2001; 108: 776–89.

Anderson JE, Held N, Wright K. Raynauds's phenomenon of the nipple: a treatable cause of painful breastfeeding. Pediatrics 2004; 113: 360–4.

Barrett ME, Heller MM, Stone HF et al. Raynaud Phenomenon of the nipple in breastfeeding mothers. An underdiagnosed cause. JAMA Dermatol 2013; 149: 300–6.

Bartels P, Hanff L, Mathot R et al. Nicardipine in pre-eclamptic patients: placental transfer and disposition in breast milk. BJOG 2006; 114: 230–3.

Begg EJ, Robson RA, Gardiner SJ et al. Quinapril and its metabolite quinaprilat in human milk. Br J Clin Pharmacol 2001; 51: 478–81.

Bennett PN (ed.). Drugs and Human Lactation. 2nd edn, Amsterdam, New York, Oxford: Elsevier 1996.

Boutroy MJ, Bianchetti G, Dubruc C et al. To nurse when receiving acebutolol: is it dangerous for the neonate? Eur J Clin Pharmacol 1986; 30: 137–9.

Bunjes R, Schaefer C, Holzinger D. Clonidine and breast-feeding. Clin Pharm 1993; 12: 178–9.

Carcas AJ, Abad-Santos F, de Rosendo JM et al. Nimodipine transfer into human breast milk and cerebrospinal fluid. Ann Pharmacother 1996; 30: 148–50.

Devlin RG, Fleiss PN. Captopril in human blood and breast milk. J Clin Pharmacol 1981; 21: 110–13.

Dugoua JJ, Mills E, Perri D et al. Safety and efficacy of ginkgo (*Ginkgo biloba*) during pregnancy and lactation. Can J Clin Pharmacol 2006; 13: e277–84.

Ehrenkranz RA, Ackermann BA, Hulse JD. Nifedipine transfer into human milk. J Pediatr 1989; 114: 478–80.

Eyal S, Kim JD, Anderson GD et al. Atenolol pharmacokinetics and excretion in breast milk during the first 6 to 8 months postpartum. J Clin Pharmacol 2010; 50: 1301–9.

Fidler J, Smith V, de Sweet M. Excretion of oxprenolol and timolol in breast milk. Br J Obstet Gynaecol 1983; 90: 961–5.

Goncalves PV, Cavalli RC, Cunha SP et al. Determination of pindolol enantiomers in amniotic fluid and breast milk by high-performance liquid chromatography: applications to pharmacokinetics in pregnant and lactating women. J Chromatogr B Analyt Technol Biomed Life Sci 2007; 852: 640–5.

Hackett LP, Wojnar-Horton RE, Dusci LJ et al. Excretion of sotalol in breast milk. Br J Clin Pharmacol 1990; 29: 277–8.

Hall CM, McCormick KP. Amiodarone and breast feeding. Arch Dis Child Fetal Neonatal Ed 2003; 88: F255.

Hartikainen-Sorri AL, Heikkinen JE, Koivisto M. Pharmacokinetics of clonidine during pregnancy and nursing. Obstet Gynecol 1987; 69: 598–600.

Hill LM, Malkasian GD Jr. The use of quinidine sulfate throughout pregnancy. Obstet Gynecol 1979; 54: 366–8.

Huttunen K, Gronhagen-Riska C, Fyhrquist F. Enalapril treatment of a nursing mother with slightly impaired renal function. Clin Nephrol 1989; 31: 278.

Jarreau PH, Le Beller C, Guillonneau M et al. Excretion of nicardipine in human milk. Paediatr Perinat Drug Ther 2000; 4: 28–30.

Jensen BP, Dalrymple JM, Begg EJ. Transfer of doxazosin into breast milk. J Hum Lact 2013; 29: 150–3.

Kaiser G, Ackermann R, Dieterle W et al. Benazepril and benazeprilat in human plasma and breast milk. IV. World Conference on Clinical Pharmacology and Therapeutics, July 1989.

Lamont RE, Elder MG. Transfer of hydralazine across the placenta and into breast milk. J Obstet Gynaecol 1986; 7: 47–8.

Lebedevs TH, Wojnar-Horton RE, Yapp P et al. Excretion of lignocaine and its metabolite monoethylglycinexylidide in breast milk following its use in a dental procedure. A case report. J Clin Periodontol 1993; 20: 606–8.

Lewis AM, Johnston A, Patel L et al. Mexiletine in human blood and breast milk. Postgrad Med J 1981; 57: 546–7.

Liedholm H, Wahlin-Boll E, Hansson A et al. Transplacental passage and breast milk concentrations of hydralazine. Eur J Clin Pharmacol 1982; 21: 417–9.

Lownes HE, Ives TJ. Mexiletine use in pregnancy and lactation. Am J Obstet Gynecol 1987; 157: 446–7.

Madadi P, Koren G, Freeman DJ et al. Timolol concentrations in breast milk of a woman treated for glaucoma: calculation of neonatal exposure. J Glaucoma 2008; 17: 329–31.

McQuinn RL, Pisani A, Wafa S et al. Flecainide excretion in human breast milk. Clin Pharmacol Ther 1990; 48: 262–7.

Manninen AK, Juhakoski A. Nifedipine concentrations in maternal and umbilical serum, amniotic fluid, breast milk and urine of mothers and offspring. Int J Clin Pharmacol Res 1991; 11: 231–6.

Miller ME, Cohn RD, Burghart PH. Hydrochlorothiazide disposition in a mother and her breast-fed infant. J Pediatr 1982; 101: 789–91.

Moretti M: Presentation at the 8th International Conference of the Organisation of Teratogen Information Services (OTIS) in San Diego, 1995.

Morselli PL, Boutroy MJ, Bianchetti G et al. Placental transfer and perinatal pharmacokinetics of betaxolol. Eur J Clin Pharmacol 1990; 38: 477–83.

Mulley BA, Parr GD, Pau WK et al. Placental transfer of chlortalidone and its elimination in maternal milk. Eur J Clin Pharmacol 1982; 13: 129–31.

Okada M, Inoue H, Nakamura Y et al. Excretion of diltiazem in human milk. N Engl J Med 1985; 312: 992–3.

Page SM, McKenna DS. Vasospasm of the nipple presenting as painful lactation. Obstet Gynecol 2006; 108: 806–8.

Penny WJ, Lewis MJ: Nifedipine is excreted in human milk. Eur J Clin Pharmacol 1989; 36: 427–8.

Phelps DL, Karim A. Spironolactone: relationship between concentrations of dethioacetylated metabolite in human serum and milk. J Pharm Sci 1977; 66: 1203.

Plomp TA, Vulsma T, de Vijlder JJM. Use of amiodarone during pregnancy. Eur J Obstet Gynecol Reprod Biol 1992; 43: 201–7.

Redman CW, Kelly JG, Cooper WD. The excretion of enalapril and enalaprilat in human breast milk. Eur J Clin Pharmacol 1990; 38: 99.

Rush JE, Snyder BA, Barrish A et al. Comment. Clin Nephrol 1991; 35: 234.

Schaefer HG, Toublanc N, Weimann HJ. The pharmacokinetics of moxonidine. Rev Contemp Pharmacother 1998; 9: 481–90.

Schimmel MS, Eidelman AJ, Wilschanski MA et al. Toxic effects of atenolol consumed during breastfeeding. J Pediatr 1989; 114: 476–8.

Sioufi A, Hillion D, Lumbroso P et al. Oxprenolol placental transfer, plasma concentrations in newborns and passage into breast milk. Br J Clin Pharmacol 1984; 18: 453–6.

Szucs KA, Axline SE, Rosenman MB. Maternal membranous glomerulonephritis and successful exclusive breastfeeding. Breastfeed Med 2010; 5: 123–6.

Tonks AM. Nimodipine levels in breast milk. Aust N Z J Surg 1995; 65: 693–4.

Valdivieso A, Valdes G, Spiro TE et al. Minoxidil in breast milk. Ann Int Med 1985; 102: 135.

Wagner X, Jouglard J, Moulin M et al. Coadministration of flecainide acetate and soltalol during pregnancy: lack of teratogenic effects, passage across the placenta, and excretion into human breast milk. Am Heart J 1990; 119: 700–2.

Wakaumi M, Tsuruoka S, Sakamoto K et al. Pilsicainide in breast milk from a mother: comparison with disopyramide and propafenone. Br J Clin Pharmacol 2005; 59: 120–2.

White WB, Yeh SC, Krol GJ. Nitrendipine in human plasma and breast milk. Eur J Clin Pharmacol 1989; 36: 531–4.

Wilson JT, Brown RD, Cherek DR et al. Drug excretion in human breast milk: principles, pharmacokinetics and projected consequences. Clin Pharmacokinet 1980; 5: 1–66.

Witter FR, Smith RV. The excretion of pentoxyfylline and its metabolites into human breast milk. Am J Obstet Gynecol 1985; 151: 1094–7.

Zeisler JA, Gaarder TD, de Mesquita SA. Lidocaine excretion in breast milk. Drug Intell Clin Pharmacol 1986; 20: 691–3.

Anticoagulants, thrombocyte aggregation inhibitors and fibrinolytics

4.7

Paul Merlob and Juliane Habermann

4.7.1	Heparin and danaparoid	725
4.7.2	Thrombin- and factor Xa-inhibitors	726
4.7.3	Thrombocyte aggregation inhibitors	726
4.7.4	Vitamin K-antagonists	727
4.7.5	Fibrinolytics	728
4.7.6	Antihemorrhagics	728
4.7.7	Volume expanders	728

Treatment with anticoagulants (heparin and derivatives), as well as with thrombin- and factor Xa-inhibitors, is acceptable during breastfeeding. Except for low dose acetylsalicylic acid, all other thrombocyte aggregation inhibitors should be used during lactation only if other alternatives are lacking. There are no human studies on the usage of fibrinolytics and antihemorrhagics during lactation.

4.7.1   Heparin and danaparoid

Heparin does not pass into the mother's milk nor is it absorbed in relevant quantities in the gastrointestinal tract. This is also expected for the low molecular-weight preparations, *certoparin, dalteparin, enoxaparin, nadroparin, reviparin* and *tinzaparin*. In a study of 15 women who received 2,500 IU dalteparin daily after caesarean section, the anti-Xa activity in the plasma of the mother and in the milk were measured as indicators for heparin effects. While a maximum of 0.308 IE/mL was measured in the plasma, the peak value in the milk was 0.037 IE/mL. The M/P ratio showed values between 0.025 and 0.224. The authors calculated, on the basis of the highest activity values in the milk, a 5.4% share of the maternal weight-related dose within 24 hours, assuming a daily intake of 250 mL milk for a newborn on the 5th day of life. If one also considers that heparin is practically not absorbed orally, no risk should be expected through the mother's milk (Richter 2001). Studies on the use of the heparin antidote protamin during breastfeeding are not available. Due to its molecular structure and the half-life of 24 minutes for the protamin-heparin complex, appreciable oral availability through the mother's milk seems unlikely.

Danaparoid apparently does not pass into the mother's milk in clinically relevant amounts. In milk samples of five patients, the anti-Xa activity was only 0–0.07 IE/mL although values in the maternal plasma between

0.15 IE/mL and 0.45 IE/mL were reached (Magnani 2010). Other case reports also describe only a minimal passage into the colostrum (Myers 2003). Even when transfer into the mother's milk cannot be completely ruled out, danaparoid is broken down by the baby's digestive enzymes.

> **Recommendation.** During treatment with unfractionated heparin, low-molecular heparins or danaparoid, breastfeeding may continue without limitation. When indicated, protamin can be used during breastfeeding. Limiting breastfeeding does not seem to be justifiable.

4.7.2   Thrombin- and factor Xa-inhibitors

A mother treated with *lepirudin* for heparin-induced thrombocytopenia received 3 months subcutaneously 2 × 50 mg daily during breastfeeding. Three hours after the lepirudin injection, a therapeutic concentration of 0.73 mg/L of *hirudin* was found in the maternal plasma. At the same time, there was no hirudin detectable (<0.1 mg/L) in the milk. The breastfed baby showed no symptoms whatsoever (Lindhoff-Last 2000). There are no clinical data available for *desirudin*. However, owing to a similar molecular structure (polypeptide with a high molecular weight) problems with the breastfed baby would hardly be expected. There are, as yet, no data on tolerance for the hirudin analog, *bivalirudin*, during breastfeeding. Due to its high molecular weight and the short half-life, an appreciable intake via the mother's milk seems unlikely. There is also, as yet, no experience with the use of *argatroban* during breastfeeding. The manufacturer refers to the transfer of the substance into the milk of rodents. It is not known whether argatroban is bioavailable orally. However, due to the molecular structure, this seems unlikely. As yet, no data have been provided on the oral thrombin inhibitor *dabigatran*. The oral bioavailability has been given as 6.5%.

Undesirable effects for the breastfed child after using the factor Xa-inhibitor *fondaparinux* have not been described up to now and seem unlikely due to the molecular structure (*pentasaccharide*). *Rivaroxaban* and *apixaban* are insufficiently researched. Data from animal experiments indicate passage of the substance into the mother's milk. Due to the high oral bioavailability (rivaroxaban 80–100%, apixaban ca. 50%) intolerance in the infant cannot be ruled out.

> **Recommendation.** With lepirudin, desirudin, bivalirudin and fondaparinux, any limitation on breastfeeding does not seem justifiable. Argatroban and the orally bioavailable medications, dabigatran, rivaroxaban and apixaban should only be used when there is a lack of alternatives. Decisions on limiting breastfeeding should be made in individual cases.

4.7.3   Thrombocyte aggregation inhibitors

Low dose *acetylsalicylic acid* (ASS; 80–300 mg/day) to inhibit thrombocyte aggregation is also well tolerated during breastfeeding (Chapter 4.1).

There are no clinical reports on the use of adenosine-diphosphate (ADP) receptor antagonists *clopidogrel, ticlopidine, prasugrel* and *ticagrelor*. Animal studies show a transfer of these substances into the animal mother's milk.

The GPIIb/IIIa antagonists, *abciximab, eptifibatide* and *tirofiban*, are insufficiently studied with respect to their use during breastfeeding. On the basis of the molecular structure it seems, at least for abciximab as a fab-fragment antibody and for the heptapeptide, eptifibatide, that an appreciable secretion into the mother's milk is unlikely. It can also be assumed that the oral bioavailability of both substances is limited. For tirofiban, secretion into the milk of rats has been established (Food and Drug Administration 2001).

Dipyridamole passes in limited amounts into the mother's milk according to the manufacturer's information.

Recommendation. Low dose acetylsalicylic acid to inhibit thrombocyte aggregation is unobjectionable. It is preferable to use it at the end of breastfeeding and not when the infant has a viral disease. Reye's syndrome may be associated with aspirin administration to infants with viral infection, but the risk of Reye's syndrome from salicylate in breast milk is unknown (Schror 2007). The use of other thrombocyte aggregation inhibitors should be critically scrutinized and only occur if other alternatives are lacking. With urgent indications, a decision about breastfeeding must be made in individual cases.

4.7.4   Vitamin K-antagonists

Coumarin derivates *acenocoumarol, phenprocoumon* and *warfarin*, as well as the *indanediones*: *fluindione* and *phenindione*, are among the Vitamin K-antagonists used as oral anticoagulants. In particular, the most widely used substances, warfarin, phenprocoumon and *acenocoumarol*, have a very high protein binding (>95%). Thus, only very small amounts would be expected in the mother's milk.

Warfarin could not be detected in the milk (overview in Bennett 1996). A small study with 11 breastfeeding mothers showed a very limited milk transfer of acenocoumarol. The dose transmitted with the milk was 500-fold lower than a therapeutic infant dose (Nava 2004).

In a woman who was treated with phenprocoumon from day 19 postpartum, 33 µg/L was measured in the 24 hours pooled sample of milk (von Kries 1993). The estimated daily phenprocoumon intake from maternal milk in a baby drinking 200 mL/kg/day was 6–8 µg/kg/day. This is only about 1/50 of the corresponding maternal plasma concentrations and much less than the average maintenance requirement in children (about 50 µg/kg/day).

Changes in coagulation parameter have not, as yet, been detected in infants who were being breastfed during their mothers' treatment with acenocoumarol, phenprocoumon or warfarin (Bennett 1996, Fondevila 1989, author's own observations) and would hardly be expected. By contrast, only about 70% of phenindione is protein-bound and a higher transfer in a therapeutic dosage for an infant has been shown. A case description refers to a breastfed baby with pathological coagulation parameters and hematomas during the mother's treatment (overview in Bennett 1996).

Lactation

4.7 Anticoagulants, thrombocyte aggregation inhibitors and fibrinolytics

> **Recommendation.** During treatment with the oral anticoagulants, acenocoumarol, phenprocoumon and warfarin, breastfeeding may continue. Reliable vitamin K prophylaxis should be ensured during the first weeks. Intramuscular administration of vitamin K is the most efficacious and cost-effective practice, reserving multidose oral prophylaxis for infants whose parents declined i.m. injection (Busfield 2013). Premature infants at least should have their coagulation status determined after a few days. The vitamin K antagonists, fluindione and phenindione, are contraindicated during breastfeeding.

4.7.5   Fibrinolytics

Clinical reports on the use of the fibrinolytics *urokinase, alteplase, tenecteplase, reteplase, anistreplase* and *streptokinase* during breastfeeding are not available. Due to the molecular structure and the very short half-life, any appreciable intake by the infant would not be expected.

> **Recommendation.** Limiting breastfeeding after use of fibrinolytics does not seem justifiable.

4.7.6   Antihemorrhagics

The antifibrinolytic, *tranexamic acid*, is secreted in limited amounts into the mother's milk. According to the manufacturer's information, the concentration in the mothers' milk, measured 1 hour after the last dose, was 1% of the maximum serum concentration after a 2 day treatment of the patients. The oral bioavailability is around 35% and the half-life is about 2 hours.

After oral administration, *p-aminomethyl-benzoic acid* is well absorbed. There are no studies available on its use during breastfeeding.

Up until now, there has been no information on the tolerance by the infant of thrombopoetin receptor agonists *romiplostim* and *eltrombopag*. According to the manufacturer, passage into the milk is likely with romiplostim. Due to the molecular structure (Fc peptide fusions protein) appreciable oral bioavailability cannot be assumed. Animal experimental data indicate that the orally bioavailable eltrombopag reaches rat pups through the mother's milk. On the use of protamine sulfate, see Section 4.7.1.

> **Recommendation.** Limitation of breastfeeding after medication with tranexamic acid is not justifiable. It is preferable to take this drug at the end of breastfeeding. P-aminomethyl-benzoic acid should only be prescribed for urgent indications. During treatment with romiplostim or eltrombopag, a decision about breastfeeding must be made in individual cases.

4.7.7   Volume expanders

Dextrans and *gelatins* while breastfeeding have not been systematically studied. Due to the structural properties of the substances, an appreciable intake by the infant would not be expected. On the use of hydroxyl ethyl starch see Chapter 4.6.

> **Recommendation.** In critical situations, the use of dextrans and gelatin is acceptable even during breastfeeding. Limitation of breastfeeding is not justifiable.

References

Bennett PN (ed). Drugs and Human Lactation. 2nd edn, Amsterdam, New York, Oxford: Elsevier 1996.

Busfield A, Samuel R, McNinch A et al. Vitamin K deficiency bleeding after NICE guidance and withdrawal of Konakion Neonatal; British Paediatric Surveillance Unit study 2006–2008. Arch Dis Child 2013; 98: 41–47.

Fondevila CG, Meschengieser S, Blanco A, et al. Effect of acenocoumarine on the breast-fed infant. Thromb Res 1989; 56: 29–36.

Food and Drug Administration. Product Information Aggrastat 2001; http://www. drugs.com/mmx/tirofiban-hydrochloride.html

Lindhoff-Last E, Willeke A, Thalhammer C. Hirudin treatment in a breastfeeding woman. Lancet 2000; 355: 467.

Magnani HN. An analysis of clinical outcomes of 91 pregnancies in 83 women treated with danaparoid (Orgaran). Thromb Res 2010; 125: 297–302.

Myers B, Westby J, Strong J. Prophylactic use of danaparoid in high-risk pregnancy with heparin-induced thrombocytopaenia-positive skin reaction. Blood Coagul Fibrinolysis 2003; 14: 485–7.

Nava LE, Gómez AB, González VM. Plasma and milk concentrations of acenocoumarin in breast-feeding women during postpartum. Ginecol Obstet Mex 2004; 72: 550–60.

Richter C, Sitzmann J, Lang P, et al. Excretion of low molecular weight heparin in human milk. Br J Clin Pharmacol 2001; 52: 708–10.

Schror K. Aspirin and Reye syndrome: review of the evidence. Paediatr Drugs 2007; 93: 195–204.

Von Kries R, Nöcker D, Schmitz-Kummer E et al. Transfer von Phenprocoumon in die Muttermilch. Monatsschr Kinderheilkd 1993; 141: 505–7.

Lactation

4.7 Anticoagulants, thrombocyte aggregation inhibitors and fibrinolytics

Antiepileptics

Paul Merlob and Christof Schaefer

4.8

| 4.8.1 | Introduction | 731 |
| 4.8.2 | Individual antiepileptics | 732 |

4.8.1 Introduction

All antiepileptics pass into the milk, albeit in differing amounts. Babies who are breastfed during maternal antiepileptic treatment apparently develop just as well as those who are not breastfed. At least, that is what was reported in one study of 82 mother–infant pairs in which breastfeeding was carried out during monotherapy with *lamotrigine, carbamazepine, phenytoin* or *valproate* by comparison to 112 non-breastfed infants of mothers undergoing antiepileptic treatment. Both groups were already exposed *in utero*. IQs were compared at the age of 3 years. The authors discuss why the experimentally observed apoptotic effect of some antiepileptics did not lead to measurable anomalies in the immature brain after exposure through the mother's milk and submit that either the intrauterine outweighed the postnatal effect (although in animal experiments, the postnatal sensitivity for such damage is no less), breastfeeding causes a counter-effect or the significantly lower concentration via the mother's milk is insufficient for such side effects (Meador 2010).

With monotherapy, nothing in most antiepileptics argues against exclusive breastfeeding. However, in individual cases, intolerance cannot be ruled out (see under the individual antiepileptics). When a combination therapy with more than one antiepileptic is required, it must be individually decided whether the baby should be supplemented or even weaned to reduce the exposure. For vitamin-K prophylaxis in the newborn period, see Chapter 2.9. For individual antiepileptics, see Chapter 4.8.2. For further information on antiepileptics, see Chapter 2.10.

Recommendation.

- The choice of an antiepileptic for readjustment during breastfeeding is also determined primarily by effectiveness, i.e. according to the type of epilepsy.
- When possible, readjustment with an antiepileptic while breastfeeding should also take into consideration tolerance during a possible new pregnancy. This argues against therapy with *valproic acid*, in particular.
- A stable adjustment during pregnancy with whatever antiepileptic should not be uncritically changed or ended after birth.

Drugs During Pregnancy and Lactation. http://dx.doi.org/10.1016/B978-0-12-408078-2.00033-0

- With good observation of the baby, monotherapy with one antiepileptic does not fundamentally argue against exclusive breastfeeding. However, antiepileptic therapy with barbiturates, *clonazepam*, *ethosuximide* or lamotrigine while breastfeeding should be critically evaluated in individual cases. This is especially the case for antiepileptic combination therapy, during which breastfeeding should be discouraged.
- If symptoms that cannot otherwise be explained, such as sedation, weak suckling and restlessness, reoccur, the concentration of the substance in the infant's serum should be determined and an embryotoxicological center should be consulted so that a decision on weaning or supplementation with infant formula can be made. Particular care should be taken in the first 2 months of life, especially with premature and sick infants. Symptoms in the first few days of life are more likely attributable to adjustment disturbances due to prenatal exposure, rather than to medication in the milk.
- As with all CNS-effective medications, there is insufficient experience available on long-term effects of maternal maintenance therapy on breastfed children. However, there is, at yet, no serious indication that breastfeeding during antiepileptic therapy leads to developmental disorders in the child.

4.8.2   Individual antiepileptics

▶ Carbamazepine

Carbamazepine has a half-life of 15–35 hours in both adults and newborns and 75% is protein bound. Studies on more than 50 milk samples showed M/P ratios of about 0.5. Including the metabolite *carbamazepinepoxide*, a relative infant dose of not more than 3–8% should be expected. In one case, however, with a maternal dose of only 250 mg daily, the relative infant dose of about 15% was determined (Shimoyama 2000). Among breastfed children, serum concentrations between 0.5 and 1.5 µg/mL – but also in one case 4.7 µg/mL (therapeutic range 5–10 µg/mL) – were measured (survey in Hägg 2000, Shimoyama 2000, Brent 1998, Wisner 1998). Individual reports describe transient toxic liver changes in infants exposed prenatally and via the mother's milk (Frey 2002, Merlob 1992). One case report describes an infant with questionable seizures and a cyanotic attack, whose mother was taking *fluoxetine* and *buspirone* in addition to carbamazepine. Further development of the baby was normal through the end of the first year of life. The authors, quite rightly, hesitate to make a connection between the medication and the symptoms (Brent 1998). Another infant had feeding difficulties and was sedated during maternal anticonvulsive combination therapy with carbamazepine, phenytoin and barbiturates (survey in Hägg 2000). Further symptoms have not been published as yet. At 3 years of age, the IQs of the children breastfed when their mothers were taking carbamazepine were not lower than the IQs of children who were given infant formula because of their mothers' carbamazepine treatment (Section 4.8.1, Meador 2010). With carbamazepine monotherapy, the baby may be breastfed, with observation for possible side-effects.

▶ Clonazepam

The half-life of *clonazepam* is 20–40 hours. Only 60% is protein-bound. In the serum of one child, 4.7 µg/L was measured. In the mother, it was between 15 and 30 µg/L (Soederman 1988). The serum of a premature infant, whose mother had long-term therapy, was found to contain 13 µg/L. In another study, apnea occurred repeatedly in a premature baby. This was seen as being related to previous exposure *in utero* (survey in Hägg 2000). In a further case, a mother took 6 mg daily (plus 1,400 mg carbamazepine), and 20 µg/L were found in the serum of this baby. In the mother, it was 50 µg/L in her serum and 12 µg/L in her milk. The baby was described as "somewhat lazy at the breast" and tired (personal observation). Due to possible side-effects in the baby, breastfeeding with clonazepam is only conditionally acceptable.

▶ Eslicarbazepine

There is insufficient experience available on eslicarbazepine while breastfeeding. Thus breastfeeding with eslicarbazepine is only conditionally acceptable.

▶ Ethosuximide and mesuximide

Ethosuximide has a half-life of 55 hours. For the newborn, it is between 32 and 38 hours. Only a limited amount is protein-bound. The M/P ratio is 1. As studies on more than 10 mothers show, the infant can receive well over 50% of a child's dose or the maternal weight-related dose. The concentration in the child's serum can reach 10–40 mg/L (therapeutic range is 40–100 mg/L). Symptoms such as irritability, weak suck and sedation have been described in individual cases (survey in Hägg 2000 as well as Bennett 1996).

There is no data on *mesuximide*. Due to possible side-effects in the baby, breastfeeding is only conditionally acceptable with ethosuximide/mesuximide.

▶ Felbamate

There is insufficient experience available on using *felbamate* while breastfeeding. Due to its potential to cause hematological side-effects and for hepatotoxic action, it is not recommended while breastfeeding (Bar-Oz 2000, Hägg 2000).

▶ Gabapentin

For *gabapentin* there is published experience with around a dozen mothers (Ohman 2005, 2009, Kristensen 2006, Hägg 2000). The M/P ratio is 1. The half-life in infancy is 14 hours.

In a casuistry by Kristensen (2006), 3% of a therapeutic child's dose via the mother's milk was calculated for an exclusively breastfed baby. Based on the data of a total of eight mother–child pairs, a relative infant dose of 1.3 to 3.8% was calculated for the exclusively breastfed child (Ohman 2005, 2009). The milk samples were taken before administration of the drug, so that the relative infant dose did not represent a maximum value. Concentrations of the substance in the serum of the clinically unremarkable babies were between 6 and 12% of the maternal values. With three babies (Ohman 2009), no medication could be detected in the serum (detection limit 0.68 μg/mL). With gabapentin monotherapy and observation for possible side-effects, breastfeeding is acceptable.

▶ Lacosamide

There is insufficient experience on the use of *lacosamide* while breast-feeding. For this reason, breastfeeding with lacosamide is only conditionally acceptable.

▶ Lamotrigine

The M/P ratio with *lamotrigine* is only 0.4–0.8 (Fotopoulou 2009, Ohman 2000). Nevertheless, significant amounts reach the breastfed baby via the milk. The most extreme value of up to 18 mg/L was found in the milk of a woman who took 800 mg daily.

The results of the largest case series to date with 30 mother–baby pairs and 210 milk samples (Newport 2008) showed that the M/P ratio is highly variable. The mean breast milk concentrations for each patient were used to calculate the mean relative infant dose which was 9.2%. Mild thrombocytosis was present in seven of eight infants at the time of serum samples (average 3.8 weeks after delivery). No other adverse events among either the mothers or their nursing infants were noted.

With four mother–child pairs in another study, 10 days after the birth, between 4.6 and 9.2 μg/mL were measured in the serum of the mothers taking a daily dose of 200–800 mg and between <1 and 2.0 μg/mL in the serum of the children. For three children, this represented 20–43% of the maternal values. After 2 months it was still 23% on average (Liporace 2004). In some other case reports and case series, concentrations of 2.6–3.3 μg/mL were measured in the child seven to 18 days after the birth (Fotopoulou 2009, Ohman 2000). In a series with six breastfed children between 2 weeks and 5 months, a maximum of just under 1 μg/mL was measured in the infants' plasma and mean relative infant dose was 7.6%. There were no reports of side-effects on the children (Page-Sharp 2006).

With one mother, who took 400 mg of lamotrigine, between 7.8 and 11.5 mg/L in the milk were measured and after the decline of the higher postpartum values, about 7 mg/L was measured in the child's serum. This represented 44–49% of the maternal values (Kacirova 2010). In a simulation model with a daily dose of 200 mg, 2 mg per day and an average serum concentration of 1 mg/L were calculated for a fully breastfed child (Cibert 2010).

A case report describes a 16-day-old, otherwise healthy, fully-breastfed child, who, after several mild apnea episodes became significantly cyanotic and had to be reanimated. At this point, therapeutic values of 4.9 μg/mL (pediatric therapeutic range: 1–5 μg/mL) were found in the child's serum. The mother took 850 mg daily at this time and had serum concentrations between 7.2 μg/mL (day 9) and 14.9 μg/mL (day 17) (Nordmo 2009). Twelve hours after birth or 20.5 hours after the mother's last pre-partum intake, 7.7 μg/mL were measured in the child. About a week after weaning due to the symptoms, the authors determined, on the basis of concentrations measured in the child then, a half-life twice as long (56 hours) as in adults. In the further course of events, the child developed unremarkably without further apnea episodes up to the age of 7.5 months.

Sixty-one informative courses of infants with lamotrigine exposure via breast milk were evaluated by Padberg (2008). In the prospective group ($n = 46$) symptoms occurred in seven infants (15.2%). In 29 infants serum levels were measured under steady state condition (later than 10 days after birth). Eighteen babies (62%) had serum levels within the therapeutic range.

Occasionally, transaminase increases have been measured in breastfed babies (Caroline 2011, Padberg 2008).

Reports were made on three children whose mothers took 200 or 250 mg of lamotrigine for bipolar disorders. Apart from an intermittently occurring skin rash, these children had all developed normally at the ages of 15 or 18 months (Wakil 2009). At the age of 3 years, the IQs of the children breastfed while their mothers took lamotrigine were not lower than the IQs of children who received infant formula due to maternal lamotrigine treatment (Section 4.8.1, Meador 2010).

Although most of the breastfed children show no symptoms, breastfeeding with lamotrigine is only conditionally acceptable due to the considerable transfer to the child. Use in the full-term infant and a maternal dose of up to 200 mg/day seems safe, but it is more important that the concentration in the child's serum be controlled and close monitoring for any side effects in the infant should be properly done.

▶ **Levetiracetam**

In the case of one individual mother–child pair with *levetiracetam* therapy (dosage not stated) a relatively pronounced transfer into the milk was determined, resulting in 99 μmol/L (16.9 mg/L) in the milk and an M/P ratio >3 (Kramer 2002). This mother was being treated simultaneously with phenytoin and valproic acid. After starting levetiracetam, the infant became hypotonic and nursed poorly. Breastfeeding was discontinued and the infant was discharged from the hospital in a healthy condition. The newborn's serum concentration 4 days after weaning was 6 μmol/L. Greenhill (2004) measured breast milk levels of levetiracetam at 4 days and 2–3 months postpartum (12 women). Breast milk levels were significantly lower than blood levels in the mother. With a further seven mother–child pairs, up to the age of 10 months, a more or less stable M/P ratio of 1, and a relative infant dose of a maximum of 7.8%, were determined. The mothers received between 1,500 and 3,500 mg daily. Only with one of the clinically unremarkable babies, could very low concentrations of the substance be detected in the serum during the breastfeeding period (Johannessen 2005). A case series with 11 mother–child pairs, in which about 13% of the maternal values were found in the plasma of the unremarkable children, similar M/P ratios and a similar relative dose were determined (Tomson 2007). The elimination half-life for the newborns was calculated as 18 hours. It is, thus, significantly longer than in adults (6–8 hours). Lopez-Fraile (2009) prospectively analyzed the variations in levetiracetam levels in five women with epilepsy during pregnancy and 2- and 12-months after delivery. The mean umbilical cord/maternal plasma ratio was 1.21 (range 0.92–1.62). However, all five patients refused to breastfeed.

In another case, a mother was advised to wean 3 days after the birth. During the pregnancy she had already taken not only levetiracetam but also *primidone*. On the following day, the baby began to have convulsions. The convulsions, which were considered to be withdrawal symptoms, ceased after resuming breastfeeding. At the age of 6 months, however, the baby was unremarkable (Rauchenzauner 2011).

Lactation

4.8 Antiepileptics

With levetiracetam monotherapy and close observation for possible side-effects, the mother can breastfeed.

▶ Oxcarbazepine

The half-life of *oxcarbazepine* in infancy, including the active metabolite, 10-hydroxy-carbazepin, is up to 20 hours. In a 5-day-old baby, only 12% of the drug and 7% of the metabolite were found despite breastfeeding, compared to the concentrations of the placentally transmitted concentrations of oxcarbazepine and metabolites measured on the first day of life (cited in Pennell 2003). With two infants, measurements at the ages of 3–4 weeks showed only 5% of the maternal concentrations of metabolites (Ohman 2009). A further case report describes an infant breastfed for 18 weeks, who developed completely unremarkably up to age 5. The mother took 2 × 300 mg oxcarbazepine (9 mg/kg) for a psychiatric illness. Eight days postpartum, 0.1 μg/mL oxcarbazepine and <0.1 μg/mL of the active metabolite,10-hydroxy-carbazepine, were measured in the blood of the breastfed infant. Twenty-three days postpartum it was <0.1 μg/mL oxcarbazepine and 0.2 μg/mL of the metabolite. The relative infant dose was calculated as 1.5% at age 8 days and 1.7% at age 23 days. The M/P ratio was 9 at age 8 days, and 5 at age 23 days. The baby's transaminases were unremarkable (Lutz 2007). Also the baby of a mother who partially breastfed for six months, while taking 1,800 mg/day, had age-appropriate development at 3 years (Eisenschenk 2006).

With oxcarbazepine monotherapy and close observation for possible side-effects, the mother can breastfeed.

▶ Phenobarbital, primidone and barbexaclone

Primidone and *barbexaclone* are metabolized to *phenobarbital* and should be evaluated as such. The half-life of phenobarbital can be up to considerably more than 100 hours in both adults and full-term newborns. Only 50% of the medication is bound to protein. In newborns it is even less. More than 160 analyzed milk samples showed an M/P ratio for phenobarbital of about 0.5 and for primidone around 0.8. A fully breastfed infant could receive a significant percentage of the substance. For phenobarbital, 50% to significantly more than 100% of the maternal weight-related dose was calculated. For primidone it was up to 38% (Pote 2004, Sugawara 1999, survey in Hägg 2000 as well as Bennett 1996). Up to 50% of the maternal concentration can be reached in the infant's serum. Sedation and resultant feeding problems have been described repeatedly. Among these descriptions is one of the oldest publications on toxic symptoms via mother's milk (Frensdorf 1926). In a report on a mother being treated with 90 mg of phenobarbital daily, the concentration in the mother's milk was more or less stable at 5 μg/mL on the 6th and 19th days postpartum (measured before taking the tablet and 2.5 hours afterwards) (Pote 2004). Maternal serum values were also stable. The child was temporarily lethargic and needed intravenous fluid therapy. In the infant's serum, the phenobarbital level reached 55 μg/mL – twice the mother's value. The death of a child was also discussed in connection with maternal phenobarbital plus primidone therapy. Here, 8.3 mg/L phenobarbital, a therapeutic concentration, was found in the baby's serum (cited in Hägg 2000).

In another case, a mother was advised to wean 3 days after the birth. During the pregnancy she had already taken not only *levetiracetam* but also primidone. On the following day, the baby began to have convulsions. The convulsions, which were considered to be withdrawal symptoms, ceased after resuming breastfeeding. At the age of 6 months, however, the baby was unremarkable (Rauchenzauner 2011).

Other barbiturates should be similarly evaluated. Depending on the half-life and the dose given, symptoms in the infant should be expected, especially when there has been more than a single dose and in combination with other anticonvulsants.

Due to the significant transfer to the baby, breastfeeding with barbiturates is only conditionally acceptable. Monitoring infant blood levels is indispensable.

▶ Phenytoin

Phenytoin has an M/P ratio of about 0.3. Studies of more than 80 milk samples have shown that a fully breastfed infant can get between 0.5 and 5%, with a maximum of 10% of the maternal weight-related dose via the mother's milk. This is normally less than 5% of a pediatric phenytoin dose (10 mg/kg) (survey in Hägg 2000). The phenytoin concentration in the serum of exposed children was, at most 1.5% of the maternal value.

The half-life of 10–40 hours does not seem to be extended in infants when they have already been exposed *in utero* (Shimoyama 1998, survey in Bennett 1996). With the exception of two case observations, side effects in breastfed babies have not been reported. These two observations describe swallowing difficulties and methemoglobinemia, as well as feeding problems and sedation, with anticonvulsive combination therapy using phenytoin plus barbiturates or with carbamazepine in addition (surveys in Shimoyama 1998 and Bennett 1996). At 3 years of age, the IQs of breastfed children exposed to phenytoin were not lower than the IQs of children who received infant formula because of maternal phenytoin therapy (Section 4.8.1, Meador 2010).

With phenytoin monotherapy, the baby may be breastfed while being closely observed for possible side-effects.

▶ Pregabalin

There is insufficient experience available on the use of *pregabalin* while breastfeeding. For this reason, breastfeeding with pregabalin is only conditionally acceptable.

▶ Rufinamide

There is insufficient experience available on the use of *rufinamide* while breastfeeding. For this reason, breastfeeding with rufinamide is only conditionally acceptable.

▶ Sultiame

There is insufficient experience available on the use of *sultiame* while breastfeeding. For this reason, breastfeeding with sultiame is only conditionally acceptable.

Lactation

4.8 Antiepileptics

▶ Tiagabine

There is insufficient experience available on the use of *tiagabine* while breastfeeding. For this reason, breastfeeding with tiagabine is only conditionally acceptable.

▶ Topiramate

It has been reported for *topiramate* that only minimal or even no amounts of the substance were measured in the serum of six breastfed unremarkable babies (Ohman 2002, 2007). Insofar as they were above the detection limit, they represented 10–20% of the maternal serum values. An M/P ratio between 0.7 and 0.9 and a relative infant dose of 3–23% were calculated. One infant who was exclusively breastfed until 8 months, with a maternal intake of 300 mg topiramate daily, developed completely unremarkably (Gentile 2009). The half-life in infancy is 24 hours. In one woman, who was stabilized on 150 mg daily, 3.1 mg/L were measured in the milk 4 hours after intake. At the age of 6 months, 3 hours after a dose that had been increased to 175 mg, the infant showed a serum concentration of 0.8 mg/L. This was 15% of the maternal value, which was measured at the same time. The baby, who was breastfed until the age of 1 year with a topiramate dose increased to 200 mg, developed normally and showed no side-effects (Fröscher 2006). With 100 mg daily, another breastfed baby developed watery, mucousy diarrhea at the age of 6 weeks. Two weeks later, the baby had been weaned to infant formula. The stool normalized within 24 hours. The milk had 5.5 mg/L topiramate (Westergren 2009).

With topiramate monotherapy, maternal doses up to 200 mg/day and close observation for possible side-effects (diarrhea, sedation) the baby can be breastfed.

▶ Valnoctamide

There is insufficient experience available on the use of *valnoctamide* while breastfeeding. For this reason, breastfeeding with valnoctamide is only conditionally acceptable.

▶ Valproic acid

The passage of *valproic acid* into the mother's milk, with an M/P ratio of about 0.05 and a relative dose of, on average, around 1% (maximum 7%) is quite limited. This has been shown in more than 40 mothers studied (survey in Hägg 2000). Even so, as a result of the decidedly longer half-life of around 47 hours, a "steady state" can develop in the blood of the breastfed newborn with 7% and more of the maternal concentration. By contrast, a further study described six children with 0.7–1.5 μg/mL serum levels representing only 0.9–2.3% of the maternal concentrations which were between 39 and 79 μg/mL (Piontek 2000). One case report describes thrombocytopenic purpura as well as anemia and reticulocytosis in a breastfed baby, whose symptoms improved after weaning. The authors discuss the abnormalities against the background of hematological side effects in treated adults (Stahl 1997). Neither these nor other symptoms are described in other publications. At 3 years of age, the IQs among valproic acid-exposed breastfed children were no lower than the IQs of children who received infant formula because of maternal valproic acid therapy (Section 4.8.1, Meador 2010).

With valproic acid monotherapy and close observation for possible side-effects (including thrombocytes count, liver enzymes) the baby can be breastfed.

▶ Vigabatrin

Vigabatrin, with an M/P ratio of about 0.3, is practically not bound to plasma protein and, due to its limited distribution volume, a quantitatively significant transfer into the mother's milk could be expected. Nevertheless, in a study on two women who received 2,000 mg daily, only about 1% of the maternal dose for the pharmacologically active substance (s-isomer) was estimated as a maximum dosage for the infant (Tran 1998).

Due to insufficient experience, breastfeeding with vigabatrin is only conditionally acceptable. Use it only with careful observation of the infants' side- effects (poor sucking, sedation, sleepiness and even apnea).

▶ Zonisamide

With 300 mg *zonisamide* daily, an average of 10.1 mg/L was measured in the maternal plasma and 9.4 mg/L in the milk. This represents an M/P ratio of just under 1. From this, an average relative infant dose of 28% can be calculated (Sugawara 1999). In a later follow-up study, three breastfed children had developed normally (Kawada 2002, Shimoyama 1999). The half-life in infancy is 60–109 hours.

Due to insufficient experience and the considerable transfer into the milk, breastfeeding with zonisamide is only conditionally acceptable.

References

Bar-Oz B, Nulman I, Koren G et al. Anticonvulsants and breastfeeding: a critical review. Peadiatr Drugs 2000; 2: 113–26.

Bennett PN (ed). Drugs and Human Lactation. 2nd edn. Amsterdam, New York, Oxford: Elsevier 1996.

Brent NB, Wisner KL. Fluoxetine and carbamazepine concentrations in a nursing mother/infant pair. Clin Pediatr 1998; 37: 41–4.

Caroline M, Precourt A. Use of lamotrigine while breastfeeding – descriptive analysis of our population and report of five cases of premature neonates {Abstract}. Birth Defects Res A 2011; 91: 414.

Cibert M, Gouraud A, Vial T et al. A physiologically based pharmacokinetic model to predict neonate exposure to drugs during breast-feeding: application to lamotrigine. Fundam Clin Pharmacol 2010; 24: 246.

Eisenschenk S. Treatment with oxcarbazepine during pregnancy. Neurologist 2006; 12: 249–54.

Frensdorf W. Übergang von Luminal in die Milch. Münch Med Wochenschr 1926; 73: 322–3.

Frey B, Braegger CP, Ghelfi D. Neonatal cholestatic hepatitis from carbamazepine exposure during pregnancy and breastfeeding. Ann Pharmacother 2002; 36: 644–7.

Fotopoulou C, Kretz R, Bauer S et al. Prospectively assessed changes in lamotrigine-concentration in women with epilepsy during pregnancy, lactation and the neonatal period. Epilepsy Res 2009; 85: 60–4.

Lactation

4.8 Antiepileptics

Fröscher W, Jürges U. Topiramateinnahme während des Stillens. Akt Neurol 2006; 33: 215–7.

Gentile S. Topiramate in pregnancy and breastfeeding. Clin Drug Investig 2009; 29: 139–41.

Greenhill L, Betts T, Yarrow H et al. Breast milk levels of levetiracetam after delivery. Epilepsia 2004; 45: 230.

Hägg S, Spigset O. Anticonvulsant use during lactation. Drug Saf 2000; 22: 425–40.

Johannessen SI, Helde G, Brodtkorb E. Levetiracetam concentrations in serum and in breast milk at birth and during lactation. Epilepsia 2005; 46: 775–7.

Kacirova I, Grundmann M, Brozmanova H. Drug interaction between lamotrigine and valproic acid used at delivery and during lactation – A case report. Klin Farmakol Farm 2010; 24: 222–5.

Kawada K, Itoh S, Kusaka T et al. Pharmacokinetics of zonisamide in perinatal period. Brain Develop 2002; 24: 95–7.

Kramer G, Hosli I, Glanzmann R et al. Levetiracetam accumulation in breast milk. Epilepsia 2002; 43: 105.

Kristensen JH, Ilett KF, Hackett LP et al. Gabapentin and breastfeeding: a case report. J Hum Lact 2006; 22: 426–8.

Liporace J, Kao A, D'Abreu A. Concerns regarding lamotrigine and breastfeeding. Epilepsy Behav 2004; 5: 102–5.

Lopez-Fraile IP, Cid AO, Juste AO et al. Levetiracetam plasma level monitoring during pregnancy, delivery, and postpartum: clinical and outcome implications. Epilepsy Behav 2009; 15: 372–5.

Lutz UC, Wiatr G, Gaertner HJ et al. Oxcarbazepine treatment during breast-feeding: a case report. J Clin Psychopharmacol 2007; 27: 730–2.

Meador KJ, Baker GA, Browning N et al. Effects of breastfeeding in children of women taking antiepileptic drugs. Neurology 2010; 75: 1954–60.

Merlob P, Mor N, Litwin A. Transient hepatic dysfunction in an infant of an epileptic mother treated with carbamazepine during pregnancy and breastfeeding. Ann Pharmacother 1992; 26: 1563–5.

Newport DJ, Pennell PB, Calamaras MR et al. Lamotrigine in breast milk and nursing infants: determination of exposure. Pediatrics 2008; 122: e223–31.

Nordmo E, Aronsen L, Wasland K et al. Severe apnea in an infant exposed to lamotrigine in breast milk. Ann Pharmacother 2009; 43: 1893–7.

Ohman I, Leuf G, Tomson T. Topiramate kinetics during lactation. Epilepsia 2007; 48: 156–7.

Ohman I, Tomson T. Pharmacokinetics of oxcarbazine in neonatal period and during lactation. Epilepsia 2009; 50: 239.

Ohman I, Vitols S, Luef G et al. Topiramate kinetics during delivery, lactation, and in the neonate: preliminary observations. Epilepsia 2002; 43: 1157–60.

Ohman I, Vitols S, Tomson T. Lamotrigine in pregnancy: pharmacokinetics during delivery, in the neonate, and during lactation. Epilepsia 2000; 41: 709–13.

Ohman I, Vitols S, Tomson T. Pharmacokinetics of gabapentin during delivery, in the neonatal period, and lactation: does a fetal accumulation occur during pregnancy? Epilepsia 2005; 46: 1621–4.

Padberg S, Weber-Schoendorfer C, Schaefer C. Lamotrigine during lactation {Abstract}. Reprod Toxicology 2008; 26: 70–1.

Page-Sharp M, Kristensen JH, Hackett LP et al. Transfer of lamotrigine into breast milk. Ann Pharmacother 2006; 40: 1470–1.

Pennell PB. Antiepileptic drug pharmacokinetics during pregnancy and lactation. Neurology 2003; 61: 35–42.

Piontek CM, Baab S, Peindl KS et al. Serum valproate levels in 6 breast-feeding mother-infant pairs. J Clin Psychiatry 2000; 61: 170–2.

Pote M, Kulkarni R, Agarwal M. Phenobarbital toxic levels in a nursing neonate. Indian Pediatr 2004; 41: 963–4.

Rauchenzauner M, Kiechl-Kohlendorfer U, Rostasy K et al. Old and new antiepileptic drugs during pregnancy and lactation – report of a case. Epilepsy Behav 2011; 20: 719–20.

Shimoyama R, Ohkubo T, Sugawara K. Monitoring of zonisamide in human breast milk and maternal plasma by solid-phase extraction HPLC method. Biomed Chromatogr 1999; 13: 370–2.

Shimoyama R, Ohkubo T, Sugawara K. Monitoring of carbamazepine and carbamazepine 10,11-epoxide in breast milk and plasma by high-performance liquid chromatography. Ann Clin Biochem 2000; 37: 210–5.

Shimoyama R, Ohkubo T, Sugawara K et al. Monitoring of phenytoin in human breast milk, maternal plasma and cord blood plasma by solid-phase extraction and liquid chromatography. J Pharm Biomed Anal 1998; 17: 863–9.

Soederman P, Matheson I. Clonazepam in breast milk. Eur J Ped 1988; 147: 212–3.

Stahl MM, Neiderud J, Vinge E. Thrombocytopenic purpura and anemia in a breast-fed infant whose mother was treated with valproic acid. J Pediatr 1997; 130: 1001–3.

Sugawara K, Shimoyama R, Ohkubo T. Determinations of psychotropic drugs and antiepileptic drugs by high-performance liquid chromatography and its monitoring in human breast milk. Hirosaki Med J 1999; 51: 81–6.

Tomson T, Palm R, Källén K et al. Pharmacokinetics of levetiracetam during pregnancy, delivery, in the neonatal period, and lactation. Epilepsia 2007; 48: 1111–6.

Tran A, O'Mahoney T, Rey E et al. Vigabatrin: placental transfer in vivo and excretion into breast milk of the enantiomers. Br J Clin Pharmacol 1998; 45: 409–11.

Wakil L, Epperson CN, Gonzalez J et al. Neonatal outcomes with the use of lamotrigine for bipolar disorder in pregnancy and breastfeeding: a case series and review of the literature. Psychopharmacol Bull 2009; 42: 91–8.

Westergren T, Hjelmeland K, Kristoffersen B et al. Topiramate-induced diarrhoea in a 2-month-old breastfed child. Drug Saf 2009; 32: 38.

Wisner KL, Perel JM. Serum levels of valproate and carbamazepine in breastfeeding mother-infant pairs. J Clin Psychopharmacol 1998; 18: 167–9.

Lactation

4.8 Antiepileptics

Psychotropic drugs

Paul Merlob and Christof Schaefer

4.9

4.9.1	Introduction	743
4.9.2	Antidepressants	743
4.9.3	Individual antidepressants	745
4.9.4	Antipsychotic	755
4.9.5	Individual antipsychotic drugs	756
4.9.6	Lithium and other antimanic drugs	762
4.9.7	Anxiolytics, hypnotics and sedatives	764
4.9.8	Benzodiazepines	764
4.9.9	Zaleplon, zolpidem and zopiclone	767
4.9.10	Other anxiolytics, hypnotics and sedatives	767
4.9.11	Psychoanaleptics	768
4.9.12	Anti-Parkinson drugs	769

4.9.1   Introduction

Psychiatric diseases frequently affect women of reproductive age and particularly during postpartum period. In the case of monotherapy, most psychopharmaceuticals are acceptable during lactation period. However, some drugs have more reassuring data than others. Therefore, careful selection should be made when a treatment is initiated. In cases of long-term therapy during pregnancy, a change of medication after birth is rarely necessary during breast feeding. However, some drugs with high transfer rates to the breastfed infant and/or poor neonatal clearance do require careful evaluation for each individual. In particular, this applies to lithium, lamotrigine, benzodiazepines. This chapter reviews all the psychopharmacological drugs in regard to their safety during breastfeeding and gives recommendations for clinical practice.

4.9.2   Antidepressants

Occurring with a frequency of approximately 10–15%, depression represents a significant problem post-delivery. Primiparae are more likely to be affected. The symptomatology of a postpartum depression can range

Drugs During Pregnancy and Lactation. http://dx.doi.org/10.1016/B978-0-12-408078-2.00034-2

from a slightly depressed mood, as a reaction to the change in the life situation and the pressures connected with that, to a deep depression with melancholic characteristics – or even a psychotic depression. Due to mechanisms that are not completely understood, most antidepressants lead to an increase in prolactin (Coker 2010), which does not necessarily lead to symptoms and does not, in principle, represent a problem during breastfeeding. Among the antidepressants selective serotonin reuptake inhibitors (SSRI) are predominantly used today. Tricyclics are used less often. With most antidepressants, there are traces in the serum of the breastfed babies. For antidepressant treatment, see the following Recommendations. For individual antidepressants see section 4.9.3. For further information on antidepressants, see Chapter 2.11.

Recommendation.

- An untreated pronounced depression can, like other serious psychiatric illnesses, lead to a disturbance in the early mother–child relationship. The need for treatment should be seriously considered from this perspective.
- Non-drug methods, such as psychotherapy, light therapy and acupuncture, are all part of an effective antidepressive treatment regimen (Chapter 2.11, Introduction).
- Readjustment of an antidepressant during breastfeeding should also include its tolerance during a possible new pregnancy.
- With a readjustment, *sertraline* is the antidepressant of first choice. *Paroxetine* and *citalopram* are also possible. However, paroxetine is not suitable for a possible new pregnancy. Among the tricyclics, *amitriptyline* and *nortriptyline* are the drugs of choice.
- *Doxepin* should be avoided because of repeatedly observed symptoms in the breastfed baby; fluoxetine should be avoided due to its long half-life and accumulation in the fetus and newborn.
- A stable adjustment during the pregnancy, with any antidepressant, should not be uncritically changed or stopped after birth. No antidepressant to which the mother was well adapted during pregnancy fundamentally requires weaning or limitation of breastfeeding. This also applies to difficult readjustments during breastfeeding.
- Should non-explainable symptoms such as sedation, weak suck or restlessness occur in the breastfed baby, a teratology information service should be consulted in addition to the pediatrician. Symptoms in the first few days of life are more likely to be adjustment disturbances due to the prenatal medication rather than to the medication in the milk.
- With some antidepressants, in particular SSRIs, peak drug concentrations in the milk can be expected up to 8 hours after intake. Thus, interruptions of breastfeeding for a few hours scarcely limit the baby's exposure. However, a nightly break in breastfeeding after taking the evening dose does make sense with most medications.
- Monotherapy is desirable. Use the lowest effective dose, preferably a single bed-time dose (if possible). Combination therapy with several psychotropic drugs should be critically reviewed before and during breastfeeding. Here, the decision about possible limitations during breastfeeding must be made on a case-by-case basis if the therapy is unavoidable.
- Ensure close medical follow-up of the breastfed infant.
- As with all psychotropic drugs, unfortunately there is insufficient experience concerning the long-term effects of ongoing therapy on breastfed babies.

4.9.3   Individual antidepressants

▶ **Agomelatine**

Agomelatine is characterized as a melatonin agent MT1/MT2-agonist and 5-HT2C-antagonist and is controversial with respect to its effectiveness. Due to the lack of sufficient data for a judgment, the better studied antidepressants are preferable.

▶ **Amitriptyline**

Amitriptyline is a tricyclic antidepressant and has a half-life of 20 hours. It is up to 95% plasma protein-bound and is rapidly metabolized to the pharmacologically equally strong *nortriptyline*. Six breastfeeding women taking 75–175 mg of amitriptyline a day were studied (survey in Weissman 2004). The M/P ratio was 1. The relative dose for an exclusively breastfed infant, including the active metabolites should not, in light of current experience, exceed 2.5%. Amitriptyline and nortriptyline could not be detected in the infants' serum, and the babies did not have any clinical symptoms.

The development in the first year of life among the 10 infants breastfed while their mothers were taking tricyclic antidepressants, did not differ from that of artificially fed infants in a control group (Yoshida 1997a). Amitriptyline is the drug of choice among the tricyclic antidepressants during breastfeeding.

▶ **Atomoxetine**

There are insufficient data on breastfeeding with atomoxetine, an SNRI. Better studied antidepressants are preferable.

▶ **Bupropion**

A case study describes *bupropion* (*amfebutamone*), which is also used for smoking cessation. It acts as a serotonin and also as a noradrenaline and dopamine blocker. The half-life is 21 hours. An M/P ratio of 8 was calculated. The relative dose, including the only half-so-effective metabolites, erythro-hydro-bupropion, hydroxybupropion, and threo-hydrobupropion, should be considered to be 1% to a maximum of 3% (survey in Weissman 2004). Neither in this child nor in three additional children (Baab 2002) was the medication detected in the serum. A further study with 10 mothers, who received 150 mg for 3 days and 300 mg for a further 4 days, reported an average of 6.75 µg/kg of bupropion daily plus 10.8, 15.75 and 68.9 µg/kg of the above-mentioned metabolites daily. Considering bupropion alone, the relative infant dose was 0.14%. Including all the metabolites, the authors calculate a transfer of about 2% (Haas 2004). With a 6-month-old baby, who was partially breastfed and whose mother had begun taking 150 mg of bupropion 3 days earlier, a questionable seizure was observed (Chaudron 2004). In another article with some printing errors, four breastfed babies whose mothers took 150 or 300 mg of bupropion daily, the recalculated weight adjusted relative infant dose was <1%, without considering the metabolites. Only in one baby was bupropion found in the urine (41 µg/L) (Davis 2009).

With a readjustment, the better studied antidepressants are preferable.

Lactation

4.9 Psychotropic drugs

▶ Citalopram

The SSRI, *citalopram*, has a half-life of about 35 hours. The activity of the metabolites, *norcitalopram* and *desmethylcitalopram*, each amounts to 13% of citalopram. On the basis of more than 65 mother–baby pairs studied (Lee 2004b, Weissman 2004, Heikkinen 2002), the following picture can be drawn: The relative dose of citalopram plus the effective metabolites for an exclusively breastfed baby is, on average, 3–5% with a maximum of 10%. The medication can either not be detected in the serum – or only in traces (Berle 2004). The highest values were ca. one-fifteenth of the therapeutic maternal concentration. Restless sleep was noted in one baby about 6 weeks old, whose mother received 40 mg a day. Citalopram (205 µg/L) was found in the milk and 12.7 µg/L in the infant's serum. A relative infant dose of 5.4% was calculated. After halving the maternal dose and introducing two feeds of infant formula, the baby's sleep pattern normalized (Schmidt 2000). In three of the 31 children studied (Lee 2004b) insignificant and non-specific symptoms were found – for example, restlessness in a 2 month old baby which appeared after his mother began therapy. As a precautionary measure, this mother weaned after 2 weeks and the restlessness improved. In individual cases, somnolence in breastfed child has been reported. With the other children described in the literature, toxic symptoms were not mentioned. Also, further development up to the age of 1 year was mostly unremarkable (Weissman 2004, Heikkinen 2002, Rampono 2000).

A mother who took 40 mg in the evening, had up to 320 µg/L in the milk. For an exclusively breastfed baby, this is up to 6.6% as a relative dose (Franssen 2006). The serum concentrations in the child corresponded to up to 1.8% of the maternal values. The abnormalities, such as irregular breathing, noted in the baby after birth, were attributed to adaptation difficulties, following intrauterine exposure. In another case, citalopram was adjusted and the baby was exclusively breastfed for 6 months. The neuropsychological development at a year and a half was judged as normal by the pediatrician (Gentile 2007). Also, in a case with 60 mg of citalopram daily, the baby developed normally to the age of 6 months with primarily mother's milk feeding (Werremeyer 2009). Citalopram can be prescribed for appropriate indications during breastfeeding.

▶ Clomipramine

Clomipramine, a tricyclic antidepressant, has a half-life of 32 hours. The pharmacologically active metabolites are N-desmethylclomipramine and two hydroxy-metabolites, 8-OH-clomipramine and 8-OH-desmethylclomipramine. Based on seven published reports on mother–child pairs, the average relative infant dose is 1.3% (survey in Weissman 2004).

In an infant who was already exposed during the pregnancy – the mother took 125 mg/day – 267 µg/L were measured in the plasma after birth. From the 7th day postpartum, the dose was increased to 150 mg/day. The maternal plasma concentration rose from 355 µg/L on day 10 to 510 µg/L on day 35. The concentration in the milk was between 270 and 624 µg/L. During the same period of time, concentrations measured in the infant's serum declined from 45 µg/L to 9.8 µg/L (this was due to the breakdown of the drug transferred prenatally.) Assuming the highest value reported in the milk, the dose for an exclusively breastfed baby – without considering the metabolites – would be approximately 4% of the maternal weight-related dose (Schimmell 1991). In another study, four mother–child pairs were reported. The mothers took between 75 and 125 mg of clomipramine daily. Milk samples were not measured. Neither clomipramine nor its metabolites could be detected in the infants' serum (< 10 µg/L; Wisner 1995).

Another study (Yoshida 1997a) reported concentrations in the milk from two women similar to those reported by Schimmell (1991). The infants did not demonstrate any adverse signs from the medication. Clomipramine can be prescribed for appropriate indications during breastfeeding.

▶ Desipramine

Desipramine, a tricyclic antidepressant, has a half-life ranging from 12 to 54 hours. It is the pharmacologically active metabolite of imipramine. Both substances are up to 95% bound to plasma proteins. On the basis of five published reports on mother–child pairs, there is an average relative infant dose of 1.6% (survey in Weissman 2004).

In a case report involving a daily dose of 300 mg, 381 µg/L of desipramine was measured in the milk. Mathematically, an infant would receive a maximum of 2.4% of the maternal weight-related dose if the metabolite, 2-hydroxydesipramine, was included (Stancer 1986). In four additional children studied, only slight traces of the drug were measured in the serum. The infants demonstrated no adverse symptoms. Desipramine can be prescribed for appropriate indications during breastfeeding.

▶ Dosulepine

Dosulepine (=*dothiepin*), a tricyclic antidepressant, has a half-life of 9 hours and is metabolized to the three pharmacologically active metabolites, *nordosulepine, dosulepine sulfoxide* and *nordosulepine sulfoxide*. In two studies, eight and 20 breastfeeding mothers respectively, receiving dosulepine therapy are reported (Buist 1993a, Ilett 1993). The M/P ratio is about 1. With daily doses up to 225 mg, a maximum of 475 µg/L dosulepine plus 1,200 µg/L of the metabolites are reported. The highest values on the same order of magnitude were reported in another study of two women (Yoshida 1997a). Based on these data, a maximum of 7% of the maternal weight-related dose was calculated for the infant when the metabolites were included. On average, however, it was less than 1% (survey in Weissman 2004). With one child, only traces of the active ingredient (4 µg/L) were detected in the serum (mother: 2.623 µg/L; Yoshida 1997a). No symptoms were reported. In a further study, prenatally exposed children aged 3 and 5 years were followed up. They demonstrated no abnormalities compared to a non-exposed control group (Buist 1995). Dosulepine can be prescribed for appropriate indications during breastfeeding.

▶ Doxepin

Doxepin, a tricyclic antidepressant, and its equally strong active metabolite *N-desmethyldoxepin*, are up to 80% bound to plasma proteins. The half-life of doxepin ranges from 8 to 25 hours; that of N-desmethyldoxepin is 33 to 81 hours. In a study of two breastfeeding mothers, one of whom

Lactation

4.9 Psychotropic drugs

received 150 mg and the other 75 mg of doxepin daily, an average of 0.3–1% of the maternal weight-related dose, including the metabolite, N-desmethyldoxepin, are reported for the infant (Kemp 1985). Another breastfed baby has been treated for depressed breathing and sedation. Values of 2.2 μg/L doxepin are measured in his plasma and – corresponding to the maternal concentration – 66 μg/L N-desmethyldoxepin are measured in the serum (Matheson 1985). The symptoms improve after changing to artificial feeding. It would seem that an accumulation must be expected in an infant. A further case report described a 9-day-old boy with a weak suck, muscular hypotonia and vomiting. His mother took 35 mg of doxepin a day. The relative infant dose reported, including the metabolite, was only 2.5%. Doxepin was found in the infant's serum just at detection level (10 μg/L). The metabolite was not detectable. The symptoms disappeared 48 hours after changing to artificial feeding (Frey 1999). During breastfeeding, better studied antidepressants should be given preference.

▶ Duloxetine

There are case reports on the SNRI, duloxetine, for eight women: After 3.5 days of taking *duloxetine* (40 mg/day), milk samples from six women who were in the process of weaning are reported. The highest value was observed about 6 hours after the last intake. A maximum of 15 μg of duloxetine was found in the total milk supply for a day. From this, the authors calculate a maximum relative infant dose of 0.25%. The M/P ratio was 0.26. The inactive metabolites were not reported (Lobo 2008). In another report on a woman taking 60 mg duloxetine daily, 64 μg/L was measured in the milk 6 hours after intake. From this, the authors calculate a 0.8% relative dose for the breastfed baby 4 hours after the last breastfeed. In turn 8 hours after the last dose, no duloxetine was detectable in the serum (detection limit 1 μg/L; Briggs 2009). A relative infant dose of 0.8% and a concentration in the breastfed baby, which also corresponds to 0.8% of the maternal concentration, was found in a further case report (Boyce 2011). During breastfeeding, the better studied antidepressants should be given preference.

▶ Escitalopram

The SSRI, *escitalopram*, is an active isomer of *citalopram* with a molecular mass of 414. At 56%, the protein binding is lower than that of citalopram (80%) and could, theoretically, facilitate a transfer to the milk. A case report describes a 3-week-old baby, whose weight gain was insufficient from the beginning of the maternal therapy until the age of 4 months and whose slightly elevated transaminases (liver enzymes), increased muscle tonus (hypertonia) in the upper extremities and frequent crying and hyperirritability were striking. The symptoms improved after supplementation in the fifth month of life (Merlob 2005). We received a report on a newborn, who begin high-pitched crying 2 hours after a breastfeed or 5 to 6 hours after maternal intake of escitalopram every afternoon. When the intake of the tablet was switched to the morning, the symptoms also occurred in the morning. This behavior improved after supplementation and disappeared after weaning.

With eight women who took 10–20 mg/day, an average of 7.6 μg/kg plus 3 μg/kg of the metabolite, *desmethylescitalopram*, was calculated for the infant under steady-state conditions. This represented a total relative infant dose of around 5%. No medication was found in the blood of three of the breastfed babies (detection limit <1 µg/L). For the other five babies, the values were under 5 µg/L. The maternal values for escitalopram and its metabolites were 24 or 20 µg/L on average. Measured against the Denver developmental tests, the children developed normally (Rampono 2006). Also, the baby of a woman who first took 5 and then 10 mg daily, had developed normally at 8 weeks. The authors calculated a relative dose of up to 7.7% (Castberg 2006). For another woman, a relative infant dose of 4.6%, including desmethylescitalopram, was reported (Hackett 2006a). This child also seemed normally developed at 9 months, according to the Denver test, as did a further baby whose mother had 20 mg daily of the therapy (Gentile 2006a). A 5-day-old baby, whose mother took 20 mg of escitalopram during the pregnancy and during breastfeeding, developed necrotizing enterocolitis after he had already been treated in the first 2 days of life for respiratory distress syndrome (Potts 2007). The authors discuss the effect of the medication on the thrombocyte function as a cause, but an effect via mother's milk should be viewed cautiously. With a readjustment, the better tested antidepressants should be given preference.

▶ **Fluoxetine**

The oldest SSRI, *fluoxetine*, and its active metabolite, *norfluoxetine*, are up to 94% bound to the plasma protein. The half-life of fluoxetine is 4 days and that of norfluoxetine is 7 days. Thereby, it has the longest half-life of the antidepressants. The M/P ratio is 0.25. Experience with 16 mother–baby pairs in two studies shows that the relative dose of fluoxetine plus norfluoxetine taken in by the breastfed baby is, on average, 6.5% with a maximum of 17%. The babies are unremarkable (Yoshida 1998a, Taddio 1996, Burch 1992). Another case report describes an infant with screaming attacks, watery stools and vomiting, whose symptoms disappeared upon weaning to infant formula. When he was put to the breast again, the symptoms reappeared (Lester 1993). The mother took 20 mg fluoxetine daily. A relative dose of around 8%, including norfluoxetine, was calculated. Fluoxetine (340 µg/L) and norfluoxetine (208 µg/L) was reported in the serum of the 10-week-old baby – therapeutic concentrations, which would be expected in an adult treated with 20 mg daily. In another case with an irritable infant (maternal dose 20 mg/day), fluoxetine (28.8 µg/L) and norfluoxetine (41.6 µg/L) were found in the milk (Isenberg 1990). From this, a dose for the baby of about 11 µg/kg/day was calculated, corresponding to 3.2% of the maternal weight-related dose. Another case report describes an infant with questionable convulsive-like symptoms and a cyanotic attack, whose mother had taken *carbamazepine* and *buspirone* in addition to fluoxetine. Further development of the child was reported to be normal up to the end of the first year of life. The authors are, with justification, hesitant to conclude that there was a connection between the medication and the symptoms (Brent 1998). Four additional children, who were followed up neurologically until the age of one, were unremarkable (Yoshida 1998a).

Chambers (1998) reports a statistically significant lower weight gain of about 9% in a group of 28 breastfed babies whose mothers were taking fluoxetine, by comparison to a control group of 34 breastfed babies without psychoactive medication. No other symptoms were reported.

Lactation

4.9 Psychotropic drugs

In a study of the serotonin metabolism, only in one of five newborns studied was any effect through fluoxetine via the mother's milk determined, measured vicariously via a lowering in whole-blood (platelet) 5-HT transporters. The affected baby did not have any symptoms (Epperson 2003). There are theoretical concerns because an SSRI-induced serotonin transport disturbance could also have an effect on the CNS with consequences for brain development.

All in all, among 80 mother–child pairs studied, five babies had symptoms for which a connection with fluoxetine was mentioned. The vast majority of the babies were unremarkable (Lanza di Scalea 2009, Weissman 2004). On the other hand, symptomatic children are even rarer with the other SSRIs. The relative infant dose is the highest with fluoxetine and the half-life is the longest. Both could contribute to a comparatively poorer tolerance by the infant. During breastfeeding, the better tolerated antidepressants are preferable.

▶ Fluvoxamine

The half-life of the SSRI, *fluvoxamine*, is 16 hours. In a breastfeeding mother who took 200 mg of fluvoxamine daily, 310 µg/L were reported in the serum and 90 µg/L in the milk. Based on this, an M/P ratio of 0.3 can be calculated. Thereby, the infant would receive 13.5 µg/kg/ fluvoxamine daily, which corresponds to 0.5% of the maternal, weight-related dose (Wright 1991). A second case report observed proportionally lower concentrations when the dose was 100 mg daily. Mathematically, this too corresponded to a relative dose of 0.5%. The cognitive and motor development of the baby, who was breastfed for 5 months, and then tested at 4 and 21 months, was unremarkable (Yoshida 1997b).

In a third mother–baby pair, with a maternal dose of 200 mg fluvoxamine daily, 48 µg/kg/ a day corresponding to a relative dose for the clinically unremarkable infant of 1.6%, was calculated (Hägg 2000a). A further group of authors reported on the determination of fluvoxamine levels in the serum of 10-week-old breastfed baby receiving a relative dose of only 0.6% based on the maximum active ingredient concentration in the milk. Nevertheless, 45% of the maternal serum concentration was measured in his serum. During the period of observation, up to 4 months of age, the baby's development was unremarkable (Arnold 2000). With five additional symptom-free children, no medication was detected in the blood (Weissman 2004, Hendrick 2001b). Fluvoxamine may be prescribed for appropriate indications during breastfeeding.

▶ Imipramine

Imipramine, a tricyclic antidepressant, has a half-life of 6 to 20 hours. It is metabolized to the pharmacologically equally strong-acting desipramine. With a dose of 200 mg /day, a maximum of 29 µg/L imipramine and 35 µg/L desipramine has been measured in the mother's milk (Sovner 1979). By contrast, in four other mothers taking 75–150 mg/day, active ingredient concentrations of up to approximately 600 µg/L has been reported. Most of the values, however, were significantly under 300 µg/L (Yoshida 1997a). A maximum value of 90 µg/L per day or 7% of the maternal weight-related dose is calculated for an infant. On average, however, it was significantly below 2% of the maternal weight-related dose (survey in Weissman 2004). Imipramine may be prescribed for appropriate indications during breastfeeding.

► **Maprotiline**

Following treatment with 100–150 mg daily of *maprotiline*, a tetracyclic antidepressant, a relative dose of 1.6% was reported, without taking into account the active metabolites (survey in Bennett 1996). With a readjustment, better tested antidepressants should be given preference.

► **Mianserin**

Mianserin is among the tetracyclic antidepressants. It is up to about 90% bound to plasma protein and it has a half-life of about 22 hours. The primary active metabolite is *desmethylmianserin*. Two breastfeeding women have been studied. They had taken 40 and 60 mg, respectively, of mianserin daily. Twenty and 80 μg/L, respectively, of mianserin and 20 or 10 μg/L of desmethylmianserin were reported in the milk. Including the metabolites, this is, mathematically, a maximum of 1.5% of the weight-related dose for an infant. No medication was detectable in the serum of the first baby. With the second baby, 12 μg/L of mianserin and 14 μg/L of desmethylmianserin were measured in the urine (Buist 1993b). With a readjustment, better tested antidepressants should be given preference.

► **Mirtazapine**

Mirtazapine, along with noradrenaline and selective serotonin-inhibitors, which resemble the tetracyclic antidepressants or mianserin, has a plasma protein binding of up to 85%. The half-life is 20–40 hours. Three weeks after the birth of her child, a mother was switched from *sertraline* to 30 mg of mirtazapine daily. After reaching steady state, a level of 25 μg/L was measured in the maternal plasma. In the milk it was a maximum of 34 μg/L and in the baby's serum, 0.2 μg/L were measured. Accordingly, the relative infant dose was a maximum of 1%. After 6 weeks of breastfeeding with this therapy, the baby was functionally normally developed, and weight gain was regular (Aichhorn 2004). With eight mothers who took between 30 and 120 mg/day, an average of 8 μg/kg/day plus 3 μg/kg of the metabolite, *desmethylmirtazapine*, were calculated for the breastfed baby. From this, a relative infant dose between 1 and 3%, including metabolites, resulted. With four of these babies, no medication was found in the serum (detection limit 1 ng/mL). With one baby, whose mother took quite a high dose of 2 mg/kg, 1.5 ng/mL were measured in the serum. By contrast, the metabolite was not detectable. Measured against the Denver test, the seven children studied for between 1.5 and 13 months had unremarkable development (Kristensen 2007). In one patient who took 22.5 mg daily, a maximum of 145 μg/L was measured in the milk (Klier 2007). Based on this maximum value, a relative dose of 6% was calculated. No active ingredient was detectable in the baby's serum. By contrast, 2 hours after the morning feed, or 14 hours after the mother had taken the medication, 10 μg/L were found in the serum of a 2-month-old baby, whose mother took 15 mg/day. This corresponded to 37% of the maternal serum concentration (Tonn 2009). No specific abnormalities were observed in these children.

Mirtazapine is acceptable during breastfeeding but careful monitoring of the infant is necessary.

▶ **Moclobemide**

The reversible MAO-inhibitor, *moclobemide*, was studied in six mother–baby pairs. An M/P ratio of 0.7 and a relative infant dose of 1.2% were reported (Pons 1990). In another study with eight mothers who took between 300 and 900 mg daily, up to 5.3 mg/L (with a daily dose of 900 mg) was measured in the milk (Buist 1998), from which a maximum relative infant dose of 2–6% was calculated. The breastfed babies were unremarkable. Also, in a further publication on four mothers, normal development of the children up to the age of 1 year was reported. Nevertheless, one mother was weaned at 2 months because of gastroesophageal reflux in her baby (Taylor 2008). With a readjustment, the better studied antidepressants should be given preference.

▶ **Nefazodone**

Nefazodone, a 5-HT2-receptor-antagonist with a half-life of 17 hours, was studied in three samples with two patients. With a daily dose of between 100 and 400 mg, concentrations of 50–700 µg/L of the active ingredient, including the active metabolite, *hydroxynefazodone*, were found in the milk. However, the sampling was done before the patients took the tablets (two single doses daily). At the time of the study, the patients had already been in treatment for at least 3 weeks (Dodd 1999). From these measurements, a relative dose for an exclusively breastfed baby of between <1 and 7% was calculated. A further case report described a premature infant who, mathematically speaking, only received 0.5% of the maternal weight-related dose (300 mg) and was still admitted to the hospital because of lethargy, weak suck and problems with temperature regulation. The symptoms improved within 72 hours after weaning (Yapp 2000). Nefazodone was taken off the market in 2003 due to a case of liver failure and thus, no longer plays any role in breastfeeding.

▶ **Nortriptyline**

Nortriptyline, a tricyclic antidepressant with a half-life of 37 hours, is the active metabolite of *amitriptyline*. Experience with a total of 27 mother–baby pairs, where the mothers were taking 50–175 mg of nortriptyline a day, showed that acute toxic symptoms among the breastfed infants would hardly be expected. The M/P ratio (about 1) and the relative infant dose (not over 2–3%) corresponded to the values with amitriptyline (survey in Weissman 2004, Spigset 1998). Only in the case of a 4-week-old baby, whose mother took 60 mg a day and had a serum concentration of only 42 µg/L, was nortriptyline measured in the serum at 10 µg/L. With other infants only minute amounts of a 10-hydroxy-metabolite were found. Nortriptyline can be prescribed for appropriate indications during breastfeeding.

▶ **Opipramol**

For *opipramol*, a tricyclic antidepressant, an older study of 10 women reported an M/P ratio of 0.1 and a relative infant dose of only 0.3% (Herrmann 1970). With a readjustment, better tested antidepressants should be given preference.

► **Paroxetine**

The half-life of the SSRI *paroxetine* is 22 hours. Based on a study of a total of 110 mother–baby pairs, the relative dose for an exclusively breastfed baby is about 1%. No paroxetine could be detected in the serum of almost all of the infants studied. No clinical abnormalities were observed (Berle 2004, Merlob 2004, Weissman 2004, Hendrick 2001b). Peak values in the milk correlated with the dose. The highest value was 101 μg/L with a maternal dose of 50 mg daily. This represents a relative infant dose of less than 2% (Stowe 2000). With a daily dose of 20 mg paroxetine, 7.6 μg per liter is found in mother's milk. For the infant, that had a value of 1.14 μg/kg/day, and this represented about 0.4% of the maternal weight-related dose (Spigset 1996). The concentrations in the serum of 16 infants, whose mothers took 10–50 mg daily, were under the detection level (<2 μg/L). In a further study with 40 mother–baby pairs and a maternal daily dose of 10–40 mg, only minimal amounts could be detected and only traces – if that – could be detected in the infants' serum. However, the concentration in the mothers' milk at 153 μg/L was more than five-fold above the average (cited in Weissman 2004, Nordeng 2001).

Merlob (2004) found no statistically significant deviations in the development and weight gain of 27 infants followed up to the age of 1, compared to a control group. Paroxetine can be prescribed for appropriate indications during breastfeeding. However, for a possible new pregnancy, it is not appropriate.

► **Reboxetine**

With four women who took between 4 and 10 mg of the SNRI, *reboxetine*, daily, the highest concentrations in the milk −10–21 μg/L – were measured, on average 4 hours after taking the medication. Correspondingly, 7–16 μg/L was found in the mothers' serum. The relative infant dose was calculated at 1.4–2.5%. Among the four babies, a maximum of 5 μg/L was found in the serum – in so far as it was detectable at all (Hackett 2006a). Three of the four children developed normally measured against the Denver test. The fourth baby had delayed development; however, this had already been noticed before the start of the maternal medication. With a readjustment, the better tested antidepressants should take precedence.

► **St. John's wort (Hypericin)**

This substance is discussed in Chapter 4.13.

► **Sertraline**

The half-life of the SSRI, *sertraline*, is 26 hours. Based on studies of about 110 mother–baby pairs, the relative dose for the breastfed baby is just under 2% of the maternal weight-related dose. In the serum of some children, traces of sertraline were measured and in three of them around 10 μg/L of the significantly less effective metabolite, *desmethylsertraline* was measured (Weissman 2004, Hendrick 2001b). In other infants, the metabolite was not detectable (Berle 2004). In one baby, the serum concentrations were 50% of the maternal values (Wisner 1998). The authors did not want to rule out direct administration of the medication to the baby as the cause. None of the babies were remarkable. Long-term studies on the development of the children with this medication are also lacking.

Stowe (1997) analyzed 148 milk samples from 12 mothers. The highest concentrations for sertraline were about 173 µg/L and for desmethylsertraline 294 µg/L. The maternal doses were between 25 and 200 mg/day. Hendrick (2001b) noted declining concentrations of desmethylsertraline in the serum of 30 infants as they grew older. A maternal dose of at least 100 mg/day was significantly more often associated with documentation of the medication in the child' serum.

With 13 babies who took part in a comparative study with nortriptyline, no sertraline was found in the serum (detection limit 2 µg/L) but in some children, desmethylsertraline was detected, with a maximum of 6 µg/L (Lanza di Scalea 2009, Wisner 2006).

In a study involving 14 mother–baby pairs on serotonin metabolism, evaluated in terms of serotonin-(5-HT-)transporter reduction in the infant's thrombocytes, no significant changes could be determined as a result of sertraline exposure via the mother's milk (Epperson 2001). Theoretically, an SSRI-induced disturbance in the serotonin transport could also lead to disturbances of the CNS development. Sertraline is among the antidepressants of first choice during breastfeeding and pregnancy.

▶ Tranylcypromine

There is insufficient experience with the use of the irreversible MAO-inhibitor, *tranylcypromine*, during breastfeeding. Better tested antidepressants should be given preference.

▶ Trazodone

Among six women who took single doses of 50 mg trazodone, which has sedating properties and differs from the other antidepressant groups, an M/P ratio of 0.14 and a child's dose of 15 µg/kg/day were calculated. This represents just under 2% of the weight-related dose. However, the pharmacologically active metabolite, 1-m-chlorophenylpiperazine was not included (Verbeek 1986). In a further case, 40 µg/L was measured in the milk with an intake of less than 75 mg of trazodone. The breastfed baby was characterized as normally developed at the age of 12 months (Misri 2006) as was another 15-week-old baby whose mother was taking 100 mg/day (Newport 2009). With a readjustment, better tested antidepressants should be given preference.

▶ Trimipramine

There is insufficient experience with *trimipramine* during breastfeeding. Very likely it should be evaluated like the other tricyclics. Trimipramine can be prescribed during breastfeeding only for appropriate indications. However, better tested antidepressants should be given preference.

▶ **Venlafaxine and desvenlafaxine**

The half-lives of the serotonin and noradrenaline reuptake inhibitor, *venlafaxine*, are 5 hours and 11 hours for its active metabolite. Based on eight mother–baby pairs, the following can be summarized: The M/P ratio is about 4. Including the 100% active metabolite, O-desmethylvenlafaxine, the exclusively breastfed baby receives on average of around 6 % and at maximum 9% of the maternal weight-related dose. The metabolite, but not venlafaxine itself, was measured in the serum of the asymptomatic baby at levels of 3.38 µg/L or, on average, 10% of the maternal values (Berle 2004, Weissman 2004, Ilett 2002, Hendrick 2001a). No abnormalities were reported among 13 babies whose mothers had taken between 37.5 and 300 mg/day. The M/P ratio was given as approximately 3. The highest values of venlafaxine and its metabolites were found in the milk eight hours after the medication is taken. The concentration of active ingredients in the baby was 57% of the value in the mother. The relative infant dose for the total substance was calculated as 8% (Newport 2009). Among 10 women who received desvenlafaxine (O-desmethylvenlafaxine), a relative infant dose of 7% was calculated. The concentrations were measured in the serum of the clinically unremarkable babies at about 5% of the maternal values (Rampono 2011). With a readjustment, the better tested antidepressants should be given precedence.

4.9.4   Antipsychotic

Although the classic neuroleptics, such as *phenothiazine* and *haloperidol* have already been used for a long time, there are only very few publications on therapy during breastfeeding. In one publication, there was speculation about whether phenothiazine increases the risk for sudden infant death and sleep apnea and whether atypical neuroleptics should have priority during breastfeeding (Hale 2004). *Clozapine*, by contrast, is associated with the risk of agranulocytosis and *olanzapine* with extrapyramidal symptoms (Gentile 2008). Yet neither this nor other serious side-effects as a result of breastfeeding while taking classic first generation neuroleptics or the newer, so-called atypical neuroleptics of the second generation, have been clearly confirmed. Only minimal concentrations of most of the active ingredients are found in mother's milk. With the phenothiazines, this is explained by, among other reasons, the high plasma protein binding. For antipsychotic treatment see the following Recommendations. For individual antipsychotic drugs see section 4.9.5. For further information on antipsychotic drugs, see Chapter 2.11.

Recommendation.

- An untreated severe psychiatric illness can lead to a disruption of the early mother–baby relationship. The necessity of therapy should also be considered from this perspective.
- Both typical as well as atypical neuroleptics can be used during breastfeeding for appropriate indications for treatment.
- Among the neuroleptics of choice during breastfeeding are the classic neuroleptics, *flupentixol, fluphenazine* and *haloperidol*, as well as the atypical neuroleptics, *quetiapine* and *olanzapine*. With a readjustment these should be given preference.

Lactation

4.9 Psychotropic drugs

- No neuroleptic to which the mother is already well-adapted during the pregnancy, requires primary weaning or a limitation of breastfeeding. This also applies to difficult readjustments during breastfeeding.
- Generally speaking, monotherapy should be the goal. A combination therapy with multiple psychotropic drugs should be viewed critically during breastfeeding. Here a decision about limitations on breastfeeding should be made on a case-by-case basis if the therapy is unavoidable.
- If symptoms recur that cannot be otherwise explained, such as sedation, weak sucking or restlessness, a Teratology Information center should be contacted in addition to the pediatrician. Symptoms in the first few days of life are more likely to be adaptation disturbances due to the prenatal medication than to medication in the milk.
- As with all psychotropic drugs, there are insufficient data on the long-term development of the children. However, the influence of medications during breastfeeding should always be evaluated against the background of the exposure that already took place during pregnancy.

4.9.5   Individual antipsychotic drugs

▶ Amisulpride

Amisulpride is among the atypical neuroleptics. With 100 mg/day, an average of 1.2 mg/L is measured in the milk and a relative infant dose of 6.1% is calculated. With a partially breastfed 5-month-old infant, 4 µg/L was found in the serum 3 hours after the last dose. This represents 3.9% of the concentration in the mother (Ilett 2010). In a further case involving 400 mg of amisulpride daily for 9 days, an average of 3.6 mg/L milk was found from which a relative infant dose of 10.7% was calculated. The 13-month-old infant was unremarkable (Teoh 2011). Due to the considerable transfer into the milk, other neuroleptics should be given preference.

▶ Aripiprazole

Aripiprazole is an atypical neuroleptic. In two women who took 15 or 18 mg daily, 13 and 39 µg/L was found in the milk (Watanabe 2011, Schlotterbeck 2007). In the 6-day-old baby of the woman taking 18 mg/day, 7.6 µg/L were measured which, however, could still have resulted from the prenatal exposure (Watanabe 2011). In a further woman taking 15 mg/day, the concentration in the milk was under the detection limit (<10 µg/L; Lutz 2010). From these case reports, relative infant doses between 0.7 and 3% was calculated. With a readjustment, better tested neuroleptics should have preference.

▶ Chlorpromazine

Chlorpromazine, a phenothiazine with a half-life of 30 hours, is absorbed at a very individual rate. According to an older study, 2 hours after a single dose of 1,200 mg (20 mg/kg) levels of 750 µg/L were measured in the mother's serum and 290 µg/L in the milk. An M/P ratio of less than 0.5 was calculated. With a dose of 600 mg, no medication could be detected in the milk (Blacker 1962). In another study of four women, levels between 7 and 98 µg/L were found in the milk (maternal serum 16–52 µg/L) – the dose of the medication was not known. Two of the children were breastfed. The first, whose mother's milk has a concentration of 7 µg/L, was unremarkable. The second baby, whose mother's milk had a concentration of 92 µg/L, was lethargic after breastfeeding, which according to the authors, may not mean anything considering the still very low concentration (Wiles 1978). Other publications confirm the very limited amount of transfer (Sugawara 1999, Yoshida 1998b). In one of these studies with five women, 0.7 µg/ mL of the active ingredient, at most, were found in the babies' serum. Acute symptoms were not observed. However, in the second year of life, mental or psychomotor developmental delays were observed in three infants whose mothers were also treated with haloperidol. The authors did not want to rule out a connection with the medication (Yoshida 1998b). With a readjustment, other neuroleptics should be given preference.

▶ **Chlorprothixene**

Chlorprothixene is among the thioxanthenes. Its chief metabolite, *chlorprothixene sulfoxide*, has no neuroleptic effect but possibly has an anticholinergic effect. Of two women studied, one had taken 200 mg/day of chlorprothixene and the second 200–400 mg/day. From the data on the concentration in the mother's milk, an average dose of 2.4 with a maximum of 4.7µg/kg/chlorprothixene a day and 3.5 to a maximum of 4.5 µg/kg chlorprothixene sulfoxide a day was calculated. Thereby, the exclusively breastfed infant takes in 0.2% of the maternal, weight-related dose of the active ingredient. No clinical abnormalities were observed (Matheson 1984). Chlorprothixene can be prescribed during breastfeeding only for appropriate indications.

▶ **Clozapine**

Clozapine is an atypical neuroleptic. With a daily dose of 50 mg, a concentration of 63.5 µg/L is measured in the first milk on the day after birth. The maternal serum value is 14.7 µg/L. One week later, with a dose of 100 mg daily, the concentration of medication in the milk has risen to 115.6 µg/L and in the serum to 41.4 µg/L (Barnas 1994). That represents an M/P ratio of 2.8. Mathematically, according to this, an infant would take in up to 17.3 µg/kg daily, about 1% of the maternal weight-related dose. In two of the case reports collected by the manufacturer, sleepiness in the breastfed babies of mothers using clozapine was reported. One mother had taken 150 mg a day, while the other had taken 12.5 mg plus 3 mg of flupenthixol. The risk of agranulocytosis was also discussed (Gentile 2008), but does not appear relevant concerning exposure via the mother's milk. In one child, disturbed speech development was reported at age 5 years. His mother had breastfed for a year while taking clozapine. Whether clozapine via the mother's milk or exposure during pregnancy or some other factor is actually a cause for the disturbance, remains open (Mendhekar 2007). With a readjustment, better tolerated neuroleptics should be given preference.

Lactation

4.9 Psychotropic drugs

Flupenthixol

The thioxanthene, *flupenthixol*, is taken orally or administered intramuscularly as a depot preparation. In the cases of three mothers who reported receiving either 2 mg flupenthixol a day or 40 mg every 2 weeks or 60 mg every 3 weeks, the concentration of the drug in the milk was the same – 1.8 µg/L (maternal serum 1.3–1.5 µg/L). On this basis, 0.27 µg/kg daily was calculated for the infant. This represents a maximum of 0.8% of the maternal weight-related flupenthixol dose (Kirk 1980). Another case description on long-term therapy, with 4 mg a day orally, also came to the same conclusion (Matheson 1988). Clinical examination of the exposed children did not reveal anything remarkable; they developed normally for their ages. Flupenthixol is among the classic neuroleptics of choice during breastfeeding using a daily dose up to 4 mg.

Fluphenazine

Fluphenazine is a phenothiazine. There are no studies available on this drug during breastfeeding. Analogous to the other phenothiazines, no significant transfer to the baby would be expected. Based on this assumption and the comprehensive use in clinical practice, fluphenazine may also be used during breastfeeding for appropriate indications and with close infant follow-up.

Haloperidol, other butyrophenones and related drugs

Among a total of 16 women who received between 1 and 40 mg of *haloperidol* a day, relative doses for the infants was 0.2–2.1%, on average, but in an extreme case about 10% was calculated (Yoshida 1998b, survey in Bennett 1996). Insofar as has been studied, breastfed infants have developed normally with monotherapy. However, in Yoshida (1998b) among three babies whose mothers were treated additionally with chlorpromazine, a mental or psychomotor developmental delay was observed in the second year of life. The authors did not rule out the possibility that these could have a connection to the medication. Three children of a mother who was treated for schizophrenia with 7.5 and 15 mg haloperidol, developed normally. They were breastfed for 6 to 8 months (Mendhekar 2011).

There are no data on other butyrophenones such as, for instance, *benperidol, bromperidol, droperidol, melperone, pipamperone* and *trifluperidol* or on the structurally related neuroleptics, *pimozide* and *fluspirilene*.

Haloperidol is among the classic neuroleptics of choice during breastfeeding. The dose should be kept as low as possible. Due to insufficient evidence, the other butyrophenones should be avoided with a new adjustment. In particular the frequently observed uncritical use of fluspirilene (as a depot injection) for non-psychotic indications should be avoided.

Levomepromazine

Levomepromazine is one of the phenothiazines. A case report describes a relative infant dose of 0.8% (Ohkubo 1993). Levomepromazine may be prescribed for appropriate indications during breastfeeding but close infant follow-up is necessary.

Olanzapine

For *olanzapine*, an atypical neuroleptic, the data from seven mother–baby pairs studied revealed a dose for the baby of about 1% of the maternal weight-related dose. The M/P ratio is 0.4. The serum concentration in the unremarkable children was under the detection limit (Gardiner 2003). Relative infant doses of under 1% were also reported in two other case reports (Lutz 2008, Whitworth 2010). A further case report described an unremarkable baby whose mother continued taking 10 mg of olanzapine daily during breastfeeding. Two and 6 weeks after birth there is no active substance detected in the baby's serum (<2 ng/mL; Kirchheiner 2000). In a study of five mother–baby pairs, an average M/P ratio of 0.5 was reported. The relative infant dose was, on average, 1.6% with a maximum of 2.5% (Croke 2002). The babies were unremarkable. With two other children, symptoms (sedation, icterus) were noticed, but were attributed to other factors (Goldstein 2000). Of 26 case reports sent to the manufacturer, four described symptomatic babies with, among other symptoms, sedation and weak suckling (cited in Gentile 2008). A direct connection has not been proven, since, to some extent, other medications were also taken. However, due to the long half-life of up to 54 hours, side-effects, particularly in very young infants, cannot be eliminated. Should sedation and weak suckling occur in the first few days of life, they are more likely to still be the consequence of drug transfer via the placenta.

One case that we observed with a daily maternal dose of 7.5 mg, produced a therapeutic serum level (0.02 µg/mL) in a symptomatic newborn on the third day of life. A relative infant dose of 1.5% via the milk (0.01 µg/mL) was calculated. At the age of 6 weeks, the infant, who continued to be breastfed, was completely unremarkable. In another case report (Whitworth 2010) the changes of plasma concentrations of olanzapine in a breast-fed infant were measured during 5 months. The results demonstrated relatively high plasma levels in the infant aged 4 months (11 ng/mL). In the following 4 months, plasma levels of olanzapine decreased to very low, even undetectable concentrations in the infant. This situation might reflect the induction of the metabolizing CYP1A2-enzyme. The baby developed normally and no side effects were observed. In a study with 22 mother–baby pairs, there was no significantly increased rate of developmental abnormalities at the ages of 1 and 2 years by comparison to a control group of non-breastfed babies whose mothers were not treated with olanzapine. The authors noted these negative results in connection with the very limited transfer via the mother's milk (Gilad 2011). Olanzapine is among the atypical neuroleptics of choice during breastfeeding.

Paliperidone

Paliperidone is an atypical neuroleptic and the active metabolite of risperidone (9-Hydroxyrisperidon). The data on paliperidone during breastfeeding are insufficient. With a readjustment, better tested neuroleptics should be given preference.

Lactation

4.9 Psychotropic drugs

▶ **Perazine**

Perazine is one of the phenothiazines. In a mother who took 25 mg daily, we report nearly constant concentrations of 30–34 µg/L in the milk during 24 hours. This corresponds to a relative dose of approximately 1% for the unremarkable infant. Perazine may be prescribed for appropriate indications during breastfeeding.

▶ **Perphenazine**

Perphenazine is one of the phenothiazines. In a study, the mother first received 24 and then 16 mg/day. There was 3.2 µg/L and, with the lower dose, 2.1 µg/L in the milk. The concentrations in the maternal serum were 4.9 and 2.0 µg/L. Mathematically, the infant would then receive 0.48 or 0.32 µg/kg/day. In both cases, this is 0.1% of the maternal weight-related dose. The exposed infant was breastfed for 3 months while his mother took the medication and demonstrated no symptoms (Olesen 1990). Perphenazine may be prescribed for appropriate indications during breastfeeding.

▶ **Promethazine**

Promethazine is a phenothiazine and low potency neuroleptic with sedative action. Frequently, it is given as an addition to the high potency neuroleptics or as an "as needed" medication as well as an alternative to tranquilizers. A weakening of the effect of oral contraceptives is possible through increased metabolism (Kuhl 2002). Analogous to the other phenothiazines, a significant transfer to the baby is not anticipated. Because of this assumption and the wide use in clinical practice, promethazine may also be prescribed during breastfeeding for appropriate indications as a low-potency neuroleptic.

▶ **Prothipendyl**

Prothipendyl is structurally related to the phenothiazines. There is insufficient experience with its use during breastfeeding. With a readjustment, better documented neuroleptics should be given preference.

▶ **Quetiapine**

For *quetiapine*, an atypical neuroleptic, there is a report on a mother in whom the highest concentration of 62 µg/L is measured in the milk 1 hour after taking 200 mg. After 2 hours, the concentration has fallen to the level measured before taking it. On average, a relative dose of just under 0.1% is calculated for the exclusively breastfed infant. An infant who was exclusively breastfed from 8 weeks after birth and followed-up at 4.5 months, developed normally (Lee 2004b).

With six mothers who took between 25 and 400 mg daily, no quetiapine was detectable in the milk of those who had taken a maximum of 75 mg (detection limit <11.5 µg/L). In the mother taking 100 mg, it was 12.3 µg/L and in the one taking 400 mg, it was 101 µg/L. Thus, the relative infant dose is significantly under 1% (Misri 2006). The mild deficiency observed in mental or psychomotor development in two of the children, measured via the Bayley test, was assessed by the authors as unlikely to be associated with the medication. In a further case with 400 mg quetiapine daily, the highest concentration in the milk (170 µg/L) was measured 1 hour after taking the medication. After 12 hours, the substance was no longer detectable. The relative dose was calculated at 0.09% (Rampono 2007); 1.4 µg/L are measured in the baby's serum. This corresponds to 6% of the maternal serum concentration. At 3 months, the baby was normal as measured via the Denver developmental test. In another study of nine mothers, who had taken between 6 and 100 mg, the simulation calculations led to relative infant doses of <0.5% and serum concentrations which were <0.6% of maternal values (Yazdani-Brojeni 2010). Other case reports describe unremarkable babies who were breastfed with quetiapine doses of up to 400 mg/day (Ritz 2005, Newport 2009, Gentile 2006b). Quetiapine is among the atypical neuroleptics of choice during breastfeeding.

▶ Risperidone

For the atypical neuroleptic, *risperidone*, a relative infant dose of 4% including active metabolites was reported for a mother–baby pair studied. No indications of symptoms were observed in the breastfed baby (Hill 2000). No abnormalities were observed in two other children who were followed up to the age of 9 months (Ratnayake 2002) and in two other publications involving three infants, none or only traces of the substance were detected in the blood. With additional mothers, relative doses of 2% to a maximum of 6% were calculated for the exclusively breastfed babies (Aichhorn 2005, Ilett 2004). There is no report of symptoms in the infants. With a mother who has taken 1 mg daily, up to 4 µg/L of the metabolite, 9-hydroxyrisperidone, were measured in the milk. Risperidone itself was not detectable. The authors calculated a relative infant dose of 4.7%. No risperidone could be detected in the baby's serum. After 3 months of full breastfeeding, the baby was unremarkable (Weggelaar 2011). Risperidone may be prescribed for appropriate indications during breastfeeding.

▶ Sertindole

Sertindole is an atypical neuroleptic. There are insufficient data on the breastfeeding period. With a readjustment, better tested neuroleptics should be given preference.

▶ Sulpiride

Sulpiride is a dopamine antagonist that stimulates the secretion of prolactin and thus, may increase the amount of milk. In two studies, the mothers received 100 mg daily. Concentrations on average of 0.97 and 0.83 mg/L – with a maximum of 1.97 or 1.46 mg/L – were measured in the milk. Based on this, an infant would receive an average of 0.135 mg/kg/a day, corresponding to 8.7% of the maternal weight-related dose. At maximum it would be 17.7%. No information on the child was published (survey in Bennett 1996). With readjustments, the better-tested neuroleptics should be given preference. Sulpiride has been tried as a stimulant to the milk production but such use is viewed critically – also with respect to its effectiveness (ABM Clinical Protocol 2011, Chapter 3.7).

Lactation

4.9 Psychotropic drugs

► **Thioridazine**

The phenothiazine, *thioridazine*, is moderately potent neuroleptic. In lower doses, it is also used for sedation. With a readjustment during breastfeeding, the better tested substances should be given preference.

► **Trifluoperazine**

Trifluoperazine is one of the phenothiazines. In two women taking 5 or 10 mg of trifluoperazine daily, an immunoassay (EIA) of the milk reported a concentration of 359 µg/L. In a chromatographic control study, the value was under the detection level. No active ingredient was found in the serum of the symptom-free babies with either method (Yoshida 1998a). With a readjustment, a better tested medication should be given preference.

► **Ziprasidone**

Ziprasidone is an atypical neuroleptic. In one woman who began 160 mg/day ziprasidone 9 days after the birth, the ziprasidone was only detectable at 11 µg/L, on one of several days before the morning dose (Schlotterbeck 2009). A relative infant dose of <0.1% was calculated from this. In another case, a report was made on an unremarkable 6-month-old baby, who was being breastfed while his mother was taking 40 mg of ziprasidone (Werremeyer 2009). When initiating neuroleptic treatment, a better tested medication should be given preference.

► **Zotepine**

Zotepine is one of the phenothiazines, but is characterized as an atypical neuroleptic. When initiating neuroleptic treatment, the better tested neuroleptics should be given preference.

► **Zuclopenthixol**

Zuclopenthixol is one of the thioxanthenes. Among eight women who received 4–50 mg daily, an average M/P ratio of 0.5 was reported. The portion transmitted through the milk was under 1% of the maternal, weight-related dose (Matheson 1988, Aaes-Jørgensen 1986). None of the exposed babies were remarkable. Zuclopenthixol can be prescribed for appropriate indications during breastfeeding with careful monitoring of the infant.

4.9.6   Lithium and other antimanic drugs

Lithium is the standard therapeutic for treating bi-polar disturbances between episodes. The half-life in adults is 8 to 45 hours (68–96 hours in newborn). The therapeutic range at 0.8–1.5 mmol/L in the serum is relatively narrow. Toxic symptoms may already occur with 2 mmol/L. The M/P ratio varies with the dose between 0.3 and 1.7 (very high maternal dosing). In older case reports, relative infant doses up to 80% was reported. According to a study of 11 mother–child pairs, the relative dose was between 0 and 30% of the maternal weight-related dose. In half of the cases, however, it was under 10% (Moretti 2003). Following the decline in high concentrations in infant sera immediately postpartum, concentrations of lithium corresponded to at most 30% of the maternal concentrations and frequently were considerably lower. Among the 11 infants mentioned above, none showed symptoms that were due to the lithium therapy. However, one publication reports on a 2-month-old infant with a tremor and abnormal pattern of movement. His serum values for lithium were twice as high as those of the mother (survey in Llewellyn 1998, Spigset 1998, Bennett 1996). In a case series with 10 mothers who had taken between 600 and 1,200 mg daily, 0.19 to 0.48 mEq/L were measured in the milk. On average, 0.16 mEq/L or 24% of the maternal serum concentration were measured in the infant's serum. At maximum it was 56%. Insofar as it is reported, the children developed normally (Viguera 2007).

Three women treated with lithium (900 mg/day) for bipolar disorder during pregnancy and lactation and their four infants provided lithium levels at 1 month postpartum. Infant levels ranged from 10 to 17% of maternal levels. Two infants had early feeding problems which were overcome with breastfeeding education and support. However, three of the four mothers had received *bupropion* or *escitalopram* in addition to the lithium (Bogen 2012).

Comparable serum concentrations, which decline in the breastfed baby up to age 6 months, were observed in other mother–baby pairs with 800 mg of lithium daily. The initially increased TSH-value in the baby normalized at the age of 2 months despite continued breastfeeding (Marin 2011). In one case, an increased TSH value was measured in a baby who had already been exposed prenatally and improved after discontinuing lithium. In another case report, apparently toxic concentrations were measured in association with very low lithium values. Such a result is seemingly caused by the coating of the blood collection tubes with lithium-heparin (Tanaka 2008).

Antiepileptics such as *carbamazepine, gabapentin, lamotrigine, levetiracetam, topiramate* and *valproic acid* have also been prescribed as episode prophylactics in bipolar affective (manic-depressive) illnesses. For the experience during breastfeeding see Chapter 4.8. *Olanzapine* and *quetiapine* are used for this indication (Section 4.9.5). There is no experience during breastfeeding for the newer medication *asenapine*.

Recommendation. With careful observation of the infant (muscle tone, tremor, involuntary movements, cyanosis, dehydration) and when the maternal lithium dose is kept as low as possible, breastfeeding can be permitted with lithium. Every exposed infant should be closely monitored (signs of dehydration, lethargy, feeding problems, weight gain) and levels of TSH should be periodically measured. At least with newly occurring suspicious symptoms, apart from the pediatrician a teratology information service should be consulted, the serum concentration should be determined in the infant and, in some cases, breastfeeding should be limited. Olanzapine and quetiapine are also acceptable. The teratogenic potential in case of a further pregnancy argues against the use of antiepileptics for psychiatric indications during breastfeeding. This applies particularly to valproic acid. The considerable transfer to the breastfed baby argues against lamotrigine even though it apparently does not have any teratogenic potential worth mentioning. Insufficient testing argues against asenapine.

Lactation

4.9 Psychotropic drugs

4.9.7   Anxiolytics, hypnotics and sedatives

Substances of various drug groups are used as sleeping medication (hypnotics). Depending on the dose, they may lead to sedation or act hypnotically. Sleep disturbances have a variety of causes and only after exhausting all alternatives should they be treated with medication. Long-term medication with sleeping pills should also be avoided during breast-feeding due to the risk of dependency.

4.9.8   Benzodiazepines

The various benzodiazepines are structurally related to one another. Moderate and long-acting benzodiazepines are primarily used as anxiolytics and sedatives. Short acting substances are available for inducing anesthesia and as hypnotics. The elimination capacity for benzodiazepine already develops in (full-term) newborns within the first week of life. An overview of the available short, medium and long-term effective benzodiazepines is in Chapter 2.11. Recently, the safety of infant exposure to benzodiazepines during lactation was studied by Kelly (2012). Adverse outcomes, specifically sedation, was observed in only 1.6% (2 of 124) of exposed infants and was not associated with benzodiazepine dose, number of hours breastfed, or any demographic trait.

In the following, the benzodiazepines for which experience during breastfeeding is available will be discussed in alphabetical order.

▶ **Alprazolam**

Alprazolam has a half-life of 12.15 hours and an M/P ratio of 0.4. In a study of eight women, an exclusively breastfed infant would receive on average 3% and a maximum of 6.7% of the maternal weight-related dose (Oo 1995). After a dose of 0.5 mg, up to 3.7 µg/L was measured in the milk. Metabolites could not be detected in the milk. Sleepiness in an infant was discussed in another publication in connection with the maternal therapy. Despite continued breastfeeding, however, the symptoms disappeared again (Anderson 1989).

▶ **Clobazam**

Clobazam, with a half-life of about 20 hours and an M/P ratio of 0.3, was measured in the milk of six women who had been treated with 30 mg/day. The maximum concentration in the milk was 330 µg/L (cited in Bennett 1996). This would lead to a relative infant dose of 10%.

▶ **Clonazepam**

For *clonazepam* see Chapter 4.8.

▶ **Diazepam**

Diazepam is 97% plasma protein-bound. The half-life is 24–48 hours and that of its active metabolite, *desmethyldiazepam*, is 30–90 hours. Among

11 women who took 10–40 mg daily, 3% to a maximum of 13% of the maternal weight-related dose, including the metabolites, was calculated for an exclusively breastfed infant (survey in Hägg 2000b, Bennett 1996). This represents just about 4% of a therapeutic infant dose of 0.5 mg/kg/day. For diazepam and desmethyldiazepam, the M/P ratio is between 0.1 and 0.3. Only traces of diazepam are detected in the serum of the breastfed babies; however, up to 46 µg/L of desmethyldiazepam has been detected. These values are significantly higher in the first few days of life if the mother has repeatedly received diazepam before the birth and the medication transmitted through the placenta has not yet been excreted by the newborn. The few case descriptions on children's symptoms such as lethargy, disinterest in suckling, sleepiness or EEG abnormalities with diazepam during breastfeeding, give the impression that only high doses of at least 30 mg/day or treatment already begun before the birth, lead to clinical abnormalities. Single maternal doses do not appear to have any effects on the infant.

▶ Flunitrazepam

With a half-life of 29 hours and an M/P ratio of 0.5, *flunitrazepam* was studied in 10 women who had taken a single oral or intravenous dose (survey in Bennett 1996). Since the active metabolites were not included, nor is the concentration under steady-state conditions known, the relative dose of a maximum of 2.5% reported here should be viewed with caution.

▶ Lorazepam

Lorazepam is among the preferred benzodiazepines today. Its half-life is 15 hours and its M/P ratio is 0.2. With less than 2.5–3.5 mg/day, 8 to 14 µg/L are found in the milk. A relative dose for the infant was calculated at up to about 5% (survey in Bennett 1996). No symptoms were observed in the baby. In one woman who had taken up to 2.5 mg lorazepam daily and, in addition, once a day, 2 mg of *lormetazepam*, which is metabolized to lorazepam to some extent, a maximum of 123 µg/L was measured in the milk (Lemmer 2007). A relative dose that can exceed 10% was calculated.

▶ Lormetazepam

Lormetazepam is up to 88% plasma protein-bound and is conjugated to pharmacologically inactive glucuronide. Its half-life is 10 hours. The M/P ratio is 0.05. In a study of five mothers who received 2 mg daily, 0.4% of the maternal weight-related dose was calculated for the baby. Only the inactive lormetazepam-glucuronide was calculated in the serum of the babies studied. The infants were clinically unremarkable (Hümpel 1982).

▶ Metaclazepam

Metaclazepam or its metabolite, *desmethylmetaclazepam* (a half-life of 11 hours and an M/P ratio of about 0.3) led to a maximum relative dose of 5.5% for 10 women who had taken a one-time dose of 20 mg (Schotter 1989).

Lactation

4.9 Psychotropic drugs

▶ Midazolam

Midazolam is a widely used short-acting hypnotic for induction of diagnostic and surgical procedures and, with its active metabolite, *hydroxymidazolam*, has a short half-life of 1.5–5 hours. The M/P ratio is significantly below 0.5. Among 12 women who either took 15 mg for 5 days or received it as a single dose, a maximum of 12 μg/L of the agent was found in milk (Matheson 1990a). From this, a maximum of 0.7% of the weight-related maternal dose was calculated. In an additional case report with intravenous administration of 6 mg, the highest concentration of 25 μg/L was reported after 30 minutes, followed by a rapid decline below the detection limit after 4 hours (Koitabashi 1997). As expected, no symptoms were observed in the breastfed babies. Among five women who received 2 mg *midazolam* as premedication for general anesthesia, a relative dose of 0.06% was calculated for the babies, which represents 0.016 μg/kg (Nitsun 2006).

▶ Nitrazepam

Nitrazepam has a half-life of just under 30 hours and an M/P ratio of 0.3. Among nine women, a maximum transfer of 2.5% was calculated. During 5 days of treatment with 5 mg an increase in the concentration in the milk from 8.4 to 13.5 μg/L was reported (Matheson 1990a).

▶ Oxazepam

Oxazepam breaks down into inactive metabolites and has a half-life of 9 hours (adults) or 20 hours (newborns). Based on the experience with three mothers, the M/P ratio was 0.2 and the relative infant dose, a maximum of 0.9% (survey in Bennett 1996).

▶ Prazepam

Prazepam is a prodrug of *desmethyldiazepam*, thus a half-life to 90 hours is anticipated. The available data argue for an evaluation similar to that for diazepam. The same applies for *pinazepam*.

▶ Quazepam

For *quazepam*, whose metabolites have a half-life of 72 hours, there is experience with four women taking a single dose of 15 mg. The M/P ratio is about 6. Including the active metabolites, a maximum of 263 μg/L is found in milk (Hilbert 1984). This means that in an extreme case, an exclusively breastfed baby could receive more than 10% of the maternal weight-related dose of active ingredients. Since the mothers studied were not breastfeeding, there are no data on the condition of the infants.

▶ Temazepam

In a study of 10 mothers took 10–20 mg daily of temazepam for at least 2 days (half-life 5 to 13 hours), only in the milk of one mother was 28 µg/L temazepam detected (detection limit 5 µg/L). The active metabolite, *oxazepam*, was not detected in any of the samples. Based on this, a relative infant dose of just under 2% can be calculated. No active ingredient was found in the serum of two babies studied. The breastfed babies were unremarkable (Lebedevs 1992).

> **Recommendation.** For sleep disturbances, the antihistamine, *diphenhydramine*, is the drug of choice. Should a benzodiazepine be needed, lormetazepam or temazepam should be chosen. Oxazepam and diazepam are acceptable as tranquilizers. These substances should also be prescribed in doses as low as possible and only for a short time. Single doses of other benzodiazepines, such as, for instance, midazolam for induction of anesthesia, do not require any limitation of breastfeeding. Generally, monotherapy should be the goal. Should unexplained symptoms such as sedation, weak suckling or restlessness occur again, a pediatrician and a teratology information center should be consulted. As with all psychoactive drugs, there is insufficient experience on long-term effects on breastfed babies of ongoing maternal therapy.

4.9.9 Zaleplon, zolpidem and zopiclone

Only traces of *zaleplon* pass into the milk (Darwish 1999).

Zolpidem has a short half-life of approximately 2 hours. The metabolites do not appear to be active. The M/P ratio was reported to be 0.1 for five women (Pons 1989). The relative dose for an exclusively breastfed baby is not be expected to exceed 1.5%.

The half-life of *zopiclone* is about 5 hours. In a study in which 12 breastfeeding women received a single dose of 7.5 mg, 80 µg/L was found in the serum and 34 µg/L was in milk. A maximum of 4% for the maternal weight-related dose was calculated for the infant (Matheson 1990b). Another study of three mothers came to similar conclusions (Gaillot 1983). A woman who took 3.75 mg of zopiclone daily, had between 24 and 47.3 µg/L in her milk. A relative infant dose of approximately 3% was calculated. Premature twins, who were primarily fed with mother's milk, had unremarkable outcomes at the age of 6 weeks (Mathieu 2010).

There is no experience during breastfeeding for *eszopiclone*, the S-enantiomere of zopiclone.

> **Recommendation.** For sleep disturbances, the antihistamine, diphenhydramine is the drug of choice. Individual doses of zopiclone are tolerable during breastfeeding. Should unexplained symptoms such as sedation, weak suckling and restlessness occur again, a pediatrician and a teratology information center should be consulted. As with all psychoactive drugs, there is insufficient experience on long-term effects on breastfed babies of ongoing maternal therapy.

4.9.10 Other anxiolytics, hypnotics and sedatives

Older, sedating antihistamines are offered, to some extent as sleep agents. Among them are *diphenhydramine*, *doxylamine* and *hydroxyzine*. In individual cases, these drugs have led to sedation or irritability in the infant. Mostly, these drugs are well-tolerated by the breastfed babies. There are no systematic studies on the breastfeeding period.

There is no indication yet that *valerian* products cause side effects in the breastfed baby. However, no data are available on the transfer of valerian into human milk.

Barbiturates were the most important sleeping medication until benzodiazepines were introduced. Since then, barbiturates have almost completely lost their importance as hypnotics. Today, only phenobarbital is still used in the treatment of epilepsy (Chapter 4.8).

Clomethiazole has a short half-life of around 5 hours. An M/P ratio of 0.9 has been reported. A relative infant dose of, on average, 0.1% with a maximum of 1.6%, has been reported for five mother–baby pairs where the mothers took 4,000 mg a day. Only in a few infant serum samples was it detectable with up to 0.018 mg/L (18 µg/L) (Tunstall 1979).

According to an older study, *glutethimide* is transferred to the infant, with a relative dose of less than 1%, after a single dose (cited in Bennett 1996).

There is no experience concerning melatonin-containing medications during breastfeeding. However, a small study has looked at the positive influence of the body's own melatonin in the mother's milk on atopic eczema in the infant. The melatonin content in the milk can be increased by laughter, with the symptoms of the children in this group improving. The study group with 24 women looked at a Charlie Chaplin film in the evening and a control group of the same size watched information on the weather (Kimata 2007).

A 2- to 4-fold higher concentration of meprobamate has been measured in milk compared with maternal serum (Wilson 1980). There are no clinical observations of children who were breastfed when their mothers were taking meprobamate.

For *buspirone, chloral hydrate, kavain* (which has been taken off the market due to hepatotoxicity), and L-*tryptophan*, there is insufficient information during breastfeeding.

Recommendation. Should sleep disturbances require treatment during breast-feeding, valerian (if possible, in a preparation without alcohol) and diphenhydramine are the drugs of choice. Long-term therapy should be avoided. Short-term treatment with doxylamine or hydroxyzine is also acceptable during breastfeeding. With clomethiazole treatment for alcoholism, it is the alcoholism that is the actual problem for the baby. Other medications should be avoided. Should unexplained symptoms, such as sedation, weak suckling and restlessness recur, a pediatrician and a teratology information center should be consulted. As with all psychoactive drugs, there is insufficient experience on long-term effects of ongoing maternal therapy on breastfed babies.

4.9.11   Psychoanaleptics

Three mothers who took 35 and 80 mg of *methylphenidate* daily for attention deficit disorder and hyperactivity (ADHS) had, on average, concentrations of 19 µg/L in the milk, or 2.9 µg/kg a day for the breastfed baby. This corresponds to a relative infant dose of 0.7% (Hackett 2005, 2006b). No methylphenidate was found in the serum of the two babies studied (detection limit 1 µg/L). In the first few months of life, the babies developed unremarkably. A relative dose of only 0.16% was calculated in another case report with a maternal dose of 15 mg of methylphenidate (Spigset 2007). In samples taken to ascertain drug exposure after different dosages, no methylphenidate was detected in the baby's blood in a recent case report (Bolea-Alamanac 2014).

There is no experience during breastfeeding for *amfetaminil, fenetylline pemoline* and *modafinil*.

> **Recommendation.** Repeated use of psychoanaleptics should be avoided during breastfeeding. When therapy is urgently required, the decision about breastfeeding should be made on a case-by-case basis. This also applies to methylphenidate for which no information on long-term effects on breastfed babies is available.

4.9.12   Anti-Parkinson drugs

There are no noteworthy toxic risks indicated for infants as a result of the occasional combination of neuroleptics or haloperidol with *biperiden*.

Unremarkable development of a breastfed baby, whose mother has taken *bromocriptine* due to a macroprolactinoma, was reported (Verma 2006).

During her three pregnancies and breastfeeding, one woman was taking 4 mg of *trihexyphenidyl* daily and breastfed her children, whose development were all unremarkable, for 6 to 8 months (Mendhekar 2011).

There is no experience on the use of *amantadin, benserazide, benzatropine bornaprin, budipin, cabergoline, carbidopa, α-dihydroergocryptine, entacapon, levodopa, lisuride, metixen, pergolide, pramipexol, pridinol, procyclidine, ropinirol, tiaprid* and on the monoamine oxidase-B(MAO-B)-inhibitors, *selegilin* and *rasagilin*.

> **Recommendation.** When urgent therapy is required, a case-by-case decision on breastfeeding must be made. Biperiden treatment during breastfeeding is probably tolerable, and the baby may also drink the milk that is still produced if treatment with *bromocriptine* or *cabergoline* is given.

References

Aaes-Jørgensen T, Bjørndal F, Bartels U. Zuclopenthixol levels in serum and breast milk. Psychopharmacology 1986; 90: 417–8.

ABM Clinical Protocol. Number 9. Use of galactogogues in initiating or augmenting the rate of maternal milk secretion (First Revision January 2011). Breastfeed Med 2011; 6: 41–9.

Aichhorn W, Stuppaeck C, Whitworth AB. Risperidone and breastfeeding. J Psychopharmacol 2005; 19: 211–3.

Aichhorn W, Whitworth AB, Weiss U et al. Mirtazapine and breastfeeding. Am J Psychiatry 2004; 161: 2325.

Anderson PO, McGuire G. Neonatal alprazolam withdrawal: possible effects on breastfeeding. Drug Intell Clin Pharm 1989; 23: 614.

Arnold LM, Lichtenstein PK, Suckow RF. Fluvoxamine concentrations in breast milk and in maternal and infant sera. J Clin Psychopharmacol 2000; 20: 491–3.

Baab SB, Peindl KS, Piontek CM et al. Serum bupropion levels in 2 breast-feeding mother-baby pairs. J Clin Psychiatry 2002; 63: 910–1.

Barnas C, Bergant A, Hummer M et al. Clozapine concentration in maternal and fetal plasma, amniotic fluid, and breast milk. Am J Psychiatry 1994; 151: 945.

Bennett PN (ed.). Drugs and Human Lactation. 2nd ed. Amsterdam, New York, Oxford: Elsevier 1996.

Berle JO, Steen VM, Aamo TO et al. Breastfeeding during maternal antidepressant treatment with serotonin reuptake inhibitors: infant exposure, clinical symptoms, and cytochrome p450 genotypes. J Clin Psychiatry 2004; 65: 1228–34.

Blacker KH, Weinstein BJ, Ellman GL. Mothers milk and chlorpromazine. Am J Psychol 1962; 114: 178–9.

Bogen DL, Sit D, Genovese A et al. Three cases of lithium exposure and exclusive breast-feeding. Arch Womens Ment Health 2012; 15: 69–72.

Bolea-Alamanac BM, Green A, Verma G et al. Methylphenidate use in pregnancy and lactation, a systematic review of evidence. Brit J Clin Pharmacology 2014; 77: 96–101.

Brent NB, Wisner KL. Fluoxetine and carbamazepine concentrations in a nursing mother/infant pair. Clin Pediatr 1998; 37: 41–4.

Briggs GG, Ambrose PJ, Ilett KF et al. Use of duloxetine in pregnancy and lactation. Ann Pharmacother 2009; 43: 1898–902.

Boyce PM, Hackett LP, Ilett KF. Duloxetine transfer across the placenta during pregnancy and into milk during lactation. Arch Womens Ment Health 2011; 14: 169–72.

Buist A, Dennerstein L, Maguire KP et al. Plasma and human milk concentrations of moclobemide in nursing mothers. Hum Psychopharmacol 1998; 13: 579–82.

Buist A, Janson H. Effect of exposure to dothiepin and northiaden in breast milk and children development. Br J Psychiatry 1995; 167: 370–3.

Buist A, Norman TR, Dennerstein L. Plasma and breast milk concentrations of dothiepin and northiaden in lactating women. Hum Psychopharmacol 1993a; 8: 29–33.

Buist A, Norman TR, Dennerstein L. Mianserin in breast milk. Br J Clin Pharmacol 1993b; 36: 133–4.

Burch KJ, Wells BG. Fluoxetine/norfluoxetine concentrations in human milk. Pediatrics 1992; 89: 676–7.

Castberg I, Spigset O. Excretion of escitalopram in breast milk. J Clin Psychopharmacol 2006; 26: 536–8.

Chambers CD, Anderson PO, Dick LM et al. Weight gain in infants breast-fed by mothers who take fluoxetine. Teratology 1998; 57: 188.

Chaudron LH, Schoenecker CJ. Bupropion and breastfeeding: a case of a possible infant seizure. J Clin Psychiatry 2004; 65: 881–2.

Coker F, Taylor D. Antidepressant-induced hyperprolactinaemia: incidence, mechanisms and management. CNS Drugs 2010; 24: 563–74.

Croke S, Buist A, Hackett LP et al. Olanzapine excretion in human breast milk; estimation of infant exposure. Int J Neuropsychopharmacol 2002; 5: 243–7.

Darwish M, Martin PT, Cevallos WH et al. Rapid disappearance of zaleplon from breast milk after oral administration to lactating women. J Clin Pharmacol 1999; 39: 670–4.

Davis MF, Miller HS, Nolan PE. Bupropion levels in breast milk for 4 mother–baby pairs: more answers to lingering questions. J Clin Psychiatry 2009; 70: 297–8.

Dodd S, Buist A, Burrows GD et al. Determination of nefazodone and its pharmacologically active metabolites in human blood plasma and breast milk by high-performance liquid chromatography. J Chromatogr B 1999; 730: 249–55.

Epperson N, Czarkowski KA, Ward-O'Brien D et al. Maternal sertraline treatment and serotonin transport in breast-feeding mother–baby pairs. Am J Psychiatry 2001; 158: 1631–7.

Epperson CN, Jatlow PI, Czarkowski K et al. Maternal fluoxetine treatment in the post-partum period: effects on platelet serotonin and plasma drug levels in breast-feeding mother–baby pairs. Pediatrics 2003; 112: 425–9.

Franssen EJ, Meijs V, Ettaher F et al. Citalopram serum and milk levels in mother and infant during lactation. Ther Drug Monit 2006; 28: 2–4.

Frey OR, Scheidt P, Brenndorff AI von. Adverse effects in a newborn infant breast-fed by a mother treated with doxepin. Ann Pharmacother 1999; 33: 690–3.

Gaillot J, Heusse D, Hougton GW et al. Pharmacokinetics and metabolism of zopiclone. Pharmacology 1983; 27: 76–91.

Gardiner SJ, Kristensen J, Begg EJ et al. Transfer of olanzapine into breast milk, calculation of infant drug dose, and effect on breast-fed infants. Am J Psychiatry 2003; 160: 1428–31.

Gentile S. Escitalopram late in pregnancy and while breast-feeding. Ann Pharmacother 2006a; 40: 1696–7.

Gentile S. Quetiapine-fluvoxamine combination during pregnancy and while breastfeeding. Arch Womens Ment Health 2006b; 9: 158–9.

Gentile S. Infant safety with antipsychotic therapy in breast-feeding: a systematic review. J Clin Psychiatry 2008; e1–e8.

Gentile S, Vozzi F. Consecutive exposure to lamotrigine and citalopram during pregnancy. Arch Womens Ment Health 2007; 10: 299–300.

Gilad O, Merlob P, Stahl B et al. Outcome of infants exposed to olanzapine during breast-feeding. Breastfeed Med 2011; 6: 55–8.

Goldstein DJ, Corbin LA, Fung MC. Olanzapine-exposed pregnancies and lactation: early experience. J Clin Psychopharmacol 2000; 20: 399–403.

Haas JS, Kaplan CP, Barenboim D et al. Bupropion in breast milk: an exposure assessment for potential treatment to prevent post-partum tobacco use. Tobacco Control 2004; 13: 52–6.

Hackett LP, Ilett KF, Kristensen JH et al. Infant dose and safety of breastfeeding for dexamphetamine and methylphenidate in mothers with attention deficit hyperactivity disorder. Ther Drug Monit 2005; 27: 220–1.

Hackett LP, Ilett KF, Rampono J et al. Transfer of reboxetine into breastmilk, its plasma concentrations and lack of adverse effects in the breastfed infant. Eur J Clin Pharmacol 2006a; 62: 633–8.

Hackett LP, Kristensen JH, Hale TW et al. Methylphenidate and breast-feeding. Ann Pharmacother 2006b; 40: 1890–1.

Hägg S, Granberg K, Carleborg L. Excretion of fluvoxamine into breast milk. Br J Clin Pharmacol 2000a; 49: 283–8.

Hägg S, Spigset O. Anticonvulsant use during lactation. Drug Saf 2000b; 22: 425–40.

Hale TW. Vortrag Jahrestagung der amerikanischen Organization of Teratogen Information Services (OTIS) 2004.

Heikkinen T, Ekblad U, Kero P et al. Citalopram in pregnancy and lactation. Clin Pharmacol Ther 2002; 72: 184–91.

Hendrick V, Altshuler L, Wertheimer A et al. Venlafaxine and breastfeeding. Am J Psychiatry 2001a; 158: 2089–90.

Hendrick V, Fukuchi A, Altshuler L et al. Use of sertraline, paroxetine and fluvoxamine by nursing women. Br J Psych 2001b; 179: 163–6.

Herrmann B, von Kobyletzki D. Opipramol in human milk? Med Welt 1970; 7: 267–9.

Hilbert JM, Gural RP, Symchowicz S et al. Excretion of quazepam into human milk. J Clin Pharmacol 1984; 24: 457–62.

Hill RC, McIvor RJ, Wojnar-Horton RE et al. Risperidone distribution and excretion into human milk: case report and estimated infant exposure during breastfeeding. J Clin Psychopharmacol 2000; 20: 285–6.

Hümpel M, Stoppeli I, Milia S et al. Pharmacokinetics and biotransformation of the new benzodiazepine, lormetazepam, in man. III. Repeated administration and transfer to neonates via breast milk. Eur J Clin Pharmacol 1982; 21: 421–5.

Ilett KF, Hackett LP, Kristensen JH et al. Transfer of risperidone and 9-hydroxy-risperidone into human milk. Ann Pharmacotherapy 2004; 38: 273–6.

Ilett KF, Kristensen JH, Hackett LP et al. Distribution and excretion of venlafaxine and its O-desmethyl metabolite in human milk and their effects in breastfed infants. Br J Clin Pharmacol 2002; 53: 17–22.

Ilett KF, Lebedevs TH, Wojnar-Horton RE et al. The excretion of dothiepin and its primary metabolites in breast milk. Br J Clin Pharmacol 1993; 33: 635–9.

Ilett KF, Watt F, Hackett LP et al. Assessment of infant dose through milk in a lactating woman taking amisulpride and desvenlafaxine for treatment-resistant depression. Ther Drug Monit 2010; 32: 704–7.

Isenberg KE. Excretion of fluoxetine in human breast milk. J Clin Psychiatry 1990; 51: 169.

Kelly LE, Poon S, Madani P et al. Neonatal benzodiazepines exposure during breastfeeding. J Pediatr 2012; 161: 448–51.

Kemp J, Ilett KF, Booth J et al. Excretion of doxepin and N-desmethyldoxepin in human milk. Br J Clin Pharmacol 1985; 20: 497–9.

Kimata H. Laughter elevates the levels of breast-milk melatonin. J Psychosom Res 2007; 62: 699–702.

Kirchheiner J, Berghofer A, Bolk-Weischedel D. Healthy outcome ander olanzapine treatment in a pregnant woman. Pharmacopsychiatry 2000; 33: 78–80.

Kirk L, Jörgensen A. Concentrations of cis(Z)-flupenthixol in maternal serum, amniotic fluid, umbilical cord serum, and milk. Psychopharmacology 1980; 72, 107–8.

Klier CM, Mossaheb N, Lee A et al. Mirtazapine and breastfeeding: maternal and infant plasma levels. Am J Psychiatry 2007; 164: 348–9.

Lactation

4.9 Psychotropic drugs

Koitabashi T, Satoh N, Takino Y. Intravenous midazolam passage into breast milk. J Anesth 1997; 11: 242–3.

Kristensen JH, Ilett KF, Rampono J et al. Transfer of the antidepressant mirtazapine into breast milk. Br J Clin Pharmacol 2007; 63: 322–7.

Kuhl H. Einfluss von Psychopharmaka auf Reproduktion and Kontrazeption. In: Kuhl H (Hrsg.) Sexualhormone and Psyche. Stuttgart: Thieme 2002, pp. 48–56.

Lanza di Scalea T, Wisner KL. Antidepressant medication use during breastfeeding. Clin Obstet Gynecol 2009; 52: 483–97.

Lebedevs TH, Wojnar-Horton RE, Tapp P et al. Excretion of temazepam in breast milk. Br J Clin Pharmacol 1992; 33: 204–6.

Lee A, Giesbrecht E, Dunn E et al. Excretion of quetiapine in breastmilk. Am J Psychiatry 2004a; 161: 1715–6.

Lee A, Woo J, Ito S. Frequency of infant adverse events that are associated with citalopram use during breastfeeding. Am J Obstet Gynecol 2004b; 190: 218–21.

Lemmer P, Schneider S, Muhe A et al. Quantification of lorazepam and lormetazepam in human breast milk using GC-MS in the negative chemical ionization mode. J Anal Toxicol 2007; 31: 224–6.

Lester BM, Cucca J, Andreozzi L et al. Possible association between fluoxetine hydrochloride and colic in an infant. J Am Acad Child Adolesc Psychiatry 1993; 32: 1253–5.

Llewellyn A, Stowe ZN, Strader JR. The use of lithium and management of women with bipolar disorder during pregnancy and lactation. J Clin Psychiatry 1998; 59 (Suppl 6): 57–64.

Lobo ED, Loghin C, Knadler MP et al. Pharmacokinetics of duloxetine in breast milk and plasma of healthy postpartum women. Clin Pharmacokinet 2008; 47: 103–9.

Lutz UC, Wiatr G, Orlikowsky T et al. Olanzapine treatment during breast feeding: a case report. Ther Drug Monit 2008; 30: 399–401.

Lutz UC, Hiemke C, Wiatr G et al. Aripiprazole in pregnancy and lactation – a case report. J Clin Psychopharmacol 2010; 30: 204–5.

Marin Gabriel MA, Olza Fernandez I, Donoso E et al. [Lithium and artificial breastmilk; or is maternal breastfeeding better?]. An Pediatr (Barc) 2011; 75: 67–68.

Matheson I, Evang A, Fredricson Overoe K et al. Presence of chlorprothixene and its metabolites in breast milk. Eur J Clin Pharmacol 1984; 27: 611–3.

Matheson I, Lunde PKM, Bredesen JE. Midazolam and nitrazepam in the maternity ward: milk concentrations and clinical effects. Br J Clin Pharmacol 1990a; 30: 787–93.

Matheson I, Sande HA, Gaillot J. The excretion of zopiclone into breast milk. Br J Clin Pharmacol 1990b; 30: 267–71.

Matheson I, Pande H, Alertsen AR. Respiratory depression caused by N-desmethyldoxepin in breast milk. Lancet 1985; 2: 1124.

Matheson I, Skjaeraasen J. Milk concentrations of flupenthixol, nortriptyline and zuclopenthixol and between-breast differences in two patients. Eur J Clin Pharmacol 1988; 35: 217–20.

Mathieu O, Masson F, Thompson MA et al. Case report: in utero exposure and safe breastfeeding in two premature twins of a chronically treated mother with high doses of zopiclone{Abstract}. Fandam Clin Pharmacol 2010; 24: 424.

Mendhekar DN. Possible delayed speech acquisition with clozapine therapy during pregnancy and lactation. J Neuropsychiatry Clin Neurosci 2007; 19: 196–7.

Mendhekar DN, Andrade C. Uneventful use of haloperidol and trihehexyphenidyl during three consecutive pregnancies. Arch Womens Ment Health 2011; 14: 83–4.

Merlob P. Use of escitalopram during lactation. 13. BELTIS Newsletter June 2005; 40–3.

Merlob P, Stahl B, Sulkes J. Paroxetine during breastfeeding: infant weight gain and maternal adherence to counsel. Eur J Pediatr 2004; 163: 135–9.

Misri S, Corral M, Wardrop AA et al. Quetiapine augmentation in lactation: a series of case reports. J Clin Psychopharmacol 2006; 26: 508–11.

Moretti ME, Koren G, Verjee Z et al. Monitoring lithium in breast milk: an individualized approach for breast-feeding mothers. Ther Drug Monit 2003; 25: 364–6.

Newport DJ, Ritchie JC, Knight BT et al. Venlafaxine in human breast milk and nursing infant plasma: determination of exposure. J Clin Psychiatry 2009; 70: 1304–10.

Nitsun M, Szokol JW, Saleh HJ et al. Pharmacokinetics of midazolam, propofol, and fentanyl transfer to human breast milk. Clin Pharmacol Ther 2006; 79: 549–57.

Nordeng H, Lindemann R, Perminov KV et al. Neonatal withdrawal syndrome after in utero exposure to selective serotonin reuptake inhibitors. Acta Paediatr 2001; 90: 288–91.

Ohkubo T, Shimoyama R, Sugawara K. High performance liquid chromatographic determination of levomepromazine in human breast milk and serum using solid phase extraction. Biomed Chromatogr 1993; 7: 227–8.

Olesen OV, Bartels U, Poulsen JH. Perphenazin in breast milk and serum. Am J Psychiatry 1990; 147: 1378–9.

Oo CY, Kuhn RJ, Desai N et al. Pharmacokinetics in lactating women: prediction of alprazolam transfer into milk. Br J Clin Pharmacol 1995; 40: 231–6.

Pons G, Francoual C, Guillet PH et al. Zolpidem excretion in breast milk. Eur J Clin Pharmacol 1989; 37: 245–8.

Pons G, Schoerlin MP, Tam YK et al. Moclobemide excretion in human breast milk. Br J Clin Pharmacol 1990; 29: 27–31.

Potts AL, Young KL, Carter BS et al. Necrotizing enterocolitis associated with in utero and breast milk exposure to the selective serotonin reuptake inhibitor, escitalopram. J Perinatol 2007; 27: 120–2.

Rampono J, Hackett LP, Kristensen JH et al. Transfer of escitalopram and its metabolite demethylescitalopram into breastmilk. Br J Clin Pharmacol 2006; 3: 316–22.

Rampono J, Kristensen JH, Hackett LP et al. Citalopram and demethylcitalopram in human milk; distribution, excretion and effects in breast-fed infants. Brit J Clin Pharmacol 2000; 50: 263–8.

Rampono J, Kristensen JH, Ilett KF et al. Quetiapine and breast feeding. Ann Pharmacother 2007; 41: 711–4.

Rampono J, Teoh S, Hackett LP et al. Estimation of desvenlafaxine transfer into milk and infant exposure during its use in lactating women with postnatal depression. Arch Womens Ment Health 2011; 14: 49–53.

Ratnayake T, Libretto SE. No complications with risperidone treatment before and throughout pregnancy and during the nursing period. J Clin Psychiatry 2002; 63: 76–7.

Ritz S. Quetiapine monotherapy in post-partum onset bipolar disorder with a mixed affective state. Eur Neuropsychopharmacol 2005; 15: S407.

Schimmell MS, Katz EZ, Shaag Y et al. Toxic neonatal effects following maternal clomipramin therapy. J Toxicol Clin Toxicol 1991; 29: 479–84.

Schlotterbeck P, Leube D, Kircher T et al. Aripiprazole in human milk. Int J Neuropsychopharmacol 2007; 10: 433.

Schlotterbeck P, Saur R, Hiemke C et al. Low concentration of ziprasidone in human milk: a case report. Int J Neuropsychopharmacol 2009; 12: 437–8.

Schmidt K, Olesen OV, Jensen PN. Citalopram and breastfeeding: serum concentration and side effects in the infant. Biol Psychiatry 2000; 47: 164–5.

Schotter A, Müller R, Günther C et al. Transfer of metaclazepam and its metabolites into breast milk. Arzneimittelforschung 1989; 39: 1468–70.

Sovner R, Orsulak PJ. Excretion of imipramine and desipramine in human breast milk. Am J Psychiatry 1979; 136: 451–2.

Spigset O, Brede WR, Zahlsen K. Excretion of methylphenidate in breast milk. Am J Psychiatry 2007; 164: 348.

Spigset O, Carleborg L, Norstrom A et al. Paroxetine level in breast milk. J Clin Psychiatry 1996; 57: 39.

Spigset O, Hägg S. Excretion of psychotropic drugs into breast milk. Pharmacokinetic overview and therapeutic implications. CNS Drugs 1998; 9:111–34.

Stancer HC, Reed KL. Desipramine and 2-hydroxydesipramine in human breast milk and the nursing infant's serum. Am J Psychiatry 1986; 143: 1597–600.

Stowe ZN, Cohen LS, Hostetter A et al. Paroxetine in human breast milk and nursing infants. Am J Psychiatry 2000; 157: 185–9.

Stowe ZN, Owens MJ, Landry JC et al. Sertraline and desmethylsertraline in human breast milk and nursing infants. Am J Psych 1997; 154: 1255–60.

Sugawara K, Shimoyama R, Ohkubo T. Determinations of psychotropic drugs and antiepileptic drugs by high-performance liquid chromatography and its monitoring in human breast milk. Hirosaki Med J 1999; 51: S81–S86.

Taddio A, Ito S, Koren G. Excretion of fluoxetine and its metabolite norfluoxetine in human breast milk. J Clin Pharmacol 1996; 36: 42–7.

Tanaka T, Moretti ME, Verjee ZH et al. A pitfall of measuring lithium levels in neonates. Ther Drug Monit 2008; 30: 752–4.

Taylor T, Kennedy D. Safety of moclobemide in pregnancy and lactation, four case reports. Birth Defects Research Part A Clin Mol Teratol 2008; 82: 413.

Lactation

4.9 Psychotropic drugs

Teoh S, Ilett KF, Hackett LP et al. Estimation of rac-amisulpride transfer into milk and of infant dose via milk during its use in a lactating woman with bipolar disorder and schizophrenia. Breastfeed Med 2011; 6: 85–8.

Tonn P, Reuter SC, Hiemke C et al. High mirtazapine plasma levels in infant after breast feeding: case report and review of the literature. J Clin Psychopharmacol 2009; 29: 191–2.

Tunstall ME, Campbell DM, Dawson BM et al. Clomethiazole treatment and breastfeeding. Br J Obstet Gynaecol 1979; 86: 793–8.

Verbeek RK, Ross SG, McKenna EA. Excretion of trazodone in breast milk. Br J Clin Pharmacol 1986; 22: 367–70.

Verma S, Shah D, Faridi MM. Breastfeeding a baby with mother on bromocriptine. Indian J Pediatr 2006; 73: 435–6.

Viguera AC, Newport DJ, Ritchie J et al. Lithium in breast milk and nursing infants: clinical implications. Am J Psychiatry 2007; 164: 342–5.

Watanabe N, Kasahara M, Sugibayashi R et al. Perinatal use of aripiprazole: a case report. J Clin Psychopharmacol 2011; 31: 377–9.

Weggelaar NM, Keijer WJ, Janssen PK. A case report of risperidone distribution and excretion into human milk: how to give good advice if you have not enough data available. J Clin Psychopharmacol 2011; 31:129–31.

Weissman AM, Levy BT, Hartz AJ et al. Pooled analysis of antidepressant levels in lactating mothers, breast milk, and nursing infants. Am J Psychiatry 2004; 161: 1066–78.

Werremeyer A. Ziprasidone and citalopram use in pregnancy and lactation in a woman with psychotic depression. Am J Psychiatry 2009; 166: 1298.

Wiles DH, Orr MW, Kolakowska T. Chlorpromazine levels in plasma and milk of nursing mothers. Br J Clin Pharmacol 1978; 5: 272.

Wilson T, Brown RD, Cherek DR et al. Drug excretion in human breast milk: principles, pharmacokinetics and projected consequences. Clin Pharmacokinet 1980; 5: 1–66.

Wisner KL, Hanusa BH, Perel JM et al. Postpartum depression: a randomized trial of sertraline versus nortriptyline. J Clin Psychopharmacol 2006; 26: 353–60.

Wisner KL, Perel M, Blumer B. Serum sertraline and N-desmethylsertraline levels in breast-feeding mother–baby pairs. Am J Psychiatry 1998; 155: 690–2.

Wisner KL, Perel M, Foglia P. Serum clomipramine and metabolite levels in four nursing mother–baby pairs. J Clin Psychiatry 1995; 56: 17–20.

Whitworth A, Stuppaeck C, Yazdi K et al. Olanzapine and breast-feeding: changes of plasma concentrations of olanzapine in a breast-fed infant over a period of 5 months. J Psychopharmacol 2010; 24: 121–3.

Wright S, Dawling S, Ashford JJ. Excretion of fluvoxamine in breast milk. Br J Clin Pharmacol 1991; 31: 209.

Yapp P, Llett KF, Kristensen H et al. Drowsiness and poor feeding in a breast-fed infant: association with nefazodone and its metabolites. Ann Pharmacother 2000; 34: 1269–72.

Yazdani-Brojeni P, Taguchi N, Garcia-Bournissen F et al. Quetiapine in human milk and simulation-based assessment of infant exposure. Clin Pharmacol Ther 2010; 87: S3–4.

Yoshida K, Smith B, Craggs M et al. Investigation of pharmacokinetics and of possible adverse effects in infants exposed to tricyclic antidepressants in breast milk. J Affect Disord 1997a; 43: 225–37.

Yoshida K, Smith B, Kumar RC. Fluvoxamine in breast milk and infant development. Br J Clin Pharmacol 1997b; 44: 210–1.

Yoshida K, Smith B, Craggs M et al. Fluoxetine in breast milk and developmental outcome of breast-fed infants. Br J Psychiatry 1998a; 172: 175–9.

Yoshida K, Smith B, Craggs M et al. Neuroleptic drugs in breast milk: a study of pharmacokinetics and of possible adverse effects in breast-fed infants. Psychol Med 1998b; 28: 81–91.

Immunomodulating and antineoplastic agents

4.10

Paul Merlob and Corinna Weber-Schöndorfer

4.10.1 Azathioprine and 6-mercaptopurine	775
4.10.2 Selective immune suppressants	776
4.10.3 Monoclonal antibodies (mAb) and other biologicals	777
4.10.4 Interferons	778
4.10.5 Other immune stimulants	779
4.10.6 Antineoplastics	779

Systemic auto-immune diseases commonly affect women during childbearing years. The control of maternal disease activity during pregnancy and lactation is imperative. With azathioprine, selective immune suppressants, some monoclonal antibodies or interferons, many breastfeeding mothers have sustained periods of disease quiescence and less disability. The evidence regarding the safety of all these medications during lactation is reviewed. With maternal antineoplastic drugs, the baby should be weaned.

4.10.1   Azathioprine and 6-mercaptopurine

Azathioprine (AZA) is quickly metabolized to *6-mercaptopurine* (6-MP), which has a lower oral bioavailability. 6-MP, in turn, is transformed into the active metabolites *6-thioguanine-nucleotide* (6-TGN) and *6-methylmercaptopurine-nucleotide* (6-MMPN).

Misgivings have frequently been raised about the use of AZA and 6-MP during breastfeeding due to its cytotoxic properties. Meanwhile, there are many reports available in which not only the development and growth of the infants, but also the concentrations of 6-MP and the active metabolites in the mother's milk were studied in the infant's and the mother's serum and, to some extent, even the genotype of thiopurine methyltransferase (TPMT) in the mother. Gene mutations can diminish the activity of TPMT, which can lead to an increase of toxic metabolites and an increase of side effects, e.g. bone marrow suppression.

The majority of observations of over 50 breastfed infants have not presented any toxic effects (Angelberger 2011, Zelinkova 2009, Christensen 2008, Gardiner 2007, Sau 2007, Moretti 2006). Only one of six children demonstrated a temporary bone marrow dysfunction (Khare 2003). Unfortunately, neither the maternal TPMT genotype nor further details were reported.

In one publication, the maternal AZA dose was between 50 and 200 mg/day. The metabolite 6-MP was not detected in the mother's milk, so that a relative infant dose of 0.09% was calculated (Moretti 2006). Gardiner (2006) considered this method to be insufficient and determined the 6-MP and 6-TGN concentrations in the serum of four mother–child pairs. While therapeutic levels were reported in the mothers, detection of the substance in the children was not successful. All of the mothers had the normal TPMT genotype. Sau (2007) also found very low concentrations of 6-MP in the milk and could not detect 6-MP and 6-TGN in the children's serum. Based upon eight mother–child pairs (maternal dose between 75 and 200 mg daily and the normal TPMT genotype), a child's maximum intake through the milk was calculated at <0.008 mg/kg per 24 hours (Christensen 2008). The metabolite, 6-MMPN, in the mother's and child's sera was also identified. While therapeutic concentrations were measured in the mother's serum, the child's serum levels were below detection (Zelinkova 2009). The development of 15 children of mothers who took an average AZA dose of 150 mg daily was compared with a similar-sized group of children from healthy mothers. The duration of breastfeeding was between 6 and 8 months and the follow-up observation was for 3.6 and 4.7 years. There were no differences in motor and intellectual development nor the frequency of in-patient hospital stays or serious infections. Somewhat more frequently, greater than two common infections per year and conjunctivitis were observed in the children of mothers treated with AZA (Angelberger 2011).

The positive experiences to date primarily comprises of mothers without the TPMT gene mutation. Therefore, safety cannot be concluded for carriers of polymorphisms with reduced TPMT activity. Because routine assessment of the genotypes is too expensive, some experts recommend that a complete blood count and liver enzymes be determined with all children.

> **Recommendation.** Breastfeeding is permitted with AZA and 6-MP treatment. A blood count to monitor for signs of immunosuppression of the child at the age of 4 weeks for instance, can be considered.

4.10.2   Selective immune suppressants

There is no information concerning the use of the *teratogenic* (see Chapter 2.12.3) *mycophenolate mofetil* (MMF) or *mycophenolic acid* (MPA) during breastfeeding.

In adults, the half-life of cyclosporine metabolites is 19 hours. All of the reports on the use of *cyclosporine* or *cyclosporine A* (CyA) during breastfeeding demonstrate normal infant growth (see, for example, Armenti 2003). Three case series (Moretti 2003, Merlob 2000, Nyberg 1998) and individual case reports (for example, Osadchy 2011, Grimer 2007), with approximately 20 mother–child pairs, reported very different drug concentrations in human milk from 14–1,016 μg/L CyA. The serum concentrations of the mothers varied between 49 and 903 μg/L. In the majority of cases, the concentrations in the children's blood were below the detection limit. However, in one case, 131 μg/L – about 70% of the maternal concentration – was reported (Moretti 2003). The mother of this clinically unremarkable child with a therapeutic CyA serum concentration (131 μg/L), showed a wide range of CyA levels in her blood and sometimes high values However, the concentration of the drug in her milk was relatively low. Summarizing all the available values in the milk, a relative dose of about 2% for the child can be expected. A later finding calculates only 0.33% of the maternal weight adjusted dose (Osadchy 2011). Neither with this child nor with others was CyA detectable in the child's serum (Morton 2011, Lahiff 2011).

In a group of 25 pregnancies treated with the immune suppressant, *tacrolimus* (after a liver transplant), the initial milk samples after birth were measured to average 0.6 µg/L. Accordingly, a fully breastfed child would receive less than 0.1 µg/kg/day. This represents a relative dose of about 0.1% (Jain 1997). French (2003) even calculates only 0.02%. By contrast, Gardiner (2006) calculates a relative dose of 0.5%. In the serum of three fully-breastfed infants of mothers receiving tacrolimus treatment, no tacrolimus was detectable. The children showed age-appropriate development, which was followed to the age of 2.5 (Gouraud 2011). One year later, Gouraud (2012) provided a longer follow-up of six children exposed to tacrolimus through breastfeeding. The median duration of follow-up was 8.5 months (range 2–30 months). No adverse effects related to tacrolimus were noted and developmental milestones were within the expected ranges. The levels of tacrolimus measured in four neonates (15–27 days after birth) were undetectable. Seven additional children with exposure during breastfeeding grew normally (Armenti 2003). Recently, Bramham (2013) assessed 14 women taking tacrolimus during pregnancy and lactation, and their 15 infants. Eleven of the children were exclusively breast-fed. Maximum estimated absorption from breast milk was 0.23% of weight-adjusted maternal dose. The authors concluded that ingestion of tacrolimus by infants via breast milk is negligible.

The amount of tacrolimus excreted in the breast milk over a 12-hour steady-state dosing interval was determined in one patient treated with 1.5 mg orally twice daily (Zheng 2013). Infant exposure to tacrolimus through the breast milk was estimated to be less than 0.3% of the mother's weight-adjusted dose. Thus, neonatal exposure to tacrolimus via breast milk is very low and does not represent a health risk to the breastfeeding infant.

Tacrolimus has a half-life of 4–57 hours. The dermal administration of tacrolimus is not problematic because little is absorbed and only low serum concentrations are achieved. The same is true for *pimecrolimus*, which is well tolerated by children from 3 to 23 months (Kapp 2002).

There are no data on *sirolimus* and *everolimus* during breastfeeding.

Recommendation. With mycophenolate mofetil (MMF) or mycophenolic acid (MPA), the mother should not breastfeed. A woman who is stably adapted to cyclosporine A (CyA) may breastfeed if the pediatrician is informed about the maternal medication. Systemic administration of tacrolimus during breastfeeding is acceptable; dermal administration is not problematic. This also holds true for pimecrolimus. Sirolimus and everolimus should not be used while breastfeeding.

4.10.3   Monoclonal antibodies (mAb) and other biologicals

Here, only those biologicals for which some experience during breast-feeding is available will be discussed.

The large molecular mass of *adalimumab* and its limited oral bio-availability make an appreciable intake via the mother's milk unlikely. This has, meanwhile, been proven. A case report describes a 100-fold

Lactation

4.10 Immunomodulating and antineoplastic agents

lower value in the mother's milk by comparison to the mother's serum (Ben-Horin 2010). In another mother's milk sample, a 1,000-fold lower value was measured and in the serum of a 2-month-old breastfed baby, no adalimumab was detectable. In a case series of eight breastfed babies nothing noteworthy was observed (Fritzsche 2011). Further case reports describe breastfed children who developed normally both during and after the maternal treatment (see, for example, Mishkin 2006, Vesga 2005).

Infliximab also has a large molecular mass and limited oral bioavailability. Förger (2004) were able only to detect traces (473 ng/mL) of *infliximab* in the mother's milk. The relative dose calculated on the basis of the values is a maximum of 0.004%. Other working groups were not able to detect infliximab in the milk (detection limit <0.10 µg/mL). Thus, Vasiliauskas (2006) found no infliximab in the mother's milk of a 6-month-old fully-breastfed infant. The high serum concentrations of the baby caused by diaplacental transfer gradually fell off during breastfeeding, although maternal therapy was continued after a brief pause. In diverse mother's milk samples of another woman having infliximab treatment, no active ingredient could be proven either. The breastfed infant developed age-appropriately (Stengel 2008). With three breastfed infants, infliximab was found neither in their serum nor in the mother's milk, but was shown in therapeutic concentrations in the mother. However, Ben-Horin (2011) found that infliximab is excreted in breast milk and its levels rose up to 101 ng/mL within 2–3 days of the infusion. These levels of infliximab in breast milk were very low (roughly 1/200th of the level in blood). Fritzsche (2012) described the first breastfed infant with detectable serum levels after maternal infliximab therapy only during lactation. Further case reports describe children who developed normally during and after maternal therapy (Correia 2010).

Due to the high molecular weight of *etanercept* and limited oral bioavailability, an appreciable intake by the breastfed child appears unlikely. The case reports confirm this. With regular injections of 25 mg etanercept twice a week, a maximum of 75 µg/mL was measured in the milk of a non-breastfeeding mother (Ostensen 2004). A relative dose of 3% is calculated from this. Other working groups found significantly lower values of <5 ng/mL in the mother's milk (see, for example, Berthelsen 2010). With another mother-child pair, etanercept was detected in the mother's serum during and after the pregnancy, in the umbilical cord blood, in the mother's milk and in the serum of the exclusively breastfed baby. Transfer to the infant via the mother's milk could be ruled out (Murashima 2009). Further works have also found minimal or no substance in the mother's milk and in the child's serum (Berthelsen 2010, Keeling 2010).

> **Recommendation.** If treatment with mAb or other biologics is indicated, the mother may breastfeed with adalimumab, etanercept and infliximab. The pediatrician should be made aware of the maternal medication.

4.10.4   Interferons

Interferons are practically unavailable with oral administration. If, following an injection to the mother, they pass into her milk to a measurable degree – which is doubtful due to their molecular mass – a toxic effect on the breastfed baby would scarcely be expected. No systematic studies of interferon therapy during breastfeeding are available.

It has been shown that *interferon-α* only passes into the mother's milk in limited amounts (Haggstrom 1996). This also applies with a maternal dose of 30 million IE of *Interferon-α2b* (Kumar 2000). The transfer of intramuscular *interferon-β1a* into human milk was studied in six women (Hale 2012). Using the highest value measured (179 pg/mL), the estimated relative infant dose would be 0.006% of the maternal dose. No side effects were noted in any of these breastfed infants. It may be assumed that passage of the other interferons is similarly low, i.e. with interferon-α2a, the pegylated interferons as well as interferon-β1a and *interferon-β1b*.

> **Recommendation.** Breastfeeding is permitted while receiving interferon treatment.

4.10.5 Other immune stimulants

▶ **Granulocyte colony-stimulating factors (G-CSF)**

Granulocyte stimulating factors are a normal component of mother's milk. *Filgrastim* has a molecular mass of 18,800 Da, a half-life of only 3.5 hours and practically no oral bioavailability, so that a relevant intake through the mother's milk seems unlikely. Calhoun (2003) concluded from a small study that recombinant G-CSF administered orally to newborns or premature infants is not absorbed. The good tolerance for filgrastim in treating premature infants is known (Canpolat 2006). The maximum relative dose of filgrastim for a breastfed baby is under 0.3% (Kaida 2007) and that of *lenograstim* is less than 0.1% (Shibata 2003). *Pegfilgrastim* should be judged similarly.

▶ **Glatiramer**

There are, as yet, no publications on the tolerance for *glatiramer acetate* during breastfeeding. Glatiramer acetate consists of four amino acids (Chapter 2.12.6). Shortly after injection, the vast majority of the amount administered has already degraded into smaller fragments in the subcutaneous tissue. Should the active ingredient actually end up in the mother's milk, this will presumably not be absorbed by the child's gastrointestinal tract.

> **Recommendation.** Breastfeeding is permitted during therapy with granulocyte colony stimulating factors. Glatiramer acetate is also acceptable.

4.10.6 Antineoplastics

There are little data on the passage of antineoplastics into the mother's milk. The results of three reports on *cisplatin* show contradictory results: Egan (1985) could not detect cisplatin in the milk, while de Vries (1989) found identical concentrations in the maternal serum and the milk. In a third case (Ben-Baruch 1992) 10-fold lower concentrations were found in the milk than in the maternal serum. Recently, Lanowska (2011) described three women with cervical cancer receiving cisplatin 20 mg/sq during pregnancy. After caesarean section and hysterectomy performed between 31 and 35 weeks of gestation, the mothers received another course of chemotherapy. Cisplatin levels in breastmilk were 0.2, 1.4, and 5.5 mg/L, which represent 0.9, 2.3 and 9% of the concentrations in maternal blood at the time of surgery.

Cyclophosphamide apparently passes into the mother's milk in possible toxic concentrations. Temporary blood count changes were observed in two breastfed infants (Bennett 1996).

A relative dose of <5% was calculated for hydroxycarbamides (*hydroxyurea, doxorubicin* and *methotrexate* (MTX); Overview in Bennett 1996). However, these antineoplastic drugs are toxic and some may be retained in infant tissues for a long time.

Four case reports describe the passage of *imatinib* into the mother's milk. Thereby, similar concentrations were measured. The highest values measured were 2,623 ng/mL (Ali 2009), 1,400 ng/mL (Gambacorti-Passerini 2007), 596 ng/mL (Russell 2007) and 1,153 ng/mL (Kronenberger 2009). The metabolite of imatinib showed a similar passage into the milk. In this case, a small fully breastfed infant would receive a maximum of 3 mg/day. This is less than 10% of a therapeutic dose. Only one of the children was breastfed. No symptoms were reported (Gambacorti-Passerini 2007).

A case report on the treatment of promyelocytic leukemia in remission showed an initially high concentration of etoposide in the milk, but after 24 hours it could no longer be detected (Azuno 1995). Concomitant mitoxantrone was measured at 129 µg/L and also persisted in high concentrations for 28 days after treatment (Azuno 1995).

There are no data available on the other antineoplastics. This also applies to the mistletoe preparation, *viscum album.*

> **Recommendation.** With maternal antineoplastic treatment, the baby should be weaned. Whether a rheumatic low-dose methotrexate treatment represents a barrier to breastfeeding, is controversial. In this case too, the majority prefer weaning. There is concern about treatment with mistletoe preparations (viscum album) while breastfeeding.

References

Ali R, Ozkalemkas F, Kimya Y et al. Imatinib use during pregnancy and breast feeding:a case report and review of the literature. Arch Gynecol Obstet 2009; 280: 169–75.

Angelberger S, Reinisch W, Messerschmidt A et al. Long-term follow-up of babies exposed to azathioprine in utero and via breastfeeding. J Crohns Colitis 2011; 5: 95–100.

Armenti VT, Radomski JS, Moritz MJ et al. Report from the national transplantation registry (NTPR): outcomes of pregnancy after transplantation. Clin Transpl 2003; 131–43.

Azuno Y, Kaku K, Fujita N. Mitoxantrone and etoposide in breast milk. Am J Hematol 1995; 48: 131–2.

Ben-Baruch G, Menczer J, Goshen R et al. Cisplatin excretion in human milk. J Natl Cancer Inst 1992; 84: 451–2.

Ben-Horin S, Yavzori M, Katz L et al. Adalimumab level in breast milk of a nursing mother. Clin Gastroenterol Hepatol 2010; 8: 475–6.

Ben-Horin S, Yavzori M, Kopylov U et al. Detection of infliximab in breast milk of nursing mothers with inflammatory bowel disease. J Crohn's Colitis 2011; 5: 555–8.

Bennett PN (ed). Drugs and Human Lactation. 2nd edn, Amsterdam, New York, Oxford: Elsevier 1996.

Berthelsen BG, Fjeldsoe-Nielsen H, Nielsen CT et al. Etanercept concentrations in maternal serum, umbilical cord serum, breast milk and child serum during breastfeeding. Rheumatology (Oxford) 2010; 49: 2225–7.

Bramham K, Chusney G, Lee J et al. Breastfeeding and tacrolimus: serial monitoring in breastfed and bottle-fed infant. Clin J Am Soc Nephrol 2013; 8: 563–7.

Calhoun DA, Maheshwari A, Christensen RD. Recombinant granulocyte colony-stimulating factor administered enterally to neonates is not absorbed. Pediatrics 2003; 112: 421–3.

Canpolat FE, Yurdakök M, Korkmaz A et al. Enteral granulocyte colony-stimulating factor for the treatment of mild (stage I) necrotizing enterocolitis: a placebo-controlled pilot study. J Pediatr Surg 2006; 41: 1134–8.

Christensen LA, Dahlerup JF, Nielsen MJ et al. Azathioprine treatment during lactation. Aliment Pharmacol Ther 2008; 28: 1209–13.

Correia LM, Bonilha DQ, Ramos JD et al. Inflammatory bowel disease and pregnancy: report of two cases treated with infliximab and a review of the literature. Eur J Gastroenterol Hepatol 2010; 22: 1260–4.

de Vries EGE, van der Zee AG, Uges DRA et al. Excretion of platinum into breast milk. Lancet 1989; 1: 497–8.

Egan PC, Costanza ME, Dodion P et al. Doxorubicin and cisplatin excretion into human milk. Cancer Treat Rep 1985; 69: 1387–89.

Förger F, Matthias T, Oppermann M et al. Infliximab in breast milk. Lupus 2004; 13: 753.

French AE, Soldin SJ, Soldin O et al. Milk transfer and neonatal safety of tacrolimus. Ann Pharmacotherapy 2003; 37: 815–8.

Fritzsche J, Mury D, Wintgens KF et al. Infliximab and adalimumab use during lactation (Abstract). Reprod Toxicol 2011; 31: 258.

Fritzsche J, Pilch A, Mury D et al. Infliximab and adalimumab use during breastfeeding. J Clin Gastroenterol 2012; 46: 718–9.

Gambacorti-Passerini CB, Tornaghi L, Marangon E et al. Imatinib concentrations in human milk. Blood 2007; 109: 1790.

Gardiner SJ, Begg EJ. Breastfeeding during tacrolimus therapy. Obstet Gynecol 2006; 107: 453–5.

Gardiner SJ, Gearry RB, Roberts RL et al. Comment: Breast-feeding during maternal use of azathioprine. Ann Pharmacother 2007; 41: 719–20.

Gouraud A, Bernard N, Millaret A et al. Serum level of tacrolimus in breastfeed infant (sic) and long-term follow-up {Abstract}. Fundam Clin Pharmacol 2011; 25: 515.

Gouraud A, Bernard N, Millaret A et al. Follow-up of tacrolimus breastfed babies. Transplantation 2012; 94: e38–40.

Grimer M. Caring for Australians with Renal Impairment (CARI): The CARI guidelines. Calcineurin inhibitors in renal transplantation: pregnancy, lactation and calcineurin inhibitors. Nephrology (Carlton) 2007; 12: S98–105.

Haggstrom J, Adriansson M, Hybbinette T et al. Two cases of CML treated with alpha-interferon during second and third trimester of pregnancy with analysis of the drug in the new-born immediately postpartum. Eur J Haematol 1996; 57: 101–2.

Hale TW, Siddiqui AA, Baker TE. Transfer of interferon beta-1a into human breastmilk. Breastfeeding Med 2012; 7: 123–5.

Jain A, Venkataramanan R, Fung JJ et al. Pregnancy after liver transplantation under tacrolimus. Transplantation 1997; 64: 559–65.

Kaida K, Ikegame K, Fujioka T et al. Kinetics of granulocyte colony-stimulating factor in the human milk of a nursing donor receiving treatment for mobilization of the peripheral blood stem cells. Acta Haematol 2007; 118: 176–7.

Kapp A, Papp K, Bingham A et al. Long-term management of atopic dermatitis in infants with topical pimecrolimus, a nonsteroid anti-inflammatory drug. J Allergy Clin Immunol 2002; 110: 277–84.

Keeling S, Wolbink GJ. Measuring multiple etanercept levels in the breast milk of a nursing mother with rheumatoid arthritis. J Rheumatol 2010; 37: 1551.

Khare MM, Lott J, Currie A et al. Is it safe to continue azathioprine in breastfeeding mothers? J Obstet Gynaecol (UK) 2003; 23: 48.

Kronenberger R, Schleyer E, Bornhäuser M et al. Imatinib in breast milk. Ann Hematol 2009; 88: 1265–6.

Kumar AR, Hale TW, Mock RE. Transfer of interferon alfa into human breast milk. J Hum Lact 2000; 16: 226–8.

Lactation

4.10 Immunomodulating and antineoplastic agents

Lahiff C, Moss AC. Cyclosporine in the management of severe ulcerative colitis while breast-feeding. Inflamm Bowel Dis 2011; 17: E78.

Lanowska M, Kohler C, Oppelt P et al. Addressing concern about cisplatin application during pregnancy. J Perinat Med 2011; 39: 279–85.

Merlob P. Cyclosporine during lactation. BELTIS, Newsletter of the Beilinson Teratology Information Service, June 2000; 67–73.

Mishkin DS, van Deinse W, Becker JM et al. Successful use of adalimumab (Humira) for Crohn's disease in pregnancy. Inflamm Bowel Dis 2006; 12: 827–8.

Moretti ME, Sgro M, Johnson DW et al. Cyclosporine excretion into breast milk. Transplantation 2003; 74: 2144–6.

Moretti ME, Verjee Z, Ito S et al. Breast-feeding during maternal use of azathioprine. Ann Pharmacother 2006; 40: 2269–72.

Morton A. Cyclosporine and lactation. Nephrology (Carlton) 2011; 16: 249.

Murashima A, Watanabe N, Ozawa N et al. Etanercept during pregnancy and lactation in a patient with rheumatoid arthritis: drug levels in maternal serum, cord blood, breast milk and the infant's serum. Ann Rheum Dis 2009; 68: 1793–4.

Nyberg G, Haljamäe U, Frisenette-Fich C et al. Breastfeeding during treatment with cyclosporine. Transplantation 1998; 65: 253–5.

Osadchy A, Koren G. Cyclosporine and lactation: when the mother is willing to breastfeed. Ther Drug Monit 2011; 33: 147–8.

Ostensen M, Eigenmann GO. Etanercept in breast milk. J Rheumatol 2004; 31: 1017–8.

Russell MA, Carpenter MW, Akhtar MS et al. Imatinib mesylate and metabolite concentrations in maternal blood, umbilical cord blood, placenta and breast milk. J Perinatol 2007; 27: 241–3.

Sau A, Clarke S, Bass J et al. Azathioprine and breastfeeding: is it safe? BJOG 2007; 114: 498–501.

Shibata H, Yamane T, Aoyama Y et al. Excretion of granulocyte colony-stimulating factor into human breast milk. Acta Haematol 2003; 110: 200–1.

Stengel JZ, Arnold HL. Is infliximab safe to use while breastfeeding? World J Gastroenterol 2008; 14: 3085–7.

Vasiliauskas EA, Church JA, Silverman N et al. Case report: evidence for transplacental transfer of maternally administered infliximab to the newborn. Clin Gastroenterol Hepatol 2006; 4: 1255–8.

Vesga L, Terdiman JP, Mahadevan U. Adalimumab use in pregnancy. Gut 2005; 54: 890.

Zelinkova Z, de Boer IP, van Dijke MJ et al. Azathioprine treatment during lactation. Aliment Pharmacol Ther 2009; 30: 90–1; author reply 91.

Zheng S, Easterling TR, Hays K et al. Tacrolimus placental transfer at delivery and neonatal exposure through breast milk. Brit J Clin Pharmacol 2013; 76: 988–96.

Hormones and hormone antagonists

4.11

Gerard H.A. Visser and Corinna Weber-Schöndorfer

4.11.1	Pituitary and hypothalamic hormones	783
4.11.2	Methylergometrine (methylergonovine)	784
4.11.3	Bromocriptine and other prolactin inhibitors	785
4.11.4	Thyroid hormones and thyroid receptor antibodies (TRAb)	785
4.11.5	Thyrostatics	786
4.11.6	Iodine	787
4.11.7	Corticosteroids	788
4.11.8	Adrenaline	789
4.11.9	Insulin and oral antidiabetics	789
4.11.10	Estrogens, gestagens, and hormonal contraceptives	790
4.11.11	Androgens and anabolics	792
4.11.12	Cyproterone acetate and other sex-hormone inhibitors	792
4.11.13	Prostaglandins	793

The hormone and hormone antagonists prescribed during lactation have such a wide variety of substances that a summary would do no justification to the different issues dealt with here.

4.11.1   Pituitary and hypothalamic hormones

Experience

There are only a few publications that discuss tolerance of hypothalamic and pituitary hormones during breastfeeding. In a series of studies on the contraceptive effect of 600 μg of buserelin, a luteinizing hormone-releasing hormone (LRH) antagonist administered nasally, a dosage of 1–2 μg was reported for the fully breastfed infant. Oral bioavailability is poor, so a toxic effect on a breastfed child is not to be expected (Fraser 1989).

The thyrotropin-releasing hormone (TRH) *protirelin* releases prolactin. Its lactation-promoting use has been discussed (Peters 1991). Toxic effects on a breastfed infant are not to be expected; however, studies are lacking.

Drugs During Pregnancy and Lactation. **http://dx.doi.org/10.1016/B978-0-12-408078-2.00036-6**

Desmopressin is found in the mother's milk in only limited amounts. *Oxytocin*, which has long been used to induce labor and for postpartum uterine involution, promotes the milk ejection reflex, and has not been shown to be toxic for the infant.

Carbetocin is a synthetic long acting analog of oxytocin, which is used intravenously and intramuscularly. It appears in the mother's milk in minimal amounts (0.00005% of the maternal weight-related dosage) (Silox 1993). There are no data on the use during breastfeeding of the other hypothalamic and pituitary hormones, or their synthetic analogs *corticorelin, sermorelin, somatorelin, cetrorelix, chorionic gonadotrophin, gonadorelin, goserelin, leuprolide acetate, menotropin, nafarelin, triptorelin, urogonadotropin, octreotide, somatostatin, tetracosactid, somatropin* (growth hormone), *follitropin-α, follitropin-β, urofollitropin, argipressin, lypressin, ornipressin, lanreotide,* and *terlipressin*. This also holds true for the oxytocin-antagonist *atosiban* and the somatropin-receptor antagonist *pegvisomant*.

Recommendation. With the exception of oxytocin, hypothalamic and pituitary hormones are seldom indicated during breastfeeding. No toxic effect on the infant has been demonstrated as yet, plus due to its limited oral bioavailability, is this to be expected. Usage for appropriate indications during breastfeeding is allowed.

4.11.2   Methylergometrine (methylergonovine)

Experience

With a maternal therapy of 2×0.125 mg *methylergometrine* up to 1.1 μg/L has been measured in the milk. This is a maximum of 0.16 μg/kg of the infant's bodyweight, or 3.1% of the maternal weight-related dosage. In a more recent study on 20 women with postpartum uterine atony, either 250 μg methylergometrine or 200 μg *misoprostol* were applied orally (see also Section 4.11.13). The maximum methylergometrine concentration in milk was reached at 2 hours. It has a half-life of 1.9 hours. Considering the maximum concentration in milk, the relative dose was 2.4%. The median M/P ratio was 0.2 (Vogel 2004).

A potentially negative influence on milk production due to prolactin antagonism is known. For breastfed infants themselves, the preparation seems to be tolerated in the overwhelming majority of cases. It should, however, be mentioned that TIS-Berlin has to date received 15 case descriptions involving ergotism-like symptoms in breastfed children (particularly restlessness, vomiting, and diarrhea) (Schaefer, personal communication). This cannot be explained in the light of the above-mentioned limited transfer. Experiences with accidental direct administration of methylergometrine to the newborn infant, due to a mix-up of the medication in the delivery room, also argue against a toxic risk via the mother's milk. In such cases, ergotism-like symptoms were first observed after a dosage that was 150–200 times above that transferred through mother's milk (Poison Control Center Berlin, unpublished observations). However, hypersensitivity, or the transfer of individual higher doses via breast milk, cannot be ruled out. In this connection, those studies on the pharmacological effects of ergotamine residue in mothers' milk substitute conducted in the 1930s are at least of historical interest (Fomina 1933).

> **Recommendation.** Single parenteral administration of methylergometrine in the delivery room is apparently unproblematic for the breastfed infant, and may be used if it is really indicated. Postpartum oral treatment with methylergometrine over several days, or even weeks, is rarely indicated in modern obstetrics. It should be considered that this agent counteracts the natural uterine involution, which normally occurs during breastfeeding via prolactin secretion. Oxytocin, which promotes the milk ejection reflex, is preferable as a medical support for uterine involution. If, however, there are sound grounds to use methylergometrine for a protracted time, there is no need for breast- feeding to be limited.

4.11.3 Bromocriptine and other prolactin inhibitors

Experience

Bromocriptine is an ergotamine derivative. As a prolactin inhibitor, it reduces the milk production and is used to treat prolactinoma. Because of the possible cardiovascular side effects in the mother, particularly the threat of cerebral angiopathy and myocardial infarction (Hopp 1996, Iffy 1996), it has been removed from the market for use in postpartum lactation suppression (Herings 1995; see also Chapter 3.7). Intolerance in the breastfed baby, even with prolactinoma treatment, has not been observed (Canales 1981). Even after an intake of 5 or 10 mg daily, no side effects via the mother's milk are to be expected in the infant.

The effect of breastfeeding on the growth of the prolactinoma appears to be more limited than that of pregnancy, so an interruption of dopamine agonist treatment with bromocriptine during breastfeeding can be considered (Rau 1996).

Cabergoline is taken less often (e.g. once a week) because of its considerably longer half-life and period of effectiveness. In addition, there seem to be fewer side effects. With respect to the other prolactin inhibitors, *lisuride, metergoline,* and *quinagolide,* experience during breastfeeding is insufficient.

> **Recommendation.** Because of maternal risks, routine prescription of bromocriptine to stop lactation is not indicated. If physical measures (and in cases of mastitis, antibiotic treatment) are insufficient, cabergoline should be preferred (see also Chapter 3.7). If a therapy with prolactin inhibitors for mastitis is considered unavoidable, the briefest and lowest dosage should be used so that milk production will not diminish. As long as milk is being produced, breastfeeding may continue, even when cabergoline is being given. In so far as other experience is available, this also applies to the other prolactin inhibitors. If the milk supply diminishes during antiprolactin treatment, relactation may be undertaken if desired.

4.11.4 Thyroid hormones and thyroid receptor antibodies (TRAb)

Experience

L-thyroxine is used as a substitute in cases of hypothyroidism (at least 1 µg/kg daily for adults) and for this reason, is not problematic. The normal

Lactation

4.11 Hormones and hormone antagonists

thyroid content of mother's milk is approximately 1 μg/L. An infant takes in about 0.15 μg/kg in 24 hours; this represents about 1% of a substitution dosage at this age (10 μg/kg daily). This amount does not influence the thyroid function of a healthy infant. The same applies for treatment (substitution) of maternal hypoparathyroidism.

This also implies that maternal L-thyroxine substitution has no therapeutic effect in cases of a neonatal congenital hypo- or athyroidism. This has to be taken into account in cases of extremely premature newborns with a higher risk for hypothyroidism. Neither breast milk nor formula contains enough thyroxine for substitution (van Wassenaer 2002).

The clinical use of thyroid receptor antibodies (TRAb) measurements for the diagnosis and follow-up of autoimmune thyroid diseases, remains a matter of controversy and differs geographically. TRAb can result in transient neonatal thyroid disease by transfer through milk from mothers treated for thyrotoxicosis. Serum TRAb concentration in neonates decreases gradually with time after birth. The calculated half-life for offspring-serum and breast-milk TRAb has been calculated as approximately 3 weeks and 2 months, respectively. Transient neonatal thyroid disease may be worse and more prolonged during breastfeeding as a consequence of TRAb in breast milk (Törnhage 2006).

Recommendation. Substitution of thyroid and parathyroid hormones establishes a physiological state, and, thus should be continued during breastfeeding if necessary. Thyroid hormones should not be given together with thyrostatics, because higher dosages of thyrostatics would then be necessary.

4.11.5   Thyrostatics

Experience

The thyrostatics include *carbimazole, propylthiouracil, thiamazol (=methimazole)*, and *sodium perchlorate*. Carbimazole is metabolized to thiamazol as the active metabolite.

The M/P quotients of carbimazole and thiamazol are about 1. With 40 mg carbimazole daily, peak methimazole values of 0.72 mg/L of milk have been measured (Cooper 1984). A maximum relative dosage of 27% carbimazole has been calculated for the breastfed infant. On average, however, 2–10% of the weight-related dosage is more likely (survey by Bennett 1996).

With 5 mg thiamazol per day, up to 65 μg/L milk could be measured. Accordingly, an infant would receive up to 9.8 μg/kg daily. This represents about 12% of the maternal dosage per kg bodyweight. In the plasma of breastfed twins, 45 and 53 μg/L – subtherapeutic levels – of thiamazol were found. The children had no symptoms, and their thyroid status was unremarkable (Rylance 1987).

A study of 46 children whose mothers received 20 mg methimazole daily for 1 month, and 42 children whose mothers started with 30 mg daily and subsequently reduced to 5–10 mg, reported normal T3, T4 and TSH values (Azizi 2002). Psychomotor development was normal at the age of 49–86 months (Azizi 2003). With treatment using 400 mg propylthiouracil, a maximum of 0.7 mg/L has been found in the mother's milk. For the infant this is at most 0.1 mg/kg, i.e. 1.5% of the maternal weight-related dosage in 24 hours. The M/P ratio is 0.1 (Kampmann 1980). In older studies in which the methodology was insufficient, M/P values of 12 were calculated. In a newer study of 11 children whose mothers took 300–750 mg daily, elevated TSH values were found in 2 children 7 days after birth. However, these values normalized in the course of time, despite a stable or increasing maternal dosage. No correlation has been found between maternal dosage or maternal thyroid hormone FT4 level on the one hand, and the infant's TSH on the other hand. Even with the highest daily dosage, there appeared to be no risk for the breast-fed baby (Momotani 2000).

All in all, the exposure of infants to thiamazol or propylthiouracil through breast milk is minimal and not clinically significant. Women with hyperthyroidism using methimazole or propylthiouracil should not be discouraged from breastfeeding, as the benefits of breastfeeding largely outweigh the theoretical minimal risks (Glatstein 2009). However, data indicate that propylthiouracil may induce severe liver damage in approximately 0.1% of exposed adults (Cassina 2012, Azizi 2011, Karras 2010). Moreover, a nationwide population-based study in 2,830 pregnant women with hyperthyroidism indicated that propylthiouracil, but not thiamazol, was associated with an increased incidence of low birth weight infants (Chen 2011). Thiamazol seems therefore, the mainstay of hyperthyroidism treatment during the second half of pregnancy and during postpartum lactation, despite its slightly higher concentration in breast milk (Cassina 2012, Azizi 2011, Karras 2010). The American Thyroid Association has recommended that PTU should not be prescribed as the first line agent in children and adolescents (Karras 2010).

Sodium perchlorate is a reserve thyrostatic. It blocks the thyroid by replacing iodine, and is used during scintigraphic studies of other organs with radioactive iodine. Sodium perchlorate also blocks the transport to the breast, where iodine accumulates (Janssen 2001). There is no experience of its use during breastfeeding.

Recommendation. Thiamazol is the thyrostatic of choice during breastfeeding, since propylthiouracil has been associated with severe liver impairment in adults (in this case lactating women). Both thiamazol and propylthiouracil result in a non-clinically significant exposure for the newborn infant. If the breastfeeding mother has been, or still is being, treated with a dosage in the upper therapeutic range, the thyroid parameter of the infant should be tested after about 3 weeks just to be safe. Sodium perchlorate should not be used during breastfeeding. Thyroid hormones should not be given together with thyrostatics, because a higher thyrostatic dosage would be necessary.

4.11.6   Iodine

Experience

While breastfeeding, the mother's *iodine* requirement is about 260 μg/day. For infants aged up to 4 months, a daily intake of 50 μg iodine is recommended; for premature infants this should be 30 μg. Iodine supplementation must be ensured during breastfeeding in areas where iodine is deficient. This can be difficult to achieve by diet with iodized salt and weekly salt-water fish meals, since the level of iodine in iodized

Lactation

4.11 Hormones and hormone antagonists

salt is only 15–25 μg/g and below the amount needed; added to which are that iodized foods are still the exception, and if regular consumption of saltwater fish does not appeal. In these cases, supplemental iodine tablets must be taken to cover the above-mentioned requirements. More recent studies have confirmed that such a supplementation significantly increases the iodine content in mother's milk, although not always to adequate levels. In case of premature infants, the amount of iodine transferred with the milk every day could only be increased to 12 μg/kg (Sukkhojaiwaratkul 2014, Seibold-Weiger 1999).

Iodine accumulates more significantly in mother's milk than any other medication studied to date. Different authors report M/P quotients between 15 and 65 with iodine products such as *povidone iodine* or the radioactive isotope *iodine[131]*. Up to 49% of the total maternal iodine[131] dosage is excreted in the milk within 24 hours!

Inhibition of the infant's thyroid function (Wolff–Chaikoff effect) caused by high iodine dosage is possible if the child's intake is 100 μg/ kg daily, or has a plasma concentration of 250 μg/L (Schönberger 1982). The use of iodine-containing disinfectants such as povidone iodine over wide areas (Chanoine 1988), or potassium iodine as an expectorant, might lead to a relatively high dosage of free iodine in the mother's milk and cause inhibition of the infant's thyroid function. In a healthy term and fully breastfed newborn, hypothyroid parameters have been diagnosed on day 17. The mother was treated with iodoform gauze because of a rectal abscess. The laboratory findings normalized after the treatment was stopped. The clinically normal infant was temporarily treated with thyroxin supplementation (l'Italien 2004).

> **Recommendation.** Sufficient iodine supplementation (about 260 μg daily) should be attempted in the interests of both mother and child. A risk of iodine overload for the infant via the mother's milk is not to be expected at this dosage level.
>
> Iodine-containing disinfectants should only be used on small wounds. Iodine-containing expectorants are contraindicated.

4.11.7   Corticosteroids

Experience

Corticosteroids are of practical significance during breastfeeding. Those that are used therapeutically include the non-fluorinated *prednisone*, *prednisolone*, and *methylprednisolone*, as well as *deflazacort, hydrocortisone* and *prednyliden*; and the fluoridated substances *amcinonide, beclomethasone, betamethasone, budesonide, cloprednol, dexamethasone, flunisolide, flumetasone, fluocortolone, fluticasone, mometasone*, and *triamcinolone*. Some preparations are used exclusively as inhalants for treating obstructive respiratory illnesses.

The M/P ratio of prednisone and prednisolone varies between 0.05 and 0.25.

One hour after parenteral administration of a single dose of 110 mg of prednisolone, a level of 760 μg/L has been measured in the milk. Four hours later it was 260 μg/L, and about 9 hours after administration the level was still 60 μg/L. Following an intravenous injection of 1 g of prednisolone, a nine-fold higher value was measured in the milk, reflecting the nine-fold higher dosage. Twenty-four hours after administration, it could no longer be detected in the milk (unpublished observation of TIS-Berlin). Other authors have reported similar or lower transfer amounts with a lower daily dosage of 10–80 mg (survey by Bennett 1996, Greenberger 1993). All in all, an average of 1–2% of the maternal weight-related dosage can be expected for the infant. In the case of the 1 g dose described above, the infant received 0.2 mg of prednisolone per kg bodyweight with the first breast feed an hour after the injection. Over 24 hours, it was 0.32 mg/kg. Even this higher maternal dosage provides only about a sixth of a therapeutic child's dosage, which is usually well tolerated (2 mg/kg per day). There is no risk for the infant from the usual short-term high-dose treatment, even when breastfed right after the injection.

Even with longer-term treatment using 80 mg daily, only a small amount of prednisolone, which does not equal 10% of the body's own cortisol production, is transferred into the milk. There are insufficient documented data on transfer with the other corticoids.

> **Recommendation.** Prednisolone, prednisone, and methylprednisolone are the corticoids of choice for systemic treatment during breastfeeding. Even high doses of up to 1 g administered once or for a few consecutive days – for example, for an asthma attack or multiple sclerosis – do not require any limitation of breastfeeding. When such high doses are given repeatedly, there should be a 3–4 hour wait for breastfeeding if that can be arranged. Other corticoids are probably also tolerated. Routine inhalation of a corticoid for asthma is no cause for concern.

4.11.8   Adrenaline

Experience

Adrenaline and noradrenaline are reserved for emergency situations, when breastfeeding is not permitted in any case. No toxic effect on the infant should be expected from the limited amount of adrenaline, which is added to local anesthesia.

> **Recommendation.** If adrenaline, noradrenaline or similar catecholamines must be administered during breastfeeding, this does not require weaning.

4.11.9   Insulin and oral antidiabetics

Experience

Insulin as a proteohormone is not secreted in the mother's milk, and is not absorbed intestinally. Any effect on the infant can therefore be ruled out.

Neither *glibenclamide* nor *glipizide* have been detected in the breastmilk of three mothers. Hypoglycemia was not observed in any of the children. In another eight women receiving a single dosage of glibenclamide, no substance was found in milk. A high protein binding of 98% may explain these results (Feig 2005).

Lactation

4.11 Hormones and hormone antagonists

Only small amounts of *metformin* are found in mothers' milk; the weight-adjusted dose for a fully breastfed child is 0.1–0.7% (Briggs 2005, Gardiner 2003, Hale 2002). Hypoglycemia has not been reported in breastfed infants. Metformin concentrations in breast milk remained stable over the time of observation. Growth, motor-social development, and illness requiring a pediatrician's visit were assessed in 61 nursing infants (21 male, 40 female), and 50 formula-fed infants (19 male, 31 female) born to 92 mothers with polycystic ovary syndrome (PCOS) taking a median of 2.55 g metformin per day throughout pregnancy and lactation. At 3 and 6 months of age, weight, height, and motor-social development did not differ between breast- and formula-fed infants. In conclusion, metformin during lactation versus formula feeding appears to have no adverse effects on the growth neither of the infant, nor on motor-social development and inter-current illnesses during the first 6 months of life (Glueck 2006).

Up to 16.2% of the weight-related dosage of tolbutamide can pass into the milk (Moiel 1967).

There are no data on the other oral *antidiabetics, acarbose, glibor-nuride, gliclazide, glimepiride, gliquidone, glisoxepide, miglitol, pioglita-zone, repaglinide,* and *rosiglitazone.* There is also insufficient experience on the antihypoglycemics *glucagon* and *diazoxide.*

Recommendation. Insulin and metformin cause no problems during breastfeeding. Glibenclamide may also be taken; however, the infant should be observed for symptoms of hypoglycemia after the start of therapy. Other oral antidiabetics should not be taken, but single doses do not require any limitation of breastfeeding.

4.11.10   Estrogens, gestagens, and hormonal contraceptives

▶ **Effect on milk production**

The amount of milk produced can decrease as a result of estrogens taken by the mother. With the older, higher-dosage contraceptives, a reduction of up to 40% has been described. Changes in the caloric, protein, nitrogen, and lipid content have also been observed, and are apparently dependent on the starting point. In normally nourished women, the alterations stay within the physiological range. However, when there is a prior milk-supply problem, the influence on milk production is unwanted, and where the mother is poorly nourished, it can be dramatic. In follow-up studies, including those on the new low-dosage preparations, the slight reductions as found in the average length of breastfeeding and milk production, as well as in a temporarily slightly reduced weight gain of the infants, did not have any effect on physical or cognitive development (survey in Bennett 1996).

▶ **Hormonal transfer to the infant via mother's milk**

Gestagens (*norethisterone, levonorgestrel, medroxyprogesterone*) as an ingredient of a mini- or combination pill or as a "3-month shot," have little or no effect on the milk supply, and only a very limited effect on its composition. In fact, many researchers found a longer period of breast-feeding in mothers with depot-medroxyprogesterone as compared to those without hormonal contraception (survey in Bennett 1996).

With a daily intake of 50 µg, *ethinylestradiol* cannot be detected in the mother's milk. Only after an oral administration of 500 µg can an infant's dose can be calculated at 0.026 µg/kg daily. This is about 0.2% of the maternal dosage per kg bodyweight.

Vaginal administration of 50 or 100 mg of estradiol also leads to negligible amounts in the mother's milk – less than 0.1% of the maternal weight-related dosage (survey by Bennett 1996).

The other estrogens, *chlorotrianisen, epimestrol, estriol, fosfestrole, mestranol,* and *polyestradiol,* have not been studied during lactation. For most of them, there is no indication for use during breastfeeding. The gestagen intake of the infant lies between 1 and 2% of the weight-related maternal dosage in a contraceptive preparation. This has been shown for "pills" with *desogestrel, megestrol, norethisterone acetate, norethynodrel* and *norgestrel* (survey by Bennett 1996, Shaaban 1991).

With 3 mg/day *drospirenon* in combination with *ethinylestradiol,* there was, on average, 3.7 ng/mL in the milk in six breastfeeding women. A fully breastfed infant would therefore receive 0.6 µg/kg per day, i.e. 1% of the weight-adjusted maternal dosage. No symptoms have been observed in any of the children (Blode 2001).

With *lynestrenol,* a relative dosage of less than 1% has been found. The transferred portion for the infant directly after injection of 150 mg depot-medroxyprogesterone acetate as a "3-month shot" was 7.5 µg/kg daily (survey by Bennett 1996).

Elcometrin, with an effectiveness of 6 months, is administered in a subdermal capsule. A maximum of 674 pmol of the active ingredient has been found in maternal serum. In the milk this was up to 640 pmol, and in the serum of individual children up to 55 pmol, while in others the serum concentration was beneath the detection limit of 13 pmol. The samples were taken 75 days following implantation. Up to the end of the first year of life, the development of the 66 participating children did not differ from those in a control group (Coutinho 1999).

Centchroman, a new nonsteroid oral contraceptive that is initially taken twice a week and later only once a week, has been studied in 13 women. With doses of 30 mg, a maximum of 122 µg/L was found in the milk. On average, however, the values were more likely to be about 50 µg/L or less. Mathematically speaking, a fully breastfed baby would receive up to 11% of a maternal weight-related dosage. The M/P ratio is between 1 and 2 (Gupta 1995).

There is no specific information on milk transfer with *chlormadinon, dydrogestone, gestonorone, gestodene, hydroxyprogesterone, levonorgestrel, medrogestone,* and *norgestimate.*

When used in oral contraceptive preparations, in gestagen-containing intrauterine pessaries, and in the "morning-after pill", these substances can probably be evaluated similarly to the above-mentioned contraceptives. Higher-dosed gestagen preparations used for other indications have not been studied with respect to their kinetics, but there are unlikely to be many indications for their use during breastfeeding.

▶ Long-term effects of hormonal contraception

The hormonal transfer from contraceptive gestagen monopreparation (the mini-pill or depot injection), and low-dosage combination "pills" into the milk does not affect the development of the infant's sexual organs. In his literature review, Truitt (2003) did not find any differences between

Lactation

4.11 Hormones and hormone antagonists

gestagen monotherapy and combination pills regarding the amount and quality of milk production. However, methodological problems in many of the evaluated studies limited his conclusions. Another study compared long-term development between 220 breastfed infants of mothers with levonorgestrel therapy, and 222 infants whose mothers used copper IUDs for contraception. Children with levonorgestrel had slightly milder respiratory tract infections, eye infections, and skin problems during the first year of life. Children whose mothers used copper IUDs more frequently showed slight psychomotor development retardation (Schiappacasse 2002). These observations should also be interpreted with caution.

Up to 6 months postpartum and in the presence of ongoing amenorrhea, the contraceptive protection from exclusive breastfeeding should be similar to that of an intrauterine pessary (IUP) or hormonal contraception (Kennedy 1992). In the so-called developing world, much more "birth control" is attributed to breastfeeding than to the other family planning measures (Hanson 1994).

> **Recommendation.** Pure gestagen preparations (mini-pills) are the oral contraceptive of choice during breastfeeding. If the mother does not tolerate them, then the low-dosage combination "pills" (ethinylestradiol plus gestagen), or gestagen depot preparations, is acceptable. If necessary, they can be started about 6–8 weeks after birth. There is no preparation among the well-established hormonal contraceptives that requires an interruption of breastfeeding.

4.11.11   Androgens and anabolics

Experience

There is no experience with the available androgens, *mesterolone, testolactone*, and *testosterone*. The same applies to the anabolics, *clostebol, metenolone* and *nandrolone*.

> **Recommendation.** Androgens and anabolics are contraindicated during breastfeeding. Accidental intake of a single dose does not require an interruption in breastfeeding.

4.11.12   Cyproterone acetate and other sex-hormone inhibitors

Experience

Following a dosage of 50 mg of *cyproterone acetate*, peak values of 260 μg/L have been measured in the milk. The infant's exposure would be 39 μg/kg/day. That is just about 5% of the maternal weight-related dosage (Stoppeli 1980). The more common daily intake of 2 mg of cyproterone acetate for acne therapy has not yet been studied.

Other antiandrogens, such as *bicalutamide* and *flutamide*, and antiestrogen-acting substances, such as *aminoglutethimide, anastrozole, formestan, raloxifene*, and *tamoxifen*, as well as the sex-hormone inhibitors *danazol* and *tibolone*, have practically no role during breast-feeding and have also not been studied.

There are also no data on *clomiphene* and the progesterone antagonist *mifepristone*. In so far as its (accidental) use during breastfeeding happens at all, a toxic effect on the infant should not be expected due to the brief exposure.

> **Recommendation.** Antiandrogens and antiestrogens are contraindicated during breastfeeding. Accidental intake of a single dose does not require an interruption of breastfeeding. However, treatment should not be continued.

4.11.13   Prostaglandins

Experience

Prostaglandins are mainly used in obstetrics for priming and inducing labor. After birth, other pharmaceuticals are used for uterine involution so that therapy during breastfeeding for obstetrical indications is not common. *Latanoprost* is administered as eye drops for glaucoma.

Prostaglandin derivatives have short half-lives ranging from a few seconds to 20–40 minutes at maximum. Both milk-promoting and milk-inhibiting effects have been noted with the various prostaglandins. In a study of 20 women with postpartum uterine atony, either 200 μg *misoprostol* or 250 μg *methylergometrine* were administered orally. The maximum misoprostol concentration in milk was reached at 1 hour, with a half-life of 0.6 hours on average, whereas methylergometrine reached the maximum at 2 hours with a half life of 1.9 hours. Considering the maximum concentration in milk, the relative dose for misoprostol was 0.04% and that of methylergometrine 2.4%. The median M/P ratios were 0.04 and 0.2, respectively (Vogel 2004).

There is no indication yet of negative effects of prostaglandins in the breastfed infant. However, documented experience is still insufficient.

> **Recommendation.** Prostaglandins should only be used for compelling treatment indications during breastfeeding. If severe glaucoma requires local treatment with latanoprost, breastfeeding can continue provided there is careful observation of the baby. Single doses of other prostaglandins, such as misoprostol for uterine atony, do not require any limitation of breastfeeding.

References

Azizi F, Amouzegan A. Management of hyperthyroidism during pregnancy and lactation. Eur J Endocrinol 2011; 164: 871–6.

Azizi F, Bahrainian M, Khamseh ME et al. Intellectual development and thyroid function in children who were breast-fed by thyrotoxic mothers taking methimazole. J Pediatr Endocr Metab 2003; 16: 1239–43.

Azizi F, Hedavati M. Thyroid function in breast-fed infants whose mothers take high doses of methimazole. J Endocrinol Invest 2002; 25: 493–6.

Bennett PN (ed.). Drugs and Human Lactation, 2nd edn, Amsterdam: Elsevier, 1996.

Blode H, Foidart JM, Heithecker R. Transfer of drospirenone to breast milk after a single oral administration of 3 mg drospirenone + 30 microg ethinylestradiol to healthy lactating women. Eur J Contracept Reprod Health Care 2001; 6: 167–71.

Briggs GG, Ambrose PJ, Nageotte MP et al. Excretion of metformin into breast milk and the effect on nursing infants. Obstet Gynecol 2005; 105: 1437–41.

Canales ES, Garcia IC, Ruiz JE et al. Bromocriptine as prophylactic therapy in prolactinoma during pregnancy. Fertil Steril 1981; 36: 524–6.

Cassina M, Dona M, Di Gianantonio et al. Pharmacological treatment of hyperthyroidism during pregnancy. Birth Defects Res A Clin Mol Teratol 2012; 94: 612–9.

Chanoine JP, Boulvain M, Bourdoux P et al. Increased recall rate at screening for congenital hypothyroidism in breast fed infants born to iodine overloaded mothers. Arch Dis Child 1988; 63: 1207–10.

Chen CH, Xirasagar S, Liu CC et al. Risk of adverse perinatal outcomes with antithyriod treatment during pregancy: a nationwide population-based study. BJOG 2011; 118: 1365–73.

Cooper DS, Bode HH, Nath B et al. Methimazole pharmacology in man: studies using a newly developed radioimmunoassay for methimazole. J Clin Endocrinol Metab 1984; 58: 473–9.

Coutinho EM, Athayde C, Dantas C et al. Use of a single implant of elcometrine (ST-1435), a non-orally active progestin, as a long acting contraceptive for postpartum nursing women. Contraception 1999; 59: 115–22.

Feig DS, Briggs GG, Kraemer JM et al. Transfer of glyburide and glipizide into breast milk. Diabetes Care 2005; 28: 1851–5.

Fomina PI. Untersuchungen über den Übergang des aktiven Agens des Mutterkorns in die Milch stillender Mütter. Archiv f Gynäkologie 1933; 157: 275–85.

Fraser HM, Dewart PJ, Smith SK et al. Luteinizing hormone releasing hormone agonist for contraception in breast-feeding women. J Clin Endocrinol Metab 1989; 69: 996–1002.

Gardiner SJ, Kirkpatrick CMJ, Begg EJ et al. Transfer of metformin into human milk. Clin Pharmacol Ther 2003; 73: 71–7.

Glatstein MM, Garcia-Bournissen F, Giglio N et al. Pharmacologic treatment of hyperthyroidism during lactation. Can Fam Physician 2009; 55: 797–8.

Glueck CJ, Salehi M, Sieve L et al. Growth, motor, and social development in breast- and formulafed infants of metformin-treated women with polycystic ovary syndrome. J Pediatr 2006; 148: 628–32.

Greenberger PA, Odeh YK, Frederiksen MC et al. Pharmacokinetics of prednisolone transfer to breast milk. Clin Pharmacol Ther 1993; 53: 324–8.

Gupta RC, Paliwal JK, Nityanand S et al. Centchroman: a new non-steroidal oral contraceptive in human milk. Contraception 1995; 52: 301–5.

Hale TW, Kristensen JH, Hackett LP et al. Transfer of metformin into human milk. Diabetologia 2002; 45: 1509–14.

Hanson LA, Ashraf R, Zaman S et al. Breast feeding is a natural contraceptive and prevents disease and death in infants, linking infant mortality and birth rates. Acta Paediatr 1994; 83: 3–6.

Herings RM, Strieker BH. Bromocriptine and suppression of postpartum lactation. Pharm World Sci 1995; 17: 133–7.

Hopp L, Haider B, Iffy L. Myocardial infarction post-partum in patients taking bromocriptine for the prevention of breast engorgement. Intl J Cardiology 1996; 57: 227–32.

Iffy L, McArdle JJ, Ganesh V. Intracerebral hemorrhage in normotensive mothers using bromocriptine postpartum. Zentralbl Gynäkol 1996; 118: 392–6.

Janssen OE, Heufelder AE, Mann K. Schilddrüsenerkrankungen. In: Ganten D. (ed.), Molekulargenetische Grundlagen von Endokrinopathien. Berlin Heidelberg: Springer Verlag, 2001, pp. 47–8.

Kampmann JP, Hansen JM, Johansen K et al. Propylthiouracil in human milk. Lancet 1980; 1: 736–8.

Karras S, Tzotza T, Kaltsas T et al. Pharmacological treatment of hyperthyroidism during lactation: a review of the literate and novel data. Padiatr Endocrinol Rev 2010; 8: 25–33.

Kennedy KI, Visness CM. Contraceptive efficacy of lactational amenorrhoea. Lancet 1992; 339: 227–30.

l'Italien A, Starceski PJ, Dixit NM. Transient hypothyroidism in a breastfed infant after maternal use of iodoform gauze. J Pediatr Endocrinol Metab 2004; 17: 665–7.

Moiel RH, Ryan RJ. Tolbutamide orinase in human breast milk. Clin Pediatr 1967; 6: 480.

Momotani N, Yamashita R, Makino F et al. Thyroid function in wholly breastfeeding infants whose mothers take high doses of propylthiouracil. Clin Endocrinol 2000; 53: 177–81.

Peters F, Schulze-Tollert J, Schuth W. Thyrotropin-releasing hormone – a lactation-promoting agent? Br J Obstet Gynecol 1991; 98: 880–5.

Rau H, Badenhoop K, Usadel KH. The treatment of prolactinomas during pregnancy and the lactation period {in German}. Dtsch Med Wschr 1996; 121: 28–32.

Rylance RY, Woods CG, Donnelly MC et al. Carbimazole and breast feeding. Lancet 1987; i: 928.

Schiappacasse V, Diaz S, Zepeda A et al. Health and growth of infants breastfed by Norplant contraceptive implants users: a six-year follow-up study. Contraception 2002; 66: 57–65.

Schönberger W, Grimm W. Transient hypothyroidism caused by iodine-containing disinfectants in the newborn {in German; author's transl}. Dtsch Med Wochenschr 1982; 107: 1222–7.

Seibold-Weiger K, Wollmann H, Rendl J et al. Iodine concentration in the breast milk of mothers of premature infants {in German}. Z Geburtsh Neonatol 1999; 203: 81–5.

Shaaban MM. Contraception with progestogens and progesterone during lactation. J Steroid Biochem Mol Biol 1991; 40: 705–10.

Silox J, Schulz P, Horbay GLA et al. Transfer of carbetocin into human breast milk. Obstet Gynecol 1993; 83: 456–9.

Stoppeli I, Rainer E, Humpel M. Transfer of cyproterone acetate to the milk of lactating women. Contraception 1980; 22: 485–93.

Sukkhojaiwaratkul D, Mahachoklertwattana P, Poomthavorn P et al. Effects of maternal iodine supplementation during pregnancy and lactation on iodine status and neonatal thyroid-stimulating hormone. J Perinatol 2014. Doi:10.1038/jp (E pub ahead of print).

Törnhage CJ, Grankvist K. Acquired neonatal thyroid disease due to TSH receptor antibodies in breast milk. J Pediatr Endocrinol Metab 2006; 19: 787–94.

Truitt ST, Fraser AB, Grimes DA et al. Hormonal contraception during lactation. Systematic review of randomized controlled trials. Contraception 2003; 68: 233–8.

van Wassenaer AG, Stulp MR, Valianpour F et al. The quantity of thyroid hormone in human milk is too low to influence plasma thyroid hormone levels in the very preterm infant. Clin Endocrinol (Oxf) 2002; 56: 621–7.

Vogel D, Burkhardt T, Rentsch K et al. Misoprostol versus methylergometrine: pharmacokinetics in human milk. Am J Obstet Gynecol 2004; 191: 2168–73.

Dermatological medication and local therapeutics

4.12

Christof Schaefer and Gudula Kirtschig

4.12.1 Topical applications and cosmetics	797
4.12.2 Essential oils	798
4.12.3 Retinoids and topicals for psoriasis, dermatitis and acne	798
4.12.4 Photochemotherapy and fumaric acid preparations	799
4.12.5 Wart removal medications	799
4.12.6 Medications for lice and scabies	799
4.12.7 Eye, nose and ear drops	800
4.12.8 Vein therapeutics and other local therapeutics	801
4.12.9 Vaginal therapeutics	801

Some of the most commonly used medications for the treatment of dermatological diseases can be safely used during lactation. However, Vitamin A derivatives/retinoids such as *isotretinoin* used in acne, or *acitretin* used in psoriasis, as well as tar preparations, should be avoided because of their toxic potential. Any topical preparation applied to the skin of the breast should be removed before breastfeeding.

4.12.1   Topical applications and cosmetics

Topical applications during breastfeeding are, in principle, acceptable as long as they are applied to a limited area of the skin and for a limited period of time. This applies to all topical treatments, as well as antiseptics and disinfectants (for iodine see Chapter 4.11), repellents, anti-infectives (topical antibiotics, antimycotics and virostatics), corticosteroids and topical anti-inflammatory drugs, astringents, antipruritics and keratolytics.

For substances not mentioned in this chapter, the Recommendations in Chapter 2.17 can serve as an orientation.

If treatment involves a large area of the skin over a long period of time, the absorption and the effects of the individual substances must be considered, and it is advised to use systemic applications of the drug as a guide (i.e. iodine and acetylsalicylic acid). If the skin of the breast needs to be treated with topicals, it should be cleaned before the baby is fed.

Cosmetics and hair preparations, including coloring and permanent waves, may be used if they improve the mother's well-being. However, absorption and transmission of its compounds through mother's milk cannot be ruled out (i.e. moschus derivatives and lead; Chapter 4.18), and particular attention needs to be paid to the ingredients of, for example, hair dyes which may contain toxic substances like lead. Even though an allergic potential of compounds of the topicals (cosmetics) used by the mother resulting in sensitization of the breastfed baby is theoretically possible, this seems a very rare and hard situation to prove.

Furthermore, avoidance of potential allergens seems not to prevent the development of atopic eczema. Studies on maternal dietary restrictions during pregnancy and lactation have led researchers to believe that antigen avoidance does not play a significant role in the prevention of atopic disease or food allergies (Gamboni 2013).

4.12.2   Essential oils

In principle, there is no reason to object to the use of essential oils. However, direct contact of the breastfed baby with the area of the treated skin should be avoided. If solutions or emulsions containing essential oils are applied to the breast, the relevant site of the skin should be thoroughly cleaned before breastfeeding (see also Chapter 2.19).

> **Recommendation.** Essential oils may only be used during breastfeeding if direct contact by the infant with the area of the treated skin is avoided.

4.12.3   Retinoids and topicals for psoriasis, dermatitis and acne

About 1% of the maternal weight-related dose of *acitretin*, which is metabolized to *etretinate*, is passed to the fully breastfed infant. This was reported for a patient who received 40 mg p.o. daily (Rollman 1990). There are no reports available on toxic symptoms in the child.

There is no experience available on *isotretinoin* and on external use of *adapalene, alitretinoin gel, tazarotene* and *tretinoin* or on *calcipotriol, dithranol* – which is sometimes combined with salicylic acid, urea, coal tar and azelaic acid preparations. However, with regard to retinoids such as *tretinoin* and its isomer *isotretinoin*, no appreciable exposure of the breastfed baby is expected following topical administration (Kong 2013, Leachman 2006, Akhavan 2003).

There is no experience on the topical use of lithium for seborrheic dermatitis during breastfeeding. However, percutaneous intake is limited (Sparsa 2004); therefore, an appreciable passage into the milk seems unlikely.

Tacrolimus and *pimecrolimus* are used for topical treatment of atopic dermatitis (Chapter 4.10).

There are also no systematic studies on the use of schist oil extracts such as *ammonium bituminosulfonate* and *sodium bituminosulfonate*; there is no hint for toxic symptoms in the breastfed baby after maternal use either.

> **Recommendation.** Systemic therapy (oral) with retinoids should not be undertaken during breastfeeding because of their toxic potential and the long half-life. This also applies to the external use of coal tar preparations because of their mutagenic and carcinogenic potential. The odd application does not require any limitation of breastfeeding. All other topical preparations mentioned are acceptable if no significant absorption is reported, which is expected for example with regular applications or if used under occlusion.

4.12.4   Photochemotherapy and fumaric acid preparations

There are no systematic studies on the use of photochemotherapy (PUVA-therapy) for psoriasis, neither with oral photosensitizers nor with topically applied methoxsalen followed by long-term UV-A-radiation, but there are no hints for toxic symptoms in the breastfed baby from case reports. This also applies to the fumaric acid preparations, dimethyl fumarate + ethyl hydrogen fumarate.

> **Recommendation.** Photochemotherapy with *methoxsalen* and UV-A radiation is acceptable during breastfeeding if required by the disease. *Fumaric acid* preparations should be avoided.

4.12.5   Wart removal medications

For toxicological considerations, topical treatment of condylomata acuminata (genital warts) should be performed with cryotherapy, laser therapy, electrocautery or trichloroacetic acid. However, with the plant-based mitosis inhibitor, *podophyllotoxin*, or the newer immune modulator and virostatic, *imiquimod*, no adverse effects in the breastfed infant are assumed given the usually limited area of application. There are, however, no studies available during breastfeeding.

Verrucae vulgares (common warts) and other warts should be treated with cryotherapy, surgical ablation or keratolytics such as salicylic acid or lactic acid. No studies are available for the cytotoxin, fluorouracil, but usually small areas are treated and no adverse effects in the breastfed infant is expected due to limited absorption.

> **Recommendation.** Treatment of choice for warts is cryotherapy, laser ablation, electrocautery or trichloric acid. Nevertheless, should other substances be urgently required, breastfeeding may be continued without limitation.

4.12.6   Medications for lice and scabies

For topical treatment of pediculosis (lice infestation), *dimeticone, coconut oil, pyrethrum, permethrin, malathion* and *allethrin I* are used. For topical treatment of scabies, *benzyl benzoate, crotamiton* and *permethrin* are available. Scabies may be treated systemically with *ivermectin* which is not licensed for this indication in all countries (Chapter 4.4). Topical medications containing *lindane* have been removed from the market in many countries.

Knowledge about the passage of medications for parasites into the mother's milk is scarce and is practically only available for the now obsolete lindane, an insecticide which is widespread in the environment. Our environment is widely contaminated with lindane; it can be detected in the mother's milk due to contaminated food, without therapeutic usage (Chapter 4.18). Studies with a 0.25% lindane solution showed dermal absorption of barely 10%. In one case, after a 3-day scabies treatment, 0.9 mg/kg (ppm) lindane was measured in the milk fat (1 liter of milk has, on average, 30–35 g of milk fat). After another one-time application it was 2.0 mg/kg. Compared to the average environmental contamination load of mother's milk, this was more than a 60-fold increase (Senger 1989). Lindane is neurotoxic; cerebral seizures after repeated topical applications in children are reported (Daud 2010). However, nothing is published on clinical effects after exposure through the mother's milk.

For the rest of the above-mentioned substances, no toxic effects by exposure via the mother's milk are expected. Pyrethrum has a shorter half-life than the synthetic *pyrethroids*. In the USA, permethrin is approved from the age of 3 months. The experience to date on therapeutic use in infants does not indicate any appreciable side-effects after breast feeding (Fölster-Holst 2000).

Recommendation. Lice infestation should be treated with dimeticone during breastfeeding. The medication of choice for scabies during breastfeeding is permethrin.

4.12.7   Eye, nose and ear drops

Eye, nose and ear drops may also be used during breastfeeding. For theoretical consideration, preparations that contain *chloramphenicol, gyrase inhibitors* or *streptomycin* should be avoided. Otherwise the recommendations formulated for pregnancy in Chapter 2.17 also apply for breastfeeding.

The carbonic anhydrase inhibitor, acetazolamide, which is related to thiazide, is prescribed p.o. for glaucoma therapy. Therapeutic doses of 1 g daily p.o. led to 2.1 mg/L in the milk. This resulted in 1.9% of the maternal weight-related dose for an infant who was described as symptom-free – 0.2–0.6 mg/L were measured in his serum (maternal serum: 5.8 mg/L) (Södermann 1984). No adverse effects are expected in the breastfed infant from eye drops that contain *brinzolamide* or *dorzolamide*.

Following maternal combination therapy for glaucoma with *timolol, dipivefrin* and *dorzolamide*, as well as sporadic systemic administration of *acetazolamide*, no adverse effects were reported in a closely monitored baby (Johnson 2001).

The American Academy of Pediatrics (2001) categorizes acetazolamide or β-blockers, e.g. timolol, *metipranolol* or *levobunolol* as acceptable for use during breastfeeding.

There are no experiences available on the other glaucoma therapeutics such as *latanoprost* and other prostaglandins as well as other ophthalmic drugs, for usage during breastfeeding. With the topical administration to the eye, toxic effects for the breastfed baby are hardly expected due to pharmacokinetic considerations. This also applies for the intravitreal injected *pegaptanib*. Due to insufficient experience, breastfeeding whilst being treated with *verteporfin* should be viewed cautiously.

4.12.8   Vein therapeutics and other local therapeutics

Aescin preparations, horse-chestnut extracts for vein problems are not known to have adverse effects in the breastfed infant; however, they are insufficiently studied and are hardly indicated for use during breastfeeding. Sclerotherapy of varicose veins, i.e. with *polidocanol*, may – if it is urgently needed – also be performed while breastfeeding.

The common topically applied hemorrhoid medications are also acceptable.

Benzydamine applications to the mouth, throat and vagina are acceptable while breastfeeding. Systematic studies on the topical use of *methenamine* treating excessive transpiration during breastfeeding are not available. Systemic absorption of larger quantities after topical application is not expected.

According to reports of the American Academy of Pediatrics (2001), no adverse effects were found in a breastfed child after maternal use of *minoxidil*, though no detailed information on the kind and duration of administration was available. The long-term use of minoxidil against hair loss should be avoided because of insufficient experience during breastfeeding (compare Chapter 2.17, postpartum effluvium).

Similarly, there is no experience reported regarding *finasteride* and topical treatment of *hirsutism* with *eflornithine*. Finasteride is not indicated in hair loss in females; it should be avoided during breastfeeding.

4.12.9   Vaginal therapeutics

Povidone iodide as vaginal suppositories and iodine rinses of the vagina are problematic due to the enrichment of free iodides in the mother's milk with potential effects on the child's thyroid function (Chapter 4.11).

There is no reason to wean treatment with other vaginal therapeutics, containing disinfectants, i.e. *dequalinium chloride salts, hexetidine, policresulen* or *estrogens*. However, a rationale for treatment with a particular drug is desired, avoiding drugs that are controversial with respect to their effectiveness. Anti-infective therapy, i.e. with *metronidazole* for *trichomoniasis* or with the nitrofurantoin *nifuratel* as well as the anti-mycotic, *chlorphenesin* should be critically considered. In the case of a proven bacterial infection, a systemic (oral) therapy should be considered, which, in general, is also compatible with breastfeeding – and more effective.

Vaginally used spermicidal contraceptives such as *nonoxinol* are no problem for the breastfed child, likewise the use of different intrauterine devices (IUD).

Lactation

4.12 Dermatological medication and local therapeutics

References

Akhavan A, Bershad S. Topical acne drugs: review of clinical properties, systemic exposure, and safety. Am J Clin Dermatol 2003; 4: 473–92.

American Academy of Pediatrics, Committee on Drugs. The transfer of drugs and other chemicals into human milk. Pediatrics 2001; 108: 776–89.

Daud Y, Daud-ur-Rehman, Farooq U. Lindane toxicity in a 7 year old boy. J Ayub Med Coll Abbottabad 2010; 22: 223.

Fölster-Holst R, Rufli T, Christophers E. Die Skabiestherapie unter besonderer Berücksichtigung des frühen Kindesalters, der Schwangerschaft und Stillzeit. Hautarzt 2000; 51: 7–13.

Gamboni SE, Allen KJ, Nixon RL. Infant feeding and the development of food allergies and atopic eczema: an update. Australas J Dermatol 2013; 54: 85–9.

Johnson SM, Martinez M, Freedman S. Management of glaucoma in pregnancy and lactation. Survey Ophthalmol 2001; 45: 449–54.

Kong YL, Tey HL. Treatment of acne vulgaris during pregnancy and lactation. Drugs 2013; 73: 779–87.

Leachman SA, Reed BR. The use of dermatologic drugs in pregnancy and lactation. Dermatol Clin 2006; 24: 167–97.

Rollman O, Pihl-Lundin I. Acitretin excretion into human breast milk. Acta Derm Venerol (Stockh) 1990; 70: 487–90.

Senger E, Menzel I, Holzmann H. Therapiebedingte Lindan-Konzentration in der Muttermilch. Dermatosen 1989; 37: 167–70.

Södermann P, Hartvig P, Fagerlund C. Acetazolamide excretion into human breast milk. Br J Clin Pharmacol 1984; 17: 599–600.

Sparsa A, Bonnetblanc JM. Lithium. Ann Dermatol Venereol 2004; 131: 255–61.

Alternative remedies, vitamins, and minerals

4.13

Ruth A. Lawrence and Eleanor Hüttel

4.13.1	Alternative remedies and phytotherapeutics	803
4.13.2	Herbal galactogogues and antigalactogogues	805
4.13.3	Topical treatment for breast problems	807
4.13.4	Vitamins, minerals, and trace elements	808
4.13.5	Biphosphonates	808
4.13.6	Exercise	809
4.13.7	Glucose 6-phosphate-dehydrogenase deficiency	809

4.13.1   Alternative remedies and phytotherapeutics

Experience

Numerous surveys in the literature report widespread use of alternative remedies with no knowledge of the risks. The interest in, and experimentation with, alternative remedies has increased in the last decades. Just as in pregnancy, there are minimal evidenced-based safety data for the use of alternative remedies and herbs in lactation; however, also as in pregnancy, history and traditional data in general support their safe use. There have, though, been case reports of unfortunate outcomes. In the United States, the Food and Drug Administration (FDA 2002) has no jurisdiction if the material is labeled with the following statement: "This product is not intended to diagnose, treat, cure or prevent any disease."

Plant preparations (in high doses) are not always harmless; contamination with pesticides and heavy metals (e.g. lead in Ayurvedic medicine or traditional Chinese herbs) has been observed (see Chapter 4.18). There are many herbs which may be used by the nursing mother for a variety of ailments, and there are very few studies regarding their efficacy. The most serious concern (beyond the obvious purity, toxicity, and efficacy) is the problem of self-diagnosis and failure to get the proper medical diagnosis and treatment. Herbs that are most commonly used include *valerian*, *hops*, and *kavain* (*kava-pyrone* from the *kava-kava root*), for nervousness and sleep disturbances; *echinacea* as an immunostimulant; *Gingko biloba* to improve general circulation; *ginseng* to improve performance; *aescin* preparations (horse-chestnut extract) for vein problems; *agnus castus* (*monk's pepper*) for gynecological indications; and *hypericin* (*St John's wort*) for depression. Black cohosh (*Cimicifuga racemosa*) is not recommended during lactation due to estrogenic effects (Dugoua 2008a, 2006b, 2006c). Systematic studies on these drugs during breastfeeding are lacking, but no damage to the infant via the mother's milk has been described, except for Kava (*Piper methysticum*). The FDA (2002) has issued a warning that links Kava to severe liver damage.

An example of a preparation that has now been banned in many countries is *comfrey* (*Symphytum officinale*), which is available both as a leaf or a root. Root preparations in general are more potent. It has the potential for causing venocclusive disease, liver failure, and death. Two neonatal deaths were reported in Canada after mothers used comfrey as a cream on the nipples; after this it was banned in Canada.

Although ethnobotanists have studied specific plant species in depth and noted some of their pharmacological properties, there are no studies, regarding herbals used during lactation, that meet pharmaceutical standards. Most of the information is derived from hearsay and experience without controls. These plants and herbals are being used, and it is important to be aware of possible side effects or even toxicities. The US Government Accountability Office (2010) has reported that 26 of 40 herbal supplements were found to have residual pesticides.

Ginkgo, echinacea, and ginseng have all been studied in blinded placebo controlled studies which failed to show a therapeutic effect. There are no known studies during lactation. Because of the disclaimer on the container, there is no guarantee that the contents are the real plant; they may not be a true mixture, or may be contaminated. Therefore, it is unwise to experiment with these products during lactation. There are many chemicals in one plant (Seely 2008, Perri 2006).

St John's wort (*Hypericum perfortum*) has been shown to be effective against mild depression. It contains 26 identifiable chemicals, one of which is 10% *hypercin*, a red dye originally credited for the therapeutic effect. For its use during lactation, see Chapter 4.9, Budzynska (2012), Dugoua (2006a), and Klier (2006).

Chastetree (*Vitex agnus-castus*) is not recommended during lactation as it may increase or decrease lactation (Dugoua 2008b; Seely 2008).

Dandelion (*Taraxcum officinate*) has been used for acute mastitis and agalactia. No studies or reports have proven its effectiveness. Dandelion contains lactones, sterols, flavonoids, and mucilages. It has been used for dysperic symptoms, liver and gall bladder disturbances and loss of appetite. Side effects are super acidic gastric complaints due to its secretion stimulant effects, and it is reported to have laxative effects although for problems in lactation there are no reports of symptoms in the infant (Thomson Healthcare 2007, Cuzzolin 2006). Fennel is in the same family, *Compositae*, and is reported to have similar effects.

Guarana (*Paullinia cupana*) is sold commercially as seeds, flowers, and roots to make a paste that is astringent and smells a bit like chocolate. It is used as a tonic for fatigue, headache, and dysmenorrhoea, and as a diuretic. It is a stimulant much like caffeine. When lactating women use it, it has been observed to cause stimulation of their infants with irritability and wakefulness. It is possible to overdose when other sources of caffeine such as coffee, tea, coke and chocolate are added (Thomson Healthcare 2007, Cuzzolin 2006, Frohne 1993).

Ginseng (*Panas ginseng*) has been reported to cause heart rate and rhythm changes (Barnes 1998) and other cardiac disorders. Ginsenosides have also been reported to cause mild oestrogen-like effects and clearly are contraindicated during lactation (Tesch 2003). It has also been associated during pregnancy and lactation with reports of fetal and neonatal androgenization (Awang 1991). Mastalgia with diffuse breast nodularity has been reported with Ginseng use (Palmer 1978), which is an important effect to be aware of at any time.

Liqorice (*Glycyrrhiza glabra*) is well known to be associated with hypertension, hyperkaliemia, and rhabdomyolysis. It is popular as a tea, as are many herbs especially during lactation. It is advised that no one take it longer than 6 weeks. Adverse effects have been reported in infants breastfed by mothers consuming liqorice tea. It is not recommended for use in lactation according to the PDR for Herbal Medicine (Thomson Healthcare 2007).

There is no systematic study of homeopathy as it relates to lactation. The doses of active principles in homeopathy, however, are minute.

Recommendation. The most common standardized preparations containing well-known phytotherapeutics (e.g. St John's wort for mild depression) are probably tolerable during lactation. Herbals and herbal products, at least those of unknown dosage and contamination, should be used with caution and obtained from a reliable source. Many plants, and especially roots, appear to be similar. Herbals should only be used with an expert herbalist's guidance. In general, therapeutic doses should be adhered to, and herbal teas should not be used excessively. If there is a choice, non-alcoholic preparations are preferable. Sensory changes in the milk can lead to feeding problems (Sachs 2013, American Academy of Pediatrics 2012).

4.13.2   Herbal galactogogues and antigalactogogues

Experience

Dozens of herbals are used as *galactogogues*, and these are the most frequently used herbals during lactation, to improve milk supply. They are usually ingested as teas, where several seeds, leaves, flowers or roots are steeped in a cup of boiling water. Taken in large quantities, some are anticoagulants and others can cause veno-occlusive disease, as with comfrey.

The best known of the herbal galactogogues is *fenugreek* (*Trigonella foenum-graecum*), also known as *greek hayseed*. It is a member of the Leguminosae family of plants, which includes peanuts, soy, and chickpeas. It has the odor of maple syrup, and is used as artificial maple flavoring. When the mother takes the usual dose (1–4 capsules 580–610 mg, 3 to 4 times daily), her milk, sweat, tears, and urine, and even her baby, smell of maple syrup. Fenugreek has been known for centuries to help some women but not all. It can cause colic in the infant, which is believed to be an allergic response. It can aggravate asthmatic symptoms. It has also been documented to lower blood sugar, and is used as a natural treatment for diabetics. In pregnancy, it can cause uterine cramps. It is available in capsule form or as seeds for teas and decoctions. It probably appears in the milk, as this usually smells of maple syrup. It is given a rating of B (minimal potential for toxicity), which is dose-related, by herbalists (Humphrey 2003).

Reports of several clinical trends involving Fenugreek were reported by Zapantis (2012) to increase milk supply. A randomized double blind placebo-controlled trial was described in Turkey. In this study clearly the fenugreek groups increased their milk supply and their babies gained more weight than the placebo (apple juice) group and the control group. No side effects were reported (Turkyılmaz 2011).

Goat's rue (*Galega officinalis*) is another plant credited as a galactogogue, but is rarely used alone. The only studies were in cows

Lactation

4.13 Alternative remedies, vitamins, and minerals

in 1900, when it was added to their feed. *Raspberry leaf* (*Rubus idaeus*) is mentioned in several mixtures, but it is astringent and may, over time, decrease milk supply. *Red clover* (*Trifolium pretense*) is also used, but often contains coumadin, which can cause bleeding. *Fennel* (*Foeniculum vulgare*) is a common constituent of galactogogue teas, and appears in the milk. The dried ripe fruit or seeds have some estrogenic effects, which have been demonstrated by increasing menses and increasing libido, and could actually decrease milk. The oil is toxic.

Alfalfa (*Medicago sativa*, a member of the pea family), which comes in tablet form, is also credited with being a galactogogue. It can cause diarrhea in both mother and baby, although it is otherwise non-toxic and increases milk production. The plant is benign, but the seeds have a potential for toxicity (Humphrey 2003).

Blessed thistle (*Cnicus benedictus*) is different from *milk thistle* (*Sitybum marianum*). It has an unjustified reputation as a galactogogue, but is not known to be toxic except for some reported gastrointestinal symptoms and allergic reactions. It contains many chemicals and volatile oils. It has many "uses," including bacteriostatic and antiseptic, and for dyspepsia. Experiments show antibacterial effects against a number of bacteria.

Milk thistle (*Silybum marianum*), however, has again become popular as a galactagogue, although the lactogenic mechanism of action is unknown (Zapantis 2012). It is commercially available as silymarin which consists of B flavonolignans (Barrette 2014, Thomson Healthcare 2007). Milk thistle has hepatoprotective effects that have been verified. Therapeutically the seeds also have an anti-inflammatory effect and a liver regenerative effect. It is known to be hepatoprotective in cirrhosis and has a regenerative ability of the liver in Deathcap mushroom poisoning from *Amanita*.

There are no known toxic effects when taken as a tea two to three times a day. A placebo controlled trial of milk thistle in the form of BIO-C[1] (micronized silymarin at 420 mg/day) was used in 50 healthy women when given 63 days of treatment. Quantity of milk was measured on days 0, 30, and 63. By day 30 milk production was increased 64% compared to the placebo group who increased from days 0 to 30 by 22%. At 63 days the silymarin group increased 86% and the control 32%. No silymarin was found in the milk nor was the composition of the milk changed. Historical evidence suggests silymarin has few side effects with a low incidence of nausea, flatulence, and diarrhea. Raw allergic reactions are reported when individuals are allergic to other plants in the Asteraceae/compositae family.

Borage (*Borage officinalis*) is a powerfully active plant that has been used to treat pain. It contains amabiline, which is a hepatotoxic *pyrrolizidine alkaloid* that can cause veno-occlusive disease. It should not be used in pregnancy or lactation, or as a galactogogue.

There are several herbs recommended for their effect in decreasing milk supply in cases of over-abundance or when weaning is desired. Occasionally, they are used inadvertently for other reasons and result in a decreased milk supply. These are *peppermint, sage, parsley*, and *agnus castus* (*monk's pepper*) (Conover 2004). *Peppermint oil* (*Menthax pierita*) contains menthol, which is the active ingredient. The oil should not be used on or near the infant. *Sage* (*Salvia officinalis*) should not be used as an essential oil, as it is concentrated thujone, which can cause seizures. Use of the cut or powdered leaves available as an herb for cooking, in small amounts, is safe, and does reduce milk supply. In larger amounts, it can cause tachycardia, dizziness, and hot flashes.

Parsley (Petroselinium crispum) will also lower milk supply when taken as leaves or juice in large amounts. The oil is toxic, as are the seeds. The popular tabbouleh salad is half parsley, and can affect milk supply.

Chasteberry (Vitex agnus-castus) from the Chaste tree is a known dopaminergic and FSH suppressive. It is also known to inhibit lactation due to the active principles *aucubin* and *agnoside* which suppress prolactin. It is used to treat PMS for this reason but is not recommended during pregnancy and only in small doses to decrease lactation postpartum. It has been used therapeutically in hyperprolactinemia.

Jasmine petals (Jasminum officinale) are very fragrant and are used to freshen rooms and people. They have been used for centuries to treat postpartum engorgement especially when the mother is not going to breastfeed. The petals and essential oils are recorded to reduce prolactin levels and are effective in decreasing milk supply.

Bromelain/trypsin complex was found to improve significantly the symptoms of painful breast engorgement during lactation (Snowden 2001).

Recommendation. The galactogogues fenugreek, goat's rue, alfalfa, and milk thistle are safe in modest doses in lactation. Sage, peppermint oil, parsley, chasteberry, Jasmine petals, and bromelain can be used to reduce milk supply in modest doses. In general, therapeutic doses should be adhered to and herbal teas should not be used excessively. If there is a choice, non-alcoholic preparations are preferable. Flavor changes in the milk can lead to feeding problems (ABM 2011, http://www.bfmed.org/Resources/Protocols.aspx). A public resource of herbs to avoid during lactation can be found at www.earthmamaangelbaby.com.

4.13.3 Topical treatment for breast problems

Experience

There are some herbs that have been used safely for topical application for breast problems in lactating women. The evidence again is historical and traditional. These include the following:

- *Green tea* – tea bags steeped in hot water and cooled are applied 4 times a day for sore or cracked nipples.
- *Calendula* ointment – this is applied topically to encourage healing and retain moisture in chafed nipples.
- *Cabbage leaf* – fresh, cool, dry cabbage leaves are applied to the breasts for 3 to 4 hours after nursing to reduce breast engorgement.
- *Jasmine* – topical application of jasmine flowers is used to suppress lactation (Section 4.13.2).

Recommendation. In any case of topical treatment, washing the breast after the application and before breastfeeding is recommended.

Lactation

4.13 Alternative remedies, vitamins, and minerals

4.13.4   Vitamins, minerals, and trace elements

Experience

A balanced nutritious diet should normally provide a good supply of vita-mins, minerals, and trace elements unless the mother has a malabsorption syndrome or other nutritional deficiency (Denham 2011). There are other circumstances that require some attention, however. Mothers who wish to diet need to consume at least 1,500 kilocalories per day. Vegetarians may have marginal intakes of the B vitamins, which are found in higher amounts in animal proteins. Strict "vegans" or macrobiotic vegetarians who exclude milk, eggs, and dairy products are at significant risk of being deficient in B vitamins, especially B_{12}. There are cases reported in the literature of meg-aloblastic anemia in breastfed infants whose mothers are vegans, due to B_{12} deficiency. Vegetarians are also at risk for inadequate mineral intake, especially iron and zinc (O'Connor 1994, Higginbottom 1978).

The issue of vitamin D has become significant because pregnant and lactating women have been noted to have reduced levels of vitamin D in their serum. With the use of sunscreen and the avoidance of sunlight, all women are converting less substrate to vitamin D because of lack of stimulation by sunshine. Cases of rickets in breastfed infants, even in sunny climates, have precipitated the recommendation of, for example, the American Academy of Pediatrics (2001), to give 400 i.u. vitamin D daily to breastfed infants (Collier 2004, Hollis 2004). Even when large doses of vitamin D (4000 i.u. daily) were given to the mother for 3 months, no ill effects were observed in the infant (Hollis 2004). Wagner (2006) discussed the option of maternal supplementation instead of giving vitamin D to the infant, since many women have low vitamin D levels and should take 1000 units per day during pregnancy and lacta-tion. Substitution of vitamins B_1, B_6, and B_{12} was also well-tolerated by the breastfed infant (American Academy of Pediatrics 2001).

> **Recommendation.** Vitamins, minerals, and trace elements can and should be used when the mother has real deficiencies. This also applies to iron. Such usage – and this also applies to *fluoride* for dental prophylaxis (Koparal 2000) – does not require lowering the infant's dosage in cases where he or she is also being treated directly. However, routine prescription of vitamin and mineral preparations during breastfeeding is not necessary if nutrition is balanced. In the interest of the future diet of the child who is still being breastfed, the mother should be made aware of the special importance of healthy nutrition, which, in the long run, can prevent the need for both her and her child to take not only substitutes but also therapeutic tablets. For iodine, see Chapter 4.11. Postpartum hair loss, which is frequently bemoaned and can be observed for many months, is physiologic and almost always improves spontaneously. The effectiveness of using mineral nutrients (for this condition) is no better proven than is the local use of estrogens (Denham 2011). An extensive review can be seen in Budzynska (2012).

4.13.5   Biphosphonates

Experience

Biphosphonates (*alendronate, clodronate, etidronate, ibandronate, pamidronate,* and *tiludronate*) are a group of chemicals that alter bone turnover and are used for various forms of osteoporosis.

Each one acts slightly differently. Inactivated by calcium ions, biphosphonates are poorly absorbed orally (between 0.1 and 0.5%) and would not be absorbed from the milk. Furthermore, in the few studies carried out, the chemical is almost undetectable in the milk (Siminoski 2000). Biphosphonates are considered to be safe during lactation (Lawrence 2010).

> **Recommendation.** Even though a direct, harmful effect on the breastfed child would not be expected, these medications should, if possible, not be used during breastfeeding. If alendronate is required during lactation, the infant should not be breastfed for 2 hours after dosing. The present forms of drug require dosing only once a week. If etidronate is necessary during lactation, breastfeeding should be delayed for more than 2 hours to avoid the peak plasma time. Pamidronate is poorly absorbed orally, so it is not considered to be a problem for the breastfed infant.

4.13.6   Exercise

Experience

Exercise studies have been conducted by a number of investigators. Lactic acid production as a result of serious exercise has been carefully studied. Lactic acid is bitter or sour in taste, and may, as a result, lead in some cases to temporary rejection of the breast milk (Wallace 1992). The levels of lactic acid in the milk rose from baseline before exercise (0.61×0.14 mM) to 1.06×33 mM after typical moderate exercise, and to 2.88×0.80 mM after maximal effort, in these same women. This is above the adult taste level of 1.6 mM. The effect lasted for 90 minutes. The impact of regular exercise on the volume and composition of breast milk as well as prolactin levels was studied. No difference was found between exercising and sedentary women (Dewey 1994). Moderate exercise sufficient to improve cardiovascular fitness without marked changes in energy expenditure, dietary intake, and bodyweight and composition does not jeopardize lactation performance (American Academy Practice 2001, Prentice 1994).

> **Recommendation.** There are no contraindications to moderate exercise while lactating.

4.13.7   Glucose 6-phosphate-dehydrogenase deficiency

Experience

Infants with glucose 6-phosphate-dehydrogenase deficiency (G 6-PD deficiency) may develop hemolytic crisis when exposed to *primaquine, salicylates, sulfonamides, nitrofurans, phenacetin, naphthalene*, some *vitamin K* derivatives (although usual neonatal vitamin K prophylaxis seems to be well tolerated), and certain foodstuffs (e.g. *fava beans*). G 6-PD deficiency is found in 10% of the black population, and in those from the Mediterranean basin (Italians, Greeks, Arabs, and Sephardic Jews). There are no data available regarding the reaction to these drugs when present in breast milk. Apparently, the dosage of the medications involved and the nutritional components in the milk are too low.

References

ABM. Academy of Breastfeeding Medicine Protocol Committee. Clinical Protocol #9: use of galactogogues in initiating or augmenting the rate of maternal mild secretion. Breastfeed Med 2011; 6: 41–9.

American Academy of Pediatrics. Section on breastfeeding, breastfeeding and the use of human milk. Pediatrics 2012; 129: e841; doi/10.1542 Peds.2011-3552.

American Academy of Pediatrics. Committee on Drugs. The transfer of drugs and other chemicals into human milk. Pediatrics 2001; 108: 776–89.

Awang DV. Maternal use of ginseng and neonatal androgenisation. JAMA 1991; 266: 363.

Barnes J, Mills SY, Abbot NC et al. Different standards for reporting ADRs to herbal remedies and conventional OTC medicines: face-to-face interviews with 515 users of herbal remedies. Br J Clin Pharmacol 1998; 45: 496–500.

Barrette EP, Basch E, Basch S. Milkthistle. Natural Standard: the Authority on Integrative Medicine (Internet) Cambridge, MA, 2014, http://www.naturalstandard.com.

Budzynska K, Gardner ZE, Dugoua JJ et al. Systematic review of breastfeeding and herbs. Breastfeed Med 2012; 7: 489–503.

Collier S, Fulhan J, Duggan C. Nutrition for the pediatric office: update on vitamins, infant feeding and food allergies. Curr Opin Pediatr 2004; 16: 314–20.

Conover E, Buehler BA. Use of herbal agents by breastfeeding women may affect infants. Pediatr Ann 2004; 33: 235–40.

Cuzzolin L, Zaffani S, Benoni G. Safety implications regarding use of phytomedicines. Euro Clin Pharmacol 2006; 62: 37–42.

Denham BE. Dietary supplements-regulatory issues and implications for public health. JAMA 2011; 306: 428–9.

Dewey KG, Lovelady CA, Nommsen-Rivers LA et al. Randomized study of the effects of aerobic exercise by lactating women on breast-milk volume and composition. N Engl J Med 1994; 330: 449–53.

Dugoua JJ, Mills E, Perri D, Koren G. Safety and efficacy of St. John's wort (hypericum) during pregnancy and lactation. Can J Clin Pharmacol 2006a; 13: e268–76.

Dugoua JJ, Mills E, Perri D, Koren G. Safety and efficacy of gingko (gingko biloba) during pregnancy and lactation. Can J Clin Pharmacol 2006b; 13: e277–84.

Dugoua JJ, Seely D, Perri D et al. Safety and efficacy of black cohosh (cimicifuga racemosa) during pregnancy and lactation. Can J Clin Pharmacol 2006c; 13: e257–61.

Dugoua JJ, Seely D, Perri D, Mills E, Koren G. Safety and efficacy of black cohosh (Caulophyllum thalictrodies) during pregnancy and lactation. Can J Clin Pharmacol 2008a; 15: e66–73.

Dugoua JJ, Seely D, Perri D, Mills E, Koren G. Safety and efficacy of chastetree (vitex agnus-cactus) during pregnancy and lactation. Can J Clin Pharmacol 2008b; 15: e74–9.

FDA. Food and Drug Administration. Consumer advisory: kava-containing dietary supplements may be associated with severe liver injury. March 25, 2002. Available at: www.fda.gov/Food/Resourcesforyou/consumers/ucm085482.htm (accessed November 26, 2012.)

Frohne D. Guarana-de neue Muntermacher, IN: DAZ 1993; 133: 218.

Higginbottom MC, Sweetman L, Nyhan WL. A syndrome of methylmalonic aciduria, homocystinuria, megaloblastic anemia and neurologic abnormalities in a vitamin B12-deficient breastfed infant of a strict vegetarian. New Engl J Med 1978; 299: 317–23.

Hollis BW, Wagner CL. Vitamin D requirements during lactation: high-dose maternal supplementation as therapy to prevent hypovitaminosis D for both the mother and the nursing infant. Am J Clin Nutr 2004; 80: 1752–8.

Humphrey S. The Nursing Mother's Herbal. Minneapolis, MN: Fairview Press, 2003.

Klier CM, Schmid-Siefel B, Schäfer MR, et al. St. Johns wort (Hypericum perforatum) and breastfeeding plasma and breast milk concentrations of hyperforin for 5 mothers and 2 infants. J Clin Psychiatr 2006; 67: 305–9.

Koparal E, Ertugrul F, Oztekin K. Fluoride levels in breast milk and infants food. J Clin Pediatr Dent 2000; 24: 299–302.

Lawrence RA, Lawrence RM. Breastfeeding: A Guide for the Medical Profession, 7th edn 2010, Philadelphia, PA: Elsevier.

O'Connor DL. Folate status during pregnancy and lactation. Adv Exp Med Biol 1994; 352: 157.

Palmer BV, Montgomery ACV, Monteiro JC. Ginseng and Mastalgia. BMJ 1978; 1: 1284.

Perri D, Dugoua JJ, Mills E, Koren G. Safety and efficacy of Echinacea (Echinacea angustafolia, E. Purperea and E. pallida) during pregnancy and lactation. Can J Clin Pharmcol 2006; 13: e262–7.

Prentice A. Should lactating women exercise? Nutr Rev 1994; 52: 358.

Sachs HC. The transfer of drugs and therapeutics into human breast milk: an update on selected topics. Pediatrics 2013; DOI:10.1542/peds.2013-1985.

Seely D, Dugoua JJ, Perri D et al. Safety and efficacy of panax ginseng during pregnancy and lactation. Can J Clin Pharmacol 2008; 15: e87–94.

Siminoski K, Fitzgerald AA, Flesch G et al. Intravenous pamidronate for treatment of reflex sympathetic dystrophy during breastfeeding. J Bone Miner Res 2000; 15: 2052–5.

Snowden HM, Renfrew MJ, Woolridge MW. Treatments for breast engorgement during lactation. Cochrane Database Syst Rev 2001; 2: CD000046.

Tesch, BJ. Herbs commonly used by women: an evidence-based review. Am J Obstetr Gynecol 2003; 188: S44–55.

Thomson Healthcare. PDR for Herbal Medicines, 4th edn, 2007, Healthcare Inc, Mondale, NJ.

Turkyılmaz C, Onal E, Hirfanoglu M. The effect of galactagogue herbal tea on breast milk production and short-term catch-up of birth weight in the first week of life. J Alern Complement Med 2011; 17: 139–42.

US Government Accountability Office. Herbal dietary supplements: examples of deceptive or questionable marketing practices and potentially dangerous advice. May 26, 2010. Available at: www.gao.gov/products/GAO-10-662T. (accessed November 26, 2012.)

Wagner CL, Hulsey TC, Fanning D et al. High-dose vitamin D3 supplementation in a cohort of breastfeeding mothers and their infants: a 6-month follow-up pilot study. Breastfeed Med 2006; 1: 59–70.

Wallace JP, Inbar G, Ernsthausen K. Infant acceptance of postexercise breast milk. Pediatrics 1992; 89: 1245–7.

Zapantis A, Steinberg JG, Schilit L. Use of herbals as galactagogues. J Pharm Pract 2012; 25: 222–31.

Contrast media, radionuclides and diagnostics 4.14

Stefanie Hultzsch

4.14.1	X-ray studies, ultrasound, and magnetic resonance imaging	813
4.14.2	Iodine-containing contrast media	813
4.14.3	Magnetic resonance contrast agents	815
4.14.4	Ultrasound contrast media	816
4.14.5	Radionuclides	816
4.14.6	Dyes	817
4.14.7	Other diagnostics	818

X-ray studies, ultrasound and magnetic resonance imaging (MRI) do not require an interruption of breastfeeding. This also applies to mammography and computer tomography without contrast media. Limitations apply for iodine- and gadolinium-containing contrast media and radioisotopes. Before applying contrast media or radioisotopes all possible alternatives should be considered. For iodine containing contrast media, breastfeeding should be interrupted for 24–48 hours if possible. For gadolinium-containing contrast media, compounds with a low risk of nephrogenic systemic fibrosis should be chosen to minimize any possible risk for the breastfed infant. The application of radioisotopes, especially ^{131}iodine, to the breastfeeding mother should be avoided.

4.14.1 X-ray studies, ultrasound, and magnetic resonance imaging

X-ray studies, ultrasound and magnetic resonance imaging (MRI) – independent of the organ being studied – do not require an interruption of breastfeeding. This also applies to mammography and computed tomography without contrast media. Limitations apply for iodine- and gadolinium-containing contrast media and radioisotopes (see below).

4.14.2 Iodine-containing contrast media

Problematic for the infant is the amount of free iodine in the contrast medium, which is normally under 1% of the total amount of contrast medium. This amount is determined by production and can increase during storage. Once administered, more free iodine may be released as a result of de-iodizing enzymes in the mother's or the infant's body. The effect of free iodide on the infant's thyroid depends on the iodine saturation before the application of contrast media. In a latent deficiency status, flooding (e.g. from the contrast medium) with iodine is more likely to lead to an effect on function than in a well-balanced iodine state.

The significance of the iodine transfer to the baby after administration of iodine containing contrast media to the breastfeeding mother cannot be adequately determined by simply measuring iodide, or contrast medium iodine in the infant's urine. The individual situation can only be precisely described with an assessment of the infant's iodine uptake and thyroid function.

Gross impairment of the breastfed infant following contrast administration to the mother is unknown. With direct diagnostic use, particularly in infants under 3 months of age, transient hypothyroidism has been described (Parravicini 1996). The effect can be due to discrete actions on the sensitive development of the brain in infancy, and usage should be avoided. However, since breastfed children only receive about 0.01% of a therapeutic infant dose of an iodine-containing contrast medium via the mother's milk, no serious consequences would be expected. In a review examining the effects on thyroid function after application of iodine-containing contrast media to neonates, the authors conclude that there is a relevant risk of hypothyroidism especially for preterm infants (Ahmet 2009). After oral application of *loxitalamic acid* 8 days postpartum to the mother, an increase in TSH (just above normal reference values) in the fully breastfed infant was noted. The level returned to normal after 10 days and no clinical abnormalities were noted in the child (unpublished data from Berlin TIS).

The water-soluble iodine-containing contrast media, *meglumine amidotrizoate* and *sodium amidotrizoate, iodamide, iohexol* and *metrizamide*, administered intravenously, appear in the milk available to a fully breastfed baby for a relative dose considerably under 1% (Nielsen 1987, Texier 1983, Fitzjohn 1982, Ilett 1981).

With iohexol and *metrizoate*, Nielsen (1987) did not expect an appreciable exposure in the breastfed infant requiring a limitation of breastfeeding. This global estimate seems questionable, since one of the four subjects in their study with ongoing high iodine concentrations of up to 141 mg/L milk, was not considered in the study summary. The authors calculated half-lives in the milk of 15–108 hours for iohexol and metrizoate. The serum half-lives of water-soluble contrast media of about 2 hours are considerably shorter. Metrizoate is no longer approved for intravenous administration.

For the fat-soluble *iopanoic acid*, used for biliary duct imaging, 7% of the maternal weight-related dose was calculated for the breastfed infant in an older study (Holmdahl 1956). Iopanoic acid is also no longer regularly used.

There are no data available on other iodine-containing contrast media such as *iobitridol, iodixanol, iomeprol, iopamidol, iopentol, iopodate, iopromide, iothalaminic acid, iotrolan, iotroxic acid, ioversol, ioxaglinic acid, loxitalamic acid, lysine amido-trizoate*.

The European Society of Urogenital Radiology (ESUR 2013) recommends that breastfeeding may be continued after application of iodine-based contrast agents to the mother. The American College of Radiology (ACR 2013) is of the same opinion; although it cautions that an informed decision to temporarily stop breastfeeding for 24 hours should be left to the mother. The guideline especially states that there is no established value to stop breastfeeding beyond 24 hours.

> **Recommendation.** When the mother is given an iodine-containing contrast medium, the possibility that the infant will absorb a significantly higher amount of free iodide than required for supplementation (Chapter 4.11.6) cannot be eliminated. Therefore, the necessity of an examination with iodine-containing contrast media and all the alternative diagnostic methods must be critically considered. With the extensive choice of other procedures, especially ultrasound, there are often safer options available. If the use of an iodine-containing contrast agent is unavoidable and the examination cannot be postponed, breastfeeding should be interrupted for 24–48 hours, at least for a fully-breastfed infant under the age of 2 months, to avoid all possible risks. This period can be bridged with milk that has been pumped ahead of time. If prior pumping of milk is not possible because of the urgency of the examination, breastfeeding can be continued, especially with an older infant. The child should then be observed for signs of hypothyroidism.

4.14.3 Magnetic resonance contrast agents

In magnetic resonance imaging, contrast agents containing *Gadolinium* are regularly used. *Gadopentetic acid* excretion into the milk was measured in a single patient over an observation time of 33 hours, 0.01% of the total administered dose of Gadolinium was found (Schmiedl 1990). In a study of 18 women, a dose was calculated for the breastfed baby, which represents less than 1% of the recommended diagnostic intravenous dose per kg of body weight (Kubik-Huch 2000).

With gadodiamide, studies on rats indicate a very limited transfer into the mother's milk (Okazaki 1996). There are no data available on other gadolinium-containing contrast media. However, it should be noted that gadolinium chelate can be degraded in the body to *gadolinium(III)* which is toxic and stored in bone (Darrah 2009).

In 2006 a causal relationship between nephrogenic systemic fibrosis (NSF), a fibrosing disease mainly of the skin and subcutaneous tissues, and gadolinium-based contrast agents was discussed (Grobner 2006). The European Society of Urogenital Radiology (Thomsen 2013) therefore recommends that breastfeeding should be interrupted for 24 hours if gadolinium-based contrast agents with a high risk for NSF are given to the mother in order to avoid any risk to the infant. Other publications advise preferentially using the more stable macrocyclic preparations, which are thought to have a lower risk for NSF in the breastfeeding woman (Fröhlich 2013). The American College of Radiology (ACR) recommends that breastfeeding does not need to be interrupted after administration of gadolinium-based contrast agents; although an informed decision to temporarily stop breastfeeding for 24 hours should be left to the mother.

Ferristen is, from a theoretical toxicological viewpoint, harmless for the breastfed infant. No human data is available on *ferucarbotran* (only available in Japan), but no transfer into mothers milk was seen in rats in 24 hours. For *ferumoxsil*, no transfer into human milk was noted.

Due to insufficient experience, no risk assessment is possible for the manganese-containing *mangafodipir*. On the other hand, the advice of the manufacturer to interrupt breastfeeding for 14 days does not seem to be justified.

> **Recommendation.** If their use cannot be delayed, continued breastfeeding is acceptable if gadolinium-containing contrast media with a low risk of NSF are used in the lowest possible dose despite insufficient experience. If a gadolinium-containing contrast agent with a higher risk of NSF has to be used, breast feeding should be interrupted for 24 hours if possible. This period can be bridged with milk that has been pumped ahead of time.
> Mangafodipir should be avoided.

4.14.4   Ultrasound contrast media

D-galactose is used as a contrast medium in ultrasound diagnostics. Galactose also occurs naturally in mother's milk. For *perflutren*, another ultrasound contrast medium, there are no data on use during breastfeeding. Perflutren is exhaled, and the naturally occurring phospholipids in the lipid microspheres are dispersed into the body's own fat depots. The synthetic component MPEG5000 is excreted renally. There are no studies on transfer into the mother's milk. However, it is conceivable that such transfer will occur with lipophilic substances. *Sulfur hexafluoride* in microspheres is used as contrast medium in ultrasound examinations. There are also no data available on use during breastfeeding. For clinical use, only very small doses are used (16 µl SF6) and the half-life is about 12 minutes (Fröhlich 2013).

> **Recommendation.** D-galactose may be used during breastfeeding. There are no data on perflutren; therefore, it should be used with caution. On sulfur hexafluoride there are also no data available, but the risk should be negligible due to the small doses used.

4.14.5   Radionuclides

131Iodine (^{131}I) accumulates in the mother's milk just like "normal" iodine (see Chapter 2.20). In a comparison of 31 radioisotopes, which can be taken in by the mother orally, or by inhalation at work or from the environment, ^{131}I accumulates the most in the milk – with 30% of the maternal dose followed by ^{45}Ca and ^{137}Cs (each 20%) as well as ^{90}Sr (10%) (Harrison 2003). In a comprehensive overview comprising 16 evaluated publications, an extensive summary of kinetic data on ^{131}I is reported (Simon 2002). The median half-life for the concentration in the milk was given by the authors as about 12 hours. If stable iodine was given as a thyroid blockade before the mother's exposure, the half-life of the ^{131}I was, on average, 8.5 hours. In both cases, the maximum value after exposure was reached about 9 hours later. Stable iodine blocks the uptake of ^{131}I by the mammary glands and the infant's thyroid, so that the intake of the radio isotope by the infant is minimized.

A comprehensive review about radiation safety for the American Thyroid Association recommends that women who are lactating, or have recently stopped breastfeeding, should not be treated with ^{131}I, since the lactating breast concentrates iodide (Sisson 2011). Breastfeeding should, therefore, be stopped at least 6 weeks prior to administration of ^{131}I to limit radiation to the breast tissue.

Bennett (1996) summarized the kinetics of many radiopharmaceuticals during breastfeeding. It is difficult to decide at what level of residual activity of these radiopharmaceuticals in the milk, can breastfeeding be permitted again. Generally a dose of 1 mSv for the infant has been considered acceptable.

In the context of the Chernobyl nuclear disaster and the concomitant radioiodine contamination, a threshold value of 500 Bq/L for infant nutrition or milk was set. Following the reactor accident in the spring of 2011 in the Fukushima region of Japan, 2.2–8 Bq/L milk were measured in some women. These values lie significantly under the highest values applicable in Japan of 100 Bq/L for radioiodine in drinking water for children (Foodwatch 2011).

The scintigraphy scans that are performed today, primarily with *technetium*, are considered much less problematic compared to iodine isotopes. An acceptable residual dose of 1 mSv is generally achieved with an interruption of breastfeeding for 10–12 hours for pumping (and discarding) of one feeding (Prince 2004, Bennett 1996).

In various studies, *18FDG* (2-deoxy-2-(18F)fluoro-D-glucose) used for positron-emission-tomography (PET), has been documented in the lactating breast (Shor 2002). Here the primary radiation load appears as a result of an increased uptake of the radiopharmaceutical into the glandular tissue of the lactating breast. 18FDG is then barely excreted into the mother's milk, so that feeding of pumped milk by a third person is possible to keep the radiation dose for the infant as low as possible (Devine 2010).

> **Recommendation.** Diagnostic or therapeutic use of radiopharmaceuticals, mostly technetium or iodine isotopes, should be postponed until the end of the breastfeeding period. For diagnostic studies that cannot be postponed, breastfeeding should be interrupted, depending on the isotope used and its dosage, until the effective dose for the child has fallen below 1 mSv. Therapeutic use of 131I requires advance weaning to minimize radiation exposure of the infant and also the breast tissue.

4.14.6   Dyes

Fluorescein is used orally and intravenously (angiography) and as a diagnostic agent for the eye. Even after use in the eye, it is detected in the milk (Mattern 1990). With intravenous use, an elimination half-life of 62 hours in the milk is anticipated. The infant would ingest, at most, a relative dose of 0.5% of the weight-related maternal dose (Maguire 1988). Toxic effects via the mother's milk are unlikely. *Indocyanine green* (sometimes with *sodium iodide*) is used for retina angiography, for measuring microcirculation and hepatic blood flow. There are no data on its use during breastfeeding. Caution is recommended if sodium iodide is included.

> **Recommendation.** Breastfeeding may continue after diagnostic administration of fluorescein. No data are available on the use of the other dyes during breastfeeding.

Lactation

4.14 Contrast media, radionuclides and diagnostics

4.14.7   Other diagnostics

Skin tests such as the *tuberculin* test, multi-test or allergy tests are considered harmless during breastfeeding (Bloch 1995).
This also applies for enzyme tests such as secretin.

> **Recommendation.** The diagnostics mentioned may be used during breastfeeding.

References

ACR (American College of Radiology) Manual on Contrast Media: http://www.acr.org/~/media/ACR/Documents/PDF/QualitySafety/Resources/Contrast%20Manual/2013_Contrast_Media.pdf.

Ahmet A, Lawson ML, Babyn P et al. Hypothyroidism in neonates post-iodinated contrast media: a systematic review. Acta Paediatr 2009; 98: 1568–74.

Bennett PN. *Drugs and Human Lactation*, 2nd edn, Amsterdam, New York, Oxford, Elsevier B.V. 1996.

Bloch AB, Advisory Council for the Elimination of Tuberculosis. Screening for tuberculosis and tuberculosis infection in high-risk populations: Recommendations of the Advisory Council for the Elimination of Tuberculosis. MMWR 1995; 44: 18–34.

Darrah T, Poreda R, Campbell E et al. The incorporation of Gd in human bone from medical contrast imaging. Geochimica et Cosmochimica Acta 2009; 73: A262.

Devine CE, Mawlawi O. Radiation safety with positron emission tomography and computed tomography. Semin Ultrasound CT MR 2010; 31: 39–45.

ESUR (European Society of Urogenital Radiology) Guidelines on Contrast Media, v8.1. http://www.esur.org/guidelines/en/index.php (accessed December 8, 2013).

Fitzjohn TP, Williams DG, Laker MF et al. Intravenous urography during lactation. Br J Radiol 1982; 55: 603–5.

Foodwatch. Calculated Fatalities from Radiation: Officially Permissible Limits for Radioactively Contaminated Food in the European Union and Japan. Table 2. http://www.fukushima-disaster.de/fileadmin/user_upload/pdf/english/calculated_fatalities_from_radiation_report_foodwatch-IPPNW.pdf, 2011.

Fröhlich JM, Kubik-Huch RA. Radiographic, MR or ultrasound contrast media in pregnant or breast-feeding women: what are the key issues? Rofo 2013; 185: 13–25.

Grobner T. Gadolinium – a specific trigger for the development of nephrogenic fibrosing dermopathy and nephrogenic systemic fibrosis? Nephrol Dial Transplant 2006; 21: 1104–8.

Harrison JD, Smith TJ, Phipps AW. Infant doses from the transfer of radionuclides in mothers' milk. Radiat Prot Dosimetry 2003; 105: 251–6.

Holmdahl KH. Cholecystography during lactation. Acta Radiol 1956; 45: 305–7.

Ilett KF, Hackett LP, Paterson JW et al. Excretion of metrizamide in milk. Br J Radiol 1981; 54: 537–8.

Kubik-Huch RA, Gottstein-Aalame NM, Frenzel T et al. Gadopentetate dimeglumine excretion into human breast milk during lactation. Radiology 2000; 216: 555–8.

Mattern J, Mayer PR. Excretion of fluorescein into breast milk. Am J Ophthalmol 1990; 109: 598–9.

Maguire, A. M., and Bennett, J. (1988). Fluorescein elimination in human breast milk. Arch. Ophthalmol. 106: 718–9.

Nielsen ST, Matheson I, Rasmussen JN et al. Excretion of iohexol and metrizoate in human breast milk. Acta Radiol 1987; 28: 523–6.

Okazaki O, Murayama N, Masubuchi N et al. Placental transfer and milk secretion of gadodiamide injection in rats. Arzneimittelforschung 1996; 46: 83–6.

Parravicini E, Fontana C, Paterlini GL et al. Iodine, thyroid function, and very low birth weight infants. Pediatrics 1996; 98: 730–4.

Prince JR, Rose MR. Measurement of radioactivity in breast milk following 99mTc-Leukoscan injection. Nucl Med Commun 2004; 25: 963–6.

Schmiedl U, Maravilla KR, Gerlach R et al. Excretion of gadopentetate dimeglumine in human breast milk. AJR Am J Roentgenol 1990; 154: 1305–6.

Shor M, Dave N, Reddy M et al. Asymmetric FDG uptake in a lactating breast. Clin Nucl Med 2002; 27: 536.

Simon SL, Luckyanov N, Bouville A et al. Transfer of ^{131}I into human breast milk and transfer coefficients for radiological dose assessments. Health Phys 2002; 82: 796–806.

Sisson JC, Freitas J, McDougall IR et al. Radiation safety in the treatment of patients with thyroid diseases by radioiodine [131]I: practice recommendations of the American Thyroid Association. Thyroid 2011; 21: 335–46.

Texier F, Roque d'Orbcastel O, Etling N. Stable iodine level in human milk after pulmonary angiography. Presse Med 1983; 12: 769.

Thomsen HS, Morcos SK, Almen T et al. Nephrogenic systemic fibrosis and gadolinium-based contrast media: updated ESUR Contrast Medium Safety Committee guidelines. Eur Radiol 2013; 23: 307–18.

Infections during breastfeeding

4.15

Bernke te Winkel and Christof Schaefer

4.15.1	Common infections	822
4.15.2	Cytomegaly	822
4.15.3	Dengue virus	823
4.15.4	Hepatitis A	823
4.15.5	Hepatitis B	824
4.15.6	Hepatitis C	824
4.15.7	Hepatitis E	824
4.15.8	Herpes simplex	825
4.15.9	Herpes zoster (shingles), chicken pox (varicella)	825
4.15.10	HIV infection	826
4.15.11	Human T-lymphotropic virus (HTLV)	827
4.15.12	Influenza	827
4.15.13	Lyme disease	828
4.15.14	Methicillin-resistant *Staphylococcus aureus* (MRSA)	828
4.15.15	Rotavirus	828
4.15.16	Tuberculosis	829
4.15.17	West Nile virus	830
4.15.18	Other infectious diseases	830

Even when the general condition of the mother with an infection would permit breastfeeding, various aspects must be considered, i.e. whether symptoms in the infant would be expected from the medication prescribed and whether transmission of the illness through the mother's milk is possible. In the final analysis, only very few infectious illnesses are transmitted through the milk. Infection after birth occurs mostly through the close contact between mother and child. Among those pathogens which can be transmitted via the milk are the human immune deficiency-virus (HIV), the human cytomegaly virus (HCMV) and the human T cell lymphotropic virus (HTLV) (Lawrence 2004).

Drugs During Pregnancy and Lactation. **http://dx.doi.org/10.1016/B978-0-12-408078-2.00040-8**

4.15.1   Common infections

> **Recommendation.** From a virological and bacteriological perspective, colds, flu-like infections, and simple gastrointestinal infections, represent no barrier to breastfeeding. There could be limitations due to the mother's general condition. General hygiene measures should be observed. Beyond that, the mother should drink sufficient fluid. This applies especially to febrile and diarrheal infections.

4.15.2   Cytomegaly

Cytomegalovirus (CMV) is a ubiquitous DNA herpesvirus that causes a wide variety of clinical manifestations. The human cytomegaly virus (HCMV) is widespread, and its prevalence varies in different populations between 40 and 100%. During the pregnancy, with a fresh HCMV infection, there may be an intrauterine infection in 40–50% of cases, while 1 to 3% is the most common congenital infection. Seven to 10% of the congenitally infected children show hematological, neurological or sensory abnormalities. A perinatal infection is not significant. Infection via the mother' milk has been documented with a reactivation of the HCMV of up to 90% in the mammary glands. HCMV-DNA has been detected in the milk, and infection of breastfed children is known. However, its course in full-term babies is asymptomatic as a rule, probably due to the passive intrauterine immunization through the placenta with IgG antibodies when a mother has had the infection. For this reason, there is no limitation on breastfeeding babies born after the 32nd week of pregnancy. Of more concern is breastfeeding or giving mother's milk to extremely prematurely born infants (<32 SSW, <1,500 g), because they have not yet developed sufficient immune competency and have not received adequate passive immunization. Inactivation by Holder pasteurization (30 minutes at 62°C) and the gentler brief pasteurization (10 seconds at 72°C) has been documented. A good alternative seems to be brief pasteurization for 5 seconds at 62°C, which was recently tested in a German study. This makes possible certain inactivation of the HCMV-virus and, at the same time, protection of the immune factors in mother's milk (Goelz 2009). Freezing at −20°C for 24 hours or longer reduces, but does not eliminate HCMV (Jim 2009, Curtis 2005, Hamprecht 2001). The infection rate of premature infants after feeding, both with previously frozen as well as fresh milk, has been evaluated in many studies – with a range from 5 to 38% (Buxmann 2009, Capretti 2009, Miron 2005). Four to 50% of the infected babies showed symptoms, while a case series described five seriously ill premature infants, among them one death (24+5 SSW) (Hamele 2010). In other studies, the babies with symptomatic infections mostly had mild courses of hematologic (*thrombocytopenia, neutropenia*) or hepatological (transaminase increase, *cholestasis*) (Jim 2009, Neuberger 2006). All of these babies recovered well with no lasting effects. In a recent meta-analysis, among 299 infants fed untreated breast milk, 19% acquired CMV infection and 4% developed CMV-associated sepsis-like syndrome (Lanzieri 2013). Among 212 infants fed frozen breast milk, there were only slightly lower rates of CMV infection, but similar rates of sepsis-like syndrome.

Long-term studies after 2 to 4 years did not find any differences in hearing tests, motor or speech development and no neurological abnormalities with CMV-infected premature infants (Capretti 2009, Doctor 2005, Miron 2005, Vollmer 2004).

To date, there are no clear guidelines nor a unified procedure for breastfeeding management of premature infants of HCMV-positive mothers (Buxmann 2010). Recommendations of pediatric societies vary from avoiding breastfeeding, through pasteurization or freezing, to feeding with fresh mother's milk.

> **Recommendation.** Newborns with a gestational age >32 weeks can be breastfed without limitation. With premature infants <32 weeks or <1,500 g, Holder or brief pasteurization may be used until the baby reaches the corrected thirty-second week of gestation.

4.15.3 Dengue virus

Dengue viruses are members of the family Flaviviridae genus Flavivirus. They are small enveloped viruses containing a single-strand RNA genome of positive polarity. Dengue is transmitted between humans by mosquitoes. Dengue virus can be vertically transmitted to the fetus in utero or to the infant at parturition (Pouliot 2010).

A case report describes breast milk as a possible route of transmission (Barthel 2013). The mother was hospitalized for preterm labor and appeared to be infected with the Dengue virus during pregnancy. The preterm infant was fed with expressed milk from day 2, then breastfed. Dengue virus was detected in the breast milk (RT-PCR positive) and the breastfeeding was stopped. On day 4 the infant developed fever and his serum tested positive for the Dengue virus. Cord blood tested negative for the Dengue virus as well as the infant's blood samples collected from day 0 and day 2. Although other routes of transmission cannot be excluded, transmission of Dengue virus through breastfeeding might be possible. Significant breast milk viral loads and breastfeeding transmission route have been described for other flavaviruses.

> **Recommendation.** Whether women should abstain from breastfeeding if they have an acute Dengue infection, must be decided in individual cases.

4.15.4 Hepatitis A

Hepatitis A virus (HAV) is a non-enveloped, icosahedral, positive-stranded RNA virus classified in the Heparnavirus genus of the Picornaviridae family. HAV is mostly spread via the fecal-oral route. Although HAV RNA can be detected in breast milk in lactating mothers with acute HAV infection, there is no indication that breastfeeding contributes to transmission of HAV from an infected mother to her child (Daudi 2012).

> **Recommendation.** If a mother is ill with hepatitis A, the newborn may be breastfed. Depending on national recommendations the infant should be immunized within 7 days when a mother becomes ill with Hepatitis A, due to close body contact and the risk of infection, just like the other members of the household.

4.15.5   Hepatitis B

Hepatitis B virus (HBV) is an enveloped DNA virus that is a member of the Hepadnaviridae family. Vertical transmission is one of the most important causes of chronic HBV infection and is the most common mode of transmission worldwide (Petrova 2010). Hepatitis B is only rarely transmitted via the placenta. Breastfeeding does not appear to increase the risk of transmission, therefore, newborns whose mothers are HBsAg- and HBeAg-positive are simultaneously immunized immediately after birth. Children of HBeAg-positive mothers have a higher risk of becoming ill. HBsAg, HBeAg and HBV-DNA have been detected in mother's milk, with the viral load correlating with that in the maternal serum (Lin 1993, Linnemann 1974). No studies have shown an increased risk of illness for the infant through breastfeeding when the mother was exclusively HBsAg positive (Gonzalez 1995, Tseng 1988). Among some 100 breastfeeding mothers with a chronic infection, of which 22% (11/51) were HBeAg positive, there was no indication of an infection via mother's milk following simultaneous immunization of the infant (Hill 2002). The authors qualified their recommendation on the safety of breastfeeding with reference to the relatively small number of mother–child pairs studied, and the uncertainty of transmission with the greater infectiousness of the HBeAg-positive mothers.

> **Recommendation.** If a mother is ill with hepatitis B, the newborn may be breastfed after simultaneous immunization (active and immunoglobulin).

4.15.6   Hepatitis C

Hepatitis C virus (HCV) is a positive-strand RNA virus. Most HCV infections are acquired through percutaneous exposure to infected blood. Sexual and household transmission of HCV does occur (Ackerman 2000). Mother-to-child (vertical) transmission is now the main route of infection in children (Tovo 2005). Fourteen cohort studies with a total of nearly 3000 mother-infant pairs found no association between breastfeeding by women infected with HVC and the risk for transmission to infants (Cottrell 2013).

The guidelines of the European Paediatric Hepatitis C Virus Network, American Academy of Pediatrics, the Centers for Disease Control and Prevention, and the US Preventive Services Task Force see no evidence for hepatitis C transmission through breastfeeding, though a minimal risk cannot be ruled out (Cottrell 2013, Pembrey 2005). They recommend not advising against breastfeeding.

> **Recommendation.** Breastfeeding is possible with a hepatitis C infection. Whether women should abstain from breastfeeding if their nipples are cracked or bleeding, must be decided in individual cases.

4.15.7   Hepatitis E

Hepatitis E virus (HEV) is a non-enveloped single-stranded RNA virus. It has been classified as the single member of the genus hepevirus in the family Hepeviridae. Vertical transmission of HEV from infected pregnant women to their newborn is well known (Aggarwal 2011). One study investigated the status of anti-HEV and HEV-RNA in the colostrum of HEV infected mothers and the possibility of transmission of HEV to their infants by breastfeeding. HEV was found in maternal milk, but none of the 86 breast-fed infants had any evidence of HEV infection until nine months of age. Formula feeding was advice given to mothers with symptomatic HEV infection, especially with high viral loads of viremia, because of the potential hazard of transmission of infection from infected breast milk, or minute maternal skin abrasions of the nipple by suckling (Chibber 2004). The available data are insufficient for a definitive evaluation of the risk.

> **Recommendation.** Breastfeeding needs not to be discouraged for infants born to asymptomatic anti-HEV positive mothers. Women with a symptomatic HEV infection, especially with high viral loads of viremia should not breastfeed.

4.15.8   Herpes simplex

Herpes simplex virus type 1 or type 2 (HSV) are double-stranded DNA-enveloped viruses. HSV is a member of the herpesvirus family. The majority of newborn infections results from intrapartum transmission (Read 2008).

HSV-DNA has been detected in the mother's milk (Kotronias 1999). With the exception of one possible infection through mother's milk, 6 days postpartum, no illness has been described (Dunkle 1979). In four case reports, an infection of the mother's breast by children with herpetic gingivostomatitis was described (Gupta 2008).

> **Recommendation.** With a local herpes simplex infection, general hygiene measures, e.g. strict hand-washing, mouth protection with herpes labialis, and avoiding direct contact with the affected area of the skin, should be carried out. If the nipple itself is affected, the infant should not be put to breast on the affected side until the lesion is healed.

4.15.9   Herpes zoster (shingles), chicken pox (varicella)

Varicella-zoster virus (VZV) is a member of the herpesvirus family and infection causes two clinically distinct forms of disease: varicella (chickenpox) and herpes zoster (shingles). Primary VZV infection results in the diffuse vesicular rash of varicella or chickenpox. DNA of the varicella-zoster viruses (VZV) has been detected in the mother's milk (Yoshida 1992). In a case report, the varicella infection of a breastfed child through the mother's milk of a woman with herpes zoster was discussed. The mother developed herpes zoster in the dermatome T 4–5 with involvement of the right breast. Separate milk samples were taken from both breasts. VZV-DNA was detected only in the right breast. Thus the authors assume an infection of the mammary glands with shedding of the virus DNA in the milk, and not over/via a hematogenic spread. This would mean that the milk from the affected side must be discarded. However, it could not be ruled out that the infection of the child occurred via direct contact with the herpes blisters on the skin (Yoshida 1995). Varicella zoster viruses were not, though, found in the mother's milk with zoster or with chicken pox (Frederick 1986).

> **Recommendation.** When a mother has a chicken pox infection in the week before and after the birth, the baby receives varicella hyperimmune globulin. The mother's milk can be pumped and fed to the baby. With a later maternal illness, the prophylactic measures are not needed and the baby can be breastfed. If the baby then becomes ill, the varicella infection generally proceeds without complications. With a zoster, the baby may continue to breastfeed, but direct contact with the affected skin area should be avoided.

4.15.10   HIV infection

HIV is a retrovirus and belongs to the family of lentiviruses. Vertical transmission can take place during pregnancy, labor and delivery, as well as postpartum through breastfeeding. The risk of transmission during breastfeeding depends on many factors, including the timing of maternal infection, maternal viral load, immune function, nutritional status of both the woman and the baby, antiretroviral use, breast health (nipple pathology, mastitis), type of breastfeeding (exclusive, mixed or replacement feeding), duration of breastfeeding and presence of oral lesions in the infant (Young 2011).

In 2011, 330,000 (280,000–390,000) children acquired HIV infection (UNAIDS 2012). This represents a 43% decline since 2003 (when 560,000 [510,000–650,000] children became newly infected (UNAIDS 2012).

Breastfeeding provides major protection against mortality from diarrhea, pneumonia and malnutrition in the first year of life in poor resource settings.

Reports from observational and controlled studies have confirmed the efficacy of combination ARVs given to HIV-infected mothers to prevent postnatal transmission (Rollins 2012). Recent reports on the implementation of the global recommendations on breastfeeding and ARVs have described improved outcomes in controlled and programmatic settings. For instance, in Zambia 1% transmission at 12 months was associated with combination maternal ARVs until the end of the breastfeeding period, compared with 12% among infants whose mothers received only antepartum and intrapartum ARVs (Gartland 2013).

An alternative method to prevent transmission during breastfeeding is heat treatment of the expressed breast milk, effectively deactivating the virus (Hoque 2013). Breastfeeding improves the survival of infants already infected with HIV (Becquet 2012).

The current WHO 2013 guidelines recommend ART for all pregnant and breastfeeding women with HIV during the period of risk of mother-to-child transmission, and continuing lifelong ART either for all women, or for the women meeting eligibility criteria for their own health. A once daily fixed dose combination of *tenofovir, lamivudine* (or *etravirene*), and *efavirenz* is the preferred first line regimen for the mother. Infants of mothers who are receiving ART and are breastfeeding should receive 6 weeks of infant prophylaxis with daily *nevirapine*. If infants are receiving replacement feeding, they should be given 4-to-6 week prophylaxis with daily nevirapine (or *zidovudine* twice daily) (WHO 2013).

Recommendation. If the mother has been diagnosed as HIV-infected, then breastfeeding should not take place in good resource settings; that is, if safe drinking water and sanitary facilities are available to the household and the community, where sufficient infant formula for adequate development of the infant is available, and the mother or caretaker can prepare the feeding cleanly and frequently enough. In poorer resource settings where these prerequisites are not in place, mothers known to be infected with HIV should exclusively breastfeed their infants for the first 6 months of life, introducing appropriate complementary food thereafter, and continue breastfeeding for the first 12 months of life. Breastfeeding should then only stop once a nutritionally adequate and safe diet without breast milk can be provided – in combination with ART treatment for mother and infant. If a mother is not receiving ART treatment, the infant prophylaxis should be prolonged until 6 weeks after maternal ART is restarted or until 1 week after breastfeeding has ended.

4.15.11   Human T-lymphotropic virus (HTLV)

HTLV-I is an enveloped, single-stranded RNA virus of the Retroviridae family, the only human pathogen of the subfamily oncovirus. This virus is the causative agent of two typically fatal diseases: adult T cell leukemia-lymphoma (ATL) and HTLV-I-associated myelopathy (HAM). After prolonged latency periods, approximately 3 to 5% of HLTV-1 infected individuals will develop either ATL or HAM (Lairmore 2011). HTLV-1 is infecting approximately 10–20 million people worldwide, particularly in southern and southeastern Japan, the Caribbean, highlands of South America, Melanesia and Equatorial Africa (Yoshimitsu 2014). HTLV-1 transmission from mother to child occurs through breastfeeding, with reported rates of 15 to 25% (Ribeiro 2012).

The mother's HTLV-1 proviral load and the duration of breastfeeding have been described as risk factors associated with vertical transmission (Ribeiro 2012).

Japanese investigators have reported that freeze-thaw processing of breast milk appeared to eliminate the infectivity of HTLV-I and prevented vertical transmission (Ando 2004).

Recommendation. In good resource settings breastfeeding is contraindicated with an HTLV infection. In poorer resource settings breastfeeding duration should be limited to 6 months if possible, to lower the risk of transmission.

4.15.12   Influenza

Whether H1N1 viruses or other influenza viruses pass into the mother's milk is not known. The primary source of infection is certainly droplet infection.

Recommendation. Breastfeeding can continue during an influenza infection in the mother.

4.15.13   Lyme disease

Lyme disease is a spirochetal infection caused by the Borrelia species and is transmitted by the bite of infected ticks. Borrelia-DNA was detected in the milk of two breastfeeding mothers with erythema migrans, and one of the two breastfed children had transient fever and vomiting. It had not been tested for Borrelia infection (Schmidt 1995). Up to now, no case of infection through breastfeeding has been described (Smith 2012).

> **Recommendation.** Breastfeeding is possible with Lyme disease. Whether this can cause an infection in the newborn is not known.

4.15.14   Methicillin-resistant *Staphylococcus aureus* (MRSA)

MRSA has been detected in mother's milk. The concentrations in previously deep-frozen milk samples in a Brazilian mother's milk bank were so low, that there was no contraindication to feeding according to Brazilian and American guidelines (Novak 2000). The increase in MRSA is also a danger for newborns. With premature babies, infection can lead to sepsis, pneumonia, necrotizing enterocolitis, skin lesions and meningitis. The transmission from mother to child probably happens through skin contact. MRSA was determined with two of eight healthy mother–child pairs (without mastitis) (Kawada 2003). Mastitis attributable to MRSA has also been described (Schoenfeld 2010). Treatment with dicloxacillin and cefalexin was not successful, with healing was only achieved with clindamycin. MRSA was also present in breast abscesses (Montalto 2009, Wilson-Clay 2008). An infection through hospital personnel probably represents the main danger, therefore before any skin contact with mother and child, strict disinfection should take place. Some authors stress the importance of early colonization of the newborn with the mother's skin germs (bonding and early breastfeeding), and the protection against hospital germs that this affords (Kitajima 2003). No MRSA infection of a newborn through the mother's milk has, as yet, been described. Breast feeding was shown to be protective against MRSA colonization in children (Chen 2011).

> **Recommendation.** Breastfeeding is permitted with MRSA. In the case of mastitis or an abscess, an adequate antibiotic should be used.

4.15.15   Rotavirus

Rotaviruses were among the first viral agents to be identified as important causes of viral gastroenteritis, and transmission occurs via the fecal-oral route. Breastfeeding reduces the risk for diarrheal diseases in infants. However, the study results are contradictory. In some studies, rotavirus infections were found to be similar in breastfed and non-breastfed infants, but the symptoms were milder in the breastfed children, i.e. less vomiting (Weinberg 1984), and the duration of the illness was shorter (Duffy 1986). In other studies, a protective effect of breastfeeding was shown, especially in the first six months of life (Gimenez-Sanchez 2010, Plenge-Bonig 2010, Dennehy 2006, Mastretta 2002). Whether rotaviruses are transmitted through mother's milk was not studied; however, various immune factors that show a protective effect – such as lactadherin, lactoferrin and specific IgA (Newburg 1998) have been documented in the milk. On the other hand, these protective factors, in particular lactoferrin, may lower the immunogenicity and efficacy of rotavirus vaccines. These inhibitory effects on the rotavirus vaccines have been shown to be stronger in Indian and South African populations than in the USA (Moon 2013), and may explain breakthrough infections in vaccinated infants (Adlhoch 2013).

> **Recommendation.** Since breastfeeding shows a positive and protective effect with rotavirus infections, breastfeeding should continue.

4.15.16   Tuberculosis

Mycobacterium tuberculosis, is an aerobic, non-spore forming, non-motile bacillus member of the Mycobacteriaceae family. Person-to-person transmission of tuberculosis (TB) occurs via inhalation of droplet nuclei. Coughing and singing facilitate formation of droplet nuclei. Neonatal TB develops following exposure of an infant to his or her mother's aerosolized respiratory secretions and not through breastfeeding.

The risk for infection is highest if a mother is diagnosed at the time of delivery or shortly thereafter. If a pregnant woman is found to have pulmonary TB shortly before delivery, then the baby, and if possible, the placenta, should be investigated for evidence of congenital TB infection and, if found, the baby treated. (Stop TB partnership childhood TB subgroup 2007).

A breastfeeding infant has a high risk of infection from a mother with smear-positive pulmonary TB, and has a high risk of developing TB. The infant should receive 6 months of *isoniazid* preventive therapy, followed by BCG immunization. Breastfeeding can be safely continued during this period. An alternative policy is to give 3 months' isoniazid, then perform a TST. If the test is negative, isoniazid should be stopped and *BCG vaccination* given. If the test is positive, isoniazid should be continued for another 3 months, after which it should be stopped and BCG given.

The American Academy of Pediatrics and the Centers for Disease Control and Prevention state that breastfeeding should not occur if the mother has active (infectious) untreated tuberculosis; however, expressed milk can be used because there is no concern about transmission through the milk. Breastfeeding can be resumed when a mother with tuberculosis is treated for a minimum of 2 weeks, and is documented that she is no longer infectious. Women with tuberculosis mastitis should breastfeed from the unaffected breast (Mathad 2012). An infection via the mother's milk with a tubercular mastitis is considered an extreme rarity and leads to an infection of the children, mostly in the tonsils. Children of mothers who are both HIV as well as TBC-positive have a higher rate of mortality (Gupta 2007).

> **Recommendation.** Breastfeeding is possible with tuberculosis. The mother must be treated and the infant should receive 6 months of isoniazid preventive therapy, followed by BCG immunization. Women with tuberculosis mastitis should breastfeed from the unaffected breast.

Lactation

4.15 Infections during breastfeeding

4.15.17   West Nile virus

West Nile viruses are members of the family Flaviviridae genus *Flavivirus*. A mosquito bite is the primary route of transmission of West Nile virus between humans.

The first possible transmission of WNV via human milk was reported to the Centers for Disease Control and Prevention (2002) in September 2002. In this case, a 40-year-old woman was transfused immediately postpartum with blood that was subsequently found to contain WNV nucleic acid. She began to breastfeed on the day of delivery and continued through day 16 after birth, her second day of hospitalization for WNV encephalitis. A sample of undiluted mother's milk from day 16 post-delivery tested positive for the presence of WNV nucleic acid and WNV-specific immunoglobin M (IgM) and IgG antibodies. Viral culture of the milk was negative for WNV. A second sample of undiluted milk collected 24 days after delivery was negative for WNV nucleic acid. This sample was positive for WNV-specific IgM antibodies when tested at a 1:400 dilution. At 25 days of age, serum from the breastfed infant tested WNV-specific IgM positive, although the child remained healthy. The mother reported that the infant had been kept primarily indoors, with no obvious exposures to mosquitoes.

Since 2003 the Centers for Disease Control have collected 10 additional cases of maternal or infant West Nile virus illness while breast-feeding (Hinckley 2007). Because the health benefits of breast-feeding are well established, available reports do not suggest that breast-feeding be discouraged in women with WNV infections.

> **Recommendation.** Breastfeeding is possible with a West Nile virus infection.

4.15.18   Other infectious diseases

With the following illnesses there is no evidence of a causal agent in the milk or an infection via breastfeeding, but preventive measures are recommended (Lawrence 2004). With a haemophilus influenza infection a 24-hour treatment of the mother is recommended before breastfeeding. With gonorrhea, breastfeeding can continue if the mother is effectively treated with, for instance, *ceftriaxon*. With a B-streptococcus-B infection during the neonatal period, i.e. with endometritis, separation of the mother and child for 24 hours and feeding the baby the expressed milk is recommended. In the case of syphilis, the mother should begin pumping and feeding it to the baby or breastfeeding only 24 hours after the start of treatment.

References

Ackerman Z, Ackerman E, Paltiel O. Intrafamilial transmission of hepatitis C virus: a systematic review. J Viral Hepat 2000; 7: 93–103.

Adlhoch C, Hoehne M, Littmann M et al. Rotavirus vaccine effectiveness and case-control study on risk factors for breakthrough infections in Germany, 2010–2011. Pediatr Infect Dis J 2013; 32: e82–9.

Aggarwal R. Clinical presentation of hepatitis E. Virus Res 2011; 161: 15–22.

Ando Y, Ekuni Y, Matsumoto Y et al. Long-term serological outcome of infants who received frozen-thawed milk from human T-lymphotropic virus type-I positive mothers. J Obstet Gynaecol Res 2004; 30: 436–8.

Barthel A, Gourinat AC, Cazorla C et al. Breast milk as a possible route of vertical transmission of dengue virus? Clin Infect Dis 2013; 57: 415–7.

Becquet R, Marston M, Dabis F et al. Children who acquire HIV infection perinatally are at higher risk of early death than those acquiring infection through breastmilk: a meta-analysis. PLoS One 2012; 7: e28510.

Buxmann H, Falk M, Goelz R et al. Feeding of very low birth weight infants born to HCMV-seropositive mothers in Germany, Austria and Switzerland. Acta Paediatr 2010; 99: 1819–23.

Buxmann H, Miljak A, Fischer D et al. Incidence and clinical outcome of cytomegalovirus transmission via breast milk in preterm infants ≤31 weeks. Acta Paediatr 2009; 98: 270–6.

Capretti MG, Lanari M, Lazzarotto T et al. Very low birth weight infants born to cytomegalovirus-seropositive mothers fed with their mother's milk: a prospective study. J Pediatr 2009; 154: 842–8.

Centers for Disease Control and Prevention. Possible West Nile virus transmission to an infant through breast-feeding – Michigan, 2002. MMWR Morb Mortal Wkly Rep 2002; 51: 877–8.

Chen CJ, Hsu KH, Lin TY et al. Factors associated with nasal colonization of methicillin-resistant Staphylococcus aureus among healthy children in Taiwan. J Clin Microbiol 2011; 49: 131–7.

Chibber RM, Usmani MA, Al-Sibai MH. Should HEV infected mothers breastfeed? Arch Gynecol Obstet 2004; 270: 15–20.

Cottrell EB, Chou R, Wasson N et al. Reducing risk for mother-to-infant transmission of hepatitis C virus: a systematic review for the U.S. Preventive Services Task Force. Ann Intern Med 2013; 158: 109–13.

Curtis N, Chau L, Garland S et al. Cytomegalovirus remains viable in naturally infected breast milk despite being frozen for 10 days. Arch Dis Child Fetal Neonatal Ed 2005; 90: F529–30.

Daudi N, Shouval D, Stein-Zamir C et al. Breastmilk hepatitis A virus RNA in nursing mothers with acute hepatitis A virus infection. Breastfeed Med 2012; 7: 313–5.

Dennehy PH, Cortese MM, Begue RE et al. A case-control study to determine risk factors for hospitalization for rotavirus gastroenteritis in U.S. children. Pediatr Infect Dis J 2006; 25: 1123–31.

Doctor S, Friedman S, Dunn MS et al. Cytomegalovirus transmission to extremely low-birthweight infants through breast milk. Acta Paediatr 2005; 94: 53–8.

Duffy LC, Byers TE, Riepenhoff-Talty M et al. The effects of infant feeding on rotavirus-induced gastroenteritis: a prospective study. Am J Public Health 1986; 76: 259–63.

Dunkle LM, Schmidt RR, O'Connor DM. Neonatal herpes simplex infection possibly acquired via maternal breast milk. Pediatrics 1979; 63: 250–1.

Frederick IB, White RJ, Braddock SW. Excretion of varicella-herpes zoster virus in breast milk. Am J Obstet Gynecol 1986; 154: 1161–7.

Gartland MG, Chintu NT, Li MS et al. Field effectiveness of combination antiretroviral prophylaxis for the prevention of mother-to-child HIV transmission in rural Zambia. AIDS 2013; 27: 1253–62.

Gimenez-Sanchez F, Delgado-Rubio A, Martinon-Torres F et al. Multicenter prospective study analysing the role of rotavirus on acute gastroenteritis in Spain. Acta Paediatr 2010; 99: 738–42.

Goelz R, Hihn E, Hamprecht K et al. Effects of different CMV-heat-inactivation-methods on growth factors in human breast milk. Pediatr Res 2009; 65: 458–61.

Gonzalez ML, Viela Sala C, Salvä Armengod F et al. Should we recommend breastfeeding to newborns of HBsAg carrier mothers. An Esp Pediatr 1995; 43: 115–9.

Gupta A, Nayak U, Ram M et al. Postpartum tuberculosis incidence and mortality among HIV-infected women and their infants in Pune, India 2002–2005. Clin Infect Dis 2007; 45: 241–9.

Gupta S, Malhotra AK, Dash SS. Child to mother transmission of herpes simplex virus-1 infection at an unusual site. J Eur Acad Dermatol Venereol 2008; 22: 878–9.

Hamele M, Flanagan R, Loomis CA et al. Severe morbidity and mortality with breast milk associated cytomegalovirus infection. Pediatr Infect Dis J 2010; 29: 84–6.

Hamprecht K, Maschmann J, Vochem M et al. Epidemiology of transmission of cytomegalo-virus from mother to preterm infant by breastfeeding. Lancet 2001; 357: 513–8.

Hill JB, Sheffield JS, Kim MJ et al. Risk of hepatitis B transmission in breast-fed infants of chronic hepatitis B carriers. Obstet Gynecol 2002; 99: 1049–52.

Hinckley AF, O'Leary DR, Hayes EB. Transmission of West Nile virus through human breast milk seems to be rare. Pediatrics 2007; 119: E666–71.

Lactation

4.15 Infections during breastfeeding

Hoque SA, Hoshino H, Anwar KS et al. Transient heating of expressed breast milk up to 65 degrees C inactivates HIV-1 in milk: a simple, rapid, and cost-effective method to prevent postnatal transmission. J Med Virol 2013; 85: 187–93.

Jim WT, Shu CH, Chiu NC et al. High cytomegalovirus load and prolonged virus excretion in breast milk increase risk for viral acquisition by very low birth weight infants. Pediatr Infect Dis J 2009; 28: 891–4.

Kawada M, Okuzumi K, Hitomi S et al. Transmission of Staphylococcus aureus between healthy, lactating mothers and their infants by breastfeeding. J Hum Lact 2003; 19: 411–7.

Kitajima H. Prevention of methicillin-resistant Staphylococcus aureus infections in neonates. Pediatr Int 2003; 45: 238–45.

Kotronias D, Kapranos N. Detection of herpes simplex virus DNA in maternal breast milk by in situ hybridization with tyramide signal amplification. In Vivo 1999; 13: 463–6.

Lairmore MD, Anupam R, Bowden N et al. Molecular determinants of human T-lymphotropic virus type 1 transmission and spread. Viruses 2011; 3: 1131–65.

Lanzieri TM, Dollard SC, Josephson CD, Schmid DS, Bialek SR. Breast milk-acquired cytomegalovirus infection and disease in VLBW and premature infants. Pediatrics 2013; 131: e1937–45.

Lawrence RM, Lawrence RA. Breast milk and infection. Clin Perinatol 2004; 31: 501–28.

Lin HH, Hsu HY, Chang MH et al. Hepatitis B virus in the colostra of HBeAg-positive carrier mothers. J Pediatr Gastroenterol Nutr 1993; 17: 207–10.

Linnemann CC Jr, Goldberg S. Letter: HBAg in breast milk. Lancet 1974; 2: 155.

Mastretta E, Longo P, Laccisaglia A et al. Effect of Lactobacillus GG and breast-feeding in the prevention of rotavirus nosocomial infection. J Pediatr Gastroenterol Nutr 2002; 35: 527–31.

Mathad JS, Gupta A. Tuberculosis in pregnant and postpartum women: epidemiology, management, and research gaps. Clin Infect Dis 2012; 55: 1532–49.

Miron D, Brosilow S, Felszer K et al. Incidence and clinical manifestations of breast milk-acquired Cytomegalovirus infection in low birth weight infants. J Perinatol 2005; 25: 299–303.

Montalto M, Lui B. MRSA as a cause of postpartum breast abscess in infant and mother. J Hum Lact 2009; 25: 448–50.

Moon SS, Tate JE, Ray P et al. Differential profiles and inhibitory effect on rotavirus vaccines of nonantibody components breast milk from mothers in developing and developed countries. Pediatr Infect Dis J 2013; 32: 863–70.

Neuberger P, Hamprecht K, Vochem M et al. Case-control study of symptoms and neonatal outcome of human milk-transmitted cytomegalovirus infection in premature infants. J Pediatr 2006; 148: 326–31.

Novak FR, da Silva AV, Hagler AN et al. Contamination of expressed human breast milk with an epidemic multiresistant Staphylococcus aureus clone. J Med Microbiol 2000; 49: 1109–17.

Pembrey L, Newell ML, Tovo PA. The management of HCV infected pregnant women and their children European paediatric HCV network. J Hepatol 2005; 43: 515–25.

Petrova M, Kamburov V. Breastfeeding and chronic HBV infection: clinical and social implications. World J Gastroenterol 2010; 16: 5042–6.

Plenge-Bonig A, Soto-Ramirez N, Karmaus W et al. Breastfeeding protects against acute gastroenteritis due to rotavirus in infants. Eur J Pediatr 2010; 169: 1471–6.

Pouliot SH, Xiong X, Harville E et al. Maternal dengue and pregnancy outcomes: A systematic review. Obstet Gynecol Surv 2010; 65: 107–18.

Read JS, Cannon MJ, Stanberry LR et al. Prevention of mother-to-child transmission of viral infections. Curr Probl Pediatr Adolesc Health Care 2008; 38: 274–97.

Ribeiro MA, Martins ML, Teixeira C et al. Blocking vertical transmission of human T cell lymphotropic virus type 1 and 2 through breastfeeding interruption. Pediatr Infect Dis J 2012; 31: 1139–43.

Rollins N, Mahy M, Becquet R et al. Estimates of peripartum and postnatal mother-to-child transmission probabilities of HIV for use in Spectrum and other population-based models. Sex Transm Infect 2012; 88: i44–51.

Schmidt BL, Aberer E, Stockenhuber C et al. Detection of Borrelia burgdorferi DNA by polymerase chain reaction in the urine and breast milk of patients with Lyme borreliosis. Diagn Microbiol Infect Dis 1995; 21: 121–8.

Schoenfeld EM, McKay MP. Mastitis and methicillin-resistant Staphylococcus aureus (MRSA): the calm before the storm? J Emerg Med 2010; 38: e31–4.

Smith GN, Gemmill I, Moore KM. Management of tick bites and lyme disease during pregnancy. J Obstet Gynaecol Can 2012; 34: 1087–91.

Stop TB partnership childhood TB subgroup. Chapter 4: Childhood contact screening and mamagement. Int J Tuberc Lung Dis 2007; 11: 12–15.

Tovo PA, Lazier L, Versace A. Hepatitis B virus and hepatitis C virus infections in children. Curr Opin Infect Dis 2005; 18: 261–6.

Tseng RYM, Lam CWK, Tam J. Breastfeeding babies of HBsAG-positive-mothers. Lancet 1988; 1: 1032.

UNAID. Report on the Global Aids Epidemic 2012; pp. 42–3, http://www.unaids.org/en/media/unaids/contentassets/documents/epidcmiology/2012/gr2012/20121120_unaids_global_report_2012_with_annexes_en.pdf

Vollmer B, Seibold-Weiger K, Schmitz-Salue C et al. Postnatally acquired cytomegalovirus infection via breast milk: effects on hearing and development in preterm infants. Pediatr Infect Dis J 2004; 23: 322–7.

Weinberg RJ, Tipton G, Klish WJ et al. Effect of breast-feeding on morbidity in rotavirus gastroenteritis. Pediatrics 1984; 74: 250–3.

WHO consolidated guidelines on the use of antiretroviral drugs for treating and preventing hiv infection recommendations for a public health approach (2013) http://apps.who.int/iris/bitstream/10665/85321/1/9789241505727_eng.pdf

Wilson-Clay B. Case report of methicillin-resistant Staphylococcus aureus (MRSA) mastitis with abscess formation in a breastfeeding woman. J Hum Lact 2008; 24: 326–9.

Yoshida M, Tezuka T, Hiruma M. Detection of varicella-zoster virus DNA in maternal breast milk from a mother with herpes zoster. Clin Diagn Virol 1995; 4: 61–5.

Yoshida M, Yamagami N, Tezuka T et al. Case report: Detection of varicella-zoster virus DNA in maternal breast milk. J Med Virol 1992; 38: 108–10.

Yoshimitsu M, White Y, Arima N. Prevention of human T-cell lymphotropic virus type 1 infection and adult T-cell leukemia/lymphoma. Recent Results Cancer Res 2014; 193: 211–25.

Young SL, Mbuya MN, Chantry CJ et al. Current knowledge and future research on infant feeding in the context of HIV: basic, clinical, behavioral, and programmatic perspectives. Adv Nutr 2011; 2: 225–43.

Lactation

4.15 Infections during breastfeeding

Recreational drugs

Mark Anderson and Marc Oppermann

4.16

4.16.1	Alcohol	835
4.16.2	Amphetamines	836
4.16.3	Caffeine	836
4.16.4	Cannabis	837
4.16.5	Cocaine	837
4.16.6	Nicotine	838
4.16.7	Opiates, including methadone	839
4.16.8	Other drugs	841

Breastfeeding mothers should avoid recreational drug use wherever possible. However, the value of breastfeeding to both mother and infant is such that it likely outweighs the risks associated with most maternal recreational drug use. The risks should be discussed on a case-by-case basis with the mother, with pragmatic advice given specific to her personal situation. Although there is evidence of deleterious short-term effects on the breastfed infant for a number of substances, there are few data relating to the long-term effects and the likely more significant exposure of the infant *in utero*, and the often-disadvantaged social background of women who use recreational drugs confound these. In general, breastfeeding is contraindicated in cases of persistent maternal use of heroin or stimulant drugs, such as amphetamine, cocaine and alcohol.

4.16.1   Alcohol

Alcohol transfers readily into breast milk leading to concentrations almost identical to those found in maternal blood. This results in the infant receiving about 10% of the mother's weight-related amount of alcohol (survey in Bennett 1996). The activity of alcohol dehydrogenase, the main route of alcohol detoxification, in the neonatal period is reduced, leading to an elimination rate around half of that measured in adults, with greater attendant risks to the infants of mothers with alcohol intake.

Despite long-held claims that alcohol is a galactagogue, there is no scientific evidence to support this view. Indeed, to the contrary, there is evidence that even moderate maternal alcohol intake may decrease breast milk production and milk ejection (Mennella 2008). Alcohol can also change the taste of the mother's milk and may lead to feeding difficulties

Drugs During Pregnancy and Lactation. **http://dx.doi.org/10.1016/B978-0-12-408078-2.00041-X**

(Mennella 1991). Consumption of more than two alcoholic drinks per day is associated with a significantly shortened duration of breastfeeding (Giglia 2008).

Other adverse effects of alcohol on infants have been reported following moderate exposure: changes in sleep behavior (Mennella 1997); potential alcohol-induced hypoglycemia (Lamminpaa 1995); mild sedation (American Academy of Pediatrics Committee on Drugs 2001); and possible mild delays in psychomotor development observed at 1 year of age (Little 1989), although the same group was not able to replicate these findings in a similar cohort at 18 months.

It is conceivable that regular excessive maternal alcohol consumption during breastfeeding may lead to significant harm to the infant. A case report details a reversible pseudo-Cushing syndrome in a child, which was attributed to the mother's massive intake of alcohol (survey in Bennett 1996).

Recommendation. Alcohol should be avoided when breastfeeding, although there is no hard evidence that occasional limited alcohol use (i.e. 1 unit of alcohol or 8 oz – equivalent to 100 mL champagne once or twice a week) causes harm to the infant. Furthermore, one drink should be consumed over a period of time (more than 30 minutes), and the mother should where possible, refrain from nursing for 2 hours thereafter to avoid any alcohol reaching the infant. With chronic or intermittent excessive alcohol consumption (binge drinking), breastfeeding should be discontinued. Alcohol use during breastfeeding also has adverse effects on the child. Babies have been found to drink less milk and to have a disturbed sleep–wake pattern for 3 hours after nursing mothers have consumed between one and two standard drinks.

4.16.2   Amphetamines

Amphetamines are transferred into the breast milk. After a regular intake of 20 mg daily, a milk to plasma (M/P) ratio of 2.8–7.5 was reported and amphetamines were detected in infant urine (Steiner 1984). No clinical symptoms were observed among 103 infants whose mothers took various amounts of amphetamines (Ayd 1973). However, irritability, poor sleeping and agitation have been described in infants breastfed by amphetamine users (American Academy of Pediatrics Committee on Drugs 2001). In four breastfeeding mothers treated with dexamphetamine for attention deficit hyperactivity disorder (ADHD), a M/P ratio was found to be maximally 5.3 with a relative infant dose of less than 10%. Normal development of the children was reported (Ilett 2007). Methamphetamine is also excreted in milk (Bartu 2009).

Recommendation. Amphetamine use during breastfeeding should be strongly discouraged. After an individual dose, an interruption of breastfeeding for at least 24 hours should be observed. In the event of regular amphetamine use, breastfeeding should be discontinued.

4.16.3   Caffeine

Methylxanthines, including *theophylline*, *caffeine*, *theobromine* and the metabolite *paraxanthin*, are considered part of the "normal" components of the milk, and arise from dietary sources as well as prescription and non-prescription medications (Blanchard 1992). The concentration in breast milk following maternal ingestion is very variable. Caffeine is metabolized by the hepatic cytochrome P450 oxidase system that is immature in the neonatal period. This results in a prolonged elimination half-life in the newborn of up to 90 hours as opposed to around 5 hours in adults. The amounts of caffeine arising in milk from usual social coffee consumption, with a milk to plasma ratio of approximately 0.6, appear to be well-tolerated by the infant. Even under controlled conditions, neither changes in heart frequency and sleep duration nor other symptoms could be detected. Regular intake of larger amounts of caffeine (daily more than four cups of coffee, eight cups of tea or relevant amounts of other caffeine-containing drinks), may lead to transitory irritability and restlessness especially in very young infants (Martín 2007).

> **Recommendation.** "Normal" caffeine consumption, i.e. a maximum of three cups of coffee or six cups of tea or 300 mg of caffeine in 24 hours, is not considered to be harmful to the infant during breastfeeding. If this amount is regularly exceeded, symptoms of irritability may occur and consumption should be reduced.

4.16.4   Cannabis

Δ9-Tetrahydrocannabinol (THC), the primary active ingredient in *cannabis*, is transferred into, and accumulates in breast milk, with an infant ingesting about 0.8% of the maternal weight-related intake of THC following a single joint in one feeding. With regular consumption of cannabis, an eight-fold higher concentration is reached in the mothers' milk than in the maternal plasma, due to the high lipophilia (Bennett 1996). Short-term effects, including sedation and lethargy have been reported in infants following THC exposure in breast milk (Liston 1998). A study of 68 infants exposed to THC via breast milk found delayed motor development at 1 year of age when compared with a control group of infants (Astley 1990).

> **Recommendation.** Cannabis use should be avoided during breastfeeding. In addition, infants should not be exposed to cannabis smoke.

4.16.5   Cocaine

Cocaine passes readily into human breast milk following maternal use, although substantial variability of the concentration in the mother's milk has been reported (Marchei 2011, Winecker 2001). Cocaine and its metabolites have been detected in the breastfed infant's urine for up to 60 hours following feeding. Adverse effects described in infants following cocaine exposure by ingestion via breast milk include seizures, tachycardia, irritability and agitation (Dickson 2001, Wiggins 1989, Chasnoff 1987).

> **Recommendation.** Cocaine use during breastfeeding should be strongly discouraged. After an individual dose, an interruption of breastfeeding for at least 24 hours should be observed. In the event of regular cocaine use, breastfeeding should be discontinued.

lactation

4.16 Recreational drugs

4.16.6   Nicotine

Nicotine and its principal metabolites pass rapidly into breast milk. Nicotine reaches a three-fold higher concentration compared with its concentration in maternal plasma and has a slightly longer half-life (Luck 1987). *Cotinine*, the major metabolite of nicotine is somewhat less concentrated than in the maternal serum, but has a significantly longer half-life than nicotine (survey in Bennett 1996). Nicotine and cotinine content in the milk increase in proportional amounts to the number of cigarettes smoked by the mother daily (Schwartz-Bickenbach 1987). Nicotine concentrations of up to 1.6 µg/L, and cotinine values of up to 20 µg/L were found in the serum of breastfed infants of smoking mothers (Luck 1987). Urinary cotinine concentrations are five to ten times higher in the urine of breastfed infants of smoking mothers than in the urine of non-breastfed infants of smoking mothers (Becker 1999). In addition, if a mother breastfeeds her baby within an hour after smoking, the nicotine transfer would appear to be particularly high. On average, a daily intake of 7 µg/kg through milk has been calculated for a fully breastfed baby of a smoking mother (Dahlström 2004).

Passive smoke inhalation is also a major source of nicotine exposure for both breastfed and non-breastfed infants. No difference with respect to hair cotinine concentration has been found in exposed children <3 years when compared with their smoking mothers (Groner 2004). The concentration of pollutants caused by passive smoking was actually higher in the children than in their mothers, even when the mothers themselves did not smoke. Dahlström (2004) found 28 and 13 µg/L of nicotine in the milk of two mothers who were only exposed to passive smoke – about half the concentration compared with that in actively smoking mothers.

Smoking has been observed to have other effects on the content of human breast milk. Other toxic and carcinogenic substances have been found in the milk of mothers who smoke. For example, *cadmium* concentrations in smoking mothers' milk are significantly higher compared with those of non-smokers (Radisch 1987). Conversely, in a comparison of 50 smoking mothers with 90 non-smokers, a lower iodine content was observed in the milk, which, according to the authors, could cause an iodine deficiency in the infants of smokers, requiring iodine supplementation (Laurberg 2004).

▶ **Effects on the infants of smokers**

Infants of mothers who smoke are more likely to suffer from infantile colic, respiratory infections, vomiting and poor weight gain though these may result from exposure to smoke passively, rather than as a result of nicotine and related substances via breast milk. Sudden unexpected death in infancy (SUDI) is also more common in infants of mothers who smoke (Bajanowski 2008).

Exposure to nicotine in breast milk may result in effects on autonomic cardiovascular control. In one study, male infants were found to suffer a decrease in heart rate variability associated with an increasing nicotine concentration in the milk (Dahlström 2008). Another small study demonstrated that 20 minutes after breastfeeding, infants of smoking mothers had significant changes in their respiratory rate and oxygen saturations compared with infants of non-smoking mothers (Stepans 1993).

In a small prospective study with 15 breastfeeding mothers, an acute episode of smoking by breastfeeding mothers detrimentally altered their infants' sleeping pattern. Infants of these mothers spent significantly less time in quiet sleep and awoke from their naps sooner (Mennella 2007).

A number of studies show that duration of breastfeeding for smoking mothers is significantly shorter than their non-smoking counterparts. Social factors are likely to be a primary issue, although there is a postulated nicotine-related reduction in prolactin production which may also play a role (Amir 2002, Letson 2002). Mothers who smoke regularly after birth give up breastfeeding prematurely up to four times more frequently than those who do not smoke or only smoke occasionally (Ratner 1999, Edwards 1998). Paternal smoking also correlates negatively with breastfeeding duration (Haug 1998).

There are no studies which document the number of cigarettes smoked by the mother, at which the advantages of breastfeeding are outweighed by the disadvantages. As a result, there is also no toxicologically grounded "threshold dose" at which breastfeeding should be avoided (Dorea 2007).

▶ Nicotine replacement therapy

Nicotine replacement products for smoking cessation also lead to exposure of the child (Schatz 1998) and, in principle, have the same risk. Nicotine patches lead to lower concentrations of nicotine in breast milk when compared with the milk of smoking mothers using 7 or 14 mg patches (Ilett 2003). Even higher nicotine concentrations were measured in the milk of two snuff-taking mothers, compared to a group of 18 smoking women (Dahlström 2004). There are no data available on the use of *bupropion*, which is also approved for weaning from smoking (see Chapter 4.9) or for *varenicline*.

Recommendation. Breastfeeding mothers should be strongly discouraged from smoking, or at least urged to reduce the number of cigarettes smoked to a minimum. Infants should be protected from passive smoking. While nicotine replacement therapy does have advantages for the breastfed baby, due to the absence of toxins from cigarette smoke in the mothers' milk, it cannot, however, be seen as harmless due to the high nicotine transfers.

Smoking women should be encouraged to breastfeed and to continue for as long as possible. Mothers who can't stop smoking should be encouraged to schedule cigarettes right after a feed so there is the longest time possible after smoking until the next feed.

4.16.7   Opiates, including methadone

▶ Heroin (diamorphine)

All opiates can be transmitted to the breastfed infant through the milk. At therapeutic doses, most are transferred into milk in only low concentrations that are unlikely to affect the infant (Sagraves 1997). Heroin, however, is excreted in sufficient amounts that may result in symptoms of withdrawal following cessation of breastfeeding (Briggs 2011). There

lactation

4.16 Recreational drugs

are other risks associated with the use of heroin, as it is often "cut" with other unknown substances that may present additional risk to the infant.

Restlessness, vomiting and poor feeding have been reported in the infants of mother's who have used heroin while breastfeeding (Cobrinik 1959).

Substitution therapy

Methadone and *levomethadone* have pharmacological properties similar to morphine, and are frequently used in opioid replacement therapy because of their relatively long half-life compared with other opioids. Methadone is transferred into breast milk, with the usual substitution dose of 10–80 mg/day leading to a relative dose for the infant of 1–6% (on average 2.8%; Begg 2001). The M/P ratio lies between 0.2 and 0.9 (Jansson 2008). The active enantiomer (levomethadone) has up to a three-fold higher concentration in the milk than the non-active one (Bogen 2011).

Maternal methadone use is generally considered to be well tolerated and usually safe for the infant, provided the mother is not using other drugs. A single case report described the death of an infant, allegedly caused by methadone in the mother's milk (Smialek 1977). However, the infant's serum methadone concentration of 400 µg/L suggests that the methadone may have been administered directly.

There is a clear correlation between the maternal daily dose and the concentration of the active ingredient in her blood and in the milk. However, even high maternal daily doses up to 130 mg (Jansson 2008, McCarthy 2000, Malpas 1999, Geraghty 1997, Wojnar-Horton 1997) appear not to be detrimental to the infant. A mother who is on a stable methadone dose and who wants to breastfeed her baby should therefore be encouraged to do so, independent of magnitude of the dose (Jansson 2009).

Symptoms of neonatal opiate withdrawal are not uncommon in infants exposed to methadone during pregnancy. Breastfeeding may protect against this. A retrospective evaluation of 437 newborns whose mothers were receiving methadone substitution treatment showed that those who were breastfed for at least 72 hours, had a 48% reduced risk for a withdrawal syndrome (Dryden 2009). In another retrospective evaluation, 62 breastfed babies of methadone treated mothers were compared with 87 bottle-fed babies of methadone treated mothers. The breastfed babies showed milder withdrawal symptoms, had a lower Finnegan score and needed pharmacological treatment less often than the bottle-fed babies (Abdel-Latif 2006). Two breastfed infants of methadone treated mothers, who had previously not required pharmacological treatment, were reported to suffer withdrawal symptoms following abrupt cessation of breastfeeding (Malpas 1999). Other authors doubt the effectiveness of withdrawal prevention via the mothers' milk with concern that the amount of methadone excreted in the milk is insufficient to prevent withdrawal (e.g. Begg 2001).

In one study of six breastfed infants from 5 to 8 days of age, whose mothers took up to 30 mg of buprenorphine daily, a M/P ratio of 1.1–2.8 and a relative dose of 0.03–0.31% was measured (median 1.7 or 0.2%). For the metabolite, *norbuprenorphine* the M/P ratio was 0.7 and the relative dose 0.12% (median). The infants showed only mild withdrawal symptoms and development in the first month of life was unremarkable

(Lindemalm 2009). A case report documented normal development up to the age of one year of the infant of a buprenorphine treated mother who breastfed for 6 months (Schindler 2003).

Recommendation. Mothers who continue to use heroin while breastfeeding should be encouraged to start on opiate replacement therapy. The risk to the infant from unidentified compounds in street heroin may be significant. Infants exposed to opiates *in utero*, may, with full breastfeeding and continued treatment of the mother with opioid replacement therapy develop milder withdrawal symptoms than a non-breastfed infant. As a result, mothers on opioid replacement therapy should be encouraged to breastfeed, provided that they are not using other drugs, and there are no other contraindications (e.g. HIV positive). The maximum daily substitution dose of methadone or buprenorphine should be decided on a case-by-case basis, with consideration of dose during pregnancy and the presence of any symptoms in the infant.

4.16.8   Other drugs

Two publications from the 1980s report on detection of *phencyclidine* (PCP) in the milk (Kaufman 1983, Nicholas 1982). *Diazepam* and its metabolites are also transferred into breast milk (Cole 1975). It is likely that the hallucinogenic amphetamines and lysergic acid diethylamide (LSD) are present in breast milk following maternal use, but no studies have been conducted to demonstrate this. There are no reports of the effects of these substances on the breastfed infant.

Recommendation. There are insufficient data upon which to base an evidence-based assessment of the risks associated with other recreational drugs. Following an individual dose, breastfeeding should be avoided for at least 24 hours. With repeated use, the decision to continue breastfeeding must be made on a case-by-case basis with a discussion of the potential risks with the mother.

References

Abdel-Latif ME, Pinner J, Clews S et al. Effects of breast milk on the severity and outcome of neonatal abstinence syndrome among infants of drug-dependent mothers. Pediatrics 2006; 117: e1163–9.

American Academy of Pediatrics Committee on Drugs. Transfer of drugs and other chemicals into human milk. Pediatrics 2001; 108:776–89.

Amir LH, Donath SM. Does maternal smoking have a negative physiological effect on breastfeeding? The epidemiological evidence. Birth 2002; 29: 112–23.

Astley S, Little RE. Maternal marijuana use during lactation and infant development at one year. Neurotoxicol Teratol 1990; 12: 161–8.

Ayd FJ. Excretion of psychotropic drugs in human milk. Int Drug Ther News Bull 1973; 8: 33–40.

Bajanowski T, Brinkmann B, Mitchell EA, et al. Nicotine and cotinine in infants dying from sudden infant death syndrome. Int J Legal Med 2008; 122: 23–8.

Bartu A, Dusci LJ, Ilett KF. Transfer of methylamphetamine and amphetamine into breast milk following recreational use of methylamphetamine. Br J Clin Pharmacol 2009; 67: 455–9.

Becker AB, Manfreda J, Ferguson AC et al. Breastfeeding and environmental tobacco smoke exposure. Arch Pediatr Adolesc Med 1999; 153: 689–91.

lactation

4.16 Recreational drugs

Begg EJ, Malpas TJ, Hackett LP et al. Distribution of R- and S-methadone into human milk during multiple, medium to high oral dosing. Br J Clin Pharmacol 2001; 52: 681–5.

Bennett PN. Drugs and Human Lactation. 2nd ed. Amsterdam, New York, Oxford: Elsevier, 1996.

Blanchard J, Weber CW, Shearer LE. Methylxanthine levels in breast milk of lactating women of different ethnic and socioeconomic classes. Biopharm Drug Dispos 1992; 13: 187–96.

Bogen DL, Perel JM, Helsel JC et al. Estimated infant exposure to enantiomer-specific methadone levels in breastmilk. Breastfeed Med 2011; 6: 377–84.

Briggs GG, Freeman RK, Yaffe SJ. Drugs in pregnancy and lactation: a reference guide to fetal and neonatal risk. 9th Edn. Philadelphia: Wolters Kluwer, Lippincott Williams & Wilkins 2011.

Chasnoff IJ, Lewis DE, Squires L. Cocaine intoxication in a breast-fed infant. Pediatrics 1987; 80: 836–8.

Cobrinik RW, Hood RT Jr, Chusid E. The effect of maternal narcotic addiction on the newborn infant; review of literature and report of 22 cases. Pediatrics 1959; 24: 288–304.

Cole AP, Hailey DM. Diazepam and active metabolite in breast milk and their transfer to the neonate. Arch Dis Child 1975; 50: 741–2.

Dahlström A, Ebersjö C, Lundell B. Nicotine exposure in breast-fed infants. Acta Paediatr 2004; 93: 810–6.

Dahlström A, Ebersjo C, Lundell B. Nicotine in breast milk influences heart rate variability in the infant. Acta Paediatr 2008; 97: 1075–9.

Dorea JG. Maternal smoking and infant feeding: breastfeeding is better and safer. Matern Child Health J 2007; 11:287–91.

Dickson PH, Lind A, Studts P, Nipper HC et al. The routine analysis of breast milk for drugs of abuse in a clinical toxicology laboratory. J Forensic Sci 2001; 46:1221–3.

Dryden C, Young D, Hepburn M et al. Maternal methadone use in pregnancy: factors associated with the development of neonatal abstinence syndrome and implications for healthcare resources. BJOG 2009; 116: 665–71.

Edwards N, Sims-Jones N, Breithaupt K. Smoking in pregnancy and postpartum: relationship to mother's choices concerning infant nutrition. Can J Nurs Res 1998; 30: 83–98.

Geraghty B, Graham EA, Logan B, Weiss EL. Methadone levels in breast milk. J Hum Lact 1997; 13: 227–30.

Giglia RC, Binns CW, Alfonso HS et al. The effect of alcohol intake on breastfeeding duration in Australian women. Acta Paediatr 2008; 97: 624–9.

Groner J, Wadwa P, Hoshaw-Woodard S et al. Active and passive tobacco smoke: a comparison of maternal and child hair cotinine levels. Nicotine Tob Res 2004; 6: 789–95.

Haug K, Irgens LM, Baste V et al. Secular trends in breastfeeding and parental smoking. Acta Paediatr 1998; 87: 1023–7.

Ilett KF, Hackett LP, Kristensen JH et al. Transfer of dexamphetamine into breast milk during treatment for attention deficit hyperactivity disorder. Br J Clin Pharmacol 2007; 63: 371–5.

Ilett KF, Hale TW, Page-Sharp M et al. Use of nicotine patches in breast-feeding mothers: transfer of nicotine and cotinine into human milk. Clin Pharmacol Ther 2003; 74: 516–24.

Jansson LM. ABM clinical protocol #21: Guidelines for breastfeeding and the drug-dependent woman. Breastfeed Med 2009; 4: 225–8.

Jansson LM, Choo R, Velez ML et al. Methadone maintenance and breastfeeding in the neonatal period. Pediatrics 2008; 121: 106–14.

Kaufman KR, Petrucha RA, Pitts FN et al. PCP in amniotic fluid and breast milk: case report. J Clin Psychiatr 1983; 44: 269–70.

Lamminpaa A. Alcohol intoxication in childhood and adolescence. Alcohol Alcohol 1995; 30: 5–12.

Laurberg P, Nøhr SB, Pedersen KM, Fuglsang E. Iodine nutrition in breast-fed infants is impaired by maternal smoking. J Clin Endocrinol Metab 2004; 89: 181–7.

Letson GW, Rosenberg KD, Wu L. Association between smoking during pregnancy and breastfeeding at about 2 weeks of age. J Hum Lact 2002; 18: 368–72.

Lindemalm S, Nydert P, Svensson JO et al. Transfer of buprenorphine into breast milk and calculation of infant drug dose. J Hum Lact 2009; 25: 199–205.

Liston J. Breastfeeding and the use of recreational drugs – alcohol, caffeine, nicotine and marijuana. Breastfeed Rev 1998; 6: 27–30.

Little RE, Anderson KW, Ervin CH et al. Maternal alcohol use during breastfeeding and infant mental and motor development at one year. N Engl J Med 1989; 321: 425–30.

Luck W, Nau H. Nicotine and cotinine concentrations in the milk of smoking mothers. Eur J Pediatr 1987; 146: 21–6.

Malpas TJ, Darlow MD. Neonatal abstinence syndrome following abrupt cessation of breast-feeding. NZ Med J 1999; 112: 12–3.

Marchei E, Escuder D, Pallas CR et al. Simultaneous analysis of frequently used licit and illicit psychoactive drugs in breast milk by liquid chromatography tandem mass spectrometry. J Pharm Biomed Anal 2011; 55: 309–16.

Martín I, López-Vílchez MA, Mur A et al. Neonatal withdrawal syndrome after chronic maternal drinking of mate. Ther Drug Monit 2007; 29: 127–9.

McCarthy JJ, Posey BL. Methadone levels in human milk. J Hum Lact 2000; 16: 115–20.

Mennella JA, Beauchamp GK. The transfer of alcohol to human milk. Effects on flavor and the infant's behavior. N Engl J Med 1991; 325: 981–5.

Mennella JA, Garcia-Gomez PL. Sleep disturbances after acute exposure to alcohol in mothers' milk. Alcohol Clin Exp Res 1997; 21: 581–5.

Mennella JA, Pepino MY. Biphasic effects of moderate drinking on prolactin during lactation. Alcohol Clin Exp Res 2008; 32: 1899–1908.

Mennella JA, Yourshaw LM, Morgan LK. Breastfeeding and smoking: short-term effects on infant feeding and sleep. Pediatrics 2007; 120: 497–502.

Nicholas JM, Lipshitz J, Schreiber EC. Phencyclidine: its transfer across the placenta as well as into breast milk. Am J Obstet Gynecol 1982; 143: 143–6.

Radisch B, Luck W, Nau H. Cadmium concentrations in milk and blood of smoking mothers. Toxicol Lett 1987; 36: 147–52.

Ratner PA, Johnson JL, Bottorff JL. Smoking relapse and early weaning among postpartum women: is there an association? Birth 1999; 26: 76–82.

Sagraves R. Drugs in breast milk: a scientific explanation. J Pediatr Health Care 1997; 11: 230–7.

Schatz BS. Nicotine replacement products: implications for the breast-feeding mother. J Hum Lact 1998; 14: 161–3.

Schindler SD, Eder H, Ortner R et al. Neonatal outcome following buprenorphine maintenance during conception and throughout pregnancy. Addiction 2003; 98: 103–10.

Schwartz-Bickenbach D, Schulte-Hobein B, Abt S et al. Smoking and passive smoking during pregnancy and early infancy. Toxicol Lett 1987; 35: 73–81.

Smialek JE, Monforte JR, Aronow R et al. Methadone deaths in children. JAMA 1977; 238: 2156–7.

Steiner E, Villén T, Hallberg et al. Amphetamine secretion in breast milk. Eur J Clin Pharmacol 1984; 27: 123–4.

Stepans MB, Wilkerson N. Physiologic effects of maternal smoking on breastfeeding infants. J Am Acad Nurse Pract 1993; 5:105–13.

Wiggins RC, Rolsten C, Ruiz B et al. Pharmacokinetics of cocaine:basic studies of route, dosage, pregnancy and lactation. Neurotoxicology 1989; 10: 367–81.

Winecker RE, Goldberger BA, Tebbett IR et al. Detection of cocaine and its metabolites in breast milk. J Forensic Sci 2001; 46: 1221–3.

Wojnar-Horton RE, Kristensen JH, Yapp P et al. Methadone distribution and excretion into breast milk of clients in a methadone maintenance programme. Br J Clin Pharmacol 1997; 44: 543–7.

Plant toxins

Ruth A. Lawrence and Christof Schaefer

4.17

Not much is known about the damage to an infant via breast milk as a result of maternal exposure to animal or plant poisons or toxins, or via the "physiological" parts of plants. There is one report (Hallebach 1985) in which an infant was harmed via his mother's milk after she had suffered *Amanita* poisoning. In another case report (Kautek 1988), it was presumed that a hemolytic crisis in an infant with congenital glucose 6-phosphate-dehydrogenase deficiency might have been caused when the mother ate *fava beans* (favism). However, this supposition is not very realistic, and has not been confirmed by other publications.

Currently, there can only be speculation about the meaning of the relatively high amounts of *aflatoxin* detected in many samples of mother's milk. Aflatoxin has been found in corn, peanuts, cotton seed, rye, barley (Ellenhorn 1997). In countries such as the Sudan or Thailand food is more highly contaminated with aflatoxins, and significant concentrations, which would exceed levels permitted in our foods, are sometimes detected in mothers' milk (Coulter 1984). However, a study in West Africa found a substantially greater contamination in infant nutrition after weaning. Their finding that children who were breastfed for longer grew better was discussed as being due to a toxic effect on children with artificial nutrition (Gong 2003). Another study also found aflatoxin M1 in the mothers' milk in a population in Australia supposed to have little exposure to contaminated food (El-Nezami 1995). High concentrations of aflatoxin B1 in mothers' milk have also been discussed in connection with the development of Kwashiorkor in breastfed children (Hendrickse 1997).

For additional information about Herbals, please see Chapter 4.13.

Recommendation. If a breastfeeding mother has symptoms caused by poisons or toxins, breastfeeding should be interrupted until symptoms have improved.

References

Coulter JBS, Lamplugh SM, Suliman GI et al. Aflatoxins in human breast milk. Ann Trop Pediatr 1984; 4: 61–6.

El-Nezami HS, Nicoletti G, Neal GE et al. Aflatoxin M1 in human breast milk samples from Victoria, Australia and Thailand. Food Chem Toxicol 1995; 33: 173–9.

Ellenhorn MJ, Barceloux DG. *Ellenhorn's Medical Toxicology: Diagnosis and treatment of human poisoning*. 2nd edn, Baltimore: Williams & Wilkins, 1997.

Gong YY, Egal S, Hounsa A et al. Determinants of aflatoxin exposure in young children from Benin and Togo, West Africa: the critical role of weaning. Int J Epidemiol 2003; 32: 556–62.

Drugs During Pregnancy and Lactation. **http://dx.doi.org/10.1016/B978-0-12-408078-2.00042-1**

Hallebach M, Kurze G, Springer S et al. Knollenblätterpilzvergiftung über Muttermilch. Z Klin Med 1985; 40: 943–5.

Hendrickse RG. Of sick turkeys, kwashiorkor, malaria, perinatal mortality, heroin addicts and food poisoning: research on the influence of aflatoxins on child health in the tropics. Ann Trop Med Parasit 1997; 91: 787–93.

Kautek L, Solem E, Böhler H. Hämolytische Krise nach Stillen! Der Kinderarzt 1988; 19: 808.

Industrial chemicals and environmental contaminants

4.18

Ruth A. Lawrence and Christof Schaefer

4.18.1	Persistent organochlorine compounds (pesticides, polychlorinated biphenyls and dioxins)	847
4.18.2	Mercury	851
4.18.3	Lead	853
4.18.4	Cadmium	855
4.18.5	Other contaminants	855
4.18.6	Breastfeeding despite environmental contaminants?	857
4.18.7	Breastfeeding and the workplace	858

4.18.1   Persistent organochlorine compounds (pesticides, polychlorinated biphenyls and dioxins)

Experience

Within this group are the classic pesticides *dichlordiphenyltrichlorethan* (DDT), *hexachlorbenzene* (HCB), *dieldrin, hexachlorcyclohexan* (HCH), and "synthetic oils" made from polychlorinated biphenyls (PCBs) as well as the polychlorinated *dioxins* and *furans*.

Dioxins are considered a group of toxic chemicals with similar chemical structures and biologic characteristics. Exposure comes from environmental contamination from forest fires, backyard burning of trash, industrial activities and previous industrial burning of waste. Degradation of dioxins is slow and residuals persist from past man-made and natural events.

Almost all living things have been exposed to dioxins. Adverse health effects depend on level of exposure as well as when, how long and how often, an individual is exposed.

Of the organochlorine pesticides, only the short-lived χ-HCH (*lindane*) is still produced today (see Chapter 4.12). Other organochlorine pesticides such as DDT have been produced since the 1970s for export only to developing countries – at present there is a DDT "renaissance" for malaria prevention in Africa. For the most part, however, organochlorine pesticides have been replaced by *carbamates, organophosphates*, and *pyrethroids*. These substances are, to some extent, significantly more toxic, but they have a lesser tendency towards persistence and accumulation in nature.

Polychlorinated biphenyls were used as softeners and color additives. Since the 1970s they may only be used in closed systems, such as hydraulic fluid and transformer or condenser filling. Since the end of the 1980s the use of polychlorinated biphenyls has been banned in most countries, but the machines installed earlier still contain large quantities of these congeners.

Polychlorinated dibenzodioxins and -furans, among which group is the quadruply-chlorinated "seveso toxin" *2,3,7,8-TCDD*, occur in connection with technical activities as by-products or impurities during the synthesis of organochlorine compounds, and when they are recycled and burned. Trash dumps and chlorinated additives in automobile fuel are among the most significant sources of dioxin in our environment.

Toxic symptoms in the infant as a result of organochlorine compounds in the mother's milk have been described only after extreme exposure. The *Turkish porphyria (Pemba–Yarda syndrome)* occurred after consumption of seed grain treated with *hexachlorbenzene*. Apart from skin rash and weight loss, there were also lethal consequences for breast-fed babies (Peters 1982). *Yusho disease* was caused by *polychlorinated biphenyls* in contaminated cooking oil. It caused muscular hypotonia, hyperexcitability, and apathy in the infants. The illness continued for many years (Miller 1977).

Concentrations in mothers' milk

Safety levels for organochlorine compounds in mothers' milk are aligned with the "no adverse effect level" (NOAEL) determined in animal studies. This is understood to be the amount of a contaminant per kg body-weight, taken in daily, that no longer causes any toxic effect (for example, a weight increase of the liver with a rise in enzyme activity in the rat). Based on the NOAEL, and taking into consideration a safety factor (SF), the acceptable daily intake (ADI) of the contaminant involved is calculated for a human being (adult or infant). The safety factor should actually be of the magnitude of 100–1,000, but in practice, for PCBs in mothers' milk, a factor of only 10 was occasionally calculated. This means that beyond a level 10 times the amount ingested by a breastfed infant per kg bodyweight daily, toxic effects can be expected in animal studies. Contamination of human milk with polychlorinated biphenyls is significantly greater than in cows' milk. The term PCB covers some 200 congeners, among which the congeners 138, 153, and 180 predominate, and are frequently presented as a proxy for the entirety of PCB contamination.

The average dioxin load in mother's milk is usually expressed in I-TEQ (International TCDD-equivalent) – i.e. the equivalent amount of seveso toxin *3,4,7,8-tetrachlordibenzodioxin* that corresponds to the total amount of all dioxin- and furan-congeners in the analyzed specimen. According to the WHO (1989), the acceptable daily intake is 1–4 pg I-TEQ/kg bodyweight per day; the American Environmental Protection Agency (EPA) allows 0.1 pg/kg per day. These values are exceeded by nursing infants by up to 100-fold or more – for example, in Germany a fully breastfed infant receives on average 55 pg I-TEQ/kg per day. However, the acceptable dosages were defined for lifelong intake and not limited to the lactation period.

Regional differences in milk contamination

The different analytical methods used in different countries must be considered when comparing contamination in mothers' milk. In general, significantly higher contamination with DDT and DDE can be observed in many so-called "developing countries" (Kunisue 2004, Minh 2004), while PCBs and dioxins are found at higher levels in industrialized countries. Corresponding differences were found between Eastern and Western Europe, with more PCBs in the West (Mehler 1994, Hesse 1981). Regional differences may also be explained by differences in nutrition of the studied cohorts (Nadal 2004).

During the 1980s, DDT/DDE concentrations of, on average, 45 mg/kg milk fat were reported in Indonesia. Levels in South Africa, Kenya, Hong Kong, and India were between 10 and 20 mg/kg; in Europe, the USA, and Australia, levels were between 1 and 2 mg/kg. Depending on the analytical methodology, the average results for PCBs in Europe, Israel, and the USA were between 0.5 and 2.5 mg/kg milk fat (survey in Bennett 1996). In industrial nations, dioxins in human milk fat were between 15 and 25 ng I-TEQ/kg milk fat. Up to 1991, some authors still observed a rise in the average contamination in mothers' milk (Mehler 1994).

Since the early 1990s, a tendency towards declining levels of persistent organochlorine compounds has been noted in the milk. Today, PCB contamination has reduced to one-third of the values measured in Europe in the 1980s – in Germany, for example, more than 30,000 samples of human milk have been analyzed (BgVV 2000) to come to this conclusion. The current data on dioxin contamination in mothers' milk show that here, too, there has been a decline, from 37 pg/g fat in 1988 to 12 pg/g fat in 2002. Nevertheless, contamination levels in the Netherlands (18 pg/g fat) and Germany are still among the highest in Europe. Lower levels have been reported in Croatia and Spain, and also in Taiwan (Chao 2004, Schuhmacher 2004).

In another German publication on the development of contamination in mothers' milk in Baden-Württemberg, it was reported that in 1988 a total of 14% of the milk samples contained at least one of the studied substances at levels above 10% of the NOAEL (mostly PCBs). In accordance with the recommendations that were in effect until 1996, mothers with such levels were advised not to breastfeed beyond 4 months. By 1996, only 2% of the milk samples exceeded this so-called SF-10 value. The number of milk samples studied every year was initially over 1000; by 1990 it reached its peak, with 1983 samples studied. By 1996, the number had declined to 280 (Seidel 1998).

Persistently high PCB levels in mother's milk were found in the Faroe Islands – the level was 2300 ng/g fat in 1987, and by 1999 it was still 1800 ng/g (Fängström 2005).

Polybrominated diphenyl ethers

Increasing levels of *polybrominated diphenyl ethers* (PBDE) were observed in mothers' milk on the Faroe Islands (rising from 2 ng/g fat in 1987 to 8 ng/g in 1999) (Fängström 2005). PBDE contamination of breast milk was also found in other countries. PBDEs are a group of more than 200 structurally similar congeners that are used as flame-retardants in electrical appliances such as television sets and computers, as well as in carpets and furniture upholstery. Because these compounds can accumulate in human tissues and, in adequate concentrations, alter metabolic and physiologic functions, the European Union (EU) banned the production, use, and import of *pentabromodiphenyl ether* and *octabromodiphenyl ether* products in 2004. *Decabromodiphenyl ether* is still in use, and its main congener, deca-BDE 209, can be detected in breast milk. A German study of 89 lactating women found, on average, 1.65 ng/g milk fat among vegetarians and a significantly higher level (2.47 ng/g) among women eating a varied diet that included meat. As with organochlorines, the levels were lower in women who had breastfed many infants. However, no significant decrease was observed between the neonatal period and 3 months after birth. A fully breastfed child ingests, on average, 10 ng/kg bodyweight and, at maximum, 50 ng/kg. Considering the NOAEL for PBDE, this corresponds to a margin of safety (MOS) of $>10^4$. Therefore, health problems are not to be expected (Vieth 2005). PBDE contamination in North America is one order of magnitude higher than that measured in Germany.

Levels measured in breastfed infants

It is estimated that breastfed infants receive one to two magnitudes more dioxins than adults. Teufel (1990) found the highest plasma concentrations after birth. At 6 months, regardless of the type of feeding, the lowest values were measured. Although the absolute amount of polychlorinated biphenyls and dioxins transferred with the milk is greater than that transferred by the placenta during pregnancy, the "dilution effect" that occurs as a result of the infant's rapidly increasing fatty tissue appears to decrease the concentration in the infant's plasma.

For dioxin, the elimination half-life of 4 months in newborns is significantly shorter than that in adults (5 years). This also contributes to the fact that although fully breastfed children have significantly higher TCDD concentrations in the blood and fatty tissue than do non-breastfed babies, the differences have completely leveled out after a few years (Kreuzer 1997). A detailed model to predict dioxin levels in the body fat of infants, dependent on the duration of breastfeeding (no breastfeeding; and after 6 weeks, 6 months, 1 year, and 2 years), was presented by Lorber (2002). According to this model that was validated with data from the study cohort of Abraham (1998), breastfed infants reach peak values during their first months of life. Up to the age of 7–10 years, however, these levels approach those found in children who were not breastfed. For PCBs, Heudorf (2002) observed no difference between breastfed and formula-fed children at the age of 12 years.

Effects of average contamination on infant development

Among the numerous studies on persistent organochlorines in the "normal" environment, some present levels in maternal and infant blood, and in breast milk (Fängström 2005, Lackmann 2005, Chao 2004, Kunisue 2004, Minh 2004, Nadal 2004, Schuhmacher 2004, Heudorf 2002). Others focus on somatic and mental development (survey in LaKind 2004). There are mainly four larger research projects which have led to several publications, i.e. the studies in North Carolina, Michigan, The Netherlands and Germany. In North Carolina, 865 infants were enrolled in around 1980 to investigate their development until the age of 5 and at puberty (Gladen 2000, 1991, 1988). Illnesses during childhood were not associated with exposure to PCB and DDE via breast milk. Furthermore, there was no significant correlation with mental and psychomotor development, or with somatic development and puberty.

The so-called Michigan study covered 240 children whose mothers regularly consumed PCB-contaminated fish from the Great Lakes (>11.8 kg over 6 years). The control group consisted of 71 children of mothers who did not consume such fish. Visual recognition at the age of 7 months was not affected. However, subtle differences of development were observed at the age of 4 years. These were more pronounced in children who had been breastfed for at least 1 year. Intelligence was not affected, at least up to the age of 11 years (Jacobson 1990, 1996, 2002).

A Dutch study with 100 breastfed and 100 formula-fed children focused on PCB and dioxins (Koopman-Esseboom 1996). Higher levels in milk were associated with elevated TSH values at birth and at 3 months, indicating disturbance of thyroid function. Neurological examinations of 400 newborns and psychomotor and cognitive tests up to the age of 4 years, revealed no persisting effects of PCBs or dioxins (survey in LaKind 2004).

A German study on mental and motor development found a negative association between PCB levels in milk and performance of the Kaufman score at the age of 42 months. Other outcome parameters were uneventful in this study, which covered in total 171 mother–child-pairs (Walkowiak 2001).

Other studies with smaller cohorts observed associations between dioxins, furans, and PCB in breast milk with lower levels of thyroid hormones, increased CD4+ lymphocytes, reduced CD8+ lymphocytes (T suppressor cells), slightly elevated liver enzymes, and lower platelet counts. In general, development was normal up to 6 months of age (survey in LaKind 2004). Even considering moderate contamination of breast milk, some authors suggest an overall positive effect of breast-feeding on psychomotor and cognitive development that compensates for potential impairments due to toxic contaminants (Vreugdenhil 2004, Ribas-Fito 2003, Boersma 2000).

State governments, industry and the Environmental Protection Agency (EPA) have worked diligently to reduce known and measurable industrial emissions of dioxin. Air emissions of dioxin have been dramatically reduced by 90% and most Americans have low level exposures. The document "Reanalysis of Key Issues Related to Dioxin Toxicity" was released in February 2012 (EPA 2012). It contains a detailed and transparent description of the underlying data and analysis. The oral reference dose (RfD) for 2,3,7,8–Tetrachlorobenzo-p-Dioxin (TCDD) is 7×10^{-10} mg/kg-day, derived from two epidemiologic studies (EPA 2012).

Recommendation. Average contamination of breast milk with persistent organochlorines does not seem to have detrimental effects on children's development. If it is assumed that any toxic effect of organochlorines is associated with their plasma level, prenatal exposure would be more relevant than intake through breast milk. All in all, breastfeeding has a positive, and probably compensatory, effect on psychomotor and cognitive development that outweighs potential toxic effects before birth and via breast milk.

4.18.2 Mercury

Experience

Elemental or metallic mercury is used in mercury thermometers and (in combination with silver and other metals) in dental amalgam. In China, dental amalgam was used to fill teeth over 1,000 years ago (cited in Drexler 1998). *Inorganic mercury*, e.g. *mercury chloride*, has been used as a disinfectant. *Organic mercury* (*ethyl mercury*) is used for the preservation of vaccines, and is accumulated in contaminated seafood (*methyl mercury*). Apart from high doses, elemental mercury is hardly absorbed via intestine (<0.01%), but 80% may reach the circulation via inhalation. Inorganic mercury (<10%) and, even more so, organic mercury (up to 95%) are orally available. The liver, kidneys, and CNS are target organs of mercury poisoning. Elemental and inorganic mercury are excreted via the kidneys, whereas organic mercury is excreted through the colon. Mercury accumulates; its half-life ranges from 6 months to several years. The mercury content in mother's milk does not reach toxic levels under normal nutritional conditions, or even in the presence of numerous amalgam fillings. Other conditions have prevailed, though – for instance, as a result of an environmental scandal in Japan, industrial waste water containing mercury heavily contaminated the fish, and led to an outbreak of Minamata disease among those who had eaten the fish and also, via their milk, among their children. The result was a spate of neurological developmental disorders, including some serious cerebral damage with spasticity. In other cases, it was mercury-contaminated seed grain, used for food (in Iran and the USSR), that caused toxic damage (Wolff 1983). In such cases, concentrations up to 540 µg/L were measured in mothers' milk.

The average mercury concentrations in Europe are 1 µg/L in the blood or 1 µg/g creatinine in the urine. In Scandinavia and Japan (Sakamoto 2002), significantly higher "normal" levels have been reported. Due to the regular intake of contaminated seafood, levels of between 16 µg/L and 40 µg/L were measured among the Inuit. Methyl mercury from contaminated seafood is measured in erythrocytes. In general, prenatal mercury exposure is more relevant than that via breast milk. Cord blood levels exceed those in maternal blood by 50–100% (Björnberg 2005, Sakamoto 2002).

Changes in the body burden of mercury in infants during early lactation compared with placental transfer was reported in 2012 (Sakamoto 2012). It was confirmed that fetal exposure to Hg strongly reflected the levels of maternal exposure. Placental transfer was remarkably high. At three months of age, however Hg had declined about 60% compared to cord blood red blood cells (RBCs) although the infants were breastfed.

Concentration in mothers' milk

In a German study of 116 women, an average of 0.9 µg/L milk (ranging from <0.25 to 20.3) was reported after birth. After 2 months of breastfeeding it was, on average, below 0.25 µg/L (ranging from <0.25 to 11.7). In the first sample, the individual value correlated with the number of fillings in the teeth, and the frequency of fish meals (there was no differentiation between fresh- and salt-water fish, and no particular information on contamination). With the second sample, which involved 84 of the 116 women in the study, there was a positive association only with the consumption of fish (Drexler 1998).

According to a study of mothers' milk samples in East Germany, more than 80% of the mercury values found were under the detection limit of 0.5 µg/L milk (Henke 1994). Similar results were found in other European countries – for example, in a recent study of 20 mother–child-pairs in Sweden, total mercury was 0.2–0.3 µg/L at 4 days, and 6 and 13 weeks after delivery (Björnberg 2005).

Ten years earlier a Swedish study of 30 women found a correlation, about 6 weeks after birth, between the number of amalgam fillings and the mercury concentration (total value and inorganic portion), both in the blood (mean value 2.3 µg/L) and in the milk (mean 0.6 µg/L). According to the authors, each filling increased the total concentration in the mother's blood by about 0.1 µg/kg and in the milk by about 0.05 µg/kg. The level of fish consumption (methyl mercury) was significantly reflected only in the contamination of the mother's blood, but not in the milk (Oskarsson 1996). A recent study from Taiwan investigated 68 healthy urban mothers, and mothers married to fishermen, in relation to fish intake (Chien 2006a). The breast milk mercury geometric mean concentration was 2.02 µg/L (0.24–9.45) in the urban group, and comparable values were found for the fishermen's group.

Based on the milk levels presented above, a fully breastfed baby would ingest up to 0.3 µg of mercury per kg daily. The ADI value set by the WHO is 0.715 µg/kg bodyweight.

According to a study of 583 children on the Faroe Islands, the mercury concentration in hair samples of 1-year-old babies is correlated with the length of breastfeeding (Grandjean 1994).

Analysis and comparisons of levels of mercury in maternal blood, cord blood, breast milk, meconium and infant hair by atomic absorption spectrophotometry were reported by Ramirez (2000). Regression analysis of cord blood levels showed a significant relationship to mother's blood, prevalence in infant's hair, gestational age, and head circumference. Of the 66 full-term infants weighing about 3,000 g at birth, those who had low head circumferences also had mercury in the meconium.

Although mercury transfer into milk is significant, levels are dependent upon mother's levels. Dental amalgams have been extensively studied but are not a significant source. Milk levels drop over the first three months of lactation (Hale 2012, Marques 2007).

Recommendation. Mercury contamination from dental amalgam does not lead to dramatic increases in heavy metal concentrations that would demand consequences such as weaning. Detoxification treatment is not indicated. In addition, chelating agents may mobilize heavy metals and in this way increase contamination of the mother's milk. On the other hand, amalgam fillings should only be removed in case of dental problems. Extensive restoration should be postponed until after the breastfeeding period. Wherever possible, amalgam should be avoided. However, at an individual level, the amalgam issue should not be stirred up into a "toxicological crisis" that puts an unjustifiable strain on the mother–child relationship.

Consumption of fish highly contaminated with mercury is not recommended during pregnancy and breastfeeding. Among such fish are shark, true eel, sturgeon, ocean perch, swordfish, perch, halibut, pike, ray, monkfish, and tuna.

4.18.3   Lead

Experience

Inorganic lead (e.g. *lead oxide*) is distinguished from *organic lead* (e.g. *tetraethyl lead*). Lead salts are absorbed via the intestine and inhalation. Sources are glazes, paints, additives in leaded fuel, lead pipes, and occupational exposure. Mainly due to the ban of leaded fuel, average lead levels in blood have substantially declined to concentrations below 10 or even 5 µg/dL during the past two decades. With a half-life of approximately 30 years in adults, >90% of lead is stored in bones.

The current authors observed a case of lead poisoning due to acid spring water (pH 5.5) which was carried through a 300 m lead pipe, resulting in tap water contaminated with 4,000 µg/L lead. At the age of 3 months, the fully breastfed infant developed serious cerebral palsy. The level in the mother's milk was 80 µg/L. It cannot be determined to what extent the prenatal exposure *in utero* and the postnatal exposure through the mother's milk caused the lead poisoning.

Concentration in mothers' milk

According to a study in West Germany in the 1980s, the average lead concentrations in mothers' milk were between 9 and 13 µg/L (Sternowsky

1985). Another study in Eastern Germany produced similar results. Interestingly, the content in mother's milk did not necessarily correlate with the industrial contaminant load in the respective region (Henke 1994). Levels were 20–50% of the ADI value of 5 µg/kg bodyweight recommended by the WHO. Significantly higher lead concentrations were found in mothers' milk in the 1980s in Tyrol (29 µg/L) and in Singapore (46 µg/L) (cited in Henke 1994), while 62 µg/L milk was measured in one worker in a factory producing storage batteries (Wolff 1983).

Corresponding to the lead levels in blood, contamination of milk has also decreased. Average levels below 5 µg/L are measured today. Even a recent report from a poor region in Ecuador where lead glazes are manufactured found mean lead levels of 4.6 µg/L (range 0.4–20.5 µg/L) as a consequence of improved working conditions (Counter 2004). This same group of mothers and children was reported again in 2006 (Counter 2007). On follow-up PbB and PbM levels in mothers were elevated but stable. Levels in children were also elevated but stable. All were consistent with the levels reported in 2003 in these same Andean villages. Among 310 women in Mexico City, 1.1 µg/L milk was measured 1 month after delivery (Ettinger 2004). A Greek study analyzed 180 specimen of colostrum for lead and found, on average, 0.5 µg/L (Leotsinidis 2005). In Croatia, 158 women had a mean contamination of 4.7 µg/L milk 4 days after birth (Ursinyova 2005).

In a Chinese study, mothers who consumed traditional Chinese herbs were compared to a control group of mothers who did not (Chien 2006b). The geometric mean of lead concentrations in all colostrum samples ($n = 72$) was 7.68 ± 8.24 µg/L. The concentration of lead in the breast milk of the consumption group was 8.59 ± 10.95 µg/L, a level significantly higher than that of 6.84 ± 2.68 µg/L found in the control group. Sixteen of the mothers provided breast milk weekly at 1–60 days postpartum. In the group that had consumed herbs ($n = 9$) the mean concentration of lead in the breast milk decreased, within days postpartum, from 9.94 µg/L in the colostrum to 2.34 µg/L in mature milk.

Analysis of data from Costa Rica (1981–1984), Chile (1991–1996) and Detroit (2002–2003) by Lozoff (2009) showed that longer breastfeeding was associated with higher infant lead concentrations in three countries and over three different decades. The settings differed in breastfeeding patterns, environmental lead sources and infant lead levels. The authors suggest that monitoring of lead levels in breastfeeding be considered.

When metal levels were measured in healthy Swedish mothers and their milk using inductively coupled plasma mass spectrometry (ICPMS), there was a correlation with fish consumption with lead showing some decline over time probably due to decreased levels in the environment (Björklund 2012).

The changes in body burden of several elements, including lead, during a three month period of breastfeeding was compared with placental transfer using maternal and cord blood (fetal) RBCs at parturition and infant RBCs at 3 months. Lead levels in cord RBCs were about 60% of maternal levels and remained consistent to the three month period.

All these data are well below the ADI for infants recommended by the WHO. However, several studies have indicated that there is no safe threshold for lead in infant's blood with respect to neurological development (e.g. reaction time, motor skills, attention, and intelligence). Even with very low blood levels of <3 µg/L, subtle correlations can be found between lead concentration and neurological test performance (Chiodo 2004).

Recommendation. Apart from extreme exposure such as that described above, lead in a mother's milk would not be expected to pose a substantial risk to her infant. Nevertheless, every unnecessary exposure to high levels of lead should be avoided (for example, ceramic vessels with lead glazing, traditional herbal medicines; see also Chapter 2.23), in order to prevent even discrete effects on the development of the central nervous system.

4.18.4   Cadmium

Experience

Moderate *cadmium* (Cd) concentrations of 6–12 µg/L were measured in mothers' milk in a German study (Henke 1994), but there were also concentrations two to three times as high, as well as those below 1 µg/L. Low concentrations (average 0.09 µg/L, range 0.02–0.73 µg/L) were also measured in a recent Austrian study that enrolled 124 women. A Greek study of 180 colostrum samples found 0.19 µg/L (Leotsinidis 2005), and a Croatian study of 158 women found 0.43 µg/L on day 4 postpartum (Ursinyova 2005). Smoking, including passive smoking, has a significant influence on the cadmium level (Radisch 1987).

Cadmium levels in Swedish women (Björklund 2012) showed a negative correlation with calcium, confirming that Cd interacts with the transport of essential micronutrients in the mammary gland. Cadmium may share common transporters with *iron* and *manganese* for transfer into breast milk, but inhibit secretion of calcium. They found low levels of Cd (median 0.07 µg/L).

In the measurements of body burden of several contaminates, Sakamoto (2012) found that the placenta acted as a barrier to Cd and that the level remained low during lactation. The Cd level in cord RBCs was about 20% of the level in maternal RBCs, and remained low during the 3-month study period [0.14 (0.06–0.22)] in infant RBCs.

The WHO ADI value for adults is 1 µg cadmium/kg bodyweight. This was exceeded by the findings in Germany (Henke 1994, cited above).

Recommendation. Toxic effects of cadmium via the mothers' milk have not, as yet, been described, and are unlikely under normal circumstances.

4.18.5   Other contaminants

Arsenic, selenium, lithium and *boron* are the most frequently measured other metals and trace elements in human milk. Analyses have been initiated because of special events in specific geographical areas. Contaminated water supply is the most common cause.

Arsenic (As) levels were measured by Björklund (2012), Sakamoto (2012), Concha (2010), and Fängström (2008). Organic but not inorganic arsenic was found in the milk of Swedish mothers which was attributed to the fish they ate (Björklund 2012). Reports of arsenic in Bangladeshi infants were found to be higher in formula fed infants that those who were breastfed. The authors state that exclusive breastfeeding protects infants from exposure to arsenic in the water supply (Fängström

Lactation

4.18 Industrial chemicals and environmental contaminants

2008). Similar contamination of the water supply was found in the Andes of Northern Argentina (Concha 2010). The placental barrier seemed to protect infants in a study of body burden that included arsenic levels at birth, and through 3 months of breastfeeding. Arsenic levels in cord blood RBCs were 60% of maternal levels at birth and remained constant for 3 months. Arsenic levels in breast milk were 1.40 (0.40–1.80) ng/mL (Sakamoto 2012).

Boron (B), a light non-metallic trace element, is found in rocks, soil and water. Boron is found in drinking water at levels less than 1–1000 μg/L in California, Germany and France and 6,000 to 15,000 μg/L in Argentina and Chile. WHO has established a level of 2,400 μg/L as an estimated NOAEL of 9.6 mgB/kg body weight/day. Harari (2012) reported that boron passes the placenta but not into milk. Breastfeeding infants have lower levels of boron than formula fed infants. High levels of boron (Concha 2010) were found in Northern Argentina in drinking water and the urine of women studied that confirm the observations by Harari (2012).

Lithium levels have also been measured by Harari (2012), Concha (2010) and found to be high in Argentina and Chile. The water supply is cited as the source of maternal contamination. The side effects of chronic lithium medication are well documented, including gastrointestinal symptoms and even renal tubular damage. Effects of long term exposure to elevated lithium levels in drinking water are unknown. Lithium passes to the fetus and through the breast milk, but non-breastfed infants are at greater risk due to increased intake of contaminated water.

Little is known about the presence of other potentially toxic elements although scattered reports also include data on *barium* (BA), *cesium* (Cs), *rubidium* (Rb), *antimony* (Sb), *selenium* (Se), *uranium* (U) and *vanadium* (V) (Björklund 2012, Concha 2010, Al-Awadi 2000, Sakamoto 2012). Contaminated water and food stuffs are identified as primary sources. These authors all recommend a wider review of water supplies worldwide.

Experience

A case report describes obstructive icteric liver disease in a breastfed baby after exposure to the volatile *organochlorine tetrachloroethene* (PER), which is used as a cleaning agent. The mother had visited her husband every day at his workplace, which was apparently strongly contaminated. This also led to neurological symptoms in the mother (Bagnell 1977). A milk sample given an hour after maternal exposure had 10 mg tetrachloroethene/L. After 24 hours, the level was still 3 mg/L. The baby's condition returned to normal after weaning. A follow-up examination at 10 years of age showed nothing remarkable. Other groups of authors have demonstrated volatile *chlorhydrocarbons* – on average 6.2 μg/L – in the milk of mothers whose exposure was not occupational. It can be 4–8 weeks after exposure before the concentration in milk of the *lipophilic tetrachloroethene* "normalizes" (Schreiber 1993). However, this should in no way be a basis for recommending weaning after "trivial" exposure. Ongoing exposure at the workplace, on the other hand, should be looked at critically during breastfeeding.

Various other contaminants, such as the organic solvents *benzene* and *toluene* (Fabietti 2004), and the bactericide *triclosan* (Adolfsson-Erici 2002), have been detected in breast milk.

Synthetic musk compounds, such as *musk xylol, musk ketone, musk ambrette*, and others, are among the nitroaromatics. These substances have a limited acute toxicity, but, like the organochlorine compounds, they seem to accumulate in the fatty tissue and persist in the environment. Current analyses of mothers' milk have indicated a mean of about 0.1 mg/kg milk fat for musk xylol. The other compounds have levels two to three times lower. Synthetic musk compounds are added to detergents and cosmetics because of their fragrance, and thus dermal absorption is a likely path for their intake. There are no indications of toxic effects as a result of intake via mothers' milk. The studies to date on general toxicity and on mutagenic and carcinogenic potential do not permit a conclusive judgment (Liebl 2000, Rimkus 1994). Since 1993, contamination of mother's milk with musk xylol has declined in Germany to about 0.02 mg/kg milk fat, following a recommendation that this substance be avoided in detergents and other cleaning agents. Since the beginning of the 1990s, musk ketone levels have remained relatively constant at 0.02 mg/kg milk fat.

There are insufficient data on the polycyclic musk compounds such as *galaxolide* and *tonalide*. These substances are also added to detergents and other cleaning agents.

In addition to these aromatics, UV-filtering substances (sunlight protection factors and sun block) are detectable in the milk (BgVV 2000).

According to a small study, silicon from breast implants was said to lead to disturbances of motility in the lower esophageal tract of breastfed infants, caused by scleroderma-like changes (Levine 1994). A definitive judgment on this hypothesis is not yet possible. A corresponding suspicion that *silicon* implants could cause collagenoses in the women themselves has not been confirmed in a meta-analysis (Janowsky 2000). Silicon compounds are used in many common medications, and exposure from these is more common than from implants.

4.18.6 Breastfeeding despite environmental contaminants?

Breast milk is a bioindicator for environmental contaminants accumulating in fat tissues (Fenton 2005). In recent years, laboratory findings in breast milk samples, combined with public pressure, have led to a declining tendency in the concentrations of contaminants. This was impressively confirmed in, for instance, the evaluation of the measurements collected over many years by the Human Milk and Dioxin Data Bank at the German Federal Institute for Consumer Health Protection and Veterinary Medicine (BgVV 2000).

Persistent organochlorine compounds are stored in the fatty tissue for life, and are only mobilized by losing weight and breastfeeding. For this reason, a low-calorie diet should be avoided while breastfeeding. Apart from a marked intake of animal fat and contaminated seafood (especially shellfish), the current dietary habits of the mother have little influence on the contamination levels in the milk. However, a primarily vegetarian diet of products having low pesticide residues does lead to a lower level of contaminants in the mother's milk.

Every breastfed child reduces the contaminant load in the fatty tissue of the mother and in the milk by about 10–20%. It could be said, somewhat cynically, that breastfeeding is the most effective detoxification technique for the mother.

Not enough is known about the long-term effect of the contaminants discussed in this chapter. There are indications that polychlorinated dioxins and furans may inhibit the immune system and promote tumor

Lactation

4.18 Industrial chemicals and environmental contaminants

development (WHO 1989, Knutsen 1984), but not yet in connection with average exposure via the mother's milk.

There is speculation as to whether so-called endocrine disruptors, i.e. contaminants with estrogenic properties (some PCBs, dioxins, phthalates), taken in via the mother's milk, may impair an infant's development (Massart 2005, Borgert 2003). What must be considered in the discussion as to whether or not to breastfeed is that the contaminants stored by the mother have already been transferred to the embryo and fetus during pregnancy.

The positive effects of breastfeeding are well documented. Poisoning of the breastfed child is mainly documented in association with severe environmental pollution (e.g. methyl mercury in Minamata) or individual intoxication of the mother. From a global standpoint, the WHO estimates that 1.3 million infant deaths below the age of 5 years can be prevented annually by breastfeeding (Jones 2003). No adverse effect on the infant as a result of the "normal" contamination of the mother's milk has been shown as yet. The recommendation, issued some years ago, of a limit on breastfeeding because of general environmental contamination, is no longer justifiable.

Due to the newer contaminant data, a contaminant analysis is no longer recommended as an aid to an individual decision on the length of breastfeeding, except in particularly contaminated regions.

Multiple studies have demonstrated that formula fed infants have higher levels of measured contaminants because of contaminated water supplies.

4.18.7   Breastfeeding and the workplace

The motto for the World Breastfeeding Week 2000 ("Breastfeeding: It's Your Right"), coined by the World Alliance for Breastfeeding Action (WABA), raised awareness that it is the responsibility of both political bodies and society at large to make it possible for women to breastfeed. Part of this responsibility is creating conditions that permit a mother to breastfeed for as long as she and her baby want to, despite her being employed outside the home. At the same time, the motto emphasized the "right" of the child to be nourished optimally – and that means the right to be breastfed.

The revised International Labor Organization Convention (ILO Convention No. 183), passed in June 2000, codifies the mother's right to retain her job, protection from being dismissed, and the adaptation of both the work and the working hours to suit the situation of the pregnant or breastfeeding mother.

Some countries have gone beyond the convention and passed legislation which provides that pregnant or breastfeeding mothers who return to their jobs after the statutory (paid) maternity leave, or at the end of their child-rearing leave, may not be required to perform certain tasks that might compromise their health or the health of their babies. Among these are regular lifting of heavy burdens, constant squatting or bending over, extreme stretching or bending, continuous standing or sitting without a break, and contact with poisonous or infectious materials, or with openly radioactive substances.

In some cases, the total working hours per day or per week are limited. Ideally, if a transfer to another workplace is necessary for any health reason, this should not involve any financial disadvantage for the pregnant or breastfeeding woman.

The ILO convention provides for paid breastfeeding breaks – at least two half-hour sessions per day. Breastfeeding breaks are not a substitute for the general breaks required by law, and nor should breastfeeding mothers be required to make up this time. These provisions have not been incorporated into labor laws in the United States.

References

Abraham K, Papke O, Gross A et al. Time course of PCDD/PCDF/PCB concentrations in breast-feeding mothers and their infants. Chemosphere 1998; 37: 1731–41.

Adolfsson-Erici M, Pettersson M, Parkkonen J et al. Triclosan, a commonly used bactericide found in human milk and in the aquatic environment in Sweden. Chemosphere 2002; 46: 1485–9.

Al-Awadi FM, Srikumar TS. Trace elements status in milk and plasma of Kuwaiti and Non-Kuwaiti mothers. Nutrition 2000; 16: 1069–73.

Bagnell PC, Ellenberger HA. Obstructive jaundice due to a chlorinated hydrocarbon in breast milk. Can Med J 1977; 117: 1047–8.

Bennett PN (ed.). Drugs and Human Lactation, 2nd edn. Amsterdam: Elsevier, 1996.

BgVV. Belastung der Bevölkerung mit Dioxinen und anderen unerwünschten Stoffen in Deutschland deutlich zurückgegangen. Trends der Rückstandsgehalte in Frauenmilch der Bundesrepublik Deutschland – Aufbau der Frauenmilch- und Dioxin-Humandatenbank am BgVV. BgVV-Pressedienst 15, 2000.

Björnberg KA, Vahter M, Berglund B et al. Transport of methylmercury and inorganic mercury to the fetus and breast-fed infant. Environ Health Perspect 2005; 113: 1381–5.

Björklund KL, Vahter M, Palm B, Grander M, Lignell S, Berglund M. Metals and trace element concentrations in breast milk of first time healthy mothers: a biological monitoring study. Environmental Health 2012; 11: 92.

Boersma ER, Lanting CI. Environmental exposure to polychlorinated biphenyls (PCBs) and dioxins. Consequences for long-term neurological and cognitive development of the child lactation. Adv Exp Med Biol 2000; 478: 271–87.

Borgert CJ, LaKind JS, Witorsch RJ. A critical review of methods for comparing estrogenic activity of endogenous and exogenous chemicals in human milk and infant formula. Environ Health Perspect 2003; 111. 1020–36.

Chao HR, Wang SL, Lee CC et al. Level of polychlorinated dibenzo-p-dioxins, dibenzo-furans and biphenyls (PCDD/Fs, PCBs) in human milk and the input to infant body burden. Food Chem Toxicol 2004; 42: 1299–308.

Chien LC, Han BC, Hsu CS et al. Analysis of the health risk of exposure to breast milk mercury in infants in Taiwan. Chemosphere 2006a; 64: 79–85.

Chien LC, Yeh CY, Lee HC et al. Effect of the mother's consumption of traditional Chinese herbs on estimated infant daily intake of lead from breast milk. Sci Total Environ 2006b; 354: 120–26.

Chiodo LM, Jacobson SW, Jacobson JL. Neurodevelopmental effects of postnatal lead exposure at very low levels. Neurotoxicol Teratol 2004; 26: 359–71.

Concha G, Broberg KI, Grandér M et al. High-level exposure to lithium, boron, cesium, and arsenic via drinking water in the Andes of northern Argentina. Environ Sci Technol 2010; 44: 6875–80.

Counter SA, Buchanan LH, Ortega F. Current pediatric and maternal lead levels in blood and breast milk in Andean inhabitants of a lead-glazing enclave. J Occup Environ Med 2004; 46: 967–73.

Counter SA, Buchanan LH, Ortega F. Lead Concentrations in Maternal Blood and Breast Milk and Pediatric Blood of Andean Villagers: 2006 follow-up investigation. J Occup Environ Med 2007; 49: 302–9.

Drexler H, Schaller KH. The mercury concentration in breast milk resulting from amalgam fillings and dietary habits. Environ Res A 1998; 77: 124–9.

Environmental Protection Agency. Reanalysis of Key Issues Related to Dioxin Toxicity and Response to NAS Comments vol. 1, Feb. 17, 2012.

Ettinger AS, Tellez-Rojo MM, Amarasiriwardena C et al. Levels of lead in breast milk and their relation to maternal blood and bone lead levels at one month postpartum. Environ Health Perspect 2004; 112: 926–31.

Lactation

4.18 Industrial chemicals and environmental contaminants

Fabietti F, Ambruzzi A, Delise M et al. Monitoring of the benzene and toluene contents in human milk. Environ Intl 2004; 30: 397–401.

Fängström B, Moore S, Nermell B et al. Breast-feeding Protects against Arsenic Exposure in Bangladeshi Infants. Environ Health Prospect 2008; 116: 963–9.

Fängström B, Strid A, Grandjean P et al. A retrospective study of PBDEs and PCBs in human milk from the Faroe Islands. Environ Health 2005; 4: 12.

Fenton SE, Condon M, Ettinger AS et al. Collection and use of exposure data from human milk biomonitoring in the United States. J Toxicol Environ Health A 2005; 68: 1691–712.

Gladen BC, Ragan NB, Rogan WJ. Pubertal growth and development and prenatal and lactational exposure to polychlorinated biphenyls and dichlorodiphenyl dichloroethene. J Pediatr 2000; 136: 490–96.

Gladen BC, Rogan WJ. Effects of perinatal polychlorinated biphenyls and dichlorodiphenyl-dichloroethene on later development. J Pediatr 1991; 119: 58–63.

Gladen BC, Rogan WJ, Hardy P et al. Development after exposure to polychlorinated biphenyls and dichlordiphenyldichlorethene transplacentally and through human milk. J Pediatr 1988; 113: 991–5.

Grandjean P, Jørgensen PJ, Weihe P. Human milk as a source of methyl mercury exposure in infants. Environ Health Perspect 1994; 102: 74–7.

Hale TW. Medications and Mothers Milk, 15th edn. Hale Publishing Amarillo, TX: 2012.

Harari F et al. Early-life exposure to lithium and boron from drinking water. Reproductive Toxicology 2012; 34: 552–60.

Henke J, Großer B, Ruick G. Konzentration von toxischen Schwermetallen in der Frauenmilch. Sozialpädiatrie 1994; 16: 544–6.

Hesse V, Gabrio T, Kirst E et al. Untersuchungen zur Kontamination von Frauenmilch, Kuhmilch und Butter in der DDR mit chlorierten Kohlenwasserstoffen. Kinderärztliche Praxis 1981; 49: 292–303.

Heudorf U, Angerer J, Drexler H. Polychlorinated biphenyls in the blood plasma: current exposure of the population in Germany. Rev Environ Health 2002; 17: 123–34.

Jacobson JL, Jacobson SW, Humphrey HEB. Effects of in utero exposure to polychlorinated biphenyls and related contaminants on cognitive functions in young children. J Pediatr 1990; 116: 38–45.

Jacobson JL, Jacobson SW. Intellectual impairment in children exposed to polychlorinated biphenyls in utero. N Engl J Med 1996; 335: 783–9.

Jacobson JL, Jacobson SW. Association of prenatal exposure to an environmental contaminant with intellectual function in childhood. J Toxicol Clin Toxicol 2002; 40: 467–75.

Janowsky E, Kupper LL, Hulka BS. Meta-analysis of the relation between silicone breast implants and the risk of connective-tissue diseases. N Engl J Med 2000; 342: 781–90.

Jones G, Steketee RW, Black RE et al. Bellagio Child Survival Study Group. How many child deaths can we prevent this year? Lancet 2003; 362: 65–71.

Knutsen AP. Immunologic effects of TCDD exposure in humans. Bull Environ Contam Toxicol 1984; 33: 673–81.

Koopman-Esseboom C, Weisglas-Kuperus N, de Ridder MAJ et al. Effects of polychlorinated biphenyl/dioxin exposure and feeding type on infants mental and psychomotor development. Pediatrics 1996; 97: 700–6.

Kreuzer PE, Csanády GyA, Baur C et al. 2,3,7,8-Tetrachlordibenzo-p-dioxin (TCDD) and congeners in infants. A toxicokinetic model of human lifetime body burden by TCDD with special emphasis on its uptake by nutrition. Arch Toxicol 1997; 71: 383–400.

Kunisue T, Someya M, Monirith I et al. Occurrence of PCBs, organochlorine insecticides, tris(4-chlorophenyl)methane, and tris(4-chlorophenyl)methanol in human breast milk collected from Cambodia. Arch Environ Contam Toxicol 2004; 46: 405–12.

Lackmann GM, Schaller KH, Angerer J. Lactational transfer of presumed carcinogenic and teratogenic organochlorine compounds within the first six months of life {in German}. Z Geburtshilfe Neonatol 2005; 209: 186–91.

LaKind JS, Amina Wilkins A, Berlin CM Jr. Environmental chemicals in human milk: a review of levels, infant exposures and health, and guidance for future research. Toxicol Appl Pharmacol 2004; 198: 184–208.

Leotsinidis M, Alexopoulos A, Kostopoulou-Farri E. Toxic and essential trace elements in human milk from Greek lactating women: association with dietary habits and other factors. Chemosphere 2005; 61: 238–47.

Levine JJ, Ilowite NT. Sclerodermalike esophageal disease in children breast-fed by mothers with silicone breast implants. J Am Med Assoc 1994; 271: 213–16.

Liebl B, Mayer R, Ommer S et al. Transition of nitro musks and polycyclic musks into human milk. Adv Exp Med Biol 2000; 478: 289–305.

Lorber M, Phillips L. Infant exposure to dioxin-like compounds in breast milk. Environ Health Perspect 2002; 110: A325–32, Figure 3.

Lozoff B, Jimenes E, Wolf A. Higher infant blood lead levels with longer duration of breast-feeding. Journal of Pediatrics 2009; 155: 663–7.

Marques RC, Dorea JG, Fonseca MF et al. Hair mercury in breast-fed infants exposed to thimerosal-preserved vaccines. Eur J Pediatrics 2007; 166: 935–41.

Massart F, Harrell JC, Federico G et al. Human breast milk and xenoestrogen exposure: a possible impact on human health. J Perinatol 2005; 25: 282–8.

Mehler HJ, Henke J, Scherbaum E et al. Pestizide, polychlorierte Biphenyle und Dioxine in Humanmilch. Sozialpädiatrie 1994; 16: 490–2.

Miller RW. Pollutants in breast milk. J Pediatr 1977; 90: 510–12.

Minh NH, Someya M, Minh TB et al. Persistent organochlorine residues in human breast milk from Hanoi and Hochiminh City, Vietnam: contamination, accumulation kinetics and risk assessment for infants. Environ Pollut 2004; 129: 431–41.

Nadal M, Espinosa G, Schuhmacher M et al. Patterns of PCDDs and PCDFs in human milk and food and their characterization by artificial neural networks. Chemosphere 2004; 54: 1375–82.

Oskarsson A, Schütz A, Skerfving S et al. Total and inorganic mercury in breast milk and blood in relation to fish consumption and amalgam fillings in lactating women. Arch Environ Health 1996; 51: 234–41.

Peters HA, Gocmen A, Cripps DJ et al. Epidemiology of hexachlorobenzene-induced porphyria in Turkey: clinical and laboratory follow-up after 25 years. Arch Neurol 1982; 39: 744–9.

Radisch B, Luck W, Nau H. Cadmium concentrations in milk and blood of smoking mothers. Toxicol Letts 1987; 36: 147–52.

Ramirez GB, Cruz CV, Pagulayan O, Ostrea E, Dalisay C. The Tagum Study I: Analysis and Clinical Correlates of Mercury in Maternal and Cord Blood, Breast Milk, Meconium and Infant's Hair. Pediatrics 2000; 106: 774–81.

Ribas-Fito N, Cardo E, Sala M et al. Breastfeeding, exposure to organochlorine compounds, and neurodevelopment in infants. Pediatrics 2003; 111: 580–85.

Rimkus G, Rimkus B, Wolf M. Nitro musks in human adipose tissue and breast milk. Chemosphere 1994; 28: 421–32.

Sakamoto M, Chan HM, Domingo JL et al. Changes in body burden of mercury, lead, arsenic cadmium and selenium in infants druing early lactation in comparison with placental transfer. Ecotoxicology and Environmental Safety 2012; 84: 179–84.

Sakamoto M, Kubota M, Matsumoto S et al. Declining risk of methylmercury exposure to infants during lactation. Environ Res 2002; 90: 185–9.

Schreiber JS. Predicted infant exposure to tetrachloroethene in human breast milk. Risk Analysis 1993; 13: 515–24.

Schuhmacher M, Domingo JL, Kiviranta H et al. Monitoring dioxins and furans in a population living near a hazardous waste incinerator: levels in breast milk. Chemosphere 2004; 57: 43–9.

Seidel HJ, Kaltenecker S, Waizenegger W. Rückgang der Belastung von Humanmilch mit ausgewählten chlororganischen Verbindungen. Umweltmed Forsch Prax 1998; 3: 83–9.

Sternowsky HJ, Wessolowski R. Lead and cadmium in breast milk. Arch Toxicol 1985; 57: 41–5.

Teufel M, Nissen KH, Sartoris J et al. Chlorinated hydrocarbons in fat tissue: analysis of residues in healthy children, tumor patients and malformed children. Arch Environ Contam Toxicol 1990; 19: 646–52.

Ursinyova M, Masanova V. Cadmium, lead and mercury in human milk from Slovakia. Food Addit Contam 2005; 22: 579–89.

Vieth B, Rüdiger T, Ostermann B et al. Rückstände von Flammschutzmitteln in Frauenmilch aus Deutschland unter besonderer Berücksichtigung von polybromierten Diphenylethern. Bericht des Umweltbundesamtes 2005.

Vreugdenhil HJ, Van Zanten GA, Brocaar MP et al. Prenatal exposure to polychlorinated biphenyls and breastfeeding: opposing effects on auditory P300 latencies in 9-year-old Dutch children. Dev Med Child Neurol 2004; 46: 398–405.

Walkowiak J, Wiener JA, Fastabend A et al. Environmental exposure to polychlorinated biphenyls and quality of the home environment: effects on psychodevelopment in early childhood. Lancet 2001; 358: 1602–7.

WHO. Polychlorinated Dibenzo-Paradioxins and Dibenzofurans; Environmental Health Criteria 88. Geneva: WHO, 1989.

Wolff S. Occupationally derived chemicals in breast milk. Am J Industr Med 1983; 4: 259–81.

Index

Note: Page numbers followed by "b" and "t" indicate recommendation boxes and tables respectively.

A

Abacavir, 152–153, 700
Abatacept, 350, 359
Abciximab, 232–233, 727
Abnormal lobe formation, 279t
Academy of Breastfeeding Medicine (ABM), 648
Acarbose, 431, 790
Acceptable daily intake (ADI), 848
ACE inhibitors (ACEI), 194, 199–200, 200b, 715
Acebutolol, 196, 711–712
Acemethacin, 657
Acenocoumarol, 233–234, 727
Acetaminophen, 27–29, 29b, 643, 646. See also Paracetamol
Acetazolamide, 486, 800
Acetic acid, 607
    derivatives, 41
Acetylcysteine, 675, 675b
Acetyldigoxin, 208
Acetylsalicylic acid (ASA), 29–32, 32b, 230, 232, 582–583, 583b, 654–655, 655b
Acipimox, 108
Acitretin, 475, 477, 478b, 797–798
Acne, 798–799
    retinoids for, 475–479, 478b
Acne gravidarum, 468
Acne treatment, 469b
Actinomycin D, 382
Activated charcoal, 362b
Acupressure, 77
Acupuncture, 77, 295b
Acyclovir, 148, 487, 697–698, 698b
Adalimumab (ADA), 103, 345–346, 346b, 359, 777–778, 778b
Adapalene, 475, 478, 478b, 798
Adefovir dipivoxil, 148
Ademethionine, 34
Adenosine, 210, 213, 719
Adrenaline, 72, 789, 789b
Adrenergic agents, 208, 208b
Adrenocorticotropic hormone (ACTH), 415
Adriamycin, 380. See also Doxorubicin
Adult T cell leukemia-lymphoma (ATL), 827
Aescin, 483, 803–804
Aflatoxins, 592, 845
Aflibercept, 350
Agar-agar, 100
Agent Orange, 612–613
Agnoside, 807

Agomelatine, 303–304, 745
Ajmaline, 211, 718
Albendazole, 144, 145b, 697
Albendazole sulfoxide, 697
Albumin, 11–12, 121, 233–234, 640t
Albumin tannate, 102
Albuterol, 66, 672
Alcohol, 469, 469b, 542–547, 601, 835–836, 836b
    binge drinking, 545–546
    fetal effects of, 547, 543–544
    fetal risk, quantifying, 544
    lactation, effects on, 647–648
    light consumption of, 545
    moderate consumption of, 545
    pharmacokinetics of, 542–547
    in pregnancy, therapeutic use of, 547, 547b
    teratogenesis, mechanism of, 542–543
Alcohol-exposed (AE), 543
Alcohol-related birth defects (ARBD), 543
Alcohol-related neurodevelopmental disorder (ARND), 543
Alcuronium, 461
Alder buckthorn, 522t
Aldesleukin, 392
Aldosterone antagonists, 216–217
Alemtuzumab, 350, 353, 386
Alendronate, 808
Alendronatic acid, 506
α-1 blockers, 202–203, 203b
α-2 blockers, 203, 203b
α-dihydroergocryptine, 330, 769
α-hexachlorocyclohexane, 610
α-methyldopa, 195–198, 196b, 647, 713–714, 713b
Alfacalcidol, 502
Alfalfa (*Medicago sativa*), 515t, 806
Alfentanil, 39, 663
Algeldrate, 94
Alginate, 94–95
Alginic acid, 94–95
Aliphatic hydrocarbons, 601
Aliskiren, 204, 204b, 716
Alitretinoin, 476, 478, 478b, 798
Alizapride, 86
Alkaloid-containing herbs, 520, 521t
Allergy, 59–61
    tests, 538
Allethrin, 481
Allethrin I, 799–800
Allopurinol, 49–50, 666–667, 667b

All-trans-retinoic acid (ATRA), 390–391
Almasilate, 94, 677–678
Almotriptan, 659
Aloe, 516t–519t
Aloin, 100–101
Alprazolam, 263, 325, 764
Alprostadil, 214
Alprostadil alfadex, 720
Alteplase, 728
Alternative remedies, 803–805, 805b
Aluminum, 483, 677–678, 678b
Aluminum aceticum, 471–472
Aluminum hydroxide, 94, 677–678
Aluminum phosphate, 94, 677–678
Amabiline, 806
Amanita, 806
    poisoning, 845
Amanita phalloides, 592, 592b
Amantadine, 150, 329, 699, 769
Ambenonium, 99
Ambrisentan, 206
Ambroxol, 70, 675, 675b
Amcinonide, 471, 788
American Academy of Pediatrics, 824, 829
    Committee on Infectious Diseases, 705
American College of Radiology (ACR), 814–815
Amezinium metilsulfate, 208, 717
Amfebutamone, 745
Amfepramone, 108, 684
Amfetaminil, 329, 769
Amikacin, 125–126, 131, 692
Amiloride, 217, 217b, 721
Aminoglutethimide, 792–793
Aminoglycosides, 125–126, 132, 692, 692b, 694
Aminophylline, 68
Aminopterin, 382
5-Aminosalicylic acid (5-ASA), 103–104, 359,
    682
Amiodarone, 209–212, 718–719
Amisulpride, 313, 315b–316b, 316, 321, 756
Amitriptyline, 302, 304, 583–584, 584b, 660b,
    744b, 745, 752
Amlodipine, 198, 714
Ammonium bitumen sulfonate, 473, 798
Ammonium sulfate, 607
Ammonium thiocyanate, 607
Ammonium thiosulfate, 607
Amodiaquine, 133–134, 134b, 695
Amorolfine, 143, 696–697
Amoxicillin, 97, 97b, 116, 679b, 688
Amphetamines, 555–556, 836, 836b
    effects on lactation, 647–648
Amphotericin B, 141, 141b, 696, 697b
Ampicillin, 116
Anabolics, 438–439, 438b, 792, 792b
Anakinra, 350, 359
Anastrozole, 389, 792–793
Androgens, 438–439, 438b, 792, 792b
Anencephaly, 121–122, 156, 279t, 283, 312, 499
Anesthetics, local, 472, 664–665
Anethole trithione, 99
Angel dust. *See* Phencyclidine piperidine (PCP)

Angelica, 520t
Angiotensin II activity, 44–45
Angiotensin II receptor antagonists (ARBs), 194,
    200–202, 201b, 715–716
Angiotensin-aldosterone system, 199
Angiotensin-converting-enzyme inhibitors. *See*
    ACE inhibitors (ACEI)
Anidulafungin, 141, 696
Anise, 683
Animal toxins, 590–592
Anistreplase, 238–239, 728
Anomaly of lacrimal duct, 279t
Antacids, 94–95, 95b, 677–678, 678b
Anterior pituitary hormones, 415–416, 416b
Anthelmintics, 144–147, 697, 697b
Anthracyclines, 373–375, 383
Anthraquinone derivatives, 100–101
Anthraquinone laxatives, 521, 522t
Anthraquinones, 100–101, 521
Antiadrenergic agents
    centrally acting, 716
    peripherally acting, 716
Antiallergics, 472
Antiarrhythmic medications, 208–213, 717–719,
    719b
    class IA, 211, 717–718
    class IB, 211, 718
    class IC, 212, 718
    class II, 212, 718. *See also* β-receptor
        blockers
    class III, 212–213, 718–719
    class IV, 213, 719
    for fetus, 209–210
    for pregnant women, 209
    pharmacology, 211–213
    toxicology, 211–213
Antiasthmatic medications, 65–74
Antibodies
    maternal antibodies, 180–181, 184–185, 706
    monoclonal antibodies, 777–778
    thyroid receptor antibodies, 785–786
Antibiotics, 487, 692–693, 797
    β-lactam, 688, 688b
    glycopeptide, 692, 692b
    local, 132, 132b, 694–695, 694b
    polypeptide, 692, 692b
Anticholinergic agents, 70
Anticholinergic spasmolytics, 681, 681b
Anticoagulants, 725–726
    indications for, 226
Anticonvulsive drugs, 16t, 211, 260, 270, 273
Antidepressants, 294–295, 295b, 743–755, 744b
    agomelatine, 745
    amitriptyline, 745
    atomoxetine, 745
    bupropion, 745
    citalopram, 746
    clomipramine, 746–747
    desipramine, 747
    desvenlafaxine, 755
    dosulepine, 747
    doxepin, 747–748

duloxetine, 748
escitalopram, 748–749
fluoxetine, 749–750
fluvoxamine, 750
imipramine, 750
maprotiline, 751
mianserin, 751
mirtazapine, 751
moclobemide, 752
nefazodone, 752
nortriptyline, 752
opipramol, 752
paroxetine, 753
reboxetine, 753
hypericin. See Hypericin
sertraline, 753–754
tranylcypromine, 754
trazodone, 754
trimipramine, 754
venlafaxine, 755
Antidiabetics, 789–790, 790b
Antidiarrheal agents, 102–103, 102b
Anti-diuretic hormone (ADH), 417
Antiemetics, 86–87, 86b, 684–685
Antiepileptic drugs (AEDs), 252–253,
      252b–253b, 324, 731–742
   classification of, 252
   contraceptive failure and, 253
   damage mechanisms, 258
   folic acid and, 259
   impact on fertility, 253–254
   mental development dysfunction, 257
   pregnancy complications associated with,
      256–257
   vitamin K and, 259–260
Antifungal agents
   systemic, 696, 696b
   topical, 696–697, 697b
Anti-galactogogues, 805–807, 807b
Antigout preparations, 49–51
Antihemorrhagics, 239–241, 240b–241b, 728,
      728b
Antihidrotica, 483–484, 484b
Antihistamines, 59–61, 78–79, 487, 591,
      671–672, 672b
Antihypertensives, 716–717, 717b
Antihypotensives, 207, 717, 717b
Anti-infective agents, 115–176, 687–704
Anti-inflammatory drugs, 797
Antimalarial medication, 695–696, 695b
Antimanic drugs, 762–764
Antimetabolites, 16t, 360
Antimony, 856
Antimycotics, 797
Antineoplastic drugs, 373–400, 779–780, 780b
   with endocrine effects, 389–390
Antipruritics, 472, 797
Antipsychotics, 313–316, 315b–316b
Antiretroviral agents, 12–13, 151–153, 153b,
      699–700, 700b
Antiretroviral therapy (ART), 151–152, 699–700.
      See also Zidovudine
Antirheumatic drugs, 41–46, 658–659
Anti-scabies, 482–483, 483b
Antiseptics, 468–471
Antithymocyte globulins, 358
Antitussives, 71–72, 675–676
Antivenom, 590–591
Antiviral agents, 697–700
   for hepatitis, 148–150
   for influenza, 150–151
Antley–Bixler syndrome, 139
Ants sting, 591–593, 591b
Anxiolytics, 324–325, 328, 764, 767–768
Apixaban, 225–226, 231
Aplasia cutis, 228, 421
   of scalp, 279t
Appetite suppressants, 108–109, 684
Apple pectin, 102
Apreomycin, 131
Aprepitant, 86
Aprotinin, 240, 240b
Arachidonic acid, 401–402
Arachnoidal cysts, 279t
Arbor vitae, 521t
Argatroban, 230, 726, 726b
l-Arginine, 206
Argipressin, 784
Aripiprazole, 313, 316, 756
Aromatherapy, 514
   diffusers, 514
Arsenic, 577–578, 578b, 616–617, 616b,
      855–856
Arsenic trioxide, 391
Artemether, 134, 136, 695
Artemisinin-based combination therapy (ACT), 134
Artemisinin derivatives, 134–135, 135b, 695
Artemotil, 134, 695
Arterial hypertension, 194–195
Artesunate, 134, 695
Articaine, 457–458, 665
Ascorbic acid. See Vitamin C
Asenapine, 313, 316, 763, 763b
Asparaginase, 391
Aspergillus oryxae, 98
Aspirin. See Acetylsalicylic acid
Astemizole, 59
Asthma treatment, anticholinergics for, 674–675,
      674b
Astringents, 471–472, 471b, 797
Atazanavir, 152, 158, 700
Atenolol, 196, 712
Atomoxetine, 304, 745
Atopic eczema, immunomodulators for, 473,
      473b
Atorvastatin, 106, 683
Atosiban, 406–408, 408b, 784
Atovaquone, 133, 135, 135b, 695
Atracurium, 461
Atrial septal defects (ASD), 546
Atropine, 98, 99b, 580–581, 581b
Atropine-like belladonna alkaloids, 98
Attention deficit hyperactivity disorder (ADHD),
      563–564, 836

Atypical antidepressants, 304
Aucubin, 807
Auranofin, 658
Aurothiomalate, 658
Autism, 5t–6t, 7, 16t, 47–48, 178–179, 544
Autism spectrum disorders (ASD), 66–67, 257, 282, 301
Autumn crocus (*Colchicum autumnale*), 50, 521t
Avitaminosis, 493
Ayurveda, 512, 803–804
Azacitidine, 384–385
Azathioprine (AZA), 94, 341–342, 342b, 352, 354, 358–359, 383, 659b, 775–776, 776b
Azelaic acid, 474, 474b
Azelastine, 59, 672
Azidocillin, 116
Azidothymidine (AZT). *See* Zidovudine
Azilsartan, 200
Azithromycin, 118, 119b, 689
Azole antifungals, 139–141, 140b
  for systemic use, 139–140
  for topical use, 140–141
Aztreonam, 688

B

Baby Friendly Hospital Initiative (BFHI), 640–641
Bacampicillin, 116
Bacitracin, 127, 692
Baclofen, 48, 666
Bacterial endotoxins, 592–593
Balsalazide, 103
Bambuterol, 67, 673, 673b
Bamipine, 59, 672
Barberry, 520t–521t
Barbexaclone, 270, 736–737
Barbiturate embryopathies, 256
Barbiturates, 731b–732b
Barium, 856
Barium sulfate contrast medium, 531
Basiliximab, 350, 358
Bath PUVA, 479, 479b
Bath salts, 556–557
Bayley Scales of Infant Development
  Second Edition (BSID-II), 300–301
  Third Edition, 300–301
BCG vaccination, 829
Beclomethasone, 67, 673, 788
Bees sting, 591–592, 591b
Belatacept, 350, 358
Belimumab, 350
Bemetizide, 215
Benazepril, 715b
Benazeprilate, 715
Bendamustine, 378–379
Bendiocarb, 609
Bendroflumethiazide, 215, 721
Benomyl, 609
Benperidol, 313, 316, 758
Benproperine, 71, 676

Benserazide, 329, 769
Benzatropine, 330, 769
Benzbromaron, 667
Benzene, 856
Benzimidazole anthelmintics, 144–145
Benzocaine, 457–458, 665, 665b
Benzodiazepines, 253, 325–327, 327b, 591, 764–767, 767b
  alprazolam, 764
  clobazam, 764
  clonazepam. *See* Clonazepam
  diazepam, 764–765
  flunitrazepam, 765
  lorazepam, 765
  lormetazepam, 765
  metaclazepam, 765
  midazolam, 766
  nitrazepam, 766
  oxazepam, 766
  prazepam, 766
  quazepam, 766
  temazepam, 766–767
Benzothiazides, 215
Benzoyl peroxide, 469, 469b
Benzydamine, 471, 801
Benzyl benzoate, 482–483, 483b, 799–800
Benzylpenicillin, 116
Betahistine, 214, 720
β-blockers, 800
β-carotene, 496, 496b
β-hexachlorocyclohexane, 610
β-lactam antibiotics, 116–117, 116b, 688, 688b
β-lactamase inhibitors, 116–117, 688b
β-receptor blockers, 196–198, 197b, 211–212, 711–713, 713b, 717b, 718
β-sympathomimetics, 406
β_2-adrenergic agonists
  non-selective, 72–73
  other agonists, 72–73
  selective, 66–67
β_2-sympathomimetics, 406–407, 406b, 672–673, 673b
Betamethasone, 210, 423, 425–426, 788
Betaxolol, 196, 712
Bethanechol, 99, 681
Bevacizumab, 350–351, 386
Bexarotene, 391
Bezafibrate, 105, 683
Bicalutamide, 792–793
Bifidobacterium, 103
Bifonazole, 140, 696
Biguanide. *See* Metformin
Bilastine, 59, 671–672
Bilateral cataract, 279t
Bilateral cryptorchidism, 49–50
Bilateral iris defect, 279t
Bilirubin, 121–122, 122b, 158, 643, 646, 689
Binge drinking, 545–546
Bioallethrin, 481
Biologicals, 480, 777–778
Biologics, 345–352
Biperiden, 318, 330, 769

Biphosphonates, 506–507, 506b, 808–809, 809b
Birth defects, smoking and, 550
Bis-(p-hydroxyphenyl)-pyridyl-2-methane
    (BHPM), 681–682, 682b
Bisacodyl, 100, 681–682
Bismuth nitrate, 679
Bismuth salts, 97, 97b
Bisoprolol, 196, 660b, 713
Bivalirudin, 230, 726, 726b
Black box warning, 374b
Black cohosh (Cimicifuga racemosa),
    803–804
Bleomycin, 377–378, 381–382, 480
Blessed thistle (Cnicus benedictus), 806
Blibornuride, 790
Blood vessel changes, 468
Blood–brain barrier, 12
Blue cohosh, 520t
Boceprevir, 149–150, 698
Borage (Borage officinalis), 806
Bornaprine, 330, 769
Boron, 856
Bortezomib, 385
Bosentan, 205–206
Botulinum neurotoxin (BoNT), 462
Botulinum toxin, 48–49, 592–593, 666, 666b
Brain-derived growth factor (BDGF), 258
Breast cancer, antineoplastic drugs for, 376,
    376b
Breastfed infants, persistent organochlorine
    compound levels in, 850
Breastfeeding
    advantages of, 639–641
    and environmental contaminants, 857–858
    support, 648
    and workplace environment, 857–858
Breastfeeding, infections during, 821–834
    B-streptococcus-B infection, 830
    common infections, 822
    cytomegaly, 822–823, 823b
    dengue virus, 823, 823b
    haemophilus influenza, 830
    hepatitis A virus, 823–824, 823b
    hepatitis B virus, 824, 824b
    hepatitis C virus, 824, 824b
    hepatitis E virus, 824–825, 825b
    herpes simplex virus, 825, 825b
    herpes zoster virus, 825–826, 826b
    HIV, 826–827, 827b
    human T-lymphotropic virus, 827, 827b
    influenza virus, 827–828, 827b
    Lyme disease, 828, 828b
    methicillin-resistant Staphylococcus
        aureus, 828, 828b
    rotavirus, 828–829, 829b
    tuberculosis, 829–830, 829b
    varicella-zoster virus, 825–826, 826b
    West Nile virus, 830, 830b
Breast problems, topical treatment for, 807,
    807b
Bright morning light therapy, 295b
Brimonidine, 486

Brinzolamide, 486, 800
British Anti-Lewisite. See Dimercaprol
Brivudine, 147, 698
Bromazepam, 325
Bromelain, 807, 807b
Bromhexine, 70, 675, 675b
Bromine, 607
Bromocriptine, 330, 416, 417b, 647–648, 769,
    769b, 785, 785b
Bromodichloromethane, 614–615
Bromperidol, 313, 316, 758
Bromsulphthalein, 537
Brotizolam, 325
B-streptococcus-B infection, during
    breastfeeding, 830
Buckhorn plantain, 70
Buclizine, 78–79
Budesonide, 103, 487, 673b, 788
Budipin, 330, 769
Bufexamac, 471
Buflomedil, 214
Bulking agents, 100
Bumetanide, 216, 721
Bunazosin, 202–203, 716
Bupivacaine, 457–458, 664
Buprenorphine, 40, 563
Bupropion, 295b, 304, 555, 745, 763, 839
Buserelin, 414, 783
Buspirone, 328, 732, 749, 768
Busulfan, 379
Butenafine, 143, 696–697
Butoconazole, 141, 696
Butylscopolamine, 98, 681, 681b
Butyrophenones, 313, 315b–316b

C

C1-esterase inhibitor deficiency, 61–62
Cabbage leaf, 807
Cabergoline, 330, 416, 417b, 769, 769b
    on lactation, 647–648
Cadmium, 617, 617b, 855
Caesarean births, 564
Caffeine, 328, 547–549, 549b, 643, 836–837, 837b
Calcipotriol, 798
Calcitonin, 506
Calcitriol, 422, 502
Calcium, 504–505, 505b
Calcium antagonists, 407, 407b, 714
Calcium carbonate, 94–95, 677–678
Calcium channel blockers (CCBs), 198–199, 199b
Calendula ointment, 807
Camphor, 472, 472b
Canakinumab, 351
Canalizumab, 51b
Cancer and pregnancy. See Malignancy and
    pregnancy
Cancer therapy, 357, 373–374
Candesartan, 200, 715
Cannabidiol, 353
Cannabis, 559–561, 560b, 837, 837b

Canrenone, 721
Capecitabine, 384–385
Capreomycin, 694
Captopril, 715b
Caraway, 683
Carbachol, 99, 681
Carbaldrate, 94, 677–678
Carbamates, 609–610, 609b, 847
Carbamazepine, 16t, 251–254, 252b–253b,
    256–264, 263b, 279, 324, 584–585, 585b,
    672, 731–732, 749, 763
  functional disturbances, 262–263
  malformation frequency, 261–262
  somatic anomalies, 262
  typical malformations, 261–263
Carbamazepineoxide, 732
Carbamic acid, 609
Carbamide preparation, 473–474, 473b
Carbapenems, 117–118, 117b
Carbendazim. *See* Benomyl
Carbenicillin, 116
Carbetocin, 784
Carbidopa, 329, 769
Carbimazole, 421, 786
Carbitocin, 404
Carbocisteine, 70, 675
Carbofuran, 485
Carbon disulfide, 603–604, 604b
Carbon monoxide (CO) poisoning, 578–579,
    579b
Carbophenothion, 610
Carboplatin, 385–386
Carboxymethyl cellulose, 100
Carcinogenic properties, 471, 520, 529, 605,
    646, 721, 799b, 838
Carcinogenicity, 49–50
Cardiac glycosides, 208, 208b
Cardiac malformation, 109, 210, 298, 303,
    306–307, 309–310, 322–323, 434–435,
    441, 588
Cardiac vasodilators, 213–214, 214b
Cardioversion, 209–210
Carminatives, 98, 98b, 683, 683b
Carmustine, 378, 386
Carteolol, 196
Caspofungin, 696
Castor oil, 101
Catecholamines, 72, 401–402, 453, 555, 789b
Catheter ablation, 209
Cathine, 108
Cathinone, 684
Catnip, 521t
Catumaxomab, 386
Cefaclor, 117
Cefadroxil, 117
Cefalexin, 688
Cefamandole, 117
Cefazolin, 117
Cefdinir, 117
Cefditoren, 117
Cefepime, 117
Cefixim, 117

Cefmetazole, 117
Cefoperazone, 117
Cefotaxime, 117
Cefotetan, 117
Cefotiam, 117
Cefoxitin, 117
Cefpirome, 117
Cefpodoxim, 117
Cefprozil, 117
Ceftaroline, 117
Ceftazidime, 117
Ceftibuten, 117
Ceftizoxime, 117
Ceftobiprole, 117
Ceftriaxone, 117, 830
Cefuroxime, 117, 688
Celecoxib, 391, 657, 658b
Celiprolol, 196
Cell/mobile phones, 625, 625b
Centchroman, 791
Center for Disease Control (CDC) vaccines,
    709–710
Cephalexin, 117
Cephalosporins, 12–13, 117, 117b, 688,
    688b–689b
Cephalotin, 117
Cephradine, 117
Cerebral atrophy, 279t, 377–378, 381, 387
Cerivastatin, 106
Certolizumab, 103
Certolizumab pegol (CZP), 346, 346b, 359
Certoparin, 227, 725
Cesium, 856
Cetirizine, 59–60, 671–672
Cetrorelix, 414–415, 784
Cetuximab, 386
Chamomile, 515t
Charcoal, 94, 102b, 683b. *See also* Medical
    charcoal
Chaste tree, 807
Chasteberry (*Vitex agnus-castus*),
    807
Chenodesoxycholic acid, 104–105, 105b, 684,
    684b
Chernobyl disaster, 623
Chicken pox, 825–826
Childhood illness, smoking and, 551–552
Children, fetal alcohol spectrum disorders in,
    547
Chinese herbs, 512, 803–804, 854
Chinese medicines, 803–804
Chinidin, 211
Chloral hydrate, 328, 768
Chlorambucil, 378
Chloramphenicol, 127–128, 128b, 132, 487,
    692–693, 693b, 800
Chlordiazepoxide, 263, 325
Chlorethane, 665
Chlorhexidine, 470
Chlorhydrate, 483
Chlorhydrocarbons, 856
Chlorinated dibenzodioxins, 613

Chlorinated drinking water by-products, 614–616, 616b
Chlorinated phenol derivatives, 470
Chlormadinon, 435, 791
Chloroform, 604, 604b
Chloroprocaine, 457–458
Chloroquine, 133–136, 135b, 358–359, 361–362, 362b, 695, 695b
Chlorothalonil, 485
Chlorotrianisen, 791
Chlorphenamine, 59, 675
Chlorphenesin, 488, 801
Chlorphenoxamine, 59, 672
Chlorpromazine, 82, 313, 317, 647, 756–757
Chlorprothixene, 313, 317, 757
Chlorprothixene sulfoxide, 757
Chlorpyrifos, 485, 580, 610–611
Chlortalidone, 215, 720, 721b
Chlortetracycline, 120
Cholera vaccination, 179, 179b
Cholestasis, 822
Cholestyramine, 683–684
Cholinergics, 99, 99b, 680–681, 681b
Chondroitin sulfate, 34, 229
Chorionic gonadotropin, 415, 784
Chorionic gonadotropin alfa, 415
Chromium, 507
Chromosomal abnormalities, 5t–6t, 51
Chronic inflammatory bowel diseases, medications for, 682–683, 683b
Chymotrypsin, 98, 240, 683
Ciclesonide, 67, 673
Ciclopirox, 143, 696–697
Ciclosporine, 342–343, 343b
Cidofovir, 147, 698
Cignoline. See Dithranol
Cilastatin, 688
Cilastin, 117
Cilazapril, 715
Cimetidine, 95–96, 678
Cinacalet, 506
Cinchocaine, 457–458, 665
Cineol, 675
Cinnarizine, 214, 720
Ciprofibrate, 105
Ciprofloxacin, 103, 123, 126, 690
Circulatory drugs, 719–720
Cisatracurium, 461
Cisplatin, 377–378, 386–387, 779–780
Citalopram, 295, 303, 305, 744b, 746
Citric acid, 607
Cladribine, 353, 383
Clarithromycin, 97, 97b, 103, 118, 119b, 679b, 689
Class IA antiarrhythmics, 211, 717–718
Class IB antiarrhythmics, 211, 718
Class IC antiarrhythmics, 212, 718
Class II antiarrhythmics, 718. See also β-receptor blockers
Class III antiarrhythmics, 212–213, 718–719
Class IV antiarrhythmics, 213, 719
Clavulanic acid, 116, 688

Cleft lip, 550, 43
Cleft palate, 37, 85, 321, 498
Clemastine, 59, 672
Clenbuterol, 67, 406, 673
Clindamycin, 119–120, 119b, 133, 409, 693, 693b
Clioquinol, 470
Clobazam, 252, 263–264, 264b, 325, 764
Clobenzorex, 108
Clobetasol propionate, 471, 471b
Clobetasone, 471
Clodronate, 808
Clodronic acid, 506
Clofarabine, 383
Clofibrate, 105
Clofibric acid derivatives and analogs, 105–106, 106b
Clomethiazole, 328, 768
Clomiphene, 440–441, 441b
Clomipramine, 302, 305, 746–747
Clonazepam, 252, 263–264, 264b, 325, 731b–732b, 732–733, 764
Clonidine, 203, 203b, 716
Clopamide, 215, 721
Clopidogrel, 230–232, 727
Clopirox, 696–697
Cloprednol, 788
Clostebol, 792
Clostridium botulinum toxin, 483–484
Clotiazepam, 325
Clotrimazole, 140, 141b, 143, 409, 696, 697b
Cloxacillin, 116
Clozapine, 313, 317, 585, 585b, 755, 757
Coagulation and pregnancy, 226. See also Fibrin; Thrombophilia
Coal tar preparations, 472–473, 473b
Coca bush (Erythroxylon coca), 557
Cocaine, 557–559, 559b, 837–838, 837b
Coconut oil, 799–800
Codeine, 37b, 71, 647, 661–662, 662b, 675
Coffee, 521t. See also Caffeine
Cognitive behavioral therapy (CBT), 555b
Cognitive development, smoking and, 553
Colbicistat, 161
Colchicine, 50–51, 585, 585b, 667, 667b
Cold remedies, 675
Colecalciferol, 502
Colesevelam, 107, 683–684, 684b
Colestipol, 107
Colestyramine, 107–108, 108b, 362b
Colistin, 127, 692
Colt's foot, 521t
Combination vaccine, 708
Comfrey (Symphytum officinale), 804
Complementary therapy, 76–78
Compositae, 804
Computerized tomography (CT), 528–529
Conduct disorder, smoking and, 553
Condylomata acuminata, 799, 480, 481b
Conestat alfa, 62
Congenital anomalies, 225–226, 233, 279t, 384

Congo red, 537
Constipation, 99–102, 102b
Consumer Labs, 513
Contrast media, 531–534
  barium sulfate, 531
  iodine-containing, 532–533, 532b, 813–815, 815b
  magnetic resonance, 533, 533b
  ultrasound/ultrasonographic, 533–534, 534b, 816, 816b
Copper, 507
Corifollitropin alfa, 415
Corneal cloudiness, 279t
Coronary therapeutic drugs, 213–214, 214b
Corticoids, 103, 358
Corticorelin, 414, 784
Corticosteroids, 94, 425, 788–789, 789b, 797
Cortisol, 423
Cosmetics, 485, 797–798
Co-trimoxazole, 128–129
Cough medications, 65–74
Coumarin, 727
  embryopathy, 234
  therapy, adverse effects of, 236
Covalent binding, 13
Cow's milk, composition of, 640t
COX inhibitors, 42–45
Coxibes, 41, 45
Cyclooxygenase-2 (COX-2) inhibitors, 45–46, 359, 657–658, 658b
Cranberry, 516t–519t
Cresol, 470
Croconazole, 141, 696
Crohn's disease, 103
Cromoglicic acid, 69, 487, 674, 674b
Crotamiton, 482–483, 483b, 799–800
Cryotherapy, 799, 799b
Cryptococcus neoformans, 142
Crystal violet, 470
Cyanescens, 561
Cyanocobalamin. *See* Vitamin B$_{12}$ (cyanocobalamin)
Cyclizine, 78–79
Cyclopentolate, 486–487
Cyclophosphamide, 358–359, 373–374, 378–381, 384, 386, 780
Cycloserine, 131, 694
Cyclosporine, 358–359, 659b, 776–777
Cyclosporine A (CyA), 342–343, 776–777, 777b
Cypermethrin, 611–612
Cyproheptadine, 59, 672
Cyproterone acetate, 438b, 439, 792–793
Cytarabine, 373–374, 383–384
Cytochalasin, 592
Cytomegaly, 822–823, 823b
Cytostatics, 385
Cytotoxic anthracycline antibiotics, 380–381

D

Dabigatran, 225–226, 726, 726b
Dabigatran etexilate, 230
Dacarbazine, 378–379, 386
Daclizumab, 351, 353
Dacthal, 485
Dalfampridine, 353–354
Dalfopristin, 129
Dalteparin, 227, 725
Danaparoid, 229, 725–726, 726b
Danazol, 61–62, 438b, 439, 792–793
Dandelion (*Taraxcum officinate*), 515t, 804
Dandy Walker anomaly, 279t
Dantrolene, 49
Dapsone, 128, 128b, 133, 694–695
Daptomycin, 127, 127b, 692
Darbepoetin alfa, 441
Darifenacin, 98, 681
Darunavir, 152, 158, 700
Dasatinib, 388
Daunorubicin, 380
Deathcap mushrooms, 806
Decabromodiphenyl ether, 849–850
Deep vein thrombosis (DVP), 228–229
Defibrillator, 213
Deflazacort, 788
Delavirdine, 152, 155–156, 700
Deltamethrin, 611–612
Demeclocycline, 120
Dengue virus infection, during breastfeeding, 823, 823b
Dequalinium chloride, 488, 801
Dequalium, 410
Dermatan sulfate, 229
Dermatitis, 798–799
Dermatological medication and local therapeutics, 797–802
  acne, 798
  dermatitis, 798–799
  essential oils, 798
  eye, nose and ear drops, 800–801
  fumaric acid preparations, 799
  lice, 799–800, 800b
  photochemotherapy, 799, 799b
  psoriasis, 798–799
  retinoids, 798–799, 799b
  scabies, 799–800, 800b
  topical applications and cosmetics, 797–798
  vein therapeutics, 801
  wart removal medications, 799, 799b
Desensitization therapy, 671, 672b
Desethylamiodarone, 718–719
Desferrioxamine, 587, 587b
Desflurane, 452, 801
Desipramine, 302, 306, 747
Desirudin, 230, 726, 726b
Desloratadine, 59, 671–672
Desmethylchloroquine, 695
Desmethylcitalopram, 746
Desmethyldiazepam, 764–766
Desmethylescitalopram, 748–749
Desmethylmetaclazepam, 765
Desmethylmianserin, 751
Desmethylmirtazapine, 751
Desmethylsertraline, 753–754

Desmopressin, 417, 417b, 784
Desogestrel, 435, 791
Desvenlafaxine, 755
Deterministic effects, 529
Developmental disorders, causes of, 14, 15t
Developmental toxic agents, mechanisms of,
    13–14
Developmental toxicology, 4–8
    drug-induced, 8–10
Dexamethasone, 210, 423–425, 788
Dexamphetamine, 836
Dexchlorpheniramine, 59, 672
Dexfenfluramin, 108–109
Dexibuprofen, 43
Dexketoprofen, 657
Dextrans, 241, 242b, 728
Dextromethorphan, 71, 675, 676b
D-galactose, 533–534, 534b, 816, 816b
Diabetes mellitus (DM), 426–428, 428b
Diacetolol, 711–712
Diacetylmorphine, 562
Diagnostic agents, 527–540
Diagnostic imaging, 527–531, 531b
    magnetic resonance imaging, 531
    radiation effects, 529–530
    ultrasound, 530–531
    X-ray examinations, 527–530
3,4-Diaminopyridine, 99
Diacetolol, 711–712
Diagnostic agents, 527–540
Diamorphine, 563, 839–840
Diarrhea, antidiarrheals for, 683
Diazepam, 263, 311–312, 325–326, 585–586,
    586b, 764–765, 767b, 841
Diazinon, 485, 580
Diazoxide, 204, 204b, 716
Dibenzepin, 302
Dibromoacetic acid, 615
Dichlordiphenyltrichlorethan (DDT), 847–849
Dichlorodiphenyldichloroethylene (DDE), 610
Dichlorodiphenyltrichlorethane (DDT), 610
Dichloromethane, 604–605, 605b
Diclectin, 685
Diclofenac, 655–656, 657b, 660b
Dicloxacillin, 116
Didanosine, 152–154, 700
Dieldrin, 610, 847
Dienogest, 435
Diethylcarbamazine, 146, 147b
Diethylenetriaminepenta acetic acid (DTPA), 607
Diethyl-m-toluamide (DEET), 485
Diethylpropion, 108
Diethylpropiorin, 684
Diethylstilbestrol (DES), 10, 437–438
Diethyltoluamide, 485
Diet manipulations, for nausea and vomiting,
    76
Digestives, 98, 98b, 683, 683b
Digitalis, 717
    glycosides, 212
    toxicity, 586, 586b
Digitoxin, 208–209
Digoxin, 212, 717, 717b

Dihydralazine, 202, 202b, 713
Dihydroartemisinin, 134, 695
Dihydrocodeine, 71
Dihydroergotamine (DHE), 47, 717
Dihydroergotamine mesylate, 208
Dihydrotachysterol, 502
Dihyralazine, 195
Diltiazem, 198, 206, 211, 714, 717b, 719
Dimenhydranate, 59, 78–79
Dimenhydrinate, 79, 684–685, 685b
Dimepranole-4-acetoamidobenzoate, 147
Dimercaprol, 577
2,3-Dimercaptopropanol, 363
Dimethicone, 683
Dimethindene, 59
Dimethoxymethylamphetamine, 555
Dimethyl fumarate, 352–353, 479–480
Dimethyltryptamine, 555
Dimeticone, 98, 481, 799–800
Dimetindene, 672
Dineprostone, 402
Dinoprostol, 402
Dioxins, 847
    in mothers' milk, 848
Diphenhydramine, 59, 78–79, 328, 684–685,
    767, 767b
Diphenhydrinate, 79–80
Diphenoxylate, 102
Diphtheria vaccination, 179–180, 180b
Dipivefrin, 486, 800
Dipyridamole, 225–226, 233, 727
Dipyrone, 655
Dirithromycin, 118–119, 689
Disease modifying antirheumatic drugs
    (DMARDs), 358–359
Disinfectants, 468–471
    alcohol, 469
    benzoyl peroxide, 469
    mercury compounds, 470
    phenol derivatives, 470
    povidone iodine, 469–470
Disopyramide, 211, 718
Distigmine, 99, 681
Dithranol, 474, 798
Diuretics, 215–217, 720–721, 721b
    effects on lactation, 647–648
    loop, 216
    thiazide, 215
Docetaxel, 385
Docosanol, 148, 698
Docusate, 101
Dolasetron, 685
Dolutegravir, 152, 161
Domperidone, 81, 647, 680, 680b
Dong quai, 520t
Dopamine agonists, 416–417, 417b,
    647–648
Doripenem, 117, 688
Dorzolamide, 486, 800
Dosulepine, 302, 747
Dosulepine sulfoxide, 747
Dothiepin, 583
Down syndrome, 505, 623

Doxazosin, 202–203, 716
Doxepin, 302, 306, 744b, 747–748
Doxorubicin, 380, 386, 780
Doxycycline, 120, 133, 689
Doxylamine, 59, 78–80, 328, 497, 685, 767, 768b
D-penicillamine, 358–359, 363–364, 659
Dried extracts, 513
Drinking water contaminants, 856
Dronedarone, 211, 213, 719
Droperidol, 81, 313, 317, 758
Drospirenon, 435, 791
Drug abuse, 555–562
  amphetamines, 555–556
  bath salts, 556–557
  cannabis, 559–561, 560b
  cocaine, 557–559, 559b
  lysergic acid diethylamide, 561
  MDMA, 556–557
  phencyclidine, 561
  psilocybin, 561–562, 562b
Drug classification, 17–18
Drug-induced reproductive/developmental toxicology, 8–10
Drug risks in pregnancy, communicating, 19–20
Ductus arteriosus (DA), 32, 32b, 43–44, 216, 279t, 583b, 589b
Duloxetine, 306, 748
Duogynon®, 437
Dydrogesterone, 435
Dydrogestone, 791
Dyes, 537–538, 537b, 817–818, 817b

E

Ear drops, 487–488, 800–801
Early human development, 2f
Ebastine, 59–60, 671–672
Ecallantide, 62
Echinacea, 516t–519t, 803–804
Echinacea purpurea, 357
Echinocandins, 141–142, 142b
Echinocandins anidulafungin, 696
Econazole, 141, 696
Eclampsia, 407, 408b
Ecstasy, 556–557
Eculizumab, 351
Edoxaban, 231
Edrophonium, 99
Efavirenz, 152, 156, 700, 826
Eflornithine, 484, 485b, 801
Elcometrin, 791
Elective termination of pregnancy (ETOP), 19
Electric shocks, 627, 627b
Electrocardioversion, 213
Electrocautery, 480, 481b, 799, 799b
Electromagnetic radiation, 625–626, 627b
Eletriptan, 659, 660b
Eltrombopag, 240, 728
Elvitegravir, 152, 161, 700, 728

Embryo/fetotoxicity, 4
  risk assessment, 15–17, 16t
Embryogenesis, 4
Emtricitabine, 152–154, 700
Enalapril, 715, 715b
(S)-enantiomer, 43
Endorphins, 34
Endothelin receptor antagonists (ERAs), 205–206
Endothion, 610
Enflurane, 452–453, 455, 665
Enfurvitide, 152, 160, 700
Enoxacin, 123, 690
Enoxaparin, 227, 725
Entacapon, 769
Entecavir, 148–149, 698
Entry inhibitors, 160–161
Environmental contaminants, 847–862
  antimony, 856
  arsenic, 855–856
  barium, 856
  boron, 856
  breastfeeding and, 857–858
  cadmium, 855
  cesium, 856
  lead, 853–855, 855b
  lithium, 856
  mercury, 851–853
  persistent organochlorine compounds, 847–851
  rubidium, 856
  selenium, 856
  uranium, 856
  vanadium, 856
Enzyme tests, 538, 818
Ephedra, 520t
Ephedrine, 72, 675. *See also* Adrenaline
Epilepsy. *See also* Seizure
  impact on fertility, 253–254
  malformations, risk of, 254–255
  teratogenicity of, 260
  typical malformations and anomalies, 256
Epimestrol, 791
Epinastine, 59, 672
Epirubicin, 380–381
Eplerenone, 216–217, 721
Epoetin alfa, 441, 442b
Epoetin beta, 441, 442b
Epoetin delta, 441
Epoetin theta, 441
Epoetin zeta, 441
Epoprostenol, 206–207
Eprosartan, 200, 715
Epsilon-aminocaproic acid, 240b
Eptifibatide, 232–233, 727
Ergocalciferol, 502
Ergot alkaloids, 404–405, 405b. *See also* Ergotamine derivatives
Ergotamine, 47, 402, 659
Ergotamine derivatives, 47–48
Ergotamine tartrate, 47, 659
Erlotinib, 388

Ertapenem, 117, 688
Erythromycin, 118–119, 119b, 688–689, 689b
Erythropoietin, 441–442, 442b
Escitalopram, 295, 306, 590, 748–749, 763
Eslicarbazepine, 252, 264, 264b, 733
Esmolol, 196
Esomeprazole, 96, 678
Essential oils, 472, 514, 514t, 521, 521t, 798
Estolate, 118
Estradiol valerate, 434
Estriol, 434, 791
Estrogens, 434–435, 790–792, 801
   effects on lactation, 647–648
   effect on milk production, 790
   hormonal transfer to infant via mother's milk,
      790–791
Eszopiclone, 327
Etanercept, 103, 346–348, 348b, 359, 778,
      778b
Ethacridine, 683
Ethacridine lactate, 102
Ethambutol, 129–130, 130b, 693
Ethanol, 579, 580b
   in pregnancy, therapeutic use of, 547
Ether (diethyl ether), 454, 454b
Ethinyl estradiol, 434, 791
Ethionamide, 131, 694
Ethosuximide, 252–253, 259, 264–265, 265b,
      731b–732b, 733
Ethyl alcohol, 409
Ethyl hydrogen fumarate, 479–480
Ethylenediamine tetra acetic acid (EDTA), 607
Ethylether, 601
Ethylmercury, 620, 851–852
Etidronate, 808
Etidronic acid, 506
Etilefrine, 208, 717
Etofenamate, 656
Etofibrate, 105, 683
Etomidate, 455–456
Etonogestrel, 435
Etoposide, 377, 379
Etravirene, 826
Etravirine, 152, 156–157, 700
Etretinate, 475, 477, 478b, 798
Eucalyptol, 70
Eucalyptus, 675
European Evaluation Food Safety Authority
      (EFSA), 512
European League Against Rheumatism (EULAR),
      359
European Medicines Agency (EMEA), 512
European Network of Teratology Information
      Services (ENTIS), 479, 495
European Paediatric Hepatitis C Virus Network,
      824
European Society of Urogenital Radiology
      (ESUR), 814–815
Evans blue, 537
Evening primrose oil, 516t–519t
Everolimus, 344, 344b, 358, 777, 777b
Ex utero intrapartum treatment, 452, 461

Exemestane, 389
Exenatide, 431
Exercise, 809, 809b
Expectorants, 70–71, 675
EXIT procedure. See Ex utero intrapartum
      treatment
Extensive laryngeal hypoplasia, 279t
Eye drops, 800–801
Ezetimibe, 108, 683

F

Factor Xa inhibitors, 231, 231b, 726
Famciclovir, 147, 698
Familial Mediterranean Fever (FMF), 50, 51b,
      667, 667b
Famotidine, 95–96, 678, 678b
Fampridine, 353–354
Famprofazone, 655
Fava beans, 809–810, 845
Febuxostat, 50
Felbamate, 252–253, 265, 265b, 733
Felodipine, 198, 714
Fenethylline, 329, 769
Fennel (Foeniculum vulgare),
      805–806
Fenofibrate, 105, 683
Fenoterol, 66, 406, 672, 673b
Fenproporex, 108
Fentanyl, 38–39, 459–460, 662–665,
      663b
Fenthion, 580–581
Fenticonazole, 141, 696
Fenugreek (Trigonella foenum-graecum),
      805
Ferristen, 533
Fertilization, 4
Ferucarbotran, 533, 533b
Ferumoxsil, 533
Fesoterodine, 98, 681
Fetal alcohol effects (FAE), 543–544
Fetal alcohol spectrum disorders (FASD),
      542–544
   in children, 547
Fetal alcohol syndrome (FAS), 543–544
Fetal anticonvulsant syndrome (FACS),
      256–257
Fetal bradycardia, 210
Fetal programming, 294
Fetal tachycardia, 209–210
Fetogenesis, 4
Fetotoxicity, 4, 15, 497b
   mechanisms of, 234–235
Feverfew, 520t
Fexofenadine, 59, 671–672
Fibromata, 468
Fibrin, 238
Fibrinolysis, 238–239, 239b
Fibrinolytics, 728, 728b
Fibroma, 468
Fidaxomicin, 128, 128b

Ficam. *See* Bendiocarb
Filgrastim, 357, 357b, 779
Finasteride, 484, 485b, 801
Fingolimod, 352–354
Fish oil, 108
Flavoxate, 98, 681
Flecainide, 209, 211–212, 717b, 718
Floppy infant syndrome, 16t, 264, 323, 326, 586b
Flouxetine, 732
Flubendazole, 144, 697
Flucloxacillin, 116
Fluconazole, 696
Flucytosine, 142, 142b, 696
Fludarabine, 383
Fludrocortisone, 423–424
Flufenamic acid, 655–656
Fluindione, 233–234, 727
Flumetasone, 471, 788
Flunarizine, 214, 720
Flunisolide, 488, 788
Flunitrazepam, 325, 765
Fluocinolone, 471
Fluocortolone, 788
Fluorescein, 537, 817
Fluorescent dyes, 537–538, 537b
Fluoride, 505–506, 505b
2-Fluoro-2-desoxy-D-glucose (FDG), 534
Fluorometholone, 488
Fluoroquinolones, 690
Fluoroscopy, 528
Fluorouracil, 480, 799
Fluoxetine, 295–296, 303–304, 306–307, 585, 749–750
Flupentixol, 313, 318, 755b–756b, 758
Fluphenazine, 313, 318, 755b–756b, 758
Flupirtine, 664
Flurazepam, 325
Flurbiprofen, 656–657
Fluspirilene, 313, 318, 758
Flutamide, 792–793
Fluticasone, 67, 471, 487, 673, 788
Fluvastatin, 106, 683
Fluvoxamine, 295, 307, 750
Folate antagonists, 382–383
Folic acid, 498–501, 498b, 500f
   and antiepileptic drugs, 259
Folinic acid, 258, 498–499
Follicle-stimulating hormone (FSH), 415
Follitropin-α, 784
Follitropin-β, 784
Follitropin alfa, 415
Follitropin beta, 415
Fomepizole, 579, 580b
Fomivirsen, 147, 698
Fondaparinux, 231, 231b, 726, 726b
Food and Drug Administration (FDA), 500, 512, 803
Food fortification, 500
Food poisoning, 592–593
Formaldehyde, 607, 607b
Formalin, 607, 607b
Formestan, 792–793
Formoterol, 67, 673, 673b

Fosamprenavir, 152, 158, 700
Fosaprepitant, 86
Foscarnet, 147–148, 698
Fosfestrole, 791
Fosfomycin, 124–125
Fosinopril, 715
Framycetin, 125–126, 692
Frovatriptan, 47, 659
Fruits, 100–101
Fukushima disaster, 623
Fulvestrant, 389
Fumaric acid preparations, 479–480, 480b, 799
Furans, 847
Furazolidone, 124, 488, 690–691
Furosemide, 216, 585, 720, 721b
Fusafungine, 132, 694
Fusidic acid, 132, 694

G

Gabapentin, 252–254, 265–266, 266b, 733–734, 763
Gadobene acid, 533
Gadodiamide, 533
Gadofosveset trisodium, 533
Gadolinium, 533, 815
Gadopentetic acid, 533
Gadoteric acid, 533
Gadoteridol, 533
Gadoversetamide, 533
Gadoxetic acid, 533
Galaxolide, 857
Gallopamil, 198, 211, 213, 714
Gamma-hydroxybutyrate (GHB), 564, 564b
Ganciclovir, 147–148, 698
Ganirelix, 414–415
Gardnerella vaginalis, 409
Garenoxacin, 123
Gastric bypass surgery, 494
Gastritis medications, 677–679
Gastrointestinal drugs, 677–686
Gastroschisis, 28, 31, 37, 42, 72, 387
Gatifloxacin, 123
Gefitinib, 388
Gelatin, 241, 242b, 728, 729b
Gemcitabine, 384
Gemeprost, 402
Gemfibrozil, 105–106, 683
General anesthesia, 451–466
Gentamicin, 125–126, 692–693
Gentian violet, 470–471
Geranium, 514t
German Commission E, 512
Gestagens, 435–437, 436b, 790–792, 792b
   effects on lactation, 648
   effect on milk production, 790
   hormonal transfer to infant via mother's milk, 790–791
Gestational diabetes mellitus (GDM), 426–429, 432

Gestodene, 435, 791
Gestonorone, 791
Ginger, 77–78, 516t–519t
Gingko biloba, 214, 720, 803–804
Ginseng, 803–804
Glatiramer acetate (GA), 356–357, 357b, 779, 779b
Glibenclamide, 431–432, 789, 790b
Gliclazide, 431, 790
Glimepiride, 431, 790
Glinides, 431
Glipizide, 789
Gliquidone, 431, 790
Glisoxepide, 790
Glitazones, 431
Glucagon, 433–434, 434b
Glucocorticoids, 86, 86b, 359, 423–426, 471, 471b, 487, 659b
Glucosamine, 34
Glucose 6-phosphate-dehydrogenase deficiency (G6-PD deficiency), 809–810
Glutethimide, 768
Glycerol, 101
Glyceryl trinitrate, 213, 719–720
Glycol ethers, 601, 607
Glycopeptide antibiotics, 126–127, 127b, 692, 692b
Glycopyrronium bromide, 98, 681
Glycylcycline, 689
Goat's rue (*Galega officinalis*), 805–806
Gold preparations, 363, 363b
Goldenseal, 520t–521t
Golimumab, 351, 359
Gonadorelin, 414, 784
Gonadotropin releasing hormone (GnRH), 414–415
Gonadotropins, 415
Gonads, 3, 535–536
Gonorrhea, 830
Goserelin, 389, 414, 784
Gout therapy, 666–667, 667b
Granisetron, 685
Granulocyte colony-stimulating factor (G-CSF), 357, 357b, 779
Grapefruit, 514t
Greek hayseed. *See* Fenugreek (*Trigonella foenum-graecum*)
Green tea, 807
Griseofulvin, 142–143, 142b, 696
Growth hormone (GH), 416
GSST1, 550
Guaifenesin, 70, 675
Guar gum, 100
Guarana (*Paullinia cupana*), 804
Gusperimus, 358
Gyrase inhibitors, 800

H

H1N1 influenza, 178–179, 182
H_2 receptor antagonists, 95–96, 96b
H_2-receptor-blocker, 678, 678b
Haemophilus influenza B (HIB) vaccination, 180, 180b
Haemophilus influenza infection, during breastfeeding, 830
Hair cosmetics, 485
Hair loss, 484, 514t, 801, 808b
Hair preparations, 797–798
Hallucinogenic amphetamines, 841
Haloacetic acids (HAA), 614–615
Halofantrine, 133, 136, 136b, 695
Halogenated inhalational anesthetic agents, 452–454, 453b
Haloperidol, 313, 318, 755, 755b–756b, 758
  effects on lactation, 647
  toxicity, 586–587, 587b
Haloprogin, 143, 696–697
Halothane, 453, 455, 665
Hazardous waste landfill sites, 622–623, 623b
Hearing deficit, 49–50, 126–127
Heart and blood medications, 193–224
Hedera helix, 675
Helicobacter pylori therapy, 97–98, 97b, 679, 679b
Hematologic malignancies, 50
Hemorrhoids, 488, 488b, 801
Heparan sulfate, 229
Heparin, 206, 227–228, 725–726, 726b
  low molecular weight heparin, 227–230, 229b, 234, 237b
  unfractionated heparin, 227–230, 229b, 237b
Heparin-induced thrombocytopenia (HIT), 227
Hepatitis, antiviral drugs for, 148–150, 698–699, 698b
Hepatitis A vaccination, 180, 180b, 706, 706b
Hepatitis A virus (HAV), infection during breastfeeding, 823–824, 823b
Hepatitis B Immune Globulin (HBIG), 709
Hepatitis B virus (HBV)
  antiviral drugs for, 148–149
  infection during breastfeeding, 824, 824b
  vaccination, 180, 180b, 706–707, 706b
Hepatitis C, antiviral drugs for, 149–150
Hepatitis E virus (HEV), infection during breastfeeding, 824–825, 825b
Herbal galactogogues, 805–807, 807b
Herbs during pregnancy, 511–526
  contraindications of, 520–522, 520t–521t
  controversies of, 515, 516t–519t
  counseling about herbs, 512–513
  essential oils, 514, 514t, 521t
  frequency of use, 514–515, 515t
  herbs, as foods, 514
  safety of, 511–512
  use of, 513
Heroin, 562, 839–840
Herpes medications, 147–148, 697–698, 698b
  for local use, 148
  for systemic use, 147–148

Herpes simplex virus (HSV)
  infection during breastfeeding, 825, 825b
  type 1, 825
  type 2, 825
Herpes zoster virus, infection during breast-
    feeding, 825–826, 826b
Hexachlorobenzene (HCB), 549–550, 610,
    847–848
Hexachlorocyclohexane (HCH), 610, 847
Hexachlorophene, 470, 470b
Hexane, 601
Hexetidine, 410, 488, 801
High-dose methotrexate, 382
Highly active antiretroviral therapy (HAART),
    151–152
Hirsutism, 801
Histone deacetylase (HDAC) deficiency, 258
Homeopathy, 512
Hops, 522t, 803–804
Horse chestnut, 483, 516t–519t, 801
Hormonal contraceptives, 790–792
  long-term effects of, 791–792
Hormones, 413–450
  anterior pituitary hormone, 415–416
  hypothalamic releasing hormone, 414–415
  parathyroid hormone, 422–423, 422b
  posterior pituitary hormone, 417, 417b
5-HT1 receptor agonist, 46
HTLV-I-associated myelopathy (HAM), 827
Human breast milk, composition of, 640t
Human chorianic somatomammotropin (HCS),
    416
Human cytomegaly virus (HCMV), infection
    during breastfeeding, 822–823
Human development, early, 2f
Human immunodeficiency virus (HIV), infection
    during breastfeeding, 826–827, 827b
Human insulin, 429–432, 430b
Human papilloma virus (HPV) vaccination,
    180–181, 181b, 707
Human placental lactogen (HPL), 416
Human T-lymphotropic virus (HTLV) infection,
    827, 827b
Hyaluronic acid, 34
Hydralazine, 195, 713, 713b
Hydrocarbon solvents, 607
Hydrochlorothiazide, 215, 720, 721b
Hydrocodone, 662, 662b
Hydrocortisone, 788
Hydrocortisone 17-butyrate, 471
Hydrocortisone acetate, 471
Hydrogen peroxide, 471
Hydromorphone, 34–35, 35b, 660–661
Hydronephrosis, 126, 266, 279t
Hydrotalcite, 94, 677–678
Hydroxycarbamides, 390, 780
Hydroxychloroquine, 358–359, 361–362, 362b,
    658–659, 659b
2-Hydroxydesipramine, 747
Hydroxyethyl starch (HES), 214, 241–242,
    242b
Hydroxylamine, 607

Hydroxymetronidazole, 691
Hydroxymidazolam, 766
Hydroxynefazodone, 752
Hydroxyprogesterone, 791
Hydroxyprogesterone caproate, 435
Hydroxyurea, 780
Hydroxyzine, 59, 78–79, 328, 672, 767,
    768b
Hymecromone, 98, 681
Hyperbaric oxygen therapy (HBO), 579
Hypercalcemia, 422
Hyperesis gravidarum, 496, 496b
Hypericin, 753, 803–804. See also St. John's
    wort
Hypericum perfortum, 804
Hyperthermia, 162, 162b
Hyperthyroidism, 419–423
Hyperuricemia, 49–50, 204
Hypervitaminosis, 493
Hypnosis, 77, 324–325, 328, 764, 767–768
Hypoglycemia, 427
  alcohol-induced, 836
Hypomagnesemia, 422
Hypoplasia of ulna or tibia, 279t
Hyposensitization therapy, 61
Hypotension, 207
Hypothalamic hormones, 783–784, 784b
Hypothalamic releasing hormones, 414–415
Hypothyroidism, 418
Hypovitaminosis, 493

I

Ibandronate, 808
Ibandronic acid, 506
Ibritumomabtiuxetan, 386
Ibuprofen, 655–656, 583b, 588, 654b–655b,
    656, 657b, 659b–660b
Icaridin, 485
Icatibant acetate, 62
Idarubicin, 379–380, 390–391
Idoxuridine, 148, 698
Ifosfamid, 379
Iloperidone, 313, 318
Iloprost, 206–207
Imatinib, 388, 780
Imipenem, 117, 688
Imipramine, 307, 750
Imiquimode, 357, 480, 799
Immune suppressants, 776–777
Immunization, maternal, 705–706
Immunoglobulins, 188, 188b, 705, 709, 709b
  in breastfed infants, efficacy of, 706
Immunomodulating agents, 775–782
  antineoplastics, 779–780, 780b
  azathioprine, 775–776, 776b
  glatiramer acetate, 779, 779b
  granulocyte colony-stimulating factors,
    779
  immune suppressants, 776–777
  interferons, 778–779, 779b

6-mercaptopurine, 775–776, 776b
monoclonal antibodies, 777–778, 778b
Immunomodulators, for atopic eczema, 473, 473b
Immunostimulatory drugs, 356–358
Immunosuppressants, 342–345
Inactivated vaccine (TIV), 707
Incretin mimetics, 431
Indacaterol, 67, 673
Indanazoline, 487
Indanediones, 727
Indapamide, 215, 721
Indicative occupational exposure limit values (IOELVs), 600
Indigo carmine, 537
Indinavir, 152, 158–159, 700
Indocyanine green, 537, 817
Indomethacin, 408, 655–656, 657b
Indian psyllium seed husks, 681–682
Indigo carmine, 527, 537
Indinavir, 152, 157–159
Industrial chemical contaminants, 847–862
  antimony, 856
  arsenic, 855–856
  barium, 856
  boron, 856
  cadmium, 855
  cesium, 856
  lead, 853–855, 855b
  lithium, 856
  mercury, 851–853
  persistent organochlorine compounds, 847–851
  rubidium, 856
  selenium, 856
  uranium, 856
  vanadium, 856
Infant development, persistent organochlorine compounds contamination, 850
Infection during breastfeeding, 824, 824b
Inflammatory bowel diseases (IBD), 94, 103–104
Infliximab (IFX), 103, 348–349, 349b, 359, 778, 778b
Influenza virus infection
  antiviral drugs for, 150–151, 699, 699b
  during breastfeeding, 827–828, 827b
  vaccination, 181–183, 183b, 707
Infusions, 513
Inhalable corticosteroids (ICS), 67–68, 673, 673b
Injection anesthetics, 455–457, 457b
Innocenti Declaration, 640
Inolimomab, 351
Inorganic lead, 617–618, 853
Inorganic mercury, 851–852
Inosin, 147
Insect stings, 61
Insulin, 428–430, 430b, 789–790, 790b
  analogs, 429
  aspart, 429–430
  detemir, 430

glargine, 430
glulisin, 430
lispro, 429
Insulin-like growth factor-1 (IGF-1), 416
Integrase inhibitors, 161
Interferon-α2b, 779
Interferon-β, 355–356, 356b
Interferon-β1a, 353, 779
Interferon-γ, 356
Interferons (IFN), 354–356, 778–779, 779b
Interferons-α, 355, 355b, 779
Interleukin-1β, 351
Intermittent preventive treatment (IPT), 133, 137–138
International Board of Lactation Consultant Examiners (IBLCE), 648
International Lactation Consultant Organization (ILCA), 648
International Society for Research in Human Milk and Lactation (ISRHML), 648
International TCDD-equivalent (I-TEQ), 848
Intravenous immunoglobulins, 352
Intrauterine devices (IUD), 410, 410b, 801
Intrauterine growth restriction (IUGR), 196–197, 226, 548
Intrauterine growth retardation, 298–299
Intrauterine pessary (IUP), 792
Iobitridol, 532, 814
Iodamide, 532, 814
Iodine, 507, 675, 787–788, 788b
  -containing contrast media, 532–533, 532b
  overdose, 16t
  Povidone, 409–410, 469–470, 469b, 488, 801
  rinses, 801
  supply, during pregnancy, 417–419
Iodixanol, 532, 814
Iodoform, 788
Iohexol, 532, 814
Iomeprol, 532, 814
Ionizing radiation, 527–528, 623
Iopamidol, 532, 814
Iopanoic acid, 532, 814
Iopentol, 532, 814
Iopodate, 532, 814
Iopromide, 532, 814
Iotalamine acid, 532
Iotalhaminic acid, 814
Iotrolan, 532, 814
Iotroxic acid, 814
Iotroxine acid, 532
Ioversol, 532, 814
Ioxagline acid, 532, 814
Ioxitalamic acid, 532, 814
Ipratropium bromide, 70, 211, 674, 674b, 719
Irbesartan, 200, 715
Irinotecan, 387, 391
Iron, 503–504, 504b, 587, 587b
Isoconazole, 141, 696
Isoflurane, 453, 665

Isoniazid, 129–130, 130b, 693, 829
Isoniazid (INH), 130
Isoniazid (+pyridoxine), 129–130, 694b
Isopropyl alcohol, 469
Isosorbide dinitrate, 213, 719–720
Isosorbide mononitrate, 213, 719–720
Isotopes
   radioactive, 534–536, 536b
   stable, 536–537, 536b
Isotretinoin (13-*cis*-retinoic acid), 475–476, 478,
   495, 797–798
Isoxsuprin, 406
Isradipine, 198, 714
Itraconazole, 139, 696
Ivabradine, 214, 720
Ivermectin, 145, 145b, 482–483, 697,
   799–800
Ivy leaves, 70

J

Jarisch-Herxheimer reaction, 116
Jasmine, 807
Jasmine petals (*Jasminum officinale*), 807
Josamycin, 118–119, 689
Juniper, 521t

K

Kanamycin, 125–126, 692
Kava (*Piper methysticum*), 803–804
Kavain, 768, 803–804
Kava-kava root, 803–804
Kava-pyrone, 803–804
Keratolytic azelaic acid, 474
Keratolytics, 473–475, 797, 799
Ketamine, 455–456
Ketamine S, 455–456
Ketanserin, 302
Keterolac, 656
Ketoconazole, 140, 696
Ketolide telithromycin, 689
Ketoprofen, 657, 657b, 660b
Ketorolac, 655–656
Ketotifen, 69
Khat-plant (*Catha edulis*), 555
Kidney development, 41, 45
K-X ray fluorescence (K-XRF), 619b–620b

L

Labetalol, 196, 712
Lacosamide, 252, 266b, 734
Lactation, drug therapy and risk during,
   639–650
   affected by medications, 647–648
   breastfeeding advantages versus medication
     risks, 639–641
   breastfeeding support, 648

   dosage calculation, 644–645
   infant characteristics, 642–643
   medication toxicity, 645–647
   medications into mother's milk, passage of,
     641–642
   milk/plasma ratio, 643–644, 645t
Lactic acid, for warts, 799
Lactitol, 100
Lactobacillus, 409
Lactoferrin, 828–829
Lactulose, 100, 681–682
La Leche League International (LLLI), 648
Lamb's tongue (*Plantago lanceolata*), 70,
   675
Lamivudine, 152–154, 698–700, 826
Lamotrigine, 251–254, 252b–253b, 257,
   267–268, 268b, 279, 324, 731b–732b, 731,
   734–735, 763
Lanreotide, 415, 784
Lansoprazole, 96, 678
Lapatinib, 388
Laquinimod, 353–354
Laser therapy, 480, 799
Latanoprost, 486, 793, 800–801
Laughing gas. *See* Nitrous oxide (N$_2$O)
Lavender, 514t
Laxatives, 681–682, 682b
Lead, 617–620, 619b–620b, 853–855, 855b
Lead oxide, 853
Leflunomide, 107, 352–353, 358–359, 362–363,
   362b, 659, 659b
Lenalidomide, 387–388
Lenograstim, 357, 779
Lepirudin, 230, 726, 726b
Lercanidipine, 198, 714
Letrozole, 389, 441
Leukemia, acute, 33, 381, 391, 482, 549
Leukotriene
   antagonists, 69
   -receptor antagonists, 673–674, 673b
Leuprolide acetate, 784
Leuprorelin, 414
Levalbuterol, 66
Levamisole, 146, 147b
Levetiracetam, 252–254, 268–269, 269b,
   735–737, 763
Levobunolol, 486, 800
Levobupivacaine, 457–458, 665
Levocabastine, 59, 672
Levocetirizine, 59, 671–672
Levodopa, 329, 769
Levodropropizine, 71, 676
Levofloxacin, 123, 690
Levomenol, 471
Levomepromazine, 313, 318, 758–759
Levomethadone, 562–563, 840
Levonorgestrel, 435, 790–791
Levopropylhexedrine, 270
Levorphanol, 675
Levothyroxine, 419
Lice, 799–800, 800b
   medications, 481–482, 482b

Licorice root extracts, 94
Lidocaine, 211, 457–459, 664, 717b, 718
Lightning strikes, 627, 627b
Lime, 675
Lincomycin, 119–120, 119b, 693, 693b
Lincosamides, 129
Lindane, 482–483, 610, 799–800, 847
Linezolid, 128, 128b, 693, 693b
Linseed, 100
Liothyronine, 419
Lipases, 98, 101, 683
Lipid lowering agents, 105–108
Lipid reducers, 683–684
Lipids peroxidation, 13
Lipopeptides antibiotics, 127, 127b
Liqorice (*Glycyrrhiza glabra*), 805
Liraglutide, 431
Lisinopril, 715
Lissencephaly, 279t
Lisuride, 330, 416, 417b, 647–648, 769, 785
Lithium, 293, 322–324, 323b–324b, 481, 481b, 762–764, 763b, 856
Lithium Baby Register, 322–323
Live-attenuated influenza vaccine (LAIV), 182, 707
Local anesthetic agents, 457–460, 460b
  combined with active substances, 459–460
Local antibiotics, 132, 132b
Lofepramine, 302
Lomefloxacin, 123, 690
Lomitapide, 108
Lomustine, 378
Long-distance travel and flights, 162–163, 163b
Loop diuretics, 216
Loperamide, 102, 683, 683b
Lophophora williamsii, 561
Lopinavir, 152, 159, 699–700
Loprazolam, 325
Loracarbef, 117
Loratadine, 59–60, 671–672
Lorazepam, 325, 765
Lormetazepam, 325, 765, 767b
Lornoxicam, 657
Losartan, 200, 715
Loteprednol, 488
Lovastatin, 106, 683
Low molecular weight heparins (LMWH), 227–230, 229b, 234, 237b, 726b
Low-dose methotrexate, 360
Low-set ears, 49–50
Lubricants, 101
Lumbar spinal, 528
Lumefantrine, 133, 136, 136b, 695
Lung hypoplasia, 14, 279t
Lurasidone, 313, 319
Luteinizing hormone-releasing hormone (LHRH), 414
Lutropin alfa, 415
Lyme disease, 828, 828b
Lynestrenol, 791
Lypressin, 784
Lysergic acid diethylamide (LSD), 561, 841

Lysine amidotrizoate, 532
Lysine amido-trizoate, 814

M

Mabs, 345, 350–352
Macrogol, 100, 681–682
Macrogol lauryl ether, 472, 483
Macrolides, 118–119, 119b, 129, 132, 688–689, 689b
Macular degeneration, 350–351, 487
Macular edema, 350–351
Magaldrate, 94, 677–678
Magnesium salts, 94
Magnesium sulfate, 100, 407–408, 408b
Magnesium sulfate IV, 204
Magnetic resonance contrast agents, 815–816, 816b
Magnetic resonance contrast media, 533, 533b
Magnetic resonance imaging (MRI), 531, 531b, 813
Major depressive disorder (MDD), 298
Malaria prophylaxis, 132–137, 133b
Malathion, 481–483, 483b, 610, 799–800
Malignancy and pregnancy, 374–376
Mandrake, 521t. *See also* Podophyllin
Mangafodipir, 533b, 815, 816b
Manganiferous mangafodipir, 533
Manidipine, 198, 714
Mannitol, 100
MAO-inhibitor, 752
Maprotiline, 302, 307, 751
Maraviroc, 160, 152, 700
Maravorioc, 160
Marijuana, 558–559
Marshmallow (*Althea officinalis*), 675
Marshmallow root, 70
Mast cell inhibitors, 674
Mast cell stabilizers, 69–70
Mastitis, 648, 667, 804, 828–829, 828b–829b
Materials Safety Data Sheets (MSDSs), 600
Maternal immunization, 705–706
m-chlorophenylpiperazine, 754
Measles vaccination, 183, 183b
Mebendazole, 144, 145b, 697, 697b
Mebeverine, 98, 681
Mecasermin, 416
Mechlorethamine, 379
Meclizine, 78–81, 685
Meclocycline, 120
Meclozine, 59
Medazepam, 325
Medical charcoal, 102
Medicinal products, maternal use of, 18–19
Medrogestone, 791
Medroxyprogesterone, 790
Medroxyprogesterone acetate, 390
Mefenamic acid, 655–656
Mefenorex, 108
Mefloquine, 133, 136–137, 136b, 695, 695b

Mefruside, 215, 721
Megestrol, 791
Megestrol acetate, 390
Meglumine amidotrizoate, 532, 814
Melanomas, 375, 437–438, 536
Melatonin, 303–304, 745, 768
Meloxicam, 657
Melperone, 313, 319, 328, 758
Menadione, 237
Menaquinone, 237
Meningitis, 139, 828
Meningococcal vaccination, 183–184, 184b
Meningomyelocele, 261
Menotropin, 415, 784
Mental development dysfunction, 257
Menthol, 43–44, 472, 806–807
Meperidine, 35–36, 36b
Mephenytoin, 273
Mepivacaine, 457–458, 665
Meprobamate, 328
Meptazinol, 35–36, 36b, 664
6-Mercaptopurine (6-MP), 103, 341–342, 342b,
    383, 775–776, 776b
Mercury, 620–622, 621b–622b, 851–853
Mercury chloride, 851–852
Mercury compounds, 470, 470b
Meropenem, 117, 688
Mesalazine, 94, 103, 682
Mescaline, 561
Mesterolone, 792
Mestranol, 791
Mesuximide, 265, 733
Metabisulfite, 457–458
Metaclazepam, 325, 765
Metals
    arsenic, 616–617
    cadmium, 617
    lead, 617–620
    mercury, 620–622
Metamizol, 32–33, 655
Metenolone, 792
Metergoline, 417, 417b, 785
Metformin, 431–433, 790, 790b
Methadone, 840
Methamidophos, 580–581
Methamphetamine, 555, 836. See also
    Methylamphetamine
Methanol, 472
    poisoning, 579–580, 580b
Methantheline, 98
Methanthelinium, 681
Methanthelinium bromide, 484
Methenamine, 801
Methenamine mandelate, 124
Methicillin-resistant *Staphylococcus aureus*
    (MRSA)
    infection during breastfeeding, 828,
        828b
Methimazole, 421, 786–787
Methinamine, 483–484
Methocarbamol, 666
Methohexital, 665

Methohexital propofol, 455–456
Methotrexate (MTX), 103, 358–359, 373–374,
    780, 780b
    high-dose, 382
    low-dose, 360–361, 361b
Methoxsalen, 479, 799b
8-Methoxypsoralen, 479, 479b
Methoxsalen, 469b, 479, 799
Methyl-(5-amino-4-oxo-pentanoate), 392
Methyl aminolevulinate, 392
Methylamphetamine, 555
Methyl cellulose, 100
Methyldopa. *See* α-methyldopa
Methylendioxymethylamphetamine (MDMA),
    556–557
Methylene blue, 537
Methylene chloride, 604–605, 605b
Methylergometrine, 402, 647–648, 784–785,
    785b, 793
Methylergonovine, 784–785
    effects on lactation, 647–648
6-Methylmercaptopurine (6-MMP), 341
6-Methylmercaptopurine-nucleotide (6-MMPN),
    775–776
Methylmercury, 620–621, 851–852
Methylnaltrexone, 101
Methylphenidate, 329, 768–769
Methylprednisolone, 103, 353, 788, 789b
Methylxanthines, 836–837
Metildigoxin, 208
Metipranolol, 486, 800
Metixen, 330, 769
Metoclopramide, 82, 647, 679, 680b, 684–685
Metolachlor, 485
Metoprolol, 195–196, 587–588, 660b, 712
Metrizamide, 532, 814
Metrizoate, 532, 814
Metronidazole, 97, 97b, 103, 125, 125b, 409,
    679b, 691, 691b, 801
Mexiletine, 211, 718
Mezlocillin, 116
Mianserin, 302, 307, 751
Micafungin, 696
Miconazole, 140, 141b, 143, 409, 696, 697b
Microsomal triglyceride transfer protein (MTTP), 108
Midazolam, 325, 756
Midecamycin, 118–119, 689
Midodrine, 208, 717
Mifepristone, 440, 440b, 793
Miglitol, 431, 790
Migraine
    attack during pregnancy, 48b
    medications, 659–660, 660b
    prophylaxis, 48b
    therapy, 46–48
Milk/plasma (M/P) ratio, 643–644
Milk contamination, regional differences in,
    848–849
Milk thistle (*Sitybum marianum*), 516t–519t,
    806
Miltefosine, 392
Minerals, 808, 808b

Minocycline, 120, 689
Minoxidil, 204, 204b, 484, 485b, 716,
    801
Mirtazapine, 308, 751
Miscarriage, 30–31, 42, 121–122, 134, 186–187,
    198, 308, 347, 507, 548–549, 575–576,
    592, 617–618
Misoprostol, 360, 402–403, 588, 679, 784, 793,
    793b
Mistletoe preparation, 780, 780b
Mitotane, 390
Mitoxantrone, 381, 780
Mivacurium, 461
Mizolastine, 59, 672
Mizoribine, 358
MMR (measles, mumps and rubella) vaccine,
    185, 708
Moclobemide, 308, 752
Modafinil, 329, 769
Modified fluid gelatin, 241
Moexipril, 715
Molsidomine, 214, 720
Mometasone, 67, 471, 673, 788
Monk's pepper (*Agnus castus*), 803–804,
    806–807
Monoacetyldapsone, 694
Monobactams, 117–118, 117b
Monoclonal antibodies, 385–386, 777–778,
    778b
Monomethylarsonic acid, 616
Montelukast, 69, 69b, 673
Morning sickness. *See* Nausea and vomiting of
    pregnancy (NVP)
Morphine, 34–35, 35b, 562, 647,
    660–661
Mothers' milk
    lead concentration in, 853–855, 855b
    mercury concentration in, 852–853
    persistent organochlorine compounds in,
        848
Motherwort, 520t
Moxifloxacin, 123, 690
Moxonidine, 203, 203b, 716
Mucolytic agents, 70–71, 675
Mugwort, 520t
Multiple sclerosis, 352–354
    medication, prenatal toxicity of, 354
    pregnancy and, 353
Multivitamin preparations, 503, 503b
Multi-test, 818
Mumps vaccination, 183, 183b
Mupirocin, 132, 694
Muromonab-CD3, 351, 358
Muscle relaxants, 36–37, 460–462, 462b
Mushrooms toxins, 592, 592b
Musk ambrette, 856–857
Musk ketone, 856–857
Musk xylol, 856–857
Mutagenicity, 3, 49–50, 125, 470, 472–473,
    479b, 506b
Myasthenia gravis, 99
Mycophenolate, 358

Mycophenolate mofetil (MMF), 343, 343b, 776,
    777b
Mycophenolic acid (MPA), 343, 776
Myotonolytics, 666, 666b
Myrtle, 675

N

Nabiximols, 353
Nabumetone, 657
N-acetylcysteine (NAC), 70
    overdose, 589, 589b
N-acetyl-p-benzoquinone imine (NAPQI), 29
Nadifloxacin, 123, 690
Nadroparin, 227, 725
Nafarelin, 414, 784
Naftidrofuryl, 214, 720
Naftifin, 143, 696–697
Nalbuphine, 664
Nalidixic acid, 690
Nalorphine, 41
Naloxone, 41, 664
Naltrexone, 41, 563, 664
Nandrolone, 792
Naphazoline, 487
Naphthalene, 809–810
Naproxen, 655–656
Naratriptan, 659
Nartograstim, 357
Nasal decongestants, 487–488
Natalizumab, 103, 349–350, 349b
Natamycin, 143, 696–697
Nateglinide, 431
National Institute for Occupational Safety and
    Health, 600
National Organization for Fetal Alcohol
    Syndrome (NOFAS), 542
Nausea and vomiting of pregnancy (NVP),
    75–92
    acupressure for, 77
    acupuncture for, 77
    antiemetics for, 86–87, 86b
    dopamine antagonists for, 81–83
    ginger for, 77–78
    glucocorticoids for, 86, 86b
    hypnosis for, 77
    pharmacological treatment for, 78–81
    pyridoxine for, 83–84, 84b
    serotonin antagonists for, 85–86
    treatment options for, 76
N-desmethylclomipramine, 746
N-desmethyldoxepin, 747–748
Nebivolol, 196
Necrotizing enterocolitis (NEC), 45
Neem oil, 481
Nefazodone, 752
Nei Guan, 77
Nelarabine, 383
Nelfinavir, 152, 159, 700
Neomycin, 125–126, 692
Neonatal development disorders, 299–300, 303

Neonates, cocaine-induced withdrawal symptoms in, 558
Neostigmine, 99, 680, 681b
Nephrogenic systemic fibrosis (NSF), 533
Nerve growth factor (NGF), 258
Netilmicin, 125–126, 692
Nettle leaf, 515t
Neural tube defects (NTDs), 499–501, 501b, 548
Neuraminidase inhibitors, 150–151
Neuroleptics, 755–756, 755b–756b
  amisulpride, 756
  aripiprazole, 756
  chlorpromazine, 756–757
  chlorprothixene, 757
  clozapine, 757
  flupenthixol, 758
  fluphenazine, 758
  haloperidol, 758
  butyrophenones, 758
  levomepromazine, 758–759
  olanzapine, 759
  paliperidone, 759
  perazine, 760
  perphenazine, 760
  promethazine, 760
  prothipendyl, 760
  quetiapine, 760–761
  risperidone, 761
  sertindole, 761
  sulpiride, 761
  thioridazine, 762
  trifluoperazine, 762
  ziprasidone, 762
  zotepine, 762
  zuclopenthixol, 762
Neutropenia, 822
Nevirapine, 152, 157, 699–700, 826
Nicardipine, 198, 407, 590, 714
Niclosamide, 145, 145b, 697, 697b
Nicotinamide. *See* Vitamin B₃
Nicotine, 838–839, 839b
  dependency, medicinal therapy for, 554–555, 555b
  effects on infants, 838–839
Nicotine replacement therapy (NRT), 549–555, 555b, 839
Nicotinic acid, 108
NICU Network Neurobehavioral Assessment Scale (NNNS), 300
Nifedipine, 195, 198, 199b, 407, 714
Nifuratel, 124, 488, 690–691
Nifurtimox, 124, 690
Nilotinib, 388
Nilvadipine, 198, 714
Nimesulide, 41, 44–45
Nimodipine, 198, 714
Nimorazole, 125, 691
Nimustine, 378
Nisoldipine, 198, 714
Nitrates, 720, 213, 214b, 719–720
Nitrazepam, 325, 766

Nitrendipine, 198, 714
Nitrofural, 124, 690–691
Nitrofurans, 132, 690–691, 691b, 809–810
Nitrofurantoin, 123–125, 125b, 690
Nitrogen mustard analog alkylators, 378–379
Nitroglycerine, 213, 719–720
Nitroimidazole antibiotics, 125, 125b, 132, 691–692, 691b
Nitrosourea alkylators, 378
Nitrous oxide (N₂O), 454–455, 454b
Nizatidine, 95–96, 678
No observed adverse effect level (NOAEL), 848–850
Non-nucleotide reverse transcriptase inhibitors (NNRTIs), 155–157
Nonoxinol, 801
Non-pharmaceutical intervention, 46
Non-steroidal anti-inflammatory drugs (NSAIDs), 41–46, 588–589, 589b, 655–657, 657b, 664b
  non-selective COX inhibitors, 42–45
  selective COX inhibitors, 45–46
Non-steroidal antirheumatics (NSAR), 359
Non-steroid antiphlogistics, 471, 471b
Noradrenaline, 196, 302, 304, 457–458, 557, 745, 751, 789, 789b
Norbuprenorphine, 840–841
Norcitalopram, 746
Nordosulepine, 747
Nordosulepine sulfoxide, 747
Norethisterone, 790
Norethisterone acetate, 791
Norethynodrel, 791
Norelgestromin, 435
Norepinephrine, 40, 307, 311, 457–458
Norethisterone, 435, 437, 790
Norethisterone acetate, 435b–436b, 437, 791
Norfloxacin, 123, 690
Norfluoxetine, 749
Norgestimate, 791
Norgestrel, 791
Norpseudoephedrine, 108, 684
Nortriptyline, 302, 308, 660b, 744b, 745, 752
Noscapine, 71, 676, 676b
Nose drops, 800–801
Nuclear accidents, 623
Nuclear industry, radiation associated with, 623–625, 624b
Nucleoside, 153–155
Nucleotide reverse transcriptase inhibitors (NRTIs), 153–155
Nutmeg, 521t
Nystatin, 143, 143b, 409, 696, 697b

O

Oats, 515t
Obesity, 108–109
Occupational exposure limits (OELs), 600, 603, 603b

Occupational exposure to anesthetic gases, 454–455, 455b
Ocrelizumab, 353
Octabromodiphenyl ether, 849–850
Octreotide, 415, 784
O-desmethyltramadol, 40
O-desmethylvenlafaxine, 312–313, 755
Ofatumumab, 386
Ofloxacin, 123, 690
OH-clomipramine, 746
OH-desmethylclomipramine, 746
Olanzapine, 313, 319, 755, 755b–756b, 759
Olestipol, 107
Oligodactyly, 279t
Olmesartan, 200, 715
Olopatadine, 59, 672
Olsalazine, 103, 682
Omalizumab, 70, 675, 675b
Omeprazole, 93, 96, 97b, 103, 678, 678b
Omoconazole, 141, 696
Omphalocele, 311
Onchocerciasis, 145
Ondansetron, 85–86, 685, 685b
Oocytes, 3
Operating room (OR) personnel, 454–455, 455b
Ophthalmic medications, 486–488, 487b
Opiate analgesics, 660b, 663b–664b
Opiates, 562–564, 839–841, 841b
  effects on lactation, 647–648
Opioid, 660–664, 660b
  agonists, 34–41
  antagonists, 34–41
Opipramol, 302, 309, 752
Opium tincture, 40, 562
Optical nerve hypoplasia, 279t
Oral antidiabetics (OAD), 430–434
Oral glucose tolerance test (OGTT), 428
Orciprenaline (metoproterenol), 72
Oregano, 561
Organic lead, 617–618
Organic mercury, 851–852
Organochlorines, 610, 610b
Organochlorine tetrachloroethene, 856
Organogenesis, 4
Organophosphates, 610–611, 611b, 847
Organophosphorus pesticides (OPs), 610–611
  poisoning, 580–581, 581b
Oritavancin, 127
Orlistat, 109
Ornidazole, 125, 691
Ornipressin, 784
Orofacial cleft, 28, 36–37, 42–43, 550
Orphenadrine, 48, 666
Oseltamivir, 150–151, 151b, 699, 699b
Oseltamivir carboxylate, 699
Osteoarthritis, 33–34, 34b
Osteolysis inhibitors, 506
Osmotic laxatives, 100
Osteoarthritis, analgesic drugs for, 33–34, 34b
Osteoporosis drugs, 506–507, 506b
Ovulation, 5t–6t, 389, 414–415, 436, 441b
Oxaceprol, 34

Oxacillin, 116
Oxaliplatin, 384–386, 391
Oxamniquine, 146, 147b
Oxazepam, 263, 325–326, 766–767, 767b
Oxcarbazepine, 252–254, 259, 264, 269–270, 270b, 324, 736
Oxicams, 41
Oxiconazole, 141, 696
Oxitropium bromide, 70
Oxprenolol, 196, 712
Oxybuprocaine, 665
Oxybutynin, 98, 681b
Oxycodone, 36–38, 37b, 662, 662b
Oxymetazoline, 487
Oxypurinol, 49–50, 666–667
Oxytetracycline, 120
Oxytocin, 402–404, 404b, 417, 417b, 585, 784
  effects on lactation, 647–648
  receptor antagonists, 408, 408b

P

Paclitaxel, 385
Paliperidone, 313, 319, 759
Palivizumab, 357
Palonosetron, 685
Pamidronate, 808
Pamidronic acid, 506
p-aminomethyl-benzoic acid (PAMBA), 238, 240b, 728
Pancreatin, 98
Pancurone, 665–666
Pancuronium, 461
Panitumumab, 386
Pantoprazole, 96, 678, 678b
Paracetamol, 27–29, 29b, 589, 589b, 646, 653–654, 654b–655b, 660b, 664h
Paraffinum subliquidum, 101
Paraquat, 581–582, 581b
Parathyroid hormone (PTH), 422–423, 422b
Paraxanthin, 836–837
Parecoxib, 658
Paricalcitol, 502
Parkinson drugs, 769
  for restless legs syndrome, 329–330, 330b
Paromomycin, 125–126, 692
Paroxetine, 295–296, 303–304, 309–311, 744b, 753
Paroxysmal nocturnal hemoglobinuria (PNH), 351
Parsley (*Petroselinium crispum*), 807
Partial agenesis of corpus callosum, 279t
Passion flower, 522t
Passive smoking, 553–554
Pediculicides, 481
Pediculosis, 481, 799–800
Pefloxacin, 123
Pegaptanib, 487, 800–801
Pegaspargase, 391
Pegfilgrastim, 357, 779
Peginterferons-α, 355, 355b
Pegloticase, 50

Pegvisomant, 416, 784
Pegylated interferon β-1a, 353
Pemba–Yarda syndrome, 848
Pemetrexed, 383
Pemoline, 769
Penbutolol, 196
Penciclovir, 148, 698
Penicillamine, 16t
Penicillins, 12–13, 116–117, 116b, 688, 688b
Pentabromodiphenyl ether, 849–850
Pentaerithritol tetranitrate, 213, 719–720
Pentamidine, 128–129, 129b
Pentasaccharide, 726
Pentazocine, 39–40
Pentosan polysulfate, 214, 720
Pentostatin, 392
Pentoxifylline, 214
Pentoxyverine, 71, 675, 676b
Peppermint, 515t
Peppermint oil (*Menthax pierita*), 806–807
Pepsin-proteinase, 98
Peramivir, 151, 151b, 699
Perazine, 313, 319, 760
Perflubutane, 533–534
Perflutren, 533–534, 816
Pergolide, 330, 647–648, 769
Perindopril, 715
Peripheral vasodilators, 214–215, 215b
Peristaltic stimulators, 679–680, 679b
Permethrin, 481–483
    for lice, 799–800
    for scabies, 799–800
Permissible exposure limits (PELs), 600, 603b
Perphenazine, 82, 313, 320, 760
Persistent organochlorine compounds, 847–851
Persistent pulmonary hypertension of the
        newborn (PPHN), 299–300, 302
Pertussis vaccination, 184, 184b
Pesticides, 608–612
Pethidine, 35–36, 36b, 663
Pharmacokinetics
    of alcohol, 542–547
    of drugs, 11–13, 11t
Phenacetin, 809–810
Phenazone, 32–33
Phencyclidine, 841
Phencyclidine piperidine (PCP), 561
Phenelzine, 309
Phenindione, 233–234, 727
Phenobarbital, 252–254, 258–259, 270–273,
        272b, 279, 328, 736–737
Phenobarbitone, 328
Phenol derivatives, 470
Phenol red, 537
Phenolsulphthalein. *See* Phenol red
Phenothiazines, 82–83, 313, 315b–316b, 647,
        755
Phenoxyacetic acid derivatives, 612–614, 613b
Phenoxybenzamine, 204, 204b, 716
Phenoxymethylpenicillin, 116
Phenprocoumon, 206, 233–234, 727
Phensuximide, 265

Phentermine, 108
Phenylbutazone, 33, 667b
Phenylbutazone derivatives, 655, 655b
3-phenylenediamine, 607
4-phenylenediamine, 607
Phenylephedrine, 72
Phenylmercuric acetate, 620
Phenylpropanolamine, 108, 684
Phenytoin, 211, 213, 252–254, 257–259,
        273–274, 274b, 279, 672, 731, 737
Phocomelia, 7–8, 15
Phosphodiesterase inhibitiors, 206
Photochemotherapy, 479, 799, 799b
Photographic/printing chemicals, 607–608,
        608b
Phylloquinone, 237
Physostigmine, 99, 681
Phytomenadione, 237
Phytonadione, 237
Phytophthora infestans, 592
Phytotherapeutics, 803–805, 805b
Pigmentation, 468
Pilocarpin, 486
Pimecrolimus, 344, 344b, 473, 473b, 798
Pimozide, 311–313, 320, 758
Pinazepam, 766
Pindolol, 196, 712
Pioglitazone, 431, 433, 790
Pipamperone, 313, 320, 758
Pipemidic acid, 123
Piperacillin, 116
Piperaquine, 133, 137, 137b, 695
Piperonyl butoxide, 481
Pirbuterol, 66
Pirenzepine, 95, 95b, 679
Piretanide, 216, 721
Piribedil, 330
Piritramide, 664
Piroxicam, 655–656, 657b
Pitavastatin, 106
Pitocin, 404
Pituitary hormones, 783–784, 784b
Pivmecillinam, 116
Placebo, 77–78, 86, 679–680
Plant preparation, 803–804. *See also* Plant
        toxins
Plant toxins, 592, 845–846
Plasmapheresis, 307, 592
Plasminogen activator inhibitors (PAI), 226
Plasmodium falciparum, 132–133
Plasmodium malariae, 135
Plasmodium ovale, 135
Plasmodium vivax, 135
Platin compounds, 386–387
Plerixafor, 357, 358b
Pneumococcal vaccination, 184, 184b
Pneumocystis pneumonia, 122, 122b, 128–129,
        135
Podophyllin, 480
Podophyllotoxin, 480, 799
    derivatives, 377–378
    toxicity, 589–590

Poisoning in pregnancy
general risk of, 575–576
medicines for, 582–590
treatment for, 576–582
Policresulen, 801
Policresulenum, 410, 488
Polidocanol, 472, 472b, 483, 801
Polio vaccine, 707–708, 708b
Poliomyelitis vaccination, 184–185, 185b
Polybrominated diphenyl ethers (PBDE), 849–850
Polychlorinated biphenyls (PCBs), 549–550, 610, 614, 614b, 847–849
contamination effects, on infant development, 850–851
in mothers' milk, 848
Polychlorinated dibenzo-dioxins, 612–614, 613b, 848
Polychlorinated dibenzofurans, 614
Polychlorinated dioxins, 847, 857–858
Polycystic ovary syndrome (PCOS), 253–254, 267, 278, 432–433
Polyestradiol, 791
Polygeline, 241
Polymyxin B, 127, 692
Polypeptide antibiotics, 127, 127b, 132, 692, 692b
Polysulfate. See Pentosan polysulfate
Pomalidomide, 387–388
Porencephaly, 278, 279t
Porfimer sodium, 392
Posaconazole, 140, 696
Positron-emission-tomography (PET), 817
Posterior pituitary hormones, 417, 417b
Postnatal adaption, 4
Postnatal adaptation disorders, 326–327
Postpartum depression, 640, 743–744
Postpartum effluvium, 468
Potassium bromide, 607
Potassium canrenoate, 216
Potassium carbonate, 607
Potassium iodate, 675
Potato blight, 592
Povidone, 487
Povidone iodinee, 409–410, 469–470, 469b, 488, 801
Prajmalium bitartrate, 211, 718
Pralidoxime, 580–581, 581b
Pramipexol, 329, 769
Pranlucast, 69
Prasugrel, 231–232, 727
Pravastatin, 683
Prazepam, 766
Praziquantel, 145–146, 146b, 697
Prazosin, 202–203, 203b, 716
Prednicarbate, 471
Prednisolone, 353, 423–424, 788, 789b
Prednisone, 103, 424, 788, 789b
Prednyliden, 252–253, 274–275, 275b, 737, 788
Pre-eclampsia, 47, 302, 344, 350–351, 358, 407, 408b, 419, 431–432, 457b, 714
Pregabalin, 252–253, 274–275, 732
Pre-gestational diabetes mellitus (PGDM), 426–428

Prenatal exposure, 28–29, 33, 35, 236, 281–282, 300–301, 326, 611, 614, 621b–622b, 756, 851b
Preterm birth, 298–299, 769
Pridinol, 330
Pridinol tetrazepam, 666
Prilocaine, 457–459, 665, 665b
Primaquine, 133, 137–139, 137b, 695, 809–810
Primidone, 253, 259, 270–273, 272b, 735–737
Primordial germ cells, 3
Pristinamycin, 129
Probarbazine, 379–380
Probenecid, 49
Probiotics, 103, 682
Procaine, 665
Procarbazine, 379–380
Prochlorperazine, 82
Procyclidine, 330, 769
Progesterone, 401–402, 435–437, 440
Progesterone compounds, 648
Proglumetacin, 657
Proguanil, 133, 135, 137–138, 137b, 695, 695b
Prolactin antagonists, 416–417, 417b
Promethazine, 82, 313, 320, 585, 760
Propafenone, 211–212, 718
Propicillin, 116
Propiverine, 98, 681
Propofol, 456–457, 665
Propoxyphene, 34
Propranolol, 196, 660b, 712
Propylthiouracil (PTU), 420, 786–787, 787b
Propyphenazone, 33
Prostacyclin, 401
Prostacyclin analogs, 206–207, 207b
Prostaglandin inhibitors, 32–33, 43–44
Prostaglandins (PG), 401–403, 403b, 793, 793b
antagonists, 408–409
effects on lactation, 647–648
Protamines, 229–230, 230b
Protease inhibitors, 157–160
Prothionamide rifabutin, 694
Prothipendyl, 313, 320, 760
Protionamide, 131
Protirelin, 414, 783
Proton pump inhibitors (PPIs), 96–97, 96b, 103, 678–679, 679b
Prucalopride, 101
Prussian blue, 582, 582b
Pseudoephedrine, 72, 675
Psilocybe semilanceata, 561
Psilocybin, 561–562, 562b
Psoriasis, 798–799
retinoids for, 475–479, 478b
Psychiatric disorder during pregnancy, 294
Psychoanaleptics, 328–329, 768–769
Psychotherapy, 295b
Psychotropic drugs, 293–340, 743–774
antidepressants. See Antidepressants
neuroleptics. See Neuroleptics
Psyllium seed husks, 100
Pteridine, 498–499
Pulmonary arterial hypertension (PAH), 205

Pulmonary hypertension, and pregnancy, 205–207, 207b
Purging buckthorn, 522t
Purine antagonists, 383
Pyoktanin, 470
Pyrantel, 146, 146b, 697
Pyrazinamide (PZA), 129–131, 131b, 693, 694b
Pyrazolone, 32–33, 655, 655b
   compounds, 32–33, 33b
Pyrethrins, 611–612, 612b
Pyrethroids, 800, 847
Pyrethrum, 481–482, 799–800
Pyridostigmine, 99, 680, 681b
Pyridoxine. See Vitamin B$_6$
Pyrimethamine, 121, 133, 137–138, 138b, 695
Pyrimidine antagonists, 383–385
Pyrvinium, 146, 146b, 697, 697b

Q

Qi, 77–78
Quazepam, 766
Quetiapine, 313, 320, 755b–756b, 760–761, 763
Quinagolide, 417, 417b, 647–648, 785
Quinapril, 715
Quinidine, 717, 717b
Quinine, 133, 136, 138–139, 139b, 695, 695b
Quinoline sulfate, 470, 471b
Quinolones, 122–123, 122b, 690, 690b
Quinupristin, 129

R

Rabeprazole, 96, 678
Rabies vaccination, 185, 185b, 708
Racecadotril, 102, 683
Radiation
   associated with nuclear industry, 623–625, 624b
   effects, of X-rays, 529–530
   electromagnetic, 625–627, 627b
   ionizing, 527–528
   -weighting factor, 527–528
Radio iodine therapy, 535
Radioactive isotopes, 534–536, 536b
Radionuclides, 816–817, 817b
Raloxifen, 506
Raloxifene, 792–793
Raltegravir, 152, 161, 700
Ramipril, 715
Ranibizumab, 351
Ranitidine, 93, 95–96, 678
Ranolazine, 214, 720
Rasagilin, 330, 769
Rasburicase, 50
Raspberry leaf (*Rubus idaeus*), 805–806
Raynaud phenomenon, 714
Reboxetine, 753
Receptor–ligand interactions, 13

Recreational drugs, 541–574, 835–844
   alcohol. See Alcohol
   amphetamines, 555–556, 836, 836b
   bath salts, 556–557
   caffeine, 547–549, 549b, 836–837, 837b
   cannabis, 559–561, 837, 837b
   cocaine, 557–559, 837–838, 837b
   diazepam, 841
   ectasy, 556–557
   LSD, 561
   mescaline, 561
   nicotine, 838–839, 839b
   opiates, 839–841, 841b
   phencyclidine, 561, 841
   psilocybin, 561–562
   sedating drugs, 562–564
   tobacco and smoking, 549–555
   xanthines, 547–549, 549b
Red clover (*Trifolium pretense*), 805–806
Red raspberry, 515t
Relative infant dose (RID), 644–645
Remifentanil, 39, 663
Renal hypoplasia, 49–50, 279t
Renal impairment, 45
Repaglinide, 431, 433, 790
Repellents, 485, 485b
Reproductive stages, 3–4, 5t–6t
Reproductive toxicology, 4–8
   drug-induced, 8–10
Reproterol, 66–67, 672
Reserpine, 203, 203b, 647, 716
Resorcin, 475, 475b
Restless legs syndrome, 329–330, 330b
Retapamulin, 132, 694
Reteplase, 238–239, 728
Retinoids, 798–799, 799b
   for acne/psoriasis, 475–479, 478b
Retinol. See Vitamin A
Reversible pseudo-Cushing syndrome, 836
Reviparin, 227, 725
Rheologics, 241–242, 242b
Rheumatoid arthritis (RA), 33, 345–348, 350–352, 358–360, 362–364
Rheumatic diseases, drugs for, 358–363
Rhubarb, 100–101
Ribavirin, 149, 698
Riboflavin. See Vitamin B$_2$
Ribostamycin, 125–126, 692
Rifabutin, 131
Rifampicin, 129–131, 131b, 694
Rifapentine, 131, 694
Rifaximin, 129, 129b
Rilonacept, 352
Rilpivirine, 152, 157, 700
Rimexolone, 488
Risedronic acid, 506
Risk communication
   of drug safety, 21
   prior to pharmacotherapeutic choice, 20
Risperidone, 313, 315b–316b, 320–321, 585, 761
   effects on lactation, 647

Ritodrine, 210, 406
Ritonavir, 152, 159, 699–700
Rituximab, 359, 386
Rivaroxaban, 225–226, 231, 726, 726b
Rizatriptan, 47, 659
Rocuronium, 461
Rocuronium bromide, 665–666
Rofecoxib, 657
Roflumilast, 70
Romiplostim, 240, 728
Ropinirole, 329, 769
Ropivacaine, 457–459, 664–665
Rose, 514t
Rosemary, 521t
Rosiglitazone, 431, 433, 790
Rosoxacin, 123
Rosuvastatin, 683
Rotavirus infection, during breastfeeding,
    828–829, 829b
Rotigotine, 329
Roxatidine, 95–96
Roxithromycin, 118, 118–119, 119b, 689
Rt-PA (recombinant tissue plasminogen
    activator), 238–239, 239b
Rubella vaccination, 185–186, 186b, 708, 708b
Rue, 520t. See also Goat's rue (Galega
    officinalis)
Rubidium, 856
Rufinamide, 252, 275, 275b, 737
Rupatadine, 59

S

S-adenosyl methionine, 34
Sage (Salvia officinalis), 806–807
St. John's wort, 516t–519t, 753, 803–804
Salazosulfapyridine, 103, 682. See also
    Sulfasalazine
Salbutamol, 66–67, 210, 406, 672, 673b
Salicylates, 809–810
    preparation, 473–474, 473b
Salicylic acid, 799
Salmeterol, 67, 673
Salves, 488
Saquinavir, 152, 160, 700
Sartan, 715–716. See also Angiotensin II
    receptor antagonists
Sativex®, 560
Saw palmetto, 522t
Saxagliptin, 431
Scabies, 799–800, 800b
Schist oil extracts, 798
Scintigraphy, 534
Sclerotherapy, 801
Scopolamine, 486–487
Second-generation antipsychotic agents (SGAs),
    315
Secondary prevention, 8, 106, 233
Secondhand smoke (SHS), 553–554
Secretin, 538, 818
Sedating drugs, 562–564
Sedatives, 324–325, 764, 767–768
Seizure. See also Epilepsy
    in pregnancy, frequency of, 254
Selective serotonin-reuptake-inhibitors (SSRI),
    295–302, 295b, 743–744, 744b
    congenital malformations, 296–298
    intrauterine growth retardation, 298–299
    long-term development, 300–301
    maternal treatment, 296–301
    neonatal development disorders, 299–300
    overdose, 590, 590b
    preterm birth, 298–299
Selegiline, 330, 769
Selenium, 507, 856
Selenium disulfide, 474, 474b
Sellafield nuclear reprocessing plant in Cumbria,
    UK, 624
Senna, 516t–519t, 522t, 682
Senna leaves, 100–101
Septum pellucidum aplasia, 279t
Sermorelin, 784
Serotonin antagonists, 85–86
Serotonin-norepinephrine reuptake inhibitors
    (SNRI), 295b
Sertaconazole, 141, 696
Sertindole, 313, 321, 761
Sertraline, 295, 303, 311, 744b, 751, 753–754
Severe acute respiratory syndrome (SARS), 149
Sevoflurane, 453–454, 665
Sex hormones, 253
Shepherd's purse, 520t
Shingles, 825–826
Short-term exposure limits (STELs), 600
Sibutramine, 109
Sildenafil, 206
Silicon, 857
Silicone, 481
Silver sulfadiazine, 121
Silymarin, 516t–519t, 806
Simeprevir, 149–150, 698
Simethicone, 98, 683
Simvastatin, 106, 683
Sirolimus, 344, 344b, 358, 777, 777b
Sitagliptin, 431
Sitaxsentan, 205
Skin changes, during pregnancy, 468
Skin glands, 468
Skin tests, 538
Slate oil preparations, 472–473, 473b
Slippery elm bark, 515t
Smallpox vaccine, 708, 708b
Smoking, 549–555
    and birth defects, 550
    and cognitive development, 553
    illness in childhood and, 551–552
    passive, 553–554
    pharmacology of, 549–550
    pregnancy complications associated with,
        550–551
Snake bites, 590–591
Sodium amidotrizoate, 532, 814
Sodium arsenate, 577, 616

Sodium arsenite, 616
Sodium aurothiomalate, 363
Sodium benzoate, 607
Sodium bicarbonate, 94–95
Sodium bituminosulfonate, 473, 798
Sodium cromoglicate, 69
Sodium hydrogen carbonate, 677–678
Sodium iodide, 537, 817
Sodium nitroprusside, 204, 204b
Sodium oxybate, 329
Sodium perchlorate, 421–422, 786–787, 787b
Sodium picosulfate, 100, 681–682, 682b
Sodium sulfate, 100
Sodium sulfite, 607
Sofosbuvir, 149–150, 698
Solifenacin, 98, 681
Solvent exposure, 601–607, 603b
Somatorelin, 414, 784
Somatostatin, 415, 784
Somatotropin, 416
Somatropin, 784
Sonic hedgehog homolog (SHH), 106
Sorafenib, 388
Sorbitol, 100
Sotalol, 209, 211–213, 713, 717b, 719
Southernwood, 520t
Sparfloxacin, 123, 690
Spectinomycin, 125–126, 692
Spermatogenesis, 3–4
Spermicide contraceptives, 410, 410b
Spider bites, 591
Spina bifida, 16t, 42, 121, 258, 278–279, 279t
Spiramycin, 118–119, 689
Spirapril, 715
Spironolactone, 216, 721, 721b
Spontaneous abortions, 5t–6t, 18–19, 181–182, 236, 343, 347, 350, 360–362, 410, 410b, 439, 455
Stable isotopes, 536–537, 536b
Statins, 106–107, 107b
Stavudine, 152–154, 699–700
Sterculia, 100
Streptococcus mutans, 241
Streptogramins, 129, 129b
Streptokinase, 238–239, 239b, 728
Streptomycin, 125–126, 131, 131b, 692, 694, 800
Striae, 468
Strontium, 506, 506b
Substitution therapy, 562–563, 840–841
Succinimides, 265
Succinylcholine, 460–461
Sucralfate, 95, 95b, 679, 679b
Sudden infant death syndrome (SIDS), 207
Sudden unexpected death in infancy (SUDI), 838
Sufentanil, 39, 459–460, 663, 663b
Sugammadex, 461
Sulbactam, 116, 688
Sulconazole, 141, 696
Sulcrafate, 677
Sulfacetamide, 121
Sulfadiazine, 121, 133, 137–138, 138b, 643
Sulfadoxine–pyrimethamine, 501

Sulfalene, 121
Sulfamerazine, 121
Sulfamethizole, 121
Sulfamethoxazole, 121, 689
Sulfanilamide, 699
Sulfasalazine, 103–104, 358–360, 659b, 682
Sulfide derivatives, 44
Sulfonamides, 121–122, 122b, 132, 682, 689–690, 690b, 809–810
Sulfonylurea derivatives, 431
Sulfur, 474–475, 475b
Sulfur containing preparations, 474–475, 475b
Sulfur dioxide, 607
Sulfur hexafluoride, 816
Sulindac, 408
Sulpiride, 313, 321, 647, 761
Sulprostone, 402
Sultiame, 252, 275, 275b, 737
Sumatriptan, 46, 659, 660b
Sunitinib, 388
Suppositories, 488
Surgical ablation, for warts, 799
Suxamethone, 665–666
Suxamethonium, 460–461
Syllium seed husks, 100
Systemic antifungal agents, 696, 696b
Systemic antihistamines, 60
Systemic autoimmune diseases, 775
Systemic corticosteroids, 49–50, 51b
Systemic lupus erythematosus (SLE), 38, 343, 387

T

Tacrolimus, 343–344, 344b, 358, 473, 473b, 777, 798
Tadalafil, 206
Talinolol, 196, 713
Tamoxifen, 378, 386, 389, 792–793
Tangerine, 514t
Tannin, 102
Tannin albuminate, 683
Tansy, 520t–521t
Tapentadol, 664
Taurolidine, 132
Taxanes, 385
Tazarotene, 798
Tazarotine, 475, 478, 478b
Tazobactam, 116, 688
Technetium, 817
Technetium-99m, 534
Teicoplanin, 126–127, 692
Telaprevir, 149–150, 698
Telavancin, 127
Telbivudine, 149, 698
Telithromycin, 118
Telmisartan, 200, 715
Telogen effluvium, 468
Temazepam, 325, 766–767, 767b
Temoporfin, 392
Temozolomide, 380
Temsirolimus, 392

Tenecteplase, 238–239, 728
Teniposide, 377–378
Tenofovir, 152–153, 155, 698, 698b, 700, 826
Teratogenesis, mechanism of, 542–543
Teratogenicity, 4
Teratogenic phenytoin, 211
Teratology information centers, 21
Terazosin, 202–203, 716
Terbinafine, 143, 143b, 696–697
Terbutaline, 66–67, 406, 672, 673b, 696–697
Terconazole, 141, 696
Terfenadine, 59
Teriflunomide, 352–354
Terizidone, 131, 694
Terlipressin, 417, 784
Tertiary prevention, 8
Testolactone, 792
Testosterone, 792
Tetanus neonatorum, 179
Tetanus vaccination, 179–180, 180b
Tethered spinal cord, 266
Tetrabenazine, 330
Tetracaine, 665
2,3,7,8-Tetrachlorodibenzo-p-dioxin (TCDD), 612
Tetrachloroethane, 601. See also
      Tetrachloroethylene
Tetrachloroethylene, 605, 605b
Tetracosactid, 415, 784
Tetracyclic antidepressants, 302–303
   congenital malformations, 302
   long-term development, 303
   maternal treatment and pregnancy
      complications, 302–303
   neonatal development disorders, 303
Tetracyclines, 120–121, 121b, 689, 689b
Tetraethyl lead, 853
Tetrahydrocannabinol, 353, 559, 560b, 837
Tetralogy of Fallot, 354
Tetramethrin, 611
Tetrathiomolybdate, 363
Tetryzoline, 487
Thalidomide, 7, 373–374, 387–388
Thallium poisoning, 582, 582b
Theobromine, 328, 547–549, 836–837
Theophylline, 68–69, 68b, 643, 674, 674b, 836–837
Thiabendazole, 144
Thiamazole, 421, 786–787, 787b
Thiamine. See Vitamin B₁
Thiazide diuretics, 194, 215
Thiethylperazine, 83
Thimerosal. See Thiomersal
Thioacetazone, 131, 694
Thioguanine, 103, 383
6-Thioguaninenucleotide (6-TGN), 341, 775–776
Thiomersal, 621
   as preservative for vaccines, 178–179
Thiopental, 455–457, 665
Thiophosphamide, 380
Thiopurine methyltransferase (TPMT), 775–776
Thioridazine, 313, 321, 762
Thioxanthenes, 313, 315b–316b
Threshold limit values (TLVs), 600

Thrombin inhibitors, 230–231, 230b
Thrombin Xa-inhibitors, 726
Thrombocyte aggregation inhibitors, 231–233,
      233b, 726–727, 727b
Thrombocytopenia, 822
Thrombophilia, 226
Thujone, 806–807
Thyme, 70, 675
Thymol, 470
Thyroid function, during pregnancy, 417–419
Thyroid hormones, 785–786
Thyroid peroxidase autoantibody (TPO-AB), 419
Thyroid receptor antibodies (TRAb), 785–786
Thyrostatics, 419–423, 786–787, 787b
Thyrotropin alfa, 416
Thyrotropin-releasing hormone (TRH), 414, 783
Thyroxin, 418
Tiagabine, 252–253, 275–276, 276b, 738
Tiaprofen, 657
Tiamphenicol, 127
Tiapride, 330, 769
Tibolone, 792–793
Ticagrelor, 232, 727
Ticarcillin, 116
Tick-borne encephalitis vaccination, 186, 186b
Ticlopidine, 231–232, 727
Tigecycline, 120, 689
Tilactase, 98
Tilidine, 40, 664
Tiludronate, 808
Tiludronic acid, 506
Time-weighted average (TWA) exposures, 600
Timolol, 196, 713, 800
Tinidazole, 125, 691
Tinzaparin, 227, 725
Tioconazole, 141, 696
Tiotropium bromide, 70, 674
Tipranavir, 152, 160, 700
Tirofiban, 232–233
Tissue plasminogen activator (t-PA), 238–239, 239b
Tizanidine, 48, 666
Tobacco, 549–555
   and birth defects, 550
   and cognitive development, 553
   illness in childhood and, 551–552
   passive, 553–554
   pharmacology of, 549–550
   pregnancy complications associated with,
      550–551
Tobramycin, 125–126, 692
Tocilizumab, 352, 359
Tocolytics, 405, 406t, 409
Tocopherol. See Vitamin E
Tofacitinib, 359
Tofisopam, 325
Tolbutamide, 790
Tolciclate, 143, 696–697
Tolfenamic acid, 41, 43
Tolnaftate, 696–697
Tolonium chloride, 537
Tolperisone, 666
Tolterodine, 98, 681

Toluene, 601, 605–607, 606b, 856
Toluidine blue, 537
Toluol, 605–606
Tolvaptan, 417
Tonalide, 857
Topical administration, 43–44, 798, 800–801
Topical antifungal agents, 143–144, 143b, 696–697, 697b
Topical applications, 797–798
Topiramate, 251–254, 259, 276–277, 277b, 738, 763
Topoisomerase inhibitors, 132
Topotecan, 391
Torasemide, 216, 721
Toremifene, 389
Toxins
    animal, 590–592
    bacterial, 592–593
    mushrooms, 592, 592b
    plant, 592
Toxoplasma, 4–7
Trabectedin, 385
Trace elements, 507, 507b, 808, 808b
Tracheomalacia, 279t
Tramadol, 40, 663, 664b
Tramazoline, 487
Trandolapril, 715
Tranexamic acid, 61–62, 238, 240b, 728
Transcobalamin II deficiency, 498
Transcranial magnetic stimulation, 295b
Transgenerational effect, 438
Transplacental carcinogenesis, 5t–6t, 10, 274, 437–438
Transplantation, 358, 358b
Tranylcypromine, 311–312, 754
Trapidil, 214, 720
Trastuzumab, 373–376, 385–386, 389
Traveling, 132–133, 708–709
Travoprost, 486
Trazodone, 312, 754
Treosulfan, 380
Treprostinil, 206–207
Tretinoin, 373–374, 390–391, 475, 477–478, 495, 798
Triamcinolone, 67, 788
Triamiphos, 610
Triamterene, 217, 217b, 721
Triarylmethanes, 100
Triazolam, 325
Tricarbocyanin, 537
Trichlor ethanol, 328
Trichloroacetic acid, 328
Trichloromethane, 604, 604b
2,4,5-Trichlorophenoxyacetic acid (2,4,5-T), 612
Trichomoniasis, 801
Triclabendazole, 144, 697
Triclosan, 856
Tricyclic antidepressants (TCA), 295b, 302–303
    congenital malformations, 302
    long-term development, 303
    maternal treatment and pregnancy
        complications, 302–303

neonatal development disorders, 303
Tricyclics, 744b
Trientine, 364
Triethylene tetramine dihydrochloride.
    See Trientine
Trifluoperazine, 82, 588, 762
Trifluperidol, 758
Trifluralin, 485
Trifluridine, 148, 698
Trigonocephaly, 278
Trihalomethanes (THM), 614–615
Trihexyphenidyl, 330
Triiodothyronine, 418
Trimethadione, 16t
Trimethobenzamide, 81, 83
Trimethoprim, 121–122, 122b, 689–690, 690b
Trimipramine, 312, 754
Triprolidine, 59, 672
Triptans, 46–47
Triptorelin, 784
Trisomy 21. See Down syndrome
Trofosfamid, 379
Troleandomycin, 118–119
Tromantadine, 148, 698
Tromethamine, 124
Tropicamide, 486–487
Trospium chloride, 98, 681
Trypaflavin, 537
L-Tryptophan, 768
Tuberculin test, 538, 818
Tuberculosis (TB), 129–132
    infection during breastfeeding, 829–830, 829b
Tuberculostatics, 131–132, 132b, 693–694, 694b
Tulobuterol, 67, 673, 673b
Tumor necrosis factor-α (TNF-α), 345, 347–348
Turkish porphyria, 848
Typhoid vaccination, 186–187, 187b
Typhoid vaccine, 708–709
Tyrosine kinase inhibitors, 388
Tyrothricin, 127, 692

U

Ulcerative colitis, 103
Ulcer medications, 677–679
Ultrasound, 530–531, 813
    contrast media, 816, 816b
Ultrasound/ultrasonographic contrast media, 533–534, 534b
Ultraviolet light therapy (UV light), 479, 479b
Unfractionated heparin (UFH), 227–230, 229b, 237b
United Kingdom, nuclear facilities, 624–625
United Nations International Children's
    Emergency Fund (UNICEF), 641
United States Pharmacopeia (USP), 513
Uranium, 856
Urea, 472, 798
Uric acid, 27, 49–50, 215
Urapidil, 202, 716

Urinary tract infections, nitrofurans for, 123–125, 125b, 690–691, 691b
Urofollitrophin, 415, 784
Urogonadotropin, 784
Urokinase, 238, 728
Ursodeoxycholic acid (UDCA), 104–105, 105b, 684, 684b
US Preventive Services Task Force, 824
Ustekinumab, 352
UV-A light therapy, 479, 479b
UV-B light therapy, 479, 479b
UV-filtering, 857

V

Vaccination. *See also* Vaccines
  cholera, 179, 179b
  diphtheria, 179–180, 180b
  haemophilus influenza B, 180, 180b
  hepatitis A, 180, 180b, 706, 706b
  hepatitis B, 180, 180b, 706–707, 706b
  HPV, 180–181, 181b, 707
  influenza, 181–183, 183b, 707
  measles, 183, 183b
  meningococcal, 183–184, 184b
  mumps, 183, 183b
  pertussis, 184, 184b
  pneumococcal, 184, 184b
  poliomyelitis, 184–185, 185b
  rabies, 185, 185b, 708
  rubella, 185–186, 186b, 708, 708b
  tetanus, 179–180, 180b
  tick-borne encephalitis, 186, 186b
  typhoid, 186–187, 187b, 708–709
  varicella, 187, 187b
  yellow fever, 187–188, 188b
Vaccines. *See also* Vaccination
  CDC recommendations for, 709–710
  inactivated, 707
  live attenuated, 707
  polio, 707–708, 708b
  smallpox, 708, 708b
  thiomersal as preservative for, 178–179
VACTERL syndrome, 347
Vaginal therapeutics, 409–410, 410b, 488
Valacyclovir, 147, 698, 698b
Valdecoxib, 657–658
Valerian, 768, 803–804
Valganciclovir, 698
Valnoctamide, 277–278, 277b, 738
Valproate, 585, 731
Valproic acid (VPA), 251–258, 252b–253b, 265–266, 282b, 293, 324, 660b, 731b–732b, 738–739, 763
  congenital anomalies linked to, 279t
  dose-response relations, 280
  frequency of majr malformations, 279–280
  mental development anomalies, 281–282
  neonatal abnormalities, 280–281
  other abnormalities, 280
  typical malformation, 278–282

Valsartan, 200, 715
Vanadium, 856
Vancomycin, 126–127, 692
Varenicline, 554, 839
Varicella vaccination, 187, 187b
Varicella Zoster Immune Globulin (VZIG), 709
Varicella-zoster virus (VZV), infection during breastfeeding, 825–826, 826b
Vasocirculatory drugs, 214–215, 215b
Vasoconstrictors, 72
Vasodilators, 719–720
Vasopressin, 417
Vecurone, 665–666
Vecuronium, 461
Vein therapeutics, 483, 484b, 801
Venlafaxine, 312–313, 755
Venous thromboembolism (VTE), 225–226
Ventricular septal defects (VSD), 546
Verapamil, 198, 210, 406, 714, 717b, 719
Vernakalant, 211
Verrucae vulgares, 799
Verteporfin, 800–801
Very low-density lipoprotein (VLDL), 108
Vigabatrin, 252–254, 259, 282–283, 283b, 739
Vildagliptin, 431
Vinblastine, 377
Vinca alkaloids and analogs, 377
Vincristine, 377
Vindesine, 377
Vinegar water, for lice, 481
Vinflunine, 377
Vinorelbine, 377, 387, 391
Virostatics, 797
Virustatics adefovir, 698
Viscum album, 780, 780b
Vitamin A (retinol), 494–496, 496b
Vitamin B_1 (thiamine), 496, 496b
  for nausea and vomiting, 84–85, 84b
Vitamin B_2 (riboflavin), 496–497, 497b
Vitamin B_3 (nicotinamide), 497, 497b
Vitamin B_6 (pyridoxine), 83–84, 84b, 497, 497b, 685, 693
Vitamin $B_{6'}$ 83–84, 84b
Vitamin B_{12} (cyanocobalamin), 497–498, 498b
Vitamin C (ascorbic acid), 498, 498b
Vitamin D, 501–502, 502b
Vitamin E (tocopherol), 502–503, 503b
Vitamin K, 237–238, 238b, 503
  antagonists, 233–237, 237b, 727–728, 728b
  antiepileptic drugs, 259–260
Vitamins, 808, 808b
Vitex. *See* Chasteberry (*Vitex agnus-castus*)
Volatile chlorhydrocarbons, 856
Vomiting. *See* Nausea and vomiting of pregnancy (NVP)
Volume expanders, 728–729, 729b
Volume replacement substances, 241–242, 242b
Voriconazole, 140, 696

W

Warfarin, 206, 225–226, 233–234, 727
Wart removal medications, 799, 799b
Wart therapeutics, 480–481, 481b
Wasp stings, 591–592, 591b
Waste incinerators, 622–623, 623b
Weight loss medications, 108–109
West Nile virus (WNV), infection during
    breastfeeding, 830, 830b
Wheat bran, 100
Wheat germ, 100
Wilson's disease, drugs for, 363–365
Wolff–Chaikoff effect, 788
Workplace environment, breastfeeding and,
    857–858
World Health Organization (WHO), 542, 640

X

Xanthines, 547–549, 549b
Xenon, 454
Xipamide, 215, 721
X-ray examinations, 527–529
    dose range, 528–529
    ionizing radiation, 527–528
    radiation effects, 529–530
X-ray studies, 813
Xylene, 601
Xylometazoline, 487

Y

Yang energy. *See* Qi
Yarrow, 520t
Yellow fever vaccination, 187–188, 188b
Yusho disease, 848

Z

Zaleplon, 327–328, 767
Zanamivir, 151, 151b, 699, 699b
Zathioprine, 103
Zefirlucast, 69
Ziconotide, 664
Zidovudine, 151–153, 155, 699–700, 826
Zilenton, 69
Zinc, 507
Zinc salts, 364–365, 364b
Zinc sulfate, 698
Zingerone, 77–78
Ziprasidone, 313, 320–321, 762
Zofenopril, 715
Zoledronic acid, 506
Zolmitriptan, 47, 659
Zolpidem, 327–328, 767
Zonisamide, 252–253, 259, 283–284, 283b,
    739
Zopiclone, 327–328, 767
Zotepine, 321, 762
Zuclopenthixol, 313, 321–322, 762

Printed and bound by CPI Group (UK) Ltd, Croydon, CR0 4YY

03/10/2024

01040419-0007